Oxford Textbook of
Community Mental Health

OXFORD TEXTBOOKS IN PSYCHIATRY

Oxford Textbook of Community Mental Health, Second Edition
Edited by Graham Thornicroft, Robert E. Drake, Oye Gureje, Kim T. Mueser, and George Szmukler

Oxford Textbook of Social Psychiatry
Edited by Dinesh Bhugra, Driss Moussaoui, and Tom J. Craig

Oxford Textbook of Migrant Psychiatry
Edited by Dinesh Bhugra

Oxford Textbook of Suicidology and Suicide Prevention, Second Edition
Edited by Danuta Wasserman

Oxford Textbook of Old Age Psychiatry, Third Edition
Edited by Tom Dening, Alan Thomas, Robert Stewart, and John-Paul Taylor

Oxford Textbook of Neuropsychiatry
Edited by Niruj Agrawal, Rafey Faruqui, and Mayur Bodani

Oxford Textbook of the Psychiatry of Intellectual Disability
Edited by Sabyasachi Bhaumik and Regi Alexander

Oxford Textbook of Inpatient Psychiatry
Edited by Alvaro Barrera, Caroline Attard, and Rob Chaplin

Oxford Textbook of Attention Deficit Hyperactivity Disorder
Edited by Tobias Banaschewski, David Coghill, and Alessandro Zuddas

Oxford Textbook of Correctional Psychiatry
Edited by Robert Trestman, Kenneth Appelbaum, and Jeffrey Metzner

Oxford Textbook of Women and Mental Health
Edited by Dora Kohen

Oxford Textbook of Community Mental Health

SECOND EDITION

EDITED BY

Graham Thornicroft

Robert E. Drake

Oye Gureje

Kim T. Mueser

George Szmukler

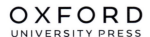

OXFORD
UNIVERSITY PRESS

Great Clarendon Street, Oxford, OX2 6DP,
United Kingdom

Oxford University Press is a department of the University of Oxford.
It furthers the University's objective of excellence in research, scholarship,
and education by publishing worldwide. Oxford is a registered trade mark of
Oxford University Press in the UK and in certain other countries

© Oxford University Press 2025

The moral rights of the authors have been asserted

First Edition published in 2011
Second Edition published in 2025

All rights reserved. No part of this publication may be reproduced, stored in
a retrieval system, or transmitted, in any form or by any means, without the
prior permission in writing of Oxford University Press, or as expressly permitted
by law, by licence or under terms agreed with the appropriate reprographics
rights organization. Enquiries concerning reproduction outside the scope of the
above should be sent to the Rights Department, Oxford University Press, at the
address above

You must not circulate this work in any other form
and you must impose this same condition on any acquirer

Published in the United States of America by Oxford University Press
198 Madison Avenue, New York, NY 10016, United States of America

British Library Cataloguing in Publication Data

Data available

Library of Congress Control Number: 2023952588

ISBN 978-0-19-889881-8

DOI: 10.1093/med/9780198898818.001.0001

Printed in the UK by
Bell & Bain Ltd., Glasgow

Oxford University Press makes no representation, express or implied, that the
drug dosages in this book are correct. Readers must therefore always check
the product information and clinical procedures with the most up-to-date
published product information and data sheets provided by the manufacturers
and the most recent codes of conduct and safety regulations. The authors and
the publishers do not accept responsibility or legal liability for any errors in the
text or for the misuse or misapplication of material in this work. Except where
otherwise stated, drug dosages and recommendations are for the non-pregnant
adult who is not breast-feeding

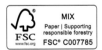

The manufacturer's authorised representative in the EU for
product safety is Oxford University Press España S.A. of el
Parque Empresarial San Fernando de Henares, Avenida de
Castilla, 2 – 28830 Madrid (www.oup.es/en).

Contents

Contributors ix

SECTION 1
Introduction

1. **Introduction to community mental health** 3
   Robert E. Drake, Oye Gureje, Kim T. Mueser, George Szmukler, and Graham Thornicroft

SECTION 2
Origins of 'community psychiatry'

2. **Historical changes in mental health practice** 11
   Nikolas Rose

3. **Mental health policy in modern America** 23
   Gerald Grob and Howard Goldman

4. **Recovery as an integrative paradigm in mental health** 33
   Mike Slade and Larry Davidson

SECTION 3
Needs: perspectives and assessment

5. **Treatment coverage for mental disorders: results from the World Health Organization World Mental Health Surveys** 45
   Daniel V. Vigo, Meredith G. Harris, Richard J. Munthali, Alan E. Kazdin, Irving Hwang, Maria Petukhova, Nancy A. Sampson, Sergio Aguilar-Gaxiola, Ali Al-Hamzawi, Jordi Alonso, Yasmin A. Altwaijri, Corina Benjet, Evelyn J. Bromet, Ronny Bruffaerts, Brendan Bunting, José Miguel Caldas-de-Almeida, Stephanie Chardoul, Giovanni De Girolamo, Peter de Jonge, Silvia Florescu, Oye Gureje, Josep Maria Haro, Chi-yi Hu, Elie G. Karam, Georges Karam, Andrzej Kiejna, Sing Lee, Fernando Navarro-Mateu, José Posada-Villa, Charlene Rapsey, Juan Carlos Stagnaro, Yolanda Torres, Maria Carmen Viana, David R. Williams, Zahari Zarkov, Philip S. Wang, and Ronald C. Kessler, on behalf of the WHO World Mental Health Survey collaborators

6. **The lived experience: focus on wellness** 57
   Margaret Swarbrick and Crystal L. Brandow

7. **Measuring mental health needs** 65
   Mike Slade and Graham Thornicroft

8. **Mental health, ethnicity, and cultural diversity: evidence and challenges** 73
   Craig Morgan

9. **The mental health challenges of immigrants and refugees** 81
   Jillian M. Stile, Quyen Ngo-Metzger, Richard F. Mollica, and Eugene F. Augusterfer

SECTION 4
Treatment and service components

10. **Early intervention for mental health and substance use disorders** 97
    Cristina Mei, Paddy Power, Gill Bedi, Sarah Maguire, Louise McCutcheon, Aswin Ratheesh, Katrina Witt, and Patrick D. McGorry

11. **Organizing the range of community mental health services** 113
    Graham Thornicroft, Michele Tansella, and Robert E. Drake

12. **Crisis and emergency services** 127
    Sonia Johnson, Justin J. Needle, Jonathan Totman, and Lorna Hobbs

13. **Early intervention for people with psychotic disorders** 141
    Paddy Power, Ellie Brown, and Patrick D. McGorry

14. **Case management and assertive community treatment** 161
    Helen Killaspy and Alan Rosen

15. **Principles and standards for medication management of individuals with serious mental illness** 171
    Thomas E. Smith and Delia C. Hendrick

16. **Psychiatric outpatient clinics** 183
    Markus Koesters, Carolin Schneider, and Thomas Becker

17. **Day hospital and partial hospitalization programmes** 187
    Aart H. Schene

18. **Inpatient treatment** 195
    Frank Holloway and Derek Tracy

19. **Residential care** 207
    Geoff Shepherd and Rob Macpherson

20. **Individual placement and support: the evidence-based practice of supported employment** 219
    Deborah R. Becker, Gary R. Bond, and Robert E. Drake

21. **Programmes to support family members and caregivers** 225
    Samantha Jankowski, Amy L. Drapalski, and Lisa B. Dixon

22. **Managing co-occurring physical disorders in mental health care** 233
    Delia C. Hendrick and Robert E. Drake

23. **Illness self-management programmes** 243
    Kim T. Mueser and Susan Gingerich

24. **Co-occurring substance use disorders** 253
    Robert E. Drake, Kim T. Mueser, and Delia C. Hendrick

25. **Behavioural health technologies and telehealth** 261
    John Torous and Elizabeth Carpenter-Song

26. **Forensic community mental health services** 271
    Lisa Wootton, Penelope Brown, and Alec Buchanan

SECTION 5
Ethical and legal aspects

27. **Ethical framework for community mental health** 283
    Abraham Rudnick, Cheryl Forchuk, and George Szmukler

28. **International human rights and community mental health** 291
    Oliver Lewis and Peter Bartlett

29. **Treatment pressures, coercion, and compulsion** 301
    George Szmukler and Paul S. Appelbaum

SECTION 6
Stigma and discrimination

30. **Public knowledge and awareness about mental illnesses** 313
    Anthony F. Jorm

31. **Reducing stigma and discriminatory behaviour** 321
    Petra C. Gronholm, Dristy Gurung, Sarah J. Parry, Nisha Mehta, and Graham Thornicroft

SECTION 7
Policies and the funding

32. **Shaping national mental health policy** 333
    Harvey Whiteford and Sandra Diminic

33. **Funding of mental health services** 341
    Dan Chisholm, Martin Knapp, and Shari Jadoolal

SECTION 8
Assessing the evidence for effectiveness

34. **Research designs and evaluating treatment interventions** 353
    Peter Tyrer

35. **Qualitative research methods in mental health** 361
    Rob Whitley

36. **Developing evidence-based mental health practices** 369
    Kim T. Mueser and Robert E. Drake

37. **Implementing guidelines** 375
    Amy Cheung, Simon Gilbody, and Jeremy Grimshaw

SECTION 9
Global mental health

38. **The global burden of disease and the mental health of communities** 389
    Daniel V. Vigo, Laura Jones, Rifat Atun, and Graham Thornicroft

39. **Planning mental health care at the national level** 401
    Nicole Votruba, Melvyn Freeman, Eleni Misganaw, Keshav Desiraju, and Charlotte Hanlon

40. **Contributions of religious, alternative, and complementary practitioners** 417
    Olatunde Ayinde and Oye Gureje

41. **Planning and implementing community services for a district: the case of PRIME** 425
    Crick Lund, Erica Breuer, Arvin Bhana, Carrie Brooke-Sumner, Mark Jordans, Nagendra Luitel, Girmay Medhin, Vaibhav Murhar, Juliet Nakku, Olivia Nalwadda, Inge Petersen, Medhin Selamu, Rahul Shidhaye, Joshua Ssebunnya, Mark Tomlinson, Charlotte Hanlon, and Vikram Patel

42. **Mental health aspects of epidemics and pandemics** 439
    Akin Ojagbemi and Oye Gureje

43. **'Mental health' in low- and middle-income countries** 449
    R. Srinivasa Murthy

44. **Overcoming impediments to community mental health in low- and middle-income countries** 461
    Benedetto Saraceno, Mark van Ommeren, and Rajaie Batniji

SECTION 10
Looking to the future

45. **Community mental health in the future** 469
    Graham Thornicroft, Robert E. Drake, Oye Gureje, Kim T. Mueser, and George Szmukler

Index 481

Contributors

Sergio Aguilar-Gaxiola Center for Reducing Health Disparities, UC Davis Health System, Sacramento, California, USA

Jordi Alonso Health Services Research Unit, IMIM-Hospital del Mar Medical Research Institut, Barcelona, Spain
CIBER en Epidemiología y Salud Pública (CIBERESP), Madrid, Spain
Pompeu Fabra University (UPF), Barcelona, Spain

Yasmin A. Altwaijri Epidemiology Section, King Faisal Specialist Hospital and Research Center, Riyadh, Saudi Arabia

Paul S. Appelbaum Dollard Professor of Psychiatry, Medicine & Law, Department of Psychiatry, Columbia University Irving Medical Center, and New York State Psychiatric Institute, New York, USA

Rifat Atun Department of Global Health and Social Medicine, Harvard Medical School, Boston, MA, USA; Department of Global Health & Population, Harvard T.H. Chan School of Public Health, Boston, MA, USA

Eugene F. Augusterfer Deputy Director, Harvard Program in Refugee Trauma, Department of Psychiatry, Massachusetts General Hospital, Boston, MA, USA

Olatunde Ayinde Senior Lecturer, Department of Psychiatry, University of Ibadan, Nigeria

Peter Bartlett Nottinghamshire Healthcare NHS Trust Professor of Mental Health Law, School of Law, University of Nottingham, Nottingham, UK

Rajaie Batniji Department of Politics and International Relations, University of Oxford, Oxford, UK

Deborah R. Becker Former Director, IPS Employment Center, Research Foundation for Mental Hygiene, Inc. (Retired)

Thomas Becker Senior Professor, Department of Psychiatry and Psychotherapy, University of Leipzig, Germany

Gill Bedi Orygen, Melbourne, Australia; Centre for Youth Mental Health, The University of Melbourne, Melbourne, Australia

Corina Benjet Department of Epidemiologic and Psychosocial Research, National Institute of Psychiatry Ramón de la Fuente Muñiz, Mexico City, Mexico

Arvin Bhana Medical Research Council, South Africa

Gary R. Bond Senior Research Associate, Westat, Inc., West Lebanon, NH, USA

Crystal L. Brandow clb strategies, LLC; Rutgers University Center of Alcohol and Substance Use Studies and Graduate School of Applied and Professional Psychology, USA

Erica Breuer College of Health, Medicine and Wellbeing, University of Newcastle, Australia

Evelyn J. Bromet Distinguished Professor of Psychiatry and Preventive Medicine, Renaissance School of Medicine at Stony Brook University, USA

Carrie Brooke-Sumner Mental health, Alcohol, Substance Use and Tobacco Research Unit (MASTRU), South African Medical Research Council, South Africa

Ellie Brown Orygen and Centre for Youth Mental Health, university of Melbourne

Penelope Brown Consultant Forensic Psychiatrist, South London and Maudsley NHS Foundation Trust, London, UK: Department of Psychological Medicine, Institute of Psychiatry, Psychology and Neuroscience, King's College London, UK

Ronny Bruffaerts Universitair Psychiatrisch Centrum - Katholieke Universiteit Leuven (UPC-KUL), Campus Gasthuisberg, Leuven, Belgium

Alec Buchanan Professor Emeritus of Psychiatry, Division of Law and Psychiatry, Department of Psychiatry, Yale University School of Medicine, New Haven, CT, USA

Brendan Bunting School of Psychology, Ulster University, Londonderry, United Kingdom

José Miguel Caldas-de-Almeida Lisbon Institute of Global Mental Health and Chronic Diseases Research Center (CEDOC), NOVA Medical School | Faculdade de Ciências Médicas, Universidade Nova de Lisboa, Lisbon, Portugal

Elizabeth Carpenter-Song Research Professor of Anthropology Dartmouth College

Stephanie Chardoul Institute for Social Research, University of Michigan, Ann Arbor, Michigan, USA

Amy Cheung Associate Professor, Department of Psychiatry, University of Toronto, Canada

Dan Chisholm Mental Health Specialist, Department of Mental Health and Substance Use, World Health Organization, Geneva, Switzerland

Larry Davidson Yale Program for Recovery and Community Health, Yale University School of Medicine, USA

Keshav Desiraju Posthumous

Sandra Diminic Principal Research Fellow, Queensland Centre for Mental Health Research, Brisbane, Australia; Adjunct Senior Fellow, School of Public Health, The University of Queensland, Brisbane, Australia

Lisa B. Dixon Professor of Psychiatry, New York State Psychiatric Institute, Columbia University Vagelos College of Physicians and Surgeons and New York-Presbyterian, Director, Division of Behavioral Health Services and Policy Research & Center for Practice Innovations

Robert E. Drake Professor of Clinical Psychiatry, Columbia University Vagelos College of Medicine and Surgery; Vice President, Westat

Amy L. Drapalski VA Capitol Health Care Network (VISN 5) Mental Illness Research, Education and Clinical Center, Baltimore, MD, USA

Silvia Florescu National School of Public Health, Management and Development, Bucharest, Romania

Cheryl Forchuk Distinguished Professor, Arthur Labatt School of Nursing, Faculty of Health Sciences, University of Western Ontario, Canada; Beryl and Richard Ivey Research Chair in Aging, Mental Health, Rehabilitation and Recovery, Lawson Health Research Institute, Parkwood Institute Research, London, ON, Canada

Melvyn Freeman Extraordinary Professor, Department of Psychology, University of Stellenbosch, South Africa

Simon Gilbody Professor, Mental Health Research Group, University of York, York, UK

Susan Gingerich Independent Trainer and Consultant

Giovanni De Girolamo Professor of Psychology and Psychiatry Department of Psychology, Catholic University, Milan, Italy

Howard Goldman Professor of Psychiatry, University of Maryland School of Medicine, Baltimore, MD, USA

Jeremy Grimshaw Senior Scientist, Clinical Epidemiology Program, Ottawa Health Research Institute, Canada; Full Professor, Department of Medicine, University of Ottawa, Canada; Canada Research Chair in Health Knowledge Transfer and Uptake

Gerald Grob Posthumous

Petra C. Gronholm Centre for Global Mental Health, Institute of Psychiatry, Psychology and Neuroscience, King's College London, UK

Contributors

Oye Gureje Professor of Psychiatry and Director, WHO Collaborating Centre for Research and Training in Mental Health, Neuroscience, Drug and Alcohol Abuse; Department of Psychiatry, University of Ibadan, Nigeria; Extraordinary Professor, Department of Psychiatry, University of Stellenbosch, South Africa

Dristy Gurung Transcultural Psychosocial Organisation, Kathmandu, Nepal

Ali Al-Hamzawi College of Medicine, University of Al-Qadisiya, Diwaniya governorate, Iraq

Charlotte Hanlon Professor of Global Mental Health Division of Psychiatry, Centre for Clinical Brain Sciences, University of Edinburgh, Edinburgh, Scotland, UK; and Department of Psychiatry, School of Medicine, College of Health Sciences, Addis Ababa University, Ethiopia

Josep Maria Haro Parc Sanitari Sant Joan de Déu, CIBERSAM, Universitat de Barcelona, Sant Boi de Llobregat, Barcelona, Spain

Meredith G. Harris School of Public Health, The University of Queensland, Brisbane, QLD, Australia

Delia C. Hendrick Psychiatrist, Co-Occurring Disorders, WestBridge, Manchester, NH, USA

Lorna Hobbs Independent consultant

Frank Holloway Emeritus Consultant Psychiatrist, South London and Maudsely NHS Foundation Trust, UK

Chi-yi Hu Shenzhen Institute of Mental Health & Shenzhen Kangning Hospital, Shenzhen, China

Irving Hwang Department of Health Care Policy, Harvard Medical School, Boston, Massachusetts, USA

Shari Jadoolal Research Assistant, Care Policy and Evaluation Centre, Department of Health Policy, London School of Economics and Political Science, UK

Samantha Jankowski Research Co-coordinator, New York State Psychiatric Institute, USA

Sonia Johnson Division of Psychiatry, UCL, London, UK

Laura Jones Department of Psychiatry, University of British Columbia, Vancouver, BC, Canada

Peter de Jonge Department of Developmental Psychology, University of Groningen, Groningen, The NetherlandsInterdisciplinary Center Psychopathology and Emotion Regulation, University Medical Center Groningen, Groningen, The Netherlands

Mark Jordans Centre for Global Mental Health, Health Service and Population Research Department, Institute of Psychiatry, Psychology and Neuroscience, King's Global Health Institute, King's College London, United Kingdom; WarChild, Netherlands

Anthony F. Jorm Centre for Mental Health and Community Wellbeing, Melbourne School of Population and Global Health, University of Melbourne, Victoria, Australia

Elie G. Karam Department of Psychiatry and Clinical Psychology, Faculty of Medicine, Balamand University, Beirut, Lebanon Department of Psychiatry and Clinical Psychology, St George Hospital University Medical Center, Beirut, Lebanon Institute for Development Research Advocacy and Applied Care (IDRAAC), Beirut, Lebanon

Georges Karam Department of Psychiatry and Clinical Psychology, Faculty of Medicine, Balamand University, Beirut, Lebanon Department of Psychiatry and Clinical Psychology, St George Hospital University Medical Center, Beirut, Lebanon Institute for Development Research Advocacy and Applied Care (IDRAAC), Beirut, Lebanon

Alan E. Kazdin, PhD, ABPP Research Professor and Sterling Professor of Psychology & Professor of Child Psychiatry (Emeritus) Henry Koerner Center New Haven, CT

Andrzej Kiejna Institute of Psychology, University of Lower Silesia, Wroclaw, Poland

Ronald C. Kessler, Ph.D. McNeil Family Professor Department of Health Care Policy Harvard Medical School Boston, MA, USA

Helen Killaspy Professor of Rehabilitation Psychiatry, Division of Psychiatry, UCL, London, UK

Martin Knapp Professor of Health and Social Care Policy, Care Policy and Evaluation Centre, Department of Health Policy, London School of Economics and Political Science, UK

Markus Kösters Center for Evidence-Based Healthcare, Faculty of Medicine and University Hospital Carl Gustav Carus, Technische Universität Dresden, Chemnitz, Germany

Sing Lee Department of Psychiatry, Chinese University of Hong Kong, Tai Po, Hong Kong

Glyn H. Lewis Professor of Epidemiological Psychiatry, UCL Division of Psychiatry, London, UK

Oliver Lewis Doughty Street Chambers, London, and School of Law, University of Leeds, UK

Nagendra Luitel TPO Nepal, Nepal

Crick Lund Co-Director, Centre for Global Mental Health, Health Service and Population Research Department, Institute of Psychiatry, Psychology and Neuroscience, King's Global Health Institute, King's College London, United Kingdom; Honorary Professor, Alan J Flisher Centre for Public Mental Health, Department of Psychiatry and Mental Health, University of Cape Town, South Africa

Rob Macpherson Consultant Psychiatrist, Gether Partnership NHS Trust, Wotton Lawn, Horton Road, Gloucester, UK

Sarah Maguire InsideOut Institute for Eating Disorders, University of Sydney, Sydney, Australia; Sydney Local Health District, NSW Health, Sydney, Australia

Louise McCutcheon Coordinator, Orygen Clinical Training, Senior Program Manager, Hype Service Development, Clinical Associate Professor, Centre for Youth Mental Health, The University of Melbourne, Australia

Patrick D. McGorry Orygen, Melbourne, Australia; Centre for Youth Mental Health, The University of Melbourne, Melbourne, Australia

Girmay Medhin Department of Psychiatry, Addis Ababa University, Ethiopia

Nisha Mehta Department of Health and Social Care, London, UK

Cristina Mei Orygen, Melbourne, Australia; Centre for Youth Mental Health, The University of Melbourne, Melbourne, Australia

Eleni Misganaw President—Mental Health Service Users Association Ethiopia (www.mhsua.org)

Richard F. Mollica Director, Harvard Program in Refugee Trauma, Department of Psychiatry, Massachusetts General Hospital, Professor of Psychiatry, Harvard Medical School, Boston, MA, USA

Craig Morgan Professor of Social Epidemiology, Co-Director, ESRC Centre for Society and Mental Health, Institute of Psychiatry, Psychology, and Neuroscience, King's College London, London, UK

Kim T. Mueser Center for Psychiatric Rehabilitation, Departments of Occupational Therapy and Psychological & Brain Sciences, Boston University, Boston, MA, USA

Richard. J. Munthali Department of Psychiatry, University of British Columbia, Vancouver, BC, Canada

Vaibhav Murhar Independent Researcher

R. Srinivasa Murthy Professor of Psychiatry (retd), Formerly of Department of Psychiatry, National Institute of Mental Health and Neurosciences, Bangalore, India

Juliet Nakku Butabika Psychiatric Hospital, Uganda

Olivia Nalwadda Founder, Uzima Ari Uganda, Researcher, Butabika National Referral Mental Hospital, Uganda

Fernando Navarro-Mateu Unidad de Docencia, Investigación y Formación en Salud Mental (UDIF-SM), Servicio Murciano de Salud, Departamento de Psicología Básica y Metodología, Universidad de Murcia, Murcia, Spain IMIB-Arrixaca, Murcia, Spain CIBER de Epidemiología y Salud Pública (CIBERESP), Madrid, Spain

Justin J. Needle School of Health & Psychological Sciences, City St George's, University of London, London, UK

Quyen Ngo-Metzger Interim Associate Dean for Faculty Affairs, Professor of Health Systems Science, Kaiser Permanente School of Medicine, Pasadena, CA, USA

Akin Ojagbemi WHO Collaborating Centre for Research and Training in Mental Health, Neuroscience, Drug and Alcohol Abuse, University of Ibadan, Ibadan, Nigeria; Department of Psychiatry, University of Ibadan, Nigeria

Mark van Ommeren Department of Mental Health and Substance Abuse, WHO, Geneva

Sarah J. Parry South London and Maudsley NHS Foundation Trust, Denmark Hill, London, UK

Contributors

Vikram Patel Harvard Medical School, USA; Sangath, Goa, India

Inge Petersen Centre for Rural Health, University of KwaZulu-Natal, South Africa

Maria Petukhova Department of Health Care Policy, Harvard Medical School, Boston, Massachusetts, USA

José Posada-Villa Colombian Institute of the Nervous System, Clinica Montserrat University Hospital, Bogotá, Colombia

Paddy Power St. Patrick's Mental Health Services, Dublin, Ireland; Trinity College Dublin, Dublin, Ireland

Charlene Rapsey Department of Psychological Medicine, University of Otago, Dunedin, Otago, New Zealand

Aswin Ratheesh Orygen, Melbourne, Australia; Centre for Youth Mental Health, The University of Melbourne, Melbourne, Australia

Nikolas Rose Honorary Professor, Institute of Advanced Studies, University College, London

Alan Rosen Professorial Fellow, Australian Health Services Research Institute [AHSRI], University of Wollongong, NSW, Clinical Associate Professor, Brain & Mind Centre, University of Sydney, NSW, Senior Psychiatrist, NSW Health, Australia

Abraham Rudnick Professor, Departments of Psychiatry and Bioethics and School of Occupational Therapy, Dalhousie University, Canada

Nancy A. Sampson Department of Health Care Policy, Harvard Medical School, Boston, Massachusetts, USA

Benedetto Saraceno Secretary General, Lisbon Institute of Global Mental Health, Portugal

Aart H. Schene Professor of Psychiatry, Faculty of Medical Sciences, Radboud University, Nijmegen, Netherlands

Caroline Schneider Research Assistant, Department of Psychiatry II, Ulm University, Günzburg, Germany

Medhin Selamu Department of Psychiatry, Addis Ababa University, Ethiopia

Geoff Shepherd Visiting Professor, Health Service and Population Research Department, Institute of Psychiatry, University of London, UK

Rahul Shidhaye Department of Psychiatry, Pravara Institute of Medical Sciences, Loni, India; Department of Health, Ethics and Society, Care and Public Health Research Institute, Maastricht University, Netherlands

Mike Slade School of Health Sciences, Institute of Mental Health, University of Nottingham, Nottingham, UK

Thomas E. Smith Chief Medical Officer, New York State Office of Mental Health, Special Lecturer, Columbia University Vagelos College of Physicians and Surgeons, New York State Psychiatric Institute, USA

Joshua Ssebunnya Butabika Psychiatric Hospital, Uganda

Juan Carlos Stagnaro Departamento de Psiquiatría y Salud Mental, Facultad de Medicina, Universidad de Buenos Aires, Argentina

Jillian M. Stile Faculty, Harvard Program in Refugee Trauma; Instructor in Clinical Psychology (in Psychiatry) Columbia University Vagelos College of Physicians & Surgeons, New York, NY, USA

Margaret Swarbrick Rutgers University Center of Alcohol and Substance Use Studies and Graduate School of Applied and Professional Psychology; Collaborative Support Programs of New Jersey Freehold NJ, USA

George Szmukler Professor of Psychiatry and Society, Institute of Psychiatry, King's College London, London, UK

Michele Tansella Posthumous

Graham Thornicroft Centre for Global Mental Health & Centre for Implementation Science, Health Service and Population Research Department, Institute of Psychiatry, Psychology and Neuroscience, King's College London, London, UK

Mark Tomlinson Institute for Life Course Health Research, Department of Global Health, Stellenbosch University, Cape Town, South Africa; School of Nursing and Midwifery, Queens University, Belfast, UK

John Torous Associate Professor of Psychiatry Harvard Medical School Boston, MA, USA

Yolanda Torres Center for Excellence on Research in Mental Health, CES University, Medellin, Colombia

Jonathan Totman University of Oxford Counselling Service, Oxford, UK

Derek Tracy Chief Medical Officer, South London and Maudsley NHS Foundation Trust; Honorary Senior Lecturer, King's, Imperial, & University College London; Editor for Public Engagement, the British Journal of Psychiatry, UK

Peter Tyrer Emeritus Professor in Community Psychiatry, Centre for Mental Health, Imperial College, London, UK

Maria Carmen Viana Department of Social Medicine, Postgraduate Program in Public Health, Federal University of Espírito Santo, Vitoria, Brazil

Daniel V. Vigo Department of Psychiatry, University of British Columbia, Vancouver, BC, Canada; Department of Global Health and Social Medicine, Harvard Medical School, Boston, MA, USA

Nicole Votruba Nuffield Department of Women's & Reproductive Health, University of Oxford & The George Institute for Global Health (UK), Imperial College London, UK

Philip S. Wang Brigham and Women's Hospital, Harvard Medical School Boston, MA, USA

Harvey Whiteford Professor of Population Mental Health, School of Public Health, The University of Queensland, Brisbane, Australia

Rob Whitley Professor, Department of Psychiatry, Douglas Research Centre, McGill University, Quebec, Canada

David R. Williams Department of Social and Behavioral Sciences, Harvard T.H. Chan School of Public Health, Boston, Massachusetts, USA

Katrina Witt Orygen, Melbourne, Australia; Centre for Youth Mental Health, The University of Melbourne, Melbourne, Australia

Lisa Wootton Consultant Forensic Psychiatrist, North London Mental Health Partnership, London, UK

Zahari Zarkov Department of Mental Health, National Center of Public Health and Analyses, Sofia, Bulgaria

Christa Zimmermann Section of Psychiatry and Clinical Psychology, University of Verona, Verona, Italy

SECTION 1
Introduction

1. **Introduction to community mental health** 3
   Robert E. Drake, Oye Gureje, Kim T. Mueser, George Szmukler, and Graham Thornicroft

Introduction to community mental health

Robert E. Drake, Oye Gureje, Kim T. Mueser, George Szmukler, and Graham Thornicroft

Community mental health has evolved as a discipline for over 65 years now. In describing this evolution as well as current approaches, this book combines traditional concepts, such as community-based interventions and an epidemiological perspective, with newer concepts, such as shared decision-making, the recovery philosophy, evidence-based practices, implementation fidelity, telemedicine, and technology tools—all of which have shaped the field over the past decade. Like community mental health care itself, the authors are multidisciplinary, international, and pluralistic. This second edition of the *Oxford Textbook of Community Mental Health* addresses recent changes and achievements, current controversies, and future challenges while emphasizing areas of convergence, where social values, health and medical sciences, and policy formation come together.

Defining community mental health

Our definition of community mental health, shown in **Box 1.1**, highlights several fundamental issues. First, community mental health assumes a public health perspective (Levin & Petrila, 1996). As summarized by Thornicroft and Tansella (2009), this approach encompasses (1) a population view; (2) patients in a socioeconomic context; (3) primary, secondary, and tertiary prevention; (4) individual as well as population-based services; (5) service provision within a wider system of care; (6) universal access to services; (7) services provided by multidisciplinary teams; (8) a long-term, life-course perspective; and (9) an emphasis on evidence-based and cost-effective interventions.

> **Box 1.1** Definition of community mental health care
>
> Community mental health care comprises the principles and practices needed to promote mental health for a local population by (1) addressing population-based needs in ways that are accessible and acceptable; (2) building on the goals and strengths of people who experience mental health conditions; (3) promoting a wide and sufficient network of supports, services, and resources; and (4) emphasizing services that are both evidence-based and recovery-oriented.

This perspective also includes a commitment to social justice by addressing the needs of traditionally underserved populations, such as racial and ethnic minorities, people who are homeless or involved with the criminal justice system, and immigrants and refugees (Eylem et al., 2020; Pathare et al., 2021; Thornicroft et al., 2010).

Second, community mental health care focuses primarily on the people who experience mental health conditions. It places less emphasis on deficits, needs, and disabilities (an illness perspective), but rather serves to stress strengths, capacities, and preferences (a recovery perspective), and the contexts in which people live, paying close attention to the social determinants of health (Rose-Clarke et al., 2020) and recognizing the potential of the syndemic approach (Singer et al., 2017). Mental health treatment and care services therefore should aim to support a person's ability to develop a positive identity, to understand and self-manage the mental health condition, and to pursue their deeply held values (Damsgaard & Angel, 2021; Drake & Whitley, 2014; Slade, 2009).

Third, community mental health care includes the community in a broadly defined sense. It emphasizes not just the reduction or reaction to environmental adversity, but also the strengths of the families, social networks, communities, and organizations that are the context of people with lived experience of mental health conditions (Patel et al., 2018; Rapp & Goscha, 2006). Mental health conditions are embedded in, and partially determined by, social and environmental contexts (Jeste & Pender, 2022). In response, services must therefore comprise a wide network of interlocking components, including physical health care, housing, supported employment, social and legal services, religious and faith organizations, peer groups, self-help organizations, and informal support systems. Because social and environmental forces impinge so strongly on people who experience mental health conditions, community mental health must attend to these larger social forces in ways that are both ethical and pragmatic (Thornicroft et al., 2016a).

Fourth, community mental health melds both the evidence-based medicine paradigm and the recovery approach. The former requires using the best available data on the effectiveness of interventions. At the same time, people who experience mental health conditions need to understand these conditions (to the extent that professionals understand them), to decide between the available options for treatment and care, including adverse or side effects, and for special regard to be given to their values and preferences in a process of shared decision-making (Drake et al., 2009a; Thornicroft & Henderson, 2016). In recent years, traditional definitions of recovery that focus on the complete remission of symptoms and illness-related deficits have been replaced by definitions that view recovery as a personally meaningful process that involves growth and achieving a satisfying life in the community, irrespective of symptoms and impairments (Damsgaard & Angel, 2021; Davidson et al., 2009; Drake & Whitley, 2014; Slade, 2009). A commitment to recovery defined in this way emphasizes helping people to deal with their symptoms and achieving their personal life goals and projects to the greatest extent possible and values their full participation with service providers and with their communities (Mueser et al., 2002). This approach to a broader sense of community mental health also recognizes the powerful and corrosive forces of stigma and discrimination against people with mental health conditions and the need to identify and put into practice effective methods for stigma reduction (Thornicroft et al., 2010, 2016b, 2022).

Community mental health care is shaped by a variety of values and forces that often conflict. Some values derive from the larger society, especially those expressed through governments' social policy on the one hand and medical science on the other, while other values derive from the smaller groups of participants directly engaged in mental health care provision—those of service users, carers, and health professionals. An analysis of community mental health therefore requires a concurrent examination of these issues from multiple perspectives. It also requires the application of the methods of a variety of academic disciplines, including the behavioural and social sciences, information technology, history, politics, and, because questions of value are so central, moral philosophy and ethics (Szmukler, 2019).

The evolution of community mental health care

In the initial phases of deinstitutionalization, attempts to recreate the hospital service environment in the community had the unintended effect of perpetuating segregation, paternalism, passivity, dependency, low expectations, stagnation, stigma, and hopelessness. At that time, early forms of community-based alternatives, such as nursing homes, group homes, day hospitals, day treatment programmes, and sheltered workshops, commonly replicated the stultifying environments of long-term hospitals. The typical 'deinstitutionalized' mental health client trudged from a supervised group home to a supervised day programme, and then perhaps to a supervised group outing. Segregation, dependence, and stigma were blatant aspects of such care. Mental health clients in these settings were often treated as though they were incompetent children who could not make their own decisions, manage their own conditions, live on their own, integrate into their communities, work competitively, and pursue friendships and leisure activities. In retrospect, community mental health care of that era can be seen as inadvertently perpetuating stigma and as continuing to socialize people into disability. Many people with mental health conditions rejected this approach, and courageous individuals with lived experience have led the recovery movement from the beginning (Deegan, 1988). These goals are consistent with the United Nations Convention on the Rights of Persons with Disabilities (2006), which has had a considerable impact in drawing attention to pervasive forms of discrimination against persons with mental health (or 'psychosocial') disabilities.

The search to improve community mental health care has steadily evolved. Over the past five decades, numerous ideas and voices have shaped this evolution. People who experience mental health conditions, their families, mental health professionals, policymakers, administrators and managers, insurers, theorists, advocates, judges, guild organizations, trades unions, for-profit industries, media, public health and safety officials, and researchers are among those who have expressed views on these issues. The voices have often been conflicting and discordant rather than unified and clear (Levine, 1981). Increases in homelessness and incarceration of people with mental health conditions have exacerbated disagreements. Consensus has rarely been achieved. And when consensus has developed, the instantiation of new models of care has often been characterized by rhetoric, inadequate funding, and failure, rather than by genuine commitment, faithful implementation, and success (Drake & Essock, 2009; Drake & Latimer, 2012).

Some ideologies, strategies, and policies have been validated by scientific evidence, but many remain largely untested. Nonetheless, these trends have strongly influenced the mental health service system and the field of community mental health. Several authors discuss these notions in detail throughout this textbook. Among the most prominent are the following:

From ethical and legal perspectives, people who experience mental health conditions have the same rights as all others in society—the same rights to pursue their own health care preferences, values, life projects, and happiness as others (United Nations, 2006; World Health Organization, 2021). Legal rights include not only freedom from arbitrary detention and abusive treatments but also freedom to live and receive services and access to social goods on an equal basis with others. They also include the right to have one's will and preferences respected in relation to life choices. In many countries, these rights can be abridged only if the individual meets specific legal standards (which may be regarded by some authorities as inconsistent with recent developments in international law). Thus, communities, clinicians, and families can no longer decide that an individual is incompetent using ad hoc criteria.

From a philosophical perspective, modern community mental health insists that people with a mental health condition are 'people first'. Neither illness nor disability should undermine personhood or define a person's identity; humanity defines personhood, and demands recognition of the inherent dignity of all human beings. Current linguistic preferences include 'a person who has a mental health condition' or 'a person with schizophrenia' rather than 'a schizophrenic or a bipolar'.

From a clinical perspective, community mental health thinking now assumes that people with even the most severe mental illnesses have the capacity to manage their own conditions and to pursue personally meaningful life goals, often despite ongoing symptoms (Davidson et al., 2009; Drake & Whitley, 2014; Slade, 2009). This is in contradistinction to older approaches which assumed the incompetence of people with, for example, any form of severe mental health condition. Current mental health philosophies and interventions thus emphasize dignity, personal values, strengths, resilience, self-management, self-agency, capability for functional recovery, and social inclusion.

From a socio-environmental perspective, the strengths of the individual's social network and community are also more salient (Rapp & Goscha, 2006). The professional view of families has transitioned from causing illness (e.g. so-called schizophrenogenic mothers), to exacerbating illness (e.g. high 'expressed emotion'), to ameliorating illness (helping a family member who experiences mental illness), and finally to invaluable allies (e.g. in the National Alliance on Mental Illness in the US). Many families provide long-term support to their relatives who experience mental health conditions, especially when the families themselves acquire appropriate education, skills, and supports. Similarly, the community environment is now viewed as a potentially empowering context, for example, in the recent development of recovery-friendly workplaces. Like others, people with mental health conditions grow and mature through participating in regular jobs, educational experiences, integrated social settings, normal housing arrangements, and routine community activities (Becker & Drake, 2003). Although the public's misperceptions about mental illness can be extremely damaging, the evidence is now clear that using the principle of social contact can effectively reduce stigma and discrimination (Thornicroft et al., 2016b, 2022).

From a psychological perspective, a recognition that helping others promotes and enhances the process of recovery from a major illness has become mainstream. Peer support and people with lived experience as mental health employees are now prominent features of the mental health system in many areas (Fortuna et al., 2022). The peer support movement continues to grow steadily, supported by numerous personal testimonies and a growing research base.

From a research perspective, community mental health continues to move steadily towards becoming a well-established domain of scientific research. Beliefs that psychotherapy cannot be studied, that theories and interventions do not need testing, and that the authority of senior clinicians and professional societies should be sufficient evidence have been fully discredited by cycles of failure and harm (Harrington, 2019). Standard scientific methods have produced a plethora of evidence-based interventions, many of which have demonstrated effectiveness in real-world settings (US Department of Health and Human Services, 2020). Rigorous research standards and transparency of systematic reviews have enhanced progress. Evidence-based medicine and evidence-based practices have largely replaced the acceptance of outpatient mental health as a cottage industry with few standards. Nevertheless, helpful debates continue regarding meaningful outcomes, appropriate research methods, and the emerging efforts to study service systems, as are addressed in many chapters of this textbook. The past two decades have also seen the growth of service users as collaborators in the research enterprise—participating in decision-making on, for example, the research questions to be asked, the most meaningful outcome measures, the acceptability to participants of research instruments to be employed, and how recruitment might be maximized (Wallcraft et al., 2009).

From a systems perspective, research on unmet needs has also expanded considerably (Substance Abuse and Mental Health Services Administration, 2020; Thornicroft, 2000). Despite increased knowledge of effective clinical interventions for most mental disorders, the gap between science and service remains large. Most of the people who experience mental health conditions are unable to access effective treatments, even in the wealthiest countries (Drake & Essock, 2009; Thornicroft et al., 2017). In the less wealthy countries, available access to treatment may be in traditional and faith healing practices where human rights violations are often common (Gureje et al., 2015). When access is not a problem, acceptability often is (Kreyenbuhl et al., 2009). Further, most mental health practitioners and systems do not use the most effective practices (Bruns et al., 2016). Continuing education programmes typically do not result in learning and using new skills, but information systems are beginning to deliver useful point-of-contact information that enhances practitioner knowledge and shared decision-making. Finally, mental health treatment systems typically record amounts of services delivered rather than quality of care and meaningful outcomes (Kruk et al., 2018). Information technology has improved these deficits but not as rapidly as promised.

From an international perspective, as globalization, climate change, migration, and cultural pluralism transform the world, community mental health systems have not often enough responded adequately to the challenges related to these trends. People from minority cultures and those who speak languages other than those of the host country have difficulty accessing services that they find personally and culturally welcoming and acceptable. Stark disparities in mental health challenges and services affect every country, and the global inequity in access to mental health care in general between countries in the high-income bracket and those in the low- and middle-income group means that the latter are even further behind in responding to these trends.

The structure of this book

We have organized this book to reflect the rich diversity of perspectives on community mental health, but also to attempt a synthesis of perspectives and views based on evidence and on personal and clinical experience. Working, studying, and reviewing community mental health across many continents for several decades, we share a remarkable convergence of ideas and inspiration. In particular, we share a commitment to the idea that community mental health should respond to the needs, goals, values, and preferences of people who experience mental health conditions.

Following this brief introduction (Chapter 1) and historical review section (Chapters 2–4), the book then provides overviews of the needs for a community mental health system (Chapters 5–9). We begin with the epidemiological data that underlie a public health approach to community mental health. People are not merely numbers, of course, and we include the perspectives of those who experience mental health conditions directly. And because we are concerned with social justice, we emphasize the needs of specific groups, such as racial, ethnic, and cultural minorities as well as immigrants and refugees, who are often overlooked in establishing generic mental health services.

Intervention science—the study of effective organization and implementation—is another critical building block for a community mental health system (Chapters 10–26). Specific components of community mental health and how are they organized constitute the heart of community mental health service provision. Ethical and legal perspectives, including the difficult issues of coercive interventions, are discussed next (Chapters 27–29). Recovery is a central organizing vision in community mental health that incorporates ethical and legal values as well as user values.

Countervailing the recovery vision are public attitudes that can be characterized by stigma and discrimination and we focus on recent evidence of how stigma and discrimination can be effectively reduced (Chapters 30 and 31). Mental health policies and financing mechanisms determine the structure of potentially available services, as we show in Chapters 32 and 33.

Within the parameters of governmental policies and funding, professionals are responsible for implementing a service system that is as effective as possible (Chapters 34–37). An entirely new section of the book covers global mental health, recognizing the long overdue recent expansion of research in this field (Chapters 38–44). Finally, we consider the future of community mental health in the global context (Chapter 45). We very much hope that this book will be useful to you in the years to come, in whatever role you play, in striving for better mental health.

REFERENCES

Becker, D. R. & Drake, R. E. (2003). *A Working Life for People with Mental Illness*. New York: Oxford University Press.

Bruns, E. J., Kerns, S. E. U., Pullmann, M. D., Hensley, S. W., Lutterman, T., & Hoagwood, K. E. (2016). Research, data, and evidence-based treatment use in the state behavioral health systems, 2001–2012. *Psychiatric Services*, **67**, 496–503.

Damsgaard, J. B. & Angel, S. (2021). Living a meaningful life while struggling with mental health: challenging aspects regarding personal recovery encountered in the mental health system. *International Journal on Environmental Research in Public Health*, **18**, 2708.

Davidson, L., Tondora, J., Lawless, M. S., O'Connell, M. J., & Rowe, M. (2009). *A Practical Guide to Recovery-Oriented Practice: Tools for Transforming Mental Health Care*. New York: Oxford University Press.

Deegan, P. E. (1988). Recovery: the lived experience of rehabilitation. *Psychosocial Rehabilitation Journal*, **11**, 11–19.

Drake, R. E., Cimpean, D., & Torrey, W. C. (2009). Shared decision making in mental health: prospects for personalized medicine. *Dialogues in Clinical Neuroscience*, **11**, 319–332.

Drake, R. E. & Essock, S. M. (2009). The science to service gap in real world schizophrenia treatment. *Schizophrenia Bulletin*, **35**, 677–678.

Drake, R. E. & Latimer, E. (2012). Lessons learned in developing community psychiatry in North America. *World Psychiatry*, **11**, 47–51.

Drake, R. E. & Whitley, R. (2014). Recovery from severe mental illness: description and analysis. *Canadian Journal of Psychiatry*, **59**, 236–242.

Eylem, O., de Wit, L., van Straten, A., Steubel, L., Melissourgaki, Z., de Vries, R., et al. (2020). Stigma for common mental disorders in racial minorities and majorities: a systematic review and meta-analysis. *BMC Public Health*, **20**, 879.

Fortuna, K. L., Solomon, P., & Rivera, J. (2022). An update of peer support/peer provided services: underlying processes, benefits, and critical ingredients. *Psychiatric Quarterly*, **93**, 571–586.

Gureje, O., Nortje, G., Makanjuola, V., Oladeji, B. D., Seedat, S., & Jenkins, R. (2015). The role of global traditional and complementary systems of medicine in the treatment of mental health disorders. *Lancet Psychiatry*, **2**, 168–177.

Harrington, A. (2019). *Mind Fixers: Psychiatry's Troubled Search for the Biology of Mental Illness*. New York: W. W. Norton.

Jeste, D., & Pender, V. (2022). Social determinants of mental health: Recommendations for research, training, practice, and policy. *JAMA Psychiatry*, **79**(4), 283–284. https://doi.org/10.1001/jamapsychiatry.2021.4385

Kreyenbuhl, J., Buchanan, R. W., Dickerson, F. B., & Dixon, L. B. (2009). The schizophrenia patient outcomes research team (PORT): updated treatment recommendations. *Schizophrenia Bulletin*, **36**, 94–103.

Kruk, M. E., Gage, A. D., Arsenault, C., Jordan, K., Leslie, H. H., Roder-DeWan, S., et al. (2018). High-quality health systems in the Sustainable Development Goals era: time for a revolution. *Lancet Global Health*, **6**, e1196–e1252.

Levin, B. & Petrila, J. (1996). *Mental Health Services: A Public Health Perspective*. Oxford: Oxford University Press.

Levine, M. (1981). *The History and Politics of Community Mental Health*. New York: Oxford University Press.

Patel, V., Saxena, S., Lund, C., Thornicroft, G., Baingana, F., Bolton, P., et al. (2018). The Lancet Commission on global mental health and sustainable development. *Lancet*, **392**, 1553–1598.

Pathare, S., Burgess, R. A., and Collins, P.Y. (2021). World Mental Health Day: prioritise social justice, not only access to care. *Lancet*, **398**, 1859–1860.

Rapp, C. & Goscha, R. (2006). *The Strengths Model: Case Management with People with Psychiatric Disabilities*. New York: Oxford University Press.

Rose-Clarke, K., Gurung, D., Brooke-Sumner, C., Burgess, R., Burns, J., Kakuma, R., et al. (2020). Rethinking research on the social determinants of global mental health. *Lancet Psychiatry*, **7**, 659–662.

Singer, M., Bulled, N., Ostrach, B., & Mendenhall, E. (2017). Syndemics and the biosocial conception of health. *Lancet*, **389**, 941–950.

Slade, M. (2009). *Personal Recovery and Mental Illness: A Guide for Mental Health Professionals*. New York: Cambridge University Press.

Substance Abuse and Mental Health Services Administration (2020). National Survey of Drug Use and Health datasets. https://www.samhsa.gov/data/release/2020-national-survey-drug-use-and-health-nsduh-releases

Szmukler, G. (2019). 'Capacity', 'best interests', 'will and preferences' and the UN Convention on the Rights of Persons with Disabilities. *World Psychiatry*, **18**, 34–41.

Thornicroft, G. (Ed.) (2000). *Measuring Mental Health Needs* (2nd ed.). London: Royal College of Psychiatrists/Gaskell.

Thornicroft, G., Alem, A., Antunes Dos Santos, R., Barley, E., Drake, R. E., Gregorio, G., et al. (2010). Lessons learned in the implementation of community mental health care. *World Psychiatry*, **9**, 67–77.

Thornicroft, G., Chatterji, S., Evans-Lacko, S., Gruber, M., Sampson, N., Aguilar-Gaxiola, S., et al. (2017). Undertreatment of people with major depressive disorder in 21 countries. *British Journal of Psychiatry*, **210**, 119–124.

Thornicroft, G., Deb, T., & Henderson, C. (2016a). Community mental health care worldwide: current status and further developments. *World Psychiatry*, **15**, 276–286.

Thornicroft, G. & Henderson, C. (2016). Joint decision making and reduced need for compulsory psychiatric admission. *JAMA Psychiatry*, **73**, 647–648.

Thornicroft, G., Mehta, N., Clement, S., Evans-Lacko, S., Doherty, M., Rose, D., et al. (2016b). Evidence for effective interventions to reduce mental-health-related stigma and discrimination. *Lancet*, **387**, 1123–1132.

Thornicroft, G., Sunkel, C., Alikhon Aliev, A., Baker, S., Brohan, E., El Chammay, R., et al. (2022). The Lancet Commission on ending stigma and discrimination in mental health. *Lancet*, **400**, 1438–1480.

Thornicroft, G. & Tansella, M. (2009). *Better Mental Health Care*. Cambridge: Cambridge University Press.

United Nations (2006). *Convention on the Rights of Persons with Disabilities*. New York: United Nations.

US Department of Health and Human Services (2020). Healthy People 2030. https://health.gov/healthypeople

Wallcraft, J., Schrank, B., & Amering, M. (2009). *Handbook of Service User Involvement in Mental Health Research*. Chichester: John Wiley & Sons.

World Health Organization (10 June 2021). New WHO guidance seeks to put an end to human rights violations in mental health care. https://www.who.int/news/item/10-06-2021-new-who-guidance-seeks-to-put-an-end-to-human-rights-violations-in-mental-health-care

SECTION 2
Origins of 'community psychiatry'

2. **Historical changes in mental health practice** 11
   Nikolas Rose

3. **Mental health policy in modern America** 23
   Gerald Grob and Howard Goldman

4. **Recovery as an integrative paradigm in mental health** 33
   Mike Slade and Larry Davidson

2

Historical changes in mental health practice

Nikolas Rose

Introduction

However we define 'community psychiatry', it is clear that, in contemporary societies, practices addressed to the mental troubles of individuals have proliferated across everyday life.[1] Psychiatric interventions occur in mental hospitals, psychiatric wards in general hospitals, special hospitals, medium secure units, day hospitals, outpatient clinics, child guidance clinics, prisons, children's homes, sheltered housing, drop-in centres, community mental health centres, domiciliary care by community psychiatric nurses, multiple forms of psychological therapies, and, of course, in the general practitioner's surgery, not least through the increasing prescription of psychiatric drugs. No phase of life is unknown to these practices: infertility, pregnancy, birth, and the postpartum period; infancy; childhood at home and at school; sexual normality, perversion, impotence, and pleasure; family life, marriage and divorce, employment and unemployment, mid-life crises, and failures to achieve; old age, terminal illness, and bereavement.

Wherever problems arise—in our homes, on the streets, in factories, schools, hospitals, the army, courtroom, or prison—experts with specialist knowledge of the nature, causes, and remedies for mental distress are on hand to provide its diagnoses and propose remedial action. And, of course, there is a wider penetration of psychiatry, broadly defined, into popular culture, as psychiatrists, mental hospitals, the mentally ill, and the problems of mental health feature daily in political and social debates, in our newspapers, in television documentaries, exposés, talk shows, and soap operas. The languages that have been disseminated have given us new vocabularies in which to think and talk about our problems—stress, trauma, depression, neuroses, compulsions, and phobias. They have also provided us with new ways of explaining, judging, and accounting for our personal miseries, of distinguishing the normal and the abnormal, identifying what is illness, and when to seek assistance and from whom. It would not, therefore, be too much of an exaggeration to say that we lived in a 'psychiatric society'.

'Community psychiatry', then, is one dimension of the 'psychiatric societies' that have taken shape over the course of the twentieth century. There have been many international variations in the historical paths followed in different national contexts, but the rationalities and practices that have taken shape are remarkably similar across the Western world. In this chapter, focusing upon the UK, I want to sketch out some of the key moments in this history.[2]

The territory of psychiatry

The early decades of the twentieth century are usually understood as a period when 'organicism' in psychiatry was in its heyday, when therapeutic pessimism dominated, and when psychiatry and its practitioners, like their patients, were entrapped within the enclosed institutional spaces that were the legacy of the asylum movement of the previous 100 years: asylums that had now become little more than vast warehouses for containment of those thought to be of unsound mind. At the outbreak of the First World War, there were nearly 140,000 patients in mental hospitals and other institutions in England and Wales, and the average county asylum housed over 1000 inmates. These figures were to increase over the subsequent four decades, reaching a peak of over 150,000 inmates by 1954 (K. Jones, 1972, Appendix 1). Conventional psychopathology by and large saw mental pathology in terms of a relation between an inherited constitution and the life stresses to which it was subject. The inherited nervous system might be insufficiently equipped with nerve cells, association fibres, or be otherwise organically flawed. After conception, including during the *in utero* period, the nervous system might be damaged by stress. The brain might be injured, or

---

[1] This is based in part on a revised and updated chapter entitled 'Psychiatry: the discipline of mental health' (N. Rose, 1986). More detailed references to original texts can be found there, and in N. Rose (1985). Thanks to Diana Rose for her advice in preparing this version. Note that at each point in the history that I describe, I have adopted the vocabulary that was used—the absence of repeated 'scare quotes' should not be taken for agreement.

[2] Except where specifically stated, reference is to developments in England and Wales.

harmed by toxins such as alcohol or by lack of nutrition or defects in the blood supply. In addition to such direct stress, the nervous system was also subject to the effects of indirect stress. Anxiety, inappropriate or over-demanding education, worries about employment or finance, intemperance or sexual excess, even religious fanaticism could adversely affect the nervous system (N. Rose, 1985, pp. 177–179; Rosen, 1959).

But this organicism still allowed psychiatry to play a role outside the asylum. Epilepsy, alcoholism, mental defect, mania, melancholia, and other personal and social ills were regarded as expressions of an inherited neuropathic constitution which might lead to antisocial and immoral conduct. Careful management of infants was essential. For those children whose families had shown pathology, this would strengthen the constitution and build up habits which would minimize the risk of onset. It was also vital in other families, for not even the strongest constitution was immune to damage. And, of course, the profligate breeding of those with severely tainted constitutions could lead to a swamping of the nation with neuropaths and a decline in national efficiency and the quality of the race. Hence the involvement of many key figures from the field of mental medicine in eugenic campaigns for the medical inspection, sterilization, or permanent segregation of mental defectives and others of the social problem group, and for their sterilization or permanent segregation (Farrall, 1985; Searle, 1976).

The wider sociopolitical role for psychiatry at this time was thus largely reactive and defensive: to help minimize and control the threat posed by insanity. But in the period following the First World War, a number of psychiatrists developed a more positive strategy. This modelled itself on the arguments of the new public health that claimed to be able to address large-scale problems concerning the size and quality of the population and its consequences (Armstrong, 1983). In this preventive medicine, the political fortunes of the nation came to be seen as dependent upon the physical health of each individual; simultaneously, individuals were thought to play a significant part in the spread of ill health through their personal conduct. Hence, reform of this conduct could promote social well-being. A complex apparatus of medical inspection, education in domestic hygiene, registration of births, infant welfare clinics, health visitors, school milk and meals, health clinics, and so forth was established to investigate these habits and to educate citizens to conduct their personal lives in a hygienic manner; and, indeed, to encourage them to want to be healthy. The new social psychiatry adopted many of these principles, and actively tried to promote mental welfare and mental hygiene. The first focus of this strategy was 'the neuroses'. This term was applied to conditions that were considered to be mild mental disturbances: they did not disable the individual completely, but were sufficient to cause social inefficiency and personal unhappiness. If left untreated, these minor troubles were thought likely to develop into more serious mental problems. And it was argued that many of those in workhouses and prisons—vagrants, criminals, delinquents, and others who were socially or industrially inefficient—suffered from mental pathology which had probably begun in a small way in treatable neurosis. Hence, the neuroses of childhood were of particular concern. They provided a fortunate early warning of troubles to come, and, given the malleability of the child, it was thought that, in the majority of cases, they could be successfully treated.

The neuroses came to light in all those sites where individuals could now be judged to fail in relation to institutional norms and expectations—in the production line routines of factory labour, in the new expectations of universal schooling, in the newly established juvenile courts, and, especially, in the unprecedented demands upon the military in the First World War. Shell shock accounted for 10% of officer casualties in the 1914–1918 war, and for 4% of casualties from other ranks. More than 80,000 such cases were estimated to have occurred over the course of the war, and some 65,000 ex-servicemen were still receiving disability pensions in 1921 because of shell shock. While senior military officers frequently regarded shell shock as merely a disguise for cowardice, organicist physicians considered the condition to be a genuine one resulting from minute cerebral haemorrhages caused by the blast (Hearnshaw, 1964, pp. 245–246; N. Rose, 1985, pp. 182–183). But doctors working in the shell shock clinics and specialized hospitals that were set up to deal with these cases were unconvinced by such organic explanations, especially given the lack of independent evidence of the postulated lesions. Versions of the therapeutic methods invented by Janet in Paris and Freud in Vienna were tried out on the shell-shocked with some success. Shell shock appeared to respond to a variety of approaches ranging from occupational training, through persuasion and a form of rational re-education, the use of suggestion, to a type of psychotherapy using hypnosis or free association. Experience with this treatment converted many to a kind of dynamic theory of the will, using concepts such as instinct and repression, and attentive to the intermixing of physical and mental symptoms. These beliefs played a key role in the mental hygiene movement: for the first time, psychiatrists would collaborate with other professionals in a strategy for the prevention, the early detection, and the voluntary treatment of mental ill health.

The rationale of mental hygiene, with its belief in a continuity between minor and major mental disorders and in the importance of early intervention for individual adjustment and social efficiency, underpinned the argument made in a series of official reports from the 1920s to the outbreak of the Second World War (discussed in detail in N. Rose, 1985, pp. 197–209). Poor mental hygiene was thought to be the cause of all sorts of social ills, preventable by education in proper techniques for mental hygiene, and by early detection of the signs of trouble followed by prompt and efficient treatment. It was believed that this was hampered by the stigma which surrounded lunacy, by the isolation of the asylum from other medical facilities, and by the legal procedures of 1890 which allowed asylums only to take patients certified through a cumbersome legal process. This discouraged individuals with mild problems from seeking help, and discouraged doctors from utilizing asylums, turning them into institutions for the incarceration of those considered beyond hope. Not only was this a counterproductive method of organizing services, it was also conceptually unwarranted. As the Royal Commission on Lunacy and Mental Disorder put it in 1926:

> insanity is, after all, only a disease like other diseases … a mind deranged can be ministered to no less effectively than a body deranged … The problem of insanity is essentially a public health problem to be dealt with on modern public health lines. (pp. 16–22)

Treatment should not require certification, compulsion, or incarceration. Facilities should be available in hospitals for outpatient and voluntary treatment to encourage easy access to help at an early stage of the disease (Rees, 1945, p. 29). This was the rationale that had led to the establishment of the Maudsley Hospital, which was completed in

1915 and the Cassel Hospital, which opened in 1919 (Barnes, 1968, pp. 10–15; K. Jones, 1972, pp. 235–236). It was for similar reasons that the Mental Treatment Act 1930 renamed asylums 'mental hospitals' and stipulated that, in the majority of cases, lunatics should be termed simply 'persons of unsound mind'. Patients could now be received for inpatient treatment on voluntary application, and local authorities were to make provision for the establishment of psychiatric outpatient clinics at general and mental hospitals.[3]

Disturbed individuals could come to the clinics themselves, once they or others were educated in the signs of mental disturbance, and now free of the fears of stigma or incurability. Others were to be referred to them from school, court, and elsewhere by statutory and voluntary agencies. In the clinics, assessment and treatment would be carried out, reports would be supplied to courts or schools, and individuals would be referred to other institutions. But the clinics would also provide the base for a system of mental hygiene which could act more widely on the lives of patients, ex-patients, and potential patients. Social workers, psychiatric social workers, probation officers, school attendance officers, and others would operate between the clinic and home, school, or courtroom, conveying information, advice, and education. The new mental hygiene was to provide the basis of a project of general public education as to the habits likely to promote mental welfare. Mental health was to be a personal responsibility and a national objective.

Community as therapy

Despite these developments, in practice the pre-Second World War psychiatric population was split between the 'neurotics'—maladjusted and delinquent children, inefficient workers, and shell-shocked soldiers and the like—and the 'psychotics'. The latter were those certified under mental health legislation, segregated from the sufferers of physical illness, and confined in the large, isolated, custodial mental hospitals. The provision of outpatient clinics was confined to a few geographical areas; only a small number of the more recently built asylums had established separate facilities for new acute patients; very few beds for inpatient treatment were provided in wards of general hospitals; and some, but not all, municipal hospitals had set up 'observation wards' where mental patients could be confined for limited periods for assessment and diagnosis before being discharged or committed to a mental hospital.

In the 1930s, mental hospitals in England and Wales had an average population of around 1200, but some contained up to 3000 patients. The majority were there for long periods—if not permanently—and active therapeutic intervention was spasmodic. It was accepted that the majority of patients were suffering from psychoses which were often hereditary in origin and mostly incurable. The old ideals of moral treatment had largely been discarded, though, for the most fortunate patients, asylums did operate as communities where they 'lived a life of contented servitude, working as orderlies, storemen, or domestic servants in a cosier world than that outside' (Clark, 1964). With the 'melancholic', 'paraphrenic', or 'deluded', certain attachments formed between staff and patients; for others, the regime varied from neglect, through surveillance and containment, to degradation and brutality.

However questionable their claims to efficacy, the new physical treatments developed in the 1930s did disrupt this stasis. They offered asylum doctors an image of themselves as healers of the sick and not merely superintendents of the institution. Waves of enthusiasm for these treatments swept through the hospitals. Physical treatments—from removal of tonsils to varieties of convulsion therapy—were selected according to the latest reports in the medical literature or the predilections of the medics. As with the claims for bleedings and purgings of the eighteenth century and for the use of sedatives such as chloral hydrate and bromides in the nineteenth century, such hopes were usually short-lived. But despite limited experimentation in asylums, or in units attached to them, the principal task of asylum doctors remained the containment of chronic patients, which often required the use of coercion, and offered few prospects for innovation other than more efficient administration.

Within mental medicine, hostility was growing between the long-established sector of asylum superintendents who dominated the Board of Control, defenders of the need for separate and distinct institutions for the treatment of the mentally ill, and physicians who sought the integration of the practice, training, and facilities of psychiatry with those of the general hospital. The future of psychiatry was being shaped outside the asylum mainstream, in specialist units in general hospitals, in outpatient clinics, in private practice, and in psychotherapy and psychoanalysis. The Second World War was decisively to shift the balance between these two wings of psychiatry (cf. Baruch & Treacher, 1978).

John Rawlings Rees, Director of the Tavistock Clinic, was appointed consulting psychiatrist to the Army, perhaps because the problems at issue in wartime were precisely those of functional nerve disorder over which the Tavistock had established its jurisdiction. In any event, the consequence was that the new tasks of psychiatry were to be thought from within the rationale of mental hygiene. Psychiatrists tried to develop methods of selection, both for the weeding out of potential problem cases and in the selection of those suitable for promotion. They tried to adjust military training techniques in order to enhance the fit between the mental and the organizational, and sought to maximize morale by methods of man-management which would promote solidarity through acting on the psychiatrically important aspects of group life. While each of these developments would have significance for the expanded role of the 'psy' professions in the post-war period, most important for psychiatry itself was the issue of treatment.[4] Psychiatrists were involved in the treatment of casualties: in the army alone they saw almost 250,000 cases during the Second World War, even discounting those referred from army intakes, those seen in selection testing and patients seen in psychiatric hospitals (Rees, 1945, p. 46). While only about 8000 of these were diagnosed as psychotic, about 130,000 were considered to be neurotic. The invaliding rate for psychiatric disabilities was over 30% of all discharges for medical causes. While military neurosis centres did manage to return about 80% of their cases

---

[3] The responsibilities of local authorities for lunacy and mental deficiency services and aftercare had already been widened by provisions of the Local Government Act of 1929 which followed the recommendations of the Royal Commission on Lunacy and Mental Disorder. cf. N. Rose (1985), pp. 158–163).

[4] On the concept of the psy professions (psychiatrists, psychologists, psychiatric social workers, and many more) see N. Rose (1996).

to duty, the results of treatment overall were poor. This emphasized the need for new treatment techniques. More fundamentally, it confirmed that psychiatry should not focus upon the confinement of the small number of deranged persons with psychosis. To fulfil the task that society required, it needed to shift its attention to the detection and treatment of those large numbers of the population who were now known to be liable to neurotic breakdown, maladjustment, inefficiency, and unemployability on the grounds of poor mental health (cf. K. Jones, 1972, pp. 262–282).

Perhaps the most significant invention in treatment concerned the institution itself. At the start of the Second World War, while confinement might have been a condition for certain types of treatment, it was not in itself considered to be therapeutic. But in the course of the war, for the first time since the heyday of moral treatment, some at least began to argue that the institution itself could be a therapeutic technology. Maxwell Jones credits Wilfred Bion with the first recognition of the principle underlying the social therapies that 'social environmental influences are themselves capable of effectively changing individual and group patterns of behaviour' (M. Jones, 1952, p. 519, cf. Kraüpl Taylor, 1958, Manning, 1976). In 1943, Bion undertook an experiment in which he treated the unruly conduct of the inmates of the Training Wing of Northfield Military Hospital through manipulating authority relations, believing that if the men themselves had to take responsibility for organizing tasks, and for defining and disciplining miscreants, they would learn that the disruption was not grounded *in* authority but in their psychological relations *to* authority.

Although the authorities terminated this experiment after 6 weeks, it was followed by a second 'Northfield experiment' in which Thomas Main sought to produce what he referred to as a 'therapeutic community' in which the hospital was to be used:

> not as an organization run by doctors in the interests of their own greater technical efficiency, but as a community with the immediate aim of full participation of all its members in its daily life and the eventual aim of the resocialisation of the neurotic individual for life in ordinary society … a spontaneous and emotionally structured (rather than medically dictated) organization in which all staff and patients engage. (Main, 1946, p. 67)

At the same time, Maxwell Jones became joint director of the Mill Hill Neurosis Unit, set up by the Ministry of Health for the treatment of 'effort syndrome' and concluded that the patient's reactions to the hospital community mirrored his reactions to the community outside, and hence that the hospital itself might be an instrument to be used to explore and improve the patient's condition.

At the end of the war, Jones was put in charge of one of the units for labour resettlement set up by the Ministry of Labour with the aim of rehabilitating ex-prisoners of war for civilian life. The techniques deployed in these 'transitional communities' for 'social reconnection' were those which had been developed in the community treatment of 'neurotic' soldiers, with the addition of attempts to connect up the 'transitional community' with the local community which surrounded it (Curle, 1947; Wilson et al., 1947; cf. Kraüpl Taylor, 1958). Where rehabilitation had previously been a mere adjunct to therapy conducted by other means—mediating between life under the dominance of medicine and life as a private matter—it was now seen as the essence of the therapeutic intervention itself. The patient was one who had lost his or her capacity to function as an adjusted social individual; treatment was to reinvest them with the rights, privileges, capacities, moralities, and responsibilities of personhood. This way of thinking, in which mental ill health is identified in terms of a failure to cope, and treatment becomes a matter of the restoration of coping capacities, would spread widely through psychiatric practice in the post-war period, and indeed would become the practical rationale of much of community psychiatry in the 1970s and beyond.

In the immediate post-war period, Jones argued that the techniques he had developed could be applied to any other socially maladjusted individuals—in particular, to 'psychopaths' (M. Jones, 1952, Introduction). In 1947, he moved to the Industrial Neurosis Unit at Belmont Hospital and applied these methods to the 'chronic unemployed neurotics' it received from all over England and included 'inadequate and aggressive psychopaths', 'schizoid personalities', 'early schizophrenics', various drug addictions, sexual perversions, and chronic psychoneurotics. Through a variety of discussion groups, intense small groups, and psychodrama, sexual, criminal, industrial or social deviants, whose behaviour was now construed as a manifestation of an underlying personality disorder, were to be managed back to a state of adjustment in which they could function smoothly within the institutional regimes which they had previously disrupted.

It required but a simple shift of perspective to see that the traditional mental hospital violated all these therapeutic maxims. Hence, in the 1950s a two-pronged attack on such institutions was mounted under the banner of the 'therapeutic community'. On the one hand, a series of research studies of psychiatric institutions confirmed the pathogenic features of their organization and management (e.g. Caudill, 1958; Stanton & Schwartz, 1954). On the other, a series of 'adventures in psychiatry' were undertaken, notably at the Cassel, Claybury, and Fulbourn hospitals, which sought to reorganize the mental hospital more or less according to the new rationale and to incorporate some or all of the new techniques of administrative therapy into their institutions, sometimes in combination with chemotherapy or psycho-analytically inspired individual therapy (Barnes, 1968, pp. 4–15; Clark, 1964; Martin, 1962). These developments were isolated and short-lived. Many psychiatrists were scandalized by the reported 'goings on' in such hospitals. They criticized the therapeutic efficacy of these attempts to use the institution as a positive element in the production of the cure, and they used arguments about the negative effects of mental hospital life in order to support their case. But, in fact, this new 'social' vision of the psychiatric institution reverberated through the system, leading to the widespread unlocking of wards throughout the 1950s, coupled with reductions in the regimentation of the lives of confined patients, and a policy of accelerated discharge.[5]

This attention to the organizational and interpersonal features of the psychiatric setting offered new opportunities for psychiatric nurses. The new therapeutic vision of the interpersonal relations of the hospital enabled them to stake a claim for a more autonomous type of expertise. Doctors could not claim special skills in the

---

[5] T. P. Rees at Warlingham Park Hospital opened the doors of 21 out of his 23 wards in the early fifties; by 1956, 22 out of 37 wards at Netherne Hospital were opened and 60% of patients were allowed out on parole within the boundaries of the estate; MacMillan opened the doors at Mapperly Hospital Nottingham in 1954, Stern did likewise at the Central Hospital Warwick in 1957 as did Mandelbrote at Coney Hill, Gloucester. Details are in Kraüpl Taylor (1958, pp. 155–156).

manipulation of the dynamic relations between members of the institutional community, yet these were now to be systematically utilized in the construction of a normal identity for the patient. At its high point, which was probably in the 1970s, this underpinned a new 'psychotherapeutic' vision of psychiatric nursing as an activity which could itself be curative through working upon the patient's relationships with the situations he or she encountered in the everyday life of the ward.

In the psychiatric wards of old mental hospitals and new psychiatric units, and in the day hospitals and half-way houses that began to proliferate, new techniques of nursing were developed and deployed. Nurses, in psychiatric and in general nursing, gradually altered their view of the patient: no longer merely a series of tasks, the patient was a sick person who needed to be actively engaged in the process of getting better.[6] These developments in nursing were accompanied by the growth of other forms of institutional therapy that owed something to the therapeutic community idea. Occupational and industrial therapies sought not only to increase muscular coordination, and hence self-confidence, but also to encourage the habits of labour. As mental disorder began to be seen, at least in part, as an inability to cope with the demands of employment, work itself began to be seen as a vital element in the treatment of mental disorder (Miller, 1986). The developing programme of hospital closure allowed these practices to develop in new psychiatric spaces—in day hospitals run by the hospital service, day centres run by local authorities, half-way houses, hostels, group homes, and a variety of other residential and non-residential institutions. In the 1970s and 1980s, these professionals and their techniques would find their homes in the new institutions of the psychiatric community.

A place would also be found for the authentic therapeutic communities. There were not only Belmont, now known as Henderson Hospital, and the Cassel, but also 'mini'-therapeutic communities (Clark, 1970; Manning & Hinshelwood, 1979). These were characterized by such techniques as large and small group meetings, projective and expressive therapies involving art and drama, occupational therapies, and individual therapies—developed in psychiatric units in general hospitals, in rehabilitative institutions in the prison system, in institutions for maladjusted, delinquent, and criminal youths, in houses for drug users and alcoholics often run by ex-patients, in the work of Richmond Fellowship, and in many other residential establishments in the public, grant-aided, charitable, and private sectors. These institutions provide a therapeutic rationale for the confinement of young neurotics and the 'personality disordered', the persistently self-damaging, the repetitively suicidal, the ostentatiously antisocial, those who continually act out, and those who are continually manipulated by others: those whose illness appears to consist only in a disruptive failure of social adjustment and whose treatment can thus be seen as co-extensive with, and exhausted by, a systematic programme of resocialization.

---

[6] Developments in nursing can be traced through the articles and letters in *Nursing Mirror* and *Nursing Times* over this period. See also Meacher (1979) and Barnes (1968). These developments in nursing are consonant with the shift in medical perception noted in Armstrong (1984).

Accounting for community psychiatry

Conventional accounts of the move of psychiatry 'into the community' in the second half of the twentieth century in the UK, the US, and much of Europe stress two factors: the discovery of genuinely effective psychotropic drugs and the recognition that confinement could be damaging. On the one hand, drugs offered the possibility of amelioration of symptoms if not cure, and did away with the necessity for long periods of institutional confinement—while also validating the medical mandate over problems of mental health. On the other, the discovery of the poor conditions within mental institutions and the pathogenic effects of confinement itself, led to a view that long periods of confinement were damaging and anti-therapeutic. In the US, Albert Deutsch documented the shameful conditions in the asylums that were reminiscent of those in the concentration camps, and Erving Goffman published his sociological account of the effects of the 'total institution' in stripping away the personality and identity of the inmate (Deutsch, 1948; Goffman, 1962). In Britain, Russell Barton diagnosed a condition he christened 'institutional neurosis'—a form of illness produced by the institution itself and John Wing demonstrated that institutionalism—apathy, resignation, dependence, depersonalization, and reliance on fantasy—was common to long-stay inmates of even well-run mental hospitals, and that reforms centring upon enriching the institutional environment were difficult to maintain in the face of institutional exigencies (Barton, 1959; Wing, 1962; see also Lomax, 1921). It appeared that the pathogenic effects of the mental hospital were intractable; the solution was not to reform the institution but to do away with it. Such accounts suggest that these developments led to changes in policy, based on the view that mental hospitals did little good but much harm, and consumed scarce resources which were better directed to more effective forms of provision. Wherever possible hospitalization should be avoided, where necessary it should be in the ordinary medical system, the length of stay should be minimized, and individuals should be maintained 'in their communities' where, rather than suffering the pathogenic consequences of institutionalization, they would be subject to the benign influences of normality.

Critics of this account of psychiatric progress point out that critiques of 'museums of madness' were nothing new, and so other factors must account for their effects at this particular moment in psychiatric history (e.g. Baruch & Treacher, 1978; Scull, 1985; Treacher & Baruch, 1981). They also dispute the significance accorded to the new discoveries in psychopharmacology, pointing to the repetitious history of enthusiastic claims for the efficacy of physical treatments of mental disorder followed by disillusionment occasioned by relapse, side effects, or other disappointments. And it is true that there is little correlation between patterns of hospital bed use and discharge rates and the use of such drugs in different areas and countries; the role of phenothiazine drugs in the 1950s was more for control within the hospital than to facilitate discharge. Thus sociologists and historians have suggested that the determinants of the move away from custodial responses to mental disorder must be found elsewhere. They suggest that what was at stake was not a desegregation of the mentally ill, but a desegregation of psychiatry—a desire of psychiatrists to end their isolation and gain access to the power, careers, and status of other medical specialisms. They regard the 'drug revolution' not as the origin of the move away from the mental hospital but as a pseudo-scientific legitimation for it (Treacher & Baruch, 1981). And they argue that the political rationale for a shift away from the custodial institution lay in a 'fiscal crisis of the state': the cost of incarceration, of maintaining the buildings, and paying the increased wages won by the unions were harder and harder to justify, in a situation where the state was finding it increasingly difficult to fund its welfare activities through the taxation system without unacceptable demands upon private profit (Scull, 1985).

The truth probably lies somewhere between these two narratives. While the cost of maintaining mental hospitals, which were largely built in the nineteenth century, was a significant factor, as we have seen, the events that led to unlocking the wards and the run-down of the mental hospital system began much earlier, predating any 'fiscal crisis'. Indeed, cross-national comparisons show no correlation between moves away from incarceration and economic prosperity or crisis. However, the development of post-war welfare states did provide crucial conditions for this shift in policy. While in the nineteenth century institutional confinement was seen as the condition for social support, in the era of the welfare state and social insurance this was no longer the case. Social insurance made it possible for individuals without wage labour to be maintained without incarceration. Public housing facilities provided the conditions for such persons to be physically sheltered outside institutions, as did the development of private and charitable housing schemes. The foundation of a comprehensive system of primary medical care enabled general practitioners to play a key role in dispensing pharmaceutical treatments without the need for hospital admission. The consolidation of medical and psychiatric social work within the local authorities and the hospitals enabled supervision of the patients outside hospitals.

However, it would be wrong to see the changes in psychiatry as merely a fortunate beneficiary of the new rationale of welfare. The post-war modernization of psychiatry was neither a mere rationalization for financial savings nor a consequence of psychopharmacology: it was the generalization of a sociopolitical strategy whose rudiments had been put in place over a 50-year period.

Blurring the boundaries of the institution

Official discussions of psychiatry in the post-Second World War period appear merely to reiterate and extend the themes concerning the need for early and voluntary treatment and the organizational and clinical similarities and interdependencies between mental and physical ills. The Royal Commission on Mental Illness and Mental Deficiency, which was set up in 1954 and reported in 1957, posed the issues in a similar way, as did the Mental Health Act 1959 which followed on from its recommendations. As the Minister put it, what was involved was a 're-orientation of mental health services away from institutional care towards care in the community'. Hence the Act extended the open-door policy, established informal admissions as the norm, extended local authority powers, encouraged liaison between health and social services, and so forth (see, for the above, K. Jones, 1972, p. 307). This strategy linked up with developments in the post-war apparatus of the welfare state. Psychiatric social work had extended from the child guidance clinics and mental hospitals into the heart of social casework (Younghusband, 1978). Psychiatric social workers were employed not only in the prison and borstal services, in care committees, and so forth, but also in the extensive work of rehabilitation of ex-service men and women, working in the mental health advisory services set up for this purpose under the National Health Service Act of 1946. And, further, psychiatrically trained social workers were now operating as Children's Officers under the Children Act of 1948: all social work now attended, to a greater or lesser extent, to the psychological investments and conflicts which underpinned even those presenting problems which were apparently entirely practical (Timms, 1964).

While the Mental Health Act of 1959 allocated considerable discretionary powers to doctors in respect of involuntary admission to mental hospital and the administration of treatment without the patient's consent, this was neither an extension of the coercive powers of the authorities nor a triumph of organicist medicine over other theories of the origin of mental disorder or other professional claims for a role in a mental health system. On the contrary, the strategy sought to minimize the role of incarceration in the social responses to mental distress, to establish links and alliances between medicine and other social agencies, to facilitate the movement of individuals among and between the different branches of the mental health system, and to encourage each of us to take responsibility for the preservation and promotion of mental health.

But despite these conceptual continuities, the transformations of the psychiatric system in the 1950s and 1960s do mark a significant shift in the spatial dispensation of psychiatry. While neither criticisms of the asylum nor claims for the efficacy of physical treatments were new, in the context of the new rationale for psychiatry as a part of public health, they enabled an extension of psychiatric modernization to those sectors of the psychiatric system which had previously been most difficult to access. On the one hand, it was now argued that the closed asylums with their populations of chronic and psychotic patients were not only sucking in social resources which were more usefully deployed in the other sectors of the system, but were also actively damaging in their effects. On the other, whatever their real efficacy, the new pharmacological technologies of treatment made it possible to imagine that people with severe psychiatric problems could be managed outside the hospital The medical complex of general practitioners, outpatient departments, and ordinary general hospitals could administer the drug-based therapeutics without the segregative institution. Social insurance and social workers could service the ill person without confinement. And madness—understood now merely as illness, unhappiness, and inefficiency—no longer constituted a fundamental threat to reason and order which required incarceration. The asylum had become unnecessary.

The policy landmarks of the new configuration are clear enough (K. Jones, 1972, pp. 321–334). Enoch Powell, Minister of Health, in his 1961 speech to the National Association of Mental Health, announced the objective of halving the number of places in hospitals for mental illness over the next 15 years, and the closure of the majority of the existing mental hospitals. The Ministry circular following this speech confirmed the decline in bed spaces, urged planning for closure of 'large, isolated and unsatisfactory buildings', and laid out the four kinds of accommodation to be provided in the new system: acute units for short-stay patients, usually in general hospitals; medium-stay units for medium-stay patients; units for long-stay patients, often in hostels or annexes of general hospitals;

and secure units provided on a regional basis. In 1962, the Hospital Plan for the next 15 years envisaged the phasing out of all specialist hospitals, such as those for the mentally ill and the chronically sick, and their incorporation into district general hospitals. In 1963, *Health and Welfare: The Development of Community Care* urged the desirability of 'community care', but did not specify what this entailed. By 1971, *Hospital Services for the Mentally Ill* proposed the complete abolition of the mental hospital system, with all inpatient, day-patient, and outpatient services provided by departments of district general hospitals, linked in to services provided by the local authority social services, general practitioners, and in consultation with the Department of Employment.

This policy was continued throughout the 1970s, irrespective of the political complexion of the government of the day. The lines of argument were similar in *Better Services for the Mentally Ill*, produced by Barbara Castle's Labour ministry in 1975, and in *Care in Action* and *Care in the Community* produced in 1981 under the aegis of the monetarist conservatism represented by Patrick Jenkin. The strategy was now more clearly developed: articulated in terms of the creation of a comprehensive psychiatric service, a continuum of care, and a community psychiatric system; prevention through education and the encouragement of practices to promote mental health; early treatment entailing the removal of stigma, ease of access, minimization of legal formalism, and the education of professionals so that they may pick up the early signs of mental disorder; outpatient treatment in clinics, sheltered housing, through domiciliary services, and with social work support; inpatient treatment to be minimized, for as short a period as possible and within the district general hospital; and aftercare on discharge provided by the outpatient services.

The psychiatric system which had taken shape in England, Europe, and the US by the 1980s was not primarily an apparatus of coercion and segregation, delineated by the mental hospital and monopolized by the medical profession. At the programmatic level, it aspired towards a 'continuum of care' which would run from custodial measures for those with major mental derangements, through voluntary treatment for minor mental troubles, to prophylactic work by propaganda, advice, and the reform of personal life in the interests of mental health. The psychiatric population was highly differentiated and distributed across a range of specialized sites: secure units, local authority group homes, specialized units for children, alcoholics, eating disorders, drug users, and so forth. And relations had been established between such institutions and other sites where psychiatric expertise was deployed: the child guidance clinic, the courtroom, the counselling centre, the prison, and the classroom. In this 'advanced' psychiatric system (Castel et al., 1982), key roles were played by non-medical professions—nursing, social work, probation, psychology, education, occupational therapy—and increasingly by quasi-professional 'voluntary' or self-help organizations.

Nor was this psychiatric complex dominated by a socially blind organicism at the level of theory or treatment. Most psychiatric professionals allowed a key role for 'social factors' in the precipitation and prevention of mental distress, sought to inject psychiatric considerations into debates over social policies, and established collaborative relations between medical treatment in hospital and the aid of other social agencies. A practical eclecticism enabled the coexistence of therapeutic ideologies and techniques which appear fundamentally opposed: from individual psychotherapy to co-counselling, from dynamic group therapy to behaviour modification, and from drug treatment to family therapy. Hospitals using psychotropic medications, therapeutic communities, feminist self-help groups, social work group homes, community nurses, and many other strange bedfellows combined to chart the domain of mental health and develop technologies for its management. The move away from the asylum extended the range of social ills seen to be flowing from psychiatric disturbance and simultaneously 'psychiatrized' new populations. Children, delinquents, criminals, vagrants and the work-shy, the aged, and unhappy marital and sexual partners all became possible objects for explanation and treatment in terms of mental disturbance. And, in the majority of cases, such treatment was not imposed coercively upon unwilling subjects but sought out by those who had come to identify their own distress in psychiatric terms.

Community and control

The shifts in psychiatric policy over the closing two decades of the twentieth century entailed a critique of many of these assumptions, and a reshaping of the practices to which they were linked. Many approaches developed over the previous 50 years fell into disrepute, as expensive, lengthy, and unproven: the demand for 'evidence-based treatments' was a key factor in displacing psychodynamically inspired therapies with interventions that sought rapid and measurable transformations in specific pathologies of thought or conduct. In this and other ways, the conceptual and practical boundaries between minor and severe mental illness were reconfigured. Many psychiatrists questioned the conception of a continuum of mental distress and argued for the need to concentrate on the severe conditions—which were increasingly thought to have an organic basis—which should be principal target of treatment and the principal concern of publicly funded psychiatric services. 'Care in the community' was criticized from all sides.[7] Critics drew attention to the neglect, homelessness, and degradation that had been produced in the name of an unrealistic policy of reduction of hospitalization, which was, in any event, hampered by inadequate funding, incompetent management, and service rivalry. Newspaper headlines focused upon the despairing plight of former mental patients isolated in bedsitters, vagrancy, homelessness, despair, and suicide and claimed that this was a policy which, under the guise of reform, amounted to abandonment. Many psychiatrists began to argue that the key factor for a successful life in the community for those with mental health problems was the maintenance of psychotropic medication: community psychiatry required not so much 'a continuum of care' but effective measures to ensure drug compliance outside the hospital.

By the close of the twentieth century, assertions that care in the community had 'failed' no longer focused on the neglect of the vulnerable in the community but on the supposed threat to 'the community' by the mentally ill in their midst. A concerted campaign of 'scare in the community' had generated a new popular conception of 'mental illness' in terms of the propensity to violence (Philo, 1996; D. Rose, 1998). Hence a new sociopolitical demand was placed on psychiatry: it should take as its principal objective the surveillance and control of the mentally ill in the name of the protection of 'the community' (cf. Crichton, 1995). The little phrase 'care in the

---

7 In this section I am drawing on my paper: N. Rose (1998).

community patient' came to identify certain persons who, because illness had stripped them of their normal moral safeguards, posed a threat to the tranquillity, order, and safety of 'the public'. The issue of homicides by those suffering from mental illness, previously a matter for a small number of forensic psychiatrists concerned with a small minority of 'dangerous individuals' who were 'mentally abnormal offenders', came to shape arguments about the sociopolitical obligations of psychiatrists and other mental health professions to secure the security of 'the public'. One word characterizes the new demands placed on psychiatry: risk (N. Rose, 1998; cf. Castel, 1991; Duggan, 1997; Steadman et al., 1993). Mechanisms for the control of risk became central to the operation of all psychiatry—identification of risk factors, risk assessment, risk registers, and risk management (Royal College of Psychiatrists, 1996).

The role of mental health professionals was less that of cure or care than of the administration of dangerous, damaged, or desperate individuals across a complex institutional field comprising institutions of various levels of security—half-way houses of various types, day centres, drop-in centres, hostels, clinics, sheltered housing, assertive outreach teams, and much more. The failures of psychiatry were now posed in terms of the failure of prediction and control of risky individuals. And there was a growing demand for the extension of coercive powers of mental health law—measures to secure drug compliance, provisions for preventive detention—in the belief that this was the only way to mitigate the dangers posed by the severely mentally ill to themselves, their families, psychiatric professionals, and 'the public' (cf. Pratt, 1995; Simon, 1998).

As concerns about risk came to the fore, so did new divisions among those who it treated: low risk, medium risk, and high risk. In the zone of low risk, quasi-therapeutic techniques of control proliferated across everyday life, regulating and reshaping individual conduct according to norms of autonomy, responsibility, competence, and self-fulfilment. Here one found counselling, mediation, conciliation, cognitive therapies, behavioural techniques, and the like within the school, the factory, the training programme for the unemployed, and in hospital clinics, tutors' studies, the work of health visitors and social workers, and, of course, the prescription of psychiatric medication from the surgeries of general practitioners. These practices for the management of the self operated in a much broader therapeutic habitat: a culture in which radio, television, and cinema offer us psychologized images of ourselves, and a whole range of practices of life shaped and organized in therapeutic terms.

The zone of medium risk was marked out by psychiatric wards in general hospitals, the practices of social workers, together with quasi public provision provided under contract by 'voluntary agencies'. Alongside this public provision, a private market opened up for the management of acute mental health problems not apparently immediately linked to danger to others. The new private arrangements were supported by the growth of private health insurance and by the emergence of market-style arrangements for the purchase of care by publicly funded health services. In this zone of medium risk, mental health was increasingly governed through the family, by means of strategies that sought to enhance, intensify, and instrumentalize the apparently 'natural' bonds of obligation between members of domestic units: the self-governing family was urged, educated, and obliged to take on itself the sociopolitical responsibility of managing its own mental health problems and its own problematic members.

The work of public agencies and state institutions increasingly came to focus on the issue of 'high risk'. Mental health professionals were given a key role within an extending apparatus charged with the obligation of the continuous and unending management of permanently problematic persons in the name of community safety. Different tactics were involved: 24-hour nursed care, community treatment orders, assertive outreach, crisis intervention, and the like. The different types of psychiatric institutions became virtually defined in terms of the need for security rather than those of therapy (Grounds, 1995). A new archipelago of islands of confinement were created: special hospitals, medium secure units, re-locked wards in psychiatric hospitals, and units for those deemed to have 'dangerous and severe personality disorders'. At the same time, new proposals were formulated for the confinement of certain 'monstrous' individuals: those who, although they may have served a sentence for their crimes, and have not been diagnosed with a treatable mental illness, were considered too risky to the general public to be allowed to go free. As the twentieth century closed, across the English-speaking world, strategies were developed for the preventive detention of sexual predators, paedophiles, and the incorrigibly antisocial—of those thought to pose a risk to the community on the basis not so much of what they have done, but of what they are and what they might do (e.g. Greig, 1997, for Australia; Pratt, 2000, for New Zealand; Scheingold et al., 1994, for the US).

The assessment and management of risk became part of the political obligation of psychiatry and the professional obligation of all those working with issues of mental health (Alberg et al., 1996; Snowden, 1997). Psychiatry and law are intrinsically bound together within these strategies of regulation and the mechanisms of law play a key role in shaping the conduct of psychiatric professionals. The shadow of the law—the real or imagined fear of prosecution or of censure by quasi-judicial public inquiries—shapes professional conduct, and provides the legitimization for the relentless task of documentation intrinsic to these risk-based psychiatric technologies. Psychiatric judgement has become enwrapped in a grid of legal and quasi-legal obligations (such as codes of practice, notes of guidance, and so forth) within a new regime of blame, in which mental health professionals operate under the threat of being held accountable for any harm to 'the community' which might result from the actions of those with whom they have been involved.

'Madness' has come to be emblematic of all the threats that are ascribed by those who think of themselves as 'normal' to those who they marginalize or exclude. Within this perception, difference is re-coded as danger, and a constant labour is required to mark out and police those differences that are no longer demarcated by the walls of an asylum or the closed doors of the hospital ward. In this new problems space, not merely those with mental health problems, not only psychiatric professionals, but everyday life itself is 'governed through madness'—that is to say, regulated and shaped in terms of the fear of those with mental health problems and the need to reduce risks. At a time when the 'users', 'consumers', and 'survivors' of psychiatry are, at last, demanding their own say in the practices of mental health, one principal challenge for psychiatrists 'in the community' lies in their capacity to manage these new tensions between their obligations to their patients and these sociopolitical demands for control.

Coda

As we reached the end of the first decade of the twenty-first century, the dilemmas of risk management in the community became intertwined with another set of dilemmas concerning the proper scope of psychiatry (N. Rose, 2006a). Epidemiological data appear to show nothing less than an 'epidemic' of mental health problems—with over one-quarter of the general population deemed to be suffering from a *Diagnostic and Statistical Manual of Mental Disorders*-diagnosable mental disorder in any one year, and around one-half across a lifetime (Kessler et al., 2005; Wittchen & Jacobi, 2005). The use of psychiatric medication continues to increase worldwide (Olfson & Marcus, 2009; N. Rose, 2006a, 2006b). Controversies flare over the increasing diagnosis of children with such conditions as autism spectrum disorder, attention deficit hyperactivity disorder, and even bipolar disorder. The profession struggles with the attempts to align definitions and classifications of disorder based on symptomatology with the belief that all psychiatric disorders are disorders of the brain, or at the very least have neural underpinnings and neural correlates (Hyman, 2007; Regier et al., 2009). The logic of prevention leads some to argue for screening of asymptomatic persons using biomarkers with the aim of early intervention to forestall the later development of psychiatric illness or antisocial conduct (Singh & Rose, 2009). Thus the questions are posed: is there really so much undiagnosed and untreated psychiatric illness, requiring greater disease awareness among professionals and public, more effective diagnosis, ready provision of psychiatric drugs, and an expanding community mental health which will reduce stigma? Or are doctors and psychiatrists too ready to diagnose disorder for variations in mood or behaviour once considered normal ups and downs of life? Are actual and potential consumers of psychiatry too ready to understand what ails them in psychiatric terms? What are the roles of the pharmaceutical companies, patient pressure groups, and psychiatrists themselves in this expansion of the territory of psychiatry? What is the proper scope of psychiatry in relation to community mental health? Perhaps we should reflect on some words of Aubrey Lewis, half a century ago, which have lost none of their relevance (Lewis, 1967):

> We can … agree that the practice of psychiatry should be limited to illness and its prevention, and that illness occurs broadly where there is disabling or distressing interference with normal function. But in the last thirty years the impatience and perhaps the credulity of public opinion has pressed upon the psychiatrist requests that he treat people who are not ill and advise on problems that are not medical. It needs no logician to detect the fallacy in the syllogism which runs: psychiatrists are experts in mental disorder; mental disorder is a form of abnormal behaviour; therefore psychiatrists are experts in abnormal behaviour of every sort. Yet in matters touching upon misbehaviour in children, vocational selection, troubles in marriage, crime, and many other tribulations, the psychiatrist has sometimes assumed responsibility, or had responsibility thrust upon him, beyond the range of his medical functions … There is no other branch of medicine which finds it so difficult to say 'no'; and is so often blamed when it says 'yes'. (pp. 277–278)

The second decade of the twenty-first century has witnessed the growth of two movements that may in time serve to significantly ameliorate the risk-focused psychiatric practice described above. First is the growth of the involvement and voice of 'service users' (or 'patients' or 'consumers') in the design of mental health services so they are more appropriate for the range of mental health problems for which help might be sought (Bombard et al., 2018; Millar et al., 2016; Omeni et al., 2014; D. Rose et al., 2016; N. Rose, 2019). In this process, there has been a struggle between moments of opposition, in part or in whole, to the powers and knowledge claims of the psychiatric apparatus from those who consider themselves 'survivors' (D. Rose & Kalathil, 2019), and attempts by psychiatrists and mental health policy makers, to incorporate the views and 'lived experience' of mental health service users into their deliberations and strategies. Formal developments in the UK include further attempts to develop alternatives to standard hospital inpatient care, even for those who previously might have been obvious cases for involuntary confinement. There have also been moves, often more rhetorical than real, to align the goals and practices of mental health services with those considered to accord with the beliefs, values, and commitments of their users, and hence there has been a growth of peer support workers, as full employees in the mental healthcare system (Lloyd-Evans et al., 2014) as well as an expansion of independent advocacy by those with experience of the mental health system. To some extent, this has led mental health professionals to give less priority to the mere alleviation of symptoms and to evaluate the extent to which an individual can 'cope' with the demands of self-management according to the conventions of everyday life in the modern world with its emphasis on autonomy and self-responsibility. However this often leaves mental health service users in thrall to a highly conditional social benefits system and its work capability assessments that are ill-suited to the lived realities of those experiencing long-term mental distress. In a related development, the 'recovery' movement, originated by service users as a radical claim against the treatment objectives and evaluations of psychiatrists, has now been transformed into a set of professional practices for mental health workers, which often has taken the form of a highly normalized 'obligation to recover' which once more places an emphasis on individual responsibility (Le Boutillier et al., 2011; D. Rose, 2014; Slade et al., 2012). Reacting to these somewhat disappointing achievements of the radical user and survivor movement in the five decades since Judi Chamberlin's pioneering book *On Our Own: Patient-Controlled Alternatives to the Mental Health System* (Chamberlin, 1978), some have argued that mental health services need to do more than listen, incorporate, and adapt, but must recognize the power of 'epistemic injustice'—that is to say the partiality of the knowledge claims underpinning psychiatry, and need for their radical revision in the light of the alternative epistemologies of mental distress arising from the mental health user and survivor movement (D. Rose, 2017; N. Rose, 2019, Ch. 8).

A parallel movement to service user involvement in service development is its increasing engagement in research, not as the subjects of the research but as collaborators with the professional research community (D. Rose, 2014; Wallcraft et al., 2009). In the UK, for example, service users now frequently sit on management committees overseeing research projects. They may have a say in the design of projects, especially in making them more user-friendly and thus more likely to be successfully completed, as well as ensuring that the questions asked are important from the service user perspective. They may be employed as researchers and often have more success than others in engaging those experiencing mental distress who are often considered 'hard to reach' yet often the research itself takes the traditional form, with scale-based quantitative evaluations prioritized over real-world, contextually rich, qualitative ethnographic approaches (Staley et al., 2013). Thus, despite the promises of rethinking that has led to the changes described above, many service users who are actively engaged with service providers in attempts to change disempowering practices continue to complain about the absence of fundamental changes in the power relations between service providers and users and the forms of knowledge that underpin conventional practices in psychiatry and mental health. Indeed, some worry that through their formal, yet often small, influence on policy formation, they may be seen to legitimize policies which they do not support (D. Rose et al., 2016).

The second movement is a growing concern with human rights, especially rights as they pertain to people with 'disabilities', including mental health disabilities. A key driver has been the United Nations (UN) Convention on the Rights of Persons with Disabilities (CRPD) in 2006 (see also Chapters 28 and 29). This treaty, ratified at the time of writing by 182 nations, has as its core principles, respect for dignity, respect for autonomy, non-discrimination and equality, and social inclusion. The Convention sets out both civil and political rights (protections against state interference) as well as social, economic, and cultural rights (that the state is obliged to provide). Of special relevance to those with mental health (or 'psychosocial') disabilities include among the former: non-discrimination (article 5); recognition before the law on an equal basis as for those without a disability (article 12); liberty and security of the person (article 14); and protection of the integrity of the person (article 17). Among the latter are the rights to live independently and be included in the community (article 19); to education (article 24); to the highest attainable standard of health (article 25); to work and employment (article 27); and to an adequate standard of living and social protection (article 28). Controversially, the UN Committee charged with oversight of the implementation of the Convention has interpreted article 12 as excluding 'substitute decision-making', that is, any decision made on behalf of a person with a disability and against the person's 'will and preferences' (Committee on the Rights of Persons with Disabilities, 2014). Thus all forms of coercive intervention are to cease, including involuntary outpatient (or community treatment) orders. While this interpretation has been contested, there has been a general recognition that coercion is seriously overused in mental healthcare and a growing number of organizations, governmental as well as non-governmental, have adopted positions calling for its minimization if not its elimination. These include, to date, a number of UN treaty bodies, including the Human Rights Committee (2014) and Human Rights Council (2017), and the World Health Organization (Funk & Drew, 2020), the World Psychiatric Association (2020), and the Parliamentary Assembly of the Council of Europe (2019). Mental health law now needs to explicitly take account of the CRPD. Relevant to rights concerning non-discrimination and social inclusion has been a growing focus on social determinants of mental illness, as well as respect for the personal values and life goals of persons with mental health disabilities (e.g. the 'Report from the Special Rapporteur on the right of everyone to the enjoyment of the highest attainable standard of physical and mental health'; United Nations Human Rights Council, 2020).

How far these movements will change the standing in society of persons with mental health disabilities remains to be seen. For that to happen, those who take law seriously must be prepared to step away from abstract debates about human rights and curb their overestimation of the powers of the law itself. No doubt rights claims have an important role in challenging the mundane humiliations that so many experience in their day-to-day dealings with authorities—humiliations that not only degrade the lives of those with mental health diagnoses, but also intensify mental distress and lead to poor mental health. But lawyers must also align themselves with the preventive strategies of social medicine, not just in the social legislation that reverses the policies that lead so many to mental distress and in the regulations governing the licencing and uses of psychopharmaceuticals, but also in the mundane world of framing regulations that can help create mental health friendly schools, workplaces, houses, and environments. For it is in this messy sociopolitical world that the injustices that lead to poor mental health are experienced, and it is here that they must be overcome.

REFERENCES

Alberg, C., Hatfied, B., & Huxley, P. (1996). *Learning Materials on Mental Health: Risk Assessment*. Manchester: University of Manchester.

Armstrong, D. (1983). *Political Anatomy of the Body: Medical Knowledge in Britain in the Twentieth Century*. Cambridge: Cambridge University Press.

Armstrong, D. (1984). The patient's view. *Social Science & Medicine*, **18**, 737–744.

Barnes, E. (Ed.) (1968). *Psychosocial Nursing: Studies from the Cassel Hospital*. London: Tavistock.

Barton, R. (1959). *Institutional Neurosis*. Bristol: Wright.

Baruch, G. & Treacher, A. (1978). *Psychiatry Observed*. London: Routledge and Kegan Paul.

Bombard, Y., Baker, G. R., Orlando, E., Fancott, C., Bhatia, P., Casalino, S., et al. (2018). Engaging patients to improve quality of care: a systematic review. *BMC Implementation Science*, **13**, 98.

Castel, R. (1991). From dangerousness to risk. In: Burchell, G., Gordon, C., & Miller, P. (Eds.), *The Foucault Effect: Studies in Governmentality* (pp. 281–298). Hemel Hempstead: Harvester Wheatsheaf.

Castel, R., Castel, F., & Lovell, A. (1982). *The Psychiatric Society* (trans. Goldhammer, A.). New York: Columbia University Press.

Caudill, W. (1958). *The Psychiatric Hospital as a Small Society*. Cambridge, MA: Harvard University Press.

Chamberlin, J. (1978). *On Our Own: Patient-Controlled Alternatives to the Mental Health System*. New York: Hawthorn Books.

Clark, D. H. (1964). *Administrative Psychiatry*. London: Tavistock.

Clark, D. H. (1970). The therapeutic community: concept, practice, future. *British Journal of Psychiatry*, **117**, 375–388.

Council of Europe (2019). Parliamentary Assembly—Resolution 2291. Ending coercion in mental health. http://assembly.coe.int/nw/xml/XRef/Xref-XML2HTML-en.asp?fileid=28038&lang=en

Crichton, J. (Ed.) (1995). *Psychiatric Patient Violence: Risk and Response*. London: Duckworth.

Curle, A. (1947). Transitional communities and social reconnection. A follow-up study of the civil resettlement of British prisoners of war. *Human Relations*, **1**, 42–68.

Deutsch, A. (1948). *The Shame of the States*. New York: Arno.

Duggan, C. (1997). Assessing risk in the mentally disordered. Introduction. *British Journal of Psychiatry. Supplement*, **32**, 1–3.

Farrall, L. A. (1985). *The Origins and Growth of the English Eugenics Movement, 1865–1925*. New York: Garland.

Funk, M. & Drew, N. (2020). WHO's QualityRights Initiative: transforming services and promoting rights in mental health. *Health and Human Rights Journal*, **22**, 69–75.

Goffman, E. (1962). *Asylums*. New York: Doubleday.

Greig, D. (1997). Shifting the boundary between psychiatry and law. *Liberty: Journal of the Victorian Council of Civil Liberties*, February.

Grounds, A. (1995). Risk assessment and management in a clinical context. In: Crichton, J. (Ed.), *Psychiatric Patient Violence: Risk and Response* (pp. 43–59). London: Duckworth.

Hearnshaw, L. S. (1964). *A Short History of British Psychology, 1840–1940*. London: Methuen.

Hyman, S. E. (2007). Can neuroscience be integrated into the DSM-V? *Nature Reviews Neuroscience*, **8**, 725–732.

Jones, K. (1972). *A History of the Mental Health Services*. London: Routledge and Kegan Paul.

Jones, M. (1952). *Social Psychiatry*. London: Tavistock.

Jones, M. (1982). Therapeutic communities past, present and future. In: Pines, M. & Rafelson, L. (Eds.), *The Individual and the Group* (Vol. 1., pp. XX–XX). London: Plenum.

Kessler, R. C., Demler, O., Frank, R. G., Olfson, M., Pincus, H. A., Walters, E. E., et al. (2005). Prevalence and treatment of mental disorders, 1990 to 2003. *New England Journal of Medicine*, **352**, 2515–2523.

Kräupl Taylor, F. (1958). A history of group and administrative therapy in Great Britain. *British Journal of Medical Psychology*, **31**, 153–173.

Le Boutillier, C., Leamy, M., Bird, V. J., Davidson, L., Williams, J., & Slade, M. (2011). What does recovery mean in practice? A qualitative analysis of international recovery-oriented practice guidance. *Psychiatric Services*, **62**, 1470–1476.

Lewis, A. J. S. (1967). Medicine and the affections of the mind. In: *The State of Psychiatry: Essays and Addresses* (pp. 273–297). London: Routledge & Kegan Paul.

Lloyd-Evans, B., Mayo-Wilson, E., Harrison, B., Istead, H., Brown, E., Pilling, S., et al. (2014). A systematic review and meta-analysis of randomised controlled trials of peer support for people with severe mental illness. *BMC Psychiatry*, **14**, 39.

Lomax, M. (1921). *Experiences of an Asylum Doctor*. London: Allen and Unwin.

Main, T. (1946). The hospital as a therapeutic institution. *Bulletin of the Menninger Clinic*, **10**, 66–70.

Manning, N. & Hinshelwood, R. (Eds.) (1979). *The Therapeutic Community: Reflections and Progress*. London: Routledge and Kegan Paul.

Manning, N. P. (1976). Innovation in social policy—the case of the therapeutic community. *Journal of Social Policy*, **5**, 265–279.

Martin, D. (1962). *Adventure in Psychiatry*. Oxford: Cassirer.

Meacher, M. (Ed.) (1979). *New Methods of Mental Health Care*. Oxford: Pergamon.

Millar, S., Chambers, M., & Giles, M. (2016). Service user involvement in mental health care: an evolutionary concept analysis. *Health Expectations*, **19**, 209–221.

Miller, P. (1986). The psychotherapy of employment and unemployment. In: Miller, P. & Rose, N. (Eds.), *The Power of Psychiatry* (pp. 143–176). Cambridge: Polity.

Olfson, M. & Marcus, S. C. (2009). National patterns in antidepressant medication treatment. *Archives of General Psychiatry*, **66**, 848–856.

Omeni, E., Barnes, M., MacDonald, D., Crawford, M., & Rose, D. (2014). Service user involvement: impact and participation: a survey of service user and staff perspectives. *BMC Health Services Research*, **14**, 491.

Philo, G. (1996). *Media and Mental Distress*. London: Longmans.

Pratt, J. (1995). Dangerousness, risk and technologies of power. *Australia and New Zealand Journal of Criminology*, **28**, 3–31.

Pratt, J. (2000). Sex crimes and the new punitiveness. *Behavioral Sciences & the Law* **18**, 135–151.

Rees, J. R. (1945). *The Shaping of Psychiatry by War*. London: Chapman and Hall.

Regier, D. A., Narrow, W. E., Kuhl, E. A., & Kupfer, D. J. (2009). The conceptual development of DSM-V. *American Journal of Psychiatry*, **166**, 645–650.

Rose, D. (1998). Television, madness and community care. *Journal of Community and Applied Social Psychology*, **8**, 213–228.

Rose, D. (2014). The mainstreaming of recovery. *Journal of Mental Health*, **23**, 217–218.

Rose, D. (2017). Service user/survivor-led research in mental health: epistemological possibilities. *Disability & Society*, **32**, 773–789.

Rose, D. & Kalathil, J. (2019). Power, privilege and knowledge: the untenable promise of co-production in mental 'health'. *Frontiers in Sociology*, **4**, 57.

Rose, D., MacDonald, D., Wilson, A., Crawford, M., Barnes, M., & Omeni, E. (2016). Service user led organisations in mental health today. *Journal of Mental Health*, **25**, 254–259.

Rose, N. (1985). *The Psychological Complex: Psychology, Politics and Society in England, 1869–1939*. London: Routledge and Kegan Paul.

Rose, N. (1989). *Governing the Soul: The Shaping of the Private Self*. London: Routledge.

Rose, N. (1996). *Inventing Ourselves: Psychology, Power and Personhood*. Cambridge, MA: Cambridge University Press.

Rose, N. (1998). Governing risky individuals: the role of psychiatry in new regimes of control. *Psychiatry, Psychology and Law*, **5**, 177–195.

Rose, N. (1999). *Powers of Freedom: Reframing Political Thought*. Cambridge: Cambridge University Press.

Rose, N. (2006a). Disorders without borders? The expanding scope of psychiatric practice. *BioSocieties*, **1**, 465–484.

Rose, N. (2006b). Psychopharmaceuticals in Europe. In: McDaid, D., Knapp, M., & Thornicroft, G. (Eds.), *Mental Health Policy and Practice in Europe* (pp. 146–187). Milton Keynes: Open University Press.

Rose, N. (2019). *Our Psychiatric Future*. Cambridge: Polity Press.

Rosen, G. (1959). Social stress and mental disease from the 18th century to the present: some origins of social psychiatry. *Millbank Memorial Fund Quarterly*, **37**, 5.

Royal College of Psychiatrists (1996). *Assessment and Clinical Management of Risk of Harm to Other People*. London: Royal College of Psychiatrists.

Royal Commission on Lunacy and Mental Disorder (1926). *Report of the Royal Commission on Lunacy and Mental Disorder* (Cmd. 2700). London: HMSO.

Scheingold, S., Pershing, J., & Olson, T. (1994). Sexual violence, victim advocacy and Republican criminology. *Law and Society Review*, **28**, 729–763.

Scull, A. (1985). *Decarceration* (2nd ed.). Cambridge: Polity.

Searle, G. R. (1976). *Eugenics and Politics in Britain, 1900–1914*. Leyden: Noordhoff.

Simon, J. (1997). Governing through crime. In: Friedman, L. & Fisher, G. (Eds.), *The Crime Conundrum: Essays on Criminal Justice* (pp. 171–190). Boulder, CO: Westview Press.

Simon, J. (1998). Managing the monstrous: sex offenders and the new penology. *Psychology, Public Policy and Law*, **4**, 1–16.

Singh, I. & Rose, N. (2009). Biomarkers in psychiatry. *Nature*, **460**, 202–207.

Slade, M., Adams, N., & O'Hagan, M. (2012). Recovery: past progress and future challenges. *International Review of Psychiatry*, **24**, 1–4.

Snowden, P. (1997). Practical aspects of clinical risk assessment and management. *British Journal of Psychiatry. Supplement*, **32**, 32–34.

Staley, K., Kabir, T., & Szmukler, G. (2013). Service users as collaborators in mental health research: less stick, more carrot. *Psychological Medicine*, **43**, 1121–1125.

Stanton, A. H. & Schwartz, M. S. (1954). *The Mental Hospital*. London: Tavistock.

Steadman, H. J., Monahan, J., Clark Robbins, P., Appelbaum, P., Grisso, T., Klassen, D., et al. (1993). From dangerousness to risk assessment: implications for appropriate research strategies. In: Hodgins, S. (Ed.), *Mental Disorder and Crime* (pp. 39–62). Newbury Park, CA: Sage.

Timms, N. (1964). *Psychiatric Social Work in Great Britain, 1939–1962*. London: Routledge and Kegan Paul.

Treacher, A. & Baruch, G. (1981). Towards a critical history of the psychiatric profession. In: Ingleby, D. (Ed.), *Critical Psychiatry* (pp. 120–159). Harmondsworth: Penguin.

United Nations (2006). Convention on the Rights of Persons with Disabilities. http://www.un.org/disabilities/documents/convention/convoptprot-e.pdf

United Nations Human Rights Committee (2014). General comment no. 35—article 9 (Liberty and security of person). CCPR/C/GC/35. https://www.refworld.org/legal/general/hrc/2014/en/104763

United Nations Human Rights Council (2017). Resolution on Mental Health and Human Rights. A/HRC/36/L.25. https://digitallibrary.un.org/record/1306486/files/A_HRC_36_L.25-EN.pdf?ln=en

United Nations Human Rights Council (2020). Report of the Special Rapporteur on the right of everyone to the enjoyment of the highest attainable standard of physical and mental health. A/HRC/44/48. https://www.ohchr.org/en/documents/thematic-reports/ahrc4448-right-everyone-enjoyment-highest-attainable-standard-physical

Wallcraft, J., Schrank, B., & Amering, M. (2009). *Handbook of Service User Involvement in Mental Health Research*. Chichester: John Wiley & Sons.

Wilson, A. T. M., Doyle, M., & Kelnar, J. (1947). Group techniques in a transitional community. *Lancet*, **1**, 735–738.

Wing, J. (1962). Institutionalism in mental hospitals. *British Journal of Social and Clinical Psychology*, **1**, 38.

Wittchen, H. U. & Jacobi, F. (2005). Size and burden of mental disorders in Europe—a critical review and appraisal of 27 studies. *European Neuropsychopharmacology*, **15**, 357–376.

World Psychiatric Association (2020). WPA position statement and call to action: implementing alternatives to coercion: a key component of improving mental health care. https://3ba346de-fde6-473f-b1da-536498661f9c.filesusr.com/ugd/e172f3_635a89af889c471683c29fcd981db0aa.pdf

Younghusband, E. (1978). *Social Work in Britain: 1950–1975*. London: George Allen and Unwin.

3

Mental health policy in modern America

Gerald Grob and Howard Goldman

In the US, a variety of factors have shaped and continuously modified mental health policy: the changing composition of the population with severe mental disorders; concepts of the aetiology and nature of mental illnesses; shifting diagnostic systems; the organization and ideology of psychiatry; funding mechanisms; and existing popular, political, social, and professional attitudes and values. Equally significant has been the structure of the American political system, which divides authority between local, state, and national government.

Few policies are formulated *de novo*, and this is particularly true of mental health. The changes that occurred during the last half of the twentieth century require an understanding of earlier developments. Before 1900, responsibility for social welfare (with the exception of a federal programme providing disability and old-age pensions for Civil War veterans and their dependents) lay largely with state governments. Beginning in the early nineteenth century, states created a vast public hospital system to care for persons with severe mental disorders. Mental health, as a matter of fact, remained the single largest item in their budgets. Many states also required local governments to contribute funds to care for their residents in state hospitals. This created an incentive to retain residents with mental disorders in almshouses where the cost of care was lower.

Towards the end of the nineteenth century, states began to assume total responsibility for funding its mental hospitals. A curious and unforeseen development followed. Local communities saw an entrepreneurial opportunity to reduce their own expenditures. In brief, they began to redefine senility in psychiatric terms, and thus to transfer aged persons from local almshouses (which in the nineteenth century served in part as old age homes) to state mental hospitals. The structural context of policymaking thus altered coverage patterns, which in turn transformed in part the mission of state hospitals by converting them into institutions that provided custodial care for large numbers of elderly disabled persons. As late as 1958 nearly one-third of all patients in state hospitals were over the age of 65 years (American Psychiatric Association, 1960; Grob, 1991).

At the end of the Second World War, the nation's public hospitals faced a crisis of unprecedented proportions. Between 1930 and 1945, state governments were preoccupied with the problems growing out of the Great Depression and the Second World War, and paid little attention to the deteriorating conditions within their public hospital system. Despite problems caused by declining appropriations, an ageing physical plant, and staff shortages, the daily census of hospitals rose steadily. In 1945, their average daily resident population was about 430,000; approximately 85,000 were first-time admissions. A decade later, the number had risen to 558,000. That elderly persons constituted a large proportion of the patient population only reinforced perceptions that such institutions were preoccupied with custodial rather than therapeutic functions (Grob, 1991).

Few public policies, however long established or stable, remain immune from broader social, economic, intellectual, and scientific currents. Beginning with the Second World War, the faith that institutionalization was the appropriate policy choice slowly began to erode. Within two decades the very legitimacy of mental hospitals had been undermined by individuals and groups committed to a new policy paradigm, namely, that the care and treatment of persons with severe mental disorders should take place in the community. By 2005, the number of institutionalized patients had fallen to slightly less than 50,000; the overwhelming majority of persons with severe disorders were now treated in general hospitals or other outpatient facilities (Atay & Foley, 2007).

What accounts for such a dramatic policy shift? The answer to this question is by no means simple. The changes in post-war mental health priorities had diverse roots. The military experiences of the Second World War allegedly demonstrated that community and outpatient treatment of persons with mental disorders was superior and more efficient. A simultaneous shift in psychiatric thinking fostered receptivity towards a psychodynamic and psychoanalytic model that emphasized life experiences, the importance of socioenvironmental factors, and psychotherapy of one form or another. The belief that early identification of individuals at risk and intervention in the community would be effective in preventing subsequent hospitalization became popular. This belief was especially encouraged by psychiatrists and other mental health professionals holding a public health orientation. They also shared a faith that psychiatry, in collaboration with other social and behavioural sciences, could ameliorate those social and environmental conditions that in their eyes played an important role in the aetiology of mental disorders. The introduction of new psychosocial and biological therapies—including but not limited to psychotropic drugs—held out the promise of a better and more productive life for persons who in the past were institutionalized. At the same time, psychiatrists began to abandon mental hospital employment for private and community practice. Finally, a series of journalistic and media exposés seemed to confirm the belief that mental hospitals were simply incarcerating persons and providing little in the way of therapy (Grob, 1991).

All of these developments, by themselves or in conjunction with each other, would surely have promoted change. Nevertheless, the entry of the federal government into the mental health policy arena proved crucial, for it altered the very ways in which policy was conceptualized and implemented. After 1945, new structural relations were forged among federal agencies; federal funding for biomedical research increased precipitously; and the role of the Public Health Service expanded dramatically. The passage of the Hill–Burton Act in 1946 provided generous subsidies for hospital construction, and third-party medical insurance programmes expanded rapidly. The emergence of a health lobby that included members of Congress and influential laypersons hastened the expansion of federal health activities.

The growing role of the federal government in health affairs did not necessarily imply that it would seek to pre-empt the traditional role of states in providing care and treatment for persons with severe mental disorders. The passage of the National Mental Health Act of 1946 and subsequent creation of the National Institute of Mental Health (NIMH), however, proved critical in hastening change (Public Law Chap. 538, 1946). The act was conceived and orchestrated through Congress by Dr Robert H. Felix, the first director of the NIMH from 1949 to 1964. One of the shrewdest and most effective federal bureaucrats of his generation, Felix worked to end institutional care and employ federal prestige and resources to create a new community-oriented policy. His underlying belief was that mental disorders represented 'a true public health problem', the resolution of which required knowledge about the aetiology and nature of mental illnesses, more effective means of prevention and treatment, and better trained personnel. Public health, according to Felix, was concerned with the 'collective health' of the community. The NIMH mental health programme was designed 'to help the individual by helping the community, to make mental health a part of the community's total health programme, to the end that all individuals will have greater assurance of an emotionally and physically healthy and satisfying life for themselves and their families'. Felix was able to frame a national agenda that assumed that community care and treatment would replace archaic and obsolete mental hospitals (Felix, 1945, 1949; Felix & Bowers, 1948).

During the 1950s, interest in community alternatives to mental hospitalization mounted. The development of psychosocial and milieu therapies, as well as the introduction of psychotropic drugs, gave impetus to the belief that early identification and treatment would obviate the need for hospitalization. Support for a community mental health programme came from a variety of constituencies. The Council of State Governments and Governors Conferences in the 1950s endorsed this approach as a means of arresting the seemingly inevitable growth of the institutionalized population. Private foundations such as the Milbank Memorial Fund as well as leading university departments of psychiatry added their voices to the chorus promoting change. The growing faith in community mental health services led New York State in 1954 and California in 1957 to enact legislation encouraging communities to expand their mental health services (Grob, 1991).

Nevertheless, activists faced a daunting problem, namely, that responsibility for policy still resided with 48 state governments. In the hope of altering intergovernmental relations and forging a national policy, they created the Joint Commission on Mental Illness and Health. A private undertaking, the commission received congressional endorsement with the passage of the Mental Health Study Act of 1955, which authorized the Public Health Service to provide federal grants. After nearly 6 years of work and the publication of nine monographs, the commission issued its final report, *Action for Mental Health*, which presented a large number of general recommendations and a plea for a dramatic increase in federal funding (Grob, 1991; Joint Commission on Mental Illness and Health, 1961).

Although President John F. Kennedy was sympathetic to *Action for Mental Health*, he faced conflicting pressures. On the one side were those pushing for legislation dealing with mental retardation; on the other side were key congressional figures determined to secure legislation dealing with mental health. Faced with a split, Kennedy sidestepped the issue by appointing an interagency task force on mental health. Because its members were not especially knowledgeable about the subject, they relied on Felix and the NIMH to guide their deliberations. Felix adroitly used his position to further his agenda. He and his staff had little use for the recommendations of the Joint Commission. Whereas the commission had emphasized the care and treatment of persons with severe disorders, the NIMH favoured a more comprehensive policy focusing on 'the improvement of the mental health of the people of the country through a continuum of services, not just upon the treatment and rehabilitative aspects of these programs'. Radical rather than incremental change was required. Felix and his staff therefore recommended the adoption of a comprehensive community programme that would make it possible 'for the mental hospital as it is now known to disappear from the scene within the next twenty-five years'. Its place would be taken by a new institution—a community mental health centre (CMHC)—that would offer comprehensive services to all Americans (National Institute of Mental Health, 1961 1962a, 1962b).

Felix's views prevailed, and in 1963 Congress enacted the Community Mental Health Centers Act, which provided a 3-year authorization of $150 million dollars for construction. Two years later it enacted legislation that offered financial support for staffing (Public Law 88-164, 1963; Public Law 89-105, 1965). The passage of this legislation, however, represented the victory of ideology over reality. The functions of a CMHC remained vague and undefined. A community programme, moreover, was based on certain assumptions: that patients had a home in the community; that a sympathetic family would assume responsibility for the care of the released patient; that the organization of the household would not impede rehabilitation; and that the patient's presence would not cause undue hardships for other family members. In 1960, however, 48% of the hospitalized population was unmarried, 12% widowed, and 13% either divorced or separated. The assumption that patients would be able to reside in the community with their families while undergoing rehabilitation was hardly supported by such data, especially since the legislation said little or nothing about income support, occupation, or housing (Kramer, 1956, 1967; Kramer et al., 1968; Pollack et al., 1959).

Nor was there evidence that CMHCs could provide care and treatment for a severely disabled population in the community. Indeed, the legislation and the subsequent regulations governing CMHCs provided no links with state hospitals. State authorities, which had administrative responsibilities for overseeing policy implementation, were also bypassed in favour of a federal–local partnership. The result was that CMHCs had considerable autonomy and freedom from state regulations. This permitted centres to focus on a new set of clients who better fitted the orientations of mental health managers and professionals trained in psychodynamic and preventive orientations. The treatment of choice at most centres was individual psychotherapy, an intervention especially adapted to a middle-class, educated clientele without severe disorders and one that was congenial to the professional staffs composed largely of social workers and clinical psychologists. In effect, CMHCs broadened the clientele of the mental health system, but did not provide services for persons with severe mental disorders. Centres, according to Donald G. Langsley (president of the American Psychiatric Association) in 1980, had 'drifted away from their original purpose' and featured 'counseling and crisis intervention for predictable problems of living'. The changing nature of staffing at CMHCs reflected its new functions; an absolute decline in the number of psychiatrists was matched by an increase in psychologists and social workers (Grob, 1991; Langsley, 1980; Musto, 1975).

In the 1960s, faith in the efficacy of prevention and community mental health reinforced the belief that institutionalization could eventually become a relic of the past. To be sure, mental hospital populations, which peaked at 558,000 in 1955, thereafter began an uneven decline. Between 1955 and 1965 state hospital populations fell by only 15%. During the following decade, the decline was 60%, although rates varied sharply from state to state. The belief that CMHCs played a role in what subsequently became known as deinstitutionalization was widespread (Mechanic & Rochefort, 1992).

In some respects, even the term 'deinstitutionalization' is somewhat of a misnomer. Indeed, the first wave of deinstitutionalization actually involved a lateral transfer of patients from state hospitals to long-term nursing facilities because states were motivated to benefit from a windfall of new federal dollars. Between 1900 and 1960, state hospitals were serving in part as old age homes. The enactment of Medicaid in 1965 encouraged the construction of nursing home beds because it provided a payment source for patients transferred from state mental hospitals or admitted to nursing homes and general hospitals. Although states were responsible for the full costs of patients in their public mental hospitals, they could transfer patients to other facilities and have the federal government assume from half to three-quarters of the cost, depending on the state's economic status. This incentive encouraged a mass transinstitutionalization of long-term patients with dementia who had been previously housed in public mental hospitals for lack of other institutional alternatives. In 1963, nursing homes cared for nearly 220,000 individuals with mental disorders, of whom 188,000 were aged 65 or older. Six years later, the comparable numbers were 427,000 and 368,000 (Goldman et al., 1983; Gronfein, 1985; Kramer, 1977; National Institute of Mental Health, 1974). Within a short time, according to a 1977 study by the General Accounting Office, Medicaid had become 'one of the largest single purchasers of mental health care and the principal federal programme funding the long-term care of the mentally disabled'. It was also the most significant 'federally sponsored programme affecting deinstitutionalization' (General Accounting Office, 1977). The shift from mental hospital to nursing facility care was a development driven by a desire to promote the use of federal resources rather than by a desire to improve the lot of elderly persons and others with a severe and persistent mental disorder.

A second wave of deinstitutionalization began in the early 1970s that included new cohorts of persons with mental disorders coming to public notice for the first time. Between 1946 and 1960 more than 59 million births were recorded. The disproportionately large size of this age cohort meant that the number of persons (most of whom were young) at risk from developing a severe mental illness was very high. They were also highly mobile and often had a dual diagnosis of a mental disorder and substance abuse. The availability of a series of federal entitlement programmes—including Social Security Disability Insurance (SSDI), Supplementary Security Income for the Aged, the Disabled, and the Blind (SSI), Medicare, and food stamps—encouraged states to make admission to mental hospitals more difficult, if only because resources for persons with severe mental disorders in the community were available.

Treatment in the community for clients with multiple needs, as compared with mental hospital care, posed severe challenges. In the community (and particularly in large urban areas), clients were widely dispersed and their successful management depended on bringing together needed services administered by a variety of bureaucracies, each with its own culture, priorities, and preferred client populations. Although there were sporadic and occasionally successful efforts to integrate these services (psychiatric care and treatment, social services, housing, social support) in meaningful ways, the results in most areas were dismal. These new patients were typically treated during short inpatient stays in general hospitals and in other outpatient settings; they had to make do with whatever services they could garner.

The decentralization of services and lack of integration made it extraordinarily difficult to deal with persons with severe disorders in the community, and many became part of the street culture where the use of alcohol and drugs was common. Individuals with a dual diagnosis of a serious mental disorder and substance abuse presented such serious problems that many mental health professionals refused to deal with them despite their growing numbers. Moreover, the decline in institutional care created a situation where the 'criminalization' of persons with serious mental illnesses became more common. If such individuals were on the streets, they were more likely to engage in acts that attracted the attention of authorities and that ended in arrest and detention. Many persons with serious mental illnesses had encounters with the police, and a significant number were caught up in the criminal justice rather than the mental health system and incarcerated in prisons. To be sure, collaboration between the two systems was possible, but often different perspectives, values, and cultures placed formidable barriers in the way of cooperation.

In the last third of the twentieth century states pursued a policy of reducing their mental hospital populations by placing barriers in the way of new admissions and only as a last resort. This policy, in conjunction with the vast expansion in the clientele and diagnoses (as exemplified in the third and subsequent editions of the American Psychiatric Association's *Diagnostic and Statistical Manual of Mental Disorders* since 1980), shifts in public attitudes and perceptions, changing treatment strategies, and social and economic factors, led to the emergence of a confusing array of organized and unorganized settings for the treatment of persons with mental illnesses. State mental health agencies, which in theory were responsible for administering the mental health system, found themselves faced with declining resources and an increasing inability to influence policy. Multiple sources of funding from a variety of federal programmes administered by independent agencies made it difficult to develop and implement comprehensive, integrated, and effective community-based services. Many of the components of community mental health care—income support, housing, social support networks—were designed for other populations and often did not fit the needs of persons with severe and cyclic persistent mental illnesses.

When the General Accounting Office prepared a comprehensive report to Congress in 1977, it laid bare the problems of a disorganized and uncoordinated mental health system. Although endorsing deinstitutionalization, the report was extraordinarily critical of the manner in which it was implemented. Responsibility for the care, support, and treatment of persons with serious disorders was 'frequently diffused among several agencies and levels of government'. The dramatic growth of federal involvement in mental health had not produced the anticipated benefits, if only because there was little or no coordination between the 135 federal programmes administered by eleven major agencies and departments (General Accounting Office, 1977).

By the 1970s, most knowledgeable observers recognized that the mental health system was in disarray. Upon taking office in early 1977, Jimmy Carter created a presidential commission to investigate the mental health system and present its recommendations to the president. After public hearings and months of deliberations, the commission presented its final report in the spring of 1978. It included more than 100 recommendations that affected not only relations among federal, state, and local governments but also public and private agencies and such federal programmes as Medicare and Medicaid. In many ways the heterogeneous character of the commission's work was influenced by a political climate in which debates were shaped by the demands of groups that defined themselves in terms of class, ethnicity, gender, and race. By that time neither state hospitals nor persons with serious and persistent mental disorders were at the centre of policy debates. The commission's final report was neither a blueprint for legislative action nor the expression of a particular group. The diversity of its recommendations could not easily be translated into legislation (Grob & Goldman, 2006; President's Commission on Mental Health, 1978).

For more than 2 years the administration and Congress struggled in an effort to draft appropriate legislation. The problem was the absence of any consensus on mental health policy. Deinstitutionalization—whatever its meaning—was coming under widespread criticism by a variety of interest groups, each with its own agenda. In October 1980, Congress finally enacted and Carter signed into law the Mental Health Systems Act. While in theory assigning the highest priority to individuals with long-term mental disorders, the legislation also recognized the claims of various other groups whose needs were quite different, including children and adolescents, the elderly, rural residents, and victims of rape. The absence of new resources and vague generalizations about the kinds of services required, however, raised doubts about the legislation's effectiveness. Indeed, in order to make it through Congress, the legislation offered something to everyone, and as a result lacked any focus. Moreover, some provisions—especially those dealing with the prevention of mental illnesses and the promotion of mental health—reflected ideology and were little more than attractive slogans that had no basis in empirical data. Nor did the legislation offer any guidelines to assist persons with severe mental disorders to negotiate a myriad of programmes administered by independent agencies (Foley & Sharfstein, 1983; Grob & Goldman, 2006; Mechanic, 1999; Public Law 96-398, 1980).

No sooner had the Mental Health Systems Act become law when its provisions were rendered moot. The inauguration of Ronald Reagan in January 1981 led to an immediate reversal of policy. In the summer of 1981, the Omnibus Budget Reconciliation Act became law. Under its provisions the federal government provided block grants to states for mental health and substance abuse services. States were given considerable leeway in spending their allocations. With but a few exceptions, the Mental Health System and CMHC Acts were repealed, thus—at least in theory—diminishing the direct role of the federal government in mental health (Public Law 97-35, 1981).

In the short run, the work of Carter's President's Commission on Mental Health appeared to have had relatively little influence on the evolution of mental health policy. Yet serendipity is often an unrecognized force in human affairs. This was particularly true of the section in the final report calling for the establishment of a national priority and a national plan to meet the needs of individuals with long-term mental illnesses. As a result of this recommendation, a Department of Health, Education and Welfare task force proposed that the secretary of the agency appoint a group to develop a 'national plan for the chronically mentally ill' (HEW Task Force, 1979; President's Commission on Mental Health, 1978). Completed in December 1980, the plan laid out a blueprint for future action (Koyanagi & Goldman, 1991a, 1991b; US Department of Health and Human Services, 1980).

In the 1980s, the Reagan administration was committed to policies that were designed to limit if not reduce the social welfare functions of the federal government. The means chosen involved sharp reductions in taxation and the transfer of many social welfare functions downward to state and local governments. Although successful to some degree, the impact of these policies was mitigated by administrative actions taken by individuals within the federal bureaucracy under pressure from advocates and members of Congress. Concerned that preoccupation with tax reductions and the shrinkage or elimination of social programmes might have devastating consequences for persons with severe and persistent mental illnesses, Congress enacted legislation that ensured that this group would retain access to resources necessary to survive in the community. Thus, the abortive effort to enact a programme of broad comprehensive reform during the Carter administration was replaced instead by an emphasis on sequential incremental change that over time at least mitigated some of the difficult conditions faced by persons whose severe and persistent mental disorders created a state of dependency.

The National Plan embodied a strategy that went beyond simple incremental change. It provided a blueprint of specific recommendations suggesting a clear direction and a sequence of steps to achieve desired changes. Specifically, it offered recommendations to change both statutes and regulations governing important mainstream health and social welfare programmes, including Medicare, Medicaid, and the disability programmes of the Social Security Administration (e.g. SSDI, SSI), which affected people with severe and persistent mental disorders. During the 1980s, many of the recommendations of the National Plan were implemented both by statutory enactments and administrative actions within the federal bureaucracy. By the 1990s, Medicaid and Medicare eclipsed state categorical dollars as a source of mental health funding. While the new federalism restored some of the lost state authority in mental health services policy, the federal government actually picked up more of the bill (Grob & Goldman, 2006).

For all of the successes of mental health policy in the 1980s, policies and programmes remained fragmented (President's New Freedom Commission on Mental Health, 2003). Federal agencies in charge of entitlement programmes were separated by bureaucratic walls from the Department of Health and Human Services and other departments with some influence on the lives of individuals experiencing a mental disorder, including the Department of Housing and Urban Development and the Departments of Labor and Education. A range of new social problems involving people with mental illnesses (homelessness, substance abuse, HIV/AIDS) created new pressures. Medicaid and Medicare may have improved mental health benefits, but these benefits had more limitations than those of general health benefits. The system remained fragmented; no single agency accepted responsibility.

In the 1990s, the gap between research and practice led to the publication of the Surgeon General's *Mental Health*. Its policy recommendations were general in scope: the necessity of building the science base; the need to overcome stigma; the importance of improving public awareness of effective treatments; the need for an adequate supply of mental health services and providers; the importance of delivering state-of-the-art treatments; the need to tailor treatment to age, sex, race, and culture; and the importance of facilitating entry into treatment as well as reducing barriers to treatment (US Department of Health and Human Services, 1999).

In 2002, George W. Bush created a President's New Freedom Commission on Mental Health. The executive order establishing the commission had limited boundaries but also reflected a wish for 'transformation'. During its deliberations the commission struggled with the tensions of encouraging change while coping with a mandate for limited resources. As Michael F. Hogan, the commission's chair observed, the nation's mental health system remained:

> fragmented, disconnected and often inadequate, frustrating the opportunity for recovery. Today's mental health care system is a patchwork relic—the result of disjointed reforms and policies. Instead of ready access to quality of care, the system presents barriers that all too often add to the burdens of mental illnesses for individuals, their families, and our communities.

The commission argued that mental health care had to be consumer and family driven. It made the concept of recovery a basic theme and outlined a number of goals for a transformed mental health system. Its recommendations, however, were not specific, nor could they be linked to federal, state, or local mental health policy. The report also came at a time when health policy occupied a very low priority for the administration, which by then was deeply involved in foreign wars (President's New Freedom Commission on Mental Health, 2003).

Both the Surgeon General and New Freedom Commission reports made the concept of 'recovery' the central theme in guiding mental health policy and practice. Nevertheless, the concept was unclear, confusing, and even contradictory. Much of its appeal was due to optimistic rhetoric rather than substance. Persons with a serious mental illness are not a homogeneous population. Some have only one episode and then return to their previous functioning. Others recover only after years of being disabled by their illness. Focusing solely on cure or recovery runs the risk of abandoning people whose serious mental illnesses leads to prolonged disability. Even when their disorder is in complete remission, such individuals do not always achieve functional recovery. Indeed, Robert P. Liberman and Alex Kopelowicz have suggested that the concept of recovery from schizophrenia is a 'concept in search of research'. A more realistic and modest definition is that recovery incorporates the important idea that careful attention to and prevention of secondary disabilities can limit some of the adverse effects of serious mental disorders and thus make it possible for persons with such disorders to realize some of their goals and have reasonable lives in the community (Liberman & Kopelowicz, 2005).

Similarly, rhetorical claims about the effectiveness of clinical interventions have often concealed underlying problems and contradictions. For more than half a century, antipsychotic drugs had been the mainstay of psychiatric practice. Though indispensable for the treatment of severe and persistent mental illnesses—especially schizophrenia—they neither cured the illness nor were their side effects negligible. Marketing and advertising by pharmaceutical companies of allegedly new and more effective drugs only exacerbated a difficult situation. Indeed, recent studies of new antipsychotic drugs failed to show any advantage over their older first-generation counterparts, to say nothing about their metabolic side effects. These new drugs, Jeffrey A. Lieberman recently observed, 'represent an incremental advance at best. This underscores the urgent need for greater progress in developing novel therapeutics for schizophrenia and related disorders' (Lieberman, 2006; Lieberman et al., 2005).

Are there 'lessons' that can be drawn from knowledge of the past? At the very least, history suggests that there is a price to be paid for implementing ideology ungrounded in empirical reality and for making exaggerated rhetorical claims. The sustained attack on a century-old institutional policy, for example, was based on a superficial if not misreading history of mental health policy in the US and was advanced as part of a campaign to justify the new community-oriented policy that became known as deinstitutionalization. The ideology of community mental health and the facile assumption that residence in the community would promote adjustment and integration was illusory and did not take into account the extent of social isolation, exposure to victimization, inducement to substance abuse, homelessness, and criminalization of persons with mental disorders. The assumption that CMHCs would assume responsibility for aftercare and rehabilitation of persons discharged from mental hospitals proved erroneous. The absence of mechanisms of control and accountability permitted CMHCs to focus on new populations of more amenable and attractive clients with far less severe disorders. Nor does the recent move to enrol persons with serious mental disorders in managed care offer assurances that the varied needs of this group will finally be met. Preliminary evidence suggests that a 'democratization' of services reduces the intensity of services for patients with more profound disabilities and needs (Mechanic & McAlpine, 1999).

Equally notable are the roles played by rhetoric and ideology in the development of mental health policy during past decades and a view of past policy that bore little relationship to reality. To dismiss rhetoric and ideology as simply forms of public posturing is to ignore their consequences. Rhetoric and ideology shape agendas and debates; they create expectations that in turn mould policies, and they inform the socialization, training, and education of those in professional occupations. The concept of community care and treatment and the corresponding attack on institutional care—all of which played significant policy roles during the last half century—were not inherently defective. But states, communities, and policy advocates lacked the foresight or commitment to ensure adequate financing and to provide needed services. In addition, optimistic claims about the prevention of mental disorders had little or no basis in empirical evidence; they represented the height of rhetorical fancy.

The history of mental health policy in the US also provides a fascinating if largely ignored case study of the interaction of political structure and ideology. In the nineteenth century, a faith in the efficacy of institutionalization led to the creation of a vast system of public hospitals that at their peak contained more than half a million patients. Yet an incremental policymaking process and intergovernmental rivalries led to a series of unanticipated consequences. By the early twentieth century, mental hospitals were providing care for a large number of elderly persons at a time when other alternatives for this group were non-existent. A half century later, dissatisfaction with the existing state of affairs led to demands that an obsolete and archaic institutional system be replaced by a new community-oriented policy. Each of these stages was shaped by intergovernmental rivalries that maximized efforts to shift costs to different levels and ideological claims that bore little relationship to reality. Moreover, the growth of a system of public welfare that included a myriad of entitlement programmes to deal with sickness and dependency had the inadvertent effect of diminishing the central policy focus on persons with severe and persistent mental illnesses. As long-term institutionalization diminished and was replaced by a variety of public programmes that focused on different populations, the latter group was faced by a fragmented system of services ill-suited to their complex needs. Americans at the beginning of the twenty-first century still faced the problem of shaping a policy that meets the needs of a people whose severe mental disorders creates dependency.

Addendum: mental health policy in the early twenty-first century (Howard H. Goldman)

There are some hopeful signs and important changes in policy since the publication of the report of the Surgeon General (US Department of Health and Human Services, 1999) and the report of the President's New Freedom Commission on Mental Health (2003). Although Americans still faced a mental health system characterized by fragmentation and inadequacies with respect to individuals with disabling mental illness, community support systems (CSSs) were implemented throughout the US by the first decade of the new century. The concept of CSSs, introduced in the late 1970s and moved forward by the Carter Commission, the Mental Health Systems Act, and the National Plan on the Chronically Mentally Ill (US Department of Health and Human Services, 1980), maintained its hold on the design of services within the public mental health system in the US. The CSS concept was focused on individuals who experienced severe and persistent mental disorders. The services within a CSS blended traditional treatment with interventions for meeting the broad social welfare needs of individuals, such as employment and housing, focused on a new concept of recovery with new effective interventions.

The reports of the Surgeon General and the President's New Freedom Commission had set forth the evidence for the effectiveness of treatments and services within a CSS, and together they ushered in a period of implementation of evidence-based practices (Drake & Goldman, 2003; Drake et al., 2001). Furthermore, the concept of recovery, which at first lacked clarity, gained an accepted meaning. Recovery implies achieving the best outcomes possible in terms of health and social participation, even while the underlying behavioural health condition might persist. Research increasingly demonstrated that, when framed this way, recovery could be achieved with new evidence-based interventions embedded within CSSs. And the CSS approach had come to dominate the public mental health services system by the turn of the century. People with severe mental disorders might continue to be impaired, but they can also achieve valued social integration and social participation (Davidson & Schmutte, 2020; Rowe & Ponce, 2020). Evidence-based practices within the CSS were the mechanism for promoting social integration and social participation.

A new initiative in evidence-based practices began within the public mental health system in the US. The report of the Surgeon General had demonstrated that there was a substantial evidence base on the effectiveness of treatments and services, but the report also found a large gap between what the research evidence recommended and actual practice. This conclusion sparked an initiative in evidence-based practice implementation that was supported by the federal Substance Abuse and Mental Health Services Administration and the Robert Wood Johnson Foundation and that was carried forward by the states (Drake et al., 2001). The journal *Psychiatric Services* published a series of papers reviewing the evidence supporting the effectiveness of specific interventions and papers focusing on implementing these services (Drake & Goldman, 2003). The series included review articles assessing the evidence on assertive community treatment, supported employment, family psychoeducation, pharmacological treatments, as well as services for individuals with comorbid substance abuse and stress-related disorders. It also discussed services across the life cycle for children and for individuals in later life, and it included papers on various aspects of implementation.

Beginning in 2014, another series of papers updating the original group of articles, called 'Assessing the Evidence Base', was published in *Psychiatric Services*. This series included reviews of 14 treatments and services, including some services that were not in the original set of papers, such as recovery housing and supported housing, services led by individuals with lived experience of mental illness, and medication assisted treatments for opiate and opioid addiction. (The series is described in Dougherty et al. (2014)). Finally, *The Palgrave Handbook of American Mental Health Policy* (Goldman et al., 2020) includes a dozen chapters on policy issues related to implementing evidence-based practices, such as those reviewed earlier but also interventions to prevent suicide, reduce gun violence, and promote citizenship and shared decision-making. Evidence-based practice implementation was the dominant theme in American mental health services policy in the first two decades of the twenty-first century.

One of the recurrent policy themes in the discussion of evidence-based practice implementation was the lack of health insurance coverage for treatment services for mental health conditions. For decades, health insurance coverage of these disorders was not on a par with coverage of other health conditions, limiting payments for specific services and requiring higher cost-sharing for similar services. Mental health insurance parity had been a goal of mental health advocates for decades, beginning in the 1970s. Parity was achieved slowly and incrementally in a sequence of opportune steps at the state and federal level (Grob & Goldman, 2006). The first steps in the process occurred in the states with mandates for insurance coverage and improved benefits; next came the changes in Medicaid and Medicare proposed in the National Plan on Chronic Mental Illness (US Department of Health and Human Services, 1980) and implemented during the 1980s (Koyanagi & Goldman, 1991a, 1991b).

The Clinton administration health insurance reform proposed a slow implementation of improved mental health benefits that would eventually result in parity coverage. Even though the whole reform was defeated, Congress passed a limited mental health parity law in 1996, which called for parity in annual and lifetime limits on coverage (Barry et al., 2010; Huskamp, 2020). At the 1999 White House Conference on Mental Health, President Clinton issued a directive to the Office of Personnel Management that all of its insurance plans in the enormous Federal Employees Health Benefits (FEHB) programme should cover in-network mental health and substance abuse services on a par with general medical and surgical services. The focus on in-network services was intended to use managed care techniques to control expenditures. A study commissioned by the federal government demonstrated that the FEHB directive resulted in improved coverage with no increase in expenditures attributable to parity coverage policy (Barry et al., 2010; Goldman et al., 2006; Grob & Goldman, 2006).

The findings of the evaluation of federal parity further encouraged advocates inside and outside the Congress to pass comprehensive parity reform, both in Medicare (MIPPA, 2008) and in private insurance, called the Mental Health Parity and Addictions Equity Act (MHPAEA, 2008). The latter law called for parity in stated benefits in the text of insurance policies that had coverage for behavioural health service, and it called for equal application of managed care techniques, in what were called 'non-quantitative treatment limitations'. However, the law did not mandate that all insurance policies provide behavioural health coverage. The final step in the sequence of incremental steps towards parity was achieved with the passage of President Obama's landmark legislation enacting the Patient Protection and Affordable Care Act (PPACA, 2010), which declared that behavioural health services were an essential benefit, which must be covered in all insurance policies whose provisions must be consistent with the parity provisions of the MHPAEA (Huskamp, 2020).

Looking forward reveals an emerging system that focuses both on the broad health and social welfare needs of individuals with disabling mental disorders and addresses the needs of those at the earliest stages of psychosis and other disorders. While CSSs that prioritize individuals already disabled by mental illness dominated the public mental health system at the end of the twentieth century, the new century introduced an initiative on early intervention with psychosis. This initiative was influenced by evidence from around the world suggesting the importance of reducing the duration of untreated psychosis coupled with evidence for the effectiveness of a suite of treatments for treating individuals in their first episode of psychosis. The hope is that early intervention will prevent or forestall the disability that has characterized the population served by the CSS (Dixon et al., 2018). For the moment, the service system will provide care for those in early stages of illness as well as those disabled by severe and persistent mental disorders.

A summary assessment of the accomplishments of mental health policy in the US following the Second World War concluded that conditions for individuals with mental disorders were 'better but not well' (Frank & Glied, 2006). The authors noted both advantages in improved medications and other evidence-based psychosocial treatments, as well as advances in insurance coverage and access to these services. At the end of the war, services had been provided predominantly by state government and the Veterans Administration for care in public mental hospitals. Over the period of more than the next half century, private and federal resources increased dramatically serving more of the population in a range of settings. The most important resources were from mainstream health and social welfare programmes, such as Medicaid, Medicare, SSDI, and SSI, as well as from private insurance. Consistent with the findings of the earlier report of the Surgeon General (US Department of Health and Human Services, 1999) and the President's New Freedom Commission on Mental Health (2003), Frank and Glied (2006) found many continuing problems and inadequacies, particularly for individuals with the most disabling conditions. These problems, including service fragmentation and limited resources to address the social determinants of care (such as underemployment and homelessness) and structural racism (over-incarceration of people of colour with mental disorders), leave much mental health policy work to be accomplished during the next decade (Goldman et al., 2020; Shim & Vinson, 2021).

REFERENCES

American Psychiatric Association (1960). *Report on Patients over 65 in Public Hospitals*. Washington, DC: American Psychiatric Association.

Atay, J. E. & Foley, D. (2007). *Background Report, Admissions and Resident Patients, State and County Mental Hospitals, United States, 2005*. Rockville, MD: Center for Mental Health Services.

Barry, C., Huskamp, H. A., & Goldman, H. H. (2010). A political history of federal mental health and addiction insurance parity. *Milbank Quarterly*, **88**, 404–433.

Davidson, L. & Schmutte, T. (2020). What is the meaning of recovery? In: Goldman, H. H., Frank, R. G., & Morrissey, J. P. (Eds.), *The Palgrave Handbook of American Mental Health Policy* (pp. 71–100). Cham: Palgrave Macmillan.

Dixon, L. B., Goldman, H. H., Srihari, V. H., & Kane, J. M. (2018). Transforming the treatment of schizophrenia in the U.S: The RAISE Initiative. *Annual Review of Clinical Psychology*, **14**, 237–258.

Dougherty R. H., Lyman, D. R., George, P., Ghose, S. S., Daniels, A. S., & Delphin-Rittmon, M. E. (2014). Assessing the evidence base for behavioral health services: introduction to the series. *Psychiatric Services*, **65**, 11–15.

Drake, R. E. & Goldman, H. H. (Eds.) (2003). *Evidence-Based Practices in Mental Health Care*. Washington, DC: American Psychiatric Association.

Drake, R. E., Goldman, H. H., Leff, H. S., Lehman, A. F., Dixon, L., Mueser, K. T., et al. (2001). Implementing evidence-based practices in routine mental health service settings. *Psychiatric Services*, **52**, 179–182.

Felix, R. H. (1945). Mental public health: a blueprint. Presentation at St. Elizabeths Hospital, April 21, 1945. In: Robert H. Felix Papers (MS C 331). Bethesda, MD: National Library of Medicine.

Felix, R. H. (1949). Mental disorders as a public health problem. *American Journal of Psychiatry*, **106**, 401–406.

Felix, R. H. & Bowers, R. V. (1948). Mental hygiene and socio-environmental factors. *Milbank Memorial Fund Quarterly*, **26**, 125–147.

Foley, H. A. & Sharfstein, S. S. (1983). *Madness and Government: Who Cares for the Mentally Ill?* Washington, DC: American Psychiatric Press.

Frank R. G. & Glied, S. A. (2006). *Better but not Well*. Baltimore, MD: The Johns Hopkins University Press.

General Accounting Office (1977). *Returning the Mentally Disabled to the Community: Government Needs to do More* (HRD-76-152). Washington, DC: General Accounting Office.

Goldman, H. H., Adams, N. H., & Taube, C. A. (1983). Deinstitutionalization: the data demythologized. *Hospital & Community Psychiatry*, **34**, 129–134.

Goldman H. H., Frank, R. G., Burnam, M. A., Huskamp, H. A., Ridgely, M. S., Normand, S. L., et al. (2006). Behavioral health insurance parity for federal employees. *New England Journal of Medicine*, **354**, 1378–1386.

Goldman, H. H., Frank, R. G., & Morrissey, J. P. (Eds.) (2020). *The Palgrave Handbook of American Mental Health Policy*. Cham: Palgrave Macmillan.

Grob, G. N. (1991). *From Asylum to Community: Mental Health Policy in Modern America*. Princeton, NJ: Princeton University Press.

Grob, G. N. & Goldman, H. H. (2006). *The Dilemma of Federal Mental Health Policy: Radical Reform or Incremental Change?* New Brunswick, NJ: Rutgers University Press.

Gronfein, W. (1985). Incentives and intentions in mental health policy: a comparison of the Medicaid and Community Mental Health Programs. *Journal of Health and Social Behavior*, **26**, 192–206.

HEW Task Force (1979). *Report of the HEW Task Force on Implementation of the Report to the President from the President's Commission on Mental Health* (DHEW Publication No. (ADM) 79-848). Rockville, MD: US Government Printing Office.

Huskamp, H. (2020). Mental health insurance parity: how full is the glass? In: Goldman, H. H., Frank, R. G., & Morrissey, J. P. (Eds.), *The Palgrave Handbook of American Mental Health Policy* (pp. 367–388). Cham: Palgrave Macmillan.

Joint Commission on Mental Illness and Health (1961). *Action for Mental Health: Final Report of the Joint Commission on Mental Illness and Health*. New York: Basic Books.

Koyanagi, C. & Goldman, H. H. (1991a). *Inching Forward: A Report on Progress Made in Federal Mental Health Policy in the 1980s*. Alexandria, VA: National Mental Health Association.

Koyanagi, C. & Goldman, H. H. (1991b). The quiet success of the national plan for the chronically mentally ill. *Hospital & Community Psychiatry*, **42**, 899–905.

Kramer, M. (1956). *Facts Needed to Assess Public Health and Social Problems in the Widespread Use of the Tranquilizing Drugs* (US Public Health Service, Publication No. 486). Washington, DC: US Public Health Service.

Kramer, M. (1967). *Some Implication of Trends in the Usage of Psychiatric Facilities for Community Mental Health Programs and Related Research* (US Public Health Service, Publication No. 1434). Washington, DC: US Public Health Service.

Kramer, M. (1977). *Psychiatric Services and the Changing Institutional Scene, 1950–1985* (DHEW Publication No. (ADM) 77-433). Washington, DC: Government Printing Office.

Kramer, M., Taube, C., & Starr, S. (1968). Patterns of use in psychiatric facilities by the aged: current status, trends, and implications. *Psychiatric Research Reports*, **23**, 89–150.

Langsley, D. G. (1980). The community mental health center: does it treat patients? *Hospital & Community Psychiatry*, **21**, 815–819.

Liberman, R. P. & Kopelowicz, A. (2005). Recovery from schizophrenia: a concept in search of research. *Psychiatric Services*, **56**, 735–742.

Lieberman, J. A. (2006). Comparative effectiveness of antipsychotic drugs. *Archives of General Psychiatry*, **63**, 1069–1072.

Lieberman, J. A., Stroup, T. S., McEvoy, J. P., Swartz, M. S., Rosenheck, R. A., Perkins, D. O., et al. (2005). Effectiveness of antipsychotic drugs in patients with chronic schizophrenia. *New England Journal of Medicine*, **353**, 1209–1223.

Mechanic, D. (1999). *Mental Health and Social Policy: The Emergence of Managed Care* (4th ed.). Boston, MA: Allyn and Bacon.

Mechanic, D. & McAlpine, D. D. (1999). Mission unfulfilled: potholes on the road to mental health parity. *Health Affairs*, **18**, 7–21.

Mechanic, D. & Rochefort, D. A. (1992). A policy of inclusion for the mentally ill. *Health Affairs*, **11**, 128–150.

MHPAEA (2008). *Mental Health Parity and Addictions Equity Act* (PL 110-343). Washington, DC: Government Publishing Office.

MIPPA (2008). *Medicare Improvements for Patients and Providers Act* (PL 110-275). Washington, DC: Government Publishing Office.

Musto, D. F. (1975). Whatever happened to community mental health? *Public Interest*, **39**, 53–79.

National Institute of Mental Health (1961). *National Institute of Mental Health Position Paper on the Report of the Joint Commission on Mental Illness and Health* (National Institute of Mental Health Records 1965–1967, Box 1, Record Group 511.2). Washington, DC: National Archives.

National Institute of Mental Health (1962a). *Preliminary Draft Report of NIMH Task Force on Implementation of Recommendations of the Report of the Joint Commission on Mental Illness and Health* (National Institute of Mental Health, Miscellaneous Records, 19561967, Box 1, Record Group 511.2). Washington, DC: National Archives.

National Institute of Mental Health (1962b). *A Proposal for a Comprehensive Mental Health Program to Implement the Findings of the report of the Joint Commission on Mental Illness and Health* (National Institute of Mental Health Miscellaneous Records, 1956–1967, Box 1, Record Group 511.2). Washington, DC: National Archives.

National Institute of Mental Health (1974). Statistical Note No. 107. Rockville, MD: National Institute of Mental Health.

Pollack, E. S., Person, P. H., Kramer, M., & Goldstein, H. (1959). *Patterns of Retention, Release, and Death of First Admissions to State Mental Hospitals* (US Public Health Service, Publication No. 672). Washington, DC: US Public Health Service.

PPACA (2010). *Patient Protection and Affordable Care Act* (PL 111-148). Washington, DC: Government Publishing Office.

President's Commission on Mental Health (1978). *Report to the President from the President's Commission on Mental Health* (4 Vols.). Washington, DC: Government Printing Office.

President's New Freedom Commission on Mental Health (2003). *Achieving the Promise: Transforming Mental Health Care in America: Final Report* (DHHS Pub. No. SMA-03-3832). Washington, DC: US Department of Health and Human Services.

Public Law Chap. 538 (1946). *U.S. Statutes at Large*, **60**, 421–426.

Public Law 88-264 (1963). *U.S. Statutes at Large*, **77**, 282–299.

Public Law 89-105 (1965). *U.S. Statutes at Large*, **79**, 427–430.

Public Law 96-398 (1980). *U.S. Statutes at Large*, **94**, 1564–1613.

Public Law 97-35 (1981). *U.S. Statutes at Large*, **95**, 535–598.

Rowe, M. & Ponce, A. N. (2020). How shall we promote citizenship social participation? In: Goldman, H. H., Frank, R. G., & Morrissey, J. P. (Eds.), *The Palgrave Handbook of American Mental Health Policy* (pp. 573–600). Cham: Palgrave Macmillan.

Shim R. S. & Vinson S. Y. (2021). *Social (In)Justice and Mental Health*. Washington, DC: American Psychiatric Association Publishing.

US Department of Health and Human Services (1980). *Steering Committee on the Chronically Mentally Ill: Toward a National Plan for the Chronically Mentally Ill*. Washington, DC: US Public Health Service.

US Department of Health and Human Services (1999). *Mental Health: A Report of the Surgeon General*. Rockville, MD: US Public Health Service.

4

Recovery as an integrative paradigm in mental health

Mike Slade and Larry Davidson

What is recovery?

The term 'recovery' is at the heart of a debate about the core purpose of mental health services. It is a contested term, with at least two meanings. We call these two meanings recovery from mental illness, or 'clinical recovery', on the one hand, and being in recovery with a mental illness, or 'personal recovery', on the other (Davidson & Roe, 2007; Slade, 2009a). Each meaning is underpinned by a set of values and creates role expectations for mental health professionals. We begin by differentiating these two meanings.

Meaning 1: clinical recovery or recovery 'from' mental illness

The first meaning of recovery has emerged from professional-led research and practice. Clinical recovery has four key features:

1. It is an outcome or a state, generally dichotomous
2. It is observable—in clinical parlance, it is objective, not subjective
3. It is rated by the expert clinician, not the patient
4. The definition of recovery is invariant across individuals.

Various definitions of this form of recovery have been proposed by mental health professionals. A widely used definition is that recovery comprises full symptom remission, full- or part-time work or education, independent living without supervision by informal carers, and having friends with whom activities can be shared, all sustained for a period of 2 years (Libermann & Kopelowicz, 2002). Defining recovery has allowed epidemiological research to establish recovery rates. In **Table 4.1** we show all 20-year or longer follow-up studies.

These empirical data, along with emerging epidemiological evidence specific to personal recovery (Simonsen et al., in press), challenge the applicability of a chronic disease model to mental illness, with its embedded assumption that conditions like schizophrenia are necessarily lifelong and have a deteriorating course.

However, deep assumptions about normality are embedded in clinical recovery. As Ruth Ralph and Patrick Corrigan comment in relation to this concept (Ralph & Corrigan, 2005):

> This kind of definition begs several questions that need to be addressed to come up with an understanding of recovery as outcome: How many goals must be achieved to be considered recovered? For that matter, how much life success is considered 'normal'? (p. 5)

As a result, and as a product of the user/survivor movement spanning the last 40 years, people who use mental health services have called for a new approach. As Ridgway (2001) argues:

> The field of psychiatric disabilities requires an enriched knowledge base and literature to guide innovation in policy and practice under a recovery paradigm. We must reach beyond our storehouse of writings that describe psychiatric disorder as a catastrophic life event. (p. 335)

The second meaning of 'recovery' provides the rubric under which such an enriched knowledge base has been accruing.

Meaning 2: personal recovery or being 'in' recovery

People personally affected by mental illness have become increasingly vocal in communicating both what their life is like with the mental illness and what helps in moving beyond the role of a patient with mental illness. Early accounts were written by individual pioneers (Coleman, 1999; Davidson & Strauss, 1992; Deegan, 1988; Fisher, 1994; O'Hagan, 1996; Ridgway, 2001). These brave, and sometimes oppositional and challenging, voices provide ecologically valid pointers to what recovery looks and feels like from the inside.

Once individual stories were more visible, compilations and syntheses of these accounts began to emerge from around the (especially Anglophone) world, such as from Australia (Andresen et al., 2003), New Zealand (Barnett & Lapsley, 2006; Goldsack et al., 2005; Lapsley et al., 2002; Mental Health Commission, 2000), Scotland (Scottish Recovery Network, 2006, 2007), the US (Davidson et al., 2005; Spaniol & Koehler, 1994), and England (Barker et al.,

Table 4.1 Recovery rates in long-term follow-up studies of psychosis

Reference	Location	Year	N	Mean length of follow-up (years)	Recovered or significantly improved (%)
Huber et al., 1975	Bonn	1975	502	22	57
Ciompi & Muller 1976	Lausanne	1976	289	37	53
Bleuler, 1978	Zurich	1978	208	23	53–68
Tsuang et al., 1979	Iowa	1979	186	35	46
Harding et al., 1987	Vermont	1987	269	32	62–68
Ogawa et al., 1987	Japan	1987	140	23	57
Marneros et al., 1989	Cologne	1989	249	25	58
DeSisto et al., 1995	Maine	1995	269	35	49
Harrison et al., 2001	18 sites	2001	776	25	56

1999; McIntosh, 2005). The understanding of recovery which has emerged from these accounts has a different focus from clinical recovery, for example, in emphasizing the centrality of hope, identity, meaning, and personal responsibility despite ongoing symptoms or impairments.

We will refer to this consumer-based understanding of recovery as *personal recovery*, to reflect its individually defined and experienced nature. To note, other distinguishing terms have also been used, including clinical recovery versus social recovery (Secker et al., 2002), scientific versus consumer models of recovery (Bellack, 2006), and organizational recovery versus personal recovery (Le Boutillier et al., 2015).

Many definitions of this form of recovery have been proposed by those who are experiencing it:

> Recovery refers to the lived or real life experience of people as they accept and overcome the challenge of the disability … they experience themselves as recovering a new sense of self and of purpose within and beyond the limits of disability. (Deegan, 1988, p. 11)

> For me, recovery means that I'm not in hospital and I'm not sitting in supported accommodation somewhere with someone looking after me. Since I've recovered, I've found that in spite of my illness I can still contribute and have an input into what goes on in my life, input that is not necessarily tied up with medication, my mental illness or other illnesses. (Scottish Recovery Network, 2006, p. 61)

The most widely cited definition, which underpins most recovery policy internationally, is by Bill Anthony (1993):

> Recovery is a deeply personal, unique process of changing one's attitudes, values, feelings, goals, skills, and/or roles. It is a way of living a satisfying, hopeful, and contributing life even within the limitations caused by illness. Recovery involves the development of new meaning and purpose in one's life as one grows beyond the catastrophic effects of mental illness. (p. 527)

It is consistent with the less widely cited but more succinct definition proposed by Retta Andresen and colleagues, that recovery involves: 'The establishment of a fulfilling, meaningful life and a positive sense of identity founded on hopefulness and self determination' (Andresen et al., 2003, p. 588).

For those who value succinctness, the definition often used in mental health services is: 'Recovery involves living as well as possible' (South London and Maudsley NHS Foundation Trust, 2010, p. 38).

The CHIME framework

To understand what personal recovery means, a systematic review was conducted to synthesize published descriptions and models of this form of recovery (Leamy et al., 2011). Five key recovery processes were identified which often occur as part of an individual's personal recovery journey: connectedness, hope and optimism, identity, meaning and purpose, and empowerment (giving the acronym CHIME). The CHIME framework was validated with people currently using mental health services (Bird et al., 2014b). Limitations of the CHIME framework include its incomplete focus on difficulties (Stuart et al., 2017), insufficient attention to relational aspects of recovery (Price-Robertson et al., 2017), and the monocultural evidence on which it is based (Slade et al., 2012).

Nonetheless, the CHIME framework is widely cited, and an independent systematic review has concluded that it is widely endorsed (van Weeghel et al., 2019). It therefore provides a strong foundation to underpin mental health policy, research, and practice. For example, it has been used so far as the gold standard to inform choice of recovery measures (Vogel et al., 2020), to explore the cross-cultural relevance of recovery (Lim et al., 2019), to investigate the impact of physical activity on recovery (Benkwitz & Healy, 2019), and to inform policy recommendations (Mental Health Coordinating Council, 2014).

Recovery as an integrative paradigm

The recovery approach to care is based on personal recovery. Personal recovery represents a paradigm shift, in which the intellectual challenge emerges from outside the dominant scientific paradigm (the understanding of recovery emerges from people who have experienced mental illness, not from mental health professionals). Previous preoccupations (e.g. risk, symptoms, and hospitalizations) become seen as a subset or special case of the new paradigm. By contrast, what was previously of peripheral interest (i.e. the patient's perspective) becomes central. This involves a reversal of some traditional clinical assumptions. Mental illness is a part of the person, rather than the person being a mental patient. Having valued social roles improves symptoms and reduces hospitalization, rather than treatment being needed before the person is ready to take on responsibilities and life roles. The recovery goals come from the patient and the support to meet these goals comes from the clinician among others, rather than traditional treatment goals being developed by the practitioner which then require compliance from the patient. Assessment focuses more on the strengths, preferences, and skills of the person than on what they cannot do. The normal human needs of work, love and play *do* apply—they are the ends to which treatment may or may not contribute. People with mental illness are fundamentally normal, that is, like everyone else in their aspirations and needs. They will over time make good decisions about their lives if they have the opportunity, support, and encouragement, rather than being people who will in general make bad decisions, so that professionals need to take responsibility for them.

Recovery is also an *integrative* paradigm, at both the personal and the system level. For the individual, it integrates the experience of mental illness with the person, by giving primacy to personhood over illness. For example, person-first language—talking about the person experiencing psychosis or the person with schizophrenia (or, even better, the person with a diagnosis of schizophrenia) rather than the schizophrenic or the schizophrenic patient—serves to remind that diagnoses classify illnesses, not people (Davidson & Flanagan, 2007). Recovery also integrates levels of experience, such as political, cultural, life events (trauma, loss, etc.), and personal values, rather than segmenting into professionally defined components of identity (Barrett, 1996). It addresses the call for culturally competent or responsive services, by highlighting the fact that a person's cultural background, affiliations, and affinities are all crucial aspects of who they are, and thereby influence help-seeking, treatment response, and ways of managing the illness.

For the mental health system, the recovery paradigm similarly involves integration of the function of traditionally separate professional disciplines in the service of action planning oriented around the individual's goals. This contrasts with care planning oriented around each discipline's specialist skills. Likewise, recovery can be used as a bridge to integrate treatment for co-occurring psychiatric and substance use disorders, or mental health and physical illnesses, rather than leaving the individual to navigate complex health and social care systems to get their needs met through fragmented or uncoordinated care (Davidson & White, 2007). Overall, a recovery-oriented system is an integrated system which wraps around the individual to meet their needs.

Finally, the relationship between recovery and other sociopolitical movements is becoming clearer, including in particular the links with human rights (Funk & Drew, 2017; Pathare et al., 2021; United Nations General Assembly, 2019), citizenship (Pelletier, 2015; Vandekinderen, 2012), and well-being (Slade et al., 2017).

We now describe a theoretical framework intended to guide mental health professionals in their efforts to support personal recovery.

The personal recovery framework

Supporting recovery will involve giving primacy to identity over illness. What is identity? Three perspectives have evolved in the humanities. Psychologists focus on personal identity—the things that make a person unique. This individuality is the reason why there cannot be one model of recovery, why professionals should be cautious about saying (or thinking) 'we do recovery', and why the individual's views on what matters to them have to be given primacy. Sociologists more commonly refer to social identity—the collection of group memberships that define the individual. Social identity is damaged when the person experiences entrapment in a low-value and stigmatized social role, such as a mental health service user. Philosophers relate identity to the existence of a persisting entity particular to a given person. Ongoing growth and transformation are central to human development, which is why the goal of returning to a premorbid state is neither attainable nor desirable. Combining these perspectives, *identity comprises those persistent characteristics which make us unique and by which we are connected to the rest of the world*. This definition underpins the personal recovery framework (Slade, 2009a) shown in **Figure 4.1**, which illustrates the identity challenges which occur for people experiencing mental illness.

The social environment comprises the world and others in it. Identity-enhancing relationships can be with the self, the mental illness, or with the social environment. Figuratively, the process of recovery involves reclaiming a positive identity in two ways (shown as arrows in **Figure 4.1**): by identity-enhancing relationships and promotion of well-being which push the mental illness into being a smaller component of identity, and by framing and self-managing which pull the mental illness part. These processes take place in a social context which provides scaffolding for the development of an identity as a person 'in recovery'.

In the personal recovery framework, the individual experiences recovery through undertaking four interrelated and overlapping recovery tasks. First, *developing a positive identity* outside of being a person with a mental illness. This process involves establishing the conditions in which it is possible to experience life as a person rather than as an illness. Second, *developing a personally satisfactory meaning* to frame the experience which professionals would understand as mental illness. This involves making sense of the experience so that it can be put in a box: framed as a part of the person but not as the whole person. This meaning might be expressed as a diagnosis or a formulation, or it may have nothing to do with clinical models—a spiritual or cultural or existential crisis. The actual meaning matters less than the degree to which it provides both a constraining frame for the experience and an impetus to move from being clinically managed to the third task of *taking personal responsibility* through self-management: being responsible for your own well-being, including seeking help and support from others when necessary. The final recovery task involves the acquisition of previous, modified, or new *valued social roles*. These normally have nothing to do with mental illness.

The job of mental health professionals

The personal recovery framework points to four ways in which practitioners can support an individual's recovery: fostering relationships, promoting well-being, offering treatments, and improving social inclusion (Slade, 2009b). Mental health services need to be oriented around these four recovery support tasks if they are to maximally support recovery.

Fostering relationships includes those with a higher being, with family and informal carers, with other people with lived experience

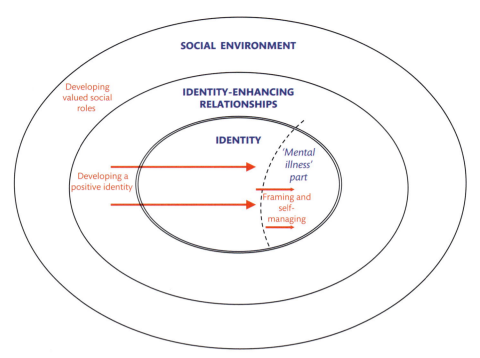

Figure 4.1 The personal recovery framework.

of mental illness, and with mental health professionals. For example, exposure to people who are further along their recovery journey may be profoundly hope-creating, and this is one reason to employ people with experience of mental illness in the mental health workforce. For the same reason, involvement in mutual self-help groups and intentional recovery communities (Whitley et al., 2008) can provide a safe space in which to create a positive personal narrative and challenge the constraints of an illness-defined identity. For professionals, the ability to connect with people during a chaotic period of their life is a recovery support when used as a springboard towards a partnership relationship, in which coaching and mentoring skills are instilled by the professional to promote self-management (Borg & Kristiansen, 2004).

Promoting well-being involves the use of expertise on mental well-being, drawing from the science of positive psychology. For example, the Authentic Happiness theory identifies different types of good life: pleasant, engaged, meaningful, and achieving (Seligman, 2002). The pleasant life (i.e. filled with positive emotions, symptom-free) is not the only type of good life, so supporting recovery also involves putting resources into, for example, spiritual development (for a meaningful life) or promoting activism (for an engaged life). The New Economics Foundation (www.neweconomics.org) identifies 'five-a-day for well-being': approaches which promote mental well-being in the same way that consuming five fruit and vegetable portions per day promotes physical well-being. Their recommended approaches are Connect, Be active, Take notice, Keep learning, and Give. Mental health services which are promoting well-being will focus efforts in these areas.

Offering treatments involves the use of evidence-based interventions, but oriented around recovery goals rather than traditional treatment goals. Treatment goals are set by the clinician, and will normally relate to avoiding bad things happening, such as relapse, hospitalization, harmful risk, etc. Recovery goals are the person's dreams and aspirations. They are unique, often idiosyncratic. They are forward-looking, although they may of course involve the past. They focus on what the person actively wants, rather than what the person wants to avoid. Recovery goals are strengths-based and orientated towards reinforcing a positive identity and developing valued social roles. They can be challenging to mental health professionals, either because they seem unrealistic or inappropriate, or because supporting them seems to lie outside the professional role. They sometimes involve effort by the professional, or they may have nothing to do with mental health services. They always require the service user to take personal responsibility and put in effort. Recovery goals are set by the service user. Treatment supports recovery when it is offered to the person in support of their recovery goals.

One evidence-based approach to supporting recovery is the REFOCUS intervention (Bird et al., 2014a), developed and evaluated (Slade et al., 2015) in the UK, and extended in Australia (Meadows et al., 2019). A second is peer support work, involving people with personal experience of mental ill health and recovery working in services to support others (White et al., 2020). A third is the Individual Placement and Support approach to obtaining and retaining mainstream employment (Brinchmann et al., 2020).

Finally, improving social inclusion is central, because hope without opportunity dies. Amartya Sen (awarded the Nobel Memorial Prize in Economic Sciences in 1998) identified the notion of substantial freedom, meaning that even where legally codified, freedom is effectively restrained when a lack of psychological, social, and financial resources make it impossible to achieve goals and live a meaningful life. The experience (and anticipation) of discrimination blights the lives of many people with mental illness. To support recovery, the focus of a clinician's role needs to enlarge beyond the level of treatment. Helping local employers to make accommodations for employees experiencing mental illness, or working with user activists to challenge discrimination, are just as much a part of the job as treating illness. Free guides for mental health professionals wishing to take up these tasks are available (Shepherd et al., 2008; Slade, 2013).

Change in values and behaviour is difficult. For people using services, this is why recovery can take a long time. For people working in services, it is just as difficult, but also just as necessary if recovery is to become a reality. We illustrate some of the implications of recovery for two concrete areas of clinical activity: person-centred care planning and prescribing of medication.

Person-centred care planning and recovery

One way of understanding the application of person-centred care planning in mental health is to place it within the context of evidence-based medicine. Evidence-based medicine is based on the confluence of four factors:

1. The empirical evidence that exists related to the effectiveness of various interventions
2. The individual practitioner's clinical experience, expertise, and judgement
3. The resources available to the person
4. Patient choice (Davidson et al., 2009b; Guyatt & Rennie, 2002; Sackett, et al., 1996).

An underlying assumption of evidence-based medicine is that all individuals have the right to make their own health care decisions (Slade, 2017). Since the person is free to ultimately make their own decisions, it becomes incumbent upon practitioners to understand this fact and to communicate with the person and their family in as accurate, informative, culturally, and personally responsive, and perhaps even persuasive, a way as possible so as to maximize outcomes. In order to do so, the practitioner needs to attend to the person's role as decision-maker, including their needs, values, and preferences, within the context of a collaborative relationship.

Person-centred care planning results from accepting and emphasizing the person's role as decision-maker and the importance of their needs, values, and preferences in the care planning process (Tondora et al., 2014). What is unique about the application of person-centred care planning in mental health is that it makes explicit the underlying assumption that people with mental illnesses are first and foremost people, and therefore more specifically, citizens of their respective societies (Rowe & Davidson, 2016). They were born with the same rights to citizenship as anyone else, and any limitations placed upon those rights will have to be justified and sanctioned by law. Beginning with this assumption means that we need not argue for or justify offering person-centred care to persons with mental illnesses as a separate population. Persons with mental illnesses are 'entitled' to person-centred care to the same degree and for the same reasons as are any other citizens: because it is in accord with the emphasis democratic societies place on autonomy and personal sovereignty. These values apply in health care as well as in other spheres of society, and they apply equally as well to persons with mental illnesses as they do to any other persons ... until, unless, and then only for as long as limitations placed on these values are justified and sanctioned by law.

That is, person-centred care, like evidence-based medicine more broadly, is considered the default condition; it should be provided unless there are clear and persuasive, and legally valid, reasons for not doing so. The onus is on those who wish to limit the applicability of this approach to any given population, whether that be persons with mental illnesses, those with developmental disabilities, those with Alzheimer's disease, those knocked unconscious by a car accident, or those with any other special considerations (e.g. forensic populations).

Understanding person-centred care planning as the default condition has both advantages and disadvantages. The advantage is that this simple understanding of person-centred care is consistent with the focus on rights and personal sovereignty emphasized above and therefore is hard to challenge based purely on principle. Few can argue that people do not want to make their own decisions or that people do not want care that is consistent with their personal values, needs, and preferences. The apparent simplicity of this explanation makes it hard to discount. Unfortunately, the disadvantage of framing this issue in this way stems precisely from this same advantage. Because it is hard to discount, person-centred care comes to be equated with 'motherhood and apple pie' (an American phrase for things that are undeniably good), and, as a result, everyone claims to be doing it already. At this vague level, it is easy for people to dismiss the challenges inherent in having to change their practice by insisting that they already practise in a person-centred way. In addition, the range of accommodations required to offer this approach to persons with mental illnesses are overlooked or underappreciated. We address a few of these below, framing questions that can be used to determine the degree to which mental health care is being provided in a person-centred fashion (Davidson et al., 2009a).

Is the care centred on an individual person?

Person-centred care can only be carried out at the level of each individual, unique person within the context of their family and life. Each person-centred care plan should look different from any others, and be based squarely on this particular person's goals, needs, values, and preferences. This does not mean that person-centred plans cannot include traditional treatments, such as taking prescribed medication or participating in cognitive behavioural psychotherapy. It does mean, however, that these interventions—and such traditional clinical goals as symptom reduction and abstinence from drugs and alcohol—are only included to the degree that the person decides to use or pursue them, which will be based on whether or not the person sees these interventions or goals as contributing to their achievement of other personally relevant recovery goals, such as attaining decent housing, getting a job, or returning to school. Relevant questions would thus include the following:

- Does the plan provide a roadmap for where the person is headed and what they are trying to do in their life, or does it merely stipulate what treatment they need?
- Can you tell from the plan what the care team is trying to accomplish, not just what they are trying to avoid?

- Does the plan address a life outside of or beyond formal mental health services, or does it remain within the boundaries of the mental health system?
- If medication is part of the plan, can you tell what the medication is to be used for?
- Is adherence an end in itself, or is it viewed as a route to some other, personally desirable end?
- Will the services being offered limit the person to the passive role of mental patient, or will they lead to some worthwhile and wished for changes in the person's life?

As mentioned above, the process begins with these goals and works backwards to what is needed for the person to advance toward their goals, rather than insisting that the person be adherent to traditional treatment goals first in order to then decide on and pursue their own personal aspirations.

Is the care based on the person's strengths?

Is it clear how the plan will utilize identified strengths, both within the person and within their social milieu? Can you tell from the plan what the person's specific interests are, and how these interests have contributed to the formulation of goals and objectives? Does the plan help to move the person towards what interests them, or does it simply move them away from problematic behaviours or activities? If substance use is identified as a problem to be addressed, for example, does the plan also address what kind of sober activities the person may want to participate in instead? Are community activities and resources identified in the plan that would support the person in pursing their interests? Are there people identified in the plan with whom the person can share these interests?

Does the plan clearly delineate the tasks and roles to be performed and the parties responsible for each? Of particular importance is, does the plan clearly identify the person's own sphere of responsibility and the tasks that they agree to take on?

This question addresses one of the more important reasons to adopt person-centred care planning in mental health; that is, recognizing and incorporating the person's own role in their recovery. What does the person need to do to promote or progress in their own recovery? What kind of support will the person need in order to do carry out these responsibilities successfully? These two questions provide the key focus of recovery-oriented care for people with mental illnesses, and require in-depth knowledge of the person, their capacities and needs, and the resources available in their social milieu. Based on this knowledge, the care team is able to identify what might be the next one or two steps in the person's recovery and to sketch out what will be involved in the person taking these next few steps. This is how the plan becomes more than a piece of paper that satisfies regulatory, accrediting, and/or reimbursing bodies by being instead more of an organic and useful work in progress.

Does the plan and the care provided change over time with the person's evolving goals and needs?

Person-centred care plans do not accept maintenance as a valid goal, as people do not want merely to be 'maintained'. It is quite possible for people to want to maintain a level of clinical stability, though, or to want to remain at a plateau of functioning for an extended period of time. Few people like change for the sake of change, and many people with mental illnesses are afraid of taking risks or trying new things out a very legitimate fear that they might suffer a setback (a fear often reinforced by caring practitioners who do not want to see people relapse). But life also does not stand still. Therefore, while containing the illness may be a very real concern and goal for some people at some times, it is not possible to do so simply by maintaining one's life, that is, by trying to stand still. Care plans therefore anticipate that change is inevitable, and that people will need to continue to adapt to new situations and new challenges, whether they like to or not. One important contribution care plans, and person-centred care more broadly, can make in such situations is to help the person identify those things that they want to keep the same while other things are changing around them.

Are the plan, and the services offered, understandable to the person?

Just as the plan needs to identify the person's own role in promoting or pursuing recovery, the plan and the care offered need to be accessible to and understandable by the person. This is one area in which psychiatric person-centred care may need to incorporate the use of tools and aids to help the person compensate for cognitive impairments or a history of educational deprivation. Does the plan address those aspects of the person's experiences that are of concern to them, and in a language that they will be able to understand (e.g. voices as opposed to auditory hallucinations, feelings of being unsafe, vulnerable, or unprotected as opposed to paranoia, etc.)? Does the person know what they have agreed to receive or participate in? Has their consent been truly informed, or will things be done to them to which they have not agreed? Even in the case of people receiving treatment involuntarily, or individuals who have legal conservators or guardians, have concerted efforts been made to inform the person of the available options and to explain what they can expect to happen, including what needs to happen for them to no longer be receiving care involuntarily or no longer need a guardian?

Finally, does the plan encourage and support the person in assuming increasing control over their life, including the power to make their own decisions?

Here, too, psychiatric person-centred care plans may need to focus specifically on these issues of control, empowerment, and decision-making more than care plans in other specialty areas of medicine. This is not only because of the impact of mental illness on the person's life, but also because of the history of mental health care and its tendency to socialize people into a passive and helpless patient role. People may need to be encouraged to take back control of certain parts of their life, the responsibility for which may have been assumed by others. They may also need to be encouraged to view themselves as capable, and as having intact domains of functioning beyond the reach of the illness. They may need to be reminded of, or introduced to, their strengths and gifts, and they may need a series of small successes, easy wins, in order to rebuild their self-confidence and sense of personal efficacy. And they may need encouragement and support in taking risks and trying new things—perhaps even some gentle prodding to get unstuck, to be liberated from the inertia of chronic illness. We turn now to our second example: the contribution of medication to personal recovery.

Medication and recovery

In a recovery-focused mental health service, a full range of psychotropic medication is available. However, the job of the service is not to get medication taken, whatever the cost. The job is to support personal recovery. This may or may not involve use of medication for an individual at a particular point in their life journey. So medication is one potential recovery support, among many. The job of the clinician is to give genuine choice and control about medication to the service user. This means that the person may decide to use medication as the prescriber recommends, or may modify the recommendations of the prescriber, or may decide not to take medication. Genuine choice is available only where any of these choices is allowable, which is why prescribing levels are a litmus test for a recovery focus (Slade et al., 2008). The content of the individual's decision about medication is in this sense irrelevant—what matters is the extent to which the person is taking personal responsibility for their well-being.

So what does a recovery-focused approach to medication look like? Of course, many clinicians will place great importance on medication. Their psychopharmacological expertise may be well developed. This is an important resource to bring to the decision-making process. The change in a recovery-focused service is that this expertise is meshed with the consumer's expertise about their own values, beliefs, goals, and preferred approaches to meeting challenges. The job of the clinician is to help people come to the best choice *for them*. Medication may or may not be necessary for recovery—the journey of recovery involves finding out whether it has a part to play. Since medication will be a tool for many people, at points in their life, it is often important to discuss. The discussion needs to focus on what will be helpful for the individual, and in order to have that discussion the first thing that needs clarifying are the person's recovery goals. Once it is clear what the person is trying to achieve in life, then the role of medication can be discussed in a more focused way. Some people will want to be prescribed medication, and it should be fully available. Some people will experience decisional uncertainty, and the clinical task is then to support decision-making through crystallizing questions, providing unbiased information, and supporting the person to plan and undertake experiments. This will involve truly shared decision-making—two experts in the room, jointly undertaking information exchange and (always) clarification of values (Slade, 2017). Decisions about medication, just like any other form of treatment, are personal not medical decisions.

How is this done? This is an area where mental health services can learn from innovative approaches to supporting the decision-making process in general medicine (e.g. www.dhmc.org/shared_decision_making.cfm, http://decisionaid.ohri.ca/odsf.html). Some of these decision-support approaches are now being evaluated in mental health services, such as CommonGround (Deegan, 2010; Finnerty et al., 2018). One such approach is to reframe medicine—in the sense of things that help you to feel better—as much more than solely pharmacological. Pat Deegan's notion of personal medicine (Deegan, 2005) includes all the things that people do to feel better: laughter, love, hope, caffeine, exercise, chocolate, etc. In other words, medicine is what you do, not just what you take. Pill medicine (i.e. psychotropic prescribed medication) is then a subset of personal medicine. This approach is, of course, already used, such as when prescribing exercise (Meyer & Broocks, 2000), nutrition therapy (Lakhan & Vieira, 2008), or bibliotherapy (Gregory et al., 2004). This has two implications.

First, the prescriber is not the arbiter of the best medicine—only the consumer can judge what medicines are helpful. This is facilitated by the development of what Deegan calls power statements which reflect the person's goals for using psychiatric medication:

> For example, a husband developed the following power statement to share with his psychiatrist:
>
> My marriage is powerful personal medicine, and is the most important thing in my life. I don't want paranoia or sexual side effects from medication to stress my marriage. You and I have to find a medication that supports me in my marriage so that my marriage can support my recovery.
>
> Notice how the power statement contextualizes the use of medication within the overarching goal for recovery. Also, notice how the power statement acts as an invitation to collaboration and shared decision-making between the prescriber and the client. (Deegan, 2007, p. 67)

Second, it highlights that finding the balance between pill medicine and other forms of personal medicine is central. If the most important medicine *to the individual* is pill medicine, then a focus on medication is appropriate. If, by contrast, the most important medicine (i.e. what gets and keeps the person well) is some other form of personal medicine, then an exclusive focus on psychopharmacology will hinder recovery.

A recovery-promoting approach is thus to view medication as an 'exchangeable protection against relapse' (Libermann, 2002, p. 339), in which pharmacological and psychosocial approaches both buffer the individual against relapse. For example, framing medication as a potential tool for sustaining well-being creates a very different dialogue (Copeland, 1999). The advantage of this view is that it creates a focus on promoting resilience (which definitely matters) rather than on medication (which may or may not matter). Resilience can be supported by working with the consumer to identify answers to the statements 'I have …' (external supports of people and resources), 'I am …' (inner personal strengths), and 'I can …' (social and interpersonal skills) (Mental Health Commission, 2001). Medication is thus one potential external support, alongside a whole range of other types of resilience-promoting supports, skills, and strengths. Finding a balance between personal medicine and pill medicine is an essential ingredient of recovery. Both prescribers and consumers will benefit from exposure to the resources which are becoming available to support people who want to come off their psychiatric medication, including websites (e.g. www.comingoff.com), booklets published by voluntary sector groups (Darton, 2005; The Icarus Project and Freedom Center, 2012) and professional groups (Guy et al., 2019), and books (Breggin & Cohen, 2007; Stastny & Lehmann, 2007; Watkins, 2007).

Conclusion

Recovery-oriented care addresses all of these things and more, helping the person to gradually piece back together a meaningful and self-determined life out of the ravages wrought by mental illness. While much work remains to be done in developing the technologies and tools that will be needed for the design and implementation of such services and supports, the fruits of these labours will more than justify the efforts involved.

KEY REFERENCES

Amering, M. & Schmolke, M. (2009). *Recovery in Mental Health: Reshaping Scientific and Clinical Responsibilities.* Chichester: Wiley.

Davidson, L., Tondora, J., Lawless, M. S., O'Connell, M., & Rowe, M. (2009). *A Practical Guide to Recovery-Oriented Practice Tools for Transforming Mental Health Care.* Oxford: Oxford University Press.

Davidson, L., Tondora, J., O'Connell, M., Bellamy, C., Pelletier, J. F., DiLeo, P., et al. (2016). Recovery and recovery-oriented practice. In: Jacobs, S. C. & Steiner, J. L. (Eds.), *Yale Textbook of Public Psychiatry* (pp. 33–47). New York: Oxford University Press.

Slade M. (2009). *Personal Recovery and Mental Illness: A Guide for Mental Health Professionals.* Cambridge: Cambridge University Press.

Slade, M., McDaid, D., Shepherd, G., Williams, S., & Repper, J. (2017). *Recovery: The Business Case.* Nottingham: ImROC.

Slade, M., Oades, L., & Jarden, A. (Eds.) (2017). *Wellbeing, Recovery and Mental Health.* Cambridge: Cambridge University Press.

Tondora, J., Miller, R., Slade, M., & Davidson, L. (2014). *Partnering for Recovery in Mental Health: A Practical Guide to Person-Centered Planning.* Chichester: John Wiley & Sons.

REFERENCES

Andresen, R., Oades, L., & Caputi, P. (2003). The experience of recovery from schizophrenia: towards an empirically-validated stage model. *Australian and New Zealand Journal of Psychiatry*, **37**, 586–594.

Anthony, W. A. (1993). Recovery from mental illness: the guiding vision of the mental health system in the 1990s. *Psychosocial Rehabilitation Journal*, **16**, 11–23.

Barker, P. J., Davidson, B., & Campbell, P. (1999). *From the Ashes of Experience.* London: Whurr Publications.

Barnett, H. & Lapsley, H. (2006). *Journeys of Despair, Journeys of Hope: Young Adults Talk About Severe Mental Distress, Mental Health Services and Recovery.* Wellington: Mental Health Commission.

Barrett, R. J. (1996). *The Psychiatric Team and the Social Definition of Schizophrenia: An Anthropological Study of Person and Illness.* London: Cambridge University Press.

Bellack, A. (2006). Scientific and consumer models of recovery in schizophrenia: concordance, contrasts, and implications. *Schizophrenia Bulletin*, **32**, 432–442.

Benkwitz, A. & Healy, L. (2019). 'Think football': exploring a football for mental health initiative delivered in the community through the lens of personal and social recovery. *Mental Health and Physical Activity*, **17**, 100292.

Bird, V., Leamy, M., Le Boutillier, C., Williams, J., & Slade, M. (2014a). *REFOCUS: Promoting Recovery in Mental Health Services* (2nd ed.). London: Rethink Mental Illness.

Bird, V., Leamy, M., Tew, J., Le Boutillier, C., Williams, J., & Slade, M. (2014b). Fit for purpose? Validation of the conceptual framework of personal recovery with current mental health service users. *Australian and New Zealand Journal of Psychiatry*, **48**, 644–653.

Bleuler, M. (1978). *The Schizophrenic Disorders.* New Haven, CT: Yale University Press.

Borg, M. & K. Kristiansen (2004). Recovery-oriented professionals: helping relationships in mental health services. *Journal of Mental Health*, **13**, 493–505.

Breggin, P. & Cohen, D. (2007). *Your Drug May Be Your Problem: How and Why to Stop Taking Psychiatric Medications.* Reading, MA: Perseus Books.

Brinchmann, B., Widding-Havneraas, T., Modini, M., Rinaldi, M., Moe, C., McDaid, D., et al. (2020). A meta-regression of the impact of policy on the efficacy of individual placement and support. *Acta Psychiatrica Scandinavica*, **141**, 206–220.

Ciompi, L. & Muller, C. (1976). *The Life-Course and Aging of Schizophrenics: A Long-Term Follow-Up Study into Old Age.* Berlin: Springer.

Coleman, R. (1999). *Recovery: An Alien Concept.* Gloucester: Hansell.

Copeland, M. E. (1999). *Wellness Recovery Action Plan.* Brattleboro, VT: Peach Press.

Darton, K. (2005). *Making Sense of Coming Off Psychiatric Drugs.* London: Mind.

Davidson, L. & Flanagan, E. H. (2007). 'Schizophrenics', 'borderlines', and the lingering legacy of misplaced concreteness: an examination of the persistent misconception that the DSM classifies people instead of disorders. *Psychiatry*, **70**, 100–112.

Davidson, L., O'Connell, M., & Tondora, J. (2009a). Conclusion: making sure the person is involved in person-centred care. In: Rudnick, A. and Roe, D. (Eds.), *Serious Mental Illness (SMI): Person-Centered Approaches* (pp. 342–363). London: Routledge.

Davidson, L. & Roe, D. (2007). Recovery from versus recovery in serious mental illness: one strategy for lessening confusion plaguing recovery. *Journal of Mental Health*, **16**, 459–470.

Davidson, L., Sells, D., Sangster, S., & O'Connell, M. (2005). Qualitative studies of recovery: what can we learn from the person? In: Ralph, R. O. and Corrigan, P. W. (Eds.), *Recovery in Mental Illness: Broadening our Understanding of Wellness* (pp. 147–170). Washington DC, American Psychological Association.

Davidson, L. & Strauss, J. (1992). Sense of self in recovery from severe mental illness. *British Journal of Medical Psychology*, **65**, 131–145.

Davidson, L., Tondora, J., Lawless, M. S., O'Connell, M., & Rowe, M. (2009b). *A Practical Guide to Recovery-Oriented Practice Tools for Transforming Mental Health Care.* Oxford: Oxford University Press.

Davidson, L. & White, W. (2007). The concept of recovery as an organizing principle for integrating mental health and addiction services. *Journal of Behavioral Health Services and Research*, **34**, 109–120.

Deegan, P. E. (1988). Recovery: the lived experience of rehabilitation. *Psychosocial Rehabilitation Journal*, **11**, 11–19.

Deegan, P. E. (2005). The importance of personal medicine. *Scandinavian Journal of Public Health*, **33**, 29–35.

Deegan, P. E. (2007). The lived experience of using psychiatric medication in the recovery process and a shared decision-making program to support it. *Psychiatric Rehabilitation Journal*, **31**, 62–69.

Deegan, P. E. (2010). A web application to support recovery and shared decision making in psychiatric medication clinics. *Psychiatric Rehabilitation Journal*, **34**, 23–28.

DeSisto, M. J., Harding, C. M., McCormick, R. V., Ashikage, T., & Brooks, G. (1995). The Maine and Vermont three-decades studies of serious mental illness: II. Longitudinal course. *British Journal of Psychiatry*, **167**, 338–342.

Finnerty, M. T., Layman, D. M., Chen, Q., Leckman-Westin, E., Bermeo, N., Ng-Mak, D. S., Rajagopalan, K., & Hoagwood, K. E. (2018). Use of a web-based shared decision-making program: impact on ongoing treatment engagement and antipsychotic adherence. *Psychiatric Services*, **69**(12), 1215–1221.

Fisher, D. V. (1994). Health care reform based on an empowerment model of recovery by people with psychiatric disabilities. *Hospital and Community Psychiatry*, **45**, 913–915.

Funk, M. & Drew, N. (2017). WHO QualityRights: transforming mental health services. *Lancet Psychiatry*, **4**, 826–827.

Goldsack, S., Reet, M., Lapsley, H., & Gingell, M. (2005). *Experiencing a Recovery-Oriented Acute Mental Health Service: Home Based Treatment from the Perspectives of Services Users, their Families and Mental Health Professionals*. Wellington: Mental Health Commission.

Gregory, R. J., Canning, S. S., Lee, T. W., & Wise, J. C. (2004). Cognitive bibliotherapy for depression: a meta-analysis. *Professional Psychology: Research and Practice*, **35**, 275–280.

Guy, A., Davies, J., & Rizq, R. (2019). *Guidance for Psychological Therapists: Enabling Conversations with Clients Taking or Withdrawing from Prescribed Psychiatric Drugs*. London: APPG for Prescribed Drug Dependence.

Guyatt, G. & Rennie, D. (2002). *Users' Guide to the Medical Literature: A Manual for Evidence-Based Clinical Practice*. Chicago, IL: American Medical Association Press.

Harding, C. M., Brooks, G., Ashikage, T., Strauss, J. S., & Brier, A. (1987). The Vermont longitudinal study of persons with severe mental illness II: long-term outcome of subjects who retrospectively met DSM-III criteria for schizophrenia. *American Journal of Psychiatry*, **144**, 727–735.

Harrison, G., Hopper, K., Craig, T., Laska, E., Siegel, C., Wanderling, J., et al. (2001). Recovery from psychotic illness: a 15- and 25-year international follow-up study. *British Journal of Psychiatry*, **178**, 506–517.

Huber, G., Gross, G., & Schuttler, R. (1975). A long-term follow-up study of schizophrenia: psychiatric course and prognosis. *Acta Psychiatrica Scandinavica*, **52**, 49–57.

Lakhan, S. E. & Vieira, K. F. (2008). Nutritional therapies for mental disorders. *Nutrition Journal*, **7**, 2.

Lapsley, H., Nikora, L. W., & Black, R. (2002). *Kia Mauri Tau! Narratives of Recovery from Disabling Mental Health Problems*. Wellington: Mental Health Commission.

Le Boutillier, C., Slade, M., Lawrence, V., Bird, V., Chandler, R., Farkas, M., et al. (2015). Competing priorities: staff perspectives on supporting recovery. *Administration and Policy in Mental Health and Mental Health Services Research*, **42**, 429–438.

Leamy, M., Bird, V., Le Boutillier, C., Williams, J., & Slade, M. (2011). A conceptual framework for personal recovery in mental health: systematic review and narrative synthesis. *British Journal of Psychiatry*, **199**, 445–452.

Libermann, R. P. (2002). Future directions for research studies and clinical work on recovery from schizophrenia: questions with some answers. *International Review of Psychiatry*, **14**, 337–342.

Libermann, R. P. & Kopelowicz, A. (2002). Recovery from schizophrenia: a challenge for the 21st century. *International Review of Psychiatry*, **14**, 242–255.

Lim, M., Li, Z., Xie, H., Tan, B., & Lee, J. (2019). An Asian study on clinical and psychological factors associated with personal recovery in people with psychosis. *BMC Psychiatry*, **19**, 256.

Marneros, A., Deister, A., Rohde, A., Steinmeyer, E.M., & Junemann, H. (1989). Long-term outcome of schizoaffective and schizophrenic disorders, a comparative study, I: definitions, methods, psychopathological and social outcome. *European Archives of Psychiatry and Clinical Neuroscience*, **238**, 118–125.

McIntosh, Z. (2005). *From Goldfish Bowl to Ocean: personal accounts of mental illness and beyond*. London: Chipmunka Publishing.

Meadows, G., Brophy, L., Shawyer, F., Enticott, J., Fossey, E., Thornton, C., et al. (2019). REFOCUS-PULSAR recovery-oriented practice training in specialist mental health care: a stepped-wedge cluster randomised controlled trial. *Lancet Psychiatry*, **6**, 103–114.

Mental Health Commission (2000). *Three Forensic Service Users and Their Families Talk about Recovery*. Wellington: Mental Health Commission.

Mental Health Commission (2001). *Recovery Competencies: Teaching Resource Kit*. Wellington: Mental Health Commission.

Mental Health Coordinating Council (2014). *Recovery for Young People: Recovery Orientation in Youth Mental Health and Child and Adolescent Mental Health Services (CAMHS): Discussion Paper*. Sydney: Mental Health Coordinating Council.

Meyer, T. & Broocks, A. (2000). Therapeutic impact of exercise on psychiatric diseases: guidelines for exercise testing and prescription. *Sports Medicine*, **30**, 269–279.

Ogawa, K., Miya, M., Watarai, A., Nakazawa, M., Yuasa, S., & Utena, H. (1987). A long-term follow-up study of schizophrenia in Japan, with special reference to the course of social adjustment. *British Journal of Psychiatry*, **151**, 758–765.

O'Hagan, M. (1996). Two accounts of mental distress. In: Read, J. & Reynolds, J. (Eds.), *Speaking Our Minds* (pp. 44–50). London: Macmillan.

Pathare, S., Funk, M., Drew Bold, N., Chauhan, A., Kalha, J., Krishnamoorthy, S., et al. (2021). Systematic evaluation of the QualityRights programme in public mental health facilities in Gujarat, India. *British Journal of Psychiatry*, **218**, 196–203.

Pelletier, J.-F., Corbière, M., Lecomte, T., Briand, C., Corrigan, P., Davidson, L., & Rowe, M. (2015). Citizenship and recovery: two intertwined concepts for civic-recovery. *BMC Psychiatry*, **15**, 37.

Price-Robertson, R., Obradovic, A., & Morgan, B. (2017). Relational recovery: beyond individualism in the recovery approach. *Advances in Mental Health*, **15**, 108–120.

Ralph, R. O. & Corrigan, P. W. (2005). *Recovery in Mental Illness: Broadening our Understanding of Wellness*. Washington, DC: American Psychological Association.

Ridgway, P. (2001). Restorying psychiatric disability: learning from first person narratives. *Psychiatric Rehabilitation Journal*, **24**, 335–343.

Rowe, M. & Davidson, L. (2016). Recovering citizenship. *Israel Journal of Psychiatry and Related Sciences*, **53**, 14–21.

Sackett, D., Rosenberg, W. M. C., Gray, J. A. M., Haynes, R. B., & Richardson, W. S. (1996). Evidence based medicine: what it is and what it isn't: it's about integrating individual clinical expertise and the best external evidence. *British Medical Journal*, **312**, 71–72.

Scottish Recovery Network (2006). *Journeys of Recovery: Stories of Hope and Recovery from Long Term Mental Health Problems*. Glasgow: Scottish Recovery Network.

Scottish Recovery Network (2007). *Routes to Recovery: Collected Wisdom from the SRN Narrative Research Project*. Glasgow: Scottish Recovery Network.

Secker, J., Membrey, H., Grove, B., & Seebohm, P. (2002). Recovering from illness or recovering your life? Implications of clinical versus social models of recovery from mental health problems for employment support services. *Disability & Society*, **17**, 403–418.

Seligman, M. (2002). *Authentic Happiness: Using the New Positive Psychology to Realize Your Potential for Lasting Fulfillment*. New York: Free Press.

Shepherd, G., Boardman, J., & Slade, M. (2008). *Making Recovery a Reality* (Briefing paper). London: Sainsbury Centre for Mental Health.

Simonsen, C., Åsbø, G., Slade, M., Wold, K., Widing, L., Flaaten, C., Engen, M., Lyngstad, S., Gardsjord, E., Bjella, T., Romm, K., Ueland, T., & Melle, I. (in press). A good life with psychosis: rate of positive outcomes in first-episode psychosis at 10-year follow-up. *Psychological Medicine*.

Slade, M. (2009a). *Personal Recovery and Mental Illness*. Cambridge: Cambridge University Press.

Slade, M. (2009b). The contribution of mental health services to recovery. *Journal of Mental Health*, **18**, 367–371.

Slade, M. (2013). *100 Ways to Support Recovery* (2nd ed.). London: Rethink Mental Illness.

Slade, M. (2017). Implementing shared decision making in routine mental health care. *World Psychiatry*, **16**, 146–153.

Slade, M., Amering, M., & Oades, L. (2008). Recovery: an international perspective. *Epidemiologia e Psichiatria Sociale*, **17**, 128–137.

Slade, M., Bird, V., Clarke, E., Le Boutillier, C., McCrone, P., Macpherson, R., Pesola, F., et al. (2015). Supporting recovery in patients with psychosis through care by community-based adult mental health teams (REFOCUS): a multisite, cluster, randomised, controlled trial. *Lancet Psychiatry*, **2**, 503–514.

Slade, M., Leamy, M., Bacon, F., Janosik, M., Le Boutillier, C., Williams, J., & Bird, V. (2012). International differences in understanding recovery: systematic review. *Epidemiology and Psychiatric Sciences*, **21**, 353–364.

Slade, M., Oades, L., & Jarden, A. (Eds.) (2017). *Wellbeing, Recovery and Mental Health*. Cambridge: Cambridge University Press.

South London and Maudsley NHS Foundation Trust (2010). *Social Inclusion and Recovery (SIR) Strategy 2010–2015*. London: SLAM.

Spaniol, L. & Koehler, M. (1994). *The Experience of Recovery*. Boston, MA: Center for Psychiatric Rehabilitation.

Stastny, P. & Lehmann, P. (2007). *Alternatives Beyond Psychiatry*. Shrewsbury: Peter Lehmann Publishing.

Stuart, S., Tansey, L., & Quayle, E. (2017). What we talk about when we talk about recovery: a systematic review and best-fit framework synthesis of qualitative literature. *Journal of Mental Health*, **26**, 291–304.

The Icarus Project and Freedom Center (2012). *Harm Reduction Guide to Coming Off Psychiatric Drugs* (2nd ed.). New York: The Icarus Project and Freedom Centre.

Tondora, J., Miller, R., Slade, M., & Davidson, L. (2014). *Partnering for Recovery in Mental Health: A Practical Guide to Person-Centered Planning*. Chichester, Wiley-Blackwell.

Tsuang, M. T., Woolson, R. F., & Fleming, J. (1979). Long-term outcome of major psychosis. *Archives of General Psychiatry*, **36**, 1295–1301.

United Nations General Assembly (2019). *Report of the Special Rapporteur on the Right of Everyone to the Enjoyment of the Highest Attainable Standard of Physical and Mental Health*. New York: Human Rights Council.

van Weeghel, J., van Zelst, C., Boertien, D., & Hasson-Ohayon, I. (2019). Conceptualizations, assessments, and implications of personal recovery in mental illness: a scoping review of systematic reviews and meta-analyses. *Psychiatric Rehabilitation Journal*, **42**, 169–181.

Vandekinderen, C., Roets, G., Roose, R., & Van Hove, G. (2012). Rediscovering recovery: reconceptualizing underlying assumptions of citizenship and interrelated notions of care and support. *Scientific World Journal*, **7**, 496579.

Vogel, J., Bruins, J., Halbersma, L., Lieben, R., de Jong, S., Van der Gaag, M., & Castelein, S. (2020). Measuring personal recovery in people with a psychotic disorder based on CHIME: a comparison of three validated measures. *International Journal of Mental Health Nursing*, **29**, 808–819.

Watkins, J. (2007). *Healing Schizophrenia: Using Medication Wisely*. Victoria: Michelle Anderson.

White, S., Foster, R., Marks, J., Morshead, R., Goldsmith, L., Barlow, S., et al. (2020). The effectiveness of one-to-one peer support in mental health services: a systematic review and meta-analysis. *BMC Psychiatry*, **20**, 534.

Whitley, R., Harris, M., Fallot, R. D., & Berley, R. W. (2008). The active ingredients of intentional recovery communities: focus group evaluation. *Journal of Mental Health*, **17**, 173–182.

SECTION 3
Needs
Perspectives and assessment

5. **Treatment coverage for mental disorders: results from the World Health Organization World Mental Health Surveys** 45

   Daniel V. Vigo, Meredith G. Harris, Richard. J. Munthali, Alan E. Kazdin, Irving Hwang, Maria Petukhova, Nancy A. Sampson, Sergio Aguilar-Gaxiola, Ali Al-Hamzawi, Jordi Alonso, Yasmin A. Altwaijri, Corina Benjet, Evelyn J. Bromet, Ronny Bruffaerts, Brendan Bunting, José Miguel Caldas-de-Almeida, Stephanie Chardoul, Giovanni De Girolamo, Peter de Jonge, Silvia Florescu, Oye Gureje, Josep Maria Haro, Chi-yi Hu, Elie G. Karam, Georges Karam, Andrzej Kiejna, Sing Lee, Fernando Navarro-Mateu, José Posada-Villa, Charlene Rapsey, Juan Carlos Stagnaro, Yolanda Torres, Maria Carmen Viana, David R. Williams, Zahari Zarkov, Philip S. Wang, and Ronald C. Kessler, on behalf of the WHO World Mental Health Survey collaborators

6. **The lived experience: focus on wellness** 57

   Margaret Swarbrick and Crystal L. Brandow

7. **Measuring mental health needs** 65

   Mike Slade and Graham Thornicroft

8. **Mental health, ethnicity, and cultural diversity: evidence and challenges** 73

   Craig Morgan

9. **The mental health challenges of immigrants and refugees** 81

   Jillian M. Stile, Quyen Ngo-Metzger, Richard F. Mollica, and Eugene F. Augusterfer

5

Treatment coverage for mental disorders
Results from the World Health Organization World Mental Health Surveys

Daniel V. Vigo, Meredith G. Harris, Richard J. Munthali, Alan E. Kazdin, Irving Hwang, Maria Petukhova, Nancy A. Sampson, Sergio Aguilar-Gaxiola, Ali Al-Hamzawi, Jordi Alonso, Yasmin A. Altwaijri, Corina Benjet, Evelyn J. Bromet, Ronny Bruffaerts, Brendan Bunting, José Miguel Caldas-de-Almeida, Stephanie Chardoul, Giovanni De Girolamo, Peter de Jonge, Silvia Florescu, Oye Gureje, Josep Maria Haro, Chi-yi Hu, Elie G. Karam, Georges Karam, Andrzej Kiejna, Sing Lee, Fernando Navarro-Mateu, José Posada-Villa, Charlene Rapsey, Juan Carlos Stagnaro, Yolanda Torres, Maria Carmen Viana, David R. Williams, Zahari Zarkov, Philip S. Wang, and Ronald C. Kessler, on behalf of the WHO World Mental Health Survey collaborators*

Introduction

As discussed in Chapters 38 and 39, mental health-related disorders are the most disabling of all disorder groupings globally (Vigo et al., 2016, 2022a), and also result in the largest economic burden of all non-communicable disorders (Bloom et al., 2011). Despite the availability of effective and cost-effective treatments (Chisholm et al., 2016), underspending on mental health care is common and the majority of individuals in need lack services (Vigo et al., 2019a). In order to measure the gap in services, the research community needs to develop valid indicators of coverage, that is, of the extent, quality, and distribution of services among the population in need.

The concept of coverage is used differently in different contexts, and several frameworks have been proposed. The Tanahashi framework developed by the World Health Organization (WHO) in 1978 spearheaded research on treatment coverage for several important areas of health care, most notably maternal and child health and primary care (Amouzou et al., 2019; Larson et al., 2016; Tanahashi, 1978). Tanahashi's effective coverage cascade distinguishes between potential and actual coverage. Potential coverage refers to the availability of services (i.e. whether they exist), their accessibility (i.e. whether barriers to utilization, such as fees or distance, hinder utilization), and whether users find them acceptable (i.e. whether services provided are culturally safe and appropriate). Actual coverage includes

---

* The WHO World Mental Health Survey collaborators are Sergio Aguilar-Gaxiola, MD, PhD; Ali Al-Hamzawi, MD; Jordi Alonso, MD, PhD; Yasmin A. Altwaijri, PhD; Laura Helena Andrade, MD, PhD; Lukoye Atwoli, MD, PhD; Corina Benjet, PhD; Guilherme Borges, ScD; Evelyn J. Bromet, PhD; Ronny Bruffaerts, PhD; Brendan Bunting, PhD; Jose Miguel Caldas-de-Almeida, MD, PhD; Graça Cardoso, MD, PhD; Stephanie Chardoul, BA; Somnath Chatterji, MD; Alfredo H. Cia, MD; Louisa Degenhardt, PhD; Koen Demyttenaere, MD, PhD; Silvia Florescu, MD, PhD; Giovanni de Girolamo, MD; Oye Gureje, MD, DSc, FRCPsych; Josep Maria Haro, MD, PhD; Meredith G. Harris, PhD; Hristo Hinkov, MD, PhD; Chi-yi Hu, MD, PhD; Peter de Jonge, PhD; Aimee Nasser Karam, PhD; Elie G. Karam, MD; Georges Karam, MD; Norito Kawakami, MD, DMSc; Ronald C. Kessler, PhD; Andrzej Kiejna, MD, PhD; Viviane Kovess-Masfety, MD, PhD; Sing Lee, MBBS; Jean-Pierre Lepine, MD; John J. McGrath, MD, PhD; Maria Elena Medina-Mora, PhD; Jacek Moskalewicz, PhD; Fernando Navarro-Mateu, MD, PhD; Marina Piazza, MPH, ScD; Jose Posada-Villa, MD; Kate M. Scott, PhD; Tim Slade, PhD; Juan Carlos Stagnaro, MD, PhD; Dan J. Stein, FRCPC, PhD; Margreet ten Have, PhD; Yolanda Torres, MPH, Dra.HC; Maria Carmen Viana, MD, PhD; Daniel V. Vigo, MD, DrPH; Harvey Whiteford, MBBS, PhD; David R. Williams, MPH, PhD; Bogdan Wojtyniak, ScD.

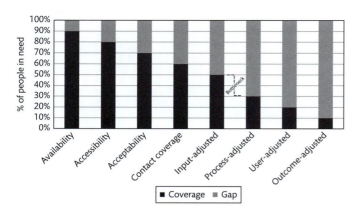

Figure 5.1 The coverage cascade.
Adapted with permission from Vigo, D., Haro, J. M., Hwang, I., Aguilar-Gaxiola, S., Alonso, J., Borges, G., et al. (2020). Toward measuring effective treatment coverage: critical bottlenecks in quality- and user-adjusted coverage for major depressive disorder. *Psychological Medicine*, 1–11.

contact coverage, which captures the percentage of people in need that utilize any services, and effective coverage, which captures the percentage of people who receive services that meet certain standards or criteria (e.g. clinical practice guideline recommendations).

Effective coverage is a complex measure that involves consideration of both the quality of services and compliance. The rationale is that if people receive care that follows guidelines to include the right human resource inputs and the right materials or processes (i.e. quality), and if users adhere to indications by the provider (i.e. compliance), they can expect a health benefit as indicated by the evidence of effectiveness. To operationalize this, effective coverage can be decomposed into a sequence of lower-order coverage indicators: contact coverage, input- and process-adjusted coverage (sometimes termed 'quality-adjusted coverage'), and finally user-adjusted coverage (i.e. effective coverage). The latter can be used as a proxy of 'outcome-adjusted coverage' (which would include a measurement of the actual health benefit obtained).

Figure 5.1 represents a hypothetical coverage cascade and shows how 'bottlenecks' in coverage can be detected (Vigo et al., 2020). Bottlenecks are indicated by large drops between two adjacent types of coverage. Bottlenecks point to critical deficits in the system, whereby large fractions of the population in need are left without services. Taken together, this representation of the coverage cascade permits nuanced study of points in care where bottlenecks in coverage occur for disorders affecting mental health, their predictors, and how these factors impact low/middle- and high-income countries.

This chapter presents an overview of treatment coverage for mental disorders based on data from the World Mental Health (WMH) Surveys Initiative, which captures detailed data on the epidemiology, impairment, and treatment associated with mental health problems across all major geographic regions of the world. Specifically, we present (1) updated estimates of contact coverage; (2) data on the different 'treatment profiles' that people access, based on the multiple provider combinations that patients come in contact with; and (3) an overview of WMH research on minimally adequate treatment (which partially includes quality adjustments) for several groups of mental disorders. Finally, we expand the previous WMH contact coverage analyses to include an estimation of (4) full effective coverage for major depressive disorder (MDD) and explore its determinants. The results for contact coverage were undertaken as described in the following 'Methods' section. The sections on treatment profiles, minimally adequate treatment, and effective coverage combine previous WMH studies with new analysis performed for this chapter.

Methods

Survey samples

Twenty-seven cross-sectional surveys were carried out in 24 countries in the following regions: Africa (Nigeria, South Africa), the Americas (Argentina, Brazil, Colombia, Mexico, US), Asia and the Pacific (New Zealand, Shenzhen in the People's Republic of China), Europe (Belgium, Bulgaria, Germany, Italy, Netherlands, Northern Ireland, Poland, Portugal, Romania, Spain, Ukraine), and the Middle East (Iraq, Israel, Lebanon, Saudi Arabia). Applying World Bank criteria (World Bank, 2003) for the year the survey was conducted, countries were classified as low/lower-middle income (Colombia/National, Iraq, Nigeria, People's Republic of China, Ukraine), higher-middle income (Brazil, Bulgaria, Colombia/Medellín, Lebanon, Mexico, Romania, South Africa), and high income (all others). Surveys were conducted face-to-face by trained lay interviewers with respondents selected using probability procedures from multistage clustered area probability household samples (Table 5.1). The total sample size of respondents aged 18 and older was 138,743 with individual country samples ranging from a low of 2357 in Romania to a high of 12,790 in New Zealand. The weighted average response rate across all countries was 72.0%, with individual country response rates ranging from a low of 50.1% in France to a high of 97.2% in Medellín, Colombia.

The interview was divided into two parts. All respondents completed Part I, which contained core diagnostic assessments and basic information about sociodemographics. All Part I respondents who met criteria for any lifetime core disorder plus a probability subsample of approximately 25% of all other Part I respondents were administered Part II, which assessed disorders of secondary interest along with predictors and consequences of disorders and service use. The Part I data were weighted to adjust for differential probabilities of selection within and between households, for non-response bias, and for residual discrepancies between the sample and census population distributions of a profile of sociodemographic and geographic variables. The Part II data were additionally weighted to adjust for the differential sampling of Part I respondents into Part II as a function of the presence of Part I core disorders. WMH weighting procedures are discussed in more detail elsewhere (Heeringa et al., 2008).

Standardized procedures were used consistently across all WMH sites for interviewer training, WHO translation and back-translation and harmonization of all study materials, and quality control of interviewer work. These procedures are described in detail elsewhere (Harkness et al., 2008; Pennell et al., 2008). Informed consent was obtained before beginning interviews in each country. Procedures for obtaining informed consent and protecting human subjects were approved and monitored by the Institutional Review Boards of the organizations coordinating the survey in each country.

Twelve-month mental disorders

Mental disorders present at any time in the 12 months before interview were assessed in the WMH Surveys with Version 3.0 of the WHO Composite International Diagnostic Interview (CIDI) (Kessler

Table 5.1 World Mental Health Survey sample characteristics by World Bank income categories

Country by income category	Survey[a]	Sample characteristics[b]	Field dates	Age range (years)	Part I	Part II	Part II and age ≤44 years[c]	Response rate[d]
I. Low- and lower-middle-income countries								
Colombia	NSMH	All urban areas of the country (approximately 73% of the total national population)	2003	18–65	4426	2381	1731	87.7
Iraq	IMHS	Nationally representative	2006–07	18–96	4332	4332	–	95.2
Nigeria	NSMHW	21 of the 36 states in the country, representing 57% of the national population. The surveys were conducted in Yoruba, Igbo, Hausa, and Efik languages	2002–04	18–100	6752	2143	1203	79.3
PRC[e]–Shenzhen[f]	Shenzhen	Shenzhen metropolitan area. Included temporary residents as well as household residents	2005–07	18–88	7132	2475	–	80.0
Ukraine	CMDPSD	Nationally representative	2002	18–91	4725	1720	541	78.3
TOTAL					(27367)	(13,051)	(3475)	82.8
II. Upper-middle-income countries								
Brazil–São Paulo	São Paulo Megacity	São Paulo Metropolitan Area	2005–08	18–93	5037	2942	–	81.3
Bulgaria	NSHS	Nationally representative	2002–06	18–98	5318	2233	741	72.0
Bulgaria 2	NSHS-2	Nationally representative	2016–17	18–91	1508	578	–	61.0
Colombia–Medellin[g]	MMHHS	Medellin metropolitan area	2011–12	19–65	3261	1673	–	97.2
Lebanon	LEBANON	Nationally representative.	2002–03	18–94	2857	1031	595	70.0
Mexico	M-NCS	All urban areas of the country (approximately 75% of the total national population)	2001–02	18–65	5782	2362	1736	76.6
Romania	RMHS	Nationally representative	2005–06	18–96	2357	2357	–	70.9
South Africa[f]	SASH	Nationally representative	2002–04	18–92	4315	4315	–	87.1
TOTAL					(30,435)	(17,491)	(3072)	77.4
III. High-income countries								
Argentina	AMHES	Eight largest urban areas of the country (approximately 50% of the total national population)	2015	18–98	3927	2116	–	77.3
Belgium	ESEMeD	Nationally representative. The sample was selected from a national register of Belgium residents	2001–02	18–95	2419	1043	486	50.6
Germany	ESEMeD	Nationally representative	2002–03	19–95	3555	1323	621	57.8
Israel	NHS	Nationally representative	2003–04	21–98	4859	4859	–	72.6
Italy	ESEMeD	Nationally representative. The sample was selected from municipality resident registries	2001–02	18–100	4712	1779	853	71.3
Netherlands	ESEMeD	Nationally representative. The sample was selected from municipal postal registries	2002–03	18–95	2372	1094	516	56.4
New Zealand[f]	NZMHS	Nationally representative	2004–05	18–98	12,790	7312	–	73.3
Northern Ireland	NISHS	Nationally representative	2005–08	18–97	4340	1986	–	68.4
Poland	EZOP	Nationally representative	2010–11	18–65	10,081	4000	2276	50.4
Portugal	NMHS	Nationally representative	2008–09	18–81	3849	2060	1070	57.3
Saudi Arabia[f]	SNMHS	Nationally representative	2013–16	18–65	3638	1793	–	61.0
Spain	ESEMeD	Nationally representative	2001–02	18–98	5473	2121	960	78.6

(continued)

Table 5.1 Continued

Country by income category	Survey[a]	Sample characteristics[b]	Field dates	Age range (years)	Part I	Part II	Part II and age ≤44 years[c]	Response rate[d]
Spain–Murcia	PEGASUS-Murcia	Murcia region. Regionally representative	2010–12	18–96	2621	1459	–	67.4
US	NCS-R	Nationally representative	2001–03	18–99	9282	5692	3197	70.9
TOTAL					(80,941)	(41,755)	(10,706)	63.4
IV. TOTAL					(138,743)	(72,297)	(17,253)	69.3

Note: World Bank (2012) data. Accessed 12 May 2012 at: http://data.worldbank.org/country. Some of the WMH countries have moved into new income categories since the surveys were conducted. The income groupings in the table reflect the status of each country at the time of data collection. The current income category of each country is available at the preceding URL.

[a] NSMH (The Colombian National Study of Mental Health); IMHS (Iraq Mental Health Survey); NSMHW (The Nigerian Survey of Mental Health and Wellbeing); CMDPSD (Comorbid Mental Disorders during Periods of Social Disruption); NSHS (Bulgaria National Survey of Health and Stress); MMHHS (Medellín Mental Health Household Study); LEBANON (Lebanese Evaluation of the Burden of Ailments and Needs of the Nation); M-NCS (The Mexico National Comorbidity Survey); RMHS (Romania Mental Health Survey); SASH (South Africa Health Survey); AMHES (Argentina Mental Health Epidemiologic Survey); ESEMeD (The European Study Of The Epidemiology Of Mental Disorders); NHS (Israel National Health Survey); WMHJ2002-2006 (World Mental Health Japan Survey); NZMHS (New Zealand Mental Health Survey); NISHS (Northern Ireland Study of Health and Stress); EZOP (Epidemiology of Mental Disorders and Access to Care Survey); NMHS (Portugal National Mental Health Survey); SNMHS (Saudi National Mental Health Survey); PEGASUS-Murcia (Psychiatric Enquiry to General Population in Southeast Spain-Murcia);NCS-R (The US National Comorbidity Survey Replication).

[b] Most WMH surveys are based on stratified multistage clustered area probability household samples in which samples of areas equivalent to counties or municipalities in the US were selected in the first stage followed by one or more subsequent stages of geographic sampling (e.g. towns within counties, blocks within towns, households within blocks) to arrive at a sample of households, in each of which a listing of household members was created and one or two people were selected from this listing to be interviewed. No substitution was allowed when the originally sampled household resident could not be interviewed. These household samples were selected from Census area data in all countries other than France (where telephone directories were used to select households) and the Netherlands (where postal registries were used to select households). Several WMH Surveys (Belgium, Germany, Italy, Poland, Spain-Murcia) used municipal, country resident or universal health care registries to select respondents without listing households. The Japanese sample is the only totally unclustered sample, with households randomly selected in each of the 11 metropolitan areas and one random respondent selected in each sample household. Twenty of the 29 surveys are based on nationally representative household samples.

[c] Argentina, Brazil, Bulgaria 2 (2016–2017), Colombia-Medellin, Iraq, Israel, Japan, New Zealand, Northern Ireland, PRC—Shenzhen, Romania, South Africa, and Spain-Murcia did not have an age restricted Part II sample. All other countries, with the exception of Nigeria and Ukraine (which were age restricted to ≤39 years) were age restricted to ≤44 years.

[d] The response rate is calculated as the ratio of the number of households in which an interview was completed to the number of households originally sampled, excluding from the denominator households known not to be eligible either because of being vacant at the time of initial contact or because the residents were unable to speak the designated languages of the survey. The weighted average response rate is 69.3%.

[e] People's Republic of China.

[f] For the purposes of cross-national comparisons we limit the sample to those aged 18+ years.

[g] Colombia moved from the 'lower- and lower-middle-income' to the 'upper-middle-income' category between 2003 (when the Colombian National Study of Mental Health was conducted) and 2010 (when the Medellin Mental Health Household Study was conducted), hence Colombia's appearance in both income categories. For more information, please see table note.

& Üstün, 2004), a fully structured diagnostic interview designed to be administered by trained lay interviewers. Disorders were defined according to the definitions and criteria of the American Psychiatric Association's *Diagnostic and Statistical Manual of Mental Disorders*, fourth edition (DSM-IV). The disorders considered in this chapter include anxiety disorders (agoraphobia with or without panic disorder, generalized anxiety disorder, panic disorder with or without agoraphobia, post-traumatic stress disorder, obsessive–compulsive disorder, social phobia, and specific phobia), mood disorders (bipolar disorder including bipolar I and II, dysthymic disorder, and MDD), impulse-control disorders (intermittent-explosive disorder, attention deficit hyperactivity disorder, oppositional defiant disorder, and conduct disorder), and substance disorders (alcohol and drug abuse with or without dependence). All diagnoses were made with CIDI organic exclusion rules. Clinical reappraisal studies of CIDI diagnoses in a number of WMH countries (Haro et al., 2006) documented generally good concordance between diagnoses based on the CIDI and diagnoses based on independent clinical interviews with the Structured Clinical Interview for DSM-IV (SCID) (First et al., 2002).

Severity of mental disorders

Disorder severity was defined using the criteria of the US Substance Abuse and Mental Health Services Administration, which defines a *severe mental illness* (SMI) as a diagnosable mental, behavioural, or emotional disorder of sufficient duration to meet DSM criteria, and that resulted in functional impairment which substantially interferes with or limits role functioning in family, work, or community activities (Substance Abuse and Mental Health Services Administration, 1993). This was operationalized in the WMH Surveys by severe role impairment due to a mental disorder in at least two areas of functioning measured by the disorder-specific Sheehan Disability Scales (SDS) (Sheehan et al., 1996), or overall functional impairment from any disorder consistent with a Global Assessment of Functioning (GAF) (Endicott et al., 1976) score of 50 or less; having either bipolar I disorder or substance dependence with a physiological dependence syndrome; or a suicide attempt in conjunction with any 12-month DSM-IV disorder. Disorders not classified as meeting criteria for SMI were classified as *moderate* in severity if the respondent had at least moderate interference in any SDS domain or substance dependence without a physiological dependence syndrome. All other disorders were classified as *mild* in severity. Some evidence for the validity of these ratings comes from statistically significant monotonic associations in the vast majority of surveys between severity and days in the prior year that respondents were totally unable to carry out normal daily activities because of these mental disorders (Druss et al., 2009).

Twelve-month mental health service use

Services received for the treatment of mental disorders in the 12 months prior to the WMH interview were assessed by asking respondents if they ever during that time period saw any of a number of different types of professionals, either as an outpatient or inpatient, for problems with emotions, nerves, mental health, or use of alcohol or drugs. Included were mental health professionals (e.g. psychiatrist, psychologist), general medical professionals (e.g. general practitioner, specialist, nurse, occupational therapist), religious counsellors (e.g. minister, sheikh), and traditional healers (e.g. herbalist, spiritualist). Examples of these types of providers were presented in a 'Respondent Booklet' as a visual recall aid and varied somewhat across countries depending on local circumstances. Follow-up questions were asked about number and duration of visits in the past 12 months.

Sociodemographic predictor variables

We examined a small number of sociodemographic correlates of treatment, including sex and family income. Family income was defined in each country in relation to within-country medians, where *low* income was defined as less than half the country median, *low average* as between low and the within-country median, *high-average* as between low-average and three times the within-country median, and *high* as more than three times the within-country average median.

Analysis procedures

Proportions of respondents with 12-month disorders were computed as well as the proportions of the latter who received any treatment in any sector within 12 months of the survey. We then examined how these patterns of service use differed across strata defined by the severity of disorders. Because the WMH data were weighted and clustered, standard errors (SEs) of parameter estimates were obtained using the Taylor series method as implemented in the SUDAAN software system (Research Triangle Institute, 2002).

Additional steps were taken for the each of the analyses presented below and are outlined in the corresponding section.

Twelve-month contact coverage for any mental disorder

The proportion of respondents (irrespective of whether they met disorder criteria or not) using any mental health services in the 12 months prior to the interview averaged 9% across surveys. This proportion varied significantly across countries, from a low of 1.6% in Nigeria to a high of 18.0% in the US, with lower proportions in low/lower-middle-income countries (3.5%) than in upper-middle-income (8.3%) or high-income countries (11.1%). Significant monotonic relationships were found between disorder severity and probability of service use in most surveys. The fraction of people with the most severe clinical presentations that received any services ranged between 4.9% in Shenzhen, PRC, and 77.1% in Northern Ireland, with an average of 43.4%. Low/lower-middle-income countries provided some coverage for 24.5% of people with severe disorders, upper-middle-income countries to 29.4%, and high-income countries to 51%. The fraction of people with moderate disorders receiving any services in low/lower-middle-income countries was 13.5%, 20.8% in upper-middle-income countries, and 32.5% in high-income countries, with an average of 27.9%. With respect to people with mild clinical presentations, 7.4% received any care in low/lower-middle-income countries, 15.9% in upper-middle-income countries, and 19.4% in high-income countries, with an average of 16.9%. As can be observed in **Table 5.2**, none of the SEs of the point estimates highlighted in this paragraph lead to overlapping estimates.

Interestingly, in many countries large fractions of the population without disorders also receive services. The largest fraction of people without any disorder receiving services is in South Africa (13.3%), and the lowest in Iraq (0.9%), with a cross-country average of 5.4%. Some countries show a very high ratio of people receiving services for mild disorders versus no disorders (Nigeria, 10:1), while others show almost no difference (Lebanon, 4:3).

Treatment profiles

Contact coverage takes different forms for different people. Mental health services are provided by a wide range of service sectors—including general medical, mental health specialist, human services, complementary/alternative, and spiritual/healer sectors—that vary in their capability to deliver mental health interventions. Some treatment seekers will receive care from a single service sector, while others will have trajectories of care involving multiple sectors, possibly reflecting multistep referral pathways or shared care arrangements (J. Wang & Patten, 2007; P. S. Wang et al., 2007). Whether individuals reach a sector of care appropriate to their level of need may depend on many factors. For example, specialist mental health care services are more scarce than general medical care services. Consequently, they tend to be allocated to people with relatively more severe and/or complex problems (Demyttenaere et al., 2004; Evans-Lacko et al., 2018). However, those in certain sociodemographic groups may be more or less likely to reach some sectors as a result of policy settings (e.g. supply and availability of services in a region), patient preferences and beliefs, and clinician decision-making (Buchan et al., 2016; Dezetter et al., 2011).

Available studies of the distribution of mental health service use across sectors have often focused on the use of individual service sectors or combinations among a small subset of sectors (Dezetter et al., 2011; Evans-Lacko et al., 2018; Fernández et al., 2021; Jackson et al., 2007; Kuramoto-Crawford et al., 2015; J. Wang & Patten, 2007). However, this approach might not describe the totality of a person's contact with services. To address this gap, we have described the most frequent combinations of sectors or 'treatment profiles' used for mental health among people with 12-month mental and substance use disorders, based on WMH data pooled across 17 high- and low/middle-income countries (Harris et al., 2022). The vast majority of service use for mental health could be captured by defining nine mutually exclusive treatment profiles. Four were single sector profiles: general medical only (including a general practitioner/primary care doctor or other medical doctor) used by 35.2% (SE 1.1) of people with contact coverage; other mental health specialty only (including a psychologist, any other mental health professional in any setting, or a social worker or counsellor in a mental health specialized setting) used by 13.8% (SE 0.7); psychiatry only, used by 11.6% (0.7); and spiritual healer only, used by 7.8% (SE 0.6). Three profiles involved the general medical sector plus either the psychiatry sector (5.1%, SE 0.4), other mental health specialty sector (10.3%, SE 0.6), or spiritual healer sector (3.3%, SE 0.4). Finally, two treatment profiles involved both psychiatry and other mental health specialty sectors, either with and without the general medical sectors, providing care to 5.9% (SE 0.5) and 7.0% (SE 0.6) of people with 12-month mental disorders, respectively.

Table 5.2 Twelve-month contact coverage for DSM-IV/CIDI disorders by severity of disorder in the World Mental Health Surveys

	Severe disorders		Moderate disorders		Mild disorders		No disorder	
	%	(SE)	%	(SE)	%	(SE)	%	(SE)
I. Low/lower-middle-income countries								
Colombia	27.7	(4.8)	10.3	(2.0)	7.8	(1.6)	3.4	(0.6)
Iraq	23.7	(6.2)	9.2	(3.2)	5.3	(2.5)	0.9	(0.2)
Nigeria	21.3	(10.2)	13.8	(7.1)	10.0	(2.7)	1.0	(0.3)
PRC–Shenzhen	4.9	(1.9)	9.2	(2.4)	5.2	(1.5)	2.5	(0.5)
Ukraine	25.7	(3.2)	21.2	(3.6)	7.6	(2.6)	4.4	(0.8)
Total	24.5	(2.8)	13.5	(1.8)	7.4	(1.1)	2.7	(0.3)
II. Upper-middle-income countries								
Brazil–São Paulo	34.5	(2.1)	21.3	(2.8)	12.7	(1.5)	4.7	(0.5)
Bulgaria	31.0	(4.6)	21.4	(3.6)	16.5	(4.7)	3.6	(0.5)
Bulgaria II	22.6	(7.4)	22.6	(7.4)	10.8	(6.3)	2.1	(0.8)
Lebanon	20.1	(5.2)	11.4	(3.1)	4.0	(1.6)	3.0	(0.7)
Mexico	25.8	(4.3)	17.9	(2.9)	11.9	(2.4)	3.2	(0.4)
Romania	36.4	(7.3)	17.4	(6.2)	14.4	(4.4)	1.8	(0.4)
Colombia–Medellin	22.0	(3.5)	18.7	(3.6)	15.4	(3.2)	3.5	(0.6)
South Africa	26.2	(3.6)	26.6	(3.9)	23.4	(3.2)	13.3	(0.9)
Total	29.4	(1.6)	20.8	(1.3)	15.9	(1.3)	5.7	(0.3)
III. High-income countries								
Argentina	30.2	(3.7)	33.0	(4.8)	21.7	(5.6)	8.7	(0.8)
Belgium	60.9	(9.1)	36.5	(8.6)	13.9	(4.3)	6.7	(1.1)
France	48.0	(6.4)	28.8	(3.9)	21.1	(3.5)	7.0	(1.1)
Germany	40.0	(8.5)	23.9	(4.6)	20.3	(5.1)	5.9	(0.9)
Israel	52.5	(3.9)	32.3	(3.7)	13.9	(3.1)	5.9	(0.4)
Italy	51.0	(6.4)	25.5	(4.1)	17.3	(4.3)	2.1	(0.4)
Japan	44.1	(11.8)	19.7	(3.8)	15.9	(4.6)	3.9	(0.6)
Netherlands	50.4	(6.8)	30.5	(7.1)	15.8	(5.9)	7.7	(1.3)
New Zealand	56.6	(2.2)	39.9	(1.9)	22.2	(1.9)	7.3	(0.5)
Northern Ireland	77.1	(4.8)	35.3	(4.1)	19.1	(4.3)	6.8	(0.8)
Portugal	66.4	(4.6)	35.0	(2.5)	18.2	(3.0)	9.0	(0.8)
Spain	58.7	(4.9)	36.9	(4.8)	17.0	(3.9)	3.9	(0.5)
Spain-Murcia	64.8	(8.7)	40.8	(6.5)	42.1	(5.1)	8.6	(0.9)
US	59.7	(2.4)	40.0	(1.3)	26.4	(1.7)	9.7	(0.6)
Poland	40.5	(5.2)	21.5	(2.9)	9.9	(1.8)	2.7	(0.3)
Saudi Arabia	21.0	(3.5)	8.9	(2.2)	13.1	(6.6)	2.7	(0.8)
Total	51.4	(1.3)	32.5	(0.9)	19.4	(0.9)	5.7	(0.2)
IV. Total	43.4	(1.0)	27.9	(0.7)	16.9	(0.6)	5.4	(0.1)

Note: see the section on measurement of 12-month disorders in the text for a description of how severity was operationalized. Treatment rates differ significantly by severity within each of the surveys, with c^2_3 values in the range 18.3–672.1, p = 0.0004 to <0.0001. Treatment rates also differ significantly across countries within each disorder severity sub-sample (c^2_{21} = 133.3–503.2, all p <0.0001, with only 22 countries with combined number of severe and moderate cases >60 used in the tests).

It also showed that certain patient characteristics tended to be associated with clusters of 'like' treatment profiles. In terms of clinical factors, for example, those with comorbid mental/substance use disorders were more likely to use multisector profiles that combined the general medical sector with either or both the psychiatry and other mental health specialty sectors. With respect to sociodemographic factors, women were more likely to use profiles that did not involve a mental health specialist, whereas men were more likely to reach the psychiatry sector. Married patients were more likely to be treated in the general medical-only sector, whereas never-married patients were generally more likely to be treated in profiles involving the other mental health specialty sector. Other characteristics were more clearly associated with specific profiles. For example, those having no (or no known) health insurance coverage were the least likely to use the psychiatry-only profile, whereas patients with state-funded/subsidized coverage were the least likely to use the other

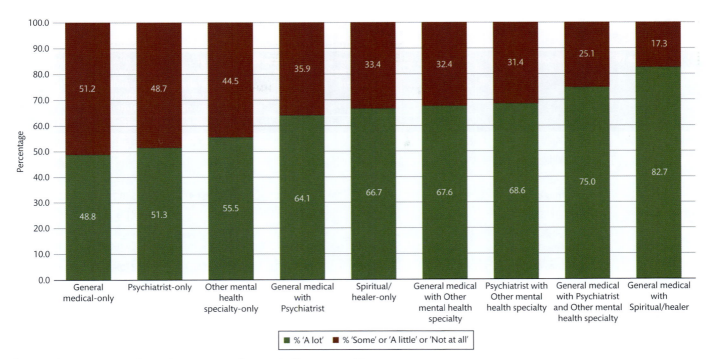

Figure 5.2 Degree to which users' perceptions of care varied by care provider.

mental health specialty-only profile. Those with lower levels of education were less likely to use the other mental health specialist-only profile but were more likely to use the general medical-only profile. The latter two findings may indicate that structural barriers to care among those at greater socioeconomic disadvantage; however, further work is needed to rule out other possible explanatory factors. With respect to user perceptions of care, high proportions of people in all treatment profiles said they were helped 'a lot', ranging from 48.8% of people seeing only a general medical provider, to 82.7% of people seeing a combination of general medical provider with spiritual providers/healers (Figure 5.2).

Twelve-month minimally adequate treatment for major depression, anxiety disorders, and substance use disorders

Previous WMH Survey reports have defined 'minimally adequate treatment' for depressive, anxiety, and substance use disorders. Minimally adequate treatment is a measure of actual coverage that partially includes quality adjustments. In the case of MDD and anxiety disorders, minimally adequate treatment was defined as either pharmacotherapy (at least 1 month of a medication plus four physician visits) or psychotherapy (at least eight sessions with any provider) (Alonso et al., 2018; Thornicroft et al., 2017). For substance use disorders, minimally adequate treatment was defined as either four visits with a specialty mental health/general medical provider or six visits with a non-medically trained professional (Degenhardt et al., 2017). Cross-national patterns of minimally adequate treatment from these reports are summarized in Table 5.3.

Across all countries combined, prevalence was highest for anxiety disorders (9.8%) and lowest for substance use disorders (2.6%). Within each disorder, prevalence was higher in high-income and upper-middle-income countries than in lower-middle-income countries (column A). In contrast to prevalence, perceived need for treatment was higher among those with MDD (56.7%) than for those with anxiety disorders (41.3%) or substance use disorders (39.1%). Within each disorder, there was a monotonic decrease in perceived need from high-income to lower-middle-income countries. That is, in high-income countries, between four and six of every ten people with disorder perceived a need for treatment, whereas in lower-middle-income countries, only three in ten perceived a need for treatment (column B). With respect to treatment, there were similar monotonic decreases in the probability of receiving any treatment among those with perceived need for it (column C), and the probability of receiving minimally adequate treatment among those with perceived need who received any treatment (column D). That is, in high-income countries, four out of every ten people who had a perceived need and received treatment got minimally adequate treatment, whereas in lower-middle-income countries, only one to two in ten did so. These patterns compounded such that, among people with disorders, only a minority received minimally adequate treatment (ranging from 16.5% for MDD down to 7.1% for substance use disorders). There was also a six- to tenfold difference in the probability of minimally adequate treatment between those in the most and least wealthy countries, with the differential being greater for substance use disorders (10.3% vs 1.0%) than for anxiety disorders (13.8% vs 2.3%) or MDD (22.4% vs 3.7%) (column E).

Twelve-month effective coverage for major depressive disorder

Building on these previous reports of minimally adequate treatment for specific mental and substance use disorders, we developed an effective coverage indicator that includes adjustments for inputs,

Table 5.3 Summary of World Mental Health Survey reports investigating minimally adequate treatment for depression, anxiety disorders, and substance use disorders

12-month DSM-IV disorder(s)	Country income category	A, % with 12-month disorder	B, % of A with perceived need for treatment	C, % of B who received any 12-month treatment	D, % of C who received minimally adequate treatment	E, % of A who received minimally adequate treatment	Number of people with 12-month disorder
		% (SE)	% (SE)	% (SE)	% (SE)	% (SE)	n
Major depressive disorder[a]	High income	5.2 (0.1)	64.9 (1.1)	77.9 (1.2)	44.2 (1.6)	22.4 (1.0)	2468
	Upper-middle income	4.7 (0.2)	52.2 (1.9)	59.6 (1.9)	36.7 (3.5)	11.4 (1.2)	1182
	Lower-middle income	3.2 (0.2)	34.6 (2.5)	52.6 (3.4)	20.5 (3.4)	3.7 (1.6)	681
	All countries combined	**4.6 (0.1)**	**56.7 (1.0)**	**71.1 (1.0)**	**41.0 (1.4)**	**16.5 (0.7)**	**4331**
Anxiety disorders[b]	High income	10.3 (0.3)	48.4 (0.9)	75.0 (1.3)	38.0 (1.4)	13.8 (0.6)	4346
	Upper-middle income	10.6 (0.3)	36.3 (1.3)	56.1 (1.9)	34.8 (2.6)	7.1 (10.7)	2169
	Lower-middle income	7.9 (0.3)	28.5 (1.6)	46.1 (3.5)	17.9 (2.7)	2.3 (0.7)	1395
	All countries combined	**9.8 (0.2)**	**41.3 (0.7)**	**66.8 (1.1)**	**35.5 (1.1)**	**9.8 (0.4)**	**7910**
Substance use disorders[c]	High income	2.6 (0.1)	43.1 (1.4)	67.5 (1.4)	35.3 (1.8)	10.3 (0.8)	1420
	Upper-middle income	3.3 (0.2)	35.6 (2.2)	59.1 (2.9)	20.3 (1.9)	4.3 (0.8)	614
	Lower-middle income	2.0 (0.2)	31.5 (2.2)	35.6 (3.1)	8.6 (2.1)	1.0 (0.4)	389
	All countries combined	**2.6 (0.1)**	**39.1 (1.1)**	**61.3 (1.3)**	**29.5 (1.4)**	**7.1 (0.5)**	**2423**

[a] Data from surveys in 24 surveys (12 high income, 6 upper-middle income, 5 lower-middle income). Source: Thornicroft et al. (2017).
[b] Data from surveys in 24 surveys (12 high income, 6 upper-middle income, 5 lower-middle income). Disorders included 12-month DSM-IV agoraphobia, generalized anxiety disorder, panic disorder, PTSD, social phobia, specific phobia, and adult separation anxiety disorder. Source: Alonso et al. (2018).
[c] Data from surveys in 28 surveys (15 high income, 7 upper-middle income, 6 lower-middle income). Disorders included 12-month DSM-IV alcohol or drug abuse or dependence. Source: Degenhardt et al. (2017).

quality, compliance, and severity, and applied it to MDD. A subset of 17 surveys were used, including 35,012 respondents in 15 countries across four continents (Argentina, Belgium, Brazil, Colombia, France, Germany, Italy, Lebanon, Mexico, the Netherlands, Nigeria, Romania, Portugal, Spain, and the US). The additional methodological steps to produce this indicator are discussed in detail in Vigo et al. (2020) and entailed the development of composite variables including the type of psychotropic received, the quality of the medication control and psychotherapy received (given by a minimum number of sessions without dropout), as well as the adherence to the medication and dose prescribed.

Across countries, contact coverage for MDD was 42%. Twenty-nine per cent of people with MDD received any psychopharmacology, 19% an adequate drug, and 16% were adequately controlled by a physician. Only 11%, in addition to receiving adequate medication and control, adhered to the indicated dose. With respect to psychotherapy, 16% of people with MDD received any psychotherapeutic support, with 14% receiving an adequate number of sessions without premature interruption or dropout. The result was that only 10% of people with MDD in the countries studied received effective coverage for MDD.

Of note, significant differences could be observed by income level. As **Figure 5.3** indicates, all indicators in high-income countries were at least double the respective indicator for low- and middle-income countries, with effective coverage in high-income countries at 12% versus 6%. An exploration of determinants of effective coverage showed that, overall, level of education, having private insurance, and being adult/middle aged are all significantly associated with increased likelihood of receiving effective coverage. Interestingly, a stratified analysis by country income level indicates that having private insurance is the only significant determinant of receiving effective coverage for MDD.

Discussion

Our studies of coverage for mental and substance use disorders yield several findings that can inform mental health systems planning. In our large and highly diverse sample of countries, 9% of people with or without a mental or substance use disorder received mental health contact coverage. In general, contact coverage showed a monotonic relationship with disorder severity. Interestingly, a fraction of people receiving mental health services do not meet disorder-level criteria. This may be due to different reasons: it may be due to misallocation of services to people without a medical need; it may reflect the failure of standard criteria to capture mental health-related needs in specific settings; or it can capture services provided to subthreshold cases to prevent new onset or recurrence. Further research is needed to understand this issue. With respect to contact coverage, country-income level also showed a monotonic relationship with coverage, with contact coverage for any severe, moderate, or mild disorder in high-income countries doubling or more the coverage received in low-income countries, a testament to the pervasive inequities in global mental health systems.

Across our samples, more than a third of people who had contact with services for any disorder were seen by the general medical sector only, which also led to the lowest level of perceived helpfulness

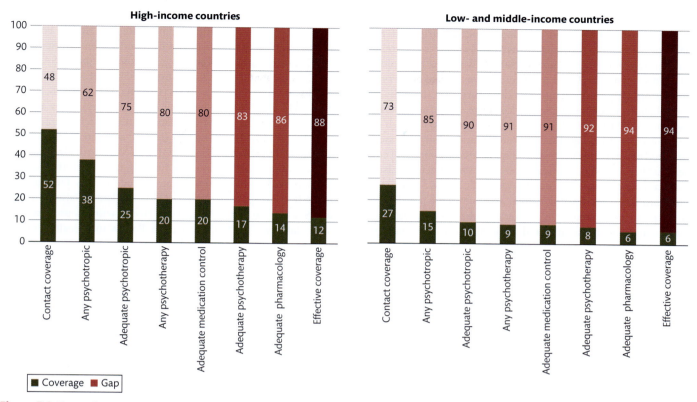

Figure 5.3 Types of treatment coverage and treatment gaps for high- versus low- and middle-income countries.

across sectors (48.8%). Next in terms of coverage were the profiles involving psychologists and other non-medical mental health specialists only (13.8%) and psychiatrists only (11.6%); more than half of people who used these profiles said they were helped a lot. The combination of a general physician plus a psychologist, social worker, or counsellor provides coverage to roughly 10% of people in need, nearly 70% of whom are highly satisfied.

The next step in our assessment of coverage, the minimally adequate treatment indicator for MDD, anxiety disorders, and substance use disorders, added specific quality adjustments, namely a minimum of sessions required with a physician or counsellor, plus medication for MDD and anxiety. Again, we found a monotonic relationship with country income level, with high-income countries providing between six and ten times more minimally adequate treatment for all of these disorders than low-income countries. Overall, minimally adequate treatment was highest for MDD (16.5%), followed by anxiety disorders (9.8%), and substance use disorders (7.1%).

Finally, our estimation of effective coverage of MDD (which in addition to quality and compliance, includes adjustments for severity) further illustrates the inequities of global mental health systems: all indicators including contact coverage, any and adequate psychopharmacology, any and adequate psychotherapy, and effective coverage, are between 2 and 2.5 times larger in high-income countries than in low- and middle-income countries. Of note, individual level effective coverage is determined overall and in high-income countries by education, insurance, and age, whereas in low- and middle-income countries the only significant determinant is having private insurance.

Several limitations have to be considered. Only residents in households were surveyed, whereas homeless, incarcerated, and hospitalized people were not assessed. These subgroups are more likely to have psychiatric disorders and, in the case of the homeless and incarcerated, less likely to receive mental health care. All questions were asked retrospectively, and recall bias cannot be ruled out. Each of the specific analyses have additional limitations that are discussed in more details elsewhere (Alonso et al., 2018; Degenhardt et al., 2017; Harris et al., 2022; Thornicroft et al., 2017; Vigo et al., 2020; P. S. Wang et al., 2007).

Despite these limitations, our results have implications for health systems planning. In general, any form of coverage in high-income countries doubles or more the coverage provided in low-income countries. In fact, contact coverage for depression in high-income countries, for example, reaches more than half the population with 12-month MDD. Keeping in mind that important fractions of people with mild disorders recover on their own, and that some people with a disorder do not perceive a need for services, contact coverage in high-income countries seems high (Boerema et al., 2017). There remain significant gaps in the quality of the services received, however, with only about a quarter of people with 12-month MDD receiving minimally adequate treatment, and about a fifth receiving effective coverage. In low- and middle-income countries, only about a quarter of people with MDD receive contact coverage, and the fraction of people receiving effective coverage is closer to one twentieth. This highlights the inequities of global health systems, and also the areas that need improvements even in high-income countries (such as training general physicians to properly manage people with mental disorders, and expanding capacity to deliver evidence-based psychotherapy). In low- and middle-income countries, the main challenge is expanding coverage, which can be achieved by training community members and non-specialists, as well as by deploying self-guided digital tools and telemedicine for service delivery and supervision. Other important areas of research are the individual determinants of obtaining effective coverage. Additional work focused on MDD suggests that being middle aged, having high education level, and having direct private insurance all increase the likelihood of receiving effective coverage across our sample of countries. Further, state-funded health care and social security also increase contact coverage in general (Vigo et al., 2022b).

In summary, coverage for mental and substance use disorders across countries is inequitable, and services that meet guidelines are scarce in high-income settings and minimal in low-income settings. Given that cost-beneficial interventions exist that, if scaled up, could improve health outcomes and economic productivity in any income setting, strategic funding of mental and substance health services based on the principles of solidarity (where high-income countries initially contribute to service scaleup in low-income countries) seems warranted both from health and economic perspective (Vigo et al., 2019b).

Funding acknowledgements

The WHO WMH Survey Initiative is supported by the US National Institute of Mental Health (NIMH; R01 MH070884), the John D. and Catherine T. MacArthur Foundation, the Pfizer Foundation, the US Public Health Service (R13-MH066849, R01-MH069864, and R01 DA016558), the Fogarty International Center (FIRCA R03-TW006481), the Pan American Health Organization, Eli Lilly and Company, Ortho-McNeil Pharmaceutical Inc., GlaxoSmithKline, and Bristol-Myers Squibb. We thank the staff of the WMH Data Collection and Data Analysis Coordination Centers for assistance with instrumentation, fieldwork, and consultation on data analysis.

None of the funders had any role in the design, analysis, interpretation of results, or preparation of this paper. The views and opinions expressed in this report are those of the authors and should not be construed to represent the views of the WHO, other sponsoring organizations, agencies, or governments.

The Argentina survey—Estudio Argentino de Epidemiología en Salud Mental (EASM)—was supported by a grant from the Argentinian Ministry of Health (Ministerio de Salud de la Nación) (Grant Number 2002-17270/13-5). The São Paulo Megacity Mental Health Survey is supported by the State of São Paulo Research Foundation (FAPESP) Thematic Project Grant 03/00204-3. The Bulgarian Epidemiological Study of common mental disorders EPIBUL is supported by the Ministry of Health and the National Center for Public Health Protection; EPIBUL 2, conducted in 2016–2017, is supported by the Ministry of Health and European Economic Area Grants. The Colombian National Study of Mental Health (NSMH) is supported by the Ministry of Social Protection. The Mental Health Study Medellín—Colombia was carried out and supported jointly by the Center for Excellence on Research in Mental Health (CES University) and the Secretary of Health of Medellín. The ESEMeD project is funded by the European Commission (Contracts QLG5-1999-01042; SANCO 2004123, and EAHC 20081308), the Piedmont Region (Italy), Fondo de Investigación Sanitaria, Instituto de Salud Carlos III, Spain (FIS 00/0028), Ministerio de Ciencia y Tecnología, Spain (SAF 2000-158-CE), Generalitat de Catalunya (2017 SGR 452; 2014 SGR 748), Instituto de Salud Carlos III (CIBER CB06/02/0046, RETICS RD06/0011 REM-TAP), and other local agencies and by an unrestricted educational grant from GlaxoSmithKline. Implementation of the Iraq Mental Health Survey (IMHS) and data entry were carried out by the staff of the Iraqi MOH and MOP with direct support from the Iraqi IMHS team with funding from both the Japanese and European Funds through the United Nations Development Group Iraq Trust Fund (UNDG ITF). The Israel National Health Survey is funded by the Ministry of Health with support from the Israel National Institute for Health Policy and Health Services Research and the National Insurance Institute of Israel. The Lebanese Evaluation of the Burden of Ailments and Needs of the Nation (LEBANON) is supported by the Lebanese Ministry of Public Health, the WHO (Lebanon), National Institute of Health/Fogarty International Center (R03 TW006481-01), anonymous private donations to IDRAAC, Lebanon, and unrestricted grants from Algorithm, AstraZeneca, Benta, Bella Pharma, Eli Lilly, Glaxo Smith Kline, Lundbeck, Novartis, OmniPharma, Pfizer, Phenicia, Servier, and UPO. The Mexican National Comorbidity Survey (MNCS) is supported by The National Institute of Psychiatry Ramon de la Fuente (INPRFMDIES 4280) and by the National Council on Science and Technology (CONACyT-G30544- H), with supplemental support from the Pan American Health Organization (PAHO). Te Rau Hinengaro: The New Zealand Mental Health Survey (NZMHS) is supported by the New Zealand Ministry of Health, Alcohol Advisory Council, and the Health Research Council. The Nigerian Survey of Mental Health and Wellbeing (NSMHW) is supported by the WHO (Geneva), the WHO (Nigeria), and the Federal Ministry of Health, Abuja, Nigeria. The Northern Ireland Study of Mental Health was funded by the Health & Social Care Research & Development Division of the Public Health Agency. The Polish project Epidemiology of Mental Health and Access to Care – EZOP Project (PL 0256) was carried out by the Institute of Psychiatry and Neurology in Warsaw in consortium with Department of Psychiatry—Medical University in Wroclaw and National Institute of Public Health–National Institute of Hygiene in Warsaw and in partnership with Psykiatrist Institut Vinderen—Universitet, Oslo. The project was funded by the European Economic Area Financial Mechanism and the Norwegian Financial Mechanism. EZOP project was co-financed by the Polish Ministry of Health. The Portuguese Mental Health Study was carried out by the Department of Mental Health, Faculty of Medical Sciences, NOVA University of Lisbon, with collaboration of the Portuguese Catholic University, and was funded by Champalimaud Foundation, Gulbenkian Foundation, Foundation for Science and Technology (FCT) and Ministry of Health. The Romania WMH study projects 'Policies in Mental Health Area' and 'National Study regarding Mental Health and Services Use' were carried out by National School of Public Health & Health Services Management (former National Institute for Research & Development in Health), with technical support of Metro Media Transilvania, the National Institute of Statistics-National Centre for Training in Statistics, SC Cheyenne Services SRL, Statistics Netherlands and were funded by Ministry of Public Health (former Ministry of Health) with supplemental support of Eli Lilly Romania SRL. The Saudi National Mental Health Survey (SNMHS) is conducted by the King Salman Center for Disability Research. It is funded by Saudi Basic Industries Corporation (SABIC), King Abdulaziz City for Science and Technology (KACST), Ministry of Health (Saudi Arabia), and King Saud University. Funding in-kind was provided by King Faisal Specialist Hospital and Research Center, and the Ministry of Economy and Planning, General Authority for Statistics. The South Africa Stress and Health Study (SASH) is supported by the US National Institute of Mental Health (R01-MH059575) and National Institute of Drug Abuse with supplemental funding from the South African Department of Health and the University of Michigan. The Shenzhen Mental Health Survey is supported by the Shenzhen Bureau of Health and the Shenzhen Bureau of Science, Technology, and Information. The Psychiatric Enquiry to General Population in Southeast Spain—Murcia (PEGASUS-Murcia) Project has been financed by the Regional Health Authorities of Murcia (Servicio Murciano de Salud and Consejería de Sanidad y Política Social) and Fundación para la Formación e Investigación Sanitarias (FFIS) of Murcia. The Ukraine Comorbid Mental Disorders during Periods of Social Disruption (CMDPSD) study is funded by the US National Institute of Mental Health (RO1-MH61905). The US National Comorbidity Survey Replication (NCS-R) is supported by the National Institute of Mental Health (NIMH; U01-MH60220) with supplemental support from the National Institute of Drug Abuse (NIDA), the Substance Abuse and Mental Health Services Administration (SAMHSA), the Robert Wood Johnson Foundation (RWJF; Grant 044708), and the John W. Alden Trust.

Conflicts of interest

Dr Harris reports consulting fees from RAND Corporation outside the submitted work.

In the past 3 years, Dr Kessler was a consultant for Datastat, Inc., Holmusk, RallyPoint Networks, Inc., and Sage Therapeutics. He has stock options in Mirah, PYM, and Roga Sciences.

REFERENCES

Alonso, J., Liu, Z., Evans-Lacko, S., Sadikova, E., Sampson, N., Chatterji, S., et al. (2018). Treatment gap for anxiety disorders is global: results of the World Mental Health Surveys in 21 countries. *Depression and Anxiety*, **35**, 195–208.

Amouzou, A., Leslie, H. H., Ram, M., Fox, M., Jiwani, S. S., Requejo, J., et al. (2019). Advances in the measurement of coverage for RMNCH and nutrition: from contact to effective coverage. *BMJ Global Health*, **4**(Suppl. 4), e001297.

Bloom, D. E., Cafiero, E. T., Jané-Llopis, E., Abrahams-Gessel, S., Bloom, L. R., Fathima, S., et al. (2011). *The Global Economic Burden of Noncommunicable Diseases*. Geneva: World Economic Forum.

Boerema, A. M., Ten Have, M., Kleiboer, A., de Graaf, R., Nuyen, J., Cuijpers, P., & Beekman, A. T. F. (2017). Demographic and need factors of early, delayed and no mental health care use in major depression: a prospective study. *BMC Psychiatry*, **17**, 367.

Buchan, H. A., Duggan, A., Hargreaves, J., Scott, I. A., & Slawomirski, L. (2016). Health care variation: time to act. *Medical Journal of Australia*, **205**, S30–S33.

Chisholm, D., Sweeny, K., Sheehan, P., Rasmussen, B., Smit, F., Cuijpers, P., & Saxena, S. (2016). Scaling-up treatment of depression and anxiety: a global return on investment analysis. *Lancet Psychiatry*, **3**, 415–424.

Degenhardt, L., Glantz, M., Evans-Lacko, S., Sadikova, E., Sampson, N., Thornicroft, G., et al. (2017). Estimating treatment coverage for people with substance use disorders: an analysis of data from the World Mental Health Surveys. *World Psychiatry*, **16**, 299–307.

Demyttenaere, K., Bruffaerts, R., Posada-Villa, J, Gasquet, I., Kovess, V., Lepine, J. P., et al. (2004). Prevalence, severity, and unmet need for treatment of mental disorders in the World Health Organization World Mental Health Surveys. *JAMA*, **291**, 2581–2590.

Dezetter, A., Briffault, X., Alonso, J., Angermeyer, M. C., Bruffaerts, R., de Girolamo, G., et al. (2011). Factors associated with use of psychiatrists and nonpsychiatrist providers by ESEMeD respondents in six European countries. *Psychiatric Services*, **62**, 143–151.

Druss, B. G., Hwang, I., Petukhova, M., Sampson, N. A., Wang, P. S., & Kessler, R. C. (2009). Impairment in role functioning in mental and chronic medical disorders in the United States: results from the National Comorbidity Survey Replication. *Molecular Psychiatry*, **14**, 728–737.

Endicott, J., Spitzer, R. L., Fleiss, J. L., & Cohen, J. (1976). The global assessment scale. A procedure for measuring overall severity of psychiatric disturbance. *Archives of General Psychiatry*, **33**, 766–771.

Evans-Lacko, S., Tachimori, H., Kovess-Masféty, V., Chatterji, S., & Thornicroft, G. (2018). Service use. In: Scott, K. M., De Jonge, P, Stein, D. J., & Kessler, R. C. (Eds.), *Mental Disorders Around the World: Facts and Figures from the WHO World Mental Health Surveys* (pp. 314–323). Cambridge: Cambridge University Press.

Fernández, D., Vigo, D., Sampson, N. A., Hwang, I., Aguilar-Gaxiola, S., Al-Hamzawi, A. O., et al. (2021). Patterns of care and dropout rates from outpatient mental healthcare in low-, middle- and high-income countries from the World Health Organization's World Mental Health Survey Initiative. *Psychological Medicine*, **51**, 2104–2116.

First, M. B., Spitzer, R. L., Gibbon, M., & Williams, J. B. W. (2002). *Structured Clinical Interview for DSM-IV-TR Axis I Disorders, Research Version, Non-patient Edition. (SCID-I/NP)*. New York: Biometrics Research, New York State Psychiatric Institute.

Harkness, J., Pennell, B. E., Villar, A., Gebler, N., Aguilar-Gaxiola, S., & Bilgen, I. (2008). Translation procedures and translation assessment in the World Mental Health Survey Initiative. In: Kessler, R. C. & Üstün, T. B. (Eds.), *The WHO World Mental Health Surveys: Global Perspectives on the Epidemiology of Mental Disorders* (pp. 91–113). New York: Cambridge University Press.

Haro, J. M., Arbabzadeh-Bouchez, S., Brugha, T. S., de Girolamo, G., Guyer, M. E., Jin, R., et al. (2006). Concordance of the Composite International Diagnostic Interview Version 3.0 (CIDI 3.0) with standardized clinical assessments in the WHO World Mental Health surveys. *International Journal of Methods in Psychiatric Research*, **15**, 167–180.

Harris, M. G., Kazdin, A. E., Munthali, R. J., Vigo, D. V., Hwang, I., Sampson, N. A., et al. (2022). Perceived helpfulness of service sectors used for mental and substance use disorders: findings from the WHO World Mental Health Surveys. *International Journal of Mental Health Systems*, **16**, 6.

Heeringa, S., Wells, J., Hubbard, F., Mneimneh, Z., Chiu, W., Sampson, N., & Berglund, P. (2008). Sample designs and sampling procedures. In: Üstün, R. K. T. (Ed.), *The WHO World Mental Health Surveys: Global Perspectives on the Epidemiology of Mental Disorders* (pp. 14–32). New York: Cambridge University Press.

Jackson, J. S., Neighbors, H. W., Torres, M., Martin, L. A., Williams, D. R., & Baser, R. (2007). Use of mental health services and subjective satisfaction with treatment among Black Caribbean immigrants: results from the National Survey of American Life. *American Journal of Public Health*, **97**, 60–67.

Kessler, R. C. & Üstün, T. B. (2004). The World Mental Health (WMH) Survey Initiative Version of the World Health Organization (WHO) Composite International Diagnostic Interview (CIDI). *International Journal of Methods in Psychiatric Research*, **13**, 93–121.

Kuramoto-Crawford, S. J., Han, B., Jacobus-Kantor, L., & Mojtabai, R. (2015). Differences in patients' perceived helpfulness of depression treatment provided by general medical providers and specialty mental health providers. *General Hospital Psychiatry*, **37**, 340–346.

Larson, E., Vail, D., Mbaruku, G. M., Mbatia, R., & Kruk, M. E. (2016). Beyond utilization: measuring effective coverage of obstetric care along the quality cascade. *International Journal for Quality in Health Care*, **29**, 104–110.

Pennell, B.-E., Mneimneh, Z., Bowers, A., Chardoul, S., Wells, J. E., Viana, M. C., et al. (2008). Implementation of the World Mental Health Surveys. In: Kessler, R. C. & Üstün, T. B. (Eds.), *The WHO World Mental Health Surveys: Global Perspectives on the Epidemiology of Mental Disorders* (pp. 33–58). New York: Cambridge University Press.

Research Triangle Institute (2002). *SUDAAN: Professional Software for Survey Data Analysis, Version 8.0.1*. Research Triangle Park, NC: Research Triangle Institute.

Sheehan, D. V., Harnett-Sheehan, K., & Raj, B. A. (1996). The measurement of disability. *International Clinical Psychopharmacology*, **11**(Suppl. 3), 89–95.

Substance Abuse and Mental Health Services Administration (1993). Final notice establishing definitions for (1) children with a serious emotional disturbance, and (2) adults with a serious mental illness. *Federal Register*, **58**, 29422–29425.

Tanahashi, T. (1978). Health service coverage and its evaluation. *Bulletin of the World Health Organization*, **56**, 295–303.

Thornicroft, G., Chatterji, S., Evans-Lacko, S., Gruber, M., Sampson, N., Aguilar-Gaxiola, S., et al. (2017). Undertreatment of people with major depressive disorder in 21 countries. *British Journal of Psychiatry*, **210**, 119–124.

Vigo, D., Haro, J. M., Hwang, I., Aguilar-Gaxiola, S., Alonso, J., Borges, G., et al. (2020). Toward measuring effective treatment coverage: critical bottlenecks in quality- and user-adjusted coverage for major depressive disorder. *Psychological Medicine*, 1–11. Advance online publication. https://doi.org/10.1017/S0033291720003797

Vigo, D., Jones, L., Atun, R., & Thornicroft, G. (2022a). The true global disease burden of mental illness: still elusive. *Lancet Psychiatry*, **9**, 98–100.

Vigo, D. V., Kazdin, A., Sampson, N., Hwang, I., Alonso, J., Andrade, L. H. (2022b). Determinants of effective treatment coverage for major depressive disorder in the WHO World Mental Health Surveys. *International Journal of Mental Health Systems*, **16**, 29.

Vigo, D. V., Kestel, D., Pendakur, K., Thornicroft, G., & Atun, R. (2019a). Disease burden and government spending on mental, neurological, and substance use disorders, and self-harm: cross-sectional, ecological study of health system response in the Americas. *Lancet Public Health*, **4**, e89–e96.

Vigo, D. V., Patel, V., Becker, A., Bloom, D., Yip, W., Raviola, G., et al. (2019b). A partnership for transforming mental health globally. *Lancet Psychiatry*, **6**, 350–356.

Vigo, D., Thornicroft, G., & Atun, R. (2016). Estimating the true global burden of mental illness. *Lancet Psychiatry*, **3**, 171–178.

Wang, J. & Patten, S. B. (2007). Perceived effectiveness of mental health care provided by primary-care physicians and mental health specialists. *Psychosomatics*, **48**, 123–127.

Wang, P. S., Aguilar-Gaxiola, S., Alonso, J., Angermeyer, M. C., Borges, G., Bruffaerts, R., et al. (2007). Use of mental health services for anxiety, mood, and substance disorders in 17 countries in the WHO world mental health surveys. *Lancet*, **370**, 841–850.

World Bank (2003). *World Development Indicators 2003*. Washington, DC: The World Bank.

6

The lived experience

Focus on wellness

Margaret Swarbrick and Crystal L. Brandow

Introduction

People who were formerly recipients of services (service users) have become architects shaping the focus, design, and delivery of community mental health practice. This chapter will examine the importance of acknowledging the lived experience from the lens of wellness, and the value of examining how viewing the lived experience can address social injustices as well as transform community mental health practice to promote wellness as a vision and outcome.

Who are service users?

There is no clear consensus regarding how to uniformly define the term 'service user'. There are a variety of terms used to designate a person who lives with a mental health condition or substance use disorder who is a past or current recipient of community mental health services. Terms include, but are not limited to, a person living with a mental disorder, patient, psychiatric survivor, ex-patient, inmate, client, recipient, mental health consumer, person in recovery, and person living with mental illness. There is much debate regarding terms. For example, many are sceptical about the term 'consumer' because this would imply a person has power and choice when most likely this is not the case. The term 'service user' is the term used internationally and generally applies to identify individuals diagnosed with a mental health condition or substance disorder who have currently, or in the past, used traditional services. This is the term that will be used throughout this chapter.

User-led movement

The self-help user-led movement (also referred to as consumer–survivor–ex-patient movement) has evolved at various paces around the world. Throughout Africa, Asia, Australia, New Zealand, and the US, public policy efforts are attempting to include service users in planning and policy development and implementation of new transformation. This movement continues to make an impact on community mental health practice. Table 6.1 summarizes key areas of focus (social justice and wellness) and contributions to system change for community mental health practice.

The service user movement is considered a political paradigm that developed out of societal discrimination based on misunderstanding and misconceptions about service users and disenchantment with the delivery of conventional medical model services. This movement viewed the conventional 'system' as dehumanizing and unresponsive to individual needs. Some factions insisted on complete liberation from psychiatry because they rejected the medical models of mental illness, professional control, and forced treatment. *Social justice* was an organizing principle of the service user-led movement. Groups organized because people were being excluded, stigmatized, and subjected to practices preventing them from having equitable access to opportunities that would support them in reaching their full potential and contributing equally within society.

Participation

People were too often limited in terms of participation in the community, as employees, students, volunteers, teachers, caregivers, parents, advisors, residents; as active citizens (National Social Inclusion Programme, 2009). Service users experienced, and

Table 6.1 Key areas of focus and contributions for community mental health practice

Focus	Contributions to system change
Social justice	Advocacy to uphold human rights, equality, and address economic and social inequities Organized to address injustices service users face in terms of social, economic, and political structures
Wellness	Strengths-focused holistic view of the individual: emotional, physical, intellectual, social, environmental, occupational, financial, and spiritual dimensions (Figure 6.1) Recognizes the effects of stigma, discrimination, racial inequities, and social determinants of health

continue to experience, this exclusion in many aspects of life—social, economic, educational, spiritual, recreational, cultural, and health. They encounter higher rates of poverty, unemployment, homelessness, poor health, inadequate access to education, and social isolation. Social justice through advocacy became the focus to correct these human rights violations. Some groups organized around the human rights violations and others acted as watchdogs to prevent people from being unnecessarily excluded from society. In the US, the initial advocacy efforts emerged from the user-led 'patient' liberation movement organized by people who experienced emotional distress, with freedoms denied by the labelling and dehumanizing and stereotypical images propagated by the mental health system and society (Zinman et al., 1987).

Service users are placing greater emphasis on issues of social inclusion/exclusion and are helping community health programmes pay greater attention to wellness dimensions (Figure 6.1) and social determinants of health, the latter of which are formidable barriers faced by many service users, as discussed further in this chapter.

Impact

The user movement has impacted the field in many ways. There have been great strides and recognition of how the personal struggles, challenges, and triumphs positively impact community mental health practice in terms of design, delivery, evaluation, and research. The lived experience of these individuals' survival and capacity to build resilience and thrive offers information to affect approaches, resources, and strategies to guide professionals and inform community mental health organizations and research.

The movement has been making efforts to help community mental health practitioners view people from their strengths and lived experiences, and not just diagnostic labels. There have been successes in terms of addressing the long-standing stigma and discrimination faced by many. The user movement has advocated for the systems to consider the 'lived experience' from the lens of wellness (Figure 6.1 and Table 6.1, described further in this chapter) to better engage, support, and empower people.

Stigma

Service users often experience stigmatization or marginalization after being labelled with a 'disorder'. Stigma is 'an attribute that is deeply discrediting' that reduces someone 'from a whole and usual person to a tainted, discounted one' (Goffman, 1963, p. 3). Stigma is a negative view attributed to a person or groups of people when their characteristics or behaviours are viewed as different from societal norms. There are three types of stigma: (1) individual stigma, (2) interpersonal stigma, and (3) structural stigma. *Structural stigma* is defined as 'societal-level conditions, cultural norms, and institutional policies that constrain the opportunities, resources, and well-being of the stigmatized' (Hatzenbuehler & Link, 2014, p. 2), and originates from the concept of institutional racism (Hatzenbuehler, 2016). *Interpersonal stigma* refers to stigma between individuals, the stigmatized and the non-stigmatized, such as the stigma that may be experienced by an employee with a mental health condition and the supervisor, or the colleagues, without mental health concerns. People may internalize that stigma as *individual stigma*.

Structural stigma

Stigma can lead to discrimination. People may feel as though they do not have the opportunity to pursue valued social roles, such as student, worker, family member, or citizen, which can be devastating. Not only may they perceive this lack of opportunity, but there may also be real barriers to pursuing health, well-being, and improved quality of life. This societal abuse (Benbow, 2009) disadvantages individuals with mental health conditions. For example,

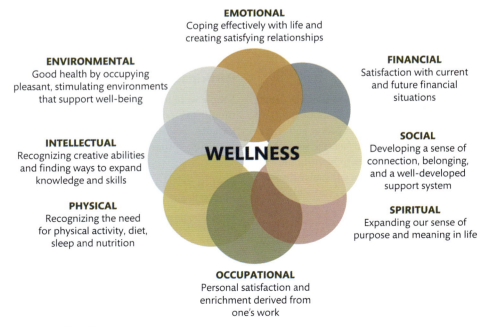

Figure 6.1 The Eight Dimensions of Wellness.
Adapted from Swarbrick, M. (2006). A wellness approach. *Psychiatric Rehabilitation Journal, 29,* 311–314.

more severe mental illness is associated with higher rates of unemployment (Luciano & Meara, 2014; Marrone & Swarbrick, 2020). Unemployment is associated with lower income, financial insecurity, limited access to social opportunities, lower sense of self-worth, and other concerns that are detrimental to one's wellness. Among the myriad of factors responsible for unemployment rates, structural stigma is one and contributes to the experience of discrimination at work. One study found employers demonstrated significant discrimination against job applicants who self-identified as having been hospitalized in the past for mental health treatment—not a culturally acceptable experience. These individuals are less likely to receive a callback following an application for a job opening (Hipes et al., 2016).

Interpersonal stigma

It is not uncommon for service users to be told that they are not fit for work, to manage their own money, or to form quality social relationships or romantic partnerships, because of a diagnosis that is referred to as 'chronic' and 'disabling'. This messaging is not strengths-based and can lead to low self-efficacy and low perceived control among service users. This can contribute to poverty and unemployment, lack of economic empowerment, social isolation, discrimination, and other life experiences that fail to support well-being and quality of life. These experiences and labels can alter the trajectory of an individual's life. They can have negative impacts on education, employment, financial self-sufficiency, supportive and intimate relationships, and opportunities to use innate talents and skills.

Individual stigma

As a response to stigma, people may internalize that stigma as individual stigma. This can lead to a diminished sense of self and of self-efficacy. *Self-stigma* is the prejudice which people adopt against themselves. According to the theoretical model of self-stigma (Watson et al., 2007), self-stigma results when an individual is (1) aware of stereotypes, (2) agrees with the stereotypes, and (3) applies those stereotypes to oneself. Self-stigma can be destructive. It can lead to shame, hopelessness, guilt, and negative self-talk—all of which can serve as significant barriers to recovery. The person may feel and act as though they have lost their previous identities, such as occupying fulfilling roles like sibling, student, caregiver, or parent. Instead, they may believe the stigmatizing views held by other society members, for example, that they can't get better, work isn't an option, or that a fulfilling life isn't possible.

Studies have examined the impact of self-stigma, as well as strategies for undercutting these beliefs. For example, researchers engaged in a quasi-experimental study of narrative enhancement and cognitive therapy to evaluate the effectiveness of the intervention in reducing self-stigma. They found that this type of treatment, which is a manualized, structured, group-based intervention, not only reduced self-stigma, but increased self-efficacy, hope, and improved quality of life (Roe et al., 2014). This programme is a 20-session intervention that combines psychoeducation to help replace stigmatizing views about mental illness and recovery with empirical findings, cognitive restructuring geared towards teaching skills to challenge negative beliefs about the self, and elements of psychotherapy focused on enhancing one's ability to narrate one's life story (Yano et al., 2011).

From the lived experience perspective, for a person to take responsibility for their personal wellness, it does not require them to accept or disclose that they have a specific diagnosis, nor does it require embracing the biomedical diagnosis. Some treatment programmes are adamant this occurs, though it is not helpful for many people. Programmes such as illness management and recovery reinforce a negative life trajectory. Rather, it is important for the person to recognize and be aware of unique difficulties that they may experience and want to address to facilitate healthful life changes and improve well-being and quality of life. Continuing to emphasize that a person has schizophrenia, or any other diagnostic categories, can continue to reinforce self-stigma, which can be very damaging. A role of providers is to help people manage difficulties and help them to make positive changes. There is a need for providers to learn to identify and guard against messages, practices, and policies that may demoralize people, engender unnecessary dependence, and perpetuate the perception of disability rather than focus on capabilities and possibilities (Ridgeway, 2001).

Experience defined

Providers should be familiar with and receptive to all lived experiences, and to recognize that all experiences are valid. The service user is the expert of their own life, and providers can be part of support systems and teams to help empower service users to embrace and activate a wellness lifestyle. This includes not only helping to combat structural stigma, identifying and ameliorating interpersonal stigma, and reversing individual stigma, but also adopting a compassionate, empathetic approach to the lived experiences of service users.

First-hand, lived experience of a mental health condition can provide insightful lessons for service users, providers, professionals, and supporters. People with lived experience are considered *experts by experience* (Vojtila et al., 2021). Historically, rather than perceive people as experts, community mental health practice has pathologized or disregarded the value of this experience. People with lived experience have experienced mental health, substance use, or trauma-related challenges. Of the significant contributions lent by this experience are the knowledge and skills associated with coping and navigating the service system. The knowledge and skills based on experience is referred to as empirical knowledge or a posteriori knowledge. This is an invaluable level of expertise which is becoming increasingly accepted, and even sought out, in mental health care.

People with lived experience (1) can be decision-makers in their own service plans, care, and treatment; (2) serve in roles such as system navigators and peer supporters; and (3) occupy leadership roles in the mental health service system (Vojtila et al., 2021). The valuable roles service users can occupy are reviewed later in this chapter.

This viewpoint of the person as the expert is quite different from the traditional Western biomedical model of treatment, which tends to view the provider as the expert. The traditional model takes a paternalistic view where the provider, who may lack first-hand experience with mental health conditions, is believed to know what is best for the individual being served. Decisions are made by the provider, and service users are expected to adhere to the decisions of the professional care team—'despite the fact that the professionals may not have fully taken into account [their] specific needs and preferences' (Pelto-Piri et al., 2013, p. 2). Allowing the individual to co-create their care with providers, engaging in shared decision-making or self-directed care, better elevates the incomparable value of lived experience. It is important to remember that personal experience is subject to an individual's *perception* and *interpretation* of their own circumstances. Therefore, when working with service users, one should tune into their *perceptual set of experiences* that have dictated how they manage their health, and how they are, or are not, maintaining quality of life and well-being.

One of the ways providers can centre an individual's experience and understand their interpretation of that experience is by encouraging cultural activation. Cultural activation is the individual's:

> recognition of the importance of providing cultural information to providers about cultural affiliations, challenges, views about, and attitudes towards behavioural health and general medical health care, as well as the consumer's confidence in his or her ability to provide this information. (Siegel et al., 2016, p. 153)

In fact, peer specialists can be helpful in facilitating the cultural activation process. Much of how people perceive and interpret their mental health is cultural (i.e. cultural stigma).

Racial and ethnic disparities

Being familiar with and receptive to all lived experiences includes an understanding about the unique experiences of oppressed racial and ethnic groups. Disparities in access to mental health support can be attributed to racism, xenophobia, and both explicit and implicit bias. They can also be attributed to lack of provider awareness and education around trauma responses and how they manifest. Structural racism, for example, is a form of trauma. Structural racism has also been illustrated as a driver of poor mental health outcomes, including psychosis. Anglin and colleagues (2021) implicate 'structural racism as a fundamental cause of the extended psychosis phenotype through group-level processes occurring at the neighbourhood level that are connected to processes occurring at the individual level (e.g., discrimination)' (p. 604). Racial discrimination is associated with subthreshold psychotic symptoms among a multi-ethnic sample (Anglin et al., 2014). Experiencing multiple traumatic experiences is associated with increased risk for psychosis (Shevlin et al., 2007).

To meaningfully engage in effective community mental health practice, providers must be equally committed to racial justice and trauma prevention and healing. To effectively work to improve individual or community mental health, attention to racial justice and trauma is necessary. Researchers studied a curriculum on racial inequities in mental health, inclusive of antiracism didactics, in a psychiatry residency programme. Of residents who participated and provided feedback, 97% indicated that discussing racism in the formal, required didactic curriculum was positive (Medlock et al., 2017). Education and training around the impact of racism and discrimination as social determinants of mental health and adverse experiences—both adverse childhood and adverse community experiences—is essential for increasing awareness of the lived experiences of oppressed groups and the impact of this oppression on mental health and substance use. A wellness lens provides a framework for addressing these concerns among individual service users.

Applying a wellness lens

'Wellness' is a powerful word and words matter! Wellness is not the absence of disease, illness, and stress but the presence of purpose in life, active involvement in satisfying activity, supportive relationships, a healthy body and living environment, and sense of contentment (Dunn, 1961; Swarbrick, 2012). Wellness is a conscious, deliberate process that requires a person to become aware of and make choices each day for a self-defined lifestyle (Swarbrick, 1997, 2012). Wellness is an active process of creating and adapting patterns of behaviour. A wellness lifestyle includes a self-defined balance of habits such as adequate sleep and rest, productivity, exercise, participation in meaningful activity, nutrition, productivity, social contact, and supportive relationships (Swarbrick, 1997, 2012). Because everyone has individual needs and preferences, this balance varies from person to person.

Wellness can be an inspiring word for people with mental and substance use conditions. The Eight Dimensions of Wellness (Swarbrick, 2006, 2012; Swarbrick & Nemec, 2016) has been embraced in recent years by the behavioural healthcare field in the US and some other countries, such as the UK. Developed by the first author of this chapter as a desire to address disparities facing people with or at risk of developing mental health conditions or substance use disorders, this model has evolved based on the lived experiences of people facing traumatic life experiences, substance use, and mental health challenges. Wellness is multidimensional, and includes physical, emotional, intellectual, social, financial, occupational, environmental, and spiritual dimensions (**Figure 6.1** and **Table 6.2**). The eight dimensions of the Wellness model have been used to craft an effective framework that focuses on the strengths and potential of individuals with mental and substance use conditions, building resilience for people to survive and thrive. It is important to focus on a person's overall wellness rather than solely on the mental illness and presenting problems.

Table 6.2 The Eight Dimensions of Wellness

Physical	Spiritual	Social	Intellectual
Maintenance of a healthy body, good health habits, and accessing health care and screening	Meaning and purpose and a sense of balance and peace	Friends, family, and the community, and having an interest in and concern for the needs of others	Lifelong learning, application of knowledge learned, and sharing knowledge
Emotional	**Occupational**	**Environmental**	**Financial**
Express feelings, enjoy life, adjust to emotional challenges, and cope with stress and traumatic life experiences	Participating in activities that provide meaning and purpose	Being and feeling physically safe, in safe and clean surroundings	Sense of control and knowledge about personal finances

Many service users have reported they can manage trauma and mental and substance use challenges by creating wellness habits, such as committing to a daily routine of medication, exercise, adequate nutrition, sleep and wake cycles, and rest (Swarbrick, 1997). The Eight Dimensions of Wellness prominently feature adjacent dimensions overlapping to convey the idea that all dimensions are connected. Each dimension can impact another, both positively and negatively. What has been the most successful aspect of this model in the authors' experiences is that it is strengths focused. For short- and long-term health and recovery, many people benefit from regularly checking in to consider what they do each day or week across each of the eight wellness dimensions, providing an opportunity to build health habits and routines on existing strengths and healthful behaviours (Swarbrick & Nemec, 2016).

Very often, people can identify what they are doing and consider how they can continue to strengthen these daily habits and routines to create balance and to manage stress, mental health or substance use symptoms, and trauma responses. The Eight Dimensions of Wellness is a very personal schema. The model recognizes that everyone has strengths—choices that help us stay healthy and well—and everyone has trouble taking good care of themselves from time to time. Addiction, trauma, and stress can impact wellness; however, wellness habits help maintain balance and well-being (Swarbrick, 2012).

Social determinants of health

The Eight Dimensions of Wellness can be applied on an individual level, as well as a community level illustrating how community-level factors influence individual well-being. On a community or neighbourhood level, the social determinants of health are often discussed as factors that influence health, including mental health. Some of the conditions practitioners conceive as 'negative social determinants of health' are adverse community experiences, or forms of structural violence (Prevention Institute, 2017). Structural violence contributes to both individual and community trauma. This is particularly the case for individuals with lived experience, and is compounded for service users who experience racism, discrimination, oppression, and poverty. For example, in the community and neighbourhood environment, 'exposure to police killings of unarmed [B]lack Americans was not associated with changes in mental health among [W]hite Americans', while they were associated with poor self-reported mental health among Black people in the general US population (Bor et al., 2018, p. 305).

Viewing community-level conditions and social determinants through a wellness lens, such as through a 'Wellness First' approach (Brandow et al., 2019), highlights the overlap between the Eight Dimensions of Wellness and social determinants of health. The World Health Organization defines the social determinants of health as 'the conditions in which people are born, grow, live, work, and age' taken together with the structural determinants (Commission on Social Determinants of Health, 2008, p. 1). Examples of social determinants offered by the World Health Organization include the health care system, early child development, employment-related conditions, community and neighbourhood environments, and social protection, among others. Across each of these domains, lack of equitable, accessible, and proper supports can harm personal wellness across each of the eight dimensions. For example, violence and crime in a community or neighbourhood will impact environmental wellness. Lack of accessible or affordable healthcare will affect physical wellness. Inadequate social protection mechanisms, leading to experiences of poverty and food insecurity, can influence emotional, spiritual, physical, and financial wellness.

Applying the wellness lens: lived experience in practice

This section will review how professionals and organizations can apply the wellness lens, including through application of available peer models and involving service users in leadership, education, and research roles.

Narrative therapy

Narratives are important resources that should be transmitted to staff and people served in every treatment setting (Legere et al., 2013). Professionals can be trained in approaches such as narrative therapy. Narrative therapy is a useful tool to embrace the lived experience from the lens of wellness. Narrative therapy challenges dominant, problematic stories that prevent people from living their best lives. Through wellness-oriented narrative therapy, negative or less than optimal views of self and unhealthy beliefs can be challenged. Service users can be guided to open their minds to new ways of living that reflect a more accurate and healthier story demonstrating their resilience and strengths.

A tenet of narrative therapy is that disorder-focused stories limit options for action (White, 2004, p. 34). These marginalizing stories pathologize and disempower people by making it seem as if their challenges define the essence of who they are. They tend to foster negative and limited ways of thinking. Often, the stories we believe about ourselves have been written by others. In passively accepting and repeating narrow and negative narratives, we unnecessarily restrict our life possibilities. Narrative therapy helps people to reclaim and take back their 'storytelling rights' (Denborough, 2014, pp. 8, 10, 22).

From a wellness perspective, people learn to find meaning in their experiences and develop a sense of purpose that draws upon their personal strengths. There is a focus on looking at the 'opportunity'. Providers ascribing to a person-centred approach can forge a collaborative relationship by attempting to know the person through their wellness lens rather than the lens of labels ascribed by others. By taking the time to listen to persons we serve, we may be able to develop better ways to support service users, driven by the perceptions of their own experiences. To apply this approach, providers and organizations can shift processes so intake includes opportunities for people to discuss wellness narratives and strengths rather than just a history of symptoms and treatments, and group and individual sessions can include discussions of wellness strategies to manage troubling symptoms and stressors, for example.

Peer providers and peer-led services

Organizations can benefit from the expertise of service users who become trained and credentialled peer providers or other peer support professionals. Employing people within community mental health practice settings is an important step towards combating stigma, increasing employment rates, and helping to create opportunities for people to contribute their strengths and talents in competitive, meaningful jobs. Peer recovery support services are increasingly offered in a range of community settings to assist individuals with substance use disorder and co-occurring mental health disorders. Peer support workers are individuals who, because of their own experiences, are experientially qualified to support peers currently experiencing substance use and associated mental health or other related problems. They offer mentoring, education, and other forms of support. Regardless of the nature of their role, peers support workers have the ability to engage the individual outside the confines of traditional clinical practice. This ability to fill critical care gaps is the most probable reason for their widespread uptake across a diverse range of treatment settings.

Peer support workers are individuals with a lived experience of a life challenge who have made a personal commitment to their own self-care and have a desire to use what was learned from one's own lived experiences to assist others with similar challenges (National Association of Peer Supporters, 2019; Substance Abuse and Mental Health Services Administration, 2015). They use their lived experience and receive training to assist others in building resilience and enhancing the quality of life of people they support. Experiential knowledge and life experience are qualities that provide a powerful message of hope that enhances engagement. Peer specialist training programmes combine the lived experience with key competencies to further enhance a peer provider's ability to assist others. Certified peer specialists are excellent clinical partners, helping to support the health and well-being of service users. There are many peer-developed and peer wellness approaches that include peer wellness coaching (Brice et al., 2014; Swarbrick et al., 2016), a peer-led financial wellness curriculum (Jiménez-Solomon et al., 2016), and other peer-led health and wellness models (Swarbrick et al., 2016).

Studies on peer support services demonstrate positive findings on measures, including reduced substance use and relapse rates, improved relationships with treatment providers and social supports, increased treatment retention, and treatment satisfaction (Eddie et al., 2019). Many have suggested more research is needed for further rigorous investigation to establish the efficacy, effectiveness, and cost–benefits. Studies are underway to solidify role definitions, identify optimal training guidelines, and establish guidance for whom and under what conditions peer recovery support services are most effective.

When engaging peer providers and other peer support professionals, it is important to avoid tokenism, or to relegate service users to menial roles. To avoid tokenism, professionals and organizations must make sure their policies, procedures, and practices are inclusive, and are supportive of hiring, maintaining, and advancing staff with lived experience in meaningful ways. Far too often, service users lack power in organizations and professional settings. With reference to the Ladder of Co-Production (National Co-production Advisory Group, 2021), service users may be involved and engaged, but are less likely to be offered equitable opportunity in co-production, which is defined as 'an equal relationship between people who use services and the people responsible for services. They work together, from design to delivery, sharing strategic decision-making about policies as well as decisions about the best way to deliver services'. An example of co production in action is illustrated through the development of the *Journey to Wellness* guide (Swarbrick et al., 2022, 2023).

Peer respite programmes

Peer respite programmes are an example of an important approach to support wellness developed by and for service users. Peer respite is 'a voluntary, short-term, overnight programme that provides community-based, non-clinical crisis support to individuals experiencing, or at risk of experiencing, a mental health crisis' (Legislative Analysis and Public Policy Association, 2021, p. 1). Peer respites were described in the 1970s (Chamberlin, 1978) as a way to avoid the distress, coercion, trauma, and potentially lengthy stay that was often a part of an inpatient stay. To accomplish this, peer respite programmes are intentionally designed as different from traditional inpatient services (Ostrow & Croft, 2014, 2015). Peer respites offer a home-like environment (Fletcher et al., 2020; Ostrow & Croft, 2014, 2015) and are designed to provide 'non-clinical peer-to-peer support' based on the view that crisis presents an opportunity for exploring and learning. Focused on multiple service goals, peer respite aims to help people feel safe at a time of crisis, find a new understanding of themselves and their situation, manage the immediate distress, and build wellness skills.

Wellness Respite is a peer-led respite programme serving adults who voluntarily agree to participate for assistance in managing acute distress that interferes with their functioning (Swarbrick, 2015). Length of stay is determined by the guest, working in collaboration with peer support staff, and is usually up to 10 days. Guests are offered a range of supports and services that can assist them in meeting wellness goals and use strategies for self-management and stress reduction (Swarbrick, 2020). Wellness Respite recognizes that crises are short term and involve a time when a person may need assistance in restoring health habits and routines, and support to manage anxiety, frustration, and depression (Swarbrick, 2015, 2020). The Wellness Respite structure and homelike environment are designed to strengthen each guest's wellness, self-care, and management of co-occurring medical or substance use issues so they can successfully manage the immediate crisis and resume valued life roles and responsibilities.

Leadership roles

Individuals with lived experience are well equipped to serve in a variety of leadership roles. Yet, roles designated for individuals with lived experience on leadership levels are not as ubiquitous as they ought to be. This creates a 'global need for lived experience leadership' (Byrne et al., 2018, p. 76). In the area of research, further discussed subsequently, lived experience research leadership is important, and can serve as a career trajectory (Jones et al., 2021). Investment in participatory research methods including service users in key leadership roles has grown significantly. Globally, there is an increase in recognition of the value of lived experience in leadership. In Australia, for example, the Queensland Mental Health Alcohol and Other Drugs Strategic Plan (2018–2023) prioritizes the engagement, participation, and leadership of individuals with lived experience in the mental health system (Queensland Mental Health Commission, 2018).

Education and research

Students, fellows, and research staff with lived experience face a unique set of emotional challenges navigating research spaces in which it is normative to speak of individuals with mental health or psychiatric diagnoses in othering, medicalized ways. Research trainees may be asked to adopt language (e.g. 'mental illness' or 'brain disorder') rejected by the advocacy community, or otherwise utilize a vernacular that does not resonate with their own experiences. These situations can easily become a significant source of personal stress. The availability of mentors who can recognize and help address these issues becomes critical as institutions respond to the call to action for advancing the role of lived experience in education and research. Mentors, department chairs, and others in community mental health leadership positions can commit to actively supporting the retention and promotion of junior faculty with lived experience. Services users can play an important role as researchers, while research and academic settings could benefit from their representation within the ranks of tenured faculty and extramurally supported primary investigators.

Early career professionals and students entering professional circles could benefit from the opportunity to hear service users' lived experiences and wellness narratives as part of their standard training programmes. First-hand wellness narratives can be woven into annual reports, communicating this lived experience with both internal and external stakeholders. In the field, at professional conferences, for example, presentations by organizations should feature content delivered by service users sharing their experiences from the lens of wellness. Relatedly, in-house professional development presentations can include these voices, thus infusing the voices of lived experience and wellness narratives into the organizational culture. These experiences are valuable educational tools. This is also highly consistent with the research on stigma reduction, which finds that first-hand accounts are highly effective at helping to dispel stigma.

Focusing on the wellness lens provides an opportunity for providers to refocus beyond the deficit perspective when collaborating with service users. There are many wellness tools (e.g. https://www.center4healthandsdc.org/integrated-health--mental-health.html) and wellness inventories (e.g. https://alcoholstudies.rutgers.edu/wellness-in-recovery/quiz/) developed by service users that can be accessed and shared as self-help resources.

Conclusion

For 30 years in community mental health, there has been recognition of the importance of building a strong user-led movement (Mosher & Burti, 1994). This chapter has highlighted how a growing movement of people around the world, once relegated to the 'patient role', are contributing their 'expertise from experience' to inform, reform, and transform community mental health practice. Narratives from the lens of wellness offer important information that can have a tremendous impact on relationships, community mental health services, and ultimately outcomes. This chapter highlights the philosophical underpinning of the service user movement; describes the value of the integration of a wellness lens into the lived experience narrative; and illustrates the connections between wellness, social determinants of health, social justice, and lived experience. Practitioners are coming to understand the valuable impact the experience of receiving services has in terms of creating responsive engagement strategies and services seen through the lens of wellness. To build new wellness-focused services, service users must play strong roles as architects of services. Professionals, researchers, and policymakers need to move from tokenism to the understanding and awareness that service users have both a right and responsibility to be fully integrated into all aspects and levels of service delivery.

REFERENCES

Anglin, D. M., Ereshefsky, S., Klaunig, M. J., Bridgwater, M. A., Niendam, T. A., Ellman, L. M., et al. (2021). From womb to neighborhood: a racial analysis of social determinants of psychosis in the United States. *American Journal of Psychiatry*, **178**, 599–610.

Anglin, D. M., Lighty, Q., Greenspoon, M., & Ellman, L. M. (2014). Racial discrimination is associated with distressing subthreshold positive psychotic symptoms among US urban ethnic minority young adults. *Social Psychiatry and Psychiatric Epidemiology*, **49**, 1545–1555.

Benbow, S. (2009). Societal abuse in the lives of individuals with mental illness. *The Canadian Nurse*, **105**, 30–32.

Bor, J., Venkataramani, A. S., Williams, D. R., & Tsai, A. C. (2018). Police killings and their spillover effects on the mental health of black Americans: a population-based, quasi-experimental study. *Lancet*, **392**, 302–310.

Brandow, C. L., Brandow, J. S., & Cave, C. (2019). A wellness first approach: a lens for improving mental health and well-being. *Ethical Human Psychology and Psychiatry*, **21**, 39–54.

Brice, G. H., Swarbrick, M. A., & Gill, K. J. (2014). Promoting wellness of peer providers through coaching. *Journal of Psychosocial Nursing and Mental Health Services*, **52**, 41–45.

Byrne, L., Stratford, A., & Davidson, L. (2018). The global need for lived experience leadership. *Psychiatric Rehabilitation Journal*, **41**, 76–79.

Chamberlin, J. (1978). *On Our Own: Patient Controlled Alternatives to the Mental Health System*. New York: McGraw-Hill.

Commission on Social Determinants of Health (2008). *Closing the Gap in a Generation: Health Equity through Action on the Social Determinants of Health. Final Report of the Commission on Social Determinants of Health*. Geneva: World Health Organization.

Dunn, H. L. (1961). *High-Level Wellness*. Arlington, VA: Beatty Press.

Eddie, D., Hoffman, L., Vilsaint, C., Abry, A., Bergman, B., Hoeppner, B., et al. (2019). Lived experience in new models of care for substance use disorder: a systematic review of peer recovery support services and recovery coaching. *Frontiers in Psychology*, **10**, 1052.

Fletcher, E., Barroso, A., & Croft, B. (2020). A case study of a peer respite's integration into a public mental health system. *Journal of Health Care for the Poor and Underserved*, **31**, 218–234.

Goffman, E. (1963). *Stigma: Notes on the Management of Spoiled Identity*. Englewood Cliffs, NJ: Prentice-Hall.

Hatzenbuehler, M. L. (2016). Structural stigma and health inequalities: research evidence and implications for psychological science. *American Psychologist*, **71**(8), 742–751.

Hatzenbuehler, M. L. & Link, B. G. (2014). Introduction to the special issue on structural stigma and health. *Social Science & Medicine*, **103**, 1–6.

Hipes, C., Lucas, J., Phelan, J. C., & White, R. C. (2016). The stigma of mental illness in the labor market. *Social Science Research*, **56**, 16–25.

Jacobs, Y. (2015, 4 June). What the research has told us about peer-run respite houses: the Second Story story. *Mad in America*. https://www.madinamerica.com/2015/06/what-the-research-has-told-us-about-peer-run-respites

Jiménez-Solomon, O. G., Méndez-Bustos, P., Swarbrick, M., Díaz, S., Silva, S., Kelley, M., et al. (2016). Peer-supported economic empowerment: a financial wellness intervention framework for people with psychiatric disabilities. *Psychiatric Rehabilitation Journal*, **39**, 222–233.

Jones, N., Atterbury, K., Byrne, L., Carras, M., Brown, M., & Phalen, P. (2021). Lived experience, research leadership, and the transformation of mental health services: building a researcher pipeline. *Psychiatric Services*, **72**, 591–593.

Legere, L., Nemec, P. B., & Swarbrick, M. (2013). Personal narrative as a teaching tool. *Psychiatric Rehabilitation Journal*, **36**, 319–321.

Legislative Analysis and Public Policy Association (2021, February). Peer respites as an alternative to hospitalization. http://legislativeanalysis.org/wp-content/uploads/2021/02/Peer-Respites-as-an-Alternative-to-Hospitilzation-FINAL.pdf

Luciano, A. & Meara, E. (2014). Employment status of people with mental illness: national survey data from 2009 and 2010. *Psychiatric Services*, **65**, 1201–1209.

Marrone, J. & Swarbrick, M. (2020). Long-term unemployment: a social determinant underaddressed within community behavioral health programs. *Psychiatric Services*, **71**, 745–748

Medlock, M., Weissman, A., Wong, S. S., Carlo, A., Zeng, M., Borba, C., et al. (2017). Racism as a unique social determinant of mental health: development of a didactic curriculum for psychiatry residents. *MedEdPORTAL*, **13**, 10618.

Mosher, L. & Burti, L. (1994). *Community Mental Health: A Practical Guide*. New York: Norton & Company.

National Association of Peer Supporters (2019). National practice guidelines for peer specialist and supervisors. https://www.peersupportworks.org/wp-content/uploads/2020/08/National-Practice-Guidelines-for-Peer-Specialists

National Co-production Advisory Group. (2021). Co-productions: it's a long term relationship [Infographic]. https://www.thinklocalactpersonal.org.uk/_assets/COPRODUCTION/Ladder-of-coproduction.pdf

National Social Inclusion Programme (2009). Vision and progress: social inclusion and mental health. http://www.socialinclusion.org.uk/publications/NSIP_Vision_and_Progress.pdf

Ostrow, L. & Croft, B. (2014). *Toolkit for Evaluating Peer Respites*. Cambridge, MA: Human Services Research Institute.

Ostrow, L. & Croft, B. (2015). Peer respites: a research and practice agenda. *Psychiatric Services*, **66**, 638–640.

Pelto-Piri, V., Engström, K., & Engström, I. (2013). Paternalism, autonomy and reciprocity: ethical perspectives in encounters with patients in psychiatric in-patient care. *BMC Medical Ethics*, **14**, 49.

Prevention Institute (2017). *What? Why? How? Answers to Frequently Asked Questions about the Adverse Community Experiences and Resilience Framework*. Oakland, CA: Prevention Institute.

Queensland Mental Health Commission (2018). Shifting minds: Queensland mental health, alcohol and other drugs strategic plan 2018–2023. https://www.qmhc.qld.gov.au/sites/default/files/files/qmhc_2018_strategic_plan.pdf

Ridgway, P. (2001). Restorying psychiatric disability: learning from first person recovery narratives. *Psychiatric Rehabilitation Journal*, **24**, 335–343.

Roe, D., Hasson-Ohayon, I., Mashiach-Eizenberg, M., Derhy, O., Lysaker, P. H., & Yanos, P. T. (2014). Narrative enhancement and cognitive therapy (NECT) effectiveness: a quasi-experimental study. *Journal of Clinical Psychology*, **70**, 303–312.

Shevlin, M., Houston, J. E., Dorahy, M. J., & Adamson, G. (2007). Cumulative traumas and psychosis: an analysis of the national comorbidity survey and the British psychiatric morbidity survey. *Schizophrenia Bulletin*, **34**, 193–199.

Siegel, C. E., Reid-Rose, L., Joseph, A. M., Hernandez, J. C., & Haugland, G. (2016). Cultural activation of consumers. *Psychiatric Services*, **67**, 153–155.

Substance Abuse and Mental Health Services Administration (2015). *Core Competencies for Peer Workers in Behavioral Health Services*. Rockville, MD: US Department of Health and Human Services, Substance Abuse and Mental Health Services Administration. http://www.samhsa.gov/sites/default/files/programs_campaigns/brss_tacs/corecompetencies.pdf

Swarbrick, M. (1997). A wellness model for clients. *Mental Health Special Interest Section Quarterly*, **20**, 1–4.

Swarbrick, M. (2006). A wellness approach. *Psychiatric Rehabilitation Journal*, **29**, 311–314.

Swarbrick, M. (2012). A wellness approach to mental health recovery. In: Rudnick, A. (Ed.), *Recovery of People with Mental Illness: Philosophical and Related Perspectives* (pp. 30–38). Oxford: Oxford University Press.

Swarbrick, M. (2015). *Peer Wellness Respite Training Manual*. Freehold, NJ: Collaborative Support Programs of New Jersey, Inc.

Swarbrick, M. (2020) *Crisis from the Lens of Wellness*. Freehold, NJ: Collaborative Support Programs of New Jersey, Inc.

Swarbrick, M., DiGioia-Laird, V., Estes, A., Kavalkovich, S., Nemec, P., Pelland, J., et al. (2022). *Journey to Wellness*. Piscataway, NJ: Center of Alcohol & Substance Use Studies, Graduate School of Applied and Professional Psychology, Rutgers University. https://alcoholstudies.rutgers.edu/wellness-in-recovery/journey-to-wellness-guide/

Swarbrick, M., Gill, K. J., & Pratt, C. W. (2016). Impact of peer delivered wellness coaching. *Psychiatric Rehabilitation Journal*, **39**, 234–238.

Swarbrick, M., Kuebler, C., Treitler, P., Estes, A., Digioia-Laird, V., Moosvi, K., & Nemec, P. (2023). Co-production: journey to wellness guide. *Journal of Psychosocial Nursing and Mental Health Services*, **61**, 24–30.

Swarbrick, M. & Nemec, P. B. (2016). Supporting the health and wellness of individuals with psychiatric disabilities. *Rehabilitation Research, Policy, and Education*, **30**, 321–333.

Swarbrick, M., Tunner, T. P., Miller, D. W., Werner, P., & Tiegreen, W. W. (2016). Promoting health and wellness through peer-delivered services: three innovative state examples. *Psychiatric Rehabilitation Journal*, **39**, 204–210.

Vojtila, L., Ashfaq, I., Ampofo, A., Dawson, D., & Selby, P. (2021). Engaging a person with lived experience of mental illness in a collaborative care model feasibility study. *Research Involvement and Engagement*, **7**, 5.

Watson, A. C., Corrigan, P., Larson, J. E., & Sells, M. (2007). Self-stigma in people with mental illness. *Schizophrenia Bulletin*, **33**, 1312–1318.

White, M. (2004). Folk psychology and narrative practices. In: Angus, L. E. & McLeod, J. (Eds). *The Handbook of Narrative and Psychotherapy* (pp. 15–51). London: Sage.

Yanos, P. T., Roe, D., & Lysaker, P. H. (2011). Narrative enhancement and cognitive therapy: a new group-based treatment for internalized stigma among persons with severe mental illness. *International Journal of Group Psychotherapy*, **61**, 576–595.

Zinman, S., Harp, H., and Budd, S. (1987). *Reaching Across: Mental Health Clients Helping Each Other*. CA: California Network of Mental Health.

Measuring mental health needs

Mike Slade and Graham Thornicroft

Introduction

The importance of needs assessment has been one of the most consistent themes to emerge from the evolution of community mental health services. The term 'need' has become especially influential in European mental health practice. In the UK, for example, national policy has for more than two decades emphasized the importance of needs assessment underpinning the planning, development, and evaluation of mental health services (Department of Health, 1999).

However, the concept of 'need' is used in different, and sometimes contradictory, ways. At the individual level, all mental health and social care should be provided on the basis of need. At the population level, funding allocation is intended to match the needs of the population, so that whether or not overall resources are adequate, efficiency and equity are achieved. The aim of this chapter is to define needs assessment, to consider different approaches to assessing needs at the individual and at the population levels, and to discuss how needs assessments can be applied in real-world settings in planning and delivering clinical care.

What are needs?

A need involves a lack of something. But of what? A categorization of needs was identified by Brewin, who grouped definitions of need within mental health care into three categories: lack of health, lack of access to services or institutions, and lack of action by mental health workers (Brewin et al., 1987). Approaches to need within each of these three categories will be reviewed.

Needs for improved health

At the individual level, the concept of need has been grounded in various theories. Maslow put forward a theory of motivation in terms of a hierarchy of needs: physiological; safety; belongingness and love; esteem; and self-actualization (Maslow, 1954). He proposed that people are motivated by the requirement to meet these needs, and that higher-level needs could only be met once the lower and more fundamental needs were met. The clinical relevance of this theory is that it implies a hierarchy of clinical priorities—interventions to meet basic physiological need (e.g. to ensure adequate food supply) should take priority over interventions to foster, for example, self-esteem.

In practice, health and social care needs are often identified in a widely defined way. In England, for example, the requirement to base the provision of services on level of need was first made explicit in the National Health Service and Community Care Act (Department of Health, 1990), which defined need as 'the requirements of individuals to enable them to achieve, maintain or restore an acceptable level of social independence or quality of life'. This definition equates need with social disablement, which occurs when a person experiences lowered psychological, social, and physical functioning in comparison with the norms of society. Three categories of social functioning measures have been identified: social attainment measures, social role performance measures, and instrumental behaviour measures (Wykes & Hurry, 1991).

Social attainments are achievements in the major life roles, such as marriage and employment. They have the advantage of being easily measurable with relatively high reliability, and so are particularly suited to large-scale, nomothetic studies and epidemiological research. For example, at a population level, significantly higher admission rates are associated with being unmarried, living alone, social deprivation, and drug misuse, and there is a large negative correlation between recovery from schizophrenia and unemployment (Warner, 2004). However, it is difficult to establish whether variables being measured are in a causal or correlative relationship.

Social role performance measures relate to how well a person is coping in their major roles of work, relationships, home, and self-care. They give a more in-depth assessment of a person's performance than social attainment measures, and cover a wide range of subdivided areas, such as instrumental and affective tasks. It can be difficult to take account of the person's social and cultural background, although this has been attempted by using consensual professional judgement (Gurland et al., 1972) or by normative scales (Cochrane & Stopes-Roe, 1977). Definitions of what constitutes pathological lack of function are culture specific, an issue recognized in taxonomic debates (Regier et al., 2009).

Instrumental measures record social behaviour, and are more suited to a detailed assessment of individual mental health service users, some of whom may not fulfil many life roles. A detailed description of behaviour allows consideration of cultural factors when analysing the data, but do not take account of the context in which behaviour takes place—the person with hygiene problems who does not have access to pleasant washing facilities. They are often designed for use with very disabled people, and so rely on staff reports which may not take account of the person's perceptions of their needs.

Best practice involves *needs-led* care planning: basing the care provided for an individual service user on an assessment of their needs. This approach offers many benefits:

- The overall level of need gives guidance about which part of the mental health system should treat the service user, for example, that people with less disabling mental disorders should be seen in primary care settings.
- Needs assessment can improve the comprehensiveness of case formulations and care plans by incorporating a broad range of health determinants, such as poor housing or lack of social support.
- Explicit identification of need can support clinician–service user discussions about care priorities, which is associated with improved treatment satisfaction (Lasalvia et al., 2005) and adherence to treatment (Gray et al., 2006).
- Identification of needs helps to identify the contribution of services outside the mental health sector.
- Needs-led care can facilitate more individualized treatment planning than diagnosis-driven approaches, by more closely matching the help offered to individual's needs.

Needs-led care planning can be differentiated from the assessment of *care* needs. Assessing care needs involves identifying whether the person will benefit from a predefined set of interventions. This will not identify all unmet needs for individual service users. Assessment of need at the individual level should therefore be a separate process from decisions about what care or treatment to provide. There are, of course, other reasons to consider needs for services, to which we now turn.

Needs for services

The second category of needs assessment schedules suggested by Brewin incorporates those measuring access to mental health services. Underlying these measures is the assumption that an unmet need indicates a lack of access to some form of psychiatric service. This category is used for informing the development of mental health services. It is less appropriate at an individual level, since it assesses needs through the filter of existing services.

At the population level, it is possible to use epidemiological methods to develop prevalence for different disorders, which can be translated into estimates of the need for services. For example, recent data from the World Mental Health Surveys show that the large majority of people with major depression disorder, anxiety disorders, and alcohol use disorder in global household survey in more than 20 countries received no minimally effective treatment (Alonso et al., 2018; Degenhardt et al., 2017; Patel et al., 2018; Thornicroft, 2007; Thornicroft et al., 2017; Wang et al., 2007) (**Figure 7.1**).

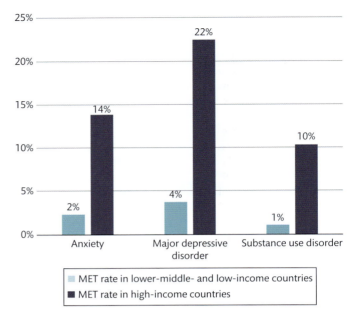

Figure 7.1 Minimally effective treatment (MET) across different resource settings.

Needs for action

Different types of need have been identified: felt (experienced), expressed (experienced and communicated), normative (judgement of professionals), and comparative (based on comparison with the position of other individuals or reference groups) (Bradshaw, 1972). This takes account of the different perceptions of need that can exist. Within health care this approach to need has been used to identify the circumstances when services should provide interventions. Need is taken to mean the ability to benefit in some way from health care, and thus distinguished from demand (what the person asks for) and supply (services given) (Stevens & Gabbay, 1991).

This raises the important topics of coverage and focusing. *Coverage* means the proportion of people who receive treatment who could benefit from it (Habicht et al., 1984). *Focusing* refers to how far those people who actually receive treatment in fact need it: do they have any form of mental disorder (Tansella, 2006)? Even in the most well-resourced countries one can find both low coverage and poor focusing (World Health Organization, 2008). From the public health perspective, therefore, the key issue is to increase both coverage and focus through the optimal use of resources, whatever the level of resources actually available.

Using this definition of need, an Australian study compared current and optimal treatment for ten high-burden mental disorders (Andrews et al., 2004). It showed that current levels of treatment at current coverage avert 13% of the overall burden attributable to these disorders. Providing optimal treatment at current coverage would avert 20% of the burden, and optimal treatment at optimal coverage would avert 28%. The development of a more robust treatment evidence base makes this innovative approach to informing public policy more possible, and the approach can be recommended for evidence-based policy initiatives.

Individual-level needs assessment measures

Several standardized approaches to the assessment of patient-level need have been developed, primarily in the UK. These have shown a transition along a continuum, from an initial focus on assessment of need as an objective state to be defined by experts following careful assessment, towards those which emphasize the subjective nature of needs assessment. Measures which focus on expert assessment include the Medical Research Council Needs for Care Assessment (NFCAS) (Brewin et al., 1987) and the Cardinal Needs Schedule (CNS) (Marshall et al., 1995), which also considers service user willingness to accept help and level of carer concern. Training is needed for using both the NFCAS and the CNS, and they are primarily used for research purposes (Kovess-Masféty et al., 2006). At the other end of this continuum are measures such as the AVON Mental Health Measure (Markovitz, 1996), the Carers and Users Experience of Services (CUES) (Lelliott et al., 2001), and the Client Assessment of Strengths, Interests and Goals (CASIG) (Lecomte et al., 2004; Wallace et al., 2001).

However, the Camberwell Assessment of Need (CAN) (Slade & Thornicroft, 2020) spans both ends of the continuum.

Camberwell Assessment of Need

The CAN is a standardized measure for assessing the needs of people experiencing severe and/or enduring mental health problems. It covers 22 health and social needs, and incorporates staff, service user, and informal carer perspectives. The CAN was developed for use by three groups:

1. Mental health workers involved in planning care for people with severe mental health problems
2. Mental health service users in rating their own needs
3. People wanting to evaluate mental health services.

Four versions of the CAN have been developed:

1. Camberwell Assessment of Need Short Appraisal Schedule (CANSAS): a version which assesses the presence of a need in the 22 CAN domains from any of service user, staff, or informal carer perspectives. CANSAS has emerged as the most useful CAN version for most clinical and research uses.
2. CANSAS—Patient-rated (CANSAS-P): a self-rated version of CANSAS, which can be self-completed with or without support. CANSAS-P is the CAN version to use where service users are self-rating their needs (Trauer et al., 2008).
3. CAN—Clinical (CAN-C): a full assessment of health and social needs, designed for clinical use. For each of the 22 CAN domains, CAN-C assesses the need rating, help received from informal carers and from services, help needed from services, and the service user's views about support needed, along with space to record a domain-specific action plan.
4. CAN—Clinical (CAN-R): a full assessment of health and social needs, designed for research use. For each of the 22 CAN domains, CAN-R assesses the need rating, help received from informal carers and from services, help needed from services, and satisfaction with the type and amount of help received.

Since the English language version was published in 1995 (Phelan et al., 1995), the CAN has been translated into 30 languages: Afrikaans, Cantonese, Czech, Danish, Dutch, French, German, Greek, Hebrew, Hindi, Hungarian, Icelandic, Indonesian, Italian, Kannada, Lithuanian, Malaysian (Bahasa), Maltese, Mandarin (mainland China), Mandarin (Taiwanese), Norwegian, Polish, Portuguese, Portuguese (Brazil), Romanian, Spanish, Swedish, Turkish, Vietnamese, and Xhosa. Contact details for CAN translators are listed on the CAN website (researchintorecovery.com/can).

Variants of the CAN have also been published, and are in widespread use for other populations:

- Older adults: Camberwell Assessment of Need for the Elderly (CANE) (Orrell & Hancock, 2004; Reynolds et al., 2000)
- People with learning or intellectual disabilities: Camberwell Assessment of Need for Developmental and Intellectual Disabilities (CANDID) (Xenitidis et al., 2000, 2003)
- Forensic patients: Camberwell Assessment of Need—Forensic (CANFOR) (Thomas et al., 2003, 2008)
- Mothers and pregnant women with mental health problems (CAN-M) (Howard et al., 2007, 2008)
- People in disaster relief situations: Humanitarian Emergency Settings Perceived Needs (HESPER) scale (Semrau et al., 2012).

Since the original psychometric evaluation of the CAN-R, many further psychometric studies have been published. Some studies have been led by the developers of the CAN, such as the evaluation of the Danish, Dutch, German, Italian, and Spanish translations of the CAN (McCrone et al., 2000) and the comparison of the performance of CAN against three other standardized measures in routine practice (Salvi et al., 2005). Others have been led by separate research groups in collaboration with the CAN developers, such as the psychometric evaluation of the CANSAS-P (Trauer et al., 2008) and of the Mandarin (Taiwanese) translation of the CAN (Yeh et al., 2006). The majority of psychometric evaluations have been conducted independently by other research groups, both in relation to the English version of the CAN (Andresen et al., 2000; Arvidsson, 2003; Bender, 2001; Wennstrom & Wiesel, 2006; Wennstrom et al., 2004, 2008) and in relation to non-English versions including the Dutch (Van der Krieke et al., 2011), Italian (Ruggeri et al., 1999), Portuguese (Brazil) (Schlithler et al., 2007), Spanish (Rosales et al., 2002), and Swedish (Hansson et al., 1995) translations.

The CAN is now the most widely used needs assessment measure in mental health systems internationally (Trauer, 2010). For example, in relation to psychosis, it is the most widely cited measure in first-episode psychosis studies (Davies et al., 2018) and a review of patient-reported outcomes in schizophrenia concluded that 'the most commonly used measures are the Camberwell Assessment of Need and the Camberwell Assessment of Need Short Appraisal Schedule' (McCabe et al., 2007, p. s22). It is also used to assess needs in diverse mental health groups (e.g. psychosis (Mascayan et al., 2019), bipolar disorder (Esan & Medubi, 2018), common mental disorders (Loranger et al., 2020)), with other clinical (e.g. neurology (Sinu et al., 2018), HIV (Durbin et al., 2017)) and non-clinical (e.g. sex trafficking (Graham et al., 2019), asylum seekers (McColl & Johnson, 2006), and non-clinical voice hearers (Jacobsen et al., 2018)) populations, and to compare the needs of different populations, such as people with and without intellectual disabilities in mental health case management services (Durbin et al., 2017). Finally, it has been used in many different service settings, specifically including inpatient (Ritsner et al., 2018) and youth mental health services (Vijverberg et al., 2018). An independent review of needs assessment measures concluded that 'only the CAN addressed a wide range of needs' (Beran, 2015, p. 6). Independent systematic reviews of measures for CAN variants have also been positive, for example 'the "CANE" qualifies best to assess the needs not only of demented individuals but of older individuals in general including those with mental illnesses' (Schmid et al., 2012, p. 339).

Empirical findings from Camberwell Assessment of Need research

Three main empirical results have emerged as consistent and replicated findings across different service setting and countries. The evidence base for these findings is presented elsewhere (Slade & Thornicroft, 2020), so here we simply identify and elaborate each finding.

- Empirical finding 1: mental health staff and service users do not rate the service user's needs in the same way, so their assessments are not interchangeable. Staff, service users, and informal carers do not assess needs in the same way, so their differing perspectives are needed for a full clinical assessment.
- Empirical finding 2: clinical care planning should be based on assessing and then meeting unmet needs identified by the service user. The service user perspective on their current serious problems ('unmet needs') is more predictive of outcome than staff assessments.
- Empirical finding 3: CAN is an approach to supporting recovery. There is international consensus about the need for a recovery orientation to be the guiding vision for mental health services (World Health Organization, 2013), and using CAN as the basis for identifying service user-rated unmet needs increases recovery support from services.

Moving from individual to population levels

In the attempt to move from considering the needs of mentally ill individuals to establishing overall community needs, these complexities are compounded in three ways. First, the needs of a wider range of individuals must be considered. These include immediate carers, people such as neighbours, and local authority staff, for example, in housing and environmental health. Second, the translation of counts of treatment-amenable problems or service needs into institutional or staff provision requirements raises questions about service design models. What sort of agency should provide particular services, in what type of setting, and how much user choice in service style should be supported by public funding authorities? Third, since reasonable requests for assistance are likely to outstrip available resources, the practical questions which emerge relate to relative rather than absolute need. Thus, we need not only to determine the existence and scale of needs, but also their importance in comparison to each other.

The overall level of needs for mental health services varies between places, reflecting differences in the prevalence of disorders. The nature of need has also changed over recent decades, reflecting developments in therapeutic capabilities, particularly in the provision of psychological therapies, changes in the extent to which severely mentally ill people's service needs have been moulded by institutionalization, and secular trends in the incidence of mental disorders.

Measures to assess population need

Measures to assess population need can be classified by the data and by the analytic approaches they use. Three types of data are commonly used. The first type of data describes the use of current mental health services. While this can be criticized as reflecting only current service provision, its ready availability and nationwide coverage mean that is extensively used.

Second, direct surveys of population-based morbidity, using epidemiological instruments, undertaken at a small or a large scale, offer a perspective independent of service activity. Simple population-based samples are very inefficient in estimating the prevalence of relatively rare conditions such as schizophrenia. Studies thus tend to use two-stage procedures, with a relatively brief initial screening process applied to a large number of people followed in-depth interviews for a selected few. 'Booster' samples, perhaps including all the known mental health service users for the areas surveyed, may be sought through mental health services (Jenkins et al., 1997). Population surveys depend on the identification of randomly sampled individuals. Some types of mental health problem, notably substance misuse, are commonly associated with socially marginal lifestyles, making it likely that sufferers will be systematically under-represented by traditional population sampling approaches.

The third type of data relates to the views of local people. Local needs assessment studies entail a structured approach to eliciting the views of service users, their carers, interested voluntary sector organizations, and all statutory agencies with responsibilities in the area. H. Smith (1998) has described how this type of study can be integrated into the overall planning process.

Government initiatives in England have tried to base the allocation of money between areas on the morbidity as well as the size of their populations. This has led to studies modelling this variation. The first widely used index was developed on the basis of consensus between general practitioners about patient-level characteristics associated with high use of primary care services (Jarman, 1983). While developed for wider purposes, this was shown to relate reasonably closely to variations in psychiatric admission. Later indices have been established by statistical modelling exercises seeking to quantify the relationship between social variables measured in censuses and either service use (McCrone et al., 2006) or population-based epidemiological findings. The variation between places in the prevalence of the less severe types of mental health issues commonly dealt with in primary care is less than that for problems usually managed by specialist mental health services, which again is much less than that observed for forensic services. Thus, models developed for one level of care should not be used to estimate patterns of need for other levels.

In practice, no single approach to assessing the needs of a population will suffice. Needs assessment at this level requires the integration of many perspectives. Examples of population-level needs assessment from the US, Canada, and New Zealand also reveal that epidemiological studies may not produce data that correspond directly to needs, and that some subpopulations, for example, particular ethnic groups, may be less well represented in such approaches, unless considerable methodological care is taken (Hanson et al., 2007; Kumar et al., 2006; Messias et al., 2007).

A set of techniques that offer considerable promise are rapid appraisal/rapid assessment techniques. These are methods to undertake brief assessments of population needs which are focused upon key focused questions, for example, on how primary care services should be augmented to treat people with depression, and examples of these approaches have been used to positive effect in South Africa (Flisher et al., 2007).

A second approach involves synthetic estimates of prevalence, which use established national case registers to estimate the prevalence of specific disorders (Martin & Wright, 2009). This approach has not been widely applied in mental health services, but in other areas of health care has been used to identify geographic inequities in service provision (Low et al., 2007).

The relationship between individual- and population-level data

At the level of individuals with mental health issues, there is a trend to increasingly involve service users/consumers in assessing needs. We have reviewed evidence that this produces a more comprehensive basis for care planning. There has been an important conceptual shift away from the view that professionals defined 'needs' while consumers stated 'demands', to a better appreciation of the many advantages to be gained from identifying, as far as possible, unmet needs in a joint and consensual way as a basis for action. If the provision of care for individuals should be based on assessment of their health and social needs, can these individual assessments be aggregated to inform service?

For population-level service planning, the key question is what types of interventions to provide, and with what capacity? Therefore, data from individual needs assessments cannot simply be aggregated to inform service development decisions. Routinely collected information about individual-level needs will be incomplete in systematic ways (and therefore non-representative), and the sample will comprise people currently using services, so does not represent the needs of the population as a whole. Even if individual needs assessments were nationally aggregated, the principal outcome of population-based needs assessment—resource allocation—is not a neat business. The diversity of views (service user, staff, carer, taxpayer) make a shared interpretation of the data problematic. Any study to identify an equitable new allocation pattern creates winners and losers. Since the results only indicate relative levels of need, losers inevitably argue that their current absolute level of resourcing is already inadequate. Political decisions are thus introduced about how fast resources should be reassigned to achieve the new idea of 'equity', and whether the shift should be achieved by actual transfer, or by differential growth. Indeed, there is an increasingly clear call from service user/consumer groups for involvement in these priority-setting planning exercises (Healthcare Quality Improvement Partnership, 2016).

Shifts of revenue resources are much easier than shifts of capital, but moving the former out of step with the latter may lead to inefficiencies. At the same time, special resources (as always) are likely to be made available to encourage implementation of currently promising service innovations. This process may push the overall distribution of funds away from the point of equity. It is rare for this dimension to be formally considered in the allocation of special allowances. Issues of timeliness, political necessity, expedience, synergy, and leadership are all also likely to influence which of the many possible service developments is eventually implemented.

The CAN has been used to inform population-level needs assessment at national and large regional levels (Trauer & Tobias, 2004). For example, the Canadian province of Ontario (population 12 million) began the Community Mental Health Common Assessment Project (CMHCAP) in 2006, with the aim of choosing and implementing a common tool for use in all 300 Ontario community mental health services (D. Smith, 2010). CMHCAP staff were recruited for relevant subject matter expertise: change management, clinical and business analysis, procurement, project management expertise, communications, consumers, technical expertise, and adult education. A central aim was to ensure that implementation was owned by, and of benefit to, community mental health services.

A second example comes from the Netherlands, where the CAN is part of the Cumulative Needs for Care Monitor (CNCM) database, a psychiatric case register system in operation since 1998, which aims to standardize and improve needs-based diagnosis in use throughout a defined catchment area in the south of the country (population 660,000) (Drukker et al., 2010). The CAN is described as 'the core instrument of the CNCM'. This project is producing clinical findings directly informing service development, for instance, they found that compared with a control region, outpatient care consumption in the CNCM region was significantly higher regardless of treatment status at baseline (Drukker et al., 2011). Similarly, a study involving 2625 assessments of 1017 people on the case register found that the transition from unmet to met need can be tracked, and that needs relating to independent living were more sensitive to treatment effects than needs related to psychopathology and daytime activities (Drukker et al., 2008).

A final example is that CANSAS was chosen for use in the Minimum Data Set of the Partners in Recovery (PIR) national programme in Australia. This programme began in 2012 and continues as part of the National Disability Insurance Scheme. The programme involves 300 consortium partner organizations to provide coordinated support for 24,000 people with severe mental disorders and complex needs. The aims are to facilitate better coordination, strengthen partnerships, improve referral pathways, and promote a community-based recovery model. The routine collection of CAN data at national level has allowed investigation of focused questions, such as the relationship between accommodation and other need domains (Isaacs et al., 2019).

Conclusion

Assessment of need can involve compromises between desirable and attainable information, and value-based judgements about how and what to measure. It is a politically, ethically, and scientifically important concept, and so assessment should be as rigorous and comprehensive as possible. For both individual- and population-level needs assessment, this means that assessment should cover a wide range of health and social domains, should take account of different perspectives (e.g. service user, staff), and should be a separate process from treatment and resourcing decisions.

KEY REFERENCES

Andrews, G. & Henderson S. (Eds.) (2000). *Unmet Need in Psychiatry*. Cambridge: Cambridge University Press.

Slade, M. & Thornicroft, G. (2020). *Camberwell Assessment of Need* (2nd ed.). Cambridge: Cambridge University Press.

Thornicroft, G. (Ed.) (2001). *Measuring Mental Health Needs* (2nd ed.). London: Gaskell.

Thornicroft, G., Becker, T., Knapp, M., Knudsen, H. C., Schene, A. H., Tansella, M., et al. (2006). *International Outcomes in Mental Health: Quality of Life, Needs, Service Satisfaction, Costs and Impact on Carers*. London: Gaskell.

REFERENCES

Alonso, J., Liu, Z., Evans-Lacko, S., Sadikova, E., Sampson, N., Chatterji, S., et al. (2018). Treatment gap for anxiety disorders is global: results of the World Mental Health Surveys in 21 countries. *Depression and Anxiety*, **35**, 195–208.

Andresen, R., Caputi, P., & Oades, L. G. (2000). Interrater reliability of the Camberwell Assessment of Need Short Appraisal Schedule. *Australian and New Zealand Journal of Psychiatry*, **34**, 856–861.

Andrews, G., Issakidis, C., Sanderson, K., Corry, J., & Lapsley, H. (2004). Utilising survey data to inform public policy: comparison of the cost-effectiveness of treatment of ten mental disorders. *British Journal of Psychiatry*, **184**, 526–533.

Arvidsson, H. (2003). Test-retest reliability of the Camberwell Assessment of Need (CAN). *Nordic Journal of Psychiatry*, **57**, 279–283.

Bender, K. (2001). The Camberwell Assessment of Need rating scales. *Australian and New Zealand Journal of Psychiatry*, **35**, 691–692.

Beran, D. (2015). Needs and needs assessments: a gap in the literature for chronic diseases. *SAGE Open*, **5**. https://doi.org/10.1177/2158244015580375

Bradshaw, J. (1972). A taxonomy of social need. In: McLachlan, J. (Ed), *Problems and Progress in Medical Care: Essays on Current Research* (pp. 69–82). Oxford: Oxford University Press.

Brewin, C., Wing, J., Mangen, S., Brugha, T., & MacCarthy, B. (1987). Principles and practice of measuring needs in the long-term mentally ill: the MRC Needs for Care Assessment. *Psychological Medicine*, **17**, 971–981.

Cochrane, R. & Stopes-Roe, M. (1977). Psychological and social adjustment of Asian immigrants to Britain: a community survey. *Social Psychiatry*, **12**, 195–206.

Davies, E., Gordon, A., Pelentsov, L., Hooper, J., & Esterman, A. (2018). Needs of individuals recovering from a first episode of mental illness: a scoping review. *International Journal of Mental Health Nursing*, **27**, 1326–1343.

Degenhardt, L., Glantz, M., Evans-Lacko, S., Sadikova, E., Sampson, N., Thornicroft, G., et al. (2017). Estimating treatment coverage for people with substance use disorders: an analysis of data from the World Mental Health Surveys. *World Psychiatry*, **16**, 299–307.

Department of Health (1990). *National Health Service and Community Care Act*. London: The Stationery Office.

Department of Health (1999). *Mental Health National Service Framework*. London: The Stationery Office.

Drukker, M., Bak, M., Campo, J. A., Driessen, G., Van Os, J., & Delespaul, P. (2010). The cumulative needs for care monitor: a unique monitoring system in the south of the Netherlands. *Social Psychiatry and Psychiatric Epidemiology*, **45**(4), 475–485.

Drukker, M., van Dillen, K., Bak, M., Mengelers, R., van Os, J., & Delespaul, P. (2008). The use of the Camberwell Assessment of Need in treatment: what unmet needs can be met? *Social Psychiatry and Psychiatric Epidemiology*, **43**, 410–417.

Drukker, M., van Os, J., Dietvorst, M., Sytema, S., Driessen, G., & Delespaul, P. (2011). Does monitoring need for care in patients diagnosed with severe mental illness impact on psychiatric service use? Comparison of monitored patients with matched controls. *BMC Psychiatry*, **11**, 45.

Durbin, A., Sirotich, F., Lunsky, Y., & Durbin, J. (2017). Unmet needs of adults in community mental health care with and without intellectual and developmental disabilities: a cross-sectional study. *Community Mental Health Journal*, **53**, 15–26.

Durbin, A., Sirotich, F., Roesslein, K., & Durbin, J. (2017). Needs among persons with human immunodeficiency virus and intellectual and developmental disabilities in community mental health care: a cross-sectional study. *Journal of Intellectual Disability Research*, **61**, 292–299.

Esan, O. & Medubi, A. (2018). The self-perceived health-care needs of patients with bipolar disorder in Nigeria. *Journal of Psychosocial Rehabilitation and Mental Health*, **5**, 159–168.

Flisher, A., Lund, C., Funk, M., Banda, M., Bhana, A., Doku, V., et al. (2007). Mental health policy development and implementation in four African countries. *Journal of Health Psychology*, **12**, 505–516.

Graham, L., Macy, R., Eckhardt, A., Rizo, C., & Jordan, B. (2019). Measures for evaluating sex trafficking after care and support services: a systematic review and resource compilation. *Aggressive and Violent Behavior*, **47**, 117–136.

Gray, R., Leese, M., Bindman, J., Becker, T., Burti, L., David, A., et al. (2006). Adherence therapy for people with schizophrenia. European multicentre randomised controlled trial. *British Journal of Psychiatry*, **189**, 508–514.

Gurland, B., Yorkstone, N., Stone, A., & Frank, J. (1972). The Structured and Scaled Interview to Assess Maladjustment (SSIAM) 1. Description, rationale and development. *Archives of General Psychiatry*, **27**, 264–267.

Habicht, J., Mason, J., & Tabatabai, H. (1984). Basic concepts for the design of evaluations during programme implementation. Methods for the Evaluation of the Impact of Food and Nutrition Programmes. In: Sahn, D. R., Lockwood, R., & Scrimshaw, N. S. (Eds.), *Methods for the Evaluation of the Impact of Food and Nutrition Programmes. Food and Nutrition Bulletin* (Suppl. 8, pp. 1–25). New York: The United Nations University.

Hanson, L., Houde, D., McDowell, M., & Dixon, L. (2007). A population-based needs assessment for mental health services. *Administration and Policy in Mental Health and Mental Health Services Research*, **34**, 233–242.

Hansson, L., Bjorkman, T., & Svensson, B. (1995). The assessment of needs in psychiatric patients. Interrater reliability of the Swedish version of the Camberwell Assessment of Needs instrument and results from a cross-sectional study. *Acta Psychiatrica Scandinavica*, **92**, 285–293.

Healthcare Quality Improvement Partnership (2016). *Patient and Public Involvement in Quality Improvement*. London: HQIP Service User Network.

Howard, L., Hunt, K., Slade, M., O'Keane, V., Senevirante, T., Leese, M., & Thornicroft, G. (2007). Assessing the needs of pregnant women and mothers with severe mental illness: the psychometric properties of the Camberwell Assessment of Need—Mothers (CAN-M). *International Journal of Methods in Psychiatric Research*, **16**, 177–185.

Howard, L., Slade, M., O'Keane, V., Seneviratne, T., Hunt, K., & Thornicroft, G. (2008). *The Camberwell Assessment of Need for Pregnant Women and Mothers with Severe Mental Illness*. London: Gaskell.

Isaacs, A., Beauchamp, A., Sutton, K., & Maybery, D. (2019). Unmet needs of persons with a severe and persistent mental illness and their relationship to unmet accommodation need's. *Health & Social Care in the Community*, **27**, e246–e256.

Jacobsen, P., Peters, E., Ward, T., Garety, P., Jackson, M., & Chadwick, P. (2018). Overgeneral autobiographical memory bias in clinical and non-clinical voice hearers. *Psychological Medicine*, **49**, 113–120.

Jarman, B. (1983). Identification of underprivileged areas. *British Medical Journal*, **286**, 1705–1709.

Jenkins, R., Bebbington, P., Brugha, T., Farrell, M., Gill, B., & Lewis, G. (1997). The National Psychiatric Morbidity Surveys of Great Britain—strategy and methods. *Psychological Medicine*, **27**, 765–774.

Kovess-Masféty, V., Wiersma, D., Xavier, M., de Almada, J., Carta, M., Dubuis, J., et al. (2006). Needs for care among patients with schizophrenia in six European countries: a one-year follow-up study. *Clinical Practice and Epidemiological Mental Health*, **2**, 22.

Kumar, S., Tse, S., Fernando, A., & Wong, S. (2006). Epidemiological studies on mental health needs of Asian population in New Zealand. *International Journal of Social Psychiatry*, **52**, 408–412.

Lasalvia, A., Bonetto, C., Malchiodi, F., Salvi, G., Parabiaghi, A., Tansella, M., & Ruggeri, M. (2005). Listening to patients' needs to improve their subjective quality of life. *Psychological Medicine*, **35**, 1655–1665.

Lecomte, T., Wallace, C. J., Caron, J., Perreault, M., & Lecomte, J. (2004). Further validation of the Client Assessment of Strengths Interests and Goals. *Schizophrenia Research*, **66**, 59–70.

Lelliott, P., Beevor, A., Hogman, J., Hohman, G., Hyslop, J., Lathlean, J., & Ward, M. (2001). Carers' and Users' Expectations of Services—User version (CUES-U): a new instrument to measure the experience of users of mental health services. *British Journal of Psychiatry*, **179**, 67–72.

Loranger, C., Bamvita, J.-L., & Fleury, M.-J. (2020). Typology of patients with mental health disorders and perceived continuity of care. *Journal of Mental Health*, **29**, 296–305.

Low, A., Unsworth, L. & Miller, I. (2007). Avoiding the danger that stop smoking services may exacerbate health inequalities: building equity into performance assessment. *BMC Public Health*, **7**, 198.

Markovitz, P. (1996). *The Avon Mental Health Measure*. Bristol: Changing Minds.

Marshall, M., Hogg, L., Gath, D. H., & Lockwood, A. (1995). The Cardinal Needs Schedule: a modified version of the MRC Needs for Care Schedule. *Psychological Medicine*, **25**, 605–617.

Martin, D. & Wright, J. A. (2009). Disease prevalence in the English population: a comparison of primary care registers and prevalence models. *Social Science & Medicine*, **2**, 266–274.

Mascayan, F., Alvarado, R., Andrews, H., Jorquera, M., Lovisi, G., de Souza, F., et al. (2019). Implementing the protocol of a pilot randomized controlled trial for the recovery-oriented intervention to people with psychoses in two Latin American cities. *Cadernos de Saúde Pública*, **35**, e00108018.

Maslow, A. (1954). *Motivation and Personality*. New York: Harper and Row.

McCabe, R., Saidi, M., & Priebe, S. (2007). Patient-reported outcomes in schizophrenia. *British Journal of Psychiatry*, **191**, s21–s28.

McColl, H. & Johnson, S. (2006). Characteristics and needs of asylum seekers and refugees in contact with London community mental health teams: a descriptive investigation. *Social Psychiatry and Psychiatric Epidemiology*, **41**, 789–795.

McCrone, P., Leese, M., Thornicroft, G., Griffiths, G., Padfield, S., Schene, A., et al. (2000). Reliability of the Camberwell Assessment of Need—European Version: EPSILON Study 6. *British Journal of Psychiatry*, **177**, 34–40.

McCrone, P., Thornicroft, G., Boyle, S., Knapp, M., & Aziz, F. (2006). The development of a Local Index of Need (LIN) and its use to explain variations in social services expenditure on mental health care in England. *Health and Social Care in the Community*, **14**, 254–263.

Messias, E., Eaton, W., Nestadt, G., Bienvenu, O., & Samuels, J. (2007). Psychiatrists' ascertained treatment needs for mental disorders in a population-based sample. *Psychiatric Services*, **58**, 373–377.

Orrell, M. & Hancock, G. (2004). *The Camberwell Assessment of Need for the Elderly (CANE)*. London: Gaskell.

Patel, V., Saxena, S., Lund, C., Thornicroft, G., Baingana, F., Bolton, P., et al. (2018). The Lancet Commission on global mental health and sustainable development. *Lancet*, **392**, 1553–1598.

Phelan, M., Slade, M., Thornicroft, G., Dunn, G., Holloway, F., Wykes, T., et al. (1995). The Camberwell Assessment of Need: the validity and reliability of an instrument to assess the needs of people with severe mental illness. *British Journal of Psychiatry*, **167**, 589–595.

Regier, D. A., Narrow, W. E., Kuhl, E. A., & Kupfer, D. J. (2009). The conceptual development of DSM-V. *American Journal of Psychiatry*, **166**, 645–650.

Reynolds, T., Thornicroft, G., Abas, M., Woods, B., Hoe, J., Leese, M., & Orrell, M. (2000). Camberwell Assessment of Need for the Elderly (CANE): development, validity, and reliability. *British Journal of Psychiatry*, **176**, 444–452.

Ritsner, M., Farkash, H., Rauchberger, B., Amrami-Weizman, A., & Zendjidjian, X. (2018). Assessment of health needs, satisfaction with care, and quality of life in compulsorily admitted patients with severe mental disorders. *Psychiatry Research*, **267**, 541–550.

Rosales, V. C., Torres, G. F., Luna Del, C. J., Jimenez, E. J., & Martinez, M. G. (2002). [Reliability of the Spanish version of the Camberwell Assessment of Needs (CAN) (Spanish version of CAN Reliability Study)]. *Actas Españolas de Psiquiatría*, **30**, 99–104.

Ruggeri, M., Lasalvia, A., Nicolaou, S., & Tansella, M. (1999). [The Italian version of the Camberwell assessment of need (CAN), an interview for the identification of needs of care]. *Epidemiologia e Psichiatria Sociale*, **8**, 135–167.

Salvi, G., Leese, M., & Slade, M. (2005). Routine use of mental health outcome assessments: choosing the measure. *British Journal of Psychiatry*, **186**, 146–152.

Schlithler, A. C., Scazufca, M., Busatto, G., Coutinho, L. M., & Menezes, P. R. (2007). Reliability of the Brazilian version of the Camberwell Assessment of Needs (CAN) in first-episode psychosis cases in Sao Paulo, Brazil. *Revista Brasileira de Psiquiatria*, **29**, 160–163.

Schmid, R., Eschen, A., Rüegger-Frey, B., & Martin, M. (2012). Instruments for comprehensive needs assessment in individuals with cognitive complaints, mild cognitive impairment or dementia: a systematic review. *International Journal of Geriatric Psychiatry*, 27, 329–341.

Semrau, M., van Ommeren, M., Blagescu, M., Griekspoor, A., Howard, L. M., Jordans, M., et al. (2012). The development and psychometric properties of the Humanitarian Emergency Settings Perceived Needs (HESPER) Scale. *American Journal of Public Health*, 102, e55–e63.

Sinu, E., Parthasarathy, B., Reddy, K., & Thomas, P. (2018). Needs of persons with neurological disorders. *Indian Journal of Psychiatric Social Work*, 9, 29–37.

Slade, M. & Thornicroft, G. (2020). *Camberwell Assessment of Need* (2nd ed.). Cambridge: Cambridge University Press.

Smith, D. (2010). Outcome measurement in Canada. In: Trauer, T. (Ed.), *Outcome Measurement in Mental Health: Theory and Practice* (pp. 116–125). Cambridge: Cambridge University Press.

Smith, H. (1998). Needs assessment in mental health services: the DISC framework. *Journal of Public Health Medicine*, 20, 154–160.

Stevens, A. & Gabbay, J. (1991). Needs assessment needs assessment. *Health Trends*, 23, 20–23.

Tansella, M. (2006). Recent advances in depression. Where are we going? *Epidemiologia e Psichiatria Sociale*, 15, 1–3.

Thomas, S., Harty, M., Parrott, J., McCrone, P., Slade, M., and Thornicroft, G. (2003). *The Forensic CAN: Camberwell Assessment of Need Forensic Version (CANFOR)*. London: Gaskell.

Thomas, S. D., Slade, M., McCrone, P., Harty, M. A., Parrott, J., Thornicroft, G., & Leese, M. (2008). The reliability and validity of the forensic Camberwell Assessment of Need (CANFOR): a needs assessment for forensic mental health service users. *International Journal of Methods in Psychiatric Research*, 17, 111–120.

Thornicroft, G. (2007). Most people with mental illness are not treated. *Lancet*, 370, 807–808.

Thornicroft, G., Chatterji, S., Evans-Lacko, S., Gruber, M., Sampson, N., Aguilar-Gaxiola, S., et al. (2017). Undertreatment of people with major depressive disorder in 21 countries. *British Journal of Psychiatry*, 210, 119–124.

Trauer, T. (2010). *Outcome Measurement in Mental Health: Theory and Practice*. Cambridge: Cambridge University Press.

Trauer, T. & Tobias, G. (2004). The Camberwell Assessment of Need and Behaviour and Symptom Identification Scale as routine outcome measures in a psychiatric disability rehabilitation and support service. *Community Mental Health Journal*, 40, 211–221.

Trauer, T., Tobias, G., & Slade, M. (2008). Development and evaluation of a patient-rated version of the Camberwell Assessment of Need Short Appraisal Schedule (CANSAS-P). *Community Mental Health Journal*, 44, 113–124.

Van der Krieke, L., Sytema, S., Wiersma, D., Tielen, H., and van Hemert, A. (2011). Evaluating the CANSAS self-report (CANSAS-P) as a screening instrument for care needs in people with psychotic and affective disorders. *Psychiatry Research*, 188, 456–458.

Vijverberg, R., Ferdinand, R., Beekman, A., & Van Meijel, B. (2018). Factors associated with treatment intensification in child and adolescent psychiatry: a cross-sectional study. *BMC Psychiatry*, 18, 291.

Wallace, C. J., Lecomte, T., Wilde, J., & Libermann, R. P. (2001). CASIG: a consumer-centered assessment for planning individualized treatment and evaluating program outcomes. *Schizophrenia Research*, 50, 105–109.

Wang, P., Aguilar-Gaxiola, S., Alonso, J., Angermeyer, M., Borges, G., Bromet, E., et al. (2007). Use of mental health services for anxiety, mood, and substance disorders in 17 countries in the WHO world mental health surveys. *Lancet*, 370, 841–850.

Warner, R. (2004). *Recovery from Schizophrenia: Psychiatry and Political Economy* (3rd ed.) New York: Brunner-Routledge.

Wennstrom, E., Berglund, L., Lindback, J., & Wiesel, F. (2008). Deconstructing the 'black box' of the Camberwell assessment of need score in mental health services evaluation. *Social Psychiatry and Psychiatric Epidemiology*, 43, 714–719.

Wennstrom, E., Sorbom, D., & Wiesel, F. (2004). Factor structure in the Camberwell Assessment of Need. *British Journal of Psychiatry*, 185, 505–510.

Wennstrom, E. & Wiesel, F. (2006). The Camberwell assessment of need as an outcome measure in routine mental health care. *Social Psychiatry and Psychiatric Epidemiology*, 41, 728–733.

World Health Organization (2008). *Mental Health Gap Action Programme (mhGAP): Scaling Up Care for Mental, Neurological and Substance Use Disorders*. Geneva: World Health Organization.

World Health Organization (2013). *Mental Health Action Plan 2013–2020*. Geneva: World Health Organization.

Wykes, T. & Hurry, J. (1991). Social behaviour and psychiatric disorders. In: Bebbington, P. (Ed.), *Social Psychiatry: Theory, Methodology, and Practice* (pp. 183–208). New Brunswick, NJ: Transaction Press.

Xenitidis, K., Slade, M., Bouras, N., & Thornicroft, G. (2003). *CANDID: Camberwell Assessment of Need for adults with Developmental and Intellectual Disabilities*. London: Gaskell.

Xenitidis, K., Thornicroft, G., Leese, M., Slade, M., Fotiadou, M., Philp, H., et al. (2000). Reliability and validity of the CANDID—a needs assessment instrument for adults with learning disabilities and mental health problems. *British Journal of Psychiatry*, 176, 473–478.

Yeh, H. S., Luh, R. L., Liu, H. J., Lee, Y. C., & Slade, M. (2006). Reliability of the Camberwell assessment of need (Chinese version) for patients with schizophrenia at a daycare center of Taiwan. *Social Psychiatry and Psychiatric Epidemiology*, 41, 75–80.

8

Mental health, ethnicity, and cultural diversity

Evidence and challenges

Craig Morgan

Migration is the primary driving force behind increasing ethnic and cultural diversity in many societies around the world. The movement of people across (and within) national boundaries, be it in search of economic prosperity or fleeing war and persecution, has been a central feature of modern history and has accelerated in recent years (de Haas et al., 2020). The most recent World Migration Report (2020) estimates the total number of migrants (i.e. persons who have lived outside their country of birth for 12 months or more) is around 281 million or 3.6% of the world's population (International Organization for Migration, 2019). This represents a threefold increase in migration over the past 50 years. These estimates do not include settled minority ethnic populations where, increasingly, the majority were born in the countries to which their parents or grandparents migrated. In the UK, for example, minority ethnic groups now form around 14% of the population (approximately 9.5 million people), with this rising to over 50% in some areas of London (e.g. Newham) (Office for National Statistics, 2011). Several trends in migration are likely to have important ongoing political, economic, and social consequences. These include the *globalization of migration* (i.e. the tendency for more countries to be affected by migration, both inward and outward); the *acceleration of migration* (i.e. the continued rise in absolute numbers of migrants in most regions of the world); and the *differentiation of migration* (i.e. the increased diversity of types and origins of migrants moving to single countries) (de Haas et al., 2020). These trends are already evident in, for example, many European countries, including the UK (Platt & Nandi, 2020). What these processes point to is an inexorable rise in ethnic and cultural diversity in many countries. This has major implications for the development and delivery of public services and, in particular, poses an ongoing challenge for mental health policy and service provision.

It is these challenges that are the focus of this chapter. Three specific aspects are considered (with examples drawn from mainly the US and the UK): (1) the extent of, and variations in, mental health needs in migrant and minority ethnic groups; (2) access to and use of mental health services among these groups; and (3) proposals for ensuring mental health services are more responsive to the needs of ethnically and culturally diverse populations. To begin with, some definitions are necessary.

Culture, ethnicity, and race

There is often confusion and imprecision in use of the terms culture, ethnicity, and race. Culture has been variously defined; for example, as shared patterns of belief, feeling, and adaptation that people carry in their minds (Leighton & Hughes, 1961), as an organized group of ideas, habits, and conditioned responses shared by members of a society (Linton, 1956), and as a blue print for living (Kluckholm, 1944). Common to most definitions is the idea of culture as a set of socially shared guidelines that shape behaviour, values, and beliefs. These are learned during childhood and adulthood through contacts with, and participation in, core institutions (e.g. education, law, religion, and medicine) and customary events and practices (e.g. rites of passage rituals, funerals, and commemorative events) (Helman, 2007). Cultures are dynamic and heterogeneous, constantly evolving as a consequence of exposure to other beliefs, values, and practices most notably through migration and, increasingly, global media (Helman, 2007). This ties to further concepts, such as acculturation, assimilation, and biculturalism, which describe the various processes whereby migrants integrate into and become comfortable with the cultural values and practices of the new society. In turn, migrant populations often bring with them novel traditions and practices which in turn impact the new society, creating a dynamic interplay in which new and modified cultural forms emerge. This is the basis for the development of multicultural societies.

The defining characteristic of ethnicity is a sense of shared identity and group belonging that emerges from, for example, a common heritage, shared language, and physical appearance. Culture, in this definition, is one element that engenders a sense of ethnic identity. What is more, common experiences, particularly of racism and discrimination, in host societies can contribute to the development of a shared identity in migrants from otherwise culturally diverse backgrounds. Fernando (1991), for example, has argued that this is a key factor that has driven the emergence of a Caribbean ethnic identity among migrants to the UK and their children from the culturally diverse islands of the Caribbean. Identity is fluid and those aspects of our heritage and background that we choose to emphasize and which feel prominent at any one point may vary according to context—migrants to the UK from the Caribbean, for example, may identify with their region of origin when in the UK and with their island of origin when in the Caribbean or when socializing with others from the Caribbean (i.e. at one moment, Caribbean; at another, Trinidadian or Jamaican, etc.). Other identities based, for example, on social position, gender, or sexuality overlay and add complexity to any sense of ethnic identity.

In Europe, at least, ethnicity has supplanted race as the primary way of talking about diverse population groups. It is now well established that certain physical characteristics, such as skin colour, do not signify biologically homogeneous groups (Jones, 1981). Nevertheless, the perception that this is the case persists and underpins frequent and far-reaching prejudice and discrimination (racism). As Fernando (1991) puts it: 'though a biological myth, race continues to be a social reality' (p. 19). Furthermore, while the language of ethnicity and ethnic groups has replaced that of race in much discourse in science and health, skin colour is often used as a short cut to defining ethnic groups (e.g. Black vs White), such that race (as a social construct) and ethnicity are frequently conflated; ethnicity (contrary to the definition above) becomes fixed (e.g. as a variable in epidemiological research), with all the fluidity, complexity, and within-group heterogeneity stripped away.

What this brief discussion emphasizes, then, are the potential pitfalls, both for research and clinical practice, of entangling culture, ethnicity, and race; it further warns against using perceived membership of an ethnic or cultural group as a shortcut to acquiring (assuming) knowledge about an individual's beliefs, values, and needs (a point considered further below).

Mental health needs

Epidemiological evidence (1): prevalence and incidence

Studies of the epidemiology of mental disorder in migrant and minority ethnic populations within countries (the majority of which have been conducted in Europe and North America) have produced some varied, some consistent, and, at times, some surprising findings.

To begin with non-psychotic disorders (for which most useable data are of prevalence), examples from the UK and the US illustrate this. Past large-scale epidemiological surveys in the US[1]—which together constitute the Collaborative Psychiatric Epidemiology Surveys with combined samples of over 15,000—have provided a wealth of data on the distribution of mental disorders by ethnic group (Williams et al., 2010). A number of broad patterns emerge. First, the following groups, compared with White Americans, all had lower rates of both lifetime and past-year mental disorders: Black American (i.e. African American, Black Caribbean), Asian American, and Latino American (with the exception of Puerto Ricans). The prevalence of lifetime disorder for White Americans was around 37% (Kessler et al., 2005) compared with 28–31% for Black Americans (Williams et al., 2007), 14–18% for Asian Americans (Takeuchi et al., 2007), and 27–28% for Latino Americans (excluding Puerto Ricans, with a prevalence similar to White Americans of around 39%) (Alegria et al., 2007).

Within the broad Black American group, further analyses by Williams et al. (2007) suggest variations by sex, with higher levels of disorder in Black Caribbean men compared with African American men. These findings are somewhat surprising, and, in many respects, add to a confusing picture. For example, the earlier Epidemiologic Catchment Area study of 23,000 individuals in five communities found higher rates of both current and lifetime disorder (assessed using the Diagnostic Interview Schedule), particularly phobic and anxiety disorders, in Black Americans (26% current; 38% lifetime) compared with White Americans (19% current; 32% lifetime) (Robins & Reiger, 1991). For Hispanic groups, rates similar to those for White Americans were reported (Robins & Reiger, 1991). Other studies, albeit methodologically weaker, have reported higher, lower, and similar rates of disorder in minority ethnic groups in the US, summarized by Williams et al. (2010, pp. 269–277). One group for which there is perhaps more consistency in findings is American Indians. Several studies, as summarized by Williams et al. (2010, p. 279), have found higher rates of mental disorder in these populations. Finally, more recent analyses of data from four US surveys of over 20,000 adults reported similar overall patterns, that is, lower lifetime prevalences in Asian (23.5%), Black (37.0%), and Latino (38.8%) populations compared with White (45.6%) (Alvarez et al., 2019).

In the UK, there have been a small number of robust population-based studies of the prevalence of mental health problems by ethnic group. In the most recent, the 2014 Adult Psychiatric Morbidity Survey (McManus et al., 2016) of over 6000 individuals, there was some evidence of modest variations by ethnic group in the prevalence of common mental disorders (operationalized as a score of 12 or more on the CIS-R) in the week prior to interview, particularly among women (Stansfield et al., 2016). For example, the age-adjusted prevalence of any common mental disorder was higher among Black/Black British women (29.3%) compared with the White British women (20.9%). There were no differences between Black/Black British and White British men (i.e. 13.5% vs 13.5%). When specific diagnostic groups were considered, there was further evidence of variations among ethnic groups. These were, compared with other ethnic groups, high prevalences of past month post-traumatic stress disorder among Black men (5.1% vs, for example, 3.5% White British men) and women (10.9% vs, for example, 4.9% White British women) (Fear et al., 2016), of past-year drug dependence among Black men (11.5% vs 2–4% in other groups) and women (4.5% vs ≤2% in other groups) (Roberts et al., 2016), and of past-year

---

[1] These are the National Comorbidity Survey Replication, the National Survey of American Life, and the National Latino and Asian American Study.

alcohol dependency among White British men (5.2% vs. 1% to 4% in other groups) (Drummond et al., 2016). There was no evidence of ethnic differences in the prevalence of other disorders, including bipolar disorder, personality disorders, and self-harm (McManus et al., 2016).

A recent systematic review of six surveys since 1999 broadly reinforces the findings from the 2014 Adult Psychiatric Morbidity Survey, finding—at most—weak evidence of variations by ethnic group for most forms of mental distress, with the possible exception of suicidality, for which there is strong evidence of a relatively low prevalence among some groups (e.g. South Asian men and Black men and women) (Rees et al., 2016). Other less robust studies further suggest high rates of self-harm and suicide in young Asian women (Bhugra et al., 1999a, 1999b) and high rates of most disorders in the Irish population (Cochrane & Bal, 1989).

The evidence for schizophrenia and other psychoses is more consistent, most of it based on incidence rather than prevalence. There is now strong evidence from studies in the UK, the Netherlands, Sweden, Denmark, Australia, and the US that the incidence of schizophrenia and other psychoses is elevated in migrant and minority ethnic populations (Morgan et al., 2019). In their recent meta-analysis of population-based incidence studies of psychoses, Selten et al. (2020) found (from a total of 49 studies) an overall relative risk (RR) for developing psychosis among migrant groups of 2.13 (95% confidence (CI) 1.99–2.27) for non-affective psychoses and 2.94 (95% CI 2.28–3.79) for affective psychoses compared with indigenous or host populations. The RR was particularly high among migrants from countries outside of Europe (RR 2.94, 95% CI 2.63–3.29) and migrants from countries where the majority population is black (RR 4.19, 95% CI 3.42–5.14). This latter finding is important, as we know that it is more visible migrant and minority groups who experience more racism and discrimination (see below).

It is important to note here that migrant, in this meta-analysis, refers to both first- and subsequent-generation migrants (i.e. including settled minority populations). What is more, the degree of increased risk is not consistent across migrant and minority ethnic groups—as hinted at in the meta-analysis conducted by Selten and colleagues (2020). For example, the ÆSOP study (a three-centre incidence and case–control study) found that in the UK, compared with White British, the incidence of all psychoses was over six times higher in Black Caribbean, around four times higher in Black African, and between 1.5 and 2 times higher in Asian and Other White (i.e. non-British) populations (Fearon et al., 2006). In a study in east London, the incidence was again found to be higher in most migrant and minority ethnic groups (Kirkbride et al., 2008). However, in Pakistani and Bangladeshi populations, this appeared to be evident for women only. In the Netherlands, the incidence appears to be highest in Moroccan migrants (Veling et al., 2006). The reasons for these variations are unclear; however, speculation has focused on differential exposure to discrimination and the buffering effects of family supports and social networks (Morgan et al., 2010).

There have been fewer studies of the prevalence of psychoses. These have tended to report smaller disparities between Black Caribbean and White British populations (e.g. the Fourth National Survey found an annual prevalence of 0.8% for White British and 1.3% for Black Caribbean (Nazroo, 1997)). The more recent Adult Psychiatric Morbidity Survey found variations by sex (Bebbington et al., 2016). There was a marked increase in past year prevalence in Black/Black British men (3.2%) compared with White British men (0.3%); no differences were found between women. As in other studies, however, the total number of individuals with a probable psychotic disorder was small and this may explain the variability between them and the divergence from what is consistently reported in incidence studies.

Asylum seekers and refugees

Most of the data summarized above relates to settled minority ethnic populations. The mental health of asylum seekers and refugees merits particular comment as prior exposure to trauma and stress is likely to be common and, at least initially, legal status and right to remain in the new country may be uncertain. The United Nations High Commission for Refugees (2021) estimates that there are over 26 million refugees worldwide. Some indication of the likely extent of mental disorder in these populations is provided in a recent systematic review of 26 studies including over 6000 refugees and asylum seekers in 14 countries (Blackmore et al., 2020). Included studies varied methodologically. The overall prevalences of post-traumatic stress disorder (31.5%) and depression (31.5%) were especially high, albeit there was considerable variation across studies. In short, there is (not surprisingly) substantial need for mental health care in refugee populations, particularly related to trauma.

Epidemiological evidence (2): ethnicity, culture, and diagnosis

The epidemiological data on rates of mental disorder in diverse populations have, so far, been presented without consideration of two critical methodological issues: (1) the use of fixed, and often crude, ethnic categories; and (2) the validity of applying diagnostic concepts and measures developed within a particular cultural framework to diverse ethnic and cultural populations. In relation to the first, it is inevitable that large-scale cross-sectional research estimating rates of disorder in populations has to rely on relatively crude variables collected at one point in time. What the definition of ethnicity discussed above suggests is that the findings have to then be treated with caution. One important consideration is that overall estimates for each ethnic group may obscure within-group variations, which are hinted at in some of the reported differences by age and sex. It is the second issue, however, which is potentially more important.

All cultures develop beliefs and practices to explain and manage ill health, and these provide socially sanctioned frameworks within which feelings of physical and mental discomfort and distress are experienced, expressed, and made sense of; they influence the responses of others and shape what help is sought, when, and from whom. In other words, culture provides us with a language or idiom for expressing and understanding distress. What this means is that the assessments and measures used in epidemiological surveys, based on Western conceptions of mental health and disorder, may not accurately capture expressions of distress that fall outside of this paradigm. A common, perhaps stereotyped, example is the distinction between those cultures that tend to 'somatize' (i.e. express emotional distress through bodily feelings such as headaches, tension, upset stomach, or palpitations) and those that tend to 'psychologize' (i.e. express emotional distress in psychological terms such as feeling sad or anxious) (Bhui et al., 2004). In so far as standard assessments (e.g. CIS-R, CIDI) focus on psychological symptoms there is a question about their capacity to accurately measure and capture mental health problems in populations that tend to 'somatize' (e.g. Asian; Lin & Cheung, 1999). In short, and efforts to validate instruments cross-culturally notwithstanding, this raises the possibility that disorder is being over- or underdiagnosed in some migrant and minority ethnic groups, potentially invalidating reported findings.

To consider a contentious example. Many commentators have forcefully argued that the repeated finding that the incidence of schizophrenia and other psychoses is high in many migrant and minority (particularly Black) ethnic groups is a function of misdiagnosis, that is, of emotional distress arising from difficult life circumstances in Black and other minority populations being misconstrued as psychosis by predominantly White psychiatrists unfamiliar with cultural idioms of distress in these populations and/or influenced by negative cultural stereotypes of Black people (Fernando, 1991; Morgan & Hutchinson, 2010). There is evidence that misdiagnosis does occur, particularly from studies in the US (Williams et al., 2010). However, studies in the UK that have sought to test this directly in the Caribbean population (which has among the highest reported rates), suggest misdiagnosis alone is not a sufficient explanation. For example, in a study at the Maudsley Hospital in London (where many of the UK studies of migration, ethnicity, and psychosis have been conducted), Hickling et al. (1999) compared diagnoses made independently by British psychiatrists and by a Jamaican psychiatrist in the same group of 66 inpatients. The authors found no difference in the percentage of Black inpatients diagnosed with schizophrenia by the British psychiatrists or the Jamaican psychiatrist.

In two other UK studies designed to investigate racial stereotyping in psychiatric assessment using case vignettes, there was no evidence that psychiatrists were more likely to diagnose schizophrenia when the ethnicity of the individual in the vignette was Black (Lewis & David, 1991; Minnis et al., 2001). What is more, studies conducted in the Caribbean by the same researchers using the same methods do not find high rates (Bhugra et al., 1996; Mahy et al., 1999), a finding which is inexplicable if these methods systematically misdiagnose Black people as suffering from psychosis when they are not. This debate highlights an significant point. Important as cultural factors are, it cannot always and simply be assumed that these underpin ethnic variations in disorder—this, in fact, would be to conflate ethnicity and culture and carries with it the risk that the social origins of important mental health disparities may be obscured and ignored.

Epidemiological evidence (3): risk and protective factors

Taken together, the findings summarized above suggest a complicated picture, one which is confused further by the methodological issues that have been noted. What is perhaps most surprising (caveats about methodological problems notwithstanding) is that rates of common mental disorders are not more consistently higher in migrant and minority ethnic groups. There are well-established associations between exposure to adverse social contexts and experiences and all common mental disorders, particularly depression and anxiety (Scheid & Wright, 2017). Many from migrant and minority ethnic groups live in economically and socially deprived areas, have poorer housing, higher rates of unemployment, poorer education, and are exposed to high levels of discrimination and racism (Barnard & Turner, 2011; Hackett et al., 2020; Joseph Rowntree Foundation, 2022; Modood et al., 1997). It may be that counter-veiling factors, such as greater access to informal social and community supports, greater resilience, and more effective coping strategies, operate to mitigate the impact of such contexts and experiences on mental health. There is, however, limited research on this, which reflects an imbalance in mental health research in general, where the focus is on risk rather than protective factors. (As an important aside, this is a significant limitation as it may be that knowledge of protective factors is more valuable in developing policies and interventions to prevent mental disorder.)

This noted, the evidence that rates of serious mental disorder (i.e. psychoses) are higher (to varying degrees) in migrant and minority ethnic groups is substantial and there is now strong evidence that these high rates are largely determined by exposure over the life course to adverse social contexts and experiences, in contexts of long-standing structural discrimination (Anglin et al., 2021; Morgan et al., 2007; 2008; 2010, 2019). This (i.e. broadly similar rates of common mental disorders, higher rates of serious mental disorders) raises a number of intriguing possibilities, including (1) that emotional distress in certain migrant and minority ethnic groups is more often expressed in the form of perceived threats (paranoia) and distorted perceptions (hallucinations); (2) that exposure to particular types of adverse social experiences involving threat and intrusion (as is common in migrant and minority ethnic groups) more often leads to symptoms of psychosis; and/or (3) that delays in seeking help for emotional distress result in unchecked movement along a continuum of mental ill health, from depression and anxiety through to paranoia, hallucinations, and thought disorder (Morgan et al., 2019). These possibilities are largely speculative, but certainly merit consideration given the potential implications for intervention. What is more, irrespective of precise aetiological relationships, it is clear that individuals from migrant and minority ethnic populations who present to mental health services will, on average, have greater social and economic needs; these are important targets for intervention both as a basis for improving engagement and promoting recovery.

Access to, and use of, mental health services

There is strong evidence of marked variations in access to and engagement with mental health services among ethnic groups. Again, examples from the US and the UK illustrate this.

In the US, the Surgeon General's comprehensive review of research on culture and mental health, conducted 20 years ago, noted a number of ethnic disparities (US Department of Health and Human Services, 2001)—disparities that largely persist. For example, despite apparently similar rates of mental disorder (psychosis notwithstanding), there is evidence that African Americans (compared with White Americans) are less likely to receive treatment (largely because of lower rates of help-seeking) and more likely to use alternative therapies. This may be, partly, related to financial barriers specific to the US health care system. There is similar evidence that Asian and Latino Americans have very low rates of mental health service utilization. Related to the discussion above, there is some evidence that the likelihood of receiving particular diagnoses varies by migrant and minority ethnic group in the US. For example, a study by Minsky et al. (2003) of around 20,000 initial contacts with inpatient and outpatient services at the University of Medicine and Dentistry of New Jersey, found that Latinos were more likely to be diagnosed with major depression, despite higher levels of self-reported psychotic symptoms (odds ratio, 1.7).

Clinically, misdiagnosis matters in so far as it contributes to the receipt of inappropriate care. There is further evidence of variations in the type and length of care received. For example, in one study Asian Americans were found to experience longer inpatient stays than White Americans (Snowden & Cheung, 1990) and in another, African Americans were found to use emergency psychiatric services more than White Americans (Snowden, 1999), a finding that mirrors research in the UK on the Black Caribbean and Black African populations (see below). Finally, there is evidence of high dropout rates among minority ethnic groups in the US—one possible important marker of the acceptability and appropriateness of mental health services to the needs of these groups.

In the UK, similar patterns are evident. For example, a significant number of studies have found that those from Black Caribbean (and increasingly Black African) ethnic groups (particularly those experiencing psychotic symptoms) access mental health services via more emergency and coercive routes, that is, fewer general practitioner referrals, more police and court referrals, and more compulsory admissions (Morgan et al., 2004). A meta-analysis of 38 studies of compulsory admissions found that, compared with White patients, those of Black Caribbean ethnicity were on average around four times more likely to be compulsorily admitted (Bhui et al., 2003). There is evidence from a further review that the likelihood of compulsory admission increases over time, in the event of further contacts (Singh et al., 2007). Further, in a 10-year follow-up of an ethnically diverse cohort of individuals with a first-episode psychosis, there was clear evidence that rates of compulsory admission were higher among Black minority groups throughout the follow-up period (Morgan et al., 2017). A more recent systematic review and meta-analysis of 40 studies found that, overall, the odds of compulsory detention were over three times higher in Black Caribbean and Black African groups compared with White or White British (Halvorsrud et al., 2018). Similar disparities were evident for police involvement in the pathway to care. What data there are suggest somewhat different patterns for Asians than for Black groups. For example, the limited available data suggests South Asians, compared with other groups, are less likely to be (re) admitted to hospital (voluntarily or compulsorily) and to secure facilities and have shorter admissions (Bhui et al., 2003). There are, however, reports that South Asians are less likely to have disorder recognized in primary care and are less likely to be referred to specialist care (Bhui et al., 2003)—findings that suggest needs are not being met.

Broadly, the data provide strong evidence (at least for the US and the UK) that pathways to and interactions with mental health services more often involve coercion among migrant and minority ethnic populations. (It is noteworthy that what limited evidence there is for asylum seekers and refugees suggests, not surprisingly, similar problems with access and engagement (McCrone et al., 2005), problems no doubt exacerbated by language barriers and mistrust.) The reasons for these ethnic variations have been the subject of considerable debate (Morgan et al., 2004). A lot of attention has focused on cultural factors, particularly beliefs about mental illness, the basic premise being that how individuals and others within their social networks make sense of and understand their experiences of distress, will shape how they respond, present their complaints, and subsequent interactions with mental health services. There is good evidence that such processes are important (Kleinman, 1980; Pescosolido, 1999). The example of somatization has already been noted; expressing distress in an idiom that is unfamiliar to Western clinicians may lead to under-recognition and a failure to provide appropriate referral and care—patterns that are evident in Asian and other (e.g. Latino) populations in the West (see above).

There is further evidence that the explanatory models individuals develop to make sense of their experiences (which are rooted in shared cultural beliefs) can inhibit help-seeking from professional mental health services and affect subsequent engagement. This may be because experiences (such as sadness, hallucinations) are not considered to be problems that fall within the ambit of medicine (or which are considered to lie beyond 'the clinical horizon') or because of the stigma that attaches to mental illness in particular communities or because of widespread mistrust of institutions of White authority (a possibility that links to the discussion below on institutional racism). It is important to note, moreover, that the kinds of beliefs that reduce the likelihood of seeking help from mental health services are not necessarily those linked to the spiritual or supernatural. Those who locate the origins of their problems in social circumstances and stress (as is common across societies, but perhaps more so in some migrant and minority ethnic groups) may equally consider professional mental health services, rooted in the medical and biological, to be inappropriate.

This emphasis on cultural beliefs, however, can obscure the role of other important processes. More generally, we know that a range of other factors influence how people come into contact and engage with mental health services, including the nature of symptoms, the range and accessibility of treatment or intervention options, practical barriers, material resources, and prior experiences (including of other family members). Kleinman and Benson (2006), in their discussion of cultural competence (see below), give the example of a Mexican man whose failure to regularly bring his HIV-positive son to clinic was interpreted by clinicians to be the consequence of a different cultural understanding of HIV. Further exploration, however, revealed that the man had a very good understanding of HIV/AIDS and its treatment; the reason for irregular attendance was that, as a low-paid bus driver who often had to work night shifts, he did not have the time to take his son to the clinic. Such practical and material barriers are more common in migrant and minority ethnic populations who, as noted above, tend to be more economically disadvantaged.

Furthermore, there has been debate about whether the patterns of access, engagement, and satisfaction in migrant and minority ethnic populations reflect institutional racism within mental health services (Norfolk, 2003; Singh & Burns, 2006). Institutional racism (a concept initially developed by Stokely Carmichael) refers to the collective norms and behaviours within organizations that systematically (and unwittingly) discriminate against those from minority ethnic groups—leading, in the case of psychiatry, to the provision of inappropriate care and insensitive practice. This has proved controversial and, in the UK, has been vigorously challenged (Singh & Burns, 2006). However, these challenges have tended to overlook—or push into the background—structural ethnic and racial inequalities that powerfully determine access to resources, opportunities, and so on, and that consequently impact both health and access to health services (Nazroo et al., 2020).

Mental health service responses

The question, then, for mental health services in multicultural societies is how to deal effectively with ethnic and cultural complexity, in the context of structural inequalities—key issues, based on the data discussed above, being recognition and engagement. In response, there have been a multitude of proposals for service development and reform to better meet the needs of diverse populations. Two broad and related responses merit particular critical consideration: (1) specialist services for minority ethnic groups, and (2) cultural competence.

In response to the perception (and evidence) that mainstream mental health services do not adequately meet the needs of diverse ethnic groups, specialist services have been developed targeted at particular populations (especially in Europe and the US). Examples abound (e.g. see Fernando and Keating (2009) for case studies on services for Chinese, African, Caribbean, and South Asian populations in the UK providing specialized forms on intervention including cultural therapy, counselling, and day services). It is, however, rare for such services to be rigorously evaluated. In the US, there is some evidence that ethnic-specific programmes for African Americans, Asian Americans, and Mexican Americans reduce dropout rates, increase use of outpatient services, reduce reliance on emergency services, and (may) improve outcomes (Walton et al., 2010). Such studies are nonetheless sparse and their generalizability to other groups and settings is unclear.

It has, moreover, been forcefully argued that the provision of separate services reinforces the perception that ethnic groups are 'other' and, by focusing on cultural difference, indirectly imply that culture is a problem that requires specialist intervention (e.g. mental health literacy education) (Bhui & Sashidharan, 2003). What such an approach assumes, moreover, is that ethnicity or culture are always the salient issues for patients from diverse groups (a potential pitfall highlighted in the example above of the Mexican man and his son who is HIV positive). A possible exception to this is specialist services for asylum seekers and refugees; it may be that the mental health needs of these groups, and the barriers to engagement with services (e.g. language, mistrust arising from experiences of persecution and trauma, etc.), are so great that appropriate care can best be delivered through dedicated services, particularly those with expertise in working with survivors of trauma.

Where the focus is on ensuring mainstream services are more able to meet the needs of diverse populations, the overarching aim has been to promote and ensure cultural competence in both individual practitioners and organizations. Indeed, this has become a near-ubiquitous guiding concept in the drive to make mental health services more responsive and there can be no doubt that, broadly, ensuring practitioners and organizations are more knowledgeable and skilled in assessing and engaging individuals from a broad range of ethnic and cultural groups is a 'good thing'. More concretely, there are significant obstacles to achieving this in practice—many related to limitations with the notion of cultural competence itself. There is, for example, no shared definition; this means the concept is difficult to operationalize and apply in such a way that interventions and forms of service delivery can be evaluated. In their review of nine evaluations of cultural competence in mental health care, Bhui et al. (2007) found that all had used different definitions. The authors of the review were able to distil from the various definitions some common components, but these were not that much more concrete (e.g. 'definitions indicate a common aim, to increase performance and the capabilities of staff when providing service to ethnic minorities' p. 4) and reflect, in briefer form, the lack of clarity in the original definitions.

What this means is that there is limited clarity about how cultural competence is to be achieved. The primary mechanism so far advocated is the provision of education and training to staff and organizations (Bhui et al., 2007). The problem, however, is that there is no consistency or agreement about the content of programmes and very few rigorous evaluations of their effectiveness (Walton et al., 2010). The result is the piecemeal development of often widely varying curricula for which, beyond specific case studies and anecdotal accounts, there is no accumulating body of knowledge about what works.

The problems with cultural competence as the guiding principle for ensuring mental health services are responsive to the needs of ethnically and culturally diverse populations may be more fundamental still. Kleinman and Benson (2006), for example, argue that the very concept of 'cultural competence' reduces culture to a technical skill that can be acquired through training; as a basis for addressing ethnic disparities, it conflates culture and ethnicity, treating them as more or less synonymous. Cultural competence, they argue, 'becomes a series of do's and don'ts that define how to treat a patient of a given ethnic background' (p. 294). What is more, as highlighted above, the emphasis on culture as the primary prism through which to think about the needs of individuals from migrant and minority ethnic groups can blind clinicians to other important factors that may relate more to social position and material resources. In response, Kleinman and Benson propose an alternative approach, based on ethnography, that seeks a fuller understanding of the local moral worlds of sufferers as a basis for engaging and intervening. Their revised cultural formulation suggests clinicians conduct mini-ethnographies, centred around understanding the following facets of individuals lives and the impact on them of the illness: (1) ethnic identity (and its importance to the individual); (2) what is at stake for individuals (i.e. what is it that illness threatens); (3) an illness narrative; and (4) exposure to psychosocial stressors. What this approach potentially offers is a broader and more individualized basis on which to negotiate engagement; the importance of culture and ethnic identity is acknowledged, but within the wider context of the individual's life—as the authors put it, their approach 'does not ask, for example, "What do Mexicans call this problem?" It asks, "What do you call this problem?"' (pp. 1675–1676).

Conclusion

The select discussions in this chapter serve to highlight a number of key ongoing challenges for mental health services in meeting the needs of migrant and minority ethnic populations. Not least among these is the need to develop conceptually sound and rigorous programmes that can be thoroughly tested and contribute to the development of a sound evidence base for what works. Appealing as Kleinman and Benson's formulation is, for example, the real test comes with attempts to formalize, implement, and evaluate this approach. This may seem demanding (and indeed it is), but it is only through this process that we will generate usable knowledge about how to most effectively organize mental health services and provide care to meet the needs of our increasingly diverse populations.

REFERENCES

Alegria, M., Mulvaney-Day, N., Woo, M., Torres, M., Gao, S., & Oddo, V. (2007). Correlates of past-year mental health service use among Latinos: results from the National Latino and Asian American Study. *American Journal of Public Health*, 97, 76–83.

Alvarez, K., Fillbrunn, M., Green, J. G., Jackson, J. S., Kessler, R. C., McLaughlin, K. A., et al. (2019). Race/ethnicity, nativity, and lifetime risk of mental disorders in US adults. *Social Psychiatry and Psychiatric Epidemiology*, 54, 553–565.

Anglin, D. M., Ereshefsky, S., Klaunig, M. J., Bridgwater, M. A., Niendam, T. A., Ellman, L. M., et al. (2021). From womb to neighborhood: a racial analysis of social determinants of psychosis in the United States. *American Journal of Psychiatry*, 178, 599–610.

Barnard, H. & Turner, C. (2011). *Poverty and Ethnicity: A Review of the Evidence*. London: Joseph Rowntree Foundation. https://www.jrf.org.uk/sites/default/files/jrf/migrated/files/poverty-ethnicity-evidence-summary.pdf

Bebbington, P., Rai, D., Strydom, A., Brugha, T., McManus, S., & Morgan, Z. (2016). Psychotic disorders. In: McManus S, Bebbington P, Jenkins R, Brugha T. (Eds.), *Mental Health and Wellbeing in England: Adult Psychiatric Morbidity Survey 2014* (pp. 132–152). Leeds: NHS Digital.

Bhugra, D., Baldwin, D. S., Desai, M., & Jacob, K. S. (1999a). Attempted suicide in west London, II. Inter-group comparisons. *Psychological Medicine*, 29, 1131–1139.

Bhugra, D., Desai, M., & Baldwin, D. S. (1999b). Attempted suicide in west London, I. Rates across ethnic communities. *Psychological Medicine*, 29, 1125–1130.

Bhugra, D., Hilwig, M., Hossein, B., Marceau, H., Neehall, J., Leff, J., Mallett, R., & Der, G. (1996). First-contact incidence rates of schizophrenia in Trinidad and one-year follow-up. *British Journal of Psychiatry*, 169, 587–592.

Bhui, K., Bhugra, D., Goldberg, D., Sauer, J., & Tylee, A. (2004). Assessing the prevalence of depression in Punjabi and English primary care attenders: the role of culture, physical illness and somatic symptoms. *Transcultural Psychiatry*, 41, 307–322.

Bhui, K., & Sashidharan, S. P. (2003). Should there be separate psychiatric services for ethnic minority groups? *British Journal of Psychiatry*, 182, 101–12.

Bhui, K., Stansfeld, S., Hull, S., Priebe, S., Mole, F., & Feder, G. (2003). Ethnic variations in pathways to and use of specialist mental health services in the UK. Systematic review. *British Journal of Psychiatry*, 182, 105–116.

Bhui, K., Warfa, N., Edonya, P., McKenzie, K., & Bhugra, D. (2007). Cultural competence in mental health care: a review of model evaluations. *BMC Health Services Research*, 7, 15.

Blackmore, R., Boyle, J. A., Fazel, M., Ranasinha, S., Gray, K. M., Fitzgerald, G., et al. (2020). The prevalence of mental illness in refugees and asylum seekers: a systematic review and meta-analysis. *PLoS Medicine*, 17, e1003337.

Cochrane, R. & Bal, S. S. (1989). Mental hospital admission rates of immigrants to England: a comparison of 1971 and 1981. *Social Psychiatry and Psychiatric Epidemiology*, 24, 2–11.

De Haas, H., Castles, S., & Miller, M. J. (2020). *The Age of Migration: International Population Movements in the Modern World* (6th ed.). New York: Guilford Press.

Drummond, C., McBride, O., Fear, N. T., & Fuller, E. (2016). Alcohol dependence. In: McManus, S., Bebbington, P., Jenkins, R., & Brugha, T. (Eds.), *Mental Health and Wellbeing in England: Adult Psychiatric Morbidity Survey 2014* (pp. 238–264). Leeds: NHS Digital.

Fear, N. T., Bridges, S., Hatch, S., Hawkins, V., & Wessely, S. (2016). Posttraumatic stress disorder. In: McManus, S., Bebbington, P., Jenkins, R., & Brugha, T. (Eds.), *Mental Health and Wellbeing in England: Adult Psychiatric Morbidity Survey 2014* (pp. 1–25). Leeds: NHS Digital.

Fearon, P., Kirkbride, J. B., Morgan, C., Dazzan, P., Morgan, K., Lloyd, T., et al. (2006). Incidence of schizophrenia and other psychoses in ethnic minority groups: results from the MRC AESOP Study. *Psychological Medicine*, 36, 1541–1550.

Fernando, S. (1991). *Mental Health, Race and Culture*. London: Macmillan.

Fernando, S. & Keating, F. (2009). *Mental Health in a Multi-Ethnic Society: A Multidisciplinary Handbook*. London: Routledge.

Halvorsrud, K., Nazroo, J., Otis, M., Hajdukova, E. B., & Bhui, K. (2018). Ethnic inequalities and pathways to care in psychosis in England: a systematic review and meta-analysis. *BMC Medicine*, 16, 223.

Hackett, R. A., Ronaldson, A., Bhui, K., Steptoe, A., & Jackson, S. E. (2020). Racial discrimination and health: a prospective study of ethnic minorities in the United Kingdom. *BMC Public Health*, 20, 1652.

Helman, C. (2007). *Culture, Health and Illness*. London: Hodder Arnold.

Hickling, F. W., McKenzie, K., Mullen, R., & Murray, R. (1999). A Jamaican psychiatrist evaluates diagnoses at a London psychiatric hospital. *British Journal of Psychiatry*, 175, 283–285.

International Organization for Migration (2019). World migration report 2020. https://publications.iom.int/system/files/pdf/wmr_2020.pdf

Jones, J. S. (1981). How different are human races? *Nature*, 293, 188–190.

Joseph Rowntree Foundation (2022). Poverty rates by ethnicity. https://www.jrf.org.uk/data/poverty-rates-ethnicity

Kessler, R. C., Berglund, P., Demler, O., Jin, R., Merikangas, K. R., & Walters, E. E. (2005). Lifetime prevalence and age-of-onset distributions of DSM-IV disorders in the National Comorbidity Survey Replication. *Archives of General Psychiatry*, 62, 593–602.

Kirkbride, J. B., Barker, D., Cowden, F., Stamps, R., Yang, M., Jones, P. B., & Coid, J. W. (2008). Psychoses, ethnicity and socio-economic status. *British Journal of Psychiatry*, 193, 18–24.

Kleinman, A. (1980). *Patients and Healers in the Context of Culture: An Exploration of the Border Land between Anthropology, Medicine, and Psychiatry*. Berkeley, CA: University of California Press.

Kleinman, A. & Benson, P. (2006). Anthropology in the clinic: the problem of cultural competency and how to fix it. *PLoS Medicine*, 3, e294.

Kluckholm, C. (1944). *Mirror for Man*. New York: McGraw-Hill.

Leighton, A. H. & Hughes, J. M. (1961). Cultures as causative of mental disorder. *Millbank Memorial Fund Quarterly*, 39, 446–470.

Lewis, G. & David, A. (1991). Racism and psychiatry. *British Journal of Psychiatry*, 158, 432–433.

Lin, K. M. & Cheung, F. (1999). Mental health issues for Asian Americans. *Psychiatric Services*, 50, 774–780.

Linton, R. (1956). *Culture and Mental Disorders*. Springfield, IL: Thomas.

Mahy, G., Mallett, R., Leff, J., & Bhugra, D. (1999). First-contact incidence of schizophrenia in Barbados. *British Journal of Psychiatry*, **175**, 28–33.

McCrone, P., Bhui, K., Craig, T., Mohamud, S., Warfa, N., Stansfeld, S. A., et al. (2005). Mental health needs, service use and costs among Somali refugees in the UK. *Acta Psychiatruca Scandinavica*, **111**, 351–357.

McManus, S., Bebbington, P., Jenkins, R., & Brugha, T. (Eds.) (2016). *Mental Health and Wellbeing in England: Adult Psychiatric Morbidity Survey 2014*. Leeds: NHS Digital.

Minnis, H., McMillan, A., Gillies, M., & Smith, S. (2001). Racial stereotyping: survey of psychiatrists in the United Kingdom. *BMJ*, **323**, 905–906.

Minsky, S., Vega, W., Miskimen, T., Gara, M., & Escobar, J. (2003). Diagnostic patterns in Latino, African American, and European American psychiatric patients. *Archives of General Psychiatry*, **60**, 637–644.

Modood, T., Berthoud, R., & Lakey, J. (1997). *Ethnic Minorities in Britain: Diversity and Disadvantage*. London: Policy Studies Institute.

Morgan, C., Charalambides, M., Hutchinson, G., & Murray, R. M. (2010). Migration, ethnicity, and psychosis: toward a sociodevelopmental model. *Schizophrenia Bulletin*, **36**, 655–664.

Morgan, C. & Hutchinson, G. (2010). The social determinants of psychosis in migrant and ethnic minority populations: a public health tragedy. *Psychological Medicine*, **40**, 705–709.

Morgan, C., Kirkbride, J., Hutchinson, G., Craig, T., Morgan, K., Dazzan, P., et al. (2008). Cumulative social disadvantage, ethnicity and first-episode psychosis: a case-control study. *Psychological Medicine*, **38**, 1701–1715.

Morgan, C., Kirkbride, J., Leff, J., Craig, T., Hutchinson, G., McKenzie, K., Morgan, K., P., et al. (2007). Parental separation, loss and psychosis in different ethnic groups: a case-control study. *Psychological Medicine*, **37**, 495–503.

Morgan, C., Knowles, G., & Hutchinson, G. (2019). Migration, ethnicity, and psychoses: evidence, models, and future directions. *World Psychiatry*, **18**, 247–258.

Morgan, C., Lappin, J., Fearon, P., Heslin, M., Donoghue, K., Lomas, B., et al. (2017). Ethnicity and long-term outcome of psychoses in a UK sample: AESOP-10 study. *British Journal of Psychiatry*, **211**, 88–94.

Morgan, C., Mallett, R., Hutchinson, G., & Leff, J. (2004). Negative pathways to psychiatric care and ethnicity: the bridge between social science and psychiatry. *Social Science & Medicine*, **5**, 739–752.

Nazroo, J. Y. (1997). *Ethnicity and Mental Health: Findings from a National Community Survey*. London: Policy Studies Institute.

Nazroo, J. Y., Bhui, K. S., & Rhodes, J. (2020). Where next for understanding race/ethnic inequalities in severe mental illness? Structural, interpersonal and institutional racism. *Sociology of Health & Illness*, **42**, 262–276.

Norfolk, Suffolk and Cambridgeshire Strategic Health Authority (2003). *Independent Inquiry into the Death of David Bennett*. Cambridge: Norfolk, Suffolk and Cambridgeshire Strategic Health Authority.

Office of National Statistics (2011). 2011 Census analysis index. https://www.ons.gov.uk/census/2011census/censusanalysisindex

Pescosolido, B. A. & Boyer, C. A. (1999). How do people come to use mental health services? Current knowledge and changing perspectives. In: Horwitz, A. V. & Scheid, T. L. (Eds.), *A Handbook for the Study of Mental Health: Social Contexts, Theories and Systems* (pp. 392–411). Cambridge: Cambridge University Press.

Platt, L. & Nandi, A. (2020). Ethnic diversity in the UK: new opportunities and changing constraints. *Journal of Ethnic and Migration Studies*, **46**, 839–856.

Rees, R., Stokes, G., Stansfield, C., Oliver, E., Kneale, D., & Thomas, J. (2016). *Prevalence of Mental Health Disorders in Adult Minority Ethnic Populations in England. A Systematic Review*. London: EPPI-Centre, Social Science Research Unit, UCL Institute of Education, University College London.

Roberts, C., Lepps, H., Strang, J., & Singleton, N. (2016). Drug use and dependence. In: McManus, S., Bebbington, P., Jenkins, R., & Brugha, T. (Eds.), *Mental Health and Wellbeing in England: Adult Psychiatric Morbidity Survey 2014* (pp. 265–293). Leeds: NHS Digital.

Robins, L. N. & Reiger, D. A. (Eds.) (1991). *Psychiatric Disorders in America: The Epidemiologic Catchment Area Study*. New York: The Free Press.

Scheid, T. L. & Wright, E. R. (2017). *A Handbook for the Study of Mental Health: Social Contexts, Theories, and Systems* (3rd ed.). Cambridge: Cambridge University Press.

Selten, J.-P., Van Der Ven, E., & Termorshuizen, F. (2020). Migration and psychosis: a meta-analysis of incidence studies. *Psychological Medicine*, **50**, 303–313.

US Department of Health and Human Services (2001). *Mental Health: Culture, Race and Ethnicity—A Supplement to Mental Health: A Report of the Surgeon General*. Rockville, MD: US Department of Health and Human Services.

Singh, S. P. & Burns, T. (2006). Race and mental health: there is more to race than racism. *BMJ*, **333**, 648–651.

Singh, S. P., Greenwood, N., White, S., & Churchill, R. (2007). Ethnicity and the Mental Health Act 1983. *British Journal of Psychiatry*, **191**, 99–105.

Snowden, L. R. (1999). African American service use for mental health problems. *Journal of Community Psychology*, **27**, 303–313.

Snowden, L. R. & Cheung, F. K. (1990). Use of inpatient mental health services by members of ethnic minority groups. *American Psychologist*, **45**, 347–355.

Stansfield, S., Clark, C., Bebbington, P., King, M., Jenkins, R., & Hinchliffe, S. (2016). Common mental disorders. In: McManus, S., Bebbington, P., Jenkins, R., & Brugha, T. (Eds.), *Mental Health and Wellbeing in England: Adult Psychiatric Morbidity Survey 2014* (pp. 37–68). Leeds: NHS Digital.

Takeuchi, D. T., Zane, N., Hong, S., Chae, D. H., Gong, F., Gee, G. C., et al. (2007). Immigration-related factors and mental disorders among Asian Americans. *American Journal of Public Health*, **97**, 84–90.

United Nations High Commission for Refugees (2021). *Global Trends: Forced Displacement in 2020*. Copenhagen: United Nations.

Veling, W., Selten, J. P., Veen, N., Laan, W., Blom, J. D., & Hoek, H. W. (2006). Incidence of schizophrenia among ethnic minorities in the Netherlands: a four-year first-contact study. *Schizophrenia Research*, **86**, 189–193.

Walton, E., Berasi, K., Takeuchi, D. T., & Uehara, E. (2010). Cultural diversity and mental health treatment. In: Schied, T. L. & Brown, T. N. (Eds.), *A Handbook for the Study of Mental Health: Social Contexts, Theories and Systems* (pp. 439–460). Cambridge: Cambridge University Press.

Williams, D. R., Haile, R., Gonzalez, H. M., Neighbors, H., Baser, R., & Jackson, J. S. (2007). The mental health of Black Caribbean immigrants: results from the National Survey of American Life. *American Journal of Public Health*, **97**, 52–59.

Williams, D. R., Costa, M., & Leavell, J. P. (2010). Race and mental health: patterns and challenges. In: Schied, T. L. & Brown, T. N. (Eds.), *A Handbook for the Study of Mental Health: Social Contexts, Theories and Systems* (pp. 268–290). Cambridge: Cambridge University Press.

9

The mental health challenges of immigrants and refugees

Jillian M. Stile, Quyen Ngo-Metzger, Richard F. Mollica, and Eugene F. Augusterfer

The magnitude of mental health and resettlement problems

In 2021, it was estimated that there were 44.9 million foreign-born people living in the US (Congressional Research Service, 2021). Since 1975, the US has resettled more than 3 million refugees (Office of Refugee Resettlement, 2021). Most immigrants and refugees come to escape poverty, mass violence, and/or political/religious oppression. Since 1960 there has been a continuous increase in immigrants coming from Latin America (from 9.4% in 1960 to 53.6% in 2007) and Asia (from 5.1% in 1960 to 26.8% in 2007). In Europe a similar trend is taking place: the European Union estimates that 28.8 million immigrants currently live in the European Union. By mid-2021, the United Nations High Commissioner for Refugees reports that there are 84 million forcibly displaced people worldwide, 48 million internally displaced people, and 26.6 million refugees (UNHCR, 2021b). According to the UNHCR, the year 2020 saw the mass movement of people within and beyond their borders, uprooted by conflict, calamity, or searching for opportunity. During 2020, several crises—some new, some long-standing, and some resurfacing after years—forced 11.2 million people to flee, compared to 11.0 million in 2019. This figure includes people displaced for the first time as well as people displaced repeatedly, both within and beyond countries' borders (UNHCR, 2021a). Patterns of both conflict and human displacement are becoming increasingly more complex. The increase in diversity of immigrant/refugee population from economically developing countries to the so-called economically developed countries has increased throughout and poses new challenges to the field of community health and mental health care.

In this chapter we will focus on describing the barriers encountered by highly traumatized immigrants and refugees from culturally diverse backgrounds and provide a model that addresses this population's specific health and mental health problems and barriers to care. Their specific medical problems have been addressed in various previous publications (Ackerman, 1997; Bhuyan & Senturia, 2005; Bikoo, 2007; Cassano & Fava, 2002; Coker et al., 2000; Culpepper, 2002; Durham et al., 2007; Fazel et al., 2005; Gavagan & Brodyaga, 1998; Lifson et al., 2002; Marshall et al., 2005; Miller, 1996; Mollica et al., 1999, 2009; Palinkas et al., 2003; Pottie et al., 2007; Roberts et al., 1998; Schillinger et al., 2002; Silberholz et al., 2017; Southeast Asian Subcommittee of the Asian American/Pacific Islander Work Group, National Diabetes Education Program, 2006; Spiegel & Nankoe, 2004; Stromme et al., 2021; Tompkins et al., 2006; Yee, 2003). This chapter will therefore focus on the new literature emerging from the areas of health disparities and refugee mental health. Health disparities is here defined as:

> a particular type of difference in health (or in the determinants of health that could be shaped by policies) in which disadvantaged social groups systematically experience worse health or more health risks than do more advantaged social groups. Disadvantaged social groups include racial/ethnic minorities, low-income people, women, or others who have persistently experienced discrimination. (Braveman, 2006; Silberholz et al., 2017)

Immigrants and refugees as both patients and communities definitely experience health disparities, such as:

- traumatic life experiences
- provider–patient communication
- socioeconomic status
- cultural differences
- levels of health literacy
- limited English proficiency (LEP).

The main setting through which to address these health care barriers is the primary health care (PHC) setting. We will first provide a model for caring for traumatized and culturally diverse patients and will then focus on an important innovation in their health care: the community health worker (CHW).

Health status of immigrant/refugee populations in the US

Historically, from 1850 until 1960, the predominant immigrants to the US were from European countries and Canada. In 1965, as part of the civil rights period, the Immigration Act abolished

European-origin preferences for immigration, and opened the door to other ethnic/racial groups (Trinh-Shevrin et al., 2009). As a result, the foreign-born population has somewhat diversified in more recent decades. The foreign-born population is defined as those who are not citizens of the US at birth. After migration to the US, some foreign-born individuals are eligible to become naturalized citizens, usually after a minimum of 5 years of legal residence. In the 2010 census, approximately half of the foreign-born population came from Latin America (21.2 million), and a quarter (11.2 million) came from Asia (Grieco et al., 2012). Twelve per cent were from Europe, and the remaining 7% were from other regions of the world (Grieco et al., 2012). Although Mexican immigration to the US is quite significant in magnitude, it is dissimilar from other migrant populations because of the shared US–Mexico border. Thus, for the scope of this chapter, we will focus on Asian immigrants to the US because they are more representative of other immigrant groups in Europe and around the world.

Asian Americans are defined according to the US census (Budiman et al., 2021), as 'people with origins in the Far East, Southeast Asia, or the Indian subcontinent' and in the US include Chinese (23%), Asian Indians (20%), Filipino (18%), Vietnamese (9%), Korean (8%), and Japanese (6%) and other small subgroups such as Cambodians, Laotians, Pakistanis, Hmong, Thai, Indonesians, and Bangladeshis. Asian Americans are extremely heterogeneous in terms of languages, cultures, and socioeconomic status. However, data on all Asian Americans are often presented in aggregate, which hides the heterogeneity within the Asian American population. Socioeconomic and health status differ widely by Asian subgroups. In addition, the myth of Asians being 'the model minority' (that all Asians succeed in American society), has hidden the plights of many Asian immigrants who have encountered significant challenges living in the US (Trinh-Shevrin et al., 2009). For example, proportionately more Asian Americans live in poverty compared to White Americans and are more likely than White Americans to have lower-wage jobs that do not provide health insurance (Trinh-Shevrin et al., 2009).

Health disparities among Asian Americans

Currently, a major cause of death among Asian Americans is cancer. Lung and breast cancers are the leading causes of death for men and women, respectively (NCI 2021. Seer Cancer Statistics Review, 2021). For women aged 40–79 years old, breast cancer mortality rates have increased among Asian Americans (and Native Americans) even though they have decreased among all other racial/ethnic groups in the US (DeSantis et al., 2019). This increased mortality may be a consequence of lack of screening, resulting in late-stage diagnosis.

Chronic diseases such as obesity, hypertension, hypercholesterolaemia, and diabetes are also increasing among immigrant populations (Trinh-Shevrin et al., 2009). The prevalence of hypercholesterolaemia and coronary heart disease are especially high among some Asian subgroups such as South Asians. Asian immigrants have increased risks of being overweight and obesity as they adopt a more sedentary lifestyle and the more calorie-dense Western diet. Higher rates of obesity exist among second-generation immigrant children when compared to first-generation children (Gong, 2019). Asian Americans are 30–50% more likely to have diabetes than White Americans (Lee et al., 2011). Compared to non-Hispanic White people, diabetes prevalence is higher among Filipinos and South Asians (Raquinio et al., 2021). Furthermore, compared to White Americans, Asian Americans are less likely to have received mental health treatment (Yang et al., 2020). Post-traumatic stress disorder (PTSD), depression, and anxiety are especially prevalent among Cambodian refugees who experienced prior traumas of war (Bogic et al., 2015). Older Asian immigrants, in particular, may experience social and linguistic isolation, increasing their risks for depression (Lai et al., 2020). Many remain untreated, or undertreated, because of language barriers and the social and cultural stigma related to mental disorders (Na et al., 2016; Snowden et al., 2011). Problems in communication between patients and their medical providers about mental health issues may exacerbate these disparities (Ngo-Metzger et al., 2007; Sorkin et al., 2009).

The health impact of trauma and immigration

Migrants typically arrive in their destination country having suffered multiple traumata. Aside from acute and chronic stressors that initially led to forced migration, there is the stress of the acculturation process itself. Refugees consistently score lower on indices of mental health than non-refugees, with pre- and post-migration conditions strongly moderating the overall effect on mental health (Porter & Haslam, 2005). Traumatic life events are associated with mental health problems, as well as lower life expectancy, and higher risks of medical problems (Friedman & Schnurr, 1995).

The trauma that people experienced in their country of origin, in addition to the acculturation stress, lead to many social, psychological, and physical problems. In a meta-analysis, it was found that, on average, refugees consistently scored lower on indices of mental health than non-refugees, with pre- and post-displacement contextual factors strongly moderating the effects of trauma on mental health (Porter & Haslam, 2005). Moreover, traumatic life events are associated with not only mental health problems, but also increased morbidity, lower life expectancy, and higher risks of medical problems (Friedman & Schnurr, 1995).

While the relationship between traumatic life experiences and mental health has been well established, recent research findings demonstrate the impact of psychological and emotionally traumatic life events on later development of chronic medical illness (Sareen et al., 2007; Sledjeski et al., 2008). For example, a relationship was found between comorbid PTSD and depression with physical health problems in Cambodian refugees resettled in the US (Berthold et al., 2014). These studies demonstrate the positive risk for physical health problems as a direct result of trauma events as well as mediated through trauma-related PTSD and depression.

Experience of traumatic life events have been highly correlated with smoking-related mortality, an increase in alcohol abuse, drug use, and other physical health problems (e.g. bruising, broken bones, or head and organ damage) as well as other chronic physical illnesses (Sareen et al., 2007). It has been well established that cumulative trauma is associated with the psychiatric diagnosis of PTSD and depression in a dose–effect relationship; that is, increasing levels of trauma lead to higher rates and severity of PTSD and depression (Mollica et al., 1998; Sledjeski et al., 2008). PTSD has been associated with physical disorders, disability, and suicidal behaviour (Sareen et al., 2007).

Over the past 25 years, major community studies (e.g. Mollica et al., 1998) have demonstrated the high rates of PTSD, depression, and physical disability in highly traumatized refugee populations. One meta-analysis showed that patients with PTSD or post-traumatic stress symptomatology reported greater general health symptoms, general medical conditions, and poorer health-related quality of life, including greater frequency and severity of pain, cardiorespiratory symptoms, and gastrointestinal complaints (Pacella et al., 2013). A RAND Corporation study of the Cambodian community in Long Beach, California, revealed prevalence rates of 62% for PTSD and 51% for depression 30 years after the Pol Pot genocide in Cambodia (Marshall et al., 2005). Data from the nationwide Canadian Community Health Survey Cycle 1.2 conducted in 2002 (N = 36,984) demonstrated that trauma-related PTSD is associated with a number of chronic medical disorders (Table 9.1) (Sareen et al., 2007).

Similarly, a large-scale community study in the US of mainstream American patients demonstrated the positive relationship between trauma events, PTSD (≥6 months) and physical illness. This study used the data from the National Comorbidity Survey—Replication (NCS-R) to examine the relationship between number of lifetime traumas, PTSD, and 15 self-reported chronic medical conditions (Table 9.2) (Sledjeski et al., 2008). The NCS-R findings reveal that:

- there is a graded relationship between trauma exposure, PTSD, and the majority of major medical conditions
- the relationship between PTSD and chronic medical conditions was explained by the number of lifetime traumas experienced.

New evidence increasingly demonstrates the health impact of depression. The fact that severe depression alone (e.g. suicide) is lethal is well recognized. Subsequent studies have shown that depression is just as lethal through its effects on chronic diseases (Cassano & Fava, 2002). People suffering from depression are two to four times more likely to develop hypertension (threefold risk), myocardial infarction (four- to six-fold increase in mortality), diabetes (15% prevalence), and stroke (25% prevalence) (Culpepper, 2002). The high prevalence of depression in resettled refugee communities in the US is most likely leading to a higher prevalence of chronic medical diseases. For example, there appears to be an epidemic of diabetes facing the Cambodian community and Cambodians are six times more likely to die of this disease if they are depressed (Carlsson et al., 2005).

Gender-based violence among migrants

Gender-based violence is perpetrated on over 30% of girls and women affecting refugees, transgender women, and women living in high conflict zones (Binagwaho et al., 2021). Overall, intimate partner violence touches the lives of one in three women (World Health Organization, 2021). Migration tends to exacerbate the stressors leading to violence. Conditions of life for women in the Covid-19 pandemic increases their exposure to gender-based violence. The isolation of women is a common tactic of perpetrators. Quarantines, lockdowns, and forced isolation restrict the movement of women outside the home, increasing their exposure to domestic violence. Escape from domestic violence is a common motivator for flight and migration; thus, one expects a high incidence of violence-related trauma in the population of female migrants.

Migrants from LGBTQ communities

Until now, there has been little research on the experience of sexual and gender minority (LGBTQ) migrants and consideration of their specific stresses. Nonetheless, it seems clear that in addition to the typical stresses associated with (usually forced) migration and persecution, LGBTQ individuals are vulnerable to additional stressors related to their sexual orientation or gender identity. This population is at risk of experiencing high levels of stigma, discrimination, and isolation both in their countries of origin and in the culture to which they migrate (Rosati et al., 2021), generating experiences of marginalization along multiple dimensions.

Previous human rights abuses in their home countries and complicated sociopolitical landscapes in their destination country may deter people from seeking access to health care services and support. Additionally, transgender individuals in the US have faced

Table 9.1 The association between PTSD and chronic physical health conditions (community sample n = 36,984, 15 years or more, response rate 77%)

	AOR	95% CI
Chronic condition (PTSD ≥ 6 months)		
Asthma	1.99	(1.38–2.88)***
Chronic bronchitis, emphysema, or chronic obstructive pulmonary disease	3.08	(2.01–4.72)***
Chronic pain conditions		
Fibromyalgia	2.59	(1.50–4.47)**;
Arthritis (excluding fibromyalgia)	3.46	(2.49–4.81)***
Back problems (excluding fibromyalgia and arthritis)	2.04	(1.51–2.74)***
Migraine headaches	2.77	(1.99–3.85)***
Cardiovascular diseases		
Hypertension	1.55	(1.09–2.20)*
Heart disease	1.69	(1.08–2.65)*
Neurological diseases		
Stroke	2.31	(0.99–5.36)
Epilepsy	1.69	(0.58–4.94)
Metabolic conditions		
Diabetes	1.58	(0.92–2.73)
Thyroid condition	1.06	(0.68–1.64)
Bowel disorder (Crohn's disease or colitis)	1.85	(1.07–3.21)*
Stomach or intestinal ulcers	1.93	(1.22–3.07)**
Chronic fatigue syndrome	5.78	(3.47–9.65)***
Cancer	2.69	(1.36–5.32)**
Multiple chemical sensitivities	3.95	(2.46–6.35)***

AOR, adjusted odds ratio; CI, confidence interval. * $p < 0.05$; ** $p < 0.01$; *** $p < 0.001$.

Table 9.2 The association between lifetime trauma and chronic medical conditions

	No trauma	Trauma	PTSD	Trauma vs no trauma		PTSD vs no trauma		PTSD vs trauma		Wald χ^2, p
	%	%	%	AOR	95% CI	AOR	95%CI	AOR	95% CI	
Arthritis/rheumatism	16.9	28.3	38.1	1.9	(1.5–2.5)*	2.8	(1.9–4.1)*	1.5	(1.2–1.8)*	28.7, 0.0001*
Back/neck pain	17.2	30.2	49.4	1.8	(1.4–2.3)*	3	(2.1–4.2)*	1.7	(1.4–2.0)*	40.9, 0.0001*
Headaches	14.8	22.1	50.3	1.6	(1.1–2.3)+	3.2	(2.1–4.9)*	2	(1.6–2.6)*	41.5, 0.0001*
Chronic pain	1.8	10.1	22.1	5.4	(3.6–7.9)*	10.1	(6.6–15.5)*	1.9	(1.5–2.4)*	113.8, 0.0001*
Heart attack	1.5	3.6	2.7	1.7	(0.6–5.0)	1.5	(0.5–4.9)	0.9	(0.4–1.7)	1.2, 0.56
Heart disease	1.3	4.9	7.5	3.1	(1.3–7.1)*	6.3	(2.3–17.2)*	2.1	(1.5–2.9)*	18.8, 0.0001*
High blood pressure	16.7	24.6	26.7	1.5	(1.0–2.3)	2	(1.3–3.2)	1.3	(1.1–1.7)	10.3, 0.006+
Seasonal allergies	27.6	39	45.2	1.7	(1.3–2.2)*	1.2	(1.1–1.4)*	1.1	(0.9–1.3)	24.7, 0.0001*
Asthma	88.1	11.9	14.1	1.5	(1.0–2.2)	1.4	(0.9–2.0)	0.9	(0.1–1.2)	4.2, 0.12
Lung disease	0.5	2.2	4.6	3.8	(1.0–15.1)	6	(1.3–27.3)	1.6	(0.8–3.0)	5.6, 0.06
Stroke	2	2.6	3.7	1	(0.6–1.9)	2	(0.9–4.6)	1.9	(1.0–3.6)	4.2, 0.12
Epilepsy	0.8	1.8	4.4	2	(0.7–6.0)	3.8	(1.1–13.8)+	1.9	(1.2–3.0)+	7.2, 0.03+
Diabetes	3.1	7.7	7.8	2.6	(1.7–4.1)*	3.1	(1.8–5.3)*	1.2	(0.8–1.7)	19.2, 0.0001*
Ulcer	4.2	9.5	17.5	1.9	(1.2–3.0)+	2.8	(1.7–4.5)*	1.5	(1.1–1.9)*	21.2, 0.0001*
Cancer	1.7	6.4	7.3	3.5	(1.7–7.3)*	4.8	(2.1–10.9)*	1.4	(0.9–2.0)	14.0, 0.0009*

Adjusted for sex, race, age, income, insurance coverage, smoking status, and lifetime diagnoses of major depressive disorder, other anxiety disorders, and substance related disorders. AOR, adjusted odds ratio; CI, confidence interval; Wald χ^2 = for the group main effect. * Significant at Bonferroni corrected p <0.003; + marginally significant at p <0.05, n = 9282.

discrimination in health care along with employment and housing (Bradford et al., 2013). Thus, many human rights violations go unspoken and health care needs go unaddressed.

LBGTQ individuals are at greater risk of exposure to complex trauma arising from migration difficulties and mental health concerns. A recent study showed that among LGBTQ asylum seekers, sexual orientation and gender identity were associated with increased psychological distress such as perceived social isolation and issues with identity disclosure (Fox et al., 2020). Another study found that among adults who have experienced trauma, LGBTQ participants who attributed their trauma to discrimination reported higher levels of psychological symptoms including attachment anxiety and avoidance, emotion dysregulation, PTSD, and dissociative symptoms (Keating et al., 2020). The intersection of multiple marginalized identities of transgender refugees (e.g. gender identity, transphobia, and post-migration stress) increases the total stress and predisposes them to mental illness.

Impact of the Covid-19 pandemic on migrants and refugees

As of March 2022, the SARS-CoV-2 (Covid-19) pandemic has resulted in over 486 million confirmed cases of infection, with over 6.14 million deaths worldwide (World Health Organization, 2022). While it is too early for firm conclusions about the impact of the Covid-19 pandemic on migrants, all signs point to a disproportionate impact on migrants, especially those who are involuntarily displaced. The Covid-19 pandemic has brought to light inequities in health and health care throughout the world. Health disparities deprive low-income and displaced populations, and people of colour of the care they need for adequate recovery, including lack of access to quality health care, and a lack of trust in the health care system, thus placing them at higher risk for developing Covid-19 infections and experiencing increase in mortality and morbidity. Moreover, poverty, unemployment, inadequate or overcrowded housing, and exposure to the virus on the job, all put migrants at high-risk (Balakrishnan, 2021; OECD, 2020).

Mental health problems have increased in the global population as a result of the Covid-19 pandemic (Wu et al., 2021). In a meta-analysis, Xiong and colleagues (2020) found that since the outbreak of Covid-19, levels of depression, anxiety, depression, PTSD, psychological distress, and stress were reported as higher than normal in the general population. The negative consequences for keeping children out of school, or dependent on remote learning without the devices they need to learn online, are likely to have a negative impact for years to come. Lack of family contact and family supports compound the isolation already experienced by migrants, depriving them of needed support and resources. Further research is urgently needed to guide efforts at prevention and treatment in this population.

Communication barriers for immigrant/refugee populations

The non-US-born immigrant and refugee population's past trauma, socioeconomic status, and limited understanding of English, the host country's culture, and health care system, puts them at an especially high risk for many health and mental health problems, as well as poor health care access and quality. Research demonstrates that language and cultural barriers negatively affect care for patients with LEP, resulting in significant and costly health disparities (Clarke et al., 2019). They are less likely to have a regular doctor, and if ill more likely to delay getting care for over a year (Derose et al., 2009). In the US, foreign-born individuals are less satisfied with the quality of care received compared to those native-born. Furthermore, those with LEP are less likely to receive mental health services if in need than non-Hispanic Whites individuals (Kim et al., 2011).

Barriers in provider–patient communication

Communicating effectively is a core component of the health care encounter and is the platform on which patients and clinicians make informed treatment decisions. Communication comprises verbal and non-verbal behaviours that serve as the foundation upon which an effective relationship is built—mutual trust, respect, and partnership. Communication includes not only question-asking and information-giving, but also many other dimensions including building rapport and paying attention (Hashim, 2017). The US National Healthcare Disparities Reports have shown that persistent disparities occur in provider–patient communication for Asian Americans, especially those who have LEP (US Department of Health and Human Services, 2019). Asian Americans were more likely than White patients to report that their doctors did not listen, spend as much time, or involve them in decisions as much as they wanted (Ngo-Metzger et al., 2004). They were also more likely than White patients to report that their doctors did not understand their backgrounds and values (Ngo-Metzger et al., 2003, 2004). This lack of communication resulted in less health education and more unmet health needs among Asian compared to White patients (Ngo-Metzger et al., 2007). In a population-based survey, older Asian Americans were more likely to report mental health needs compared to older White Americans but were less likely than White Americans to have their medical providers discuss their mental health problems with them (Sorkin et al., 2008). Other research has found that Asian American women were less likely to receive cancer screening compared to their White counterparts (Wang et al., 2008). Furthermore, Asian American women diagnosed with breast cancer were less likely to receive breast-conserving surgery compared to White women (Goel et al., 2005). Asian Americans with end-stage cancer were also less likely to receive hospice care compared to White patients (Ngo-Metzger et al., 2008). These health disparities may be a consequence of communication barriers. A number of barriers to effective provider–patient communication may exist. These barriers include (1) socioeconomic differences, (2) cultural differences, (3) LEP, and (4) low levels of health literacy.

Socioeconomic differences

Immigrants in the US are more likely to have lower socioeconomic status compared to native citizens. Individuals with lower socioeconomic status are more likely to report physicians spending less time with them and poor communication (Verlinde et al., 2012). Research has found that physicians' information-giving was positively influenced by the patient's communication style, such as question-asking and expressiveness (Street, 1991). Patients' levels of verbal expressiveness were strongly related to their levels of education. After controlling for the patient's communication style, evidence suggested that physicians gave more information to particular types of patients: more educated patients received more health information than their less educated counterparts (Verlinde et al., 2012). Providers spent a larger proportion of their time in the physical examination of patients with lower education and less time assessing health knowledge and answering patients' questions (Verlinde et al., 2012). These findings persisted across racial/ethnic groups, suggesting that providers associated patients' higher education levels with higher health literacy and competency, and thus gave them more health-related information.

Cultural differences

In addition to socioeconomic differences, providers and patients from different cultural backgrounds may have different explanations of health and illness. Most Western providers belong to a 'biomedical' culture that views diseases as having natural, mechanistic causes that can often be treated by repairing organs or manipulating chemical pathways (Kagawa-Singer & Kassim-Lakha, 2003). In contrast, patients from different cultures may have different needs, beliefs, and values (Ibeneme, et al., 2017). If the provider insists that the Western biomedical view of disease as the only 'right way', and discounts the patient's views on their illness, miscommunication may occur. When providers and patients can understand and appreciate each other's perspectives on the illness, they are more likely to communicate effectively and be able to negotiate differences. Effective communication and negotiation are especially important in order to avoid frustration and misunderstanding, and to arrive at an acceptable treatment plan.

Asian cultures encourage showing deference to authority and avoiding conflict in order to 'save face'. Asian people also tend to be less direct and show less emotion compared to individuals from Western cultures, which may lead medical providers to assume that they do not have questions or concerns. Thus, Asian Americans may be less likely to openly question medical professionals, even when they do not understand or disagree. Yet, Asian American patients may leave the medical visit with unresolved questions or unmet expectations. Furthermore, Asian Americans are also more likely to use Eastern herbal or traditional folk medicine, or other Asian complementary and alternative medicine (CAM) (Ahn et al., 2006). These herbs may interact with prescription medications and lead to life-threatening complications (Boullatta & Nace, 2000). In a national study of 3258 Chinese and Vietnamese American patients seen at 11 community health clinics, two-thirds reported that they used CAM while also receiving Western medical care (Ahn et al., 2006). Yet only 7% reported that their doctors discussed CAM use with them. Patients whose doctors discussed the use of CAM with them were more satisfied compared to those whose doctors failed to understand or discuss their CAM use (Ahn et al., 2006).

Limited English-language proficiency

In the US, 67.3 million people speak languages other than English at home, with the most common other language being Spanish. Languages with more than a million people who speak it at home in 2018 were Spanish (41.5 million), Chinese (3.5 million), Tagalog (1.8 million), Vietnamese (1.5 million), Arabic (1.3 million), French (1.2 million), and Korean (1.1 million) (US Census Bureau, 2019). Approximately 4 million Asian Americans have LEP and encounter language barriers when communicating with their medical providers (Trinh-Shevrin et al., 2009). LEP individuals often have problems accessing medical care (Berdahl et al., 2019) and tend to experience more medical communication errors than

English-proficient patients (Wasserman et al., 2014). Language barriers result in less health information given to patients (Clarke et al., 2019; Ngo-Metzger et al., 2007), worse provider–patient communication (Weech-Maldonado et al., 2003), and longer hospital stays (Lindholm et al., 2012). Having access to trained, professional interpreters during health care visits can alleviate some, but not all, of the health disparities associated with language barriers (Ngo-Metzger et al., 2007). Because of the cultural stigma surrounding mental health issues, Asian Americans may be particularly reluctant to discuss their mental health needs in the presence of an interpreter (Ngo-Metzger et al., 2007). Thus, having a medical or mental health provider who can speak the patient's native language is still optimal.

Even among Asian Americans with higher education who can speak English, those who are non-native English speakers may still encounter serious health literacy challenges. They may lack knowledge about how to navigate the complex and fragmented medical and health insurance systems in the US. Thus, patients whose native language is not English may encounter obstacles in obtaining health care and are at risk for poor health (Sentell & Braun, 2012).

Levels of health literacy

Health literacy is defined as the 'degree to which individuals have the ability to find, understand, and use information and services to inform health-related decisions and actions for themselves and others' (Office of Disease Prevention and Health Promotion, 2021). Health literacy is not confined to just basic reading and writing skills, but is also comprised of listening skills and the ability to understand and use health information. Patients with low health literacy have more problems with medication adherence (Kalichman et al., 1999), are more likely to take medications incorrectly, and have worse health outcomes (McDonald & Shenkman, 2018). Health literacy is often associated with individuals' education, income, race, age, and country of birth (Chesser et al., 2016). Immigrants, older individuals, and those who are racial/ethnic minorities are more likely to have lower health literacy compared to White individuals.

Approximately 25 million people in the US are LEP. When LEP patients receive care from physicians who are truly language concordant, some evidence show that language disparities are reduced. Seventy-six per cent (25/33) of the studies demonstrated that at least one of the outcomes assessed was better for patients receiving language-concordant care (Diamond et al., 2019).

The processes by which health literacy affect health outcomes are still under intense study (Weiss et al., 2003). However, poor doctor–patient communication may be a fundamental factor. Poor communication impacts all components of the health care encounter, from taking an accurate medical history to explanations of diagnoses and treatments. Physicians often use medical jargon that patients do not understand. Furthermore, time pressures created by the 15-minute general medical visit may result in doctors providing information quickly, with little time to answer patients' questions (Linzer et al., 2015). This problem can be exacerbated since patients with lower health literacy tend not to ask questions (Menendez et al., 2017). Previous research has shown that patients with low health literacy are often ashamed to ask for help from providers, even though they do not understand instructions on how to take medications (Easton et al., 2013). Also, it is well established that language barriers contribute to health disparities and that the use of ad hoc interpretation by untrained family members results in substandard care (Carlson et al., 2022).

The role of primary health care

The Institute of Medicine defines PHC as 'integrated and accessible care by clinicians who are responsible for addressing a majority of personal health needs through a sustained partnership with patients and practising in a family and community context' (Institute of Medicine, 1996).

Access to PHC is essential for the acute and long-term care of refugees over their entire lifetime. Mishori and his colleagues (2017) comprehensively review the health and mental health needs of refugees resettled in the US (Table 9.3). Refugees have higher rates of chronic pain compared to the general population; also, much higher rates of PTSD and depression. Chronic non-communicable diseases such as diabetes mellitus and hypertension, and the threatened onset decades later of stroke and heart disease, are highly prevalent. All refugees, by definition, have suffered human rights violations and many have been tortured. Certainly, the extensive traumatic life experiences of refugees dramatically contribute to their poorer health status over time.

The traumatic life history of the refugee must be a central focus of primary healthcare. The conceptual model in **Figure 9.1** looks at trauma and health and mental health risks for the traumatized refugee/immigrant patient from diverse cultural backgrounds. In this model, traumatic life events are directly linked to physical health, as well as indirectly linked to physical health through the mediation of depression and PTSD. Mental health and physical illness are directly related to major lifestyle factors such as diet, smoking, obesity, lack of exercise, and alcohol/substance abuse that can be directly improved though community-based interventions.

The new focus on trauma as a major health and mental health risk factor highlights the need for a new prevention and intervention

Table 9.3 Common presenting health problems in refugees

Mental health problems	Pain
Adjustment disorder	Abdominal pain
Anxiety	Headache
Depression	Musculoskeletal pain
PTSD	Pelvic pain in females
Sleep problems	**Undiagnosed chronic conditions**
Social isolation	Asthma
Nutritional problems	Chronic obstructive pulmonary disease
Anaemia	Diabetes mellitus
Overweight/obesity	Dyslipidaemia
Vitamin B_{12} deficiency	Hypertension
Vitamin D deficiency	Impaired fasting glucose levels
	Oral/dental problems

Adapted with permission from Eckstein, B. (2011). Primary care for refugees. *American Family Physician*, 83, 432. Mishori, R., Aleinikoff, S., & Davis, D. M. (2017). Primary care for refugees: challenges and opportunities. *American Family Physician*, 96, 112–120.

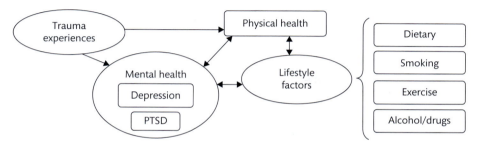

Figure 9.1 Conceptual model: trauma, PTSD, depression, and physical health.
Wagner, E. H. (1998). Chronic disease management: what will it take to improve care for chronic illness? *Effective Clinical Practice*, 1, 2–4.

strategies in the community-based health care of these populations. In this model, trauma risk assessment is essential to the identification and treatment of major health and mental health problems. Furthermore, treatment must be extended to addressing major lifestyle through health promotion activities that need to occur in addition to more conventional reliance on medication and/or counselling (Mollica, 2006).

PHC is considered an ideal health care environment for addressing the health and mental health needs of traumatized persons from culturally diverse communities. PHC serves as the initial point of contact for patients with trauma related health and psychiatric problems (Barrett et al., 1988). Domestic violence, for example, is associated with a wide range of adverse health impacts, but it is often not identified by PHC providers (Fraser, 2003). A study, for example, of 150 women seen consequently in PHC by a female physician revealed that a history of physical and mental abuse (unacknowledged by the primary care provider (PCPs)) was associated with an increase in all measures of health care utilization (Sansone et al., 1997). As in the case of all traumatized patients, victims of domestic violence as well as refugees and other traumatized patient groups do not often seek care just for trauma-related injuries but for health-related problems which appear unrelated to the trauma events. It is, therefore, essential that there is an adequate risk assessment of trauma events in PHC so that the patient's PCP can connect the dots between risk and medical illness.

The usual care by PCPs may be less than optimal with studies indicating the recognition of trauma-related distress as less than 40% (Barrett et al., 1988), diagnosis of PTSD as low as 2% (Taubman-Ben-Ari et al., 2001), and depression less than 50% (Pignone et al., 2002). In PHC veteran clinics where PTSD and depression should be routinely diagnosed, less than 50% of diagnosable patients were identified (Magruder et al., 2005). Underdiagnosis and undertreatment for historically disadvantaged ethnic groups (e.g. African Americans), those with language barriers (e.g. Hispanics), and special highly traumatized populations (e.g. resettled refugees) may be especially high (Alim et al., 2006; Feldman, 2006; Miranda et al., 2003). For example, Davis et al. (2008) have recently revealed that low-income African Americans in urban PHC clinics were at a high risk for trauma, with PTSD rates of 22% but only 13.3% of the latter received trauma-focused treatment interventions. The identification and treatment of trauma-related health and mental health disorders in low-income culturally diverse communities in PHC must be developed and evaluated.

The interest PCPs have in a patient's traumatic life history is extremely limited even when the PCPs are caring for patients such as refugees where a history of violence is very common. The fast pace of the PHC visit creates barriers to exploring a patient's traumatic life history and major psychosocial issues. PCPs may also not be aware of the new findings relating traumatic life experiences such as refugee trauma, domestic violence, and history of child abuse to the patient's medical problems.

Despite the inherent and current limitations of primary care, it remains the ideal place for diagnosis and treatment of health and mental health problems in the immigrant and refugee population. Firstly, it is their first point of access. For mental health problems, PHC can be less stigmatizing than special mental health clinics and, despite the many barriers, can meet the person's entire spectrum of mental health and medical needs (Carey et al., 2003). Furthermore, mental health units called behavioural health that are staffed by mental health practitioners and are embedded within the primary care setting are in position to maximize the psychosocial treatment of torture survivors.

A major qualitative community-based study was conducted in the UK in 2018 to describe the barriers refugees and asylum seekers had accessing primary healthcare. The major barriers for refugees are identified and presented in **Box 9.1** (Kang et al., 2019). This study, according to the authors, draws attention to the importance of good basic PHC and the human cost of poor access.

In order to integrate mental health into primary healthcare, the time pressure that leads to short clinical visits, and the health care practitioner's limited knowledge of the importance of identifying the traumatic life experiences of the patient need to be overcome. While it is true that the fast pace of the PHC visit creates

---

Box 9.1 Barriers to refugees utilizing primary healthcare

- Language and interpretation
- Knowledge about eligibility for care
- Navigating and negotiating the primary healthcare system
- Difficulty paying for medication
- Difficulty paying for dental treatment
- Difficulty paying for transportation
- Long waiting times for appointments
- Short appointment times
- Negative experiences in medical consultations
- Discrimination on grounds of race, religion, and immigration status.

Kang, C., Tomkow, L., & Farrington, R. (2019). Access to primary health care for asylum seekers and refugees: a qualitative study of service user experiences in the UK. *British Journal of General Practice*, 69, e537–e545. https://doi.org/10.3399/bjgp19X701309

barriers to exploring a patient's traumatic life history and major psychosocial issues, it is paramount to take that time. Although the majority of immigrants usually seek help in the primary care setting, most PCPs (i.e. doctors, nurses, and mental health practitioners) still need to be trained in order to effectively identify and treat survivors of mass violence and natural disasters (Henderson et al., 2005). PCPs may not be aware of the new findings relating traumatic life experiences such as refugee trauma, domestic violence, and history of child abuse to the patient's medical problems. Even if the doctor knows of the importance of trauma in the patient's health, they may be lacking the skill necessary to have that discussion with their patients, let alone diagnose and treat in a culturally appropriate manner. Culture- and evidence-based services provided in community clinics are seen as ideal for immigrants who may or may not be survivors of mass violence. Such an integrated setting can also improve their quality of life through the management of possible chronic medical and psychiatric conditions.

At the clinical level, Berthold and her colleagues (2020) provide an expanded complex care approach illustrated by the case study of a refugee torture survivor resettled in the US. In their approach, the chronic case model, which focuses on transforming daily care of patients with chronic illnesses from acute and reactive clinical care to proactive comprehensive long-term care of the refugee patient. The latter includes using within PHC five domains of diagnosis and treatment: the trauma story, bio-medical, psychological, social, and spiritual domains. **Figure 9.2** demonstrates this new clinical approach at the macro-level (Daniels et al., 2009; Wagner, 1998).

This chronic care model promoted by Wagner (1998) reinforces the conceptual framework described above for the care of immigrants and is consistent with the report on American health care by the Institute of Medicine (2001). Most importantly, an informed active patient and a trained clinical provider team is necessary for improved outcomes. In this model, patient self-management and self-care is essential. For the latter reason, there has been a small but growing movement advancing health promotion, community, and family support, and the enhancement of an immigrant's self-healing, resiliency and coping responses (Mollica, 2006). In addition to training PCPs, the use of CHWs can bring forth Wagner's model of the activated and empowered patient. CHWs can utilize a community's existing social networks to maximize and facilitate health education, identification and treatment of common health and mental health problems among immigrant populations.

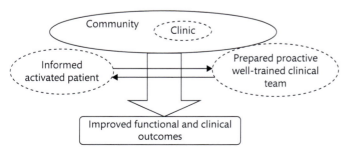

Figure 9.2 Integrated chronic care model.

Use of community health workers as part of the health care team

For immigrant and minority populations, the use of CHWs is an effective approach for promoting access to health services and increasing health-related knowledge. CHWs have been defined as 'community members who work almost exclusively in community settings and who serve as connectors between ... consumers and providers to promote health among groups that have traditionally lacked access to adequate health care' (Norris et al., 2006). They are usually members of the immigrant or minority communities who are lay persons trained to provide advocacy, support, counselling, and information to the target community. A substantial literature suggests that with careful training and monitoring, lay health workers can be effective in health promotion (Hodgins et al., 2016). For example, effective CHW interventions have been conducted among racial/ethnic minority adults (Verhagen et al., 2014). The goals of these interventions can often be classified as (1) increasing access to services, (2) increasing health-related knowledge, or (3) changing health behaviours. For example, Vietnamese-speaking CHWs successfully increased rates of cervical cancer screening among Vietnamese Americans (Ma et al., 2015).

A key component to successful CHW interventions includes cultural tailoring. Cultural tailoring refers to adapting the interventions to reach the target groups' values, beliefs, and practices, but also takes into account individualized personal preferences in order to avoid stereotyping (Fisher et al., 2007). These interventions often rely on the cultural expertise of the CHWs to inform the programmes (Katigbak et al., 2015). Community health interventions have been most successful at increasing access to screening, enhancing disease prevention, and improving chronic disease management (Malcarney et al., 2017).

Conclusion

The high risk of health and mental health problems associated with trauma and acculturation stress compounded with low access to care inhibit the recovery of immigrants and refugees and exacerbates existing health disparities. Increasing the knowledge and skills in PHC is paramount, as is improving outreach efforts that include community-based strategies and partnerships and build upon the already existing social and cultural supports of the community. The use of CHWs can be extremely effective in achieving these goals through a culturally and scientifically based approach. Only by creating activated doctors and patients working together in a partnership can we make a real change in the way that immigrants/refugees are able to access and receive health and mental health services.

REFERENCES

Ackerman, L. K. (1997). Health problems of refugees. *Journal of the American Board of Family Practice*, **10**, 337–348.

Ahn, A. C., Ngo-Metzger, Q., Legedza, A. T., Massagli, M. P., Clarridge, B. R., & Phillips, R. S. (2006). Complementary and alternative medical therapy use among Chinese and Vietnamese Americans: prevalence, associated factors, and effects of patient-clinician communication. *American Journal of Public Health*, **96**, 647–653.

Alim, T., Graves, E., Mellman, T., Aigbogun, N., Gray, E., Lawson, W., et al. (2006). Trauma exposure, posttraumatic stress disorder and depression in an African American primary care population. *Journal of the National Medical Association*, **98**, 1630–1636.

Andrews, J. O., Felton, G., Wewers, M. E., & Heath, J. (2004). Use of community health workers in research with ethnic minority women. *Journal of Nursing Scholarship*, **36**, 358–365.

Balakrishnan, V. S. (2021). Impact of COVID-19 on migrants and refugees. *Lancet Infectious Diseases*, **21**, 1076–1077.

Barnes, J. S. & Bennett, C. E. (2002). *The Asian population: 2000*. C2KBR/01-16. Washington, DC: US Census Bureau.

Barrett, J., Barrett, H., Oxman, T., & Gerber, P. (1988). The prevalence of psychiatric disorders in a primary care practice. *Archives of General Psychiatry*, **45**, 1100–1106.

Berdahl, T. A. & Kirby, J. B. (2019). Patient-provider communication disparities by limited English proficiency (LEP): trends from the US Medical Expenditure Panel Survey, 2006–2015. *Journal of General Internal Medicine*, **34**, 1434–1440.

Berthold, S. M., Kong, S., Mollica, R. F., Theanvy Kuoch, T., Scully, M., & Franke, T. (2014). Comorbid mental and physical health and health access in Cambodian refugees in the US. *Journal of Community Health*, **39**, 1045–1052.

Berthold, S. M., Polatin, P., Mollica, R., Higson-Smith, C., Streets, F. J., Kelly, C. M., & Lavelle, J. (2020). The complex care of a torture survivor in the United States: the case of Joshua. *Torture: Quarterly Journal on Rehabilitation of Torture Victims and Prevention of Torture*, **30**, 23–39.

Bhuyan, R. & Senturia, K. (2005). Understanding domestic violence resource utilization and survivor solutions among immigrant and refugee women: introduction to the special issue. *Journal of Interpersonal Violence*, **20**, 895–901.

Bikoo, M. (2007). Female genital mutilation: classification and management. *Nursing Standard*, **22**, 43–49.

Binagwaho, A., Ngarambe, B., & Yohannes, T. (2021). Gender-based violence against women. *JAMA Health Forum*, **2**, e210868.

Bird, J. A., McPhee, S. J., Ha, N. T., Le, B., Davis, T., & Jenkins, C. N. H. (1998). Opening pathways to cancer screening for Vietnamese American women: lay health workers hold a key. *Preventive Medicine*, **27**, 821–829.

Bogic, M., Njoku, A., & Priebe, S. (2015). Long-term mental health of war-refugees: a systematic literature review. *BMC International Health and Human Rights*, **15**, 29.

Boullatta, J. I. & Nace, A. M. (2000). Safety issues with herbal medicine. *Pharmacotherapy*, **20**, 257–269.

Bradford, J., Reisner, S. L., Honnold, J. A., & Xavier, J. (2013). Experiences of transgender-related discrimination and implications for health: results from the Virginia Transgender Health Initiative Study. *American Journal of Public Health*, **103**, 1820–1829.

Braveman, P. (2006). Health disparities and health equity: concepts and measurement. *Annual Review of Public Health*, **27**, 167–194.

Budiman, A. & Ruiz, N. G. (2021). Key facts about Asian Americans, a diverse and growing population. Pew Research Center. https://www.pewresearch.org/fact-tank/2021/04/29/key-facts-about-asian-americans/

Carey, P. D., Stein, D. J., Zungu-Dirwayi, N., & Seedat, S. (2003). Trauma and posttraumatic stress disorder in an urban Xhosa primary care population: prevalence, comorbidity, and service use patterns. *Journal of Nervous and Mental Disease*, **191**, 230–236.

Carlson, E. S., Barriga, T. M., Lobo, D., Garcia, G., Sanchez, D., & Fitz, M. (2022). Overcoming the language barrier: a novel curriculum for training medical students as volunteer medical interpreters. *BMC Medical Education*, **22**, 27.

Carlsson, J. M., Mortensen, E. L., & Kastrup, M. (2005). A follow-up study of mental health and health-related quality of life in tortured refugees in multidisciplinary treatment. *Journal of Nervous and Mental Disease*, **193**, 651–657.

Cassano, P. & Fava, M. (2002). Depression and public health: an overview. *Journal of Psychosomatic Research*, **53**, 849–857.

Chesser, A. K., Keene Woods, N., Smothers, K., & Rogers, N. (2016). Health literacy and older adults: a systematic review. *Gerontology & Geriatric Medicine*, **2**, 2333721416630492.

Clarke, S. K., Jaffe, J., & Mutch, R. (2019). Overcoming communication barriers in refugee health care. *Pediatric Clinics of North America*, **66**, 669–686.

Coker, A. L., Smith, P. H., Bethea, L., King, M. R., & McKeown, R. E. (2000). Physical health consequences of physical and psychological intimate partner violence. *Archives of Family Medicine*, **9**, 451–457.

Congressional Research Service (2021). Citizenship, and immigration of the U.S. foreign born population, 2021. https://www.cbo.gov/publication/58939

Culpepper, L. (2002). Depression and chronic medical illness: diabetes as a model. *Psychiatric Annals*, **32**, 528–534.

Daniels, A., Adams, N., Carroll, C., & Beinecke, R. (2009). A conceptual model for behavioral health and primary care integration: emerging challenges and strategies for improving international mental health services. *International Journal of Mental Health*, **38**, 100–112.

Davis, R., Kessler, K., & Schwartz, A. (2008). Treatment barriers for low-income, urban African Americans with undiagnosed post-traumatic stress disorder. *Journal of Traumatic Stress*, **2**, 218–222.

De Alba, I., Ngo-Metzger, Q., Sweningson, J. M., & Hubbell, F. A. (2005). Pap smear use in California: are we closing the racial/ethnic gap? *Preventative Medicine*, **40**, 747–755.

Derose, K., Bahney, B., Lurie, N., & Escarce, J. (2009). Immigrants and health care access, quality, and cost. *Medical Care Research and Review*, **66**, 355–408.

DeSantis, C. E., Ma, J., Gaudet, M. M., Newman, L. A., Miller, K. D., Goding Sauer, A., et al. (2019), Breast cancer statistics, 2019. *CA: A Cancer Journal for Clinicians*, **69**, 438–451.

Diamond, L., Izquierdo, K., Canfield, D., Matsoukas, K., & Gany, F. (2019). A systematic review of the impact of patient-physician non-English language concordance on quality of care and outcomes. *Journal of General Internal Medicine*, **34**, 1591–1606.

Dietrich, S., & Hernandez, E. (2022). *American Community Survey Reports: Language Use in the United States: 2019*. U.S. Census Bureau.

Divi, C., Koss, R., Schmaltz, S., & Loeb, J. (2007). Language proficiency and adverse events in US hospitals: a pilot study. *International Journal for Quality in Health Care*, **19**, 60–67.

Durham, J., Gillieatt, S., & Ellies, P. (2007). An evaluability assessment of a nutrition promotion project for newly arrived refugees. *Health Promotion Journal of Australia*, **18**, 43–49.

Easton, P., Entwistle, V. A., & Williams, B. (2013). How the stigma of low literacy can impair patient-professional spoken interactions and affect health: insights from a qualitative investigation. *BMC Health Services Research*, **13**, 319.

Fazel, M., Wheeler, J., & Danesh, J. (2005). Prevalence of serious mental disorder in 7000 refugees resettled in western countries: a systematic review. *Lancet*, **365**, 1309–1314.

Feldman, R. (2006). Primary health care for refugees and asylum seekers: a review of the literature and a framework for services. *Public Health*, **120**, 809–816.

Fiscella, K., Goodwin, M. A., & Stange, K. C. (2002). Does patient educational level affect office visits to family physicians? *Journal of the National Medical Association*, **94**, 157–165.

Fisher, T. L., Burnet, D. L., Huang, E. S., Chin, M. H., & Cagney, K. A. (2007). Cultural leverage: interventions using culture to narrow racial disparities in health care. *Medical Care Research and Review*, **64**(Suppl. 5), 243S–282S.

Fox, S. D., Griffin, R. H., & Pachankis, J. E. (2020). Minority stress, social integration, and the mental health needs of LGBTQ asylum seekers in North America. *Social Science & Medicine*, **246**, 112727.

Fraser, K. (2003). *Domestic Violence and Women's Physical Health*. Canberra: Australian Domestic & Family Violence Clearinghouse.

Friedman, M. J. & Schnurr, P. P. (1995). The relationship between trauma, post-traumatic stress disorder, and physical health. In: Friedman, M. J., Charney, D. S., & Deutch, A. Y. (Eds.), *Neurobiological and Clinical Consequences of Stress: From Normal Adaptation to Post-Traumatic Stress Disorder* (pp. 507–524). Philadelphia, PA: Lippincott Williams & Wilkins Publishers.

Gavagan, T. & Brodyaga, L. (1998). Medical care for immigrants and refugees. *American Family Physician*, **57**, 1061–1068.

Goel, M. S., Burns, R. B., Phillips, R. S., Davis, R. B., Ngo-Metzger, Q., & McCarthy, E. P. (2005). Trends in breast conserving surgery among Asian Americans and Pacific Islanders, 1992–2000. *Journal of General Internal Medicine*, **20**, 604–611.

Gong, S., Wang, K., Li, Y., & Alamian, A. (2019). The influence of immigrant generation on obesity among Asian Americans in California from 2013 to 2014. *PLOS ONE, 14*(2), e0212740. https://doi.org/10.1371/journal.pone.0212740

Goodman, R. (2001). Psychometric properties of the strengths and difficulties questionnaire. *Journal of the American Academy of Child and Adolescent Psychiatry*, **40**, 1337–1345.

Greenfield, S., Kaplan, S., & Ware, J. E., Jr. (1985). Expanding patient involvement in care. Effects on patient outcomes. *Annals of Internal Medicine*, **102**, 520–528.

Greenfield, S., Kaplan, S. H., Ware, J. E., Jr., Yano, E. M., & Frank, H. J. (1988). Patients' participation in medical care: effects on blood sugar control and quality of life in diabetes. *Journal of General Internal Medicine*, **3**, 448–457.

Grieco, E. M., Acosta, Y., & De La Cruz, G. P. (2012). *The Foreign-Born Population in the United States: 2010*. US Department of Commerce, Economics and Statistics Administration, US Census Bureau.

Hampers, L. C. & McNulty, J. E. (2002). Professional interpreters and bilingual physicians in a pediatric emergency department: effect on resource utilization. *Archives of Pediatric & Adolescent Medicine*, **156**, 1108–1113.

Harris, R. M., Bausell, R. B., Scott, D. E., Hetherington, S. E., & Kavanagh, K. H. (1998). An intervention for changing high-risk HIV behaviors of African American drug-dependent women. *Research in Nursing & Health*, **21**, 239–250.

Hashim M. J. (2017). Patient-centered communication: basic skills. *American Family Physician*, **95**, 29–34.

Henderson, D. C., Mollica, R. F., Tor, S., Lavelle, J., & Culhane, M. A., & Hayden D. (2005). Building primary care practitioners' attitudes and confidence in mental health skills in a post-conflict society: a Cambodian example. *Journal of Nervous and Mental Disease*, **193**, 551–559.

Hodgins, F., Gnich, W., Ross, A. J., Sherriff, A., & Worlledge-Andrew, H. (2016). How lay health workers tailor in effective health behaviour change interventions: a protocol for a systematic review. *Systematic Reviews*, **5**, 102.

Ibeneme, S., Eni, G., Ezuma, A., & Fortwengel, G. (2017). Roads to health in developing countries: understanding the intersection of culture and healing. *Current Therapeutic Research, Clinical and Experimental*, **86**, 13–18.

Institute of Medicine (1996). *Primary Care: America's Health in a New Era*. Washington, DC: National Academy Press.

Institute of Medicine (2001). *Crossing the Quality Chasm: A New Health System for the 21st Century*. Washington, DC: National Academic Press.

Kagawa-Singer, M. & Kassim-Lakha, S. (2003). A strategy to reduce cross-cultural miscommunication and increase the likelihood of improving health outcomes. *Academic Medicine*, **78**, 577–587.

Kalichman, S. C. Ramachandran, B., & Catz, S. (1999). Adherence to combination antiretroviral therapies in HIV patients of low health literacy. *Journal of General Internal Medicine*, **14**, 267–273.

Kang, C., Tomkow, L., & Farrington, R. (2019). Access to primary health care for asylum seekers and refugees: a qualitative study of service user experiences in the UK. *British Journal of General Practice*, **69**, e537–e545.

Katigbak, C., Van Devanter, N., Islam, N., & Trinh-Shevrin, C. (2015). Partners in health: a conceptual framework for the role of community health workers in facilitating patients' adoption of healthy behaviors. *American Journal of Public Health*, **105**, 872–880.

Keating, L. & Muller, R. T. (2020). LGBTQ+ based discrimination is associated with PTSD symptoms, dissociation, emotion dysregulation, and attachment insecurity among LGBTQ+ adults who have experienced trauma. *Journal of Trauma & Dissociation*, **21**, 124–141.

Kim, G., Aguado Loi, C. X., Chiriboga, D. A., Jang, Y., Parmelee, P., & Allen, R. S. (2011). Limited English proficiency as a barrier to mental health service use: a study of Latino and Asian immigrants with psychiatric disorders. *Journal of Psychiatric Research*, **45**, 104–110.

Lai, D., Li, J., Ou, X., & Li, C. (2020). Effectiveness of a peer-based intervention on loneliness and social isolation of older Chinese immigrants in Canada: a randomized controlled trial. *BMC Geriatrics*, **20**, 356.

Lapham, S. C., Hall, M., & Skipper, B. (1995). Homelessness and substance use among alcohol abusers following participation in Project H&ART. *Journal of Addictive Diseases*, **14**, 41–55.

Lee, J. W., Brancati, F. L., & Yeh, H. C. (2011). Trends in the prevalence of type 2 diabetes in Asians versus whites: results from the United States National Health Interview Survey, 1997–2008. *Diabetes Care*, **34**, 353–357.

Leigh, G., Hodgins, D. C., Milne, R., & Gerrish, R. (1999). Volunteer assistants in the treatment of chronic alcoholism. *American Journal of Drug and Alcohol Abuse*, **25**, 543–559.

Lewin, S. A., Dick, J., Pond, P., Zwarenstein, M., Aja, G., van Wyk, B. E., et al. (2005). Lay health workers in primary and community health care. *Cochrane Database of Systematic Reviews*, **1**, CD004015.

Lifson, A. R., Thai, D., O'Fallon, A., Mills, W. A., & Hang, K. (2002). Prevalence of tuberculosis, hepatitis B virus, and intestinal parasitic infections among refugees to Minnesota. *Public Health Reports*, **117**, 69–77.

Lindholm, M., Hargraves, J. L., Ferguson, W. J., & Reed, G. (2012). Professional language interpretation and inpatient length of stay and readmission rates. *Journal of General Internal Medicine*, **27**, 1294–1299.

Linzer, M., Bitton, A., Tu, S. P., Plews-Ogan, M., Horowitz, K. R., Schwartz, M. D., et al. (2015). The end of the 15–20 minute primary care visit. *Journal of General Internal Medicine*, **30**, 1584–1586.

Ma, G. X., Fang, C., Tan, Y., Feng, Z., Ge, S., & Nguyen, C. (2015). Increasing cervical cancer screening among Vietnamese Americans: a community-based intervention trial. *Journal of Health Care for the Poor and Underserved*, **26**(2 Suppl.), 36–52.

Magruder, K. M., Frueh, B., Knapp, R. G., Davis, L., Hamner, M. B., Martin, R. H., et al. (2005). Prevalence of post-traumatic stress disorder in veterans' affairs primary health care clinics. *General Hospital Psychiatry*, **27**, 169–179.

Malcarney, M. B., Pittman, P., Quigley, L., Horton, K., & Seiler, N. (2017). The changing roles of community health workers. *Health Services Research*, **52**(Suppl. 1), 360–382.

Marshall, G., Schell, T. L., Elliot, M. N., Bethold, S. M., & Chun, C. (2005). Mental health and Cambodian refugees 2 decades after resettlement in the United States. *Journal of the American Medical Association*, **294**, 571–579.

McDonald, M. & Shenkman, L. J. (2018). Health literacy and health outcomes of adults in the United States: implications for providers. *Internet Journal of Allied Health Sciences and Practice*, **16**, Article 2.

McNeely, M. J. & Boyko, E. J. (2004). Type 2 diabetes prevalence in Asian Americans: results of a national health survey. *Diabetes Care*, **27**, 66–69.

Menendez, M. E., van Hoorn, B. T., Mackert, M., Donovan, E. E., Chen, N. C., & Ring, D. (2017). Patients with limited health literacy ask fewer questions during office visits with hand surgeons. *Clinical Orthopaedics and Related Research*, **475**, 1291–1297.

Miller, B., Kolonel, L., Bernstein, J., & Young, J. (1996). *Racial/Ethnic Patterns of Cancer in the United States 1988–1992. The Unequal Burden of Cancer among Asian Americans*. Bethesda, MD: Asian American Network for Cancer Awareness, Research and Training (AANCART).

Miranda, J., Duan, N., Sherbourne, C., Schoenbaum, M., Lagomasino, I., Jackson-Triche, M., et al. (2003). Improving care for minorities: can quality improvement interventions improve care and outcomes for depressed minorities? Results of a randomized, controlled trial. *Health Services Research*, **38**, 613–630.

Miranda, J., Lawson, W., & Escobar, J. (2002). Ethnic minorities. *Mental Health Services Research*, **4**, 231–237. Mishori, R., Aleinikoff, S., & Davis, D. M. (2017). Primary care for refugees: challenges and opportunities. *American Family Physician*, **96**, 112–120.

Mollica, R. F. (2006). *Healing Invisible Wounds: Paths to Hope and Recovery in a Violent World*. Orlando, FL: Harcourt Press.

Mollica, R. F., Cardozo, B. L., Osofsky, H. J., Raphael, B., Ager, A., & Salama, P. (2004). Mental health in complex emergencies. *Lancet*, **364**, 2058–2067.

Mollica, R. F., Lyoo, I. K., Chernoff, M. C., Bui, H. X., Lavelle, J., Yoon, S. J., et al. (2009). Brain structural abnormalities and mental health sequelae in South Vietnamese ex–political detainees who survived traumatic head injury and torture. *Archives of General Psychiatry*, **66**, 1221–1232.

Mollica, R. F., McInnes, K., Pham, T., Smith Fawzi, M. C., Murphy, E., & Lin, L. (1998). The dose-effect relationships between torture and psychiatric symptoms in Vietnamese ex-political detainees and a comparison group. *Journal of Nervous and Mental Disease*, **186**, 543–553.

Mollica, R. F., McInnes, K., Sarajlic, N., Lavelle, J., Sarajlic, I., & Massagli, M. P. (1999). Disability associated with psychiatric co-morbidity and health status in Bosnian refugees living in Croatia. *Journal of the American Medical Association*, **282**, 433–439.

Mui, A. C. & Kang, S. Y. (2006). Acculturation stress and depression among Asian immigrant elders. *Social Work*, **51**, 243–255.

Na, S., Ryder, A. G., & Kirmayer, L. J. (2016). Toward a culturally responsive model of mental health literacy: facilitating help-seeking among East Asian immigrants to North America. *American Journal of Community Psychology*, **58**, 211–225.

Ngo-Metzger, Q., Legedza, A. T. R., & Phillips, R. S. (2004). Asian Americans' reports of their health care experiences: results of a national survey. *Journal of General Internal Medicine*, **19**, 111–119.

Ngo-Metzger, Q., Massagli, M. P., Clarridge, B. R., Manocchia, M., Davis, R. B., Iezzoni, L. I., et al. (2003). Linguistic and cultural barriers to care: perspectives of Chinese and Vietnamese immigrants. *Journal of General Internal Medicine*, **18**, 44–52. Ngo-Metzger, Q., Phillips, R. S., & McCarthy, E. P. (2008). Ethnic disparities in hospice use among Asian-American and Pacific Islander patients dying with cancer. *Journal of the American Geriatrics Society*, **56**, 139–144.

Ngo-Metzger, Q., Sorkin, D. H., Phillips, R. S., Greenfield, S., Massagli, M. P., Clarridge, B., et al. (2007). Providing high-quality care for limited English proficient patients: the importance of language concordance and interpreter use. *Journal of General Internal Medicine*, **22**, 324–330.

Norris, S. L., Chowdhury, F. M., Van Le, K., Armour, T., Brownstein, J. N., Zhang, X., et al. (2006). Effectiveness of community health workers in the care of persons with diabetes. *Diabetic Medicine*, **23**, 544–556.

Nyamathi, A., Flaskerud, J. H., Leake, B., Dixon, E. L., & Lu, A. (2001). Evaluating the impact of peer, nurse case-managed, and standard HIV risk-reduction programs on psychosocial and health promoting behavioral outcomes among homeless women. *Research in Nursing & Health*, **24**, 410–422.

OECD (2020), *International Migration Outlook 2020*, OECD Publishing, Paris, https://doi.org/10.1787/ec98f531-en.

Office of Disease Prevention and Health Promotion (2021). Health literacy in healthy people 2030. Health.gov. https://health.gov/our-work/national-health-initiatives/healthy-people/healthy-people-2030/health-literacy-healthy-people-2030

Office of Refugee Resettlement (2008). *History*. Washington, DC: Office of Refugee Resettlement.

Pacella, M. L., Bryce, H., & Delahanty, D. L. (2013). The physical health consequences of PTSD and PTSD symptoms: a meta-analytic review. *Journal of Anxiety Disorders*, **27**, 33–46.

Palinkas, L. A., Pickwell, S. M., Brandstein, K., Clark, T. J., Hill, L. L., Moser, R. J., et al. (2003). The journey to wellness: stages of refugee health promotion and disease prevention. *Journal of Immigrant Health*, **5**, 19–28.

Pang, K. Y. (2000). Symptom expression and somatization among elderly Korean immigrants. *Journal of Clinical Geropsychology*, **6**, 199–212.

Pignone, M., Gaynes, B., & Rushton, J. (2002). Screening for depression in adults: a summary of the evidence for the U.S. Preventive Services Task Force. *Annals of Internal Medicine*, **136**, 760–764.

Popkin, B. M. & Udry, J. R. (1998). Adolescent obesity increases significantly in second and third generations US immigrants: the National Longitudinal Study of Adolescent of Health. *Journal of Nutrition*, **128**, 701–706.

Porter, M. & Haslam, N. (2005). Pre-displacement and post-displacement factors associated with mental health of refugees and internally displaced persons. *Journal of the American Medical Association*, **294**, 602–612.

Pottie, K., Janakiram, P., Topp, P., & McCarthy, A. (2007). Prevalence of selected preventable and treatable diseases among government-assisted refugees: implications for primary care providers. *Canadian Family Physician Medecin de Famille Canadien*, **53**, 1928–1934.

Raquinio, P., Maskarinec, G., Dela Cruz, R., Setiawan, V. W., Kristal, B. S., Wilkens, L. R., & Le Marchand, L. (2021). Type 2 diabetes among Filipino American adults in the multiethnic cohort. *Preventing Chronic Disease*, **18**, E98.

Roberts, G. L., Williams, G. M., Lawrence, J. M., & Raphael, B. (1998). How does domestic violence affect women's mental health? *Women & Health*, **28**, 117–129.

Rosati, F., Coletta, V., Pistella, J., Scandurra, C., Laghi, F., & Baiocco, R. (2021). Experiences of life and intersectionality of transgender refugees living in Italy: a qualitative approach. *International Journal of Environmental Research and Public Health*, **18**, 12385.

Roter, D. L., Hall, J. A., & Katz, N. R. (1988). Patient-physician communication: a descriptive summary of the literature. *Patient Education and Counseling*, **12**, 99–119.

Rudd, R. E., Moeykens, B. A., & Colton, T. C. (2000). Health and literacy: a review of medical and public health literature. In: Comings, J., Garners, B., & Smith, C. (Eds.), *Annual Review of Adult Learning and Literacy* (pp. 158–199). San Francisco, CA: Jossey-Bass.

Sansone, R. A., Wiederman, M., & Sansone, L. (1997). Health care utilization and history of trauma among women in a primary care setting. *Violence and Victims*, **12**, 165–172.

Sareen, J., Cox, B., Stein, M., Afifi, T., Fleet, C., & Asmundso, G. (2007). Physical and mental comorbidity, disability, and suicidal behavior associated with posttraumatic stress disorder in a large community sample. *Psychosomatic Medicine*, **69**, 242–248.

Schillinger, D., Grumbach, K., Piette, J., Wang, C., Wilson, C., Daher, K., et al. (2002). Association of health literacy with diabetes outcomes. *Journal of the American Medical Association*, **288**, 475–482.

Schmidley, A. (2001). *U.S. Census Bureau, Current Population Reports, Series P23-206, Profile of the Foreign-Born Population in the United States: 2000*. Washington, DC: US Census Bureau, US Government Printing Office.

Sentell, T. & Braun, K. L. (2012). Low health literacy, limited English proficiency, and health status in Asians, Latinos, and other racial/ethnic groups in California. *Journal of Health Communication*, **17**(Suppl. 3), 82–99.

Silberholz, E. A., Brodie, N., Spector, N. D., & Pattishall, A. E. (2017) Disparities in access to care in marginalized populations. *Current Opinion in Pediatrics*, **29**, 718–727.

Sledjeski, E. M., Speisman, B., & Dierker, L. (2008). Does number of lifetime traumas explain the relationship between PTSD and chronic medical conditions? Answers from the National Comorbidity Survey-Replication (NCS-R). *Journal of Behavioral Medicine*, **31**, 341–349.

Snowden, L. R., Masland, M. C., Peng, C. J., Wei-Mien Lou, C., & Wallace, N. T. (2011). Limited English proficient Asian Americans: threshold language policy and access to mental health treatment. *Social Science & Medicine*, **72**, 230–237.

Sorkin, D. H., Pham, E., & Ngo-Metzger, Q. (2009). Racial and ethnic differences in the mental health needs and access to care of older adults in California. *Journal of the American Geriatric Society*, **57**, 2311–2317.

Sorkin, D. H., Tan, A., Hays, R. D., Mangione, C. M., & Ngo-Metzger, Q. (2008). Self-reported health status of older Vietnamese and non-Hispanic whites in California. *Journal of the American Geriatric Society*, **56**, 1543–1548.

Southeast Asian Subcommittee of the Asian American/Pacific Islander Work Group, National Diabetes Education Program (2006). *Silent Trauma: Diabetes, Health Status, and the Refugee. Southeast Asians in the United States*. Washington, DC: Department of Health and Human Services and National Diabetes Education Program. https://www.aapcho.org/wp/wp-content/uploads/2006/06/SilentTrauma.pdf

Spiegel, P. & Nankoe, A. (2004). UNHCR, HIV/AIDS and refugees: lessons learned. *Forced Migration Review*, **19**, 21–23.

Street, R. L., Jr. (1991). Information-giving in medical consultations: the influence of patients' communicative styles and personal characteristics. *Social Science & Medicine*, **32**, 541–548.

Stromme, E. M., Igland, J., Haj-Younes, J., Kumar, B. N., Fadnes, L. T., Hasha, W., & Diaz, E. (2021). Chronic pain, and mental health problems among Syrian refugees: associations, predictors, and use of medication over time: a prospective cohort study. *BMJ Open*, **11**, e046454.

Suarez-Almazor M. E. (2004). Patient-physician communication. *Current Opinion in Rheumatology*, **16**, 91–95.

Surveillance, Epidemiology, and End Results Program. (n.d.). *Cancer Disparities*. National Cancer Institute. https://seer.cancer.gov/statfacts/html/disparities.html

Taubman-Ben-Ari, O., Rabinowitz, J., Feldman, D., & Vaturi, R. (2001). Post-traumatic stress disorder in the primary care medical setting. *Psychological Medicine*, **31**, 555–560.

Tompkins, M., Smith, L., Jones, K., & Swindells, S. (2006). HIV education needs among Sudanese immigrants and refugees in the Midwestern United States. *AIDS and Behaviour*, **10**, 319–323.

Trinh-Shevrin, C., Islam, N. S., & Rey, M. J. (2009). *Asian American Communities and Health*. San Francisco, CA: John Wiley & Sons.

UNHCR (2021a). Global trends: forced displacement. https://www.unhcr.org/uk/global-trends

UNHCR (2021b, November). Refugee data finder. https://www.unhcr.org/refugee-statistics/download/

US Census Bureau (2000). *Census 2000 Summary File 3, Matrices P19, P20, PCT13, and PCT14*. Washington, DC: US Census Bureau.

US Census Bureau (2007). *American Community Survey*. Washington, DC: US Census Bureau.

US Census Bureau (2013). *Language Use in the United States: 2011*. Washington, DC: US Census Bureau.

US Department of Health and Human Services (2020). 2019 National healthcare quality and disparities report. Agency for Healthcare Research and Quality, AHRQ Publication 20(21)-0045-EF. https://www.ahrq.gov/research/findings/nhqrdr/nhqdr19/index.htmlVerhagen, I., Steunenberg, B., de Wit, N. J., & Ros, W. J. (2014). Community health worker interventions to improve access to health care services for older adults from ethnic minorities: a systematic review. *BMC Health Services Research*, **14**, 497.

Verlinde, E., De Laender, N., De Maesschalck, S., Deveugele, M., & Willems, S. (2012). The social gradient in doctor-patient communication. *International Journal for Equity in Health*, **11**, 12.

Wagner, E. H. (1998). Chronic disease management: what will it take to improve care for chronic illness? *Effective Clinical Practice*, **1**, 2–4.

Wang, J. H., Sheppard, V. B., Schwartz, M. D., Liang, W., & Mandelblatt, J. S. (2008). Disparities in cervical cancer screening between Asian American and Non-Hispanic white women. *Cancer Epidemiology, Biomarkers & Prevention*, **17**, 1968–1973.

Washington, O. G. M. & Moxley, D. P. (2003). Group interventions with low-income African American women recovering from chemical dependency. *Health & Social Work*, **28**, 146–157.

Wasserman, M., Renfrew, M. R., Green, A. R., Lopez, L., Tan-McGrory, A., Brach, C., & Betancourt, J. R. (2014). Identifying and preventing medical errors in patients with limited English proficiency: key findings and tools for the field. *Journal for Healthcare Quality*, **36**, 5–16.

Weech-Maldonado, R., Morales, L. S., Elliott, M., Spritzer, K., Marshall, G., & Hays, R. D. (2003). Race/ethnicity, language, and patients' assessments of care in Medicaid managed care. *Health Services Research*, **38**, 789–808.

Weiss, B. D., Schwartzberg, J., Davis, T., Parker, R., Williams, M., and Wang, C. (2003). *Health Literacy: A Manual for Clinicians*. Chicago, IL: AMA Foundation.

Williams, M. V., Davis, T., Parker, R. M., & Weiss, B. D. (2002). The role of health literacy in patient-physician communication. *Family Medicine*, **34**, 383–389.

World Health Organization (2021). *Addressing Violence Against Women in Health and Multisectoral Policies: A Global Status Report.* Geneva: World Health Organization.

World Health Organization (2022). WHO COVID-19 dashboard. https://covid19.who.int/

Wu, T., Jia, X., Shi, H., Niu, J., Yin, X., Xie, J., & Wang, X. (2021). Prevalence of mental health problems during the COVID-19 pandemic: a systematic review and meta-analysis. *Journal of Affective Disorders*, **281**, 91–98.

Xiong, J., Lipsitz, O., Nasri, F., Lui, L. M. W., Gill, H., Phan, L., et al. (2020). Impact of COVID-19 pandemic on mental health in the general population: a systematic review. *Journal of Affective Disorders*, **277**, 55–64.

Yang, K. G., Rodgers, C., Lee, E., & Lê Cook, B. (2020). Disparities in mental health care utilization and perceived need among Asian Americans: 2012–2016. *Psychiatric Services*, **71**, 21–27.

Yee, B. (2003). *Health and Health Care of Southeast Asian American Elders: Vietnamese, Cambodian, Hmong, and Laotian Elders.* Department of Health Promotion and Gerontology, University of Texas Medical Branch, Galveston, Texas Consortium of Geriatric Education Centers.

Yee, B. W. K. (2004). *Health and Health Care of Southeast Asian American Elders: Vietnamese, Cambodian, Hmong, and Laotian elders.* ResearchGate.

Zeidan, A. J., Khatri, U. G., Munyikwa, M., Barden, A., & Samuels-Kalow, M. (2019). Barriers to accessing acute care for newly arrived refugees. *Western Journal of Emergency Medicine*, **20**, 842–850.

SECTION 4
Treatment and service components

10. **Early intervention for mental health and substance use disorders** 97
    Cristina Mei, Paddy Power, Gill Bedi, Sarah Maguire, Louise McCutcheon, Aswin Ratheesh, Katrina Witt, and Patrick D. McGorry

11. **Organizing the range of community mental health services** 113
    Graham Thornicroft, Michele Tansella, and Robert E. Drake

12. **Crisis and emergency services** 127
    Sonia Johnson, Justin J. Needle, Jonathan Totman, and Lorna Hobbs

13. **Early intervention for people with psychotic disorders** 141
    Paddy Power, Ellie Brown, and Patrick D. McGorry

14. **Case management and assertive community treatment** 161
    Helen Killaspy and Alan Rosen

15. **Principles and standards for medication management of individuals with serious mental illness** 171
    Thomas E. Smith and Delia C. Hendrick

16. **Psychiatric outpatient clinics** 183
    Markus Koesters, Carolin Schneider, and Thomas Becker

17. **Day hospital and partial hospitalization programmes** 187
    Aart H. Schene

18. **Inpatient treatment** 195
    Frank Holloway and Derek Tracy

19. **Residential care** 207
    Geoff Shepherd and Rob Macpherson

20. **Individual placement and support: the evidence-based practice of supported employment** 219
    Deborah R. Becker, Gary R. Bond, and Robert E. Drake

21. **Programmes to support family members and caregivers** 225
    Samantha Jankowski, Amy L. Drapalski, and Lisa B. Dixon

22. **Managing co-occurring physical disorders in mental health care** 233
    Delia C. Hendrick and Robert E. Drake

23. **Illness self-management programmes** 243
    Kim T. Mueser and Susan Gingerich

24. **Co-occurring substance use disorders** 253
    Robert E. Drake, Kim T. Mueser, and Delia C. Hendrick

25. **Behavioural health technologies and telehealth** 261
    John Torous and Elizabeth Carpenter-Song

26. **Forensic community mental health services** 271
    Lisa Wootton, Penelope Brown, and Alec Buchanan

10

Early intervention for mental health and substance use disorders

Cristina Mei, Paddy Power, Gill Bedi, Sarah Maguire, Louise McCutcheon, Aswin Ratheesh, Katrina Witt, and Patrick D. McGorry

Introduction

The case for early intervention

One of the most significant recent reforms in mental health care is the creation of early intervention services for psychosis, pioneered in Australia in the early 1990s (Malla & McGorry, 2019). As outlined in Chapter 13, these services have been scaled up in many countries and have been shown to be highly effective in controlled trials (Correll et al., 2018), real-world settings (Posselt et al., 2021), and in economic analyses (Mihalopoulos et al., 2009). This proof of concept has provided the foundation for a broader early intervention model that encompasses the full range of mental ill health (e.g. anxiety and mood disorders, personality disorders (PDs), eating disorders (EDs), and substance use disorders (SUDs)), with a strong focus on young people (approximately 12–25 years of age), as detailed in the current chapter (McGorry et al., 2022).

Young people are disproportionately affected by mental ill health: 50% of adult-type mental disorders have their onset by 14 years of age and 75% by 24 years (Kessler et al., 2005). Mental ill health is the leading cause of disability in young people, accounting for 45% of the overall burden of disease between the ages of 10 and 24 years (Gore et al., 2011). The emergence of mental ill health during adolescence or early adulthood can substantially disrupt a young person's trajectory and their potential in terms of education, social and workforce participation, and economic security (Copeland et al., 2015; Dalsgaard et al., 2020; Gardner et al., 2019; Weavers et al., 2021). Early intervention is critical for modifying the course of mental illness, mitigating its disabling impacts, and strengthening the productivity of young people (McGorry et al., 2022). Childhood-onset disorders—notably, autism and attention deficit hyperactivity disorder—are another important subgroup that can further impact the transition to adulthood and require early detection and sustained intervention, beginning in early childhood.

A key goal of early intervention services is to reduce the duration of untreated illness and to deliver effective evidence-based care during the critical years following illness onset (Malla, 2022).

The recognition and characterization of subthreshold stages of illness has brought forward the timing of early intervention. Learnings from the early psychosis model demonstrated that the duration of untreated psychosis is a strong indicator of prognosis, with a longer duration predicting poorer symptomatic and functional recovery, and a decreased likelihood of remission (Drake et al., 2020; Howes et al., 2021). Similarly, other mental disorders have shown an association between a long duration of untreated illness and poor clinical outcome (Altamura et al., 2015; Austin et al., 2021; Ghio et al., 2014). Adding weight to the case for early intervention is the damaging effect that illness progression (e.g. brain or neurocognitive changes) can have on recovery (Abé et al., 2022; Hermens et al., 2013; Sapolsky, 2000; Treasure et al., 2015a). This is recognized by the clinical staging model (described below and in Chapter 13); that is, intervention delivered early in the illness course is more likely to be effective than during later stages of illness when neurobiological impairment and functional disability are more entrenched (McGorry & Mei, 2021).

There are also strong economic arguments in favour of early intervention and prevention (Campion & Knapp, 2018). Mental ill health is the dominant contributor to the global economic burden of non-communicable diseases, with the cost estimated to reach US $16 trillion by 2030 (Bloom et al., 2011). This economic impact is largely driven by the early age of onset of mental ill health and the subsequent loss of productivity due to diminished health, disability, and premature death, including by suicide. Investment in mental health care can generate a strong return on investment: for every $1 spent towards the treatment of depression and anxiety, there is a $4–$5 return in better health and enhanced productivity (Chisholm et al., 2016).

Despite the above arguments and the moral imperative of early intervention, structural and cultural flaws within traditional systems of mental health care have impeded early intervention efforts during the peak onset period for mental illness. This has contributed to low rates of service use among young people and high rates of service discontinuity during the transition from child to adult services

(McGorry et al., 2022; Singh et al., 2010). This largely reflects the adoption of a paediatric–adult model of health care that mainly focuses on young children and older adults and is misaligned to the epidemiology of mental illness and the developmental needs of young people (McGorry et al., 2022). Under-resourcing and underfunding are also major contributors. A paediatric–adult service delivery spilt is also incompatible with developmental and societal shifts that have altered and protracted the transition to mature adulthood (Arnett et al., 2014; Sawyer et al., 2018). This all supports the need for a youth mental health subspecialty that is tailored to the needs of young people, eliminates ill-placed age boundaries across service streams, and reduces barriers to early intervention (McGorry et al., 2022).

Integrated youth mental health care services

The successful implementation of the early psychosis service model provided the basis for a broader youth mental health reform agenda that has gained momentum—predominately in high-income countries—to respond to the high unmet need among adolescents and young adults (McGorry et al., 2022). The reform process began in Australia in 2006 following an extensive advocacy campaign that led to the creation of 'headspace', an enhanced primary mental health care model for young people aged 12–25 years (McGorry et al., 2014, 2019; Rickwood et al., 2019). Headspace is a high-capacity platform that provides proportional and stage-specific care, with supported transitions (e.g. to secondary and tertiary services) for young people who require more intensive, long-term, or complex care (Rickwood et al., 2019). A multidisciplinary team (clinical and non-clinical staff, including peer workers) provides the young person and their family with the full cycle of care in a 'one-stop shop' location, with integration of mental health, physical and sexual health, alcohol and other drug, and vocational support (McGorry et al., 2019). From an initial ten centres, the headspace platform has been scaled up to 136 centres across Australia (to reach 164 by 2023) that are accessed by more than 100,000 young people each year (headspace, 2021). Its digital services (eheadspace) are accessed by more than 25,000 young people per annum (headspace, 2021).

The headspace model of care has inspired similar platforms internationally (e.g. headspace in Denmark and Israel, Jigsaw in Ireland, Access Open Minds in Canada, allcove in the US, @ease in the Netherlands, and Youthspace and Forward Thinking Birmingham in England), which offer stigma-free, youth-friendly, and a low threshold ('no wrong door') entry to care (McGorry et al., 2022). The development of headspace and similar international models has been guided by the principles of co-design and youth participation (McGorry et al., 2022). While as yet there is no single model constituting best practice for integrated youth mental health care (Hetrick et al., 2017), core principles have been defined (Box 10.1) that can be locally adapted and tailored according to factors such as available workforce and resources, culture, and funding (Killackey et al., 2020; McGorry et al., 2022). Many of these principles (e.g. co-design, low-stigma, peer workers) are transferable to mental health services that target adults aged 26 and over (Department of Health, 2020).

Young people accessing integrated youth mental health services vary in terms of level of need and presentation (Hetrick et al., 2017). In Australia, the majority of young people accessing headspace are in the very early stages of illness (i.e. distress disorder with or without subthreshold specificity, stages 1a and 1b), although a proportion are seeking care for full-threshold (stage 2) or more advanced stages

> **Box 10.1** Principles of integrated youth mental health care
>
> *Rapid, easy, and affordable access*: services should be in low-stigma and easy-to-access locations, and care should be provided in a timely manner at no or minimal cost.
>
> *Youth-specific care*: services should be co-designed, inclusive, and youth-friendly, acknowledging young people's developmental period and the impact of mental ill health on this life stage.
>
> *Awareness, engagement, and integration*: these elements require strong knowledge of and relationship with relevant stakeholders; education of referrers and community members on early detection, when to refer, and how to advocate for young people; and integration of youth mental health services with other health and social services.
>
> *Early intervention*: intervention should be provided at the earliest opportunity to improve prognosis and may be facilitated by locating services in community/youth-appropriate settings; engaging with groups at high-risk of mental illness; and community outreach, education, and training to promote early identification and provide crisis intervention for suicide risk.
>
> *Youth partnership*: young people should be empowered to meaningfully contribute to services and be partners in all service elements.
>
> *Family engagement and support*: support should be provided to the young person's family (broadly defined) via a range of approaches (e.g. family peer workers, psychoeducation, family therapy).
>
> *Continuous improvement*: there should be a commitment to improvement and learning, including via workforce development and training, auditing, and actively seeking and responding to feedback from young people and families.
>
> *Prevention*: services should promote the prevention of mental illness, which may involve health promotion activities, anti-stigma measures, suicide prevention, identifying and targeting high-risk groups, and identifying and addressing local social determinants of health.
>
> Source: Killackey et al. (2020); McGorry et al. (2022).

of illness (i.e. recurrent or treatment resistant illness, stages 3 and 4) (Filia et al., 2021; Iorfino et al., 2019; Purcell et al., 2015). While headspace and similar integrated models of care have demonstrated positive outcomes, including improvements in access to care, symptomatic and functional recovery, and client satisfaction (Hetrick et al., 2017), a subgroup of young people—who have been termed the 'missing middle'—present with more complex and sustained mental illness and may not benefit from the brief episodes of care that these services are typically designed to deliver (McGorry, 2022). For these individuals, a specialist multidisciplinary backup system is needed, which has commenced for early psychosis (Brown et al., 2022) and has potential to be scaled up and extended to cover the diagnostic spectrum.

Delivering safe and effective early intervention, that is matched to level of need and risk of illness progression, is facilitated by a clinical staging approach, which ensures that the type, intensity, and duration of intervention is stage specific and guided by patient choice and risk–benefit considerations (McGorry & Hickie, 2019). Within this framework, early stages of mental ill health are characterized by non-specific and ambiguous symptoms that may progress to diagnosable syndromes. Reflecting this, interventions are offered in a stepwise manner; simple and benign interventions are deployed early in the illness course, while more intensive and specific approaches that may also pose greater risk are offered during later stages. Clinical staging can be applied to any disorder that tends to or may progress, as outlined below in relation to anxiety, mood, personality, and EDs, and in Chapter 13 for psychotic disorders.

Early intervention for mental and substance use disorders

Providing appropriate and stage-based early intervention requires a highly skilled and diverse workforce that can manage the range of illness presentations and complexity (Rickwood et al., 2019). This section details the application of early detection and intervention for specific presentations that commonly emerge during adolescence and young adulthood. For details on early intervention for psychotic disorders, see Chapter 13.

Mood and anxiety disorders

Epidemiology

In early detection and intervention for mood and anxiety disorders, the range of conditions that fall within this broad umbrella needs consideration. The scope of this section will be aligned with that specified by the International Classification of Diseases, 11th revision (ICD-11), which includes depression, bipolar disorder (BD), phobias, specific and generalized anxiety disorders, and selective mutism, while disorders of traumatic stress and obsessive–compulsive disorders will not be included. Several mood and anxiety disorders may also be considered to be on a continuum with various degrees of overlap. In dimensional approaches to psychopathology, particularly in younger children, it is not uncommon for mood and anxiety disorders to be combined into 'internalizing disorders' given their high degree of overlap. This is supported by data on the comorbidity between mood and anxiety disorders. The World Mental Health Surveys indicate that 45% of those with depression also experience anxiety (Kessler et al., 2007), while birth cohort studies suggest lifetime comorbidity rates of up to 70% (Moffitt et al., 2007). Much of this comorbidity is sequential and typically highest in the 1–5 years after diagnosis of one disorder (Plana-Ripoll et al., 2019).

In community samples, depression and anxiety are highly prevalent and contribute to significant burden. The interquartile range for lifetime prevalence of anxiety and depressive disorders across the world are roughly similar at 10–17% (Kessler et al., 2007), admittedly with large intercountry variations. Similarly, the World Mental Health Surveys indicate that the interquartile range for age of onset for some anxiety disorders such as phobias and separation anxiety is early (7–14 years), while that for other anxiety and mood disorders is in the late twenties through to the forties. However, other approaches (particularly birth cohort studies) indicate a much higher prevalence and an earlier age of onset (Caspi et al., 2020). In the Dunedin cohort, by the age of 26 years, 26% had a diagnosis of an anxiety disorder while 18% had had a depressive episode (Kim-Cohen et al., 2003). Data from birth cohort and other longitudinal studies indicate that those with early onset of anxiety and mood disorders are at an increased risk for other mental disorders (Plana-Ripoll et al., 2019). This has meant that staging models for more severe mood disorders such as BD (Berk et al., 2017; Power, 2015) or transdiagnostic models for youth (Shah et al., 2020) include these symptoms as 'non-specific' or early stages (stage 1a) in the evolution of youth mental ill health. More severe disorders such as BD are also less prevalent (1–2%) (Merikangas et al., 2011), and have a narrower age of onset earlier than that of depression and generalized anxiety disorder (Lin et al., 2006).

Course and prognosis

Mood and anxiety disorders typically have a remitting course. For example, 60–90% of adolescents with depression remit within a year (Dunn & Goodyer, 2006; March et al., 2004). However, in such youth, 33–50% will have had a recurrence after remission (Dunn & Goodyer, 2006; Lewinsohn et al., 1994). Suicidality is a significant concern in youth depression, with nearly half of those attempting suicide in adolescence estimated to have had a recent depressive episode (Hawton & van Heeringen, 2009). Youth anxiety disorders have a variable course depending on the type of disorder, treatment and duration of follow-up (Ginsburg et al., 2011), with at least half responding to psychological treatments (James et al., 2020). The early onset, high prevalence, and poor outcomes in at least a proportion mean that the global burden of depression and anxiety is high, with a peak impact in young adult years. Approximately 7% of all years of life lost to disability is attributable to these disorders in childhood, which rises to 12% in young adulthood into mid-life (Institute for Health Metrics and Evaluation, 2015). This provides a compelling argument for considering early identification, and intervention for mood and anxiety disorders in adolescents and young adults.

Early detection

Early detection of disorders such as depression and anxiety may include both *screening* (i.e. better detection of previously undiagnosed disorder) and *prediction* (i.e. identification of factors that occur temporally earlier that help diagnose the disorder at a later point in time). With respect to the latter, there have been relatively few replicated prediction models for youth mood disorders with methodological factors contributing to difficulties in generalizing models (Rocha et al., 2021). There are emerging risk calculators using prediction models for those with BD (Hafeman et al., 2017) but these require replication.

Data on screening are substantially stronger. In screening for youth depression, the recommendations include targeted screening for those considered at higher risk in the general population, or annual universal screening for asymptomatic youth aged 12 and over in primary care (Zuckerbrot et al., 2018). Tools include the 2-item Patient Health Questionnaire (Kroenke et al., 2003), or the 25-item Strengths and Difficulties questionnaire (Goodman, 1997). However, there is no evidence to indicate improved health outcomes with screening for depression in youth (Roseman et al., 2017). With even fewer supporting data, the utility of routine screening for BD in young people is less clear. For anxiety disorders, current guidelines recommend screening (Connolly et al., 2007), with measures such as the Multidimensional Anxiety Scale for Children (March et al., 1999) useful for those over 8 years. In addition to screening, a clinical assessment of severity, impairment, comorbidity, family and contextual factors, as well as trauma or life events is important for intervention planning.

Early intervention

Early interventions for youth depression and anxiety may include universal, targeted, or indicated prevention programmes (typically referring to stages 0, 1a, and 1b) as well as clinical interventions, typically psychological, family-based, or pharmacological interventions (typically referring to stages 1b–2). There has been a wealth of research into efforts to prevent depression and anxiety in youth, with meta-analyses indicating that universal, targeted and indicated prevention strategies decrease the risk of new onset depression or anxiety (relative risk 0.47–0.61) in youth (Stockings et al., 2016b). Group based cognitive behavioural therapy (CBT) has shown promising effects (Ssegonja et al., 2019). Once significant depression or anxiety is identified, prompt treatment is essential, particularly given the risks associated with these disorders including impairment and suicidality. For young people with anxiety disorders, CBT with or without mindfulness training, as well as selective serotonin reuptake inhibitors have a high level of evidence and are recommended treatments (Connolly et al., 2007). For young people with depression, CBT and interpersonal therapy are evidence based, while fluoxetine and escitalopram have some evidence of efficacy, particularly for moderate to severe depression. School-based intervention programmes also have small to medium effects for targeting depression and anxiety but with limited maintenance of effects (Gee et al., 2020). Not surprisingly given the comorbidity and the shared interventions that are effective for youth depression and anxiety, randomized controlled trials of one disorder also indicate cross-over benefit for the other (Garber et al., 2016). Finally, given the prevalence of depression and anxiety in the pre-onset stages of BD, early intervention for mood and anxiety disorders can also serve as preventive interventions for BD. This is particularly relevant given the relative absence of direct evidence for early interventions in BD. Thus, depression and anxiety disorders are strong candidates for early intervention particularly for youth (Davey & McGorry, 2019). At an individual level however, risks of interventions need to be weighed against the possibility of harms (e.g. the use of stimulants or antidepressants in those at high risk for BD may trigger a manic episode) (DelBello et al., 2001; Strawn et al., 2014).

Personality disorders

Epidemiology

Although it is accepted that PDs emerge during adolescence and young adulthood, early detection and intervention for this group of disorders remains controversial (Chanen & Nicol, 2021). The longitudinal Children in the Community study estimated the prevalence of PDs in community and primary care settings to be 17%, peaking at 12/13 years of age (Cohen et al., 2005). By 24 years, the cumulative prevalence for any PD is 25.7%, with 20% of these experiencing severe PD (Johnson et al., 2008).

Borderline personality disorder (BPD) is the most common PD presenting in primary care and tertiary mental health settings and is associated with a wide range of severe and persistent negative outcomes, including significant morbidity and mortality (Chanen et al., 2017). The estimated prevalence of BPD in community-dwelling youth is approximately 3% and is equally distributed between males and females. However, the prevalence of BPD increases to 20–25% among help-seeking young people, and at least three-quarters of these are usually female (Chanen & Nicol, 2021). Considering its high prevalence and negative long-term outcomes we focus primarily on BPD in this section.

Course and prognosis

There is a normative increase in borderline pathology following puberty, that peaks around mid-adolescence, coinciding with the peak period of onset of the major mental disorders (Chanen & Thompson, 2019; Thompson et al., 2019). BPD features in adolescence and young adulthood have been associated with increased risk of other mental health conditions (mood and anxiety, EDs, and SUDs), physical health complications, recurrent self-harm, and a two-decade reduction in life expectancy (Chanen et al., 2020; Fok et al., 2012; Levine et al., 2021). Young people with BPD features experience marked functional disability due to disruption of educational/vocation pathways, and impairment in peer and intimate relationships (Kaess et al., 2017; Videler et al., 2019). Even decades after the diagnostic features of BPD have resolved, functioning remains stubbornly low (Álvarez-Tomás et al., 2019). Up to two-thirds of adults with BPD are unemployed and do not engage in regular vocational activities (Ng et al., 2016).

Considerable psychopathology, disrupted functioning, distress, and high rates of help-seeking are associated with both a full diagnosis of BPD (five or more features in the Diagnostic and Statistical Manual of Mental Illnesses, fifth edition (DSM-5)), as well as subthreshold syndrome (less than five DSM-5 features) (Kaess et al., 2017; Moran et al., 2016; Thompson et al., 2019). Therefore, the concept of clinical staging in which the intensity of interventions is matched to the stage of illness is useful for guiding prevention and early intervention for BPD (Chanen et al., 2016, 2020; Hutsebaut et al., 2019). In particular, meta-diagnostic concepts such as the Clinical High At Risk Mental State (CHARMS), which includes BPD features along with other forms of psychopathology, allow for consideration of the combination of difficulties as well as their impact on functioning and development in young people (McGorry et al., 2018), with the aim of early intervention for BPD to alter the whole life course trajectory (Chanen & McCutcheon, 2013).

Early detection

Two decades of scientific literature have demonstrated the reliability and validity of the BPD diagnosis in young people, with suitable screening tools and structured clinical interviews available (Chanen et al., 2020). However, misguided beliefs and fear about exposing young people to the stigma and discrimination associated with a diagnosis of PD often result in well-intentioned health professionals avoiding or delaying the diagnosis in those aged under 18 (Chanen, 2021). This delays access to appropriate treatments and systems of care until iatrogenic complications have set in and problems have become entrenched (Chanen & Nicol, 2021; Sharp & Wall, 2018).

Early intervention

Most young people experience barriers to accessing early intervention for PD (Chanen & Nicol, 2021). Specialized PD programmes are rare and often have rigid and/or restrictive entry criteria, thereby excluding the majority with PD features (Storebø et al., 2020). Young people with mild to moderate PD, or who are in the early stages of PD, infrequently receive consistent or evidence-based approaches when accepted into primary care (O'Dwyer et al., 2020). Overall, little has changed over the past decade, and youth mental health services have failed to develop the range of service options necessary to meet the demand across different illness stages (Chanen & Nicol, 2021).

Nevertheless, the evidence base for effective interventions for young people with BPD features is growing (Bo et al., 2021; Storebø et al., 2020). Some randomized controlled trials have specifically targeted early intervention samples in which most of the participants had some BPD features or full threshold BPD (Chanen et al., 2008, 2022; Beck et al., 2020), while others have focused on self-harm outcomes without specifying illness stage (McCauley et al., 2018; Mehlum et al., 2019; Rossouw & Fonagy, 2012). In most cases, the structured treatments outperformed their comparison conditions (treatment as usual) in terms of the rate of improvement and/or the extent of improvement on the primary outcomes. Further, when simple, structured treatments have been compared to specialized psychotherapies, regardless of theoretical model, they have produced similar outcomes (Storebø et al., 2020). However, outcomes following structured psychosocial interventions are still relatively modest and not sustained in the long-term (Chanen et al., 2020; Storebø et al., 2020; Storebø et al., 2020).

Trials to date have shown that interventions developed for adults with BPD can be successfully adapted for young people and that good outcomes can be achieved with briefer, less intensive treatments than previously thought, even for young people with a severe disorder (Chanen et al., 2022). Early illness stages are likely to be suitable for more generic treatment strategies, such as online psychoeducation and peer worker initiatives. For later and severe stages of disorder, the role played by different components of treatment is unclear (e.g. family interventions, individual and group dialectical behaviour therapy skills programmes, other psychotherapies, or service models) as is how digital and virtual reality initiatives can be integrated. However, a recent study demonstrated better outcomes for young adults with BPD if they attended a dialectical behaviour therapy programme specifically designed for young adults compared to one for all ages (Lyng et al., 2020).

Eating disorders

Epidemiology

EDs—anorexia nervosa (AN), bulimia nervosa (BN), binge eating disorder (BED), and other specific feeding and eating disorders (OSFED)—are relatively common problems, but detection rates in the healthcare system are low (Ivancic et al., 2021) and few receive adequate care (Hart et al., 2011). EDs affect both sexes (although females are disproportionally represented) and all cultural groups. Recent Australian research suggests there may be particularly high rates in Indigenous populations (Burt et al., 2020) although culturally specific diagnostic strategies are lacking. While the prevalence of EDs is higher in Western countries, increasing rates have been found in non-Western countries (Galmiche et al., 2019). The true community incidence of EDs is unknown but best evidence suggests AN is the least common of the disorders with a lifetime prevalence of approximately 1.4% for women and 0.2% for men, followed by BN at 1.9% for women and 0.6% for men, BED at 2.8% for women and 1.0% for men, while lifetime prevalence for OSFED across sexes is about 3.2% (Galmiche et al., 2019). There has been a surge in the incidence of EDs with the recent Covid-19 lockdown restrictions (Taquet et al., 2021).

EDs occur across the lifespan, with onset as early as 5 years of age (Madden et al., 2009) and as late as the eighth decade of life (Gowers & Crisp, 1990). The incidence and prevalence of EDs peak during adolescence and emerging adulthood; periods of intense psychosocial development. Best estimates of mean age of onset for AN, BN, and OSFED is between 13 and 19 years, while BED typically onsets slightly later (Micali et al., 2013; Mitchison et al., 2020; Steinhausen & Jensen, 2015). Studies suggest risk for onset of EDs in females increases steadily from age 12 to 22 (the peak occurring between 16 and 19 years) (Silén et al., 2020). Very recent examination of point prevalence rates for EDs in Australian adolescents indicates approximately 22% of adolescents have an ED, with no difference in the rate of illness between younger and older adolescents for most ED diagnostic categories (Mitchison et al., 2020). Even higher rates of disordered eating behaviours are found in the Australian general population (Aouad et al., 2021; Mitchison et al., 2020), including between 31.6% and 51.7% of adolescents (Lawrence et al., 2016; Sparti et al., 2019; Wilksch et al., 2020).

Course and prognosis

There is sparse and conflicting data on the natural course of EDs from prodrome to recovery or entrenched chronic illness. Once an ED emerges, the average duration of AN and BN is long; recent long-term follow-up data of people who received specialist treatment indicate that at 9 years, 31.4% of participants with AN and 68.2% with BN are recovered, while at 22 year follow-up the rates are 62.8% and 68.2%, respectively (Eddy et al., 2017). Of those who had not recovered at 9 years, 50.6% (AN) and 44.1% (BN) recovered at 22 years. Relapse rates at 22 years were 10.5% for AN and 20.5% for BN. Less is known about long-term outcomes for BED and other EDs, but treatment is important as spontaneous remission appears to be low and early symptom change is the best predictor of outcome across all EDs (Vall & Wade, 2015). Mortality is elevated in both AN and BN with an increased mortality risk of more than five and two times, respectively (Smink et al., 2012).

Illness stages have been mostly examined in AN (Maguire et al., 2008; Treasure et al., 2015b), with a four-stage model of early illness through to severe and enduring illness having been developed and tested (Maguire et al., 2017). Markers in the later stages include perceiving the disorder as part of one's identify, rigidity of routine, obsessions, and compulsions (Maguire et al., 2012). Staging models are consistent with the theoretical rationale for general early intervention approaches to EDs (Grange & Loeb, 2007; Loeb & le Grange, 2013; Schmidt et al., 2016). Unlike staging models in other areas of psychiatry, the 'prodrome' stage of illness and characteristics of distinct stages have not been well studied or conceptualized, even for AN where the evidence is still emerging.

We know there are high levels of disordered eating behaviours and subthreshold illness in the general community and research indicates at least half of these cases transition to full syndrome illness (Grange & Loeb, 2007). Other research suggests that the pathway to development of an ED may start even earlier; large longitudinal studies suggest anxiety symptoms and disorders in childhood are associated with later development of an ED (Schaumberg et al., 2019; Swinbourne & Touyz, 2007). Depression in childhood and early adolescence has also been found to be a potent predictor of the later onset of an ED (Jacobi et al., 2011; Ranta et al., 2017).

Recent longitudinal analyses of high-risk teenagers have revealed there may be unique risk processes and prodrome sequences for the four EDs (Stice et al., 2017, 2021). For example, in AN over-evaluation of weight and shape in one's self-worth emerged first, followed by feelings of fatness and fear of weight gain, while for the other EDs all three seemed to emerge simultaneously. Behaviourally, for both AN and BN, compensatory weight control behaviours were more likely to emerge before binge eating (61–73% of the time), whereas in individuals who developed BED, binge eating emerged before any compensatory behaviours. Two prodromal symptoms—weight/shape overvaluation and fear of weight gain—significantly predicted onset of all four disorders (Stice et al., 2021). The authors concluded that the incorporation of prodromal symptoms into aetiological models would be useful. Recent network analysis of illness seems to confirm this pattern of symptom emergence with cognitive symptoms more dominant in the early stage of illness, and behavioural later (Christian et al., 2020).

Early detection

In Australia, the general practitioner is still the best place for EDs to be identified early and referred to care. That said, analysis of the last decades of Australian primary care data reveals detection rates are low, and referral to services once detected are even lower (Ivancic et al., 2021). There is strong evidence to suggest screening for EDs should be routinely implemented in the care of the high-risk groups, including individuals with diabetes, women seeking reproductive healthcare and youth (Bryant et al., 2022). There is evidence of utility in screening in primary care, although considerations include the diverse populations seen in this setting, increasingly heterogeneous presentation, and significant overlap of symptoms between the disorders (Bryant et al., 2022).

Online screening initiatives appear to prompt some improvement in rates of help-seeking but screening alone will not address low treatment rates, with many individuals failing to seek support even after a positive screen and referral (likely due to a combination of factors including service-related barriers, cost and ambivalence) (Fitzsimmons-Craft et al., 2020a, 2020b). Other barriers include lack of clinician knowledge and training (including primary and reproductive healthcare personnel), concerns about stigma and taboo (both on the part of the patient and professional), and lack of time. Individuals with a high body mass index, males, transgender/gender diverse, and ethnic minorities, face additional barriers and are less likely to be identified by a healthcare professional (Bryant et al., 2022).

Early intervention

In terms of a staged intervention approach to EDs, it is a story more of gaps in the service continuum than of tailored treatment options. There have been a number of promising trials of targeted preventive approaches addressing ED risk factors and behaviours (e.g. media literacy programmes that empower individuals to critically evaluate media content and unrealistic images, cognitive dissonance interventions that target thin-ideal internalization, and CBT to reduce risk factors such as body dissatisfaction and dieting), but it is unclear whether these actually lower ED incidence (Le et al., 2017) or whether they cause harm.

Beyond prevention, 'early-stage' ED is, at this time, defined as the first 3 years after onset of full-criteria illness. Treatments with an evidence base to be delivered in this window are few, except for AN. The Maudsley Family-Based Treatment was designed to be delivered during the first 3 years after onset of AN and full remission rates between 50% and 80% have been reported in clinical trials (Rienecke, 2017). An adapted Maudsley Family-Based Treatment delivered in the prodrome of AN has been recently piloted with promising results (Loeb et al., 2020). The FREED early intervention programme for all ED diagnostic groups is also to be delivered within the first 3 years, with outcome data available only on AN presentations to date (Fukutomi et al., 2020; McClelland et al., 2018). Beyond these three treatments, very little has been tested. Of course, the issue remains that if the great body of literature on early intervention across the other mental illnesses is any indication, what we currently describe as early intervention in EDs may not be early enough.

Substance use disorders

Epidemiology

SUDs are differentiated from non-problematic substance use by outcome: in people with SUDs, use causes escalating negative social and health impacts and continues despite awareness of such impacts. The prevalence of SUD varies markedly by country (GBD 2016 Alcohol and Drug Use Collaborators, 2018; Glantz et al., 2020) and as a function of the changing legal and sociocultural status of individual substances (Hasin et al., 2019). Internationally, 2.6% of adults are estimated to have an SUD annually, with higher prevalence rates in upper-middle-income countries like South Africa (5.8%; Degenhardt et al., 2017). Lifetime SUD prevalence ranges from 1.3% to 15% of the population, also depending on the country of estimate (Kessler et al., 2007). There are reliable sex differences in SUD prevalence, with males more likely to have an SUD than females (Hughto et al., 2021). This gap may be narrowing in higher-income countries due to increasing rates of SUD in women (McHugh et al., 2018). Transgender individuals have rates of SUD around three times greater than their cisgender peers (Hughto et al., 2021).

The prevalence of SUDs peaks during early adulthood and declines steadily thereafter (Degenhardt et al., 2019; Vasilenko et al., 2017), with a median age of onset between 18 and 29 (Kessler et al., 2007). Recent evidence suggests that young people are delaying initial use of a range of substances in high-income countries like the US (Alcover & Thompson, 2020) and Australia (Livingston et al., 2020). This may reduce the prevalence of SUDs in younger age cohorts in some countries in coming years.

Course and prognosis

Experimentation with substances including alcohol, tobacco, cannabis, opioids, hallucinogens, and psychostimulants typically starts in mid to late adolescence, with onset of illicit drug use (e.g. cannabis, psychostimulants) slightly later than initiation of alcohol and tobacco (Degenhardt et al., 2016). Numerous factors—sociocultural (e.g. substance availability), contextual (e.g. neighbourhood and family characteristics), and individual (e.g. stressful life events)—contribute to the risk of substance use onset in young people (Degenhardt et al., 2016).

SUDs develop after transition from experimentation to more regular use. Rates of transition from first use to SUD depend on the substance: using a nationally representative sample of US adults, one estimate found that 67.5% of those who use nicotine, 22.7% of those who use alcohol, 20.9% of people who use cocaine, and 8.9% of cannabis users go on to develop dependence (Lopez-Quintero et al., 2011). Data from the National Comorbidity Survey revealed similar findings: progression from first use to dependence occurred in approximately 23–24% of those who used alcohol, 20% who used cocaine, and 10% who used cannabis (Wagner & Anthony, 2002). SUDs also take a range of trajectories depending on the substance, the sociocultural context, and the individual involved.

While there is substantial variability, some groups of young people are at particularly high risk for transition to problematic use and associated poor outcomes. Early onset substance use is a reliable risk factor for SUD development and poorer prognosis (Volkow et al., 2021). Women tend to initiate substance use later than men; however, there is evidence that they may progress from use to SUD more rapidly than males (McHugh et al., 2018). Mental illness, LGBTQI+ status, criminal justice system involvement, being Indigenous or homeless, and injecting drug use have all been identified as conferring greater risk for SUDs and associated problems in young people (Lopez-Quintero et al., 2011).

SUDs vary in severity, with higher severity associated with a more chronic course of illness (Sarvet & Hasin, 2016). Comorbid personality pathology predicts greater persistence in SUDs (Sarvet & Hasin, 2016). Differences across substances also exist: in a community cohort of young people with cannabis use disorders followed longitudinally until age 30, over 80% achieved sustained remission (>12 months), with some third of those who recovered having a second cannabis use disorders episode within the study period (Farmer et al., 2015). Conversely, problematic use of heroin, cocaine, and methamphetamine appear to be more persistent (Hser et al., 2008).

Early detection

The majority of people with SUDs do not seek treatment for their problematic use. Indeed, internationally, most people with SUDs do not perceive a need for treatment. Consistent with this, few people with an SUD receive treatment: data from the World Health Organization World Mental Health Surveys indicate that only one in every nine individuals with a past-year SUD received SUD-specific treatment within that time frame (Harris et al., 2019).

In this context, early detection and referral for treatment may be particularly important. Yet screening for illicit drug use in primary care remains uncommon. A recent evidence synthesis for the US Preventative Services Task Force found that while brief screening instruments with acceptable accuracy to detect drug use exist, there is no direct evidence of harms or benefits of such screening in adolescents or adults. Moreover, most evidence regarding the efficacy of pharmacological and psychosocial interventions for SUDs is derived from studies of treatment-seeking individuals rather than those referred after detection via screening (Patnode et al., 2020). Despite this relative lack of evidence, in practice guidelines the Preventative Services Task Force recommended that where diagnostic and treatment referral options are available, adults should be screened for drug use in primary care settings (US Preventive Services Task Force, 2020). Conversely, the Task Force recommended against screening in adolescents, arguing that evidence was insufficient to implement routine screening.

An earlier evidence synthesis for the Preventative Services Task Force examined evidence regarding screening and brief counselling interventions for unhealthy alcohol use in primary care and college settings (O'Connor et al., 2018). The report concluded that multiple instruments were available to detect unhealthy alcohol use with reasonable accuracy in such settings, and that brief psychosocial interventions reduced aspects of alcohol use related to usual care in those identified via screening. On this basis, the Task Force recommended that screening for alcohol use be undertaken in adults, with brief intervention and referral offered as needed. Due to a lack of evidence, the Task Force again recommended against routine screening for young people under 18 years (US Preventive Services Task Force, 2018). While understandable given potential stigma and other risks associated with identification of alcohol and other substance use in young people, it substantially constrains early intervention opportunities (Williams & Levin, 2020).

Early intervention

Numerous school-based universal programmes have been implemented to prevent substance use in young people. Early approaches, such as Drug Abuse Resistance Education—offered to primary school age students—showed little effect (Ennett et al., 1994). More recent approaches include school curricula offered to young high school students prior to onset of substance use. Curricula that combine information about drugs with interactive social competence training (e.g. to improve social and coping skills) and social norm training—to challenge young people's assumptions about drug use—have been shown to prevent onset of drug use compared to usual teaching (Faggiano et al., 2014).

Targeted prevention efforts include personality-based interventions (Edalati & Conrod, 2019). These programmes are based on links between certain personality characteristics (e.g. hopelessness, impulsivity) and elevated risk for substance use onset. Evidence suggests that programmes offered in early secondary school to young people identified as high-risk on the basis of these personality characteristics can reduce alcohol and other drug use by around 50%, while also reducing onset of mental ill health (Edalati & Conrod, 2019).

Evidence regarding indicated prevention and early interventions for SUDs is limited (Stockings et al., 2016a). Given the stigma associated with substance use, one potentially beneficial approach may be opportunistic interventions offered at times when individuals may be more open to considering changes in their substance use. A recent randomized controlled trial combined motivational enhancement with personality-targeted intervention, offered to young people accessing emergency department or rest/recovery services for alcohol-related injuries or illness (Hides et al., 2021). The intervention reduced alcohol use at 12 months compared to two control conditions.

Motivational interviewing, which explicitly considers the stage of presentation of the individual with regards to their readiness for change, is well suited to early intervention because it is responsive to any stage of the change process. Unfortunately, evidence to date has not suggested strong effects of motivational interviewing on substance use in young people (Foxcroft et al., 2016; Li et al., 2016). Further research is needed to assess the benefits of motivational interventions in early-stage SUDs.

A range of psychosocial interventions have been found to be efficacious for young people with existing SUDs, including CBT, family therapy, and multicomponent approaches, and adolescent community reinforcement approach (Fadus et al., 2019). Of note, while in adults best practice treatment for SUDs is combined psychotherapy and pharmacotherapy (where available for the primary drug used) (Ray et al., 2020), there is limited evidence as to the efficacy and risks of pharmacotherapy in younger people, suggesting that further research is needed to confirm the efficacy and safety of SUD medications in adolescents and young adults.

Self-harm and suicide

Epidemiology

Suicide and self-harm in young people are a growing public health concern. Worldwide, suicide is the third leading cause of death for children (10–14 years), and the second leading cause of death among adolescents (15–19 years) and young adults (20–24 years) (World Health Organization, 2018a). Non-fatal self-harm, which includes all intentional acts of self-injury or self-poisoning irrespective of motivation and/or degree of suicidal intent (Hawton et al., 2003), is very common. One in five young people report engaging in self-harm at least once in their lifetime (Lim et al., 2019).

Suicide and self-harm show age, gender/sex, and geographic patterns. Suicide and self-harm in children are rare. Rates are generally higher in adolescents and young adults (Gillies et al., 2018; Glenn et al., 2020). Suicide rates are also higher in young males, although there are some exceptions to this general pattern in Asia (World Health Organization, 2018a). In contrast, rates of self-harm are generally higher in young females in most countries (Diggins et al., 2017; Griffin et al., 2018). Rates of both suicide and self-harm also vary by country (Gillies et al., 2018; Glenn et al., 2020).

Course and prognosis

Self-harm and suicidal behaviour typically have their onset in adolescence, with prevalence peaking in those aged 16 years, before declining with advancing age (Gillies et al., 2018). For most young people, self-harm and suicidal behaviour resolve by young adulthood (Moran et al., 2012; Plener et al., 2015). Nevertheless, self-harm during adolescence is associated with a number of adverse outcomes in adulthood: increased risk of mental ill health, substance misuse, further self-harm (Borschmann et al., 2017; Mars et al., 2014), and premature death, including by suicide (Finkelstein et al., 2015).

Early detection

Early detection has the potential to improve outcomes by linking those at risk of self-harm and suicide with appropriate care before these patterns of behaviour become established. For young people, much of this work has occurred within school and other educational settings by implementing screening programmes to detect those at risk of suicide using questionnaire-style instruments. While these programmes have been found to be effective in improving the identification of young people who have not previously been in contact with services (Peña & Caine, 2006), their effects on referrals, service use and engagement are less clear.

Early intervention

Early intervention programmes generally identify young people after their first episode of self-harm. The aim is to reduce the risks of further self-harm and suicide by linking young people with effective care. For young people, this is sometimes achieved via training 'community gatekeepers' (i.e. teachers, parents, and others in the community who have regular contact with young people and may be well placed to notice changes in a young person's mood or behaviour that could indicate increasing risk) (Steeg et al., 2014).

Once a young person presents to hospital, further early interventions should include the provision of a full psychosocial risk/needs assessment to identify potential risk and/or protective factors, timely referral to other services as required, and the provision of adequate support over the post-discharge period as this represents the peak risk period for further self-harm and suicide. Several jurisdictions internationally are currently implementing aftercare services to achieve this, by providing early and assertive follow-up (generally within 72 hours), 24-hour crisis support, and brief contact-based interventions. Together, these programmes may help foster a sense of ongoing connection with services, improve treatment engagement, and reduce distress, suicidal thinking, and self-harm (Steeg et al., 2014).

Postvention as prevention/early intervention

Given that the risks of both self-harm and suicide are raised in young people who have been bereaved by the suicide of another person (Hill et al., 2020), the World Health Organization now specifically recommends that postvention interventions should be implemented to prevent self-harm and/or suicidal behaviour in those bereaved (World Health Organization, 2018b). While there is limited evidence of effectiveness for these programmes on levels of grief, anxiety, depression, and suicidal ideation, and none to date on self-harm or suicide, there have been relatively few studies on the potential benefit of postvention as prevention/early intervention, and fewer still have been investigated outcomes for young people specifically (Andriessen et al., 2019).

Nevertheless, postvention interventions are likely to be an important component of any comprehensive programme to reduce self-harm and suicide and should include, at a minimum, supportive, therapeutic, and educational components delivered by trained facilitators (Andriessen et al., 2019). For young people specifically, these programmes should be implemented in both community and school/educational settings to ensure maximal reach.

Early intervention across the lifespan

Mental health conditions emerge and often evolve and accumulate in diverse ways across the lifespan (Caspi et al., 2020), beginning with developmental disorders in early childhood, emotional and behavioural disorders in mid-childhood, and anxiety disorders, mood disorders, psychotic disorders, PDs, EDs, and SUDs in adolescence and young adulthood. While the main focus of this chapter has been on early intervention for disorders that have their peak onset during adolescence and young adulthood (de Girolamo et al., 2019), age of onset is distributed across the lifespan and early intervention may be indicated at other key onset periods during adulthood: postpartum (Munk-Olsen et al., 2006), menopause (Riecher-Rössler, 2017), mid-life (Harvey et al., 2018), and later adulthood or old age (Robinson et al., 2015). Additionally, prevention strategies that target maternal health and fetal development (Freedman et al., 2018) as well as key risk factors during early development (Arango et al., 2018) are required to bring forward the timing of early intervention and reduce the risk of developing a mental illness later in life (Vieta & Berk, 2022). Thus, in additional to early intervention for young people, there is a need to invest in early intervention strategies for younger children (e.g. for attention deficit hyperactivity disorder, anxiety and conduct disorders), mature adults (e.g. community mental health hubs; Department of Health, 2020), and older adults (e.g. for the dementias and other mental health issues). As with mental disorders that emerge earlier in life, there are considerable economic benefits of early detection and intervention for dementia (Barnett et al., 2014), and the best models of care have not been adequately implemented or scaled-up (Kenigsberg et al., 2015). Across the lifespan and the diagnostic spectrum of mental disorders, early detection and intervention models require more refined and dynamic approaches to prevent or alleviate the burden of mental disorders (de Girolamo et al., 2019). In addition to being guided by age of onset, these models should be developmentally appropriate, with separate streams for children, young people, adults, and older adults while ensuring seamless care across the lifespan.

Conclusion

The onset of mental ill health between childhood and young adulthood has the potential to disrupt major developmental tasks and the successful transition to mature adulthood, with lifelong consequences. This life stage represents a crucial opportunity to 'bend the curve' and modify the course of illness through early intervention. Over the last two decades, substantial progress has been achieved in expanding the focus of early intervention to the full spectrum of mental ill health and in developing youth-specific early intervention services, although gaps remain in low- and middle-resource settings. Even in high-income settings, greater urgency and investment is needed to scale-up services and strengthen integration with specialist mental health care for complex and persistent conditions. While evidence for early intervention continues to build, early detection and intervention of adult-type mental illnesses that have their peak onset during youth is feasible and offers substantial benefits. The high rates of comorbidity between mental illnesses and their non-specific and overlapping early clinical phenotypes support an integrative, rather than siloed, approach to early intervention. Stage-based care supports such a strategy and guides the delivery of pre-emptive intervention that has potential to modify the course of illness and mitigate the social and economic impacts of mental ill health.

REFERENCES

Abé, C., Ching, C. R. K., Liberg, B., Lebedev, A. V., Agartz, I., Akudjedu, T. N., et al. (2022). Longitudinal structural brain changes in bipolar disorder: a multicenter neuroimaging study of 1,232 individuals by the ENIGMA Bipolar Disorder Working Group. *Biological Psychiatry*, **91**, 582–592.

Alcover, K. C. & Thompson, C. L. (2020). Patterns of mean age at drug use initiation among adolescents and emerging adults, 2004–2017. *JAMA Pediatrics*, **174**, 725–727.

Altamura, A. C., Buoli, M., Caldiroli, A., Caron, L., Cumerlato Melter, C., Dobrea, C., et al. (2015). Misdiagnosis, duration of untreated illness (DUI) and outcome in bipolar patients with psychotic symptoms: a naturalistic study. *Journal of Affective Disorders*, **182**, 70–75.

Álvarez-Tomás, I., Ruiz, J., Guilera, G., & Bados, A. (2019). Long-term clinical and functional course of borderline personality disorder: a meta-analysis of prospective studies. *European Psychiatry*, **56**, 75–83.

Andriessen, K., Krysinska, K., Hill, N., Reifels, L., Robinson, J., Reavley, N., & Pirkis, J. (2019). Effectiveness of interventions for people bereaved through suicide: a systematic review of controlled studies of grief, psychosocial and suicide-related outcomes. *BMC Psychiatry*, **19**, 49.

Aouad, P., Hay, P., Soh, N., Touyz, S., Mannan, H., & Mitchison, D. (2021). Chew and spit (CHSP) in a large adolescent sample: prevalence, impact on health-related quality of life, and relation to other disordered eating features. *Eating Disorders*, **29**, 509–522.

Arango, C., Díaz-Caneja, C. M., McGorry, P. D., Rapoport, J., Sommer, I. E., Vorstman, J. A., et al. (2018). Preventive strategies for mental health. *Lancet Psychiatry*, **5**, 591–604.

Arnett, J. J., Žukauskienė, R., & Sugimura, K. (2014). The new life stage of emerging adulthood at ages 18–29 years: implications for mental health. *Lancet Psychiatry*, **1**, 569–576.

Austin, A., Flynn, M., Richards, K., Hodsoll, J., Duarte, T. A., Robinson, P., et al. (2021). Duration of untreated eating disorder and relationship to outcomes: a systematic review of the literature. *European Eating Disorders Review*, **29**, 329–345.

Barnett, J. H., Lewis, L., Blackwell, A. D., & Taylor, M. (2014). Early intervention in Alzheimer's disease: a health economic study of the effects of diagnostic timing. *BMC Neurology*, **14**, 101.

Beck, E., Bo, S., Jørgensen, M. S., Poulsen, S., Storebø, O. J., Fjellerad Andersen, C., et al. (2020). Mentalization-based treatment in groups for adolescents with borderline personality disorder: a randomized controlled trial. *Journal of Child Psychology and Psychiatry and Allied Disciplines*, **61**, 594–604.

Berk, M., Post, R., Ratheesh, A., Gliddon, E., Singh, A., Vieta, E., et al. (2017). Staging in bipolar disorder: from theoretical framework to clinical utility. *World Psychiatry*, **16**, 236–244.

Bloom, D. E., Cafiero, E. T., Jané-Llopis, E., Abrahams-Gessel, S., Bloom, L. R., Fathima, S., et al. (2011). *The Global Economic Burden of Noncommunicable Diseases*. Geneva: World Economic Forum.

Bo, S., Vilmar, J. W., Jensen, S. L., Jørgensen, M. S., Kongerslev, M., Lind, M., & Fonagy, P. (2021). What works for adolescents with borderline personality disorder: towards a developmentally informed understanding and structured treatment model. *Current Opinion in Psychology*, **37**, 7–12.

Borschmann, R., Becker, D., Coffey, C., Spry, E., Moreno-Betancur, M., Moran, P., & Patton, G. C. (2017). 20-year outcomes in adolescents who self-harm: a population-based cohort study. *Lancet Child and Adolescent Health*, **1**, 195–202.

Brown, E., Gao, C. X., Staveley, H., et al. (2022). The clinical and functional outcomes of a large naturalistic cohort of young people accessing national early psychosis services. *Australian and New Zealand Journal of Psychiatry*, **56**, 1265–1276.

Bryant, E., Spielman, K., Le, A., Marks, P., National Eating Disorder Research Consortium, et al. (2022). Screening, assessment and diagnosis in the eating disorders: findings from a rapid review. *Journal of Eating Disorders*, **10**, 78.

Burt, A., Mannan, H., Touyz, S., & Hay, P. (2020). Prevalence of DSM-5 diagnostic threshold eating disorders and features amongst Aboriginal and Torres Strait islander peoples (First Australians). *BMC Psychiatry*, **20**, 449.

Campion, J. & Knapp, M. (2018). The economic case for improved coverage of public mental health interventions. *Lancet Psychiatry*, **5**, 103–105.

Caspi, A., Houts, R. M., Ambler, A., Danese, A., Elliott, M. L., Hariri, A., et al. (2020). Longitudinal assessment of mental health disorders and comorbidities across 4 decades among participants in the Dunedin birth cohort study. *JAMA Network Open*, **3**, e203221.

Chanen, A. M. (2021). Bigotry and borderline personality disorder. *Australasian Psychiatry*, **29**, 579–580.

Chanen, A. M., Berk, M., & Thompson, K. (2016). Integrating early intervention for borderline personality disorder and mood disorders. *Harvard Review of Psychiatry*, **24**, 330–341.

Chanen, A. M., Betts, J. K., Jackson, H., Cotton, S. M., Gleeson, J., Davey, C. G., et al. (2022). Effect of 3 forms of early intervention for young people with borderline personality disorder: the MOBY randomized clinical trial. *JAMA Psychiatry*, **79**, 109–119.

Chanen, A. M., Jackson, H. J., McCutcheon, L. K., Jovev, M., Dudgeon, P., Yuen, H. P., et al. (2008). Early intervention for adolescents with borderline personality disorder using cognitive analytic therapy: randomised controlled trial. *British Journal of Psychiatry*, **193**, 477–484.

Chanen, A. M. & McCutcheon, L. (2013). Prevention and early intervention for borderline personality disorder: current status and recent evidence. *British Journal of Psychiatry*, **202**, s24–s29.

Chanen, A. M. & Nicol, K. (2021). Five failures and five challenges for prevention and early intervention for personality disorder. *Current Opinion in Psychology*, **37**, 134–138.

Chanen, A. M., Nicol, K., Betts, J. K., & Thompson, K. N. (2020). Diagnosis and treatment of borderline personality disorder in young people. *Current Psychiatry Reports*, **22**, 25.

Chanen, A., Sharp, C., Hoffman, P., & Global Alliance for Prevention Early Intervention for Borderline Personality Disorder. (2017). Prevention and early intervention for borderline personality disorder: a novel public health priority. *World Psychiatry*, **16**, 215–216.

Chanen, A. M. & Thompson, K. N. (2019). The age of onset of personality disorders. In: de Girolamo, G., McGorry, P. D. & Sartorius, N. (Eds.), *Age of Onset of Mental Disorders: Etiopathogenetic and treatment implications* (pp. 183–201). Cham: Springer.

Chisholm, D., Sweeny, K., Sheehan, P., Rasmussen, B., Smit, F., Cuijpers, P., & Saxena, S. (2016). Scaling-up treatment of depression and anxiety: a global return on investment analysis. *Lancet Psychiatry*, **3**, 415–424.

Christian, C., Perko, V. L., Vanzhula, I. A., Tregarthen, J. P., Forbush, K. T., & Levinson, C. A. (2020). Eating disorder core symptoms and symptom pathways across developmental stages: a network analysis. *Journal of Abnormal Psychology*, **129**, 177–190.

Cohen, P., Crawford, T. N., Johnson, J. G., & Kasen, S. (2005). The children in the community study of developmental course of personality disorder. *Journal of Personality Disorders*, **19**, 466–486.

Connolly, S. D., Bernstein, G. A., & Work Group on Quality Issues (2007). Practice parameter for the assessment and treatment of children and adolescents with anxiety disorders. *Journal of the American Academy of Child and Adolescent Psychiatry*, **46**, 267–83.

Copeland, W. E., Wolke, D., Shanahan, L., & Costello, E. J. (2015). Adult functional outcomes of common childhood psychiatric problems: a prospective, longitudinal study. *JAMA Psychiatry*, **72**, 892–899.

Correll, C. U., Galling, B., Pawar, A., Krivko, A., Bonetto, C., Ruggeri, M., et al. (2018). Comparison of early intervention services vs treatment as usual for early-phase psychosis: a systematic review, meta-analysis, and meta-regression. *JAMA Psychiatry*, **75**, 555–565.

Dalsgaard, S., McGrath, J., Østergaard, S. D., Wray, N. R., Pedersen, C. B., Mortensen, P. B., & Petersen, L. (2020). Association of mental disorder in childhood and adolescence with subsequent educational achievement. *JAMA Psychiatry*, **77**, 797–805.

Davey, C. G. & McGorry, P. D. (2019). Early intervention for depression in young people: a blind spot in mental health care. *Lancet Psychiatry*, **6**, 267–272.

de Girolamo, G., McGorry, P. D., & Sartorius, N. (Eds.) (2019). *Age of Onset of Mental Disorders: Etiopathogenetic and Treatment Implications*. Cham: Springer.

Degenhardt, L., Bharat, C., Glantz, M. D., Sampson, N. A., Scott, K., Lim, C. C. W., et al. (2019). The epidemiology of drug use disorders cross-nationally: findings from the WHO's World Mental Health Surveys. *International Journal of Drug Policy*, **71**, 103–112.

Degenhardt, L., Glantz, M., Evans-Lacko, S., Sadikova, E., Sampson, N., Thornicroft, G., et al. (2017). Estimating treatment coverage for people with substance use disorders: an analysis of data from the World Mental Health Surveys. *World Psychiatry*, **16**, 299–307.

Degenhardt, L., Stockings, E., Patton, G., Hall, W. D., & Lynskey, M. (2016). The increasing global health priority of substance use in young people. *Lancet Psychiatry*, **3**, 251–264.

DelBello, M.P., Soutullo, C. A., Hendricks, W., Niemeier, R. T., McElroy, S. L., & Strakowski, S. M. (2001). Prior stimulant treatment in adolescents with bipolar disorder: association with age at onset. *Bipolar Disorders*, **3**, 53–57.

Department of Health (2020). Service model for adult mental health centres. https://consultations.health.gov.au/mental-health-services/adult-mental-health-centres/.

Diggins, E., Kelley, R., Cottrell, D., House, A., & Owens, D. (2017). Age-related differences in self-harm presentations and subsequent management of adolescents and young adults at the emergency department. *Journal of Adolescent Health*, **66**, 470–77.

Drake, R. J., Husain, N., Marshall, M., Lewis, S. W., Tomenson, B., Chaudhry, I. B., et al. (2020). Effect of delaying treatment of first-episode psychosis on symptoms and social outcomes: a longitudinal analysis and modelling study. *Lancet Psychiatry*, **7**, 602–610.

Dunn, V. & Goodyer, I. M. (2006). Longitudinal investigation into childhood- and adolescence-onset depression: psychiatric outcome in early adulthood. *British Journal of Psychiatry*, **188**, 216–222.

Edalati, H. & Conrod, P. J. (2019). A review of personality-targeted interventions for prevention of substance misuse and related harm in community samples of adolescents. *Frontiers in Psychiatry*, **9**, 770.

Eddy, K. T., Tabri, N., Thomas, J. J., Murray, H. B., Keshaviah, A., Hastings, E., et al. (2017). Recovery from anorexia nervosa and bulimia nervosa at 22-year follow-up. *Journal of Clinical Psychiatry*, **78**, 184–189.

Ennett, S. T., Tobler, N. S., Ringwalt, C. L., & Flewelling, R. L. (1994). How effective is drug abuse resistance education? A meta-analysis of Project DARE outcome evaluations. *American Journal of Public Health*, **84**, 1394–1401.

Fadus, M. C., Squeglia, L. M., Valadez, E. A., Tomko, R. L., Bryant, B. E., & Gray, K. M. (2019). Adolescent substance use disorder treatment: an update on evidence-based strategies. *Current Psychiatry Reports*, **21**, 96.

Faggiano, F., Minozzi, S., Versino, E., & Buscemi, D. (2014). Universal school-based prevention for illicit drug use. *Cochrane Database of Systematic Reviews*, **12**, CD003020.

Farmer, R. F., Kosty, D. B., Seeley, J. R., Duncan, S. C., Lynskey, M. T., Rohde, P., et al. (2015). Natural course of cannabis use disorders. *Psychological Medicine*, **45**, 63–72.

Filia, K., Rickwood, D., Menssink, J., Gao, C. X., Hetrick, S., Parker, A., et al. (2021). Clinical and functional characteristics of a subsample of young people presenting for primary mental healthcare at headspace services across Australia. *Social Psychiatry and Psychiatric Epidemiology*, **56**, 1311–1323.

Finkelstein, Y., Macdonald, E., Hollands, S., Hutson, J. R., Sivilotti, M. L., Mamdani, M. M., et al. (2015). Long-term outcomes following self-poisoning in adolescents: a population-based cohort study. *Lancet Psychiatry*, **2**, 532–539.

Fitzsimmons-Craft, E. E., Balantekin, K. N., Graham, A. K., DePietro, B., Laing, O., Firebaugh, M. L., et al. (2020a). Preliminary data on help-seeking intentions and behaviors of individuals completing a widely available online screen for eating disorders in the United States. *International Journal of Eating Disorders*, **53**, 1556–1562.

Fitzsimmons-Craft, E. E., Eichen, D. M., Monterubio, G. E., Firebaugh, M. L., Goel, N. J., Taylor, C. B., & Wilfley, D. E. (2020b). Longer-term follow-up of college students screening positive for anorexia nervosa: psychopathology, help seeking, and barriers to treatment. *Eating Disorders*, **28**, 549–565.

Fok, M. L. Y., Hayes, R. D., Chang, C. K., Stewart, R., Callard, F. J., & Moran, P. (2012). Life expectancy at birth and all-cause mortality among people with personality disorder. *Journal of Psychosomatic Research*, **73**, 104–107.

Foxcroft, D.R., Coombes, L., Wood, S., Allen, D., Almeida Santimano, N.M.L., & Moreira, M.T. (2016). Motivational interviewing for the prevention of alcohol misuse in young adults. *Cochrane Database of Systematic Reviews*, **7**, CD007025.

Freedman, R., Hunter, S. K., & Hoffman, M. C. (2018). Prenatal primary prevention of mental illness by micronutrient supplements in pregnancy. *American Journal of Psychiatry*, **175**, 607–619.

Fukutomi, A., Austin, A., McClelland, J., Brown, A., Glennon, D., Mountford, V., et al. (2020). First episode rapid early intervention for eating disorders: a two-year follow-up. *Early Intervention in Psychiatry*, **14**, 137–141.

Galmiche, M., Déchelotte, P., Lambert, G., & Tavolacci, M.P. (2019). Prevalence of eating disorders over the 2000–2018 period: a systematic literature review. *American Journal of Clinical Nutrition*, **109**, 1402–1413.

Garber, J., Brunwasser, S. M., Zerr, A. A., Schwartz, K. T. G., Sova, K., & Weersing, V. R. (2016). Treatment and prevention of depression and anxiety in youth: test of cross-over effects. *Depression and Anxiety*, **33**, 939–959.

Gardner, A., Cotton, S., O'Donoghue, B., Killackey, E., Norton, P., & Filia, K. (2019). Group differences in social inclusion between young adults aged 18 to 25 with serious mental illness and same-aged peers from the general community. *International Journal of Social Psychiatry*, **65**, 631–642.

GBD 2016 Alcohol and Drug Use Collaborators (2018). The global burden of disease attributable to alcohol and drug use in 195 countries and territories, 1990–2016: a systematic analysis for the Global Burden of Disease Study 2016. *Lancet Psychiatry*, **5**, 987–1012.

Gee, B., Reynolds, S., Carroll, B., Orchard, F., Clarke, T., Martin, D., et al. (2020). Practitioner review: effectiveness of indicated school-based interventions for adolescent depression and anxiety—a meta-analytic review. *Journal of Child Psychology and Psychiatry*, **61**, 739–756.

Ghio, L., Gotelli, S., Marcenaro, M., Amore, M., & Natta, W. (2014). Duration of untreated illness and outcomes in unipolar depression: a systematic review and meta-analysis. *Journal of Affective Disorders*, **152–154**, 45–51.

Gillies, D., Christou, M. A., Dixon, A. C., Featherston, O. J., Rapti, I., Garcia-Anguita, A., et al. (2018). Prevalence and characteristics of self-harm in adolescents: meta-analyses of community-based studies 1990–2015. *Journal of the American Academy of Child and Adolescent Psychiatry*, **57**, 733–41.

Ginsburg, G. S., Kendall, P. C., Sakolsky, D., Compton, S. N., Piacentini, J., Albano, A. M., et al. (2011). Remission after acute treatment in children and adolescents with anxiety disorders: findings from the CAMS. *Journal of Consulting and Clinical Psychology*, **79**, 806–813.

Glantz, M. D., Bharat, C., Degenhardt, L., Sampson, N. A., Scott, K. M., Lim, C. C. W., et al. (2020). The epidemiology of alcohol use disorders cross-nationally: findings from the World Mental Health Surveys. *Addictive Behaviors*, **102**, 106128.

Glenn, C., Kleiman, E., Kellerman, J., Pollak, O., Cha, C. B., Esposito, E. C., et al. (2020). Annual research review: a meta-analytic review of worldwide suicide rates in adolescents. *Journal of Child Psychology and Psychiatry*, **61**, 294–308.

Goodman, R. (1997). The Strengths and Difficulties Questionnaire: a research note. *Journal of Child Psychology and Psychiatry*, **38**, 581–586.

Gore, F. M., Bloem, P. J. N., Patton, G. C., Ferguson, J., Joseph, V., Coffey, C., et al. (2011). Global burden of disease in young people aged 10–24 years: a systematic analysis. *Lancet*, **377**, 2093–2102.

Gowers, S. G. & Crisp, A. H. (1990). Anorexia nervosa in an 80-year-old woman. *British Journal of Psychiatry*, **157**, 754–757.

Grange, D. & Loeb, K. L. (2007). Early identification and treatment of eating disorders: prodrome to syndrome. *Early Intervention in Psychiatry*, **1**, 27–39.

Griffin, E., McMahon, E., McNicholas, F., Corcoran, P., Perry, I., & Arensman, E. (2018). Increasing rates of self-harm among children, adolescents and young adults: a 10-year national registry study 2007–2016. *Social Psychiatry and Psychiatric Epidemiology*, **53**, 663–671.

Hafeman, D. M., Merranko, J., Goldstein, T. R., Axelson, D., Goldstein, B. I., Monk, K., et al. (2017). Assessment of a person-level risk calculator to predict new-onset bipolar spectrum disorder in youth at familial risk. *JAMA Psychiatry*, **74**, 841–847.

Harris, M. G., Bharat, C., Glantz, M. D., Sampson, N. A., Al-Hamzawi, A., Alonso, J., et al. (2019). Cross-national patterns of substance use disorder treatment and associations with mental disorder comorbidity in the WHO World Mental Health Surveys. *Addiction*, **114**, 1446–1459.

Hart, L. M., Granillo, M. T., Jorm, A. F., & Paxton, S. J. (2011). Unmet need for treatment in the eating disorders: a systematic review of eating disorder specific treatment seeking among community cases. *Clinical Psychology Review*, **31**, 727–735.

Harvey, S. B., Sellahewa, D. A., Wang, M.-J., Milligan-Saville, J., Bryan, B. T., Henderson, M., et al. (2018). The role of job strain in understanding midlife common mental disorder: a national birth cohort study. *Lancet Psychiatry*, **5**, 498–506.

Hasin, D. S., Shmulewitz, D., & Sarvet, A. L. (2019). Time trends in US cannabis use and cannabis use disorders overall and by sociodemographic subgroups: a narrative review and new findings. *American Journal of Drug and Alcohol Abuse*, **45**, 623–643.

Hawton, K. & van Heeringen, K. (2009). Suicide. *Lancet*, **373**, 1372–1381.

Hawton, K., Zahl, D., & Weatherall, R. (2003). Suicide following deliberate self-harm: long-term follow-up of patients who presented to a general hospital. *British Journal of Psychiatry*, **182**, 537–542.

headspace (2021). *headspace Annual Report 2020–2021*. Melbourne: headspace National Youth Mental Health Foundation.

Hermens, D. F., Lagopoulos, J., Tobias-Webb, J., De Regt, T., Dore, G., Juckes, L., et al. (2013). Pathways to alcohol-induced brain impairment in young people: a review. *Cortex*, **49**, 3–17.

Hetrick, S. E., Bailey, A. P., Smith, K. E., Malla, A., Mathias, S., Singh, S. P., et al. (2017). Integrated (one-stop shop) youth health care: best available evidence and future directions. *Medical Journal of Australia*, **207**, S5–S18.

Hides, L., Quinn, C., Chan, G., Cotton, S., Pocuca, N., Connor, J. P., et al. (2021). Telephone-based motivational interviewing enhanced with individualised personality-specific coping skills training for young people with alcohol-related injuries and illnesses accessing emergency or rest/recovery services: a randomized controlled trial (QuikFix). *Addiction*, **116**, 474–484.

Hill, N., Robinson, J., Pirkis, J., Andriessen, K., Krysinska, K., Payne, A., et al. (2020). Association of suicidal behavior with exposure to suicide and suicide attempt: a systematic review and multilevel meta-analysis. *PLoS Medicine*, **17**, e1003074.

Howes, O. D., Whitehurst, T., Shatalina, E., Townsend, L., Onwordi, E. C., Mak, T. L. A., et al. (2021). The clinical significance of duration of untreated psychosis: an umbrella review and random-effects meta-analysis. *World Psychiatry*, **20**, 75–95.

Hser, Y.-I., Huang, D., Brecht, M.-L., Li, L., & Evans, E. (2008). Contrasting trajectories of heroin, cocaine, and methamphetamine use. *Journal of Addictive Diseases*, **27**, 13–21.

Hughto, J. M. W., Quinn, E. K., Dunbar, M. S., Rose, A. J., Shireman, T. I., & Jasuja, G. K. (2021). Prevalence and co-occurrence of alcohol, nicotine, and other substance use disorder diagnoses among US transgender and cisgender adults. *JAMA Network Open*, **4**, e2036512.

Hutsebaut, J., Videler, A. C., Verheul, R., & Van Alphen, S. P. J. (2019). Managing borderline personality disorder from a life course perspective: clinical staging and health management. *Personality Disorders: Theory, Research, and Treatment*, **10**, 309–316.

Institute for Health Metrics and Evaluation (2015). *GBD Compare*. Seattle, WA: IHME, University of Washington.

Iorfino, F., Scott, E. M., Carpenter, J.S., Cross, S. P., Hermens, D. F., Killedar, M., et al. (2019). Clinical stage transitions in persons aged 12 to 25 years presenting to early intervention mental health services with anxiety, mood, and psychotic disorders. *JAMA Psychiatry*, **76**, 1167–1175.

Ivancic, L., Maguire, S., Miskovic-Wheatley, J., Harrison, C., & Nassar, N. (2021). Prevalence and management of people with eating disorders presenting to primary care: a national study. *Australian and New Zealand Journal of Psychiatry*, **55**, 1089–1100.

Jacobi, C., Fittig, E., Bryson, S. W., Wilfley, D., Kraemer, H. C., & Taylor, C. B. (2011). Who is really at risk? Identifying risk factors for subthreshold and full syndrome eating disorders in a high-risk sample. *Psychological Medicine*, **41**, 1939–1949.

James, A. C., Reardon, T., Soler, A., James, G., & Creswell, C. (2020). Cognitive behavioural therapy for anxiety disorders in children and adolescents. *Cochrane Database of Systematic Reviews*, **11**, CD013162.

Johnson, J. G., Cohen, P., Kasen, S., Skodol, A. E., & Oldham, J. M. (2008). Cumulative prevalence of personality disorders between adolescence and adulthood. *Acta Psychiatrica Scandinavica*, **118**, 410–413.

Kaess, M., Fischer-Waldschmidt, G., Resch, F., & Koenig, J. (2017). Health related quality of life and psychopathological distress in risk taking and self-harming adolescents with full-syndrome, subthreshold and without borderline personality disorder: rethinking the clinical cut-off? *Borderline Personality Disorder and Emotion Dysregulation*, **4**, 7.

Kenigsberg, P.-A., Aquino, J.-P., Bérard, A., Gzil, F., Andrieu, S., Banerjee, S., et al. (2015). Dementia beyond 2025: knowledge and uncertainties. *Dementia*, **15**, 6–21.

Kessler, R. C., Angermeyer, M., Anthony, J. C., De Graaf, R., Demyttenaere, K., Gasquet, I., et al. (2007). Lifetime prevalence and age-of-onset distributions of mental disorders in the World Health Organization's World Mental Health Survey Initiative. *World Psychiatry*, **6**, 168–176.

Kessler, R. C., Berglund, P., Demler, O., Jin, R., Merikangas, K. R., & Walters, E. E. (2005). Lifetime prevalence and age-of-onset distributions of DSM-IV disorders in the National Comorbidity Survey Replication. *Archives of General Psychiatry*, **62**, 593–602.

Killackey, E., Hodges, C., Browne, V., Gow, E., Varnum, P., McGorry, P., & Purcell, R. (2020). *A Global Framework for Youth Mental Health: Investing in Future Mental Capital for Individuals, Communities and Economies*. Geneva: World Economic Forum.

Kim-Cohen, J., Caspi, A., Moffitt, T. E., Harrington, H., Milne, B. J., & Poulton, R. (2003). Prior juvenile diagnoses in adults with mental disorder: developmental follow-back of a prospective-longitudinal cohort. *Archives of General Psychiatry*, **60**, 709–717.

Kroenke, K., Spitzer, R. L., & Williams, J. B.W. (2003). The Patient Health Questionnaire-2: validity of a two-item depression screener. *Medical Care*, **41**, 1284–1292.

Lawrence, D., Hafekost, J., Johnson, S. E., Saw, S., Buckingham, W. J., Sawyer, M. G., et al. (2016). Key findings from the second Australian Child and Adolescent Survey of Mental Health and Wellbeing. *Australian and New Zealand Journal of Psychiatry*, **50**, 876–886.

Le, L. K. D., Barendregt, J. J., Hay, P., & Mihalopoulos, C. (2017). Prevention of eating disorders: a systematic review and meta-analysis. *Clinical Psychology Review*, **53**, 46–58.

Levine, G. N., Cohen, B. E., Commodore-Mensah, Y., Fleury, J., Huffman, J. C., Khalid, U., et al. (2021). Psychological health, well-being, and the mind-heart-body connection: a scientific statement from the American Heart Association. *Circulation*, **143**, e763–e783.

Lewinsohn, P. M., Clarke, G. N., Seeley, J. R., & Rohde, P. (1994). Major depression in community adolescents: age at onset, episode duration, and time to recurrence. *Journal of the American Academy of Child and Adolescent Psychiatry*, **33**, 809–818.

Li, L., Zhu, S., Tse, N., Tse, S., & Wong, P. (2016). Effectiveness of motivational interviewing to reduce illicit drug use in adolescents: a systematic review and meta-analysis. *Addiction*, **111**, 795–805.

Lim, K.-S., Wong, C., McIntyre, R., Wang, J., Zhang, Z., Tran, B. X., et al. (2019). Global lifetime and 12-month prevalence of suicidal behavior, deliberate self-harm and non-suicidal self-injury in children and adolescents between 1989 and 2018: a meta-analysis. *International Journal of Environmental Research and Public Health*, **16**, 4581.

Lin, P.-I., McInnis, M. G., Potash, J. B., Willour, V., MacKinnon, D. F., DePaulo, J. R., & Zandi, P. P. (2006). Clinical correlates and familial aggregation of age at onset in bipolar disorder. *American Journal of Psychiatry*, **163**, 240–246.

Livingston, M., Holmes, J., Oldham, M., Vashishtha, R., & Pennay, A. (2020). Trends in the sequence of first alcohol, cannabis and cigarette use in Australia, 2001–2016. *Drug and Alcohol Dependence*, **207**, 107821.

Loeb, K. L. & le Grange, D. (2013). Family-based treatment for adolescent eating disorders: current status, new applications and future directions. *International Journal of Child and Adolescent Health*, **2**, 243–254.

Loeb, K. L., Weissman, R. S., Marcus, S., Pattanayak, C., Hail, L., Kung, K. C., et al. (2020). Family-based treatment for anorexia nervosa symptoms in high-risk youth: a partially-randomized preference-design study. *Frontiers in Psychiatry*, **10**, 985.

Lopez-Quintero, C., Pérez de los Cobos, J., Hasin, D. S., Okuda, M., Wang, S., Grant, B. F., et al. (2011). Probability and predictors of transition from first use to dependence on nicotine, alcohol, cannabis, and cocaine: results of the National Epidemiologic Survey on Alcohol and Related Conditions (NESARC). *Drug and Alcohol Dependence*, **115**, 120–130.

Lyng, J., Swales, M. A., Hastings, R. P., Millar, T., & Duffy, D. J. (2020). Outcomes for 18 to 25-year-olds with borderline personality disorder in a dedicated young adult only DBT programme compared to a general adult DBT programme for all ages 18+. *Early Intervention in Psychiatry*, **14**, 61–68.

Madden, S., Morris, A., Zurynski, Y. A., Kohn, M., & Elliot, E. J. (2009). Burden of eating disorders in 5–13-year-old children in Australia. *Medical Journal of Australia*, 190, 410–414.

Maguire, S., Le Grange, D., Surgenor, L., Marks, P., Lacey, H., & Touyz, S. (2008). Staging anorexia nervosa: conceptualizing illness severity. *Early Intervention in Psychiatry*, 2, 3–10.

Maguire, S., Surgenor, L. J., Le Grange, D., Lacey, H., Crosby, R. D., Engel, S. G., et al. (2017). Examining a staging model for anorexia nervosa: empirical exploration of a four stage model of severity. *Journal of Eating Disorders*, 5, 41.

Maguire, S., Touyz, S., Surgenor, L., Crosby, R. D., Engel, S. G., Lacey, H., et al. (2012). The clinician administered staging instrument for anorexia nervosa: development and psychometric properties. *International Journal of Eating Disorders*, 45, 390–399.

Malla, A. (2022). Reducing duration of untreated psychosis: the neglected dimension of early intervention services. *American Journal of Psychiatry*, 179, 259–261.

Malla, A. & McGorry, P. (2019). Early intervention in psychosis in young people: a population and public health perspective. *American Journal of Public Health*, 109(Suppl. 3), S181–S184.

March, J. S., Conners, C., Arnold, G., Epstein, J., Parker, J., Hinshaw, S., et al. (1999). The Multidimensional Anxiety Scale for Children (MASC): confirmatory factor analysis in a pediatric ADHD sample. *Journal of Attention Disorders*, 3, 85–89.

March, J., Silva, S., Petrycki, S., Curry, J., Wells, K., Fairbank, J., et al. (2004). Fluoxetine, cognitive-behavioral therapy, and their combination for adolescents with depression: Treatment for Adolescents with Depression Study (TADS) randomized controlled trial. *JAMA*, 292, 807–20.

Mars, B., Heron, J., Crane, C., Hawton, K., Lewis, G., Macleod, J., et al. (2014). Clinical and social outcomes of adolescent self harm: population based birth cohort study. *BMJ*, 349, g5954.

McCauley, E., Berk, M. S., Asarnow, J. R., Adrian, M., Cohen, J., Korslund, K., et al. (2018). Efficacy of dialectical behavior therapy for adolescents at high risk for suicide a randomized clinical trial. *JAMA Psychiatry*, 75, 777–785.

McClelland, J., Hodsoll, J., Brown, A., Lang, K., Boysen, E., Flynn, M., et al. (2018). A pilot evaluation of a novel First Episode and Rapid Early Intervention service for Eating Disorders (FREED). *European Eating Disorders Review*, 26, 129–140.

McGorry, P. D. (2022). The reality of mental health care for young people, and the urgent need for solutions. *Medical Journal of Australia*, 216, 78–79.

McGorry, P. D., Goldstone, S. D., Parker, A. G., Rickwood, D. J., & Hickie, I. B. (2014). Cultures for mental health care of young people: an Australian blueprint for reform. *Lancet Psychiatry*, 1, 559–568.

McGorry, P. D., Hartmann, J. A., Spooner, R., & Nelson, B. (2018). Beyond the 'at risk mental state' concept: transitioning to transdiagnostic psychiatry. *World Psychiatry*, 17, 133–142.

McGorry, P. D. & Hickie, I. B. (Eds.) (2019). *Clinical Staging in Psychiatry: Making Diagnosis Work for Research and Treatment*. Cambridge: Cambridge University Press.

McGorry, P. D. & Mei, C. (2021). Clinical staging for youth mental disorders: progress in reforming diagnosis and clinical care. *Annual Review of Developmental Psychology*, 3, 15–39.

McGorry, P. D., Mei, C., Chanen, A., Hodges, C., Alvarez-Jimenez, M., & Killackey, E. (2022). Designing and scaling up integrated youth mental health care. *World Psychiatry*, 21, 61–76.

McGorry, P., Trethowan, J., & Rickwood, D. (2019). Creating headspace for integrated youth mental health care. *World Psychiatry*, 18, 140–141.

McHugh, R. K., Votaw, V. R., Sugarman, D. E., & Greenfield, S. F. (2018). Sex and gender differences in substance use disorders. *Clinical Psychology Review*, 66, 12–23.

Mehlum, L., Ramleth, R. K., Tørmoen, A. J., Haga, E., Diep, L. M., Stanley, B. H., et al. (2019). Long term effectiveness of dialectical behavior therapy versus enhanced usual care for adolescents with self-harming and suicidal behavior. *Journal of Child Psychology and Psychiatry and Allied Disciplines*, 60, 1112–1122.

Merikangas, K. R., Jin, R., He, J.-P., Kessler, R. C., Lee, S., Sampson, N. A., et al. (2011). Prevalence and correlates of bipolar spectrum disorder in the world mental health survey initiative. *Archives of General Psychiatry*, 68, 241–251.

Micali, N., Hagberg, K. W., Petersen, I., & Treasure, J. L. (2013). The incidence of eating disorders in the UK in 2000–2009: findings from the General Practice Research Database. *BMJ Open*, 3, e002646.

Mihalopoulos, C., Harris, M., Henry, L., Harrigan, S., & McGorry, P. (2009). Is early intervention in psychosis cost-effective over the long term? *Schizophrenia Bulletin*, 35, 909–918.

Mitchison, D., Mond, J., Bussey, K., Griffiths, S., Trompeter, N., Lonergan, A., et al. (2020). DSM-5 full syndrome, other specified, and unspecified eating disorders in Australian adolescents: prevalence and clinical significance. *Psychological Medicine*, 50, 981–990.

Moffitt, T. E., Harrington, H., Caspi, A., Kim-Cohen, J., Goldberg, D., Gregory, A. M., & Poulton, R. (2007). Depression and generalized anxiety disorder: cumulative and sequential comorbidity in a birth cohort followed prospectively to age 32 years. *Archives of General Psychiatry*, 64, 651–660.

Moran, P., Coffey, C., Romaniuk, H., Olsson, C., Borschmann, R., Carlin, J. B., & Patton, G. C. (2012). The natural history of self-harm from adolescence to young adulthood: a population-based cohort study. *Lancet*, 379, 236–243.

Moran, P., Romaniuk, H., Coffey, C., Chanen, A., Degenhardt, L., Borschmann, R., & Patton, G. C. (2016). The influence of personality disorder on the future mental health and social adjustment of young adults: a population-based, longitudinal cohort study. *Lancet Psychiatry*, 3, 636–645.

Munk-Olsen, T., Laursen, T. M., Pedersen, C. B., Mors, O., & Mortensen, P. B. (2006). New parents and mental disorders: a population-based register study. *JAMA*, 296, 2582–2589.

Ng, F. Y. Y., Bourke, M. E., & Grenyer, B. F. S. (2016). Recovery from borderline personality disorder: a systematic review of the perspectives of consumers, clinicians, family and carers. *PLoS One*, 11, e0160515.

O'Dwyer, N., Rickwood, D., Buckmaster, D., & Watsford, C. (2020). Therapeutic interventions in Australian primary care, youth mental health settings for young people with borderline personality disorder or borderline traits. *Borderline Personality Disorder and Emotion Dysregulation*, 7, 23.

O'Connor, E. A., Perdue, L. A., Senger, C. A., Rushkin, M., Patnode, C. D., Bean, S. I., & Jonas, D. E. (2018). Screening and behavioral counseling interventions to reduce unhealthy alcohol use in adolescents and adults: updated evidence report and systematic review for the US Preventive Services Task Force. *JAMA*, 320, 1910–1928.

Patnode, C. D., Perdue, L. A., Rushkin, M., Dana, T., Blazina, I., Bougatsos, C., et al. (2020). Screening for unhealthy drug use: updated evidence report and systematic review for the US Preventive Services Task Force. *JAMA*, 323, 2310–2328.

Peña, J. & Caine, E. (2006). Screening as an approach for adolescent suicide prevention. *Suicide and Life-Threatening Behavior*, 36, 614–637.

Plana-Ripoll, O., Pedersen, C. B., Holtz, Y., Benros, M. E., Dalsgaard, S., de Jonge, P., et al. (2019). Exploring comorbidity within mental disorders among a Danish national population. *JAMA Psychiatry*, **76**, 259–270.

Plener, P., Schumacher, T., Munz, L., & Groschwitz, R. (2015). The longitudinal course of non-suicidal self-injury and deliberate self-harm: a systematic review of the literature. *Borderline Personality Disorder and Emotion Dysregulation*, **2**, 2.

Posselt, C. M., Albert, N., Nordentoft, M., & Hjorthøj, C. (2021). The Danish OPUS early intervention services for first-episode psychosis: a phase 4 prospective cohort study with comparison of randomized trial and real-world data. *American Journal of Psychiatry*, **178**, 941–951.

Power, P. (2015). Intervening early in bipolar disorder in young people: a review of the clinical staging model. *Irish Journal of Psychological Medicine*, **32**, 31–43.

Purcell, R., Jorm, A. F., Hickie, I. B., Yung, A. R., Pantelis, C., Amminger, G. P., et al. (2015). Demographic and clinical characteristics of young people seeking help at youth mental health services: baseline findings of the Transitions Study. *Early Intervention in Psychiatry*, **9**, 487–497.

Ranta, K., Väänänen, J., Fröjd, S., Isomaa, R., Kaltiala-Heino, R., & Marttunen, M. (2017). Social phobia, depression and eating disorders during middle adolescence: longitudinal associations and treatment seeking. *Nordic Journal of Psychiatry*, **71**, 605–613.

Ray, L. A., Meredith, L. R., Kiluk, B. D., Walthers, J., Carroll, K. M., & Magill, M. (2020). Combined pharmacotherapy and cognitive behavioral therapy for adults with alcohol or substance use disorders: a systematic review and meta-analysis. *JAMA Network Open*, **3**, e208279.

Rickwood, D., Paraskakis, M., Quin, D., Hobbs, N., Ryall, V., Trethowan, J., & McGorry, P. (2019). Australia's innovation in youth mental health care: the headspace centre model. *Early Intervention in Psychiatry*, **13**, 159–166.

Riecher-Rössler, A. (2017). Oestrogens, prolactin, hypothalamic-pituitary-gonadal axis, and schizophrenic psychoses. *Lancet Psychiatry*, **4**, 63–72.

Rienecke, R. D. (2017). Family-based treatment of eating disorders in adolescents: current insights. *Adolescent Health, Medicine and Therapeutics*, **8**, 69–79.

Robinson, L., Tang, E., & Taylor, J. P. (2015). Dementia: timely diagnosis and early intervention. *BMJ*, **350**, h3029.

Rocha, T. B.-M., Fisher, H. L., Caye, A., Anselmi, L., Arseneault, L., Barros, F. C., et al. (2021). Identifying adolescents at risk for depression: a prediction score performance in cohorts based in 3 different continents. *Journal of the American Academy of Child and Adolescent Psychiatry*, **60**, 262–273.

Roseman, M., Saadat, N., Riehm, K. E., Kloda, L. A., Boruff, J., Ickowicz, A., et al. (2017). Depression screening and health outcomes in children and adolescents: a systematic review. *Canadian Journal of Psychiatry*, **62**, 813–817.

Rossouw, T. I. & Fonagy, P. (2012). Mentalization-based treatment for self-harm in adolescents: a randomized controlled trial. *Journal of the American Academy of Child and Adolescent Psychiatry*, **51**, 1304–1313.

Sapolsky, R. M. (2000). The possibility of neurotoxicity in the hippocampus in major depression: a primer on neuron death. *Biological Psychiatry*, **48**, 755–765.

Sarvet, A. L. & Hasin, D. (2016). The natural history of substance use disorders. *Current Opinion in Psychiatry*, **29**, 250–257.

Sawyer, S. M., Azzopardi, P. S., Wickremarathne, D., & Patton, G. C. (2018). The age of adolescence. *Lancet Child and Adolescent Health*, **2**, 223–228.

Schaumberg, K., Zerwas, S., Goodman, E., Yilmaz, Z., Bulik, C. M., & Micali, N. (2019). Anxiety disorder symptoms at age 10 predict eating disorder symptoms and diagnoses in adolescence. *Journal of Child Psychology and Psychiatry and Allied Disciplines*, **60**, 686–696.

Schmidt, U., Adan, R., Böhm, I., Campbell, I. C., Dingemans, A., Ehrlich, S., et al. (2016). Eating disorders: the big issue. *Lancet Psychiatry*, **3**, 313–315.

Shah, J. L., Scott, J., McGorry, P. D., Cross, S. P. M., Keshavan, M. S., Nelson, B., et al. (2020). Transdiagnostic clinical staging in youth mental health: a first international consensus statement. *World Psychiatry*, **19**, 233–242.

Sharp, C. & Wall, K. (2018). Personality pathology grows up: adolescence as a sensitive period. *Current Opinion in Psychology*, **21**, 111–116.

Silén, Y., Sipilä, P. N., Raevuori, A., Mustelin, L., Marttunen, M., Kaprio, J., & Keski-Rahkonen, A. (2020). DSM-5 eating disorders among adolescents and young adults in Finland: a public health concern. *International Journal of Eating Disorders*, **53**, 520–531.

Singh, S. P., Paul, M., Ford, T., Kramer, T., Weaver, T., McLaren, S., et al. (2010). Process, outcome and experience of transition from child to adult mental healthcare: multiperspective study. *British Journal of Psychiatry*, **197**, 305–312.

Smink, F. R. E., Van Hoeken, D., & Hoek, H. W. (2012). Epidemiology of eating disorders: incidence, prevalence and mortality rates. *Current Psychiatry Reports*, **14**, 406–414.

Sparti, C., Santomauro, D., Cruwys, T., Burgess, P., & Harris, M. (2019). Disordered eating among Australian adolescents: prevalence, functioning, and help received. *International Journal of Eating Disorders*, **52**, 246–254.

Ssegonja, R., Nystrand, C., Feldman, I., Sarkadi, A., Langenskiöld, S., & Jonsson, U. (2019). Indicated preventive interventions for depression in children and adolescents: a meta-analysis and meta-regression. *Preventive Medicine*, **118**, 7–15.

Steeg, S., Coopner, J., & Kapur, N. (2014). Early intervention for self-harm and suicidality. In: Byrne, P. & Rosen, A. (Eds.), *Early Intervention in Psychiatry: EI of Nearly Everthing for Better Mental Health* (pp. 255–266). Chichester: John Wiley & Sons.

Steinhausen, H. C. & Jensen, C. M. (2015). Time trends in lifetime incidence rates of first-time diagnosed anorexia nervosa and bulimia nervosa across 16 years in a danish nationwide psychiatric registry study. *International Journal of Eating Disorders*, **48**, 845–850.

Stice, E., Desjardins, C. D., Rohde, P., & Shaw, H. (2021). Sequencing of symptom emergence in anorexia nervosa, bulimia nervosa, binge eating disorder, and purging disorder and relations of prodromal symptoms to future onset of these disorders. *Journal of Abnormal Psychology*, **130**, 377–387.

Stice, E., Gau, J. M., Rohde, P., & Shaw, H. (2017). Risk factors that predict future onset of each DSM-5 eating disorder: predictive specificity in high-risk adolescent females. *Journal of Abnormal Psychology*, **126**, 38–51.

Stockings, E., Hall, W. D., Lynskey, M., Morley, K. I., Reavley, N., Strang, J., et al. (2016a). Prevention, early intervention, harm reduction, and treatment of substance use in young people. *Lancet Psychiatry*, **3**, 280–296.

Stockings, E. A., Degenhardt, L., Dobbins, T., Lee, Y. Y., Erskine, H. E., Whiteford, H. A., & Patton, G. (2016b). Preventing depression and anxiety in young people: a review of the joint efficacy of universal, selective and indicated prevention. *Psychological Medicine*, **46**, 11–26.

Storebø, O. J., Stoffers-Winterling, J. M., Völlm, B. A., Kongerslev, M. T., Mattivi, J. T., Jørgensen, M. S., et al. (2020). Psychological therapies for people with borderline personality disorder. *Cochrane Database of Systematic Reviews*, **5**, CD012955.

Strawn, J. R., Adler, C. M., McNamara, R. K., Welge, J. A., Bitter, S. M., Mills, et al. (2014). Antidepressant tolerability in anxious and depressed youth at high risk for bipolar disorder: a prospective naturalistic treatment study. *Bipolar Disorders*, **16**, 523–530.

Swinbourne, J. M. & Touyz, S. W. (2007). The co-morbidity of eating disorders and anxiety disorders: a review. *European Eating Disorders Review*, **15**, 253–274.

Taquet, M., Geddes, J. R., Luciano, S., & Harrison, P. J. (2021). Incidence and outcomes of eating disorders during the COVID-19 pandemic. *British Journal of Psychiatry*, **220**, 1–3.

Thompson, K. N., Jackson, H., Cavelti, M., Betts, J., McCutcheon, L., Jovev, M., & Chanen, A. M. (2019). The clinical significance of subthreshold borderline personality disorder features in outpatient youth. *Journal of Personality Disorders*, **33**, 71–81.

Treasure, J., Cardi, V., Leppanen, J., & Turton, R. (2015a). New treatment approaches for severe and enduring eating disorders. *Physiology and Behavior*, **152**, 456–465.

Treasure, J., Stein, D., & Maguire, S. (2015b). Has the time come for a staging model to map the course of eating disorders from high risk to severe enduring illness? An examination of the evidence. *Early Intervention in Psychiatry*, **9**, 173–184.

US Preventive Services Task Force (2018). Screening and behavioral counseling interventions to reduce unhealthy alcohol use in adolescents and adults: US Preventive Services Task Force recommendation statement. *JAMA*, **320**, 1899–1909.

US Preventive Services Task Force (2020). Screening for unhealthy drug use: US Preventive Services Task Force recommendation statement. *JAMA*, **323**, 2301–2309.

Vall, E. & Wade, T.D. (2015). Predictors of treatment outcome in individuals with eating disorders: a systematic review and meta-analysis. *International Journal of Eating Disorders*, **48**, 946–971.

Vasilenko, S. A., Evans-Polce, R. J., & Lanza, S. T. (2017). Age trends in rates of substance use disorders across ages 18–90: differences by gender and race/ethnicity. *Drug and Alcohol Dependence*, **180**, 260–264.

Videler, A. C., Hutsebaut, J., Schulkens, J. E. M., Sobczak, S., & van Alphen, S. P. J. (2019). A life span perspective on borderline personality disorder. *Current Psychiatry Reports*, **21**, 51.

Vieta, E. & Berk, M. (2022). Early intervention comes late. *European Neuropsychopharmacology*, **59**, 1–3.

Volkow, N. D., Han, B., Einstein, E. B., & Compton, W. M. (2021). Prevalence of substance use disorders by time since first substance use among young people in the US. *JAMA Pediatrics*, **175**, 640–643.

Wagner, F. A. & Anthony, J. C. (2002). From first drug use to drug dependence: developmental periods of risk for dependence upon marijuana, cocaine, and alcohol. *Neuropsychopharmacology*, **26**, 479–488.

Weavers, B., Heron, J., Thapar, A. K., Stephens, A., Lennon, J., Bevan Jones, R., et al. (2021). The antecedents and outcomes of persistent and remitting adolescent depressive symptom trajectories: a longitudinal, population-based English study. *Lancet Psychiatry*, **8**, 1053–1061.

Wilksch, S. M., O'Shea, A., Ho, P., Byrne, S., & Wade, T. D. (2020). The relationship between social media use and disordered eating in young adolescents. *International Journal of Eating Disorders*, **53**, 96–106.

Williams, A. R. & Levin, F. R. (2020). The perils of screening for unhealthy drug use are a call to action for the mental health workforce. *JAMA Psychiatry*, **77**, 1101–1102.

World Health Organization (2018a). Global Health Observatory Data repository: suicide rate estimates, crude, 5-year age groups up to 29 years. https://apps.who.int/gho/data/node.main.MHSUICIDE5YEARAGEGROUPS?lang=en

World Health Organization (2018b). *National Suicide Prevention Strategies: Progress, Examples and Indicators*. Geneva: World Health Organization.

Zuckerbrot, R. A., Cheung, A., Jensen, P. S., Stein, R. E. K., Laraque, D., & GLAD-PC Steering Group (2018). Guidelines for Adolescent Depression in Primary Care (GLAD-PC): part I. Practice preparation, identification, assessment, and initial management. *Pediatrics*, **141**, e20174081.

11

Organizing the range of community mental health services

Graham Thornicroft, Michele Tansella, and Robert E. Drake

Introduction

In discussing the organization of the full range of community mental health services in this chapter, we shall first consider some important pre-conditions, namely (1) the scale of needs in any given population, (2) the degree of treatment coverage of these needs by services, (3) the quantity and quality of available resources, and (4) how far the attitudes of staff and the population at large promote or hinder a service primarily focused upon the needs of service users. We go on to describe the 'balanced care' model, which includes both hospital-based and community-based care, and its application in low-, medium-, and high-resource countries and settings. We then summarize our own experience in developing community care to draw out the key lessons learned, including the need to include a wide range of stakeholder groups. Finally, we discuss the main barriers that can impede the implementation of the balanced care model, and methods to overcome these types of resistance.

The pre-conditions for organizing community mental health services

Population needs, treatment coverage, and focusing

To plan community mental health services, we must first understand both the levels of need in the local area and population, and the available resources. Figure 11.1 shows the relationship between true prevalence and treated prevalence. True prevalence means the total number of cases of people with a particular mental health condition in a defined area, or population. Treated prevalence, by contrast, refers to the proportion of this number of people who receive care. In the National Comorbidity Survey Replication study, for example, a survey of 4319 participants representative of the general population in the US (shown as A in Figure 11.1, 100%), the true prevalence of all emotional disorders was 30.5% (B) of those surveyed, while 20.1% of all participants received treatment for any mental disorder (C) (Kessler et al., 2005). Notably, among group C, half of these individuals did not have an emotional disorder at the time of treatment, and typically sought psychotherapeutic help for other reasons. Table 11.1 summarizes this information numerically.

In a similar study in six European countries, using the same methods as the National Comorbidity Survey Replication study, among 7731 participants, the true prevalence of all emotional disorders was estimated to be 11.7%, and the treated prevalence rate was 6.1% among all respondents (Alonso et al., 2007). Interestingly, among those who were treated, the majority had no clearly identified mental illness. Therefore, despite the large differences in total prevalence rates between the US and Europe, possibly due to methodological differences between these studies, mental health services did not focus their limited resources upon people with clear mental

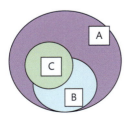

Figure 11.1 Relationship between true prevalence and treated prevalence. Key: A = total adult population, B = true prevalence, C = treated prevalence.

Table 11.1 National Comorbidity Survey Replication study data for true and treated annual prevalence rates of emotional disorders among adults in the general population

	Treated	Not treated	Total
Emotional disorder	10.07%	20.43%	30.50% (1/3 of cases treated: poor coverage[a])
No emotional disorder	10.03% (1/2 of those treated are not cases: poor focusing[b])	59.47%	69.50%
Total	20.10%	79.90%	100%

[a] *Coverage* is the percentage of people who could benefit from treatment and actually receive it.
[b] *Focusing* refers to whether those people actually receiving treatment need it.

disorders, nor upon people with more severe or more disabling conditions. These findings highlight the important issues of coverage and focusing. *Coverage* means the proportion of people could benefit from treatment who actually receive it (Alonso et al., 2007).

Evidence-based practices, implementation, and cultural issues

In addition to the problems of coverage and focus, real-world mental health systems, even in the richest countries, typically fail to assure the consistent quality of services (Institute of Medicine (US) Committee, 2006). They do so in three critical ways, by failing to (1) provide effective, or evidence-based, treatments; (2) implement evidence-based interventions with sufficient fidelity to improve outcomes; and (3) provide services in culturally sensitive ways that would enhance access and acceptability for people from ethnic-racial and other minority backgrounds. The evidence for each of these problems is robust. In the US, for example, most people with a diagnosis of serious mental illness get no mental health care, and most of those who do receive care get ineffective or harmful interventions (Wang et al., 2002). Probably fewer than 5% of people with a serious mental illness in the US receive the effective psychosocial services that would benefit them (Drake & Essock, 2009). The reasons are legion: access and acceptability problems for people from minority backgrounds, dropouts due to services that are clinician centred rather than client centred, poor alignment between payment systems and evidence-based practices, clinicians' inability or unwillingness to adopt new interventions, inadequate implementation processes, and misinformation from vested interest groups (Drake et al., 2009; Fixsen et al., 2009; Kreyenbuhl et al., 2009; Mojtabai et al., 2009).

Social determinants of health

Social determinants of health refer to environmental conditions that affect health, functioning, and quality of life (Allen et al., 2014; Rose-Clarke et al., 2020). Numerous social determinants disproportionately affect patients with mental health conditions (Jeste & Pender, 2022). Common social determinants for this population include poverty, lack of safe housing, unemployment, pervasive stigma, victimization, lack of insurance parity, inappropriate use of incarceration, homelessness, and many more.

Social determinants typically explain more of the variance in outcomes than treatment (Hood et al., 2016). Furthermore, mental health treatments for social problems are generally ineffective and costly (Alegria et al., 2017). Examples are abundant: providing psychiatric hospitalization rather than supportive housing for mentally ill people who are homeless, day treatment rather than supported employment for those who are unemployed, incarceration for disruptive behaviour related to mental illness and/or substance use disorder, polypharmacy for people living in abusive situations, and many more. Addressing social determinants by using preventive public health interventions can be more effective and less expensive than traditional mental health treatments (Drake & Bond, 2021). European countries generally provide greater prevention and greater safety net services for people with mental illness than the US. In all countries, however, prevention is more likely to mitigate personal, familial, community, and societal suffering and costs.

In all countries, people from disadvantaged groups, such as race, ethic, or gender minorities, are even more prone to experience negative social determinants, including difficulties accessing high-quality mental health care. Thus, movements to address diversity, equity, and inclusion are prioritizing increased efforts to increase access to care and opportunities for social and health success for these groups (Rose-Clarke et al., 2020).

Staff attitudes

A further important pre-condition to understand before organizing mental health services is the nature of staff attitudes towards service users and towards community-based models of care. Moving from a mental health system dependent upon hospitals to one which is a balance of hospital and community services implies far more than only a physical relocation of treatment sites, because it also requires a fundamental reorientation of perspective. Table 11.2 shows staff attitudes typical for the two approaches. Within institutions, hierarchical and traditional structures predominate, with a focus on control, order, routine, and the medicalization of treatment and care. Within the balanced care model, there is a refocusing upon strengths, recovery, individualized care, involving service users and family members in care decisions, and staff of all disciplines having a greater degree of professional autonomy than is common in traditional hospital settings, within the context of multidisciplinary teamwork.

Further, therapeutic orientation will vary according to the care setting, as shown in Table 11.3. For example, staff in community-based services will often tend to pay greater attention to assessing and treating people with mental illness in their own homes, and will assess a wider range of their clinical and social needs. More fundamentally,

Table 11.2 Differences in staff attitudes between institutional and community perspectives

	Institutional perspective	Community perspective
Staff attitudes	Seeing service users (usually referred to as patients within institutional settings) within the hospital context Focus on symptoms and behavioural control Planned/routine contacts Guidance from set policies and procedures Hierarchical decision-making and authority structure (often biomedical model) Stronger reliance on pharmacological treatments View that service users with severe symptoms should remain in hospital Paternalistic attitude that staff are responsible for the behaviour of service users View that service users in hospital are not responsible for their own antisocial behaviour and that these should not be reported to police	Seeing service user within the home, family, and community context Belief in individual recovery goals Attention to social determinants of health Helping the family to receive and provide support Flexibility: planned and unplanned contacts Responses to changing needs and goals of service users Emphasis on shared decision-making and negotiation (between staff, and between staff and service users) Combining pharmacological, psychological, and social interventions View that symptoms do not necessarily determine the correct care setting for each person Empowering emphasis on the responsibilities of service users along with their choices and consequences Service users assumed to be responsible for their behaviour and to undergo due legal process if committing a crime

Table 11.3 Differences in therapeutic orientation between the institutional and community perspectives

	Institutional perspective	Community perspective
Therapeutic orientation	Emphasis on symptom relief Improved facilities and expertise for physical assessment, investigation, procedures, and treatment Hierarchical decisions Focus on control of violent behaviour Standardized treatment for groups of individuals Regulated timetable Separated short-term treatment and rehabilitation Culture which tends to avoid risk taking Clinical and administrative leadership by medical doctors (which may maintain closer links with other medical specialities)	Greater focus on service user empowerment Linkages to physical health care More autonomy for staff in different disciplines Sees behaviour more often within specific contexts More individualized treatment and care Flexibility in when and where service users are treated Recognizing the importance of social determinants Integration of clinical and social interventions Culture of new approaches to services and care plans Leadership can be exercised by any discipline (which may be seen to make mental health services distinct and distant from other medical specialities)

the community orientation seeks to assist people with mental illness in leading their own lives according to their own specific priorities and recovery goals (putting staff in a facilitatory or supportive role), rather than maintaining the traditional attitudes of dependence, paternalism, and low expectations. It may also be true that staff in regions that have moved beyond deinstitutionalization will still have challenges regarding issues such as evidence-based practices, inclusion of people with lived experience, and equity for minority groups.

Implementing the balanced care model

Evidence for a balance of hospital and community care

In this section we argue for a balanced care model for adult mental health services and present the evidence for this approach. Many scientific reviews of specific community mental health services are presented in other chapters of this book, and guidelines are updated regularly by government and other agencies (e.g. National Institute for Health and Care Excellence, Cochrane, and Substance Abuse and Mental Health Services Administration). In our view, it is also the case that even in countries that are post-deinstitutionalization the issues of structure, organization, intervention choice, and financing are all critical issues. We discuss below service models that are suitable for areas with low, medium and high levels of resources (Thornicroft & Tansella, 2013a, 2013b). Both the balanced scheme and the three types of resource level are clearly oversimplified but intended to make complex realities more manageable.

Table 11.4 indicates that areas with low level of resources (column 1) can afford to provide most of their mental health care in primary health care settings, delivered by primary care and community health worker staff. Indeed, community and lay health workers are common in many low- and middle-income countries and have been

Table 11.4 Mental health service components in low-, medium-, and high-resource settings: the balanced care model

1. Low level of resource setting	2. Medium level of resource setting	3. High level of resource setting
(Step A) Primary mental health care with specialist back-up	(Step A) Primary mental health care with specialist back-up *and*	(Step A) Primary mental health care with specialist back-up *and*
		(Step B) General adult mental health care *and*
	(Step B) General adult mental health care	(Step C) Specialized mental health care
Screening and assessment by primary care staff Talking treatments including counselling and advice Pharmacological treatment Liaison and training with mental health specialist staff, when available Limited specialist back-up available for: • training • consultation for complex cases • inpatient assessment and treatment for cases which cannot be managed in primary care, e.g. in general hospitals	1. Outpatient/ambulatory clinics	1. Specialized clinics for specific disorders or patient groups including: • children and adolescents • eating disorders • co-occurring substance use disorder • treatment-resistant affective disorders • severe personality disorders • justice-system involvement
	2. Community mental health teams	2. Specialized community mental health teams including: • early intervention teams • assertive community treatment
	3. Acute inpatient care	3. Alternatives to acute hospital admission including: • home treatment/crisis resolution teams • crisis/respite houses • acute day hospitals
	4. Long-term community-based residential care	4. Alternative types of long-stay community residential care including: • intensive 24-hour staffed residential provision • less intensively staffed accommodation • independent accommodation
	5. Rehabilitation, occupation, and work	5. Alternative forms of rehabilitation, occupation, and work: such as individual placement and support

shown to complement the usual medical model of care (Chatterjee et al., 2014). The very limited specialist back-up can then offer training, consultation for complex cases, and inpatient assessment and treatment for cases which cannot be managed in primary care (Saxena & Maulik, 2003). Some low-resource countries may in fact be in a pre-asylum stage (Njenga, 2002), in which apparent community care represents widespread neglect or abuse of mentally ill people. Where asylums do exist, policymakers face difficult choices about whether to upgrade the quality of care they offer (Njenga, 2002) or convert the resources of the larger hospitals into decentralized services instead (Alem, 2002).

We have deliberately separated the types of care into these three schemes because the differences in mental health care which are possible in low- and high-resource areas (both between and within countries) are vast (World Health Organization, 2020). Areas (countries or regions) with a medium level of resources may first establish the service components shown in column 2, and later, as resources allow, chose to add some of the wider range of specialized services indicated in column 3. The choice of which of these more specialized services to develop first depends upon local factors including service traditions and specific circumstances; consumer, carer, and staff preferences; existing services strengths and weaknesses; and the way in which evidence is interpreted and used. A more detailed consideration of specific types of mental health service provision in low-, medium-, and high-resource countries and settings is given in the chapters in Section 9 of this book on global mental health.

In Latin American countries, nearly all of which are classified as middle-income countries in 2022, health care systems are implementing, albeit it slowly, community-based mental health treatments and rehabilitation programmes (Cubillos et al., 2020; Marsch et al., 2022; Mascayana et al., 2022). As these countries implement and plan new services, key questions involve cultural adaptations of evidence-based practices, implementation in real-world settings, and financing of community services. Leaders also should avoid some of the mistakes made in high-income countries like the US during deinstitutionalization (Cubillos et al., 2020). For example, can these countries skip over the step of community segregation in group homes and day centres between institutionalization and community integration?

This balanced care model also indicates that the forms of care relevant and affordable to areas with a high level of resources will be elements from column 3 in addition to the components in columns 1 and 2 in Table 11.4, which will usually already be present. The model is therefore *additive* and *sequential* in that new resources allow extra levels of service to be provided over time, in terms of mixtures of the components within each step, when the provision of the components in each previous step is complete.

Primary mental health care with specialist back-up

Well-defined psychological conditions that cause disability are common in general health care and primary health care settings in every country. In areas with a low level of resources (column 1 in Table 11.4), the large majority of cases of mental disorders should be recognized and treated within primary health care (Desjarlais et al., 1995). The World Health Organization has suggested that the integration of essential mental health treatments within primary health care in these countries is feasible (World Health Organization, 2022).

General adult mental health care

The recognition and treatment of most people with mental illnesses, especially depression and anxiety-related disorders, remains a task for primary care. General adult mental health care refers to a range of service components in areas that can afford specialty mental health care. The elements necessary in such a basic form of a comprehensive mental health service comprise an amalgam of the following five core components:

Outpatient/ambulatory clinics

These vary according to whether people can self-refer or need to be referred by other agencies such as primary care; whether there are fixed appointment times or open access assessments; if doctors alone or other disciplines also provide clinical contact; if direct or indirect payment is made; if there are methods to enhance attendance rates; the response to non-attenders; and the frequency and duration of clinical contacts. Despite little evidence on these key characteristics of outpatient care (Becker, 2001), many countries share a strong clinical consensus that such clinics are a relatively efficient way to organize the provision of evidence-based assessment and treatment, providing that the clinic sites are accessible to local populations. These clinics are of course simply methods of arranging clinical contact between staff and patients, and the key issue is the *content and balance* of the clinical interventions, that is, the amount and proportion of different evidence-based interventions.

Community mental health teams

Community mental health teams (CMHTs) are the basic building block for community mental health services. The simplest model of provision of community care is for generic (non-specialized) CMHTs to provide the full range of interventions (including the contributions of psychiatrists, community psychiatric nurses, social workers, psychologists, and occupational therapists), usually prioritizing adults with severe mental illness, for a locally defined geographical catchment area (Department of Health, 2002; Thornicroft et al., 1999). A series of studies and systematic reviews, comparing CMHTs with a variety of hospital-based services, suggest clear benefits to the introduction of generic community-based multidisciplinary teams: they can improve engagement with services, increase user satisfaction, increase met needs, and improve adherence to treatment, although they do not improve symptoms or social function (Burns, 2001; Simmonds et al., 2001; Thornicroft et al., 1998; Tyrer et al., 1998, 2003). In addition, continuity of care and service flexibility have been shown to be more developed where a CMHT model is in place.

Case management is a method of *delivering* care rather than a clinical intervention in its own right, and at this stage the evidence suggests that it can most usefully be implemented within the context of CMHTs (Holloway & Carson, 2001). It is a style of working which has been described as the 'co-ordination, integration and allocation of individualised care within limited resources' (Thornicroft, 1991, p. 141). A considerable literature shows that case management can be moderately effective in improving continuity of care, quality of life, and patient satisfaction, but there is conflicting evidence on whether it has any impact on the use of inpatient services (Mueser et al., 1998; Ziguras & Stuart, 2000; Ziguras et al., 2002). Case management needs to be carefully distinguished from the much more specific and more intensive *assertive community treatment*. Case management of all types has generally become more strengths-based and less deficit-based (Rapp & Goscha, 2004).

Acute inpatient care

A balanced system of mental health care requires acute inpatient beds, but the amount and type of beds remain controversial (Drake & Wallach, 2019; O'Reilly et al., 2019). A 2005–2015 longitudinal study of 171 countries showed that the number of beds has decreased at a rate of 8% per year (Metcalfe & Drake, 2019). A higher Human Development Index was still associated with more mental hospital beds. The number of beds undoubtedly depends on local population characteristics and the amount and quality of community-based services. The quality of inpatient services also varies widely. Large institutions characterized by neglect and over-reliance on medications continue to exist in many regions, while some European countries, such as Italy, have developed a strong system of shifting mental hospital beds to local general hospitals to counter stigma (Barbui et al., 2018; Tansella, 1986).

Alternative services (such as home treatment teams, crisis house, and acute day hospital care, see 'Alternatives to acute inpatient care') can offer realistic alternative care for some voluntary patients (Howard et al., 2008; Johnson et al., 2005a, 2005b). Nevertheless, those who need urgent medical assessment, or those with severe and comorbid medical and psychiatric conditions, severe psychiatric relapse and behavioural disturbance, high levels of suicidality or assaultativeness, acute neuropsychiatric conditions, or elderly people with concomitant severe physical disorders, will usually require high-intensity immediate support in acute inpatient hospital units.

There is a relatively weak evidence base for many aspects of inpatient care, and most studies are descriptive accounts (Szmukler & Holloway, 2001). There are few systematic reviews in this field, one of which found that there were no differences in outcomes between routine admissions and planned short hospital stays (Johnstone & Zolese, 1999). More generally, although there is a consensus that acute inpatient units are necessary, the number of beds required is highly contingent upon which other services exist locally and upon local social and cultural characteristics (Drake & Wallach, 2019; Thornicroft & Tansella, 1999). For example, per capita annual mental health spending varies across US states more than tenfold, from $37 to $375 (Open Minds, 2020), which means that community-based services are rarely available in some states. Acute inpatient care commonly absorbs most of the mental health budget (Knapp & Wong, 2020). Therefore, minimizing the use of bed-days, for example, by reducing the average length of stay, may be an important goal, if the resources released in this way can be used for other service components. A related policy issue concerns how to provide acute beds in a humane and less institutionalized way that is acceptable to patients, for example, in general hospital units (Barbui et al., 2018).

Long-term community-based residential care

It is important to know whether people with severe and long-term disabilities should be still cared for in larger, traditional institutions or be transferred to long-term community-based residential care. The evidence here, for medium- and high-resource level areas, is clear. When deinstitutionalization is carefully carried out, for those who have previously received long-term inpatient care for many years, then the outcomes are more favourable for most people who are discharged to community care (Shepherd & Murray, 2001; Thornicroft & Bebbington, 1989). The Team for the Assessment of Psychiatric Services (TAPS) study in London (Leff, 1997), for example, completed a 5-year follow-up on over 95% of 670 discharged long-stay non-demented people and found that community services were more cost-effective (Knapp et al., 1990). In many high-income countries, the effects of hospital closure are now such that very few long-stay hospital beds remain within the mental health system.

Rehabilitation, occupation, and work

Rates of unemployment among people with mental disorders are usually much higher than in the general population, and are also higher than among people with severe physical disabilities (Virgolino et al., 2022). Traditional methods of vocational rehabilitation included day centres, psychiatric rehabilitation centres, and other forms of pre-employment training (Drake et al., 2012; Rosen & Barfoot, 2001). Over the past 20 years, supported employment designed specifically for people with mental health conditions has emerged as an evidence-based practice, demonstrating effectiveness and cost-effectiveness compared to previous models (Bond et al., 2020; Knapp & Wong, 2020). Chapter 20 in this volume reviews the findings from 28 randomized controlled trials of the individual placement and support model.

Specialized mental health services

The balanced care model suggests that areas with high levels of resources may already provide all or most of the service components in Steps A and B and are able to offer additional components from the options shown in Step C in **Table 11.4**.

Outpatient/ambulatory clinics

Specialized outpatient facilities for particular disorders or patient groups are common in many high-resource areas and may include, for example, services dedicated to people with eating disorders; people with anxiety disorders; people with dual diagnosis (psychotic disorders and substance abuse); cases of treatment-resistant affective or psychotic disorders; people requiring specialized forms of psychotherapy, such as those with severe personality disorders; mentally disordered offenders; mentally ill mothers and their babies; and those with other specific disorders (such as post-traumatic stress disorder). Local decisions about whether to establish such specialized clinics will depend upon several factors, including their relative priority in relation to the other specialized services described below, identified services gaps, and the financial opportunities available.

Community mental health teams

These are by far the most researched of all the components of balanced care, and most randomized controlled trials and systematic reviews in this field refer to such teams (Mueser et al., 1998). Two types of specialized CMHT have been particularly well developed as adjuncts to generic CMHTs: assertive community treatment (ACT) teams and early intervention teams.

ACT teams

These provide a form of specialized mobile outreach treatment for people with more disabling mental disorders, and have been clearly characterized (Killaspy et al., 2006, 2009; Scott & Lehman,

2001; Teague et al., 1998). There is now strong evidence that ACT can produce the following advantages in high level of resource areas: (1) reducing admissions to hospital and the use of acute beds, (2) reducing homelessness, (3) improving accommodation status, and (4) increasing service user satisfaction. ACT has not been shown to produce improvements in mental state or social functioning. ACT can reduce the cost of inpatient services, but does not change the overall costs of care (Latimer, 1999; Marshall & Lockwood, 2003; McCrone et al., 2009; Phillips et al., 2001). Nevertheless, it is not known how far ACT is cross-culturally relevant and indeed there is evidence that ACT may be less effective where usual services already offer high levels of integration and continuity of care, for example, in the UK, than in settings where the treatment-as-usual control condition may offer little to people with severe mental illnesses (Burns, 2009). ACT has been extended to people with justice system involvement (Morrissey et al., 2016) and substance use disorder (Penzenstadler et al., 2019), but the outcomes of randomized controlled trials are thus far mixed. More details about the provision of ACT services are given in Chapter 14.

Early intervention teams

There has been considerable interest in the prompt identification and treatment of first or early episode cases of psychosis. Much of this research has focused upon the time between first clear onset of symptoms and the beginning of treatment, referred to as the 'duration of untreated psychosis', while other studies have placed more emphasis upon providing family interventions when a young person's psychosis is first identified (Addington et al., 2003; Raune et al., 2004). There is now emerging evidence that a longer duration of untreated psychosis is a predictor of worse outcome for psychosis; in other words, if patients wait a long time after developing a psychotic condition before they receive treatment, then they may take longer to recover and have a less favourable long-term prognosis.

Despite widespread enthusiasm for and adoption of early intervention teams for psychosis since the early 2000s, few rigorous studies exist. A 2020 Cochrane review concluded that these teams may provide modest benefits to participants during treatment compared to usual care (Puntis et al., 2020). The potential benefits include fewer dropouts from services, small reductions in hospitalizations, small increases in functioning, and increases in service satisfaction, but these advantages may disappear when special services end. How, when, and whom to transfer to usual care remain open questions.

Alternatives to acute inpatient care

Three main alternatives to acute inpatient care include acute day hospitals, crisis residences, and in-home treatment/crisis resolution teams. *Acute day hospitals* offer programmes of day treatment for those with acute and severe psychiatric problems as an alternative to admission to inpatient units. A systematic review of nine randomized controlled trials established that acute day hospital care is suitable for about 30% of people who would otherwise be admitted to hospital, offering advantages in terms of faster improvement and lower cost. Thus, acute day hospital care is probably an effective option when demand for inpatient beds is high (Marshall et al., 2001).

Crisis houses are residences in community settings staffed by trained mental health professionals and offering admission for some people who would otherwise be admitted to hospital. A wide variety of respite houses, havens, and refuges have been developed, but crisis house is used here to mean facilities that are alternatives to non-compulsory hospital admission. The little available research evidence suggests that they are very acceptable to their residents (Szmukler & Holloway, 2001), may be able to offer an alternative to hospital admission for about a quarter of otherwise admitted patients, and may be more cost-effective than hospital admission (Mosher, 1999; Sledge et al., 1996). Nevertheless, evidence suggests that female patients in particular prefer non-hospital alternatives (such as single-sex crisis houses) to acute inpatient treatment, perhaps reflecting the lack of perceived safety in some hospitals (Johnson et al., 2009; Killaspy et al., 2000). According to a more recent review, crisis houses offer a cost-effective alternative to inpatient admission and are potentially less frightening, stigmatizing, and socially dislocating (Lloyd-Evans & Johnson, 2019). However, little consensus exists regarding the most effective service components and configurations.

Home treatment/crisis resolution teams are mobile CMHTs offering assessment for people in psychiatric crises and providing intensive treatment and care at home. The key active ingredients appear to be regular home visits, and the combined provision of health and social care (Johnson et al., 2008). A Cochrane systematic review (Catty et al., 2002) found that most of the research evidence is from the US or the UK, and concluded that home treatment teams reduce days spent in hospital, especially if the teams make regular home visits and have responsibility for both health and social care (Joy et al., 1998). A national study in England between 1998 and 2003 found that hospital admissions were reduced by 10% in areas which had crisis resolution teams, and by 23% where these teams offered a 24-hour on-call system (Glover et al., 2006). Intensive home treatment aims to reduce the negative psychological effects in usual care, but a recent study in the Netherlands found that intensive home treatment did not improve self-efficacy when compared to usual care (Barakat et al., 2021).

Crisis plans and advance directives: a Joint Crisis Plan (JCP) aims to empower the holder and to facilitate early detection and treatment of relapse (Sutherby et al., 1999). It is developed by a patient together with mental health staff. Held by the patient, it contains their choice of information, which can include an advance agreement for treatment preferences for any future emergency, when they might be too unwell to express coherent views. The JCP format was developed after consultation with national user groups, interviews with organizations and individuals using crisis cards (Sutherby & Szmukler, 1998), and detailed development work with service users in South London. The results of the pilot study (Sutherby et al., 1999) showed that (at 6–12-month follow-up) 57% of participating patients felt more involved in their care, 60% felt more positive about their situation, 51% felt more in control of their mental health problem and 41% were more likely to continue treatment. The JCP may have direct and indirect effects: family doctors and carers may be able to react earlier to a relapse, while emergency department staff may make better decisions when informed by the JCP. Negotiating the content may clarify treatment issues and build consensus between patients and staff, potentially reducing future compulsion in treatment and care. Recent research has shown that JCPs are able to halve the rates of compulsory treatment in hospital (Henderson et al., 2004), and are cost-effective (Flood et al., 2006).

Psychiatric advance directives enable an individual to document preferences for future treatment at times if and when they are unable to make decisions (Thornicroft & Henderson, 2016). A Cochrane Collaborative review included only two trials involving 321 people with severe mental illnesses and found no significant difference in hospital admission (n = 160, one randomized controlled trial, relative risk 0.69, 95% confidence interval 0.5–1.0), or number of psychiatric outpatient attendances between participants given advanced treatment directives or usual care. Similarly, no significant differences were found for compliance with treatment, self-harm, or number of arrests (Campbell et al., 2009). A review of several studies showed a mixed picture and concluded that advance directives can potentially support empowerment, minimize experienced coercion, and improve coping strategies (Khazaal et al., 2014). The impact on inpatient service use is uncertain, although some studies have indicated the potential to reduce compulsory hospitalizations (Barrett et al., 2013; Henderson et al., 2004, Thornicroft et al., 2013).

Alternative types of long-stay community residential care

As described above, these are usually replacements for long-stay wards in psychiatric institutions (Shepherd & Murray, 2001). Three categories of such residential care can be identified: (1) *24-hour staffed residential care* (high-staffed hostels, residential care homes, or nursing homes, depending on whether the staff have professional qualifications), (2) *day-staffed residential places* (hostels or residential homes which are staffed during the day), and (3) *lower supported accommodation* (minimally supported hostels or residential homes with visiting staff). There is limited evidence on the cost-effectiveness of these types of residential care, and no completed systematic reviews (Chilvers et al., 2003). Policymakers must therefore decide upon the need for such services with local stakeholders (Rosen & Barfoot, 2001; Thornicroft, 2001). More information is provided about supported accommodation in Chapter 19.

Alternative forms of rehabilitation, occupation, and work

Although vocational rehabilitation has been offered in various forms to people with severe mental illnesses for over a century, its role has weakened because of discouraging results, financial disincentives to work, and pessimism about outcomes for these patients (Cook et al., 2005; Latimer et al., 2006; Lehman et al., 1995). However, recent alternative forms of occupation and vocational rehabilitation have again raised employment as an outcome priority. Consumer and carer advocacy groups have set work and occupation as one of their highest priorities, to enhance both functional status and quality of life (Chamberlin, 2005; Thornicroft et al., 2002). As described above and elsewhere in this volume (see Chapter 20), individual placement and support-supported employment has emerged as an evidence-based practice, and insurers are beginning to recognize that individual placement and support is a cost-effective mental health intervention that improves self-esteem and quality of life as well as employment and earnings (Drake & Wallach, 2020).

The importance of community-level support

The balanced care model recognizes the importance of community support for people with mental health problems. As **Figure 11.2** indicates, in many circumstances it will be more appropriate for people with early or mild mental health problems to seek help from local and community groups and organizations rather than health services. Depending on the setting and the resource level, these community-based supports can include children and parenting groups, work and employment centres, women's groups, leisure and sports facilities, community development and faith-based organizations, and self-help groups as well as social media platforms that can give assistance to people with mental health problems not severe or complex enough to need a health service intervention. Such services need to be integrated within the wider system of care and to direct those people who develop higher levels of acuity or need to more intense sources of support.

Engagement with local stakeholders

Organizing the range of community-based mental health services effectively requires making links with key figures and stakeholders in the local community. They will most often include not only family doctors, general hospital, and other health service clinicians, but also the whole range of interests shown in **Box 11.1**. But a wider array of stakeholders may also wish to have their interests represented and taken into account in decision-making. These constituencies may include neighbourhood or resident associations, local school staff, governors and parents, representatives of different cultural and ethnic communities, shopkeepers and members of local business, and church ministers and elders of other faith communities. The importance of these stakeholders emerges particularly at times when plans are being developed to open new mental health facilities, and meaningful consultations at this stage may prevent local opposition that could prevent implementation of community services.

Lessons learned in organizing community mental health services

What are the overall lessons learned from taking part in the development of community mental health care over the last 20–30 years? The following specific issues are common (Thornicroft et al., 2008):

- Anxiety and uncertainty in the process of change
- Needing to compensate for a possible lack of structure in community services
- Uncertainty about how to initiate new developments
- Managing opposition within the mental health system
- Dealing with opposition from neighbours
- Maximizing and managing a clearly identified budget
- Ensuring that rigidities in the old system are made more flexible
- Creating practical way to minimize the dysfunctional effects of boundaries between different service components
- Needing to support staff education, training, and morale during change
- Implementing evidence-based practices with sufficient fidelity
- Expecting outside experts to provide answers rather than accepting responsibility for making decisions to suit local circumstances.

Beyond these challenges, we have provisionally concluded that the following overall lessons often apply when developing community care. First, it takes time to make service changes robust. Part of the reason for this is that staff will need to be persuaded that change is likely to bring improvements for patients, and indeed their scepticism is a positive asset, to act as a buffer against changes that are

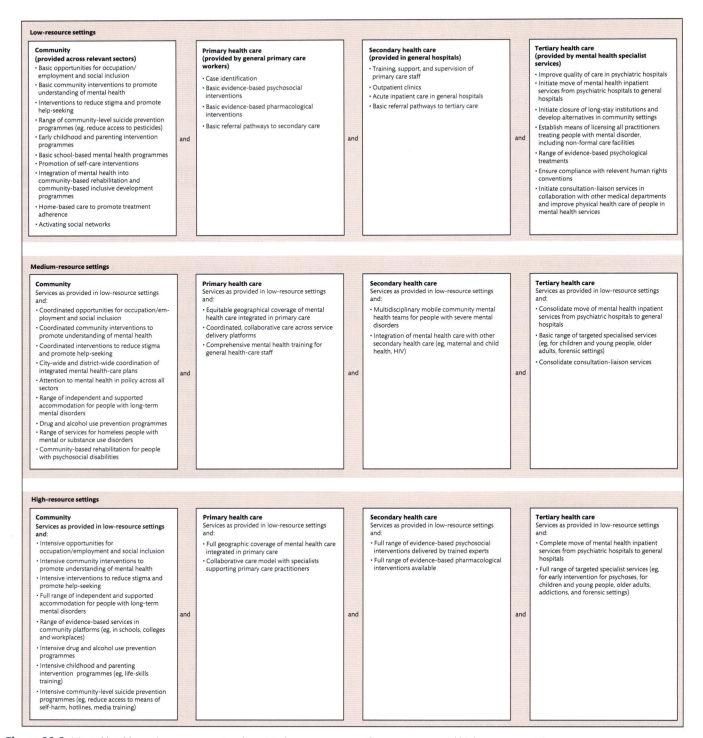

Figure 11.2 Mental health service components relevant to low-resource, medium-resource, and high-resource settings.
Reproduced with permission from Patel, V., Saxena, S., Lund, C., Thornicroft, G., Baingana, F., Bolton, P., Chisholm, D., Collins, P. Y., Cooper, J. L., Eaton, J., Herrman, H., Herzallah, M. M., Huang, Y., Jordans, M. J. D., Kleinman, A., Medina-Mora, M. E., Morgan, E., Niaz, U., Omigbodun, O., Prince, M., Rahman, A., Saraceno, B., Sarkar, B. K., De Silva, M., Singh, I., Stein, D. J., Sunkel, C. & Unutzer, J. (2018). The Lancet Commission on global mental health and sustainable development. *Lancet*, 392, 1553–1598.

too rapid, too frequent, or implausible. The next reason for not rushing change is that, to succeed, it is likely to need the support of many organizations and agencies, and they need to be identified and included gradually, at the start of each cycle of service changes. Those which are, or which feel, excluded are likely to oppose change, sometimes successfully. Further, in situations where health service changes may be a topic for political debate, it is usually necessary to build a cross-party consensus on the mental health strategy so that it will continue intact if the government changes. Again, this will often take time to achieve.

> **Box 11.1** Key stakeholders at the local level
> - Service users/consumers
> - Family members/carers
> - Health care professionals (mental health and primary care staff)
> - Other public services agencies (e.g. police and housing)
> - Other service provider groups (e.g. non-governmental organizations, church and charitable groups)
> - Policymakers: politicians, political advisers, and officials
> - Service planners and commissioners
> - Advocacy groups
> - Local media (e.g. newspaper and radio).

Time is also needed to progress from the initiation stage of a change to the *consolidation phase*. In the early stages of service reform, a charismatic individual or small group typically champions the main proposals and recruits support from stakeholder groups and others with influence within the health care system. In Eastern European countries, for example, the medical director/superintendents of the psychiatric hospital will in practice hold a veto for or against change (Thornicroft & Tansella, 2009). An example of the timescale required is the pattern of services changes in Verona in Italy over the last 30 years, derived from the local case register, as shown in **Figure 11.3**. As the number of psychiatric beds has progressively declined, so the provision of day care, residential care, and outpatient and community contacts has steadily increased over many years. It is notable that while the provision of some of the service components has fluctuated year by year, that the long-term pattern over time is clear—a move from inpatient towards more community care.

The second overall lesson is that it is essential to listen to users' and families' experiences and perspectives (Thornicroft & Tansella, 2009). Everyone involved needs to keep a clear focus on the fact that the primary purpose of mental health services is to improve outcomes that are valued by people with mental illnesses themselves. The intended beneficiaries of care therefore need to be—in some sense—in charge when planning and delivering treatment and care. This is a profound transformation, changing from a traditional and paternalistic perspective, in which staff were expected to make all important decisions in the best interests of patients, to an approach in which people with mental illness work, to a far greater extent, in partnership with care providers.

The third lesson is that the team managing such a process needs clear expertise and authority to manage the whole budget, recognizing that the risks are high that services changes will be used as an occasion for budget cuts. Having a protected budget is necessary but not sufficient as it is also vital to be able to exercise flexibility within the overall budget, typically to transfer funds from reducing the use of inpatient beds to CMHTs, occupational services, or residential options. When such a financial boundary for mental health funds is not established and fiercely maintained, money can easily be diverted to other areas of health care. In other words, financial mechanisms need to be created to ensure that money will follow the patients into the community, where such service transformations take place.

The next key point is something of a paradox: as mental health care is progressively deinstitutionalized, so some aspects of the mental health system need to be institutionalized! For example, pre-qualification-level professional teaching and training curricula will need to be redesigned to include theoretical and practical aspects of delivering care in community settings and codified in training curricula. Similarly, post-qualifying training courses need to be taught on a regular basis, particularly in the early stages for staff making the transition from hospital to community clinical

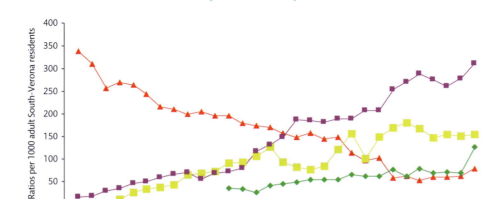

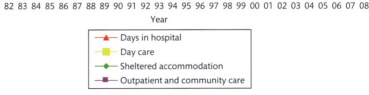

Figure 11.3 Patterns of mental health service provision in Verona, 1979–2008.

Table 11.5 Key barriers and challenges to better mental health care

Barriers	Challenges to overcoming barriers
1. Insufficient funding for mental health services	<ul><li>Inconsistent and unclear advocacy</li><li>Perception that mental health indicators are weak</li><li>People with mental disorders are not a powerful lobby</li><li>Lack of general public interest in mental health</li><li>Social stigma</li><li>Belief that mental health care is not cost-effective</li><li>Lack of insurance parity for mental health care</li></ul>
2. Mental health resources centralized in and near big cities and in large institutions	<ul><li>Historical reliance on mental hospitals</li><li>Fragmentation of mental health responsibilities between different government departments</li><li>Differences between central and provincial government priorities</li><li>Vested interests of staff in continuing large hospitals</li><li>Political risks associated with trade union protests</li><li>Need for transitional funding to move to community-based care</li></ul>
3. Complexities of integrating mental health care effectively in primary care services	<ul><li>Primary care workers already overburdened</li><li>Lack of training, supervision, and ongoing specialized support</li><li>Lack of continuous supply of relevant medications in primary care</li></ul>
4. Low numbers and limited types of health workers trained and supervised in mental health care	<ul><li>Poor working conditions in public mental health services</li><li>Lack of incentives for staff to work in rural areas</li><li>Professional establishment opposes expanded role for non-specialists in mental health workforce</li><li>Medical students and psychiatrists trained primarily in mental hospitals</li><li>Inadequate training of general health workforce</li><li>Mental health specialists have minimal time for training and supervising others</li><li>Lack of infrastructure to enable community-based supervision</li></ul>
5. Mental health leaders often deficient in public health skills and experience	<ul><li>Those who rise to leadership positions often only trained in clinical management of individuals, not population health</li><li>Public health training does not include mental health</li><li>Lack of training courses in public mental health</li><li>Mental health clinical leaders overburdened by clinical and management responsibilities and private practice</li></ul>
6. Fragmentation between mental health advocacy groups	<ul><li>Conceptual and practical differences between consumers and mental health staff, especially about diagnoses and treatments</li><li>Divisions between consumer and family member groups</li><li>Politicians therefore find it easy to ignore an incoherent message</li></ul>
7. Information systems	<ul><li>Absence of information systems, implementation standards, and outcomes monitoring (Drake et al., 2009, 2010)</li></ul>
8. Difficulties in adjusting to the challenges of modernized mental health services	<ul><li>Objections to evidence-based practices</li><li>The burden of documentation</li><li>The newness of digital technologies (see Chapter 25)</li><li>Accepting users as colleagues</li></ul>

Adapted from Saraceno et al. (2007).

duties. A further issue is that new forms of legal provision, such as mental health or legal capacity laws, may be needed so that they are relevant to the context where most clinical contacts between staff and people with mental illnesses take place outside hospitals. A further consideration is that standards of quality for the implementation of evidence-based practices must be put in place in ways that are perceived as helpful guides, rather than burdens, by clinicians and users.

Understanding barriers to change

We have argued that serious but surmountable barriers face those who wish to develop a balanced care model. To enact such a vision means eroding, quickly or slowly, forms of resistance that have often prevented meaningful improvement in mental health care across the globe. The key barriers have been identified as shown in **Table 11.5** (Saraceno et al., 2007).

Finally, we reaffirm the central importance of learning from experience—primarily the experience of people with lived mental illness and their family members. Our central contention in this book is that the primary aim of mental health care (at all levels) is to support the achievement of better outcomes for all people with mental health conditions. As the intended beneficiaries, people with such conditions need to have a central voice in what services are planned, how they are provided, and how their impact is assessed—namely in every aspect of care (Chamberlin, 2005). If there is one defining characteristic that we wish to see embodied in the future, it is that service users are actually included as full partners in directly contributing to better mental health care.

REFERENCES

Addington, J., Coldham, E. L., Jones, B., Ko, T., & Addington, D. (2003). The first episode of psychosis: the experience of relatives. *Acta Psychiatrica Scandinavica*, **108**, 285–289.

Alem, A. (2002). Community-based vs. hospital-based mental health care: the case of Africa. *World Psychiatry*, **1**, 99–100.

Alegria, M., Drake, R. E., Kang, H., Metcalfe, J., Liu, J., Dimarzio, K. A., & Ali, N. (2017). Integrating social services within mental health care. *Health Affairs*, **36**, 1024–1031.

Allen, J., Balfour, R., Bell, R., & Marmot, M. (2014). Social determinants of mental health. *International Review of Psychiatry*, **26**, 392–407.

Alonso, J., Codony, M., Kovess, V., Angermeyer, M. C., Katz, S. J., Haro, J. M., et al. (2007). Population level of unmet need for mental healthcare in Europe. *British Journal of Psychiatry*, **190**, 299–306.

Barakat, A., Blankers, M., Cornelis, J. E., Lommerse, N. M., Beekman, A. T. F., & Dekker, J. J. M. (2021). The effects of intensive home treatment on self-efficacy in patients recovering from a psychiatric crisis. *International Journal of Mental Health Systems*, **15**, 1.

Barbui, C., Papola, D., & Saraceno, B. (2018). Forty years without mental hospitals in Italy. *International Journal of Mental Health Systems*, **12**, 43.

Barrett, B., Waheed, W., Farrelly, S., Birchwood, M., Dunn, G., Flach, C., et al. (2013). Randomised controlled trial of joint crisis plans to reduce compulsory treatment for people with psychosis: economic outcomes. *PLoS One*, **8**, e74210.

Becker, T. (2001). Out-patient psychiatric services. In: Thornicroft, G. & Szmukler, G. (Eds.), *Textbook of Community Psychiatry* (pp. 277–282). Oxford: Oxford University Press.

Becker, T. & Vazquez-Barquero, J. L. (2001). The European perspective of psychiatric reform. *Acta Psychiatrica Scandinavica Supplementum*, **410**, 8–14.

Bond, G. R. & Drake, R. E. (2020). Assessing the fidelity of evidence-based practices: history and current status of a standardized measurement methodology. *Administration and Policy in Mental Health*, **47**, 874–884.

Bond, G. R., Drake, R. E., & Becker, D. R. (2008). An update on randomized controlled trials of evidence-based supported employment. *Psychiatric Rehabilitation Journal*, **31**, 280–290.

Bond, G. R., Drake, R. E., & Becker, D. R. (2020). An update on IPS supported employment. *World Psychiatry*, **19**, 190–191.

Bond, G. R., Drake, R. E., & Pogue, J. (2019). Expanding IPS supported employment to new populations. *Psychiatric Services*, **70**, 488–498.

Burns, T. (2001). Generic versus specialist mental health teams. In: Thornicroft, G. & Szmukler, G. (Eds.), *Textbook of Community Psychiatry* (pp. 231–241). Oxford: Oxford University Press.

Burns, T. (2009). End of the road for treatment-as-usual studies? *British Journal of Psychiatry*, **195**, 5–6.

Campbell, L. A., Kisely, S. R., & Cochrane Schizophrenia Group (2009). Advance treatment directives for people with severe mental illness. *Cochrane Database of Systematic Reviews*, **1**, CD005963.

Catty, J., Burns, T., Knapp, M., Watt, H., Wright, C., Henderson, J., & Healey, A. (2002). Home treatment for mental health problems: a systematic review. *Psychological Medicine*, **32**, 383–401.

Chamberlin, J. (2005). User/consumer involvement in mental health service delivery. *Epidemiologia e Psichiatria Sociale*, **14**, 10–14.

Chatterjee, S., Naik, S., John, S., Dabholkar, H., Balaji, M., Koschorke, M., et al. (2014). Effectiveness of a community-based intervention for people with schizophrenia and their caregivers in India (COPSI): a randomised controlled trial. *Lancet*, **383**, 1385–1394.

Chilvers, R., Macdonald, G., & Hayes, A. (2003). Supported housing for people with severe mental disorders. *Cochrane Database of Systematic Reviews*, **4**, CD000453.

Cook, J. A., Leff, H. S., Blyler, C. R., Gold, P. B., Goldberg, R. W., Mueser, K. T., et al. (2005). Results of a multisite randomized trial of supported employment interventions for individuals with severe mental illness. *Archives of General Psychiatry*, **62**, 505–512.

Cubillos, L., Muñoz, J., Caballero, J., Mendoza, M., Adriana Pulido, A., Carpio, K., et al. (2020). Addressing severe mental illness rehabilitation in Colombia, Costa Rica, and Peru. *Psychiatric Services*, **71**, 378–384.

Department of Health (2002). *Community Mental Health Teams, Policy Implementation Guidance*. London: Department of Health.

Desjarlais, R., Eisenberg, L., Good, B., & Kleinman, A. (1995). *World Mental Health: Problems and Priorities in Low Income Countries*. Oxford: Oxford University Press.

Drake, R. E. & Bond, G. R. (2008). Supported employment: 1998 to 2008. *Psychiatric Rehabilitation Journal*, **31**, 274–276.

Drake, R. E. & Bond, G. R. (2021). Psychiatric crisis care and the more is less paradox. *Community Mental Health Journal*, **57**, 1230–1236.

Drake, R. E., Deegan, P., Woltmann, E., Haslett, W., Drake, T., & Rapp, C. (2010). Comprehensive electronic decision support systems. *Psychiatric Services*, **61**, 714–717.

Drake, R. E. & Essock, S. M. (2009). The science to service gap in real world schizophrenia treatment. *Schizophrenia Bulletin*, **35**, 677–678.

Drake, R. E., Essock, S. M., & Bond, G. R. (2009). Implementing evidence-based practices for the treatment of schizophrenia patients. *Schizophrenia Bulletin*, **35**, 704–713.

Drake, R. E., Bond, G. R., & Becker, D. R. (2012). *Individual Placement and Support: An Evidence-based Approach to Supported Employment*. Oxford: Oxford University Press.

Drake, R. E., Meara, E. R., & Bond, G. R. (2019). Employment for people with serious mental illness: policy issues. In: Goldman, H. H., Frank, R. G., & Morrissey, J. P. (Eds.), *Handbook of U.S. Mental Health Policy* (pp. 449–470). Washington, DC: American Psychiatric Press.

Drake, R. E. & Wallach, M. A. (2019). Assessing the optimal number of beds for a region. *Administration and Policy in Mental Health*, **46**, 696–700.

Drake, R. E. & Wallach, M. A. (2020). Employment is a critical mental health intervention. *Epidemiology and Psychiatric Sciences*, **29**, 178.

Fixsen, D., Naoom, S., Blase, K., Friedman, R., & Wallace, F. (2009). *Implementation Research: A Synthesis of the Literature*. Tampa, FL: University of South Florida.

Flood, C., Byford, S., Henderson, C., Leese, M., Thornicroft, G., Sutherby, K., & Szmukler, G. (2006). Joint crisis plans for people with psychosis: economic evaluation of a randomised controlled trial. *BMJ*, **333**, 729–732.

Glover, G., Arts, G., & Babu, K. S. (2006). Crisis resolution/home treatment teams and psychiatric admission rates in England. *British Journal of Psychiatry*, **189**, 441–445.

Henderson, C., Flood, C., Leese, M., Thornicroft, G., Sutherby, K., & Szmukler, G. (2004). Effect of joint crisis plans on use of compulsory treatment in psychiatry: single blind randomised controlled trial. *BMJ*, **329**, 136.

Holloway, F. & Carson, J. (2001). Case management: an update. *International Journal of Social Psychiatry*, **47**, 21–31.

Hood, C. M., Gennusp, K. P., Swain, G. R., & Catlin, B. B. (2016). County health rankings: relationships between determinant factors and health outcomes. *American Journal of Preventive Medicine*, **50**, 129–135.

Howard, L. M., Rigon, E., Cole, L., Lawlor, C., & Johnson, S. (2008). Admission to women's crisis houses or to psychiatric wards: women's pathways to admission. *Psychiatric Services*, **59**, 1443–1449.

Institute of Medicine (US) Committee on Crossing the Quality Chasm: Adaptation to Mental Health and Addictive Disorders (2006). *Improving the Quality of Health Care for Mental and Substance-Use Conditions*. Washington, DC: National Academy Press.

Jeste, D. V. & Pender, V. B. (2022). Social determinants of mental health: recommendations for research, training, practice, and policy. *JAMA Psychiatry*, **79**, 283–284.

Johnson, S., Needle, J., Bindman, J., & Thornicroft, G. (2008). *Crisis Resolution and Home Treatment in Mental Health*. Cambridge: Cambridge University Press.

Johnson, S., Gilburt, H., Lloyd-Evans, B., Osborn, D. P., Boardman, J., Leese, M., et al. (2009). In-patient and residential alternatives to standard acute psychiatric wards in England. *British Journal of Psychiatry*, **194**, 456–463.

Johnson, S., Nolan, F., Hoult, J., White, I. R., Bebbington, P., Sandor, A., et al. (2005a). Outcomes of crises before and after introduction of a crisis resolution team. *British Journal of Psychiatry*, **187**, 68–75.

Johnson, S., Nolan, F., Pilling, S., Sandor, A., Hoult, J., McKenzie, N., et al. (2005b). Randomised controlled trial of acute mental health care by a crisis resolution team: the north Islington crisis study. *BMJ*, **331**, 599.

Johnstone, P. & Zolese, G. (1999). Systematic review of the effectiveness of planned short hospital stays for mental health care. *BMJ*, **318**, 1387–1390.

Joy, C., Adams, C., & Rice, K. (1998). Crisis intervention for people with severe mental illness. *Cochrane Database of Systematic Reviews*, **2**, CD001087.

Kessler, R. C., Demler, O., Frank, R. G., Olfson, M., Pincus, H. A., Walters, E. E., et al. (2005). Prevalence and treatment of mental disorders, 1990 to 2003. *New England Journal of Medicine*, **352**, 2515–2523.

Khazaal, Y., Manghi, R., Dalahaye, M., Machado, A., Penzenstadler, L., & Molodynski, A. (2014). Psychiatric advance directives, a possible way to overcome coercion and promote empowerment. *Frontiers in Public Health*, **2**, 37.

Killaspy, H., Bebbington, P., Blizard, R., Johnson, S., Nolan, F., Pilling, S., & King, M. (2006). The REACT study: randomised evaluation of assertive community treatment in north London. *BMJ*, **332**, 815–820.

Killaspy, H., Dalton, J., McNicholas, S., & Johnson, S. (2000). Drayton Park, an alternative to hospital admission for women in acute mental health crisis. *Psychiatric Bulletin*, **24**, 101–104.

Killaspy, H., Kingett, S., Bebbington, P., Blizard, R., Johnson, S., Nolan, F., Pilling, S., & King, M. (2009). Randomised evaluation of assertive community treatment: 3-year outcomes. *British Journal of Psychiatry*, **195**, 81–82.

Knapp, M., Beecham, J., Anderson, J., Dayson, D., Leff, J., Margolius, O., O'Driscoll, C., & Wills, W. (1990). The TAPS project. 3: predicting the community costs of closing psychiatric hospitals. *British Journal of Psychiatry*, **157**, 661–670.

Knapp, M. & Wong, G. (2020). Economics and mental health: the current scenario. *World Psychiatry*, **19**, 3–14.

Kreyenbuhl, J., Buchanan, R. W., Dickerson, F. B., & Dixon, L. B. (2009). The schizophrenia patient outcomes research team (PORT): updated treatment recommendations. *Schizophrenia Bulletin*, **36**, 94–103.

Latimer, E. A. (1999). Economic impacts of assertive community treatment: a review of the literature. *Canadian Journal of Psychiatry*, **44**, 443–454.

Latimer, E. A., Lecomte, T., Becker, D. R., Drake, R. E., Duclos, I., Piat, M., et al. (2006). Generalisability of the individual placement and support model of supported employment: results of a Canadian randomised controlled trial. *British Journal of Psychiatry*, **189**, 65–73.

Leff, J. (1997). *Care in the Community: Illusion or Reality?* London: Wiley.

Lehman, A. F., Carpenter, W. T., Jr., Goldman, H. H., & Steinwachs, D. M. (1995). Treatment outcomes in schizophrenia: implications for practice, policy, and research. *Schizophrenia Bulletin*, **21**, 669–675.

Lloyd-Evans, B. & Johnson, S. (2019). Community alternatives to in-patient admissions in psychiatry. *World Psychiatry*, **18**, 31–32.

Marsh, L. A., Gomez-Restrepo, C., Bartels, S. M., Bell, K., Camblor, P. M., Castro, S., et al. (2022). Scaling up science-based care for depression and unhealthy alcohol use in Colombia: an implementation science project. *Psychiatric Services*, **73**, 196–205.

Marshall, M., Crowther, R., Almaraz-Serrano, A., Creed, F., Sledge, W., Kluiter, H., et al. (2001). Systematic reviews of the effectiveness of day care for people with severe mental disorders: (1) acute day hospital versus admission; (2) vocational rehabilitation; (3) day hospital versus outpatient care. *Health Technology Assessment*, **5**, 1–75.

Marshall, M. & Lockwood, A. (2003). Assertive community treatment for people with severe mental disorders. *Cochrane Database of Systematic Reviews*, **2**, CD001089.

Mascayano, F., Alvarado, R., Andrews, H. F., Jorquera, M. J., Lovisi, G. M., Souza, F. M., et al. (2022). A recovery-oriented intervention for people with psychoses: a pilot randomized controlled trial in two Latin American cities. *Psychiatric Services*, **35**, e00108018.

McCrone, P., Killaspy, H., Bebbington, P., Johnson, S., Nolan, F., Pilling, S., & King, M. (2009). The REACT study: cost-effectiveness analysis of assertive community treatment in north London. *Psychiatric Services*, **60**, 908–913.

Metcalfe, J. & Drake, R. E. (2020). National levels of human development and number of psychiatric beds. *Epidemiology and Psychiatric Sciences*, **29**, e167.

Mojtabai, R., Fochtmann, L., Chang, S., Kotov, R., Craig, T. J., & Bromet, E. (2009). Unmet need for mental health care in schizophrenia: an overview of literature and new data from a first-admission study. *Schizophrenia Bulletin*, **35**, 679–695.

Morrissey, J. P., Domino, M. E., & Cuddeback, G. S. (2016). Expedited Medicaid enrollment, mental health service use, and criminal recidivism among released prisoners with severe mental illness. *Psychiatric Services*, **67**, 842–849.

Mosher, L. R. (1999). Soteria and other alternatives to acute psychiatric hospitalization: a personal and professional review. *Journal of Nervous & Mental Disease*, **187**, 142–149.

Mueser, K. T., Bond, G. R., Drake, R. E., & Resnick, S. G. (1998). Models of community care for severe mental illness: a review of research on case management. *Schizophrenia Bulletin*, **24**, 37–74.

Njenga, F. (2002). Challenges of balanced care in Africa. *World Psychiatry*, **1**, 96–98.

Open Minds (2020). Mental health spending by state across the U.S. https://store.SAMHSA.gov

O'Reilly, R., Allison, S., & Bastiampiallai, T. (2019). Observed outcomes: an approach to calculate the optimum number of psychiatric beds. *Administration and Policy in Mental Health*, **46**, 507–517.

Patel, V., Saxena, S., Lund, C., Thornicroft, G., Baingana, F., Bolton, P., et al. (2018). The Lancet Commission on global mental health and sustainable development. *Lancet*, **392**, 1553–1598.

Penzenstadler, L., Soares, C., Anci, E., Molodynski, A., & Khazaal, Y. (2019). Effect of assertive community treatment for patients with substance use disorder: a systematic review. *European Addiction Research*, **25**, 56–67.

Petersen, L., Jeppesen, P., Thorup, A., Abel, M. B., Ohlenschlaeger, J., Christensen, T. O., et al. (2005). A randomised multicentre trial of integrated versus standard treatment for patients with a first episode of psychotic illness. *BMJ*, **331**, 602.

Phillips, S. D., Burns, B. J., Edgar, E. R., Mueser, K. T., Linkins, K. W., Rosenheck, R. A., et al. (2001). Moving assertive community treatment into standard practice. *Psychiatric Services*, **52**, 771–779.

Puntis, S., Minichino, A., De Crescenzo, F., Harrison, R., Cipriani, A., & Lennox, B. (2020). Specialised early intervention teams for recent-onset psychosis. *Cochrane Database of Systematic Reviews*, **11**, CD013288.

Rapp, C. A. & Goscha, R. J. (2004). The principles of effective case management of mental health services. *Psychiatric Rehabilitation Journal*, **27**, 319–333.

Raune, D., Kuipers, E., & Bebbington, P. E. (2004). Expressed emotion at first-episode psychosis: investigating a carer appraisal model. *British Journal of Psychiatry*, **184**, 321–326.

Rose-Clarke, K., Gurung, D., Brooke-Sumner, C., Burgess, R., Burns, J., Kakuma, R., et al. (2020). Rethinking research on the social determinants of global mental health. *Lancet Psychiatry*, **7**, 659–662.

Rosen, A. & Barfoot, K. (2001). Day care and occupation: structured rehabilitation and recovery programmes and work. In: Thornicroft, G. & Szmukler, G. (Eds.), *Textbook of Community Psychiatry* (pp. 296–308). Oxford: Oxford University Press.

Saraceno, B., Van, O. M., Batniji, R., Cohen, A., Gureje, O., Mahoney, J., et al. (2007). Barriers to improvement of mental health services in low-income and middle-income countries. *Lancet*, **370**, 1164–1174.

Saxena, S. & Maulik, P. (2003). Mental health services in low and middle income countries: an overview. *Current Opinion in Psychiatry*, **16**, 437–442.

Scott, J. & Lehman, A. (2001). Case management and assertive community treatment. In: Thornicroft, G. & Szmukler, G. (Eds.), *Textbook of Community Psychiatry* (pp. 253–264). Oxford: Oxford University Press.

Shepherd, G. & Murray, A. (2001). Residential care. In: Thornicroft, G. & Szmukler, G. (Eds.), *Textbook of Community Psychiatry* (pp. 309–320). Oxford: Oxford University Press.

Simmonds, S., Coid, J., Joseph, P., Marriott, S., & Tyrer, P. (2001). Community mental health team management in severe mental illness: a systematic review. *British Journal of Psychiatry*, **178**, 497–502.

Sledge, W. H., Tebes, J., Rakfeldt, J., Davidson, L., Lyons, L., & Druss, B. (1996). Day hospital/crisis respite care versus inpatient care, part I: clinical outcomes. *American Journal of Psychiatry*, **153**, 1065–1073.

Sutherby, K. & Szmukler, G. I. (1998). Crisis cards and self-help crisis initiatives. *Psychiatric Bulletin*, **22**, 4–7.

Sutherby, K., Szmukler, G. I., Halpern, A., Alexander, M., Thornicroft, G., Johnson, C., & Wright, S. (1999). A study of 'crisis cards' in a community psychiatric service. *Acta Psychiatrica Scandinavica*, **100**, 56–61.

Szmukler, G. & Holloway, F. (2001). In-patient treatment. In: Thornicroft, G. & Szmukler, G. (Eds.), *Textbook of Community Psychiatry* (pp. 321–337). Oxford: Oxford University Press.

Tansella, M. (1986). Community psychiatry without mental hospitals—the Italian experience—a review. *Journal of the Royal Society of Medicine* **79**, 664–669.

Teague, G. B., Bond, G. R., & Drake, R. E. (1998). Program fidelity in assertive community treatment: development and use of a measure. *American Journal of Orthopsychiatry*, **68**, 216–232.

Thornicroft, G. (1991). The concept of case management for long-term mental illness. *International Review of Psychiatry*, **3**, 125–132.

Thornicroft, G. (2001). *Measuring Mental Health Needs* (2nd ed.). London: Royal College of Psychiatrists, Gaskell.

Thornicroft, G. & Bebbington, P. (1989). Deinstitutionalisation—from hospital closure to service development. *British Journal of Psychiatry*, **155**, 739–753.

Thornicroft, G., Becker, T., Holloway, F., Johnson, S., Leese, M., McCrone, P., et al. (1999). Community mental health teams: evidence or belief? *British Journal of Psychiatry*, **175**, 508–513.

Thornicroft, G. & Henderson, C. (2016). Joint decision making and reduced need for compulsory psychiatric admission. *JAMA Psychiatry*, **73**, 647–648.

Thornicroft, G., Rose, D., Huxley, P., Dale, G., & Wykes, T. (2002). What are the research priorities of mental health service users? *Journal of Mental Health*, **11**, 1–5.

Thornicroft, G. & Tansella, M. (1999). *The Mental Health Matrix: A Manual to Improve Services*. Cambridge: Cambridge University Press.

Thornicroft, G. & Tansella, M. (2009). *Better Mental Health Care*. Cambridge: Cambridge University Press.

Thornicroft, G. & Tansella, M. (2013a). The balanced care model for global mental health. *Psychological Medicine*, **43**, 849–863.

Thornicroft, G. & Tansella, M. (2013b). The balanced care model: the case for both hospital- and community-based mental healthcare. *British Journal of Psychiatry*, **202**, 246–248.

Thornicroft, G., Tansella, M., & Law, A. (2008). Steps, challenges and lessons in developing community mental health care. *World Psychiatry*, **7**, 87–92.

Thornicroft, G., Wykes, T., Holloway, F., Johnson, S., & Szmukler, G. (1998). From efficacy to effectiveness in community mental health services. PRiSM Psychosis Study. 10. *British Journal of Psychiatry*, **173**, 423–427.

Tyrer, P., Evans, K., Gandhi, N., Lamont, A., Harrison-Read, P., & Johnson, T. (1998). Randomised controlled trial of two models of care for discharged psychiatric patients. *BMJ*, **316**, 106–109.

Tyrer, S., Coid, J., Simmonds, S., Joseph, P., & Marriott, S. (2003). Community mental health teams (CMHTs) for people with severe mental illnesses and disordered personality. *Cochrane Database of Systematic Reviews*, **2**, CD000270.

Virgolino, A., Costa, J., Santos, O., Pereira, M. E., Antunes, R., Ambrosio, S., et al. (2022). Lost in transition: a systematic review of the association between unemployment and mental health. *Journal of Mental Health*, **31**, 432–444.

Wang, P. S., Demler, O., & Kessler, R. C. (2002). Adequacy of treatment for serious mental illness in the United States. *American Journal of Public Health*, **92**, 92–98.

World Bank (2002). *World Development Report 2002: Building Institutions for Markets*. Washington, DC: World Bank.

World Health Organization (2020). *Mental Health Atlas 2020*. Geneva: World Health Organisation.

World Health Organization (2022). *World Mental Health Report*. Geneva: World Health Organization.

Ziguras, S. J. & Stuart, G. W. (2000). A meta-analysis of the effectiveness of mental health case management over 20 years. *Psychiatric Services*, **51**, 1410–1421.

Ziguras, S. J., Stuart, G. W., & Jackson, A. C. (2002). Assessing the evidence on case management. *British Journal of Psychiatry*, **181**, 17–21.

12

Crisis and emergency services

Sonia Johnson, Justin J. Needle, Jonathan Totman, and Lorna Hobbs

Introduction: acute care outside the inpatient unit

Our primary focus in this chapter is on services that are delivered mainly by mental health professionals and intended to support people with significant mental illnesses who are experiencing an exacerbation of their mental health or social problems of such severity that they reach the threshold for inpatient admission, or else seem likely very soon to reach this threshold unless pre-emptive action is taken. Acute care for people close to the threshold of admission has a particular importance in economic, pragmatic, and policy terms, in that clinicians, service users, service planners, and policymakers all tend to prioritize avoiding psychiatric hospital admission wherever possible. However, most acute and crisis mental health services in practice assess and manage people with a wide range of needs and circumstances, even if they are intended to focus primarily on hospital diversion (Johnson et al., 2022). Conversely, community and voluntary sector services whose remit includes responding to a variety of life crises often include people with significant mental illnesses among their clients, and can have an especially significant role for those who have disengaged from statutory mental health services (Newbigging et al., 2020).

From the perspective of service users and carers, easy and prompt access to helpful and acceptable crisis services to help them at the times when they are most distressed is consistently rated as very important, with avoiding inpatient admission whenever possible also often identified as an important priority (Rose, 2001). From an economic and policy point of view, acute care, especially in hospital, consumes a large share of the mental health budget in most countries (see Holloway and Tracy, Chapter 18, this volume), making it very desirable that optimal outcomes are achieved as efficiently as possible.

Given these major reasons for regarding acute care as a priority, the evidence base is surprisingly weak. For example, none of the 2009 recommendations of the Schizophrenia Patient Outcomes Research Team (PORT) (Dixon et al., 2010) related to models of acute care delivery, and the only firm recommendations that the National Institute for Health and Care Excellence guidelines on schizophrenia and bipolar disorder make in relation to acute care are that crisis resolution and home treatment teams (CRHTTs) should be available. Despite this lack of robust evidence, mental health crises and, in particular, models aimed at diverting people from hospital admission, have been the focus of considerable innovative service development in the past few decades. In this chapter, we complement Holloway and Tracy's discussion of inpatient care by reviewing models of community and acute care that do not involve psychiatric admission. We include services aimed primarily at initial assessment and triage (mental health care in the general hospital emergency department, standalone emergency assessment services, services aimed at reducing contacts with the police, and those aimed at extended initial triage and assessment), a service model that combines assessment with provision of a community alternative to acute admission (CRHTTs), and one mainly aimed at providing an alternative to admission (community residential crisis services). Finally, we discuss the need to focus on local acute care systems as a whole, and on the extent to which flexibility and a range of options and pathways is available to meet the wide range of needs with which service users in crisis present.

Acute day care is not covered in this chapter as it is the focus of Chapter 17, but it should also be seen as a potentially important element in the delivery of integrated mental health care, catering especially for people who can safely remain at home during a crisis but have needs for social, therapy, and activity not met by home-based services such as CRHTTs (Osborn et al., 2021).

Acute mental health care in the emergency department

While the other models we discuss have to varying degrees been intentionally designed to improve crisis care, the general hospital emergency department (ED), also known in the US as the emergency room and in the UK as the accident and emergency (A&E) or casualty department, has remained by default a mainstay of emergency mental health care. Increasing use of EDs by mental health patients has been documented in several countries, despite endeavours to create other forms of readily accessible crisis care (NHS England, 2014; Santillanes et al., 2020; Tran et al., 2020). A fall in presentations early in the Covid-19 pandemic (March/April 2020) was reported to be followed by a rebound (Sampson et al., 2022). Apart from rising numbers, reasons for focusing on ED presentations among people with mental health problems include that ED attenders include individuals with significant mental health difficulties who do not engage with other mental health services (Barratt et al., 2016), and that a substantial proportion of people who go on to commit suicide have been found to have attended EDs in the preceding year (Ahmedani et al., 2014; Da Cruz et al., 2011).

Despite the almost universal use of EDs as a setting for at least preliminary assessment of mental health problems, there is substantial evidence that neither service users nor clinicians find the interactions that take place there satisfactory. Based on action research in a London hospital, Crowley (2000) suggests there is a 'clash of cultures' between the ED, with its focus on immediate stabilization, and the needs of psychiatric patients for more individualized care, with time needed to pinpoint the principal issues that need attention. Multiple logistical factors contribute to further delays in assessment and treatment, including availability of on-call psychiatric liaison staff, communication with other teams, lack of inpatient beds, and (in the case of assessments under mental health legislation) legal directives (Henderson et al., 2003; Healthcare Safety Investigation Branch, 2018). In the hectic environment of the ED, where speed and timeliness are central, psychiatric emergencies may be seen as difficult and burdensome. Further, the environment may exacerbate service users' symptoms: the noisy, chaotic, and clinical nature of the environment, lack of privacy, and the distressing sights and sounds sometimes experienced may all contribute to increased distress among service users, reported in a number of countries (Carstensen et al., 2017; Sacre et al., 2022).

Findings from various countries converge to suggest that clinicians, especially those not trained in mental health, have more negative attitudes towards service users presenting with mental health problems, particularly those who repeatedly self-harm or abuse alcohol or drugs, than to other patients. They are more likely to perceive such service users as disingenuous, dangerous, or unpredictable, and to lack confidence in their skills and ability to assess and treat them, especially where there is a lack of effective follow-up care (Clarke et al., 2014; Saunders et al., 2012). This may well be due in part to the constraints imposed by the ED environment itself; indeed, there is evidence that assessments carried out by psychiatrically trained personnel are of less good quality than elsewhere (Taggart et al., 2006), and that patients assessed in these settings are more likely to be admitted to hospital than if assessed elsewhere (Cotton et al., 2007).

Given these problems with quality and appropriateness of care in relation to the environment, it is not surprising that service users' experiences of attending the ED for a mental health crisis are largely negative (Sacre et al., 2022). Stigmatizing, discriminatory, and punitive attitudes, especially towards repeat attenders following self-harm and towards people who have received a 'personality disorder' diagnosis (DeLeo et al., 2022), have been widely reported. Other negative attitudes, such as lack of empathy and compassion, can leave service users feeling unwanted, rejected, and disrespected. Service users have reported being denied treatment (including pain relief following self-harm) or told that their attendance at the ED was inappropriate, although certain conditions, such as psychosis, tend to be regarded as more 'valid' than others. Long waiting times can lead to a sense of feeling forgotten, exacerbated by limited communication and poor interpersonal skills among staff. Other issues, such as poor interprofessional and interagency communication, lack of information sharing, exclusion from decision-making about their care, lack of reference to pre-existing care plans, lack of discharge planning and options for follow-up, restrictive practices, and fear of being legally detained, have been widely identified as having a negative impact on service user experience and as exacerbating symptoms and distress (Dombagolla et al., 2019; Quinivan et al., 2021).

In view of these long-standing challenges in addressing the needs of people with mental health difficulties in general hospital EDs, there is an obvious rationale for diverting people away from this setting: alternative forms of crisis care that may allow this are discussed below. However, in most settings, general hospital EDs continue to play a major role within the mental health care system: patients tend to present there in substantial numbers even where other local alternatives are available, and the availability of both physical and mental health interventions, for example, for people with comorbid illnesses or who need physical care for consequences of self-harm, is not matched elsewhere.

Strategies for enhancing and improving care delivered in general EDs are thus of high importance. A long-established approach to this is through employing specialist psychiatric personnel (Wand & White, 2007), most often in the form of a consultation-liaison service. A review of published literature on such models (Evans et al., 2019) identified several models of provision of mental health staff, including integration of mental health staff into the ED team, delivery of a psychiatric liaison service working across the ED and the general hospital as a whole, and establishing a contract between the ED and a psychiatric service within the same hospital allowing referrals to be made from ED. High-quality evidence is limited, but various benefits are reported for such models at the level of service user indicators, such as improved satisfaction and reduced readmission rates, waiting times, use of restraints, and unplanned departures from ED (Paton et al., 2016; Wand & White, 2007).

Other approaches to improving quality of care for people who have mental health difficulties and attend the ED have involved training for staff or specifically designed interventions for assessment or brief treatment. A systematic review (Zarska et al., 2023) of training interventions for generalist ED staff and psychosocial interventions delivered by such staff for patients who self-harm concluded that, in pre–post comparisons, training appeared to be followed by an increase in staff knowledge and, in some studies, skills, confidence, and attitudes, though no evidence was found on patient outcomes. Psychosocial interventions (safety planning and follow-up contact) were followed in pre–post comparisons by reduction in suicide attempts. A scoping review of interventions for people presenting in EDs with mental health problems (Johnston et al., 2019) assessed the evidence on a wide range of intervention types (including pharmacological, psychological, triage/assessment/screening, educational, case management, and referral/follow-up). It identified a substantial evidence base on the use of ED interventions, although this was found to be highly heterogeneous and of variable quality, limiting generalizable conclusions about their effectiveness. Few interventions focused on families or carers. A review focused on interventions to reduce repeat attendance in EDs, frequently associated with mental health problems, identified evidence on three types of intervention: case management, individualized care plans, and information sharing (Soril et al., 2015). Most studies of case management interventions reported modest reductions in number of ED visits. Only one study evaluated individualized care plans and found no change in ED visits, and evidence from the two studies evaluating information sharing was mixed. The relative effectiveness of case management approaches in reducing ED visits, as well as costs, has been confirmed by other reviews (Hudon et al., 2016; Van den Heede & Van de Voorde, 2016), although further adequately powered and better targeted studies to determine which specific aspects of case management are most effective are still needed.

If the ED is to continue acting as a last resort for those in crisis and an access point into mental health services for people previously not engaged, it is essential for it to work collaboratively with other teams and organizations. Effective communication is particularly important for the ED, which straddles mental health and acute care trusts and sees such a diverse range of patients. Ensuring better continuity of care is a key challenge for acute mental health systems in all countries. Where CRHTTs and other forms of community-based crisis assessment and home treatment services are available, the relationship between these services and the ED is crucial for continuity, as well as to other services that may be entry points to the mental health care system, such as early intervention teams for psychosis and assessment teams.

Extended assessment and diversion following emergency department attendance

As well as the limited efforts described above to enhance the quality of mental health interventions in the ED, a number of service models have been developed that extend the period of mental health assessment in an environment intended to be more calming and conducive to good-quality mental health care than the ED.

A range of such approaches has been developed and described internationally. In the US, an American Psychiatric Association Task Force recommended in 2002 the provision of dedicated psychiatric emergency services (PESs) in general hospitals with at least 3000 visits per year (Allen et al., 2002). This model became prominent against a background of difficulties in sustaining a network of comprehensive community services in many areas (Allen, 2007). PESs vary in structure and organization but essentially operate on the principle that more effective care is provided by separating, to some degree, physical and mental health services. The American Psychiatric Association Task Force report (Allen et al., 2002) outlines the advantages of a separate PES facility, both for patient care and economic efficiency: 'In a separate space and with appropriate staff, a controlled and supportive milieu can develop despite high levels of disturbance and rapid turnover' (p. 10).

PES (for which other names include comprehensive psychiatric emergency programme (CPEP) and emergency psychiatric assessment, treatment and healing, EmPATH) are widespread in the US, where emergency psychiatry is a distinct subspecialty, and in Canada. They are generally linked to one or more EDs (Zeller, 2019) and staffed by multidisciplinary psychiatric teams, including mental health nurses and psychiatrists (available on-call if not on-site), usually providing 24-hour access. Unlike the standard ED approach of triage and transfer, PESs have extra capability to observe and provide intensive treatment, typically for a period of up to 24 hours, aiming to stabilize the crisis within this time and reduce the need for admission. Routine data on the impact of a PES serving a large area of California and linked to several EDs indicated that it substantially reduced both ED waiting times and admission rates (Zeller et al., 2014), and in a rural mid-western area, admissions for people with suicidal ideation fell substantially following introduction of an EmPATH unit (Kim et al., 2022).

Psychiatric decision units have been established in a small number of centres in the UK (Goldsmith et al., 2021) with the aim of assessing selected referrals from the ED in an environment more conducive to thorough psychosocial assessment and holistic care planning via psychiatric liaison teams in the ED. They offer a stay of between 12 and 72 hours, providing recliner chairs rather than beds (subject to some criticism) and aiming to provide a calming environment, psychosocial assessment, brief interventions, and onward referrals. Despite promising reports of impacts on service use, substantial evaluations of extended assessment and triage services following ED attendance are few, and impacts on patient experience need to be better understood. A UK cohort study found no clear effect on admission from psychiatric decision unit introduction (Goldsmith et al., 2023). Brief admission or triage wards, though not community based, are a further model trialled at various times and places over the past few decades with the aim of offering intensive treatment assessment and planning, sometimes closely linked to EDs. Some earlier trials, for example, from the 1970s, showed promise but the benefits of this model have not more recently been established (Anderson et al., 2022; Lloyd-Evans et al., 2009; Williams et al., 2014).

Crisis assessment outside the general hospital

An early innovative model for management of mental health crises was the walk-in clinic offering assessment combined with triage and, in some cases, brief treatment to people experiencing mental health crises. In the US in the 1950s and 1960s, these clinics were closely allied to crisis intervention theory (Caplan, 1964), in which a crisis was regarded not as a manifestation of psychiatric illness but a general human response to severe psychosocial stress, presenting challenges but also opportunities for growth if the crisis was negotiated in an adaptive way. In the heyday of the theory, walk-in crisis clinics proliferated in casualty departments and, later, community mental health centres. Failure to recruit many otherwise mentally healthy individuals to brief crisis interventions, a concern that the needs of the severely mentally ill were not being addressed, and funding restrictions contributed to the waning of this model in the US in the 1970s and 1980s (Goldfinger & Lipton, 1985).

As walk-in crisis intervention services declined in the US, similar services proliferated in Europe, especially in the Netherlands and German-speaking countries (Häfner, 1977; Katschnig et al., 1993). As in the US, European services tended not to attract the generally healthy population originally envisaged (Katschnig et al., 1993), and doubts were in any case increasing about the extent to which they, as opposed to the severely mentally ill, were an appropriate target group. Dissatisfaction also grew with the capacity of these services to prevent hospital admission. In Holland, for example, ambulatory mental health services providing walk-in emergency care to a wide range of people were believed to have caused a marked increase in psychiatric admissions during the 1980s (Gersons, 1996).

Currently, there are a range of examples around the world of mental health crisis assessment centres away from general hospitals, based in psychiatric hospitals, community mental health premises, or freestanding community locations. Some employ relatively conventional models of clinical assessment and intervention not dissimilar to ED services, while others deliver care and support of a more non-clinical and sometimes socially focused nature. The PESs discussed above may be located away from general hospital premises, even though they retain close links with EDs. Some types of crisis assessment service have been established to prevent people in crisis being referred directly for assessment on mental health wards, as assessment on wards has been linked to high rates of subsequent admission (Stulz et al., 2015).

During the Covid-19 pandemic, concerns about overcrowding in EDs and infection control considerations resulted in the development in some countries of new crisis assessment centres located away from the general hospital. For example, in England, 80% of provider mental health trusts reported in 2020 that they had established a crisis assessment centre (crisis hub was another popular description as an alternative to the ED) (Parmar & Bolton, 2020). Where such services remained in place, they appeared to continue to divert some referrals from EDs, potentially resulting in assessment in a better environment (Health Innovation Network, 2022; Sampson et al., 2022). However, a full evaluation of their impacts on the acute mental health care system still needs to be carried out, one concern being that removing mental health professionals from EDs may increase stigma among acute hospital staff and negatively affect care for the many people with both physical and mental health problems. Another example of crisis care innovation in response to Covid-19 is the shift towards greater crisis care provision in community mental health centres in Italy following the onset of the pandemic (Di Lorenzo et al., 2021).

Some mental health crisis centres in the community aim to offer crisis support and, to some extent, assessment that is clearly distinct from standard clinical approaches. An emerging model in England is the crisis café. Such services, sometimes referred to as 'safe havens' or 'sanctuaries', provide walk-in assessment, support, and triage for people experiencing a mental health crisis (Dalton-Locke et al., 2021). They are intended to provide a less formal and clinical environment and, whether based in the voluntary or statutory sector, tend to be delivered by staff who do not have formal mental health professional qualifications, although they often have considerable relevant experience, including lived experience of mental health crises (Dalton-Locke et al., 2021; Molodynski et al., 2020). Opening times are usually outside standard office hours when other forms of support are not available. People experiencing a crisis can usually access immediate support without a referral, sometimes with an initial call to a phone line, which may prevent escalation to a point where ED attendance or admission are required. Similar walk-in services with a more informal approach exist in a variety of other countries under a variety of names (Kalb et al., 2022), and the upsurge of interest in them might be seen as to some extent a return to the walk-in emergency services of the late twentieth century.

Informal drop-in crisis services with a less clinical approach have potential to improve access and choice, especially for people who do not appear well served by conventional clinical models, such as people with a 'personality disorder' diagnosis (DeLeo et al., 2022), but research evaluating their effectiveness and safety and their role in local crisis care systems is so far lacking and would be a useful future research focus.

Initiatives to facilitate assessment following police contact

The police may become involved in mental health crises in various ways, including through response to violent or disturbed behaviour, when someone experiencing a mental health crisis is a victim, when their assistance is requested because someone about whom there are concerns is missing or unreachable, or when someone is identified as at risk of imminent suicide (Huey et al., 2021). A 2016 literature review estimated that police were involved in the pathway to mental health care for around one in ten individuals, although, while the author searched for all English language studies, only studies from North America were found (Livingston, 2016). Potential adverse consequences of police involvement in mental health crises, especially if officers lack relevant training or support, include increased trauma and coercion, unnecessary arrests and legal processes, unjustified transfers to hospital, and inappropriately punitive responses to people in mental health crisis, even resulting, in some cases, in vulnerable people being killed by the police, especially if they are from racially minoritized groups (DeGue et al., 2016; Huey et al., 2021; Isselbacher, 2020). A review of qualitative literature on stakeholder experiences of police and ambulance first responses to mental health crises (Xanthopoulou et al., 2022) identified stigmatizing attitudes among first responders, lack of understanding of relevant law and services, and the arbitrary nature of training as barriers to effective and empathic responses. Difficulties were reported to be frequently exacerbated by failures of mental health services to respond promptly and effectively both to people in crisis and their families and to first responders. Focused training and first responder personal or family experience of mental health problems were perceived as improving responses.

Various service models have been developed to improve outcomes for people in mental health crisis following contact with the police. They usually consist of police and mental health staff responding to mental health-related emergency calls together, ranging from telephone liaison to 24-hour joint response, although in other models of mobile crisis response, the aim is for mental health staff rather than police to attend wherever possible (Waters, 2021).

A systematic review of models involving joint mental health worker and police response (Puntis et al., 2018) found studies carried out in Australia, Canada, the UK, and the US. Some evidence was found for associations between such co-responder services and reduced use of police powers to detain people under mental health legislation, and of police custody. A more recent review (Marcus & Stergiopoulos, 2022) also concluded that there was a certain amount of evidence that models involving co-responses by both police and mental health professionals result in better immediate outcomes and experiences than police-only responses, but noted that findings were mixed and the evidence overall of low quality. In studies of stakeholder experiences and perspectives, co-responder models tend to be perceived by service users, mental health workers, and police as preferable to police-only response, with plain clothes police and unmarked vehicles improving experiences (Puntis et al., 2018; Waters, 2021). However, significant challenges remain in coordination and collaboration between agencies with very different procedures, roles and values, and limited resources for onward referral and resolving a crisis are also frequently reported impediments to effective triage.

A concern regarding co-response models is that some may result in greater police involvement overall in the management of mental health crises; the aim in some models is thus to avoid police involvement as far as is feasible, with some observational studies reporting that avoidance of restraint or legislative processes is feasible in many mobile crisis responses without police involvement (Marcus & Stergiopoulos, 2022; Waters, 2021).

Home-based acute services

Services that provide some combination of acute assessment outside a hospital context and intensive treatment based in patients' homes have been an element in deinstitutionalization from the beginning: terms used to describe them have included CRHTT, intensive home treatment team, crisis assessment and treatment team, and mobile crisis service. The first such service to be widely written about and discussed was that established by Arie Querido in Amsterdam in the 1930s (Querido, 1935). Querido was influenced by ideas about the importance of social environment arising from the mental hygiene movement in the US in the early twentieth century (Salmon, 1916). Responding also to economic pressure during the Great Depression to save on hospital costs, he instituted a city-wide system of home visiting by a psychiatrist and a social worker whenever a patient was referred for admission. An alternative treatment plan, sometimes involving further home visits, was implemented whenever possible. In the UK, community visits in crises were instituted in some areas as early as the 1950s, as in the Worthing experiment: initiated in 1956, this involved home visits by a psychiatrist and a social worker to all those referred for acute admission and was reported to result in falls in admission of 55% and 79% to two local hospitals (Carse et al., 1958).

Very early home-visiting initiatives, such as the Worthing experiment, tended to form part of a shift throughout a catchment area's services towards greater community working: they were not distinct specialist teams. In the 1960s and early 1970s, specialist acute community teams with a focus on preventing admissions were established and evaluated in various countries. One of the most extensive of these initiatives was the network of services developed by Paul Polak in Denver, Colorado, in the 1970s (Polak & Kirby, 1976). Polak's innovations included a team which assessed all individuals referred for admission at home and offered 24-hour home treatment whenever feasible, integration of hospital and community treatment teams, and a network of family sponsor homes, in which families were paid to accommodate up to two patients in crisis, supported by the home treatment team.

Some of the working practices of current CRHTTs can be traced back to two services that share the somewhat confusing distinction of being cited in support of two major innovative models: assertive outreach teams (AOTs) and CRHTTs (see Chapter 14). The Training in Community Living service, established by Leonard Stein and colleagues in Madison, Wisconsin, in the late 1970s (Stein & Test, 1980), and the service established by John Hoult and his colleagues in Sydney in 1979 (Hoult, 1991) resembled current CRHTTs in recruiting patients at the point of acute admission during a crisis and diverting them wherever possible to home treatment. However, like AOTs and unlike CRHTTs, the initial Madison and Sydney teams continued to treat people intensively in the community once the initial crisis had resolved, with the long-term goals of improving their stability in the community and their social functioning. Following these initial experiments, Leonard Stein and John Hoult both concluded that the crisis treatment function would be better split off from continuing care, as it seemed to them difficult for a single team to have both functions (Johnson & Thornicroft, 2008a).

In the US, the term 'mobile crisis service' has been used to describe a wide range of services in which home visits in crisis are an element (Geller et al., 1995; Heath, 2005), some primarily providing a visit and then onwards triage, others providing some initial intervention at home (Zeller & Kircher, 2020). The mobile crisis service model has in many areas developed a significant focus on partnership with the police and avoiding unnecessary and potentially even lethal police involvement in mental health crises, as described above (Isselbacher, 2020). The research base regarding outcomes of this model and the characteristics of the model associated with best outcomes and service user experiences remains limited (Zeller & Kircher, 2020).

Evolution of the crisis resolution and home treatment team

The model of community-based crisis assessment and intensive home treatment that has received the most attention in research literature is the CRHTT. This has been implemented nationwide in both England and Norway (Hasselberg et al., 2011; Johnson, 2013) and more locally in several other countries in the past two decades, and a substantial, though not definitive, evidence base has accumulated (Holgersen et al., 2022). While the most substantial and thoroughly evaluated implementation of the model has been in the UK, the immediate precursors were in Australia, where state policy, first in New South Wales in the 1980s and then in the state of Victoria in the 1990s, required the adoption of the crisis assessment and treatment team model, operating 24 hours and serving adults of working age during office hours and the whole population out of hours (Carroll et al., 2001). These teams in most respects resemble the CRHTT model subsequently introduced throughout England (Johnson & Thornicroft, 2008a).

Implementation of the crisis resolution and home treatment team model

Most early UK experiments with home-based care in crises involved a service delivered as part of the range of functions of a community mental health team, as in the Worthing experiment described above. In the 1990s, concern grew that community mental health teams operating in office hours 5 days a week could not offer an effective alternative to admission, and experimentation with specialist team models of crisis assessment and home treatment began in a few centres, notably Birmingham (Dean et al., 1993). In 1995, John Hoult, an Australian pioneer of crisis assessment and treatment team development, moved to Birmingham, UK, and established the Yardley Psychiatric Emergency Team there (Minghella et al., 1998), with replications following in centres including Islington (London) and Bradford.

Early implementations of the CRHTT model were seen as successful and, against the background of a perceived 'crisis in acute care' (Appleby, 2003), with unmet demand for inpatient beds and considerable user dissatisfaction with hospital care, CRHTT introduction was adopted as national policy in the NHS Plan for England in 2000 (Department of Health, 2000, 2001). The development of 335 CRHTTs across England was mandated. Each was expected to carry a caseload of 20–30 at a time, to see around 300 people a year in total, and to be available 24 hours a day, 7 days a week. This extensive shift in the national community mental health care system has largely been maintained, with almost all English provider catchment areas still having CRHTTs two decades later (Dalton-Locke et al., 2021).

Norway has followed England in adopting the CRHTT model as a national requirement (Gråwe et al., 2005; Hasselberg et al., 2011), although the focus seems to be less on severe mental health problems than in the UK implementation. Implementations of the model are also reported in countries including Germany (Kilian et al., 2016), Switzerland (Stulz et al., 2020), Ireland (Hannigan, 2013), Spain (Martin-Iñigo et al., 2022), and Greece (Koureta et al., 2023).

Principles and practice of crisis resolution and home treatment teams

The evolution of the CRHTT model has tended at least until recently to be pragmatic rather than theoretically driven. A feature of their initial development was that they tended to be established by energetic pioneers as a pragmatic response to difficulties they identified in the service systems in which they worked, rather than on the basis of a well-defined theoretical model. As well as a view that psychiatric admission is often best avoided, both on economic grounds and for patients' well-being, autonomy, and good social functioning, core working principles have tended to be that home treatment allows a greater focus on social milieu than is possible in hospital, with services aiming to engage social networks and to address the social triggers and perpetuating factors for crises (Johnson & Needle, 2008).

The relatively loosely defined nature of the model, which might be seen more as a vehicle for delivering care than a distinct form of treatment, accommodates a range of treatment styles and philosophies. However, a substantial consensus supports a set of core organizational characteristics and interventions for CRHTTs. Box 12.1 summarizes these. The focus exclusively on severe crises that would otherwise result in admission has been seen as important if the CRHTT is to have the resources to divert patients from hospital: these guidelines are influenced by previous experiences of community crisis intervention services that have tended to drift towards mainly recruiting a 'worried well' population who might not otherwise be seen by secondary mental health services (Katschnig & Cooper, 1991). In practice, most CRHTTs are also likely to be carrying out a certain amount of pre-emptive work, accepting patients who appear very likely to meet the threshold for hospital admission in the very near future unless another highly intensive intervention, such as intensive home treatment by a CRHTT, is instituted.

Box 12.1 Key organizational characteristics of CRHTTs

- A multidisciplinary team capable of delivering a full range of emergency psychiatric interventions in the community
- Senior psychiatrists work within the team alongside members of the other main mental health professions
- Target group is people who, in the absence of the CRHTT, would require admission to an acute hospital bed
- Rapid assessment is offered in the community, with a response within an hour when this is needed
- Intensive home treatment offered rather than hospital admission whenever initial assessment indicates this is feasible
- When patients are admitted, contact maintained and early discharge to home treatment takes place whenever feasible
- Low patient–staff ratios allow visits two or three times daily when required
- Twenty-four-hour availability (though staff may be on call from home during the night)
- For patients already on the caseload of other community services (e.g. community mental health teams), the team works in partnership with these services
- Team approach, with caseload shared between clinicians and at least daily handover meetings for review of patients
- Gatekeeping role: team controls access to all local acute inpatient beds
- Intensive home treatment programme is short term, with most patients discharged to continuing care services (if needed) within 6 weeks.

Wheeler et al. (2015) reviewed the literature on ingredients associated with good outcomes in CRHTTs, concluding that extended opening hours and the presence of a psychiatrist within the team may increase capacity to prevent admissions. Evidence on stakeholder perspectives and guidelines tended to prioritize 24-hour availability, a gatekeeping role, with patients admitted to acute beds only if the CRHTT has assessed and agreed that this is necessary, and a multidisciplinary team, allowing a full range of psychological, social, and biological perspectives on assessment and interventions to be available. Bespoke training also emerged as a priority in this review, with many of the skills required by CRHTT staff specific to the CRHTT worker role rather than to a particular profession.

Core interventions

Expert consensus and various guidelines on CRHTTs identify a core range of interventions to be delivered by CRHTTs, although the details of many of these are not highly specified (Crompton & Daniel, 2007; Department of Health, 2001; Johnson & Needle, 2008). Box 12.2 summarizes a set of core interventions identified as key components in CRHTT care.

Assessment is necessarily a core task for CRHTT practitioners: all need to feel confident in assessing and reassessing risk, suitability for home treatment, symptoms and their response to treatment, substance misuse, social difficulties that may have triggered or be perpetuating the crisis, and psychological and social resources for coping with the crisis. Other core interventions include engaging and supporting social networks, helping address immediate practical difficulties that are an obstacle to recovery, and prescribing and managing medication, often key to trying to reduce quickly the severity of initial symptoms and disturbance so that home treatment

> **Box 12.2** Core CRHTT interventions
>
> - Comprehensive initial assessment, including risk, symptoms, social circumstances, stressors and relationships, substance use, and physical health status
> - Opportunities to talk through current problems with staff, brief interventions aimed at increasing problem-solving abilities, and daily living skills
> - Education about mental health problems for patients and social network
> - Engagement—intensive attempts to establish a relationship and negotiate a treatment plan which is acceptable to patients
> - Symptom management, including starting or adjusting medication, and brief psychological interventions
> - Medication administered to patients in the community and their adherence encouraged and supervised, twice daily if needed
> - Practical help—support with pressing financial, housing, or childcare problems, getting home into a habitable state, and obtaining food
> - Identification and discussion of potential triggers to the crisis, including difficulties in family and other important relationships; may include 'systems' work
> - Discharge planning beginning at an early stage, so that continuing care services are available as soon as the crisis has resolved.

remains feasible. Beyond these simple but essential activities of engaging, assessing, monitoring, supporting, educating, and ensuring appropriate medication is received, a standard array of CRHTT interventions has not been established, and practice is likely to vary depending on the skills, interests, and approaches of clinicians and managers in each team. As already discussed, the idea that the antecedents to crises are often social and can more readily be addressed in patients' own homes has been important in the development of CRHTTs. Many CRHTTs thus aim to intervene with patients' social networks in some way, identifying and addressing some of these social triggers. Bridgett and Polak (2003a, 2003b) describe a relatively structured approach to social systems intervention, involving the early use of social systems meetings at which problems in the system are identified and the participants encouraged to find solutions. Other forms of intervention that may be useful within CRHTTs include brief psychological interventions focusing on symptoms or substance use, structured work on relapse prevention or developing crisis plans to be implemented in any future crisis, and interventions focusing on problem-solving or medication adherence.

Responding to variability in outcomes and service user experiences, the CORE fidelity scale for CRHTTs advances on these principles with the development of a 39-item scale intended to measure good practice from the perspectives of service users, clinicians, and experts (Lloyd-Evans et al., 2016). Additions to this beyond the core elements so far described include service user involvement, integration with other services, and measures to address inequalities in service delivery.

Current evidence on community-based crisis assessment and home treatment

When CRHTTs first became national policy in the UK, they were criticized for their scanty evidence base (Pelosi & Jackson, 2000), derived mainly from older studies in which neither experimental nor control group were very comparable with current models (Johnson & Thornicroft, 2008b). Subsequently, evidence has emerged, primarily from the UK but more recently from several other countries, that hospital diversion is achievable with good-quality implementation of the model. Randomized controlled evidence (Johnson et al., 2005b; Murphy et al., 2015; Paton et al., 2016; Stulz et al., 2020) suggests that CRHTTs and similar models reduce admissions and costs, tend to be more acceptable to service users, and probably achieve similar clinical outcomes to other forms of acute care. Observational studies, including some at catchment area level, have also tended to support the finding that hospital admissions can be reduced by introducing the model (Carpenter et al., 2013; Jethwa et al., 2007; Johnson et al., 2005a; Keown et al., 2007; McCrone et al., 2009a, 2009b). This effect probably relates more to voluntary than compulsory admissions (Furminger & Webber, 2009; Johnson et al., 2005a, 2005b; Keown et al., 2007). The workforce implications of this reorganization of the acute care system are also important: UK data have been reassuring, suggesting fairly good satisfaction and low burnout among CRHTT compared with other mental health staff (Johnson et al., 2012; Nelson et al., 2009).

While CRHTTs have appeared a useful model in planned evaluations, important reservations have also emerged about its wider implementation. Service users in qualitative studies and in national surveys (Johnson, 2013; Morant et al., 2017) tend to favour being supported at home rather than in hospital if possible. However, they also report negative experiences related to aspects of the model, including continuity of care, quality of therapeutic relationships, responsiveness, and provision of interventions other than medication delivery and monitoring. While admissions appear reduced in the relatively good-quality implementations of the model that have tended to be the focus of research studies, it is not clear that this has been reliably achieved at a national level in the UK.

Discrepancies between the results of planned evaluations of the model and wider introduction in routine settings are likely to be explained by difficulties in implementing the models as intended. Surveys of English and Norwegian CRHTTs using the CORE fidelity scale suggested low to moderate fidelity in routine settings without regular fidelity monitoring (Hasselberg et al., 2021; Lamb et al., 2020). A cluster randomized trial of a multi-component toolkit designed to improve CRHTT model fidelity (Lloyd-Evans et al., 2020) found the introduction of the toolkit to be associated with both a rise in model fidelity and some evidence of reduced admissions. The CORE fidelity scale is now recommended in NHS policy and is potentially useful in getting this model right in practice.

Community-based crisis residential services

Staying at home during a crisis is preferred by many service users but is not always practical or desirable. The risk of harm to self or others is too great for some patients to be left alone for extended periods of time without supervision. Others may be severely functionally impaired, have no fixed abode, or live in environments that exacerbate their difficulties (e.g. those in abusive relationships). A further impediment to home treatment is that some carers may feel unable to sustain their role in supporting someone at home. Where these difficulties are severe, hospital may be indicated: however, where they are available, residential services outside hospital provide a further potential solution to unmet needs for containment, company, or respite.

Residential alternatives have a history spanning many decades but have yet to become a standard component in catchment area services in any country. This is despite strong advocacy from service user groups and a view that they may provide a recovery environment that is less stigmatizing, coercive, and institutionalized than inpatient hospital care (Howard et al., 2009). Models of residential crisis service provision in the community include free-standing crisis houses, family sponsor homes, and hybrid services in which acute beds are combined with another service type in the community.

Crisis houses

Crisis houses are usually unlocked, standalone community units that are based in converted residential premises (Davies et al., 1994). They typically serve up to 15 patients at a time. A comprehensive UK survey carried out as part of the Alternatives Study identified several subtypes of free-standing community residential service (Johnson et al., 2009). Clinical crisis houses included mental health professionals among their staff and overlapped considerably with acute wards in the types of care provided. Crisis team beds were small clusters of beds very closely linked to a CRHTT, which usually managed the service and controlled admission to the beds. The final group of services identified were non-clinical alternatives, characteristically managed by voluntary sector organizations and aiming to offer a range of interventions significantly different from those provided in hospital, though most services were closely integrated into local catchment area service systems and little evidence of radically different treatment models was found.

In the US, crisis houses also vary in the degree to which they adhere to conventional clinical practices and staffing patterns, but some more distinctive models, including user-led services, have been described (Greenfield et al., 2008). One of the earlier and more radical crisis house alternatives was Loren Mosher's Soteria service, which operated from 1971 to 1983. The service aimed to manage first- or second-episode psychosis in a crisis house setting with minimal reliance on antipsychotic medication. A small randomized controlled trial suggested similar or better outcomes for Soteria patients as compared to hospitalized patients, including lower subsequent use of antipsychotic medication. Furthermore, 43% of Soteria patients reported being well after 2 years without ever having received medication (Bola & Mosher, 2002). Despite these encouraging results, uptake of the Soteria model has been minimal in the US, but similar services have been established in Switzerland, Germany, Sweden, Hungary, and Finland (Calton et al., 2008; Ciompi et al., 1992). Other US crisis house alternatives have adhered to more conventional clinical models, and Warner (2010) suggested that this led in some places to a pressure to establish relatively large facilities that admit compulsorily detained patients and provide a low-cost alternative to scarce and expensive acute beds: this may make it difficult to meet the aspiration to provide care that is tranquil and domestic in atmosphere and individualized in character. Elsewhere, a variety of crisis house models have been described, from clinical alternatives to hospital to service-user led models aiming to adopt very different values from those seen as underpinning standard acute care. Community residential alternatives have continued to attract considerable interest from service planners and to be frequently advocated by service users without having become mandatory or consistently available in any country. A survey of English mental health catchment areas (Dalton-Locke et al., 2021) found that their provision was increasing, with some access to such services in at least half of catchment areas.

Can crisis houses act as a substitute for admission?

Two types of evidence are available regarding the extent to which crisis houses are a true substitute for acute admission. Randomized controlled trial evidence on the extent to which patients referred for acute admission can instead be treated in a crisis house setting was reviewed by Lloyd-Evans et al. (2009) and Thomas and Rickwood (2013). No relevant trials appear to have been published in the past decade, but earlier trials suggest that community residential alternatives can provide care for at least a proportion of those otherwise destined for hospital, generally at lower overall cost. Other evidence comes from observational studies comparing crisis residential service and hospital users. In the Alternatives Study (Johnson et al., 2010), similarities outweighed differences in a comparison between users of four community crisis residential services and local acute hospital wards, but users of the community services were more likely to be help-seekers, more often already known to mental health services, and less likely to be seen as posing a risk to others. Qualitative interviews with local managers, clinicians, and service users indicated that they saw the roles of community alternatives as distinct but overlapping, with community alternatives able to provide acute care for some, but not all, potential acute inpatients and also to relieve pressure on acute wards through early discharge and by admitting pre-emptively some patients who would be likely otherwise to require hospitalization at a later stage.

Do community residential alternatives have any advantages over acute wards?

As in most areas of acute care, the evidence comparing community residential alternatives with hospitals in terms of outcomes is relatively insubstantial. However, most findings indicate greater service user satisfaction with the community alternatives, accompanied by relatively few differences on other measured outcomes (Fenton et al., 1998; Gilburt et al., 2010; Howard et al., 2010; Lloyd-Evans et al., 2009; Osborn et al., 2010; Slade et al., 2010). Sweeney et al. (2014) found that service user satisfaction, therapeutic relationship, and perceived peer support were all greater in a crisis house than acute ward environment, with quantitative findings suggesting service users experienced crisis house staff as kinder and more compassionate, and value having greater freedom and autonomy. Greenfield et al. (2008) are unusual in reporting greater symptomatic improvement as well as greater service satisfaction: the relatively large size of their trial and distinctive consumer-led nature of their model are potential explanations for this. Given the relative equipoise on other outcomes and the advantages in terms of service user acceptability, cost becomes a very important consideration: community residential crisis services vary widely in cost, but are often reported to be less expensive than hospital, especially because of their shorter length of stay (Byford et al., 2010; Greenfield et al., 2008; Warner, 2010). This may help ensure that this continues to be a model of interest, even in straitened economic circumstances, although more robust evidence about which models work for whom and how to optimize experiences and outcomes in this setting is still desirable.

Crisis family placements

In crisis family placements, families are selected and trained to provide short-term crisis accommodation and support (Brook, 1980). Supported by community mental health services, crisis family placements aim to prevent hospitalization and facilitate community reintegration by offering a safe and normative family environment in which patients can recover from immediate crisis (Brook, 1980). Like crisis houses, crisis family placements have a long history. However, the model seems currently to be used relatively little. Polak's original Denver acute service network (see above) included crisis family placements, and a US survey indicated that such homes were the most widely available form of residential alternative crisis care during the 1970s (Stroul, 1988). Crisis family placements have continued to operate in Madison, Wisconsin (Bennett, 1995; Warner, 2010), but we are aware of no published evaluations of such services in the US since the original Denver study.

In the UK, there seem to be only very few instances of this model (Johnson et al., 2009), but the Accredited Accommodation Scheme in Powys, Wales (Readhead et al., 2002) and the Host Families scheme in Hertfordshire (International Mental Health Collaborating Network, n.d.; Kamera, 2013) are both examples, and a Crisis Family Placement scheme is part of the strategy for improving care for Black people in South West London (South West London Integrated Care System, 2022). Initially, the scheme aimed to provide crisis care, but in practice it was expanded to provide planned periods of respite and rehabilitative social care. Elsewhere in Europe, Denmark has a long history of placing adults in family care as an alternative to hospitalization. Small naturalistic studies of Danish crisis family placements, modelled on US programmes, provide some level of support for their effectiveness in terms of patient/family satisfaction and reductions in readmissions and bed days (Aagaard et al., 2008). Thus, despite its long history and the appealing normalization principles on which it is based, the capacity of this form of care to substitute for acute hospital admission is yet to be robustly tested.

Beyond crisis mental health service models

The aim of the current chapter has primarily been to delineate the main models in which specialist mental health professionals respond to crises among people with significant mental health problems. However, the range of settings in which people experiencing such crises may seek help is much wider than the boundaries of such services. In particular, the voluntary sector provides a wide range of services, some explicitly for people experiencing crises of various types (including the crisis café and crisis house models discussed above), others for a wider group of people with mental health and social needs. People who are disengaged and perhaps disillusioned with mainstream mental health care are an important group of recipients of crisis care in the voluntary sector, as are members of minorities at particular risk of negative experiences of mental health services, such as members of racially minoritized groups or gender and sexual minorities, or people with especially stigmatized diagnoses, such as 'borderline personality disorder' (Newbigging et al., 2020). Approaches tend to be more informal, flexible, non-hierarchical, and embedded in local communities than in statutory mental health services. Involvement and sometimes leadership by people with relevant personal experience is also more frequent in this sector, as is peer support (Faulkner, 2020). We have also focused primarily in this chapter on models found in high-income countries: in low- and middle-income countries, crisis responses rely more on non-governmental organizations and grassroots community organizations and networks (Johnson et al., 2022). Given the negative experiences some service users report in statutory crisis services, the different approaches pursued in the voluntary sector potentially provide valuable learning.

Our focus on crisis response should not obscure the need to focus on preventing such crises if at all possible. In a rapid evidence synthesis, Paton et al. (2016) identified a number of interventions with supporting evidence of effectiveness in preventing crises and/or relapses of illness. These include early intervention services for psychosis, intensive case management models, and a range of pharmacological and psychological interventions for psychosis and bipolar disorder. Investing in the full implementation of such models has potential to reduce crisis care use. Beyond such clinical models, social stressors and adverse social circumstances are contributors to crises, and a comprehensive programme to reduce adversity and inequality, as well as to implement interventions for severe mental illness that are clearly evidence based, is arguably the optimal approach to crisis prevention (Drake & Bond, 2021).

Conclusion: towards an integrated and evidence-based acute care system

The current chapter and other chapters in this textbook together delineate the key components of local acute care systems. Some, like acute inpatient beds and services in EDs, are apparently indispensable and inescapable elements in all areas; others are additional components introduced to achieve better quality of care. Indeed inpatient services have been called the Cinderella of contemporary mental health services: this description can readily be extended to acute psychiatry in general (Johnson et al., 2022). The ethical and practical difficulties of doing research with severely ill individuals at the time of a crisis are considerable (Howard et al., 2009). Slow development of clearly defined models of care in this area has both contributed to and been perpetuated by the limited research base. While in other areas of mental health service provision, such as assertive community treatment, supported employment, and early intervention for psychosis, there are theory-driven and clearly defined models of care, with fidelity measures often available to evaluate them, in acute care most approaches have been pragmatic and ad hoc, with the exception of the recent development of fidelity standards for CRHTTs. Large variations in service models such as crisis houses, home treatment teams, and indeed acute inpatient wards make conventional evaluative research difficult to conduct, although realist approaches, with their focus on 'what works, for whom, under what circumstances, and why' (Duncan et al., 2018, p. 452), may have potential.

While we have focused on service models with a specific role, what matters from a service user perspective is their pathway through the acute care system as a whole, and whether care that effectively meets their needs is available at each stage of the crisis, with smooth transitions and coordination between components of the service system. Continuity of care is especially crucial within the acute care system, as needs must be assessed and the right services mobilized rapidly to support acutely distressed service users and their social networks, while periods of treatment with particular acute services are brief, making it necessary to organize coordination between services and planning of the next stage in the patient's journey very quickly. While most of the relevant literature focuses on single components in the acute care pathway, mechanisms for achieving effective coordination and continuity of care between them need to be major foci for future service planning and research that places service user perspectives at the centre of service delivery and evaluation. Thus, a goal for further research and service planning in this area is to progress towards an integrated acute care pathway, aiming to establish clearly defined and evidence-based models of care that include mechanisms for maximizing continuity of care. There is no shortage of work still to be done to achieve this.

REFERENCES

Aagaard, J., Freiesleben, M., & Foldager, L. (2008). Crisis homes for adult psychiatric patients. *Social Psychiatry and Psychiatric Epidemiology*, **43**, 403–409.

Ahmedani, B. K., Simon, G. E., Stewart, C., Beck, A., Waitzfelder, B. E., Rossom, R., et al. (2014). Health care contacts in the year before suicide death. *Journal of General Internal Medicine*, **29**, 870–877.

Allen, M. H. (2007). The organization of psychiatric emergency services and related differences in restraint practices. *General Hospital Psychiatry*, **29**, 467–469.

Allen, M. H., Forster, P., Zealberg, J., & Currier, G. (2002). *Report and Recommendations Regarding Psychiatric Emergency Services*. Washington, DC: American Psychiatric Association Task Force on Psychiatric Emergency Services.

Anderson, K., Goldsmith, L. P., Lomani, J., Ali, Z., Clarke, G., Crowe, C., et al. (2022). Short-stay crisis units for mental health patients on crisis care pathways: systematic review and meta-analysis. *BJPsych Open*, **8**, e144.

Appleby, L. (2003). So, are things getting better? *Psychiatric Bulletin*, **27**, 441–442.

Barratt, H., Rojas-García, A., Clarke, K., Moore, A., Whittington, C., Stockton, S., et al. (2016). Epidemiology of mental health attendances at emergency departments: systematic review and meta-analysis. *PLoS One*, **11**, e0154449.

Bennett, R. (1995). The crisis home program of Dane County. In: Warner, R. (Ed.), *Alternatives to the Hospital for Acute Psychiatric Treatment* (pp. 213–223). Washington, DC: American Psychiatric Press.

Bola, J. R. & Mosher, L. R. (2002). Predicting drug-free treatment response in acute psychosis from the Soteria project. *Schizophrenia Bulletin*, **28**, 559–575.

Bridgett, C. & Polak, P. (2003a). Social systems intervention and crisis resolution. Part 1: assessment. *Advances in Psychiatric Treatment*, **9**, 424–431.

Bridgett, C. & Polak, P. (2003b). Social systems intervention and crisis resolution. Part 2: intervention. *Advances in Psychiatric Treatment*, **9**, 432–438.

Brook, B. D. (1980). Community families: a seven-year program perspective. *Journal of Community Psychology*, **8**, 147–151.

Byford, S., Sharac, J., Lloyd-Evans, B., Gilburt, H., Osborn, D. P., Leese, M., et al. (2010). Alternatives to standard acute in-patient care in England: readmissions, service use and cost after discharge. *British Journal of Psychiatry. Supplement*, **53**, s20–s25.

Calton, T., Ferriter, M., Huband, N., & Spandler, H. (2008). A systematic review of the Soteria paradigm for the treatment of people diagnosed with schizophrenia. *Schizophrenia Bulletin*, **34**, 181–192.

Caplan, G. (1964). *Principles of Preventive Psychiatry*. New York: Basic Books.

Carpenter, R., Falkenburg, J., White, T., & Tracy, D. (2013). Crisis teams: systematic review of their effectiveness in practice. *The Psychiatrist*, **37**, 232–237.

Carroll, A., Pickworth, J., & Protheroe, D. (2001). Service innovations: an Australian approach to community care—the Northern Crisis Assessment and Treatment Team. *Psychiatric Bulletin*, **25**, 439–441.

Carse, J., Panton, N. E., & Watt, A. (1958). A district mental health service: the Worthing experiment. *Lancet*, **1**, 39–41.

Carstensen, K., Lou, S., Groth Jensen, L., Konstantin Nissen, N., Ortenblad, L., Pfau, M., and Vedel Ankersen, P. (2017). Psychiatric service users' experiences of emergency departments: a CERQual review of qualitative studies. *Nordic Journal of Psychiatry*, **71**, 315–323.

Ciompi, L., Dauwalder, H. P., Maier, C., Aebi, E., Trutsch K., Kupper Z., et al. (1992). The pilot project 'Soteria Berne'. Clinical experiences and results. *British Journal of Psychiatry*, **161**, 145–153.

Clarke, D., Usick, R., Sanderson, A., Giles-Smith, L., and Baker, J. (2014). Emergency department staff attitudes towards mental health consumers: a literature review and thematic content analysis. *International Journal of Mental Health Nursing*, **23**, 273–284.

Cotton, M. A., Johnson, S., Bindman, J., Sandor, A., White, I. R., Thornicroft, G., et al. (2007). An investigation of factors associated with psychiatric hospital admission despite the presence of crisis resolution teams. *BMC Psychiatry*, **7**, 52.

Crompton, N. & Daniel, D. (2007). *Guidance Statement on Fidelity and Best Practice for Crisis Services*. London: Department of Health/Care Services Improvement Partnership.

Crowley, J. J. (2000). A clash of cultures: A&E and mental health. *Accident and Emergency Nursing*, **8**, 2–8.

Da Cruz, D., Pearson, A., Saini, P., Miles, C., While, D., Swinson, N., et al. (2011). Emergency department contact prior to suicide in mental health patients. *Emergency Medicine Journal: EMJ*, **28**, 467–471.

Dalton-Locke, C., Johnson, S., Harju-Seppänen, J., Lyons, N., Sheridan Rains, L., Stuart, R., et al. (2021). Emerging models and trends in mental health crisis care in England: a national investigation of crisis care systems. *BMC Health Services Research*, **21**, 1174.

Davies, S., Presilla, B., Strathdee, G., & Thornicroft, G. (1994). Community beds: the future for mental health care? *Social Psychiatry and Psychiatric Epidemiology*, **29**, 241–243.

Dean, C., Phillips, J., Gadd, E., Joseph, M., & England, S. (1993). Comparison of community based service with hospital based service for people with acute, severe psychiatric illness. *British Medical Journal*, **307**, 473–426.

DeGue, S., Fowler, K. A., & Calkins, C. (2016). Deaths due to use of lethal force by law enforcement: findings from the national violent death reporting system, 17 U.S. States, 2009–2012. *American Journal of Preventive Medicine*, **51**(5 Suppl. 3), S173–S187.

DeLeo, K., Maconick, L., McCabe, R., Broeckelmann, E., Sheridan Rains, L., Rowe, S., & Johnson, S. (2022). Experiences of crisis care among service users with complex emotional needs or a diagnosis of 'personality disorder', and other stakeholders: systematic review and meta-synthesis of the qualitative literature. *BJPsych Open*, **8**, e53.

Department of Health (2000). *The NHS Plan*. London: The Stationery Office.

Department of Health (2001). *Crisis Resolution/Home Treatment Teams: The Mental Health Policy Implementation Guide*. London: Department of Health.

Di Lorenzo, R., Frattini, N., Dragone, D., Farina, R., Luisi, F., Ferrari, S., et al. (2021). Psychiatric emergencies during the Covid-19 pandemic: a 6-month observational study. *Neuropsychiatric Disease and Treatment*, **17**, 1763–1778.

Dixon, L., Dickerson, L. Bellack, A., Bennett., M., Dickinson, W., Goldberg, R. W., et al. (2010). The 2010 Schizophrenia PORT Psychosocial Treatment Recommendations and Summary Statements. *Schizophrenia Bulletin*, **36**, 48–70.

Dombagolla, M. H. K., Kant, J. A., Lai, F. W. Y., Hendarto, A., & Taylor, D. M. (2019). Barriers to providing optimal management of psychiatric patients in the emergency department (psychiatric patient management). *Australasian Emergency Care*, **22**, 8–12.

Drake, R. E., and Bond, G. R. (2021). Psychiatric crisis care and the more is less paradox. *Community Mental Health Journal*, **57**, 1230–1236.

Duncan, C., Weich, S., Fenton, S. J., Twigg, L., Moon, G., Madan, J., et al. (2018). A realist approach to the evaluation of complex mental health interventions. *British Journal of Psychiatry*, **213**, 451–453.

Evans, R., Connell, J., Ablard, S., Rimmer, M., O'Keeffe, C., & Mason, S. (2019). The impact of different liaison psychiatry models on the emergency department: a systematic review of the international evidence. *Journal of Psychosomatic Research*, **119**, 53–64.

Faulkner, A. (2020). *Peer Support: Working with the Voluntary, Community and Social Enterprise Sector*. London: National Survivor User Network (NSUN).

Fenton, W. S., Mosher, L. R., Herrell, J. M., & Blyler, C. R. (1998). Randomized trial of general hospital and residential alternative care for patients with severe and persistent mental illness. *American Journal of Psychiatry*, **155**, 516–522.

Furminger, E. & Webber, M. (2009). The effect of crisis resolution and home treatment on assessments under the 1983 Mental Health Act: an increased workload for approved social workers? *British Journal of Social Work*, **39**, 901–917.

Geller, J. L., Fisher, W. H., & McDermeit, M. (1995). A national survey of mobile crisis services and their evaluation. *Psychiatric Services*, **46**, 893–897.

Gersons, B. P. (1996). From emergency to social psychiatric service centers; the Amsterdam experience. *European Psychiatry*, **11**, 192.

Gilburt, H., Slade, M., Rose, D., Lloyd-Evans, B., Johnson, S., & Osborn, D. P. J. (2010). Service users' experiences of residential alternatives to standard acute wards: qualitative study of similarities and differences. *British Journal of Psychiatry*, **197**(Suppl. 53), s26–s31.

Goldfinger, S. M. & Lipton, F. R. (1985). Emergency psychiatry at the crossroads. *New Directions for Mental Health Services*, **28**, 107–110.

Goldsmith, L. P., Anderson, K., Clarke, G., Crowe, C., Jarman, H., Johnson, S., et al. (2021). The psychiatric decision unit as an emerging model in mental health crisis care: a national survey in England. *International Journal of Mental Health Nursing*, **30**, 955–962.

Goldsmith, L. P., Anderson, K., Clarke, G., Crowe, C., Jarman, H., Johnson, S., et al. (2023). Service use preceding and following first referral for psychiatric emergency care at a short-stay crisis unit: a cohort study across three cities and one rural area in England. *International Journal of Social Psychiatry*, **69**, 928–941.

Gråwe, R. W., Ruud, T., & Bjørngaard, H. (2005). Alternative interventions in acute mental health care. *Tidsskrift for Den Norske Lægeforening*, **125**, 3265–3268.

Greenfield, T. K., Stoneking, B. C., Humphreys, K., Sundby, E., & Bond, J. (2008). A randomized trial of a mental health consumer-managed alternative to civil commitment for acute psychiatric crisis. *American Journal of Community Psychology*, **42**, 135–144.

Häfner, H. (1977). Psychiatric crisis intervention—a change in psychiatric organization. Report on developmental trends in the Western European countries and in the USA. *Psychiatria Clinica*, **10**, 27–63.

Hannigan, B. (2013). Connections and consequences in complex systems: insights from a case study of the emergence and local impact of crisis resolution and home treatment services. *Social Science & Medicine*, **93**, 212–219.

Hasselberg, N., Gråwe, R. W., Johnson, S., & Ruud, T. (2011). An implementation study of the crisis resolution team model in Norway: are the crisis resolution teams fulfilling their role? *BMC Health Services Research*, **11**, 96.

Hasselberg, N., Holgersen, K. H., Uverud, G. M., Siqveland, J., Lloyd-Evans, B., Johnson, S., & Ruud, T. (2021). Fidelity to an evidence-based model for crisis resolution teams: a cross-sectional multicentre study in Norway. *BMC Psychiatry*, **21**, 231.

Healthcare Commission (2008). *The Pathway to Recovery: A Review of Acute Inpatient Mental Health Services*. London: The Healthcare Commission.

Health Innovation Network (2022). *Evaluating NHS Mental Health Crisis Hubs in London: Final Report*. London: NHS England. https://healthinnovationnetwork.com/wp-content/uploads/2022/11/MH-Crisis-Hubs-Evaluation-Final-Report.pdf

Healthcare Safety Investigation Branch. (2018). *Investigation into the Provision of Mental Health Care to Patients Presenting at the Emergency Department* (I2017/006). Farnborough: Healthcare Safety Investigation Branch.

Heath, D. S. (2005). *Home Treatment for Acute Mental Disorders*. New York: Brunner-Routledge.

Henderson, M. J., Hicks, A. E., and Hotopf, M. H. (2003). Reforming emergency care: implications for psychiatry. *Psychiatric Bulletin*, **27**, 81–82.

Holgersen, K. H., Pedersen, S. A., Brattland, H., & Hynnekleiv, T. (2022). A scoping review of studies into crisis resolution teams in community mental health services. *Nordic Journal of Psychiatry*, **76**, 565–574.

Hoult, J. (1991). Home treatment in New South Wales. In: Hall, P. & Brockington, I. F. (Eds.), *The Closure of Mental Hospitals* (pp. 107–114). London: Gaskell/Royal College of Psychiatrists.

Howard, L. M., Flach, C., Leese, M., Byford, S., Killaspy, H., Cole, L., et al. (2010). The effectiveness and cost effectiveness of admissions to women's crisis houses compared with traditional psychiatric wards–a pilot patient preference randomized controlled trial. *British Journal of Psychiatry*, **197**(Suppl. 53), s32–s40.

Howard, L. M., Leese, M., Byford, S., Killaspy, H., Cole, L., Lawlor, C., et al. (2009). Methodological challenges in evaluating the effectiveness of women's crisis houses compared with psychiatric wards. *Journal of Nervous Mental Disorders*, **197**, 722–727.

Hudon, C., Chouinard, M. C., Lambert, M., Dufour, I., & Krieg, C. (2016). Effectiveness of case management interventions for frequent users of healthcare services: a scoping review. *BMJ Open*, **6**, e012353.

Huey, L., Ferguson, L., & Vaughan, A. D. (2021). The limits of our knowledge: tracking the size and scope of police involvement with persons with mental illness. *FACETS*, **6**, 424–448.

International Mental Health Collaborating Network (n.d.). Host families. https://imhcn.org/bibliography/recent-innovations-and-good-practices/host-families-6/

Isselbacher, J. (2020). As mobile mental health teams work to de-escalate crises, some warn their models still rely on police partnerships. *STAT*, 29 July.

Jethwa, K., Galappathie, N., & Hewson, P. (2007). Effects of a crisis resolution and home treatment team on in-patient admissions. *Psychiatric Bulletin*, **31**, 170–172.

Johnson, S. (2013). Crisis resolution and home treatment teams: an evolving model. *Advances in Psychiatric Treatment*, **19**, 115–123.

Johnson, S., Dalton-Locke, C., Baker, J., Hanlon, C., Salisbury, T. T., Fossey, M., et al. (2022). Acute psychiatric care: approaches to increasing the range of services and improving access and quality of care. *World Psychiatry*, **21**, 220–236.

Johnson, S., Gilburt, H., Lloyd-Evans, B. et al. (2009). Inpatient and residential alternatives to standard acute wards in England. *British Journal of Psychiatry*, **194**, 456–463.

Johnson, S., Lloyd-Evans, B., Morant, N., Gilburt, H., Shepherd, G., Slade, M., et al. (2010). Alternatives to standard acute in-patient care in England: roles and populations served. *British Journal of Psychiatry. Supplement*, **53**, s6–s13.

Johnson, S. & Needle, J. J. (2008). Crisis resolution teams: rationale and core model. In: Johnson, S., Needle, J. J., Bindman, J., & Thornicroft, G. (Eds.), *Crisis Resolution and Home Treatment in Mental Health* (pp. 67–84). Cambridge: Cambridge University Press.

Johnson, S., Nolan, F., Hoult, J., White, I. R., Bebbington, P., McKenzie, N., et al. (2005a). Outcomes of crises before and after introduction of a crisis resolution team. *British Journal of Psychiatry*, **187**, 68–75.

Johnson, S., Nolan, F., Pilling, S., Sandor, A., Hoult, J., McKenzie, N., et al. (2005b). Randomised controlled trial of acute mental health care by a crisis resolution team: the north Islington crisis study. *British Medical Journal*, **331**, 599.

Johnson, S., Osborn, D. P., Araya, R., Wearn, E., Paul, M., Stafford, M., et al. (2012). Morale in the English mental health workforce: questionnaire survey. *British Journal of Psychiatry*, **201**, 239–246.

Johnson, S. & Thornicroft, G. (2008a). The development of crisis resolution and home treatment teams. In: Johnson, S., Needle, J. J., Bindman, J., & Thornicroft, G. (Eds.), *Crisis Resolution and Home Treatment in Mental Health* (pp. 9–22). Cambridge: Cambridge University Press.

Johnson, S. & Thornicroft, G. (2008b). The classic home treatment studies. In: Johnson, S., Needle, J. J., Bindman, J., & Thornicroft, G. (Eds.), *Crisis Resolution and Home Treatment in Mental Health* (pp. 37–50). Cambridge: Cambridge University Press.

Johnston, A. N., Spencer, M., Wallis, M., Kinner, S. A., Broadbent, M., Young, J. T., et al. (2019). Review article: interventions for people presenting to emergency departments with a mental health problem: a systematic scoping review. *Emergency Medicine Australasia: EMA*, **31**, 715–729.

Kalb, L. G., Holingue, C., Stapp, E. K., Van Eck, K., & Thrul, J. (2022). Trends and geographic availability of emergency psychiatric walk-in and crisis services in the United States. *Psychiatric Services*, **73**, 26–31.

Kamera, N. (2013). A family affair. *Mental Health Today*, November/December, 28–29.

Katschnig, H. & Cooper, J. (1991). Psychiatric emergency and crisis intervention services. In: Bennett, D. H. & Freeman, H. L. (Eds.), *Community Psychiatry: The Principles* (pp. 517–542). Edinburgh: Churchill Livingstone.

Katschnig, H., Konieczna, T., & Cooper, J. (1993). *Emergency Psychiatric and Crisis Intervention Services in Europe: A Report Based on Visits to Services in Seventeen Countries*. Geneva: World Health Organization.

Keown, P., Tacchi, M. J., Niemiec, S., & Hughes J. (2007). Changes to mental healthcare for working age adults: impact of a crisis team and an assertive outreach team. *Psychiatric Bulletin*, **31**, 288–292.

Kilian, R., Becker, T., & Frasch, K. (2016). Effectiveness and cost-effectiveness of home treatment compared with inpatient care for patients with acute mental disorders in a rural catchment area in Germany. *Neurology, Psychiatry and Brain Research*, **22**, 81–86.

Kim, A. K., Vakkalanka, J. P., Van Heukelom, P., Tate, T., & Lee, S. (2022). Emergency psychiatric assessment, treatment, and healing (EmPATH) unit decreases hospital admission for patients presenting with suicidal ideation in rural America. *Academic Emergency Medicine*, **29**, 142–149.

Koureta, A., Papageorgiou, C., Asimopoulos, C., Bismbiki, E., Grigoriadou, M., Xidia, S., et al. (2023). Effectiveness of a community-based crisis resolution team for patients with severe mental illness in Greece: a prospective observational study. *Community Mental Health Journal*, **59**, 14–24.

Lamb, D., Lloyd-Evans, B., Fullarton, K., Kelly, K., Goater, N., Mason, O., et al. (2020). Crisis resolution and home treatment in the UK: a survey of model fidelity using a novel review methodology. *International Journal of Mental Health Nursing*, **29**, 187–201.

Livingston, J. D. (2016). Contact between police and people with mental disorders: a review of rates. *Psychiatric Services*, **67**, 850–857.

Lloyd-Evans, B., Bond, G. R., Ruud, T., Ivanecka, A., Gray, R., Osborn, D., et al. (2016). Development of a measure of model fidelity for mental health crisis resolution teams. *BMC Psychiatry*, **16**, 427.

Lloyd-Evans, B., Osborn, D., Marston, L., Lamb, D., Ambler, G., Hunter, R., et al. (2020). The CORE service improvement programme for mental health crisis resolution teams: results from a cluster-randomised trial. *British Journal of Psychiatry*, **216**, 314–322.

Lloyd-Evans, B., Slade, M., Jagielska, D., & Johnson, S. (2009). Residential alternatives to acute psychiatric hospital admission: systematic review. *British Journal of Psychiatry*, **195**, 109–117.

Marcus, N. & Stergiopoulos, V. (2022). Re-examining mental health crisis intervention: a rapid review comparing outcomes across police, co-responder and non-police models. *Health & Social Care in the Community*, **30**, 1665–1679.

Martin-Iñigo, L., Ortiz, S., Urbano, D., Teba Pérez, S., Contaldo, S. F., Alvarós, J., et al. (2022). Assessment of the efficacy of a Crisis Intervention Team (CIT): experience in the Esplugues Mental Health Center (Barcelona). *Social Psychiatry and Psychiatric Epidemiology*, **57**, 2109–2117.

McCrone, P., Johnson, S., Nolan, F., Pilling, S., Sandor, A., Hoult, J., et al. (2009a). Economic evaluation of a crisis resolution service: a randomised controlled trial. *Epidemiologia e Psichiatria Sociale*, **18**, 54–58.

McCrone, P., Johnson, S., Nolan, F., Sandor, A., Hoult, J., Pilling, S., et al. (2009b). Impact of a crisis resolution team on service costs in the UK. *Psychiatric Bulletin*, **33**, 17–19.

Minghella, E., Ford, R., Freeman, T., Hoult, J., McGlynn, P., & O'Halloran, P. (1998). *Open All Hours: 24-Hour Response for People with Mental Health Emergencies*. London: Sainsbury Centre for Mental Health.

Molodynski, A., Puntis, S., Mcallister, E., Wheeler, H., & Cooper, K. (2020). Supporting people in mental health crisis in 21st-century Britain. *BJPsych Bulletin*, **44**, 231–232.

Morant, N., Lloyd-Evans, B., Lamb, D., Fullarton, K., Brown, E., Paterson, B., et al. (2017). Crisis resolution and home treatment: stakeholders' views on critical ingredients and implementation in England. *BMC Psychiatry*, **17**, 254.

Murphy, S. M., Irving, C. B., Adams, C. E., & Waqar, M. (2015). Crisis intervention for people with severe mental illnesses. *Cochrane Database of Systematic Reviews*, **12**, CD001087.

Nelson, T., Johnson, S., & Bebbington, P. (2009). Satisfaction and burnout among staff of crisis resolution, assertive outreach and community mental health teams. *Social Psychiatry and Psychiatric Epidemiology*, **44**, 541–549.

Newbigging, K., Rees, J., Ince, R., Mohan, J., Joseph, D., Ashman, M., et al. (2020). *The Contribution of the Voluntary Sector to Mental Health Crisis Care: A Mixed-Methods Study*. Southampton: NIHR Journals Library (*Health Services and Delivery Research*, No. 8.29).

NHS England (2014). *NHS Five Year Forward View*. London: NHS England.

Osborn, D. P. J., Favarato, G., Lamb, D., et al. (2021). Readmission after discharge from acute mental healthcare among 231 988 people in England: cohort study exploring predictors of readmission including availability of acute day units in local areas. *BJPsych Open*, **7**(4), e136. doi:10.1192/bjo.2021.961 [published Online First: 2021/07/20].

Osborn, D. P., Lloyd-Evans, B., Johnson, S., Gilburt, H., Byford, S., Leese, M., & Slade, M. (2010). Residential alternatives to acute inpatient care in England: satisfaction, ward atmosphere and service user experiences. *British Journal of Psychiatry. Supplement*, **197**(Suppl. 53), s41–s45.

Parmar, N. & Bolton, J. (2020). *Alternatives to Emergency Departments for Mental Health Assessments during the COVID-19 Pandemic*. London: Faculty of Liaison Psychiatry, Royal College of Psychiatrists.

Paton, F., Wright, K., Ayre, N., Dare, C., Johnson, S., Lloyd-Evans, B., et al. (2016). Improving outcomes for people in mental health crisis: a rapid synthesis of the evidence for available models of care. *Health Technology Assessment*, **20**, 1–162.

Pelosi, A. J., & Jackson, G. A. (2000). Home treatment—engimas and fantasies. *British Medical Journal*, **320**, 308–309.

Polak, P. R. & Kirby, M. W. (1976). A model to replace psychiatric hospitals. *Journal of Nervous and Mental Disease*, **162**, 13–22.

Puntis, S., Perfect, D., Kirubarajan, A., Bolton, S., Davies, F., Hayes, A., et al. (2018). A systematic review of co-responder models of police mental health 'street' triage. *BMC Psychiatry*, **18**, 256.

Querido, A. (1935). Community mental hygiene in the city of Amsterdam. *Mental Hygiene*, **19**, 177–195.

Quinlivan, L. M., Gorman, L., Littlewood, D. L., Monaghan, E., Barlow, S. J., & Campbell, S. M. (2021). 'Relieved to be seen'—patient and carer experiences of psychosocial assessment in the emergency department following self-harm: qualitative analysis of 102 free-text survey responses. BMJ Open, **11**, e044434.

Readhead, C., Henderson, R., Hughes, G., & Nickless, J. (2002). Accredited accommodation: an alternative to inpatient care in rural north Powys. *Psychiatric Bulletin*, **26**, 264–265.

Rose, D. (2001). *Users' Voices: The Perspectives of Mental Health Service Users on Community and Hospital Care*. London: The Sainsbury Centre for Mental Health.

Sacre, M., Albert, R., & Hoe, J. (2022). What are the experiences and the perceptions of service users attending emergency department for a mental health crisis? A systematic review. *International Journal of Mental Health Nursing*, **31**, 400–423.

Salmon, T. W. (1916). Mental hygiene. In: Milton, J. & Rosenau, J. (Eds.), *Preventive Medicine and Hygiene* (pp. 331–61). New York: D. Appleton and Co. [As reprinted in the *American Journal of Public Health*, 2006, 96, 1740–1742.]

Sampson, E. L., Wright, J., Dove, J., & Mukadam, N. (2022). Psychiatric liaison service referral patterns during the UK COVID-19 pandemic: an observational study. *European Journal of Psychiatry*, **36**, 35–42.

Santillanes, G., Axeen, S., Lam, C. N., & Menchine, M. (2020). National trends in mental health-related emergency department visits by children and adults, 2009–2015. *American Journal of Emergency Medicine*, **38**, 2536–2544.

Saunders, K. E., Hawton, K., Fortune, S., & Farrell, S. (2012). Attitudes and knowledge of clinical staff regarding people who self-harm: a systematic review. *Journal of Affective Disorders*, **139**, 205–216.

Slade, M., Byford, S., Barrett, B., Lloyd-Evans, B., Osborn, D. P. J., Skinner, R., et al. (2010). Alternatives to standard acute inpatient care in England: short term clinical outcomes and cost-effectiveness. *British Journal of Psychiatry*, **197**(Suppl. 53), s14–s19.

Soril, L. J., Leggett, L. E., Lorenzetti, D. L., Noseworthy, T. W., & Clement, F. M. (2015). Reducing frequent visits to the emergency department: a systematic review of interventions. *PLoS One*, **10**, e0123660.

South West London Integrated Care System (2022). Addressing inequalities inequalities in mental health linked to ethnicity. https://www.southwestlondonics.org.uk/local-stories/addressing-inequalities-in-mental-health-linked-to-ethnicity-in-wandsworth/

Stein, L. I. & Test, M. A. (1980). Alternative to mental hospital treatment. Conceptual model, treatment program, and clinical evaluation. *Archives of General Psychiatry*, **37**, 392–397.

Stroul, B. A. (1988). Residential crisis services: a review. *Hospital and Community Psychiatry*, **39**, 1095–1099.

Stulz, N., Nevely, A., Hilpert, M., Bielinski, D., Spisla, C., Maeck, L., and Hepp, U. (2015). Referral to inpatient treatment does not necessarily imply a need for inpatient treatment. *Administration and Policy in Mental Health*, **42**, 474–483.

Stulz, N., Wyder, L., Maeck, L., Hilpert, M., Lerzer, H., Zander, E., et al. (2020). Home treatment for acute mental healthcare: randomised controlled trial. *British Journal of Psychiatry*, **216**, 323–330.

Sweeney, A., Fahmy, S., Nolan, F., Morant, N., Fox, Z., Lloyd-Evans, B., et al. (2014). The relationship between therapeutic alliance and service user satisfaction in mental health inpatient wards and crisis house alternatives: a cross-sectional study. *PLoS One*, **9**, e100153.

Taggart, C., O'Grady, J., Stevenson, M., Hand, E., McClelland, R., & Kelly, C. (2006). Accuracy of diagnosis at routine psychiatric assessment in patients presenting to an accident and emergency department. *General Hospital Psychiatry*, **28**, 330–335.

Thomas, K. A. & Rickwood, D. (2013). Clinical and cost-effectiveness of acute and subacute residential mental health services: a systematic review. *Psychiatric Services*, **64**, 1140–1149.

Tran, Q. N., Lambeth, L. G., Sanderson, K., de Graaff, B., Breslin, M., Huckerby, E. J., et al. (2020). Trend of emergency department presentations with a mental health diagnosis in Australia by diagnostic group, 2004–05 to 2016–17. *Emergency Medicine Australasia: EMA*, **32**, 190–201.

Van den Heede, K. & Van de Voorde, C. (2016). Interventions to reduce emergency department utilisation: a review of reviews. *Health Policy*, **120**, 1337–1349.

Wand, T. & White, K. (2007). Examining models of mental health service delivery in the emergency department. *Australian and New Zealand Journal of Psychiatry*, **41**, 784–791.

Warner, R. (2010). The roots of hospital alternative care (Editorial). *British Journal of Psychiatry*, **197**(Suppl. 53), s4–s5.

Waters, R. (2021). Enlisting mental health workers, not cops, in mobile crisis response. *Health Affairs*, **40**, 864–869.

Wheeler, C., Lloyd-Evans, B., Churchard, A., Fitzgerald, C., Fullarton, K., Mosse, L., et al. (2015). Implementation of the crisis resolution team model in adult mental health settings: a systematic review. *BMC Psychiatry*, **15**, 74.

Williams, P., Csipke, E., Rose, D., Koeser, L., McCrone, P., Tulloch, A. D., et al. (2014). Efficacy of a triage system to reduce length of hospital stay. *British Journal of Psychiatry*, **204**, 480–485.

Xanthopoulou, P., Thomas, C., & Dooley, J. (2022). Subjective experiences of the first response to mental health crises in the community: a qualitative systematic review. *BMJ Open*, **12**, e055393.

Zarska, A., Barnicot, K., Lavelle, M., Dorey, T., & McCabe, R. (2023). A systematic review of training interventions for emergency department providers and psychosocial interventions delivered by emergency department providers for patients who self-harm. *Archives of Suicide Research*, **27**, 829–850.

Zeller, S. (2019). Hospital-based psychiatric emergency programs: the missing link for mental health systems. *Psychiatric Times*, **36**, 1–31.

Zeller, S., Calma, N., & Stone, A. (2014). Effects of a dedicated regional psychiatric emergency service on boarding of psychiatric patients in area emergency departments. *Western Journal of Emergency Medicine*, **15**, 1–6.

Zeller, S. & Kircher, E. (2020). Understanding crisis services: what they are and when to access them. *Psychiatric Times*, 6 August. https://www.psychiatrictimes.com/view/understanding-crisis-services-what-they-are-when-access-them

13

Early intervention for people with psychotic disorders

Paddy Power, Ellie Brown, and Patrick D. McGorry

Introduction

Early intervention in psychosis (EIP) has established itself as the cornerstone of service provision in psychosis over the last three decades (Correll et al., 2018). It is the latest key development in the management of psychotic disorders over the last 70 years, following from the introduction of antipsychotic medication, de-institutionalization, community care, and more effective psychosocial interventions. It borrows from principles that have emerged over the last few decades in other areas of medicine, social care, and education. Its focus is on early detection, prevention, and intervention in young people with emerging first-episode psychosis (FEP). It has become a social movement in its own right, developing its own national and international associations (e.g. the International Early Psychosis Association; www.iepa.org.au), World Health Organization-endorsed principles (Bertolote & McGorry, 2005) and attracting considerable political, media, financial, and community support. It has reformed services and become a model of care for other areas of psychiatry.

This explosion of interest in EIP over the past three decades has established it as the gold standard in treating psychotic disorders (National Institute for Health and Care Excellence (NICE), 2014). Countries such as the UK, Canada, Australia, New Zealand, Denmark, and Ireland have committed to funding national roll-outs of these services. This has been further supported by economic evaluations highlighting the substantial health savings involved (Aceituno et al., 2019; McCrone et al., 2008).

Over the past two decades, the early intervention field has expanded into other forms of mental disorders (see Chapter 11), not only in conditions typically affecting young people but even into old age psychiatry (Naismith et al., 2009). The International Early Psychosis Association has broadened its remit to include all mental health generally and not just psychosis. However, questions remain regarding the long-term benefits of early intervention (Allison et al., 2019; Bertelsen et al., 2008; Gafoor et al., 2010; Pelosi, 2009) and there is much to discover about the true extent of its merits. There is still uncertainty about the ideal model. Should they be available for all age groups not just youth (Lappin et al., 2016), or for all forms of psychoses not just non-affective psychosis (Mei et al., 2021), or provided separately from generic services or integrated with them? However, when there is good fidelity to its key components, EIP delivers reliable good outcomes (Brown et al., 2021a).

What is the aim of intervention in psychosis?

The aim of EIP is not only to focus on early detection, intervention, recovery, and prevention at an age when people are most likely to develop psychosis, but also on maintaining this approach throughout the 'critical period' (the first 3 years of recovery) that determines long-term outcome (Birchwood et al., 1998). Investing in services at this early stage will not only ameliorate and prevent unnecessary suffering but it will also maximize the chances of a full recovery (Correll et al., 2018) and minimize the risk of relapse, thereby reducing the overall suffering, burden, and costs for individuals, families, and society (Aceituno et al., 2019).

Why does intervention in psychosis matter?

Psychotic disorders, such as schizophrenia and mood disorders (with psychosis) affect about 3% of the population in their lifetime. They are a major source of suffering and disability in society. Schizophrenia is estimated to affect 21 million globally and is ranked 12th in the global burden of disease (Charlson et al., 2018). Bipolar disorder incurs a similar burden and is ranked even higher in young people. Tragically, life expectancy is reduced by an average of 15 years in schizophrenia (Hjorthoj et al., 2017) and by 8–12 years in bipolar disorder (Kessing et al., 2015).

There is now substantive evidence that people developing psychotic disorders experience long delays in accessing treatment and this contributes significantly to more severe symptoms, poorer outcome, and premature death (Drake et al., 2020; Howes et al., 2021; O'Keeffe et al., 2022). This relationship appears to be curvilinear/logarithmic with poorer outcomes becoming entrenched relatively quickly within the first few months of psychosis onset

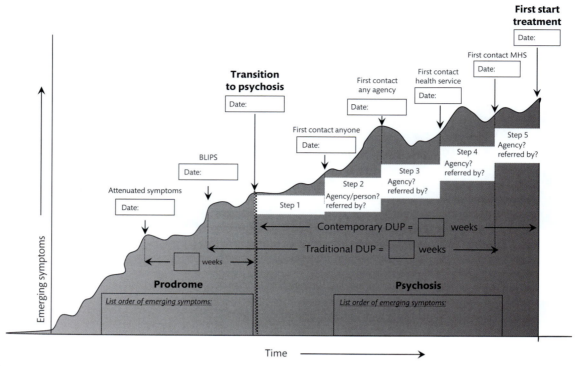

Figure 13.1 Duration of untreated psychosis and steps in the pathways to care. BLIP, brief limited intermittent psychotic symptoms; MHS, mental health service.

(Drake et al., 2020). Delays can occur at each step in the pathways to care (**Figure 13.1**). A measure of the overall delay is the duration of untreated psychosis (DUP). Historically, it averages 1 year (median 10 weeks) in studies with half of this delay happening after first contact with health services (Power et al., 2007a).

These long delays and DUP significantly reduce the effectiveness of treatment and one's capacity to return to normal functioning (Drake et al., 2020; Marshall et al., 2009; Perkins et al., 2005). It is particularly debilitating because these disorders usually emerge at an age when people are trying to establish their own independence and consolidate their personal, educational, social, and vocational trajectories. Prolonged periods of illness can seriously dislocate individuals from these developmental trajectories, making it very difficult to regain their premorbid functioning even if antipsychotic treatment is effective. The high rates of suicide (approximately 1% per year during the first 5 years) and depression attest to the extent of suffering individuals experience in their early years of illness (Power & Robinson, 2009).

At a neurobiological level, there is evidence that neuronal connectivity and glial cell function may be disrupted in a dynamic way during the emergence of psychosis, compromising the brain's 'information processing' systems and leading to restricted cognitive capacity and functioning (McGlashan, 2006; Parellada & Gasso, 2021). Associated changes in brain structure and volume (e.g. hippocampal regions) may emerge early and reach a plateau within several years of illness onset in those who develop schizophrenia (McHugo et al., 2020; Velakoulis et al., 2006). A similar plateau is reached as symptoms and cognitive deficits become entrenched. The earlier one intervenes, the greater the potential to reverse this process. Antipsychotic medication and psychosocial interventions may operate by extinguishing the 'chemical firestorm' of psychosis and allowing a return to the normal processes of neuronal plasticity and connectivity. Through relearning and reconnectivity, a gradual return to normal functioning can be achieved (McGlashan, 2006). Neuroprotective strategies may ultimately have an important role to play in future therapeutics (Conus, 2016).

Who is intervention in psychosis for?

EIP targets those who have developed a first episode of psychosis and those at incipient risk of developing psychosis. Psychotic disorders (**Figure 13.2**) have a pooled incidence of 26.6 per 100,000 person-years (Jongsma et al., 2019). Most psychotic disorders emerge between the mid-teens and late twenties (Kessler et al., 2005) during a critical phase of neurobiological and psychosocial maturation when the accumulating effects of predisposing and precipitating factors (such as genetics, brain maturation, drugs, and stress) come to a head.

Young adults

Almost half of all FEP presentations to mental health services are aged 16–35 years old (Reay et al., 2010). Young adults with psychosis are twice as likely to be male than female (Fusar-Poli et al., 2020a). Non-affective psychosis accounts for about two-thirds of presentations in this age group (Fusar-Poli et al., 2020b). Affective disorder with psychosis (bipolar and depressive disorders with psychosis) accounts for about a fifth and the rest include a rather diverse collection of relatively rare conditions including organic psychoses etc. In the developing world, organic factors (e.g. AIDS and other illnesses) contribute to a much greater proportion (Mbewe et al., 2006).

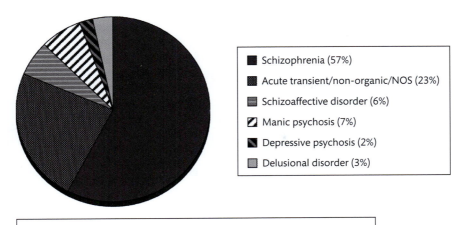

Diagnostic categories using OPCRIT (at 1 month post initial first diagnosis of psychosis) in sample of 150 cases attending LEO service (LEO CAT trial).

Figure 13.2 International Classification of Diseases, tenth revision, diagnostic distribution in FEP population aged 16–35. LEO CAT, Lambeth Early Onset Crisis Assessment Team; NOS, not otherwise specified; OPCRIT, Operational Criteria Checklist.
Adapted from Coentre, R., Blanco, P., Fontes, S., & Power, P. (2011). Initial diagnosis and treatment in first-episode psychosis: can an operationalized diagnostic classification system enhance treating clinicians' diagnosis and the treatment chosen? *Early Intervention in Psychiatry*, 5, 132–139.

Children and adolescent populations

About 10% of FEP are diagnosed by Child and Adolescent Mental Health Services (Fusar-Poli et al., 2020a; Singh et al., 2003). They tend to have more severe symptoms, poorer functioning, higher levels of comorbidity (50% have neurodevelopmental disorders such as autism spectrum disorder or intellectual disability), more frequent and longer hospitalizations, and poorer outcomes. These more complex dynamic presentations are more challenging to diagnose (Correll et al., 2022). This is complicated by the higher prevalence of brief attenuated psychotic symptoms in younger children (Kelleher et al., 2012).

Older adults

While psychosis is predominately a condition of young people, a relatively smaller cohort (30%) of the FEP population will first present between the ages of 35 and 65 (Greenfield et al., 2018) with so-called late-stage psychosis. They are distinguished by being female, married, having children, trauma histories, physical comorbidity (Greenfield et al., 2018), cognitive deficits (Vahia et al., 2010), and psychotic depression (Reay et al., 2010). A further peak in psychosis emerges later in life in the over 65-year-olds during the involutional phase of life when dementia, physical illnesses, depression, and alcohol-related psychoses (accounting for 54%, 15%, 12%, and 6%, respectively), become much more prevalent than schizophrenia spectrum disorders (4%) (Reimann & Hafner, 1973). In these late-onset populations, the sex disparity of 2:1 (males:females) seen in younger populations is reversed, even in schizophrenia-spectrum psychoses (Reeves et al., 2002).

What actually is first-episode psychosis?

The rather broad inclusion of disorders under the rubric of 'psychosis' begs the question what exactly is 'psychosis'? Traditionally, it is defined as a syndrome characterized by hallucinations, delusions, or thought disorder. However, as these appear to be ubiquitous experiences even in normal healthy adult populations, they would only be considered pathological when they become frequent, pervasive, persistent, severe, distressing, and/or disabling. In simple terms, they could be viewed along a continuum with 'normality' in much the same way as one might view depression, anxiety, and a host of other syndromes (**Figure 13.3**). Schizophrenia-spectrum disorders might be at one extreme of this continuum, the ultra-high-risk group being one stage earlier and psychotic experiences in the general population (McGrath et al., 2015) being at the other end.

Defining exactly when psychotic experiences become pathological is more challenging, particularly as one's subjective appraisal plays a significant role in whether the experiences become distressing or disabling. For some individuals, such psychotic experiences might even be appraised as life-affirming. In certain cultural or social settings, transient psychotic experiences are actively sought as a rite of passage or expansion of consciousness, deliberately induced by mind-altering substances or sensory stimulation/deprivation (Wießner et al., 2021).

Psychotic experiences in the general population are relatively common. Almost one-fifth of the general population admit to lifetime experiences of psychotic symptoms (van Os et al., 2001). The incidence rate is about 3% and the point prevalence about 5% (van Os et al., 2009). When clinically assessed, only a fraction (1.5–2% general population) actually meet clinical criteria for a 'psychotic disorder'. However, subclinical psychosis is associated with similar demographic factors to those in clinical populations, that is males, migrants, ethnic minorities, unemployed, unmarried, and being less educated (van Os et al., 2009). Despite the relative 'normality' of fleeting psychotic experiences, they do represent a heightened risk of subsequent psychotic as well as other disorders (Krabbendam et al., 2005). In addition, psychotic experiences are commonly seen in 11–24% of other 'non-psychotic' disorders such as anxiety disorders, depression, and borderline personality disorder (Kelleher & DeVylder, 2017). When exposed to additional risk factors, these subgroups appear to be at greater risk of progressing into a disabling

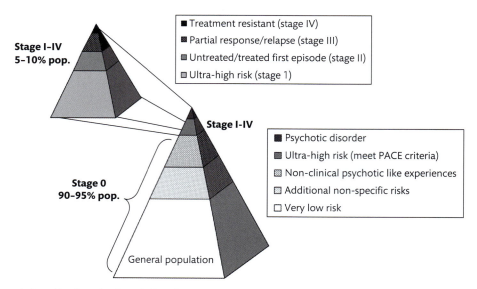

Figure 13.3 General population risk of psychosis and clinical staging I–IV. PACE, Personal Assessment and Crisis Evaluation.

and persistent psychotic disorder. Hence these psychotic-like experiences can be viewed as warning signs of future sustained and complex mental disorder, whether psychotic or otherwise. While some will never require help, there are others who will need clinical care well before their condition reaches the threshold for a psychotic disorder (van Os et al., 2009). If they do become psychotic, this period would traditionally be reframed as the 'prodrome' of their psychosis.

Until the 1990s, there were few, if any, consistent definitions of when someone has crossed the boundary from the prodromal phase to full-threshold psychosis (Breitborde et al., 2009). This posed a considerable dilemma in the past for practitioners working in early psychosis, not only when faced with trying to detect who actually is at highest risk but also knowing when to start treatments for psychosis.

For the purposes of EIP services, an internationally agreed definition has been pragmatically derived to define the point at which a psychotic prodrome ends and an 'acute psychotic episode' begins. This point of 'transition to psychosis' is based on the upper cut-off of the 'at-risk mental state' (ARMS) (Yung et al., 2005). In approximate terms, this is when someone has experienced unremitting frank psychotic symptoms for more than a week. Prior to this 'transition' point, the evidence suggests that psychotic experiences are more likely than not to either remit spontaneously or fail to progress (Yung et al., 2009). It is also the point when one would traditionally advise antipsychotic medication with consideration given to compulsory treatment if the risks were high.

However, this definition of an acute psychotic episode still does not sit particularly well with our international diagnostic criteria, for example, an acute and transient psychotic disorder (International Classification of Diseases, 11th revision) requires at least 2 weeks' duration, schizophrenia at least a month (Gaebel et al., 2020). A manic or depressive episode with psychosis accepts any duration of psychosis, however fleeting. Earlier stages of the emerging psychoses (e.g. the ARMS) are also not well covered by existing international diagnostic systems, though the *Diagnostic and Statistical Manual of Mental Disorders*, fifth edition (DSM-5), did controversially consider introducing the 'Psychosis Risk Syndrome' (Carpenter, 2009). Excluding this 'at-risk' diagnostic category may leave people waiting to receive much needed care until they reach official 'thresholds'.

Distinguishing the type of first-episode psychosis

Once a *'psychotic episode'* is confirmed, the question remains *what kind* of psychosis is the person experiencing? In EIP, the approach to diagnosis challenges the traditional and deterministic views of psychotic disorders such as 'schizophrenia' and opens the doors to a better understanding of the gene–environment interactions underpinning the onset and course of the illness (McGorry et al., 2006). No longer is there a simplistic categorization into schizophrenia, brief psychotic episodes, drug-induced psychosis, and stress-induced psychosis but instead psychosis is viewed along a spectrum. Substance use or stress are seen as just one of many predisposing and precipitating environmental factors that interact in a dynamic way with other underlying genetic or developmental vulnerabilities to precipitate an episode of psychosis in much the same way as cholesterol, cigarette smoking, stress, hypertension, obesity, and diet might each conspire to 'cause' a heart attack. The severity and outcome of the episode depend largely on the interaction of these factors as well as how early the condition is caught. The central treatment of psychoses remains the same except in adjusting for stage of illness (see stages in following sections). If any diagnostic distinction is to be made, it is between the affective, non-affective, and organic psychoses. The others (e.g. drugs, stress, trauma, and personality traits) are viewed as complicating comorbidities with the potential to worsen prognosis rather than reasons for withholding treatment—relapse rates are actually higher in first-episode patients with complicating substance use disorders (Schoeler et al., 2016).

Most psychotic disorders fall into two main types: non-affective psychosis (schizophrenia spectrum disorders) and affective psychosis (manic psychosis and depressive psychosis). Not only are non-affective psychoses subtypes distinguished by how long the psychosis lasts (**Figure 13.4**), but there is considerable overlap between the

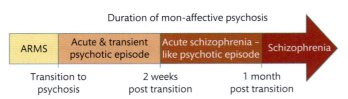

Figure 13.4 Diagnostic distinctions with duration of non-affective psychosis.

different subtypes. A more pragmatic alternative is to view them on a spectrum.

Affective subtypes (Figure 13.5) likewise depend on duration, as well as the severity and character of mood states.

The clinical staging model of psychosis: stages 0–4

To address these conceptual challenges, a clinical staging model of psychosis (Figure 13.6) has been proposed, similar in principle to the staging of cancers and other medical illnesses (McGorry & Hickie, 2019). The advantage of this model is that each stage better describes the emergence, course, progression, prognosis, and the potential for recovery and remission with or without treatment. It also guides the choice and provision of more appropriate stage-specific interventions and services (Fusar-Poli et al., 2017).

As in other medical conditions, there is an explicit assumption that a certain percentage of individuals will naturally progress from a more benign stage to a more severe stage of illness if untreated. The earlier a stage that treatment is started, typically the better the prognosis. Broadly, the effectiveness of interventions at different stages can be measured by their ability to prevent further progression and achieve recovery. However, as with all types of health intervention, there is a balance to be struck as not every case will naturally progress to the next stage, meaning that an awareness of the number needed to treat in order to prevent one case progressing to the next stage is needed.

In recent years, major advances have been made in identifying who will progress or who will benefit most from treatments at different stages. Nonetheless, prognostic indicators at the individual

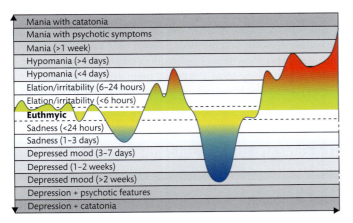

Figure 13.5 Course and diagnostic distinctions in affective psychosis. Example of emerging first-episode manic psychosis (meeting criteria for bipolar disorder).

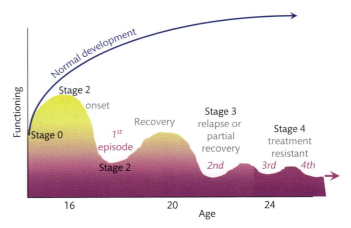

Figure 13.6 Developmental timelines/trajectories and clinical staging of psychosis.

level remain crude. There is still considerable scope for refinement using biomarkers and other measures of prognosis. Ideally, treatment regimens could be individually tailored not only to the stage of illness but also to a person's (and their circumstance's) unique constellation of risk and protective factors.

Stage 0: asymptomatic at-risk group

This group is clinically asymptomatic but carries a significantly greater risk of psychosis than the general population (e.g. relatives of affected cases). As yet, there is no accurate 'universal' screening tool to identify this group. Genetic and developmental factors are clearly some of the most important predisposing risks (Weinberger & Berger, 2009). However, the interaction with environmental factors plays a major role (Barnett & Jones, 2008; van Os & Poulton, 2009). Not everyone carrying a high genetic risk will develop psychosis—only a fifth of individuals with psychosis have an affected first-degree relative (Faridi et al., 2009).

At an individual level, accurately attributing risk to all these factors remains a considerable challenge and, to date, predictive models have not been possible. Nonetheless, for those at particularly high risk, for example, having two affected first-degree relatives (Johnstone et al., 2005), non-invasive preventative strategies may be warranted such as improving mental health literacy and advice about particular risks (e.g. drug use).

At a community level, certain populations are recognized as being at much greater risk of psychosis. 'Hot spots' of psychosis exist in inner city areas, particularly in neighbourhoods with high levels of social deprivation (Kirkbride et al., 2007). Again, at a public health level, it may be possible to reduce the risk of psychosis by targeting high-risk subgroups, but the question remains of what to target them with.

Stage 1a: mild symptomatic (non-specific) clinical high-risk group

This stage includes mild subclinical populations with mild or non-specific symptoms including neurocognitive deficits or mild functional decline. The likelihood of spontaneous remission is high and only a small proportion progress to the next stage of illness—not necessarily psychosis. Interventions at this stage should be benign and non-specific (e.g. information, support, and general counselling services, etc.).

Stage 1b: clinical high-risk group with subthreshold/prodromal symptoms

This stage refers to a clinical high risk for psychosis (CHR-P) population at ultra-high risk for psychosis. They are a group who are experiencing distress and functional decline, prompting them to actively seek help, and who meet clinical criteria (known as 'PACE criteria', based on the Personal Assessment and Crisis Evaluation (PACE) clinic in Orygen, Melbourne, Australia). Individuals meeting these criteria are at ultra-high risk of becoming psychotic (Yung et al., 2009). These criteria are supported by several similar well-developed rating scales/structured interviews, for example, the Comprehensive Assessment of At-Risk Mental States (CAARMS) (Yung et al., 2005), Structured Interview for Prodromal Symptoms (SIPS) and Scale of Prodromal Symptoms (SOPS) (Miller et al., 2003), and Schizophrenia Proneness Instrument-Adult (SPIA) (Gross, 1989) which have been internationally validated (Fusar-Poli et al., 2015).

The criteria, using the CAARMS (Yung et al., 2005), describes a clinical population of young people (aged 14–30) with one or more of the following features:

1. Attenuated positive psychotic features in the last year
2. Brief limited intermittent psychotic symptoms (BLIPS—self-remitting psychotic symptoms lasting less than a week)
3. Trait and state risk factor group (schizotypal personality disorder or first-degree relative with psychosis) plus a significant deterioration in functioning in the last year.

In a recent meta-analysis of 'transition' rates to psychosis (Salazar de Pablo et al., 2021) found that on average the rate of progression from CHR-P to FEP at 6 months was 9%, 15% at 1 year, 20% at 2 years, and 26% at 4 years. Traditionally, only a small fraction (<5%) of FEP individuals are picked up by mental health services during this 'prodromal' period. Though this figure increases to 10% when youth mental health services were included (Brown et al., 2021a), it is still a missed opportunity to intervene.

Stage 2: first-episode psychosis

This stage refers to those who have transitioned to a first episode of psychosis (see above). It covers the course of the ARMS, DUP, and the subsequent treatment/recovery period. Worryingly, about a third of people worldwide with schizophrenia are never treated (Thornicroft, 2007). This increases to half of cases in developing countries (Kurihara et al., 2005).

At a primary care level about 50% of FEP patients will be seen by their general practitioners (GPs) during their DUP but only 50% are referred by them to mental health services (Power et al., 2007a). At the next level of secondary care, detection of psychosis by mental health clinicians is much closer to 100% but engagement in treatment still falls well short of this, with at least 10% failing to engage even in well-resourced EIPs. For those who do engage, initial diagnostic dilemmas are common and changes in diagnosis (even to non-psychotic disorders) are not unusual.

Once individuals with FEP engage in evidence-based treatment, the prospect of remission of positive symptoms is good (Brown et al., 2021a). About 60% of first-episode patients will achieve full remission from psychosis within the first 18 months of follow-up and another 30% will achieve partial remission (Lally et al., 2017). Treatment resistance is relatively uncommon in the first episode but does affect about 10% of this populations (Bozzatello et al., 2019; Huber & Lambert, 2009). Factors that may predict a good response to treatment include female sex, later age of illness onset, good premorbid functioning, absence of magnetic resonance imaging (MRI) abnormalities, and adherence to medication. However, these predictors do not typically survive meta-regression analysis (Catalan et al., 2021), highlighting the intrinsic heterogeneity of FEP cohorts. However, the effect of DUP does survive this and continues to do so even to outcomes 20 years later (O'Keeffe et al., 2022), highlighting the need for services to address shortening DUP as a primary focus of intervention (Malla, 2022).

Stage 3: incomplete/partial remission and relapse

Stage 3 is reserved for FEP patients whose psychosis responds but fails to remit fully with treatment or later relapses. About 40% of FEP patients either partially remit or fail to remit altogether after a year of treatment. For the other 60% of FEP patients who do remit completely from their first episode, about two-thirds will eventually relapse within 5 years, giving an overall rate of relapse of 80% for all first-episode patients (Robinson et al., 1999). Few (16%) relapse within the first year of treatment. The majority (60%) relapse between the end of the first year and the third year. Furthermore, up to 80% of patients who relapse will relapse again within the first 5 years of follow-up. Remission is generally slower and less complete with each relapse. Predictors of relapse include non-adherence to treatment, poor premorbid functioning, long DUP, substance use, stress, life events, and high expressed emotion (Alvarez-Jimenez et al., 2012; Gleeson et al., 2009; Robinson et al., 1999). Relapse rates are significantly lower for those attending EIP services (Craig et al., 2004).

Stage 4: severe, persistent, unremitting, treatment-refractory psychosis

Stage 4 includes those whose psychosis has become persistent and unresponsive to treatment. Less than 10% of FEP patients respond poorly to treatment of their first episode (Bozzatello et al., 2019; Edwards et al., 1998; Thien et al., 2018). However, with each subsequent relapse of FEP patients in earlier stages of illness, treatment refractory rates accumulate so that by the fifth year about 55% of patients with non-affective psychosis end up with stage 4 persistent psychotic symptoms (Robinson et al., 1999). Predictors of poor response are similar to stage 3 (Bozzatello et al., 2019). Levels of impaired psychosocial functioning are high (Vita & Barlati, 2018).

This pattern suggests that, in the initial years, psychotic disorders are usually episodic and for most patients only becoming more enduring and chronic with each subsequent relapse. One of the cornerstones of good long-term treatment therefore is sustaining initial recovery and preventing relapse in the critical initial 3–5 years of follow-up.

The clinical pathway: guidelines for assessment and treatment

Initial assessment, formulation, diagnosis, and treatment plan

Regardless of location, rapid access to comprehensive high-quality multidisciplinary mental health assessment is critical for EIP. This should be supported by a clearly agreed and standardized triage/referral pathway for all referrals, for example, in England there are the official guidances from the NHS (NHS England, 2016) (incorporating the NICE guidelines) and the standards set by the Royal College of Psychiatrists (Chandra et al., 2018). This initial clinical assessment forms the basis of a biopsychosocial formulation, the staging of the illness, and the development of an individually tailored, stage-specific, agreed package of interventions, including recommendations for carers and any other agencies. Comorbidities should be identified early and care plans put in place to address them (e.g. alcohol and drug use, trauma, and developmental disorders). Some may be better addressed quickly (e.g. addictions) and some are best addressed when the young person has recovered from their psychosis (e.g. trauma issues and developmental disorders).

The initial clinical assessment is best undertaken by specially trained mental health clinicians with enhanced understanding of young people with psychosis and their families. One of the main initial aims is to determine whether the person is experiencing a psychotic episode and what treatments/services would be of benefit to them. It may take several sessions to complete. A more comprehensive diagnostic formulation (see below) may need to wait until the consultant psychiatrist and other members of the multidisciplinary team (MDT) have had a chance to assess the person and their circumstances.

Ideally, the assessment should incorporate elements of an adolescent assessment with its developmental perspective, involvement of carers, and feedback from agencies such as GPs and teachers (Box 13.1). This is greatly enhanced by including a developmental trajectory/timeline and the patient's life story, outlining the quality and extent of personal psychosocial development, stresses, emotional maturity, and functioning. It maps the onset, course, and impact of the illness, linking together key events along the way (Figure 13.6).

If FEP is confirmed at the initial assessment, then the standard practice is to appoint a keyworker or case manager. This clinician's role is to engage, ensure care planning, provide interventions, and coordinate with other staff and agencies throughout the patient's time with the EIP service. This role extends to supporting families who are often highly stressed on first contact. They should be interviewed as early as possible to provide reassurance and explanations, obtain collateral details, communicate risk, clarify family medical and mental health histories, and assess their own needs. It may be appropriate to connect them with other carer supports or family peer workers.

Finally, if no psychotic symptoms can be elicited then further observation and collateral may be appropriate if some patients are very guarded or unable to provide an accurate history. It would not be unusual for them to reveal later that they were hearing voices all along. Others may have already been on antipsychotic treatment with good effect by the time they are assessed by the early intervention service (EIS), leaving assessors to rely on the observations of previous clinicians. For those who never experienced psychosis then one should consider whether they might meet criteria for CHR-P. A referral for a CAARMS or SIPS/SOPS assessment by clinicians trained in these assessments may then be appropriate.

The mental state examination

When presenting at this early stage of FEP, people may not bear the hallmarks of a more chronic picture of psychosis, particularly as emotional and social functioning may still be relatively well preserved. Mood may be less blunted but more unstable. Delusions tend to be more fluid, less systematized, entrenched, or complex. Similarly, hallucinations tend to be less well formed and some insight might be retained. About 30% of people are experiencing suicidal ideation at the time they first present to EIP services, representing a time of particularly high risk (Pelizza et al., 2020). The first episode of psychosis is the highest risk period for homicide associated with mental illness (Neilssen & Large, 2010). Finally, neurocognitive functioning may be less impaired at this stage and long-term side effects of pharmacological treatments (extrapyramidal symptoms and weight gain) may yet to have become entrenched.

Use of standardized assessment tools

A common diagnostic tool is the Structured Clinical Interview for DSM-5 (SCID). Supplementing this are a range of measures specific to psychosis, for example, the Nottingham Onset Scale, the SAPS, the Brief Negative Symptom Scale, and finally more general measures of functioning (e.g. SOFAS or CGAS). Measures screening for axis II disorders are best postponed until the person has made a good recovery as the effects of acute psychosis will invalidate the results. When timely, then it might be helpful to screen for autism spectrum disorder with the RAADS and AQ, for attention deficit hyperactivity disorder with the ASRS, for post-traumatic stress disorder with the PCL-5, and personality disorders with the SCID-R.

Physical examination and investigations

A physical examination and standardized medical investigations are an essential part of the initial assessment (Freudenreich et al., 2009; Skikic & Arriola, 2020). This is for several reasons: (1) to rule out/identify any organic factors contributing to the psychotic episode; (2) to identify any pre-existing or potential medical conditions; (3) to establish a baseline prior to the emergence of side effects from medication treatment (e.g. metabolic syndrome); and (4) to start of process of physical health/lifestyle monitoring and education

---

Box 13.1 Core details in the clinical history assessment

Core details in the clinical history should include:
1. A detailed timeline of the emerging psychosis: the onset, course, duration, severity, related mood changes, triggers, aggravating factors, alleviating factors, appraisal, and reactions
2. Duration of prodrome, date of transition to psychosis, and DUP
3. Pathways to care, help-seeking, and engagement
4. Interventions/treatments, effectiveness, periods of non-adherence, duration to response/remission
5. Course and nature of side effects
6. Comorbidities: axis I and II disorders (course and any treatments)
7. Risk behaviours (e.g. suicidality, forensic issues, neglect, and disengagement)
8. Medical conditions (including treatments and allergies)
9. Family history, context/dynamics, reaction, understanding of psychosis, and care elicited
10. Personal and social development, milestones, education and occupational functioning, premorbid adjustment, traumas, responsibilities and aspirations, and personality traits
11. Lifestyle/health factors such as diet, weight, sleep, exercise, smoking, daily routine.

Table 13.1 Biological investigations: standard list of investigations during initial assessment

Type of test	Test
Routine bloods	Haematology Erythrocyte sedimentation rate Liver function tests Urea & electrolytes Thyroid function test Serum calcium and phosphate Fasting blood glucose and HbA1c Fasting lipid profile Prolactin levels
Blood tests if indicated	Autoantibody screen Hepatitis screen HIV
Urine	Drug screen Pregnancy test
Imaging and neurophysiology	Electrocardiogram MRI or computed tomography scan
Extra tests if indicated	Electroencephalogram Lumbar puncture

Adapted from Freudenreich, O., et al. (2009).

regarding diet, weight, exercise, sleep hygiene, smoking, alcohol and drug use, and sexual health.

Monitoring the physical health of individuals with FEP is an essential part of early intervention care—lifespans for people schizophrenia are 15–20 years shorter than their peers (Hjorthøj et al., 2017). The leading cause of this mortality is cardiovascular disease (Hjorthøj et al., 2017) with high rates of obesity (50%), hyperglycaemia (19%), hypertension (39%), metabolic syndrome (33%), and smoking (60–70%) (Cooper et al., 2012; Mitchell et al., 2013). This is further aggravated by the poor level of physical health care and monitoring they receive (Shiers et al., 2009).

The initial physical investigations are listed in Table 13.1. Some are essential while others rely on clinical indication and may not be possible until the person is well enough to tolerate the procedure (e.g. MRI brain scan).

There are no reliable biological/genetic markers that one can be recommend as diagnostic or prognostic aids in FEP. While many genetic variants predictive of schizophrenia have been found (Trubetskoy et al., 2022), their effect is too small individually to be reliable predictors clinically (Cardno, 2014). Earlier suspected genetic markers of risk such as *AKT1*, *COMT*, and *FAAH* variants have not been proven by more recent studies (Hindocha et al., 2020). However, there is potential benefit in identifying fast or slow metabolizers of certain antipsychotic medications or particular risk for side effects (e.g. diabetes and hypercholesterolaemia). Work continues on identifying reliable genetic markers of risk for psychosis, treatment response, and side effects but their use currently in clinical settings remains minimal (Arranz et al., 2021).

Formulation and diagnosis

Though the type of psychotic disorder (Figures 13.3 and 13.4) is important to diagnose, the clinical formulation is a far more useful description. It provides the foundation for building the person's care plan. It aims to explain (1) the type of psychosis, its severity, stage, complications, and impact; (2) the predisposing, precipitating, and aggravation factors; (3) the complications and comorbidities; (4) risks; (5) the context of the person's life circumstances; (6) the person's understanding, reaction to it, and likely willingness to engage in treatments and supports offered; and (7) the levels of care, understanding, and support needed and available.

The diagnostic formulation should routinely involve a face-to-face evaluation by the responsible consultant psychiatrist, before the diagnoses are confirmed and conveyed sensitively and positively to the patient and family, and before the comprehensive treatment plan is agreed upon. This should be summarized in an individual care plan with copies forwarded (if appropriate) to all agencies involved including copies to the individual and their carers.

Discussion about treatment options should occur early on and outline anticipated timelines, obstacles, and expected outcomes, while conveying optimism about recovery. The risk of relapse should be highlighted and it is also important to be frank and honest about the prognosis with and without treatment.

Comorbid axis I and II conditions are common in individuals with FEP and may require additional focus and targeted interventions. For example, anxiety and depression are present for around 30% and 20%, respectively (Wilson et al., 2020). Substance use disorder is also present for around 40% of these individuals (Hunt et al., 2018). Developmental disorders such as attention deficit hyperactivity disorder and autism spectrum disorder are more common than in the general population, with rates of autism spectrum disorder diagnosis being identified around 3–4% (Sunwoo et al., 2020). Trauma and child adversity is also more than twice as common than in the general population (Morgan et al., 2020). Although helpful to identify these comorbid conditions early, more formal assessments and treatments are best postponed until the person has recovered from their psychotic episode.

A final important part of the formulation is the risk assessment and management plan—given the high prevalence of suicidality and violence during the first episode. It should include checking access to potentially fatal means (e.g. tablets, ropes, car, and firearms). It should also take into account the influence of protective factors. One commonly used risk measure for violence is the HCR-20 (Douglas et al., 2013). It separates factors into (1) actuarial historical factors (e.g. demographics, previous incidents, family history), (2) current reversible mental state factors (e.g. agitation, paranoia, command hallucinations), and (3) risk management future 'what-if' scenarios (e.g. exposure to destabilizers, disengagement, loss of supports, etc.). This approach has been adapted for use in suicide risk assessment (Power & McGowan, 2011).

Finally, patients and carers benefit greatly from a personalized orientation to services with an explanation of the remit of the service, after-hours/crisis access details, the interventions available, and the roles of different health professionals on the team with information resources (pamphlets, medication pamphlets, websites, staff photo charts, etc.). Additional resources should be offered to patients or carers with special needs or conditions.

Stage-specific interventions

Once the initial assessment has been completed, and stage of psychosis confirmed, then the most appropriate treatment for that stage should be recommended (Fusar-Poli et al., 2017). Patients and carers may need time to process the options and they should be given relevant information to assist in their decision, for example, medication comparison charts (www.choiceandmedication.org).

Stage 1 interventions in the CHR-P group

Pharmacological treatments at this CHR-P stage remain controversial (Fusar-Poli et al., 2019a). However, people attending these CHR-P clinics are help-seeking and have a demonstrable need for clinical care. Typically, they present with high levels of distress, impaired functioning (Brown et al., 2021a), and generally meet criteria for non-psychotic mental disorders (e.g. anxiety, depression, or personality disorder). These conditions will require treatment in their own right, so the key issue is what additional treatments to offer to reduce the risk of progression to psychosis.

For those meeting criteria for CHR-P, evidence-based treatment recommendations have been developed by the European Psychiatric Association (Schmidt et al., 2015) and are summarized below.

Non-specific interventions

Given the high levels of comorbidity with CHR-P, evidence-based psychosocial interventions should be provided aiming at an optimal psychosocial recovery and involving carers throughout the process. Interventions should not be limited to preventing the development of psychosis though they may have a common goal. The delivery of cognitive behavioural case management by CHR-P services is one such model that shows promise in the early stages of help-seeking (Nelson et al., 2018). Targeting substance use during the CHR-P phase may have significant benefits to an individual's long-term outcome (Carney et al., 2017). With other comorbid conditions one needs to intervene with caution as evidence-based treatments may have the potential to increase the risk of psychosis or mania, for example, stimulants in those with attention deficit hyperactivity disorder and antidepressants in those with a strong family history of bipolar disorder (Patel et al., 2015; Zalpuri & Singh, 2017).

Monitoring for emerging psychotic symptoms

Monitoring for emerging psychotic symptoms over a follow-up period of at least 2 years will reduce the DUP markedly if FEP treatments are provided quickly. This alone has been shown to reduce admissions and improve outcomes (Valmaggia et al., 2015).

Specific psychological interventions for CHR-P

Cognitive behavioural therapy (CBT) has been the most widely evaluated therapy and has been shown to significantly reduce transition rates (Mei et al., 2021). The effect appears to be sustained a year later. The recommended course should be at least 15–30 sessions with a minimum of 12 months.

Specific medication interventions

Antipsychotic medication is not recommended as a first-line treatment as studies have shown psychological therapies to be as effective and more enduring. However, if these are not proving beneficial or if attenuated psychotic/BLIP symptomatology is worsening then low-dose second-generation antipsychotics are recommended for a limited period in combination with CBT. Long-term antipsychotic treatment alone to prevent transition is not recommended. A more benign medical intervention with omega-3 fish oils shows limited benefits in this population (Susai et al., 2022). More recent trials of cannabidiol in CHR-P are pending (Amminger et al., 2021). As yet, there is very little evidence to guide preventative treatments in those of ultra-high risk of bipolar disorder (Zalpuri & Singh, 2017).

Stage 2 interventions in the first episode of psychosis

Pharmacotherapy

Treatment guidelines recommend antipsychotic medication as soon as a diagnosis of an acute episode of psychosis is confirmed. Treatment response in FEP is often quicker and likely to happen at a lower dose in FEP (Barnes et al., 2011), particularly if the DUP is short (Drake et al., 2020). Ideally, the choice of antipsychotic medication should be based on patient preference, determined by the side effect profile. A meta-analysis (Zhang et al., 2013) comparing first-generation (FGAs) and second-generation antipsychotics (SGAs) in the first episode revealed that SGAs (particularly olanzapine, amisulpride, and, less so, risperidone and quetiapine) significantly outperformed FGAs with lower discontinuation rates, negative symptoms, cognition deficits, and extrapyramidal side effects. However, weight gain and metabolic changes were greater with SGAs (olanzapine, risperidone, and clozapine). Certain SGAs (risperidone and olanzapine) may protect against grey matter changes commonly seen in the emerging first episode (Girgis et al., 2006; Lieberman et al., 2005). Low-dose risperidone is also more effective than haloperidol in preventing relapse (Schooler et al., 2005). For these reasons, the SGAs are preferable in most cases (Kahn et al., 2008).

FEP patients are particularly prone to extrapyramidal side effects at standard doses, especially with FGAs (Kahn et al., 2008). This commonly leads to non-compliance (Fleischhacker et al., 2003). Children and adolescents are even more susceptible to side effects. So, low doses are preferable. Low doses (e.g. risperidone 2 mg/day) are effective and safe in the majority of first-episode patients (McGorry et al., 2010; Merlo et al., 2002). For younger patients, James and Broome (2017) recommend either quetiapine, risperidone, or aripiprazole. The advice is to 'start low and go slow' increasing every 2–3 weeks if no therapeutic response is seen (Figure 13.7). If no response is seen after the third increment, the medication should be switched to another atypical agent starting at a mid-range dose and increasing also if no response is seen. In cases of treatment resistance by the fourth month, serious consideration should be given to clozapine once a formal MDT case review has addressed all contributing factors (see 'Stage 4 interventions'). Benzodiazepines are recommended in the short term for anxiety, agitation, and insomnia.

If the psychosis is driven primarily by affective disturbance (manic, depressive, or mixed mood) then the advice is to promptly add a mood stabilizer in acute manic psychosis or an antidepressant in acute depressive psychosis to the above antipsychotic regimen unless the psychotic features are very mild and fleeting. Doses of mood stabilizers and antidepressants need to be titrated up to relatively high doses given that affective psychosis represents the more severe end of the affective spectrum. Doses of both antipsychotic and mood stabilizer or antidepressant need to be adjusted downwards after the acute episode to prophylactic levels to minimize the risk of side effects during the recovery. In women, mood stabilizers pose additional risks (e.g. polycystic ovarian disease with valproate and teratogenic effects with lithium).

Unfortunately, there are no clear guidelines about how long to continue treatment after the first episode. Standard practice in

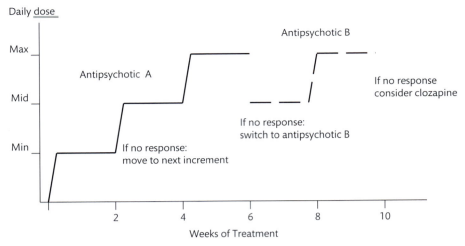

Figure 13.7 Antipsychotic medication regimen in first-episode psychosis. *In depressive psychosis*: add antidepressant at start and titrate upwards until response. *In manic psychosis*: add mood stabilizer at start and titrate upwards to anti-manic dose.

uncomplicated non-affective psychosis is to continue antipsychotic medication for at least a year after remission. However, is important to remember that relapse is most likely to occur between the first and third years of follow-up and that suggests a longer period of prophylactic medication (e.g. 3 years minimum post remission) would be far more protective (Chen et al., 2008; Wunderink et al., 2007). This is particularly important in those with adverse prognostic indicators (e.g. family history, younger age of onset, long DUP, etc.) or high levels of risk behaviours when unwell.

For typical manic psychoses, common practice is to gradually withdraw the antipsychotic several months after remission but to continue the mood stabilizer for a minimum of 18 months depending on the illness duration and severity. Antidepressants should be prescribed very cautiously if post-manic depression develops.

Medication side effects should be monitored regularly during follow-up and a formal physical review performed with blood tests to check for medication complications such as weight gain, metabolic syndrome, diabetes, and extrapyramidal symptoms.

Useful treatment guidelines in FEP

Medication prescribing guidelines in FEP are outlined below and reflect the recommendations made above. They include the following:

- 'International clinical practice guidelines for early psychosis' (International Early Psychosis Association Writing Group, 2005)
- 'Psychosis and schizophrenia in adults: prevention and management' (Clinical guideline CG178) (NICE, 2014)
- 'Psychosis and schizophrenia in children and young people: recognition and management' (Clinical guideline CG155) (NICE, 2013)
- *Medical Management in Early Psychosis: A Guide for Medical Practitioners* (ENSP Medical Management Writing Group, 2014)
- *Practical Management of Bipolar Disorder* (Young et al., 2010).

Psychological interventions

There is now a wealth of modularized CBT and psychosocial packages, catering for different aspects of the first episode and comorbidities. Ideally, all individuals with FEP patients should be offered individual therapy sessions. However, timing is crucial as many are not able to benefit from formal sessions until they have recovered sufficiently from the acute psychotic episode. Initial therapy sessions during the acute episode are best tailored towards engagement, support, reassurance, and psychoeducation, leaving more formal CBT interventions until the individual can make more rational appraisals of their psychotic experiences (Jackson et al., 2008). CBT sessions may become necessary after the acute psychotic episode stabilizes, and adjustment difficulties during their recovery become more present. This can include becoming social anxious, experiencing low mood, persistent negative symptoms, or attentional deficits. Relapse prevention should be provided routinely during the recovery phase to help patients recognize their own early warning signs/relapse signatures and develop contingency plans to manage relapses (Gleeson et al., 2013).

There is increasing recognition of the value of CBT in FEP and it is now recommended as standard practice in treatment guidelines (NICE, 2014). Other psychological interventions trialled in individuals with FEP with a less well established evidence base include mindfulness (Jansen et al., 2020) and acceptance and commitment therapy (Brown et al., 2021b). Though controversial, intensive cognitive behaviour case management without antipsychotic medication may be suitable for a small minority with short DUPs (Francey et al., 2020).

Family interventions

The needs of carers should be considered from the outset (NICE, 2014). Most young people with FEP are still living at home when they enter EIP services and families will often have been struggling for months trying to cope. Relationships will have become strained and levels of expressed emotion high. During the recovery phase of FEP, families are expected to become carers and often do not anticipate the extent of burden this might place on them. The broad aim of family interventions is to support and educate families about psychosis, equip them with skills to become effective carers, limit the burden, and reduce levels of expressed emotions. Family interventions have been shown to be effective at reducing relapse, duration of hospitalizations, and psychotic symptoms, and increase functioning in both the short and long term (Camacho-Gomez & Castellvi, 2020; Pharoah et al., 2010). Most families, however, manage with limited need for formal family therapy and most services limit this to psychoeducation sessions and regular care planning sessions (McNab & Linszen, 2009).

Vocational/educational/psychosocial interventions

Many individuals experiencing FEP are already disadvantaged by their socioeconomic circumstances which have impacted their education and work histories, before the effects of the illness contributing further. Ensuring a focus on vocational strategies can go a long way to reversing this and rebuilding self-esteem and resilience. Individual Placement and Support (IPS) which focuses on (re)engaging individuals with work as well also education, appears to be the most appropriate and effective approach with young first-episode patients (Killackey et al., 2019). IPS is adaptable to different sociopolitical settings and appears to have better outcomes than other models of vocational rehabilitation. New digital/online interventions (e.g. Horyzons) have been shown to be effective in improving vocational or educational attainment (Alvarez-Jimenez et al., 2019).

Group programmes

Group psychosocial programmes in FEP have a particular role in providing patients with an opportunity to meet others going through similar experiences and offering support, education about psychosis, structure and routine to facilitate recovery. They can be delivered by clinicians or peer workers and examples include groups with a focus on psychoeducation, healthy living, lifestyle issues, diet, stress management, parenting, and recreational activities, cooking, art, and exercise groups (Somaiya et al., 2022).

Stage 3 interventions

Antipsychotic medication is a major factor in relapse following FEP (Taipale et al., 2022). Cessation is associated with a 77% risk of relapse within 1 year and 90% risk within 2 years. This is in contrast with a 3% risk on medication (Zipursky et al., 2014). With each relapse, the risk of further relapse increases, the effectiveness of antipsychotic deteriorates, and higher doses are required (Taipale et al., 2022). There is no definitive guidance about how long to continue antipsychotic medication but 3 years after remission from the FEP and 5 years from remission of that last relapse would seem a reasonable recommendation.

It is essential to ascertain why relapse has occurred and review the reasons why with the patient and their family. Drug use, stress, non-adherence due to negative symptoms, memory deficits, and side effects may all be implicated and need addressing in their own right (e.g. drug counselling, supervision of medications by carers, etc.). Relapse prevention counselling should be routinely offered either individually or in a group psychoeducation format. Relapses can be a source of great disappointment and frustration for the individual and their family. They need time and support to readjust and process what has happened. Complicating depression and suicidality may need specific treatment.

For those relapsing after a planned withdrawal of medication then simply restarting the same antipsychotic at the previous or slightly higher dose may be enough to achieve remission again. However, for those relapsing while on stable doses, then one should follow the incremental steps outlined in the treatment of stage 2 (see earlier section).

If the relapse is that of bipolar or schizoaffective disorder then consideration should be given to combined medications (antipsychotic plus mood stabilizer) or the addition of a second mood stabilizer.

If relapse has resulted from repeated non-adherence to medication despite the best efforts of all involved, then depot antipsychotic medication should be considered as an alternative to oral medication. Ideally, this should be an SGA antipsychotic that was already effective and well tolerated in oral form. Oral medication should be continued for several weeks after the depot is started to allow it to reach a steady state.

Stage 4 interventions

Stage 4 interventions are for those who don't achieve remission (after the first and subsequent episodes of psychosis) despite adequate trials of at least two antipsychotic medications at top doses. As with stage 3, a formal MDT reassessment (including a medication review) should be undertaken to determine why the patient's psychosis is treatment refractory and what additional interventions might be helpful. Baseline measures of psychopathology and functioning should be part of this review.

Clozapine is recommended for all patients with treatment-resistant schizophrenia and who are likely to adhere to the treatment protocols. Though clozapine is a major step to take (it generally implies continuing treatment indefinitely), avoidable delays are far too common (Thien & O'Donoghue, 2019). Before commencing, patients and carers should have a formal counselling session explaining the pros and cons of clozapine. A standard pre-clozapine medical work-up and side effect monitoring protocols should be in place. Initiation should be slow with small increments until therapeutic blood levels are reached. Side effects are generally the norm and a quarter of FEP patients end up discontinuing clozapine mostly because of cardiac complications (Thien et al., 2018). However, clozapine has a 76% chance of producing remission in treatment refractory FEP (Thien et al., 2018).

Stage 4 psychosocial interventions should routinely include more intensive psychosocial interventions including CBT for psychosis which has been shown to complement the response to clozapine (Edwards et al., 2011). For those with severe negative and enduring positive symptoms despite clozapine, there should be serious consideration of whether the patient would be better served by specialist care from residential/daycare/community-based rehabilitation services.

Discharge and long-term follow-up

Most EIP services are time limited to 3 years. By then, discharge to primary care may be adequate for the 40–54% (stage 2) of people who achieve full remission from FEP without relapse (Catalan et al., 2021; Power et al., 2007b). However, the rest (stage 3 and 4) will require a longer follow-up and transfer to continuing care mental health services. Adequate time needs to be given to preparing patients for discharge/transfer, equipping them and their carers with the knowledge that they need to carry with them into the future about their condition, its treatment, how to minimize the risk of relapse, and practical advice about what to say to future health professionals, prospective employers, insurers, partners, and friends. Patients should be given copies of service discharge summaries with their relapse prevention plans and recommendations for future management. These recommendations and risks should be made clear to follow-up services like GPs.

Long-term outcomes

Though there is consistent evidence that outcomes while attending EIP services are significantly better than those obtained in standard services, these benefits diminish upon discharge from EIP services when assessed at 5- or 10-year follow-up (Chan et al., 2019). This raises the question of whether EIP services should be continued for longer (e.g. 5 years), or up to a certain age (e.g. 25 years of age). Perhaps this should be the case for some patients (e.g. stages 3 and 4) but it may not be necessary for patients with better outcomes. A meta-analysis of three randomized controlled trials of extended EIS beyond 2 years is not conclusive (Puntis et al., 2020), perhaps because including stage 2 cases diluted the benefits of extended EIS for stage 3 and 4 cases.

Predicting longer-term outcome is not helped by the lack of sophisticated prognostic indicators. Existing ones are still quite crude and poorly validated. But early examples with machine learning show promise (Leighton et al., 2019). Until there is more evidence about outcomes in the longer term, it is clear that in the short term, FEP patients fare better in EIP services than generic services. With the advent of Big Data and better designed outcome studies, there is the real possibility of being able to develop prognostic tools that can map and compare potential outcomes for individuals depending on their treatment and lifestyle choices (e.g. the relative risk of stopping medication and using cannabis).

What do early intervention in psychosis services look like?

EIP services vary greatly in design across the world, from 'stand-alone' teams whose sole purpose is EIP, to generic community mental health teams enhanced with embedded EIP staff/interventions (Health Service Executive, 2019). Between these two extremes, there is the 'hub and spoke' model. Some EIP services are age specific, such as Child and Adolescent Mental Health Services, young adult, and older adult while others extend to the full adult age range (as in England over the last decade). Although there is a very rich amount of local variation, most EIP services start off or end up being 'stand-alone' (Pinfold et al., 2007). Only a very small number of EIP services provide dedicated FEP inpatient care (Craig & Power, 2010).

In a systematic review of EIS models, Behan et al. (2017) found the evidence base was strongest for 'stand-alone' EIP services, less so for hub and spoke models, and no evidence in favour of augmented community mental health teams. The hub and spoke model can work well within rural areas where the incidence of psychosis is low and cases/services are dispersed across wide distances (Cheng et al., 2014; Fowler et al., 2009). This is not the case in urban areas where the incidence of psychosis is often several times higher and complicated by high levels of comorbidity/risk in deprived inner-city populations. For these urban areas, stand-alone specialist EIP services are logistically more functional, robust, and effective.

Individual EIP teams generally cater for relatively large catchment areas (e.g. >250,000 population). They should promote early detection by referrers such as GPs, fast-track referrals, promote engagement, assessment, home-based acute care treatment, and in-reach for those needing hospitalization. They provide the mainstay of community mental health services and intensive psychosocial interventions needed for optimal recovery over the first 2–3 years of follow-up. Staff-to-patient ratios are typically relatively high (e.g. 1:15) to cater for these demands. In addition to their clinical role, EIP services have a long tradition of close ties with research and evaluation. It is from these studies that a strong evidence base supporting EIP has emerged (McGorry et al., 2010).

Virtually all EIP services target those with non-affective psychoses (schizophrenia, schizoaffective disorder, schizophreniform psychosis, brief psychotic episodes, delusional disorders), most include affective psychoses (manic psychosis, depressive psychosis) and drug-induced psychoses (**Figure 13.1** describes the diagnostic distribution). Some specifically exclude those with certain comorbid conditions such as learning disability, personality disorders, and organic psychoses.

Despite the prominence of research in the CHR-P population for psychosis, only a small minority of EIP services cater for these clients (see below) and often via a separate specialist CHR-P clinic operating in primary care settings.

Key components of early intervention services

There are at least six core service components in EISs. Few services possess all these components or are at various stages of development. The first component aims to reduce DUP, the second addresses the CHR-P population, and the third aims to improve the quality of inpatient and community care and recovery from FEP. The remaining components aim to support, train, develop, evaluate, and ensure fidelity to the early intervention model.

In terms of the evolution of EISs, the first component is a surprisingly neglected area despite its importance in determining outcome (Malla, 2022). The second component is still viewed as lower priority and is absent from most services. The community aspect of the third component is the main focus of most EIS while the inpatient aspect is rarely mentioned. The remaining components tend to lag behind in development and are introduced in stages.

The first EIS component: reducing the duration of untreated psychosis

Reducing the DUP requires two main strategies: (1) improving early detection and prompt referral by referrers to mental health services and (2) ensuring a rapid and effective response by front-end mental health services to referrals.

Education campaigns: raising awareness and signposting for referrers

The goal of these campaigns is to raise awareness of the early signs of psychosis and to signpost prompt access to appropriate services, thereby reducing the DUP. These campaigns are generally provided by the EIS but others are run by health educators, training programmes, colleges, etc. They are targeted at different steps in the pathways to care starting with the general population, school-based programmes, non-health professionals, health professionals, and mental health professionals. Such health education programmes do need to be carefully designed for the specific needs of their audience in order to maximize the potential for appropriate referrals.

Broad public health campaigns may be very effective in reducing the DUP, for example, from a median of 16 weeks to 5 weeks in the TIPPS programme (Melle et al., 2004) but they may also generate high numbers of inappropriate referrals (eight referrals to one FEP case) (Johannessen et al., 2005). This contrasts with the much lower ratio (two referrals to one FEP case) when education campaigns are limited to primary care health professionals (Power et al., 2007b). GPs will recognize and refer about 50% of FEP patients presenting to them with untreated FEP. With specific GP education training this proportion can be increased to 80% (Power et al., 2007b).

Improving front-end access to EIS: early detection and assessment clinics/teams

Mapping local pathways to care for first-episode patients is a very revealing exercise and helps expose the barriers to access, engagement assessment, and treatment in FEP. Some of these barriers can be easily remedied by simple promotion of front-end services and closer links with referrers such as education, primary care, social services, correctional services, etc. Others are more complicated and steeped in cultural prejudices. This stigma can be partially addressed by relatively simple investment into the visual appeal and reception of these clinics or locating them in primary health care or youth-friendly settings. Providing extended-hours services and capacity for outreach/home assessments go a long way to minimizing the risk of contact with traditional emergency services, police, A&E departments, and hospitals. However, it is essential that these front-end services are well resourced with properly trained clinicians experienced in the complex subtleties and risks of presentations of patients with early psychosis. They need to be very responsive and timely in triaging and assessing referrals properly to achieve the waiting time standards set, such as by the NHS (NHS England, 2016).

Finally, most EIP services don't have early detection teams/clinics, so instead work closely with generic front-end services to access referrals (e.g. from acute inpatient units, crisis assessment, and home-based treatment teams). This relies on a considerable degree of cooperation to triage and fast-track potential early psychosis cases. One solution is to broaden the remit of early detection across all front-end mental health services, for example, the youth assessment team and headspace clinics that form the front end into Orygen Youth Health services in Melbourne, Australia (www.oyh.org.au).

The second EIS component: CHR-P clinics

Dozens of CHR-P clinics have sprung up over the past four decades specifically focusing on a clinical population at ultra-high risk for psychosis. At least five have been established in London (Fusar-Poli et al., 2019b) covering a population of over 2 million. Many of these clinics were established with research funding with the aim of enhancing the screening process and undertaking trials of interventions to reduce the transition to psychosis. Some of the clinics have morphed into mainstream clinical services situated in primary care settings but still have a large research component. One of the earliest is the PACE clinic set up in 1995 in Melbourne, Australia, as part of the EPPIC service (Yung et al., 2009). In practice, CHR-P clinics only manage to attract a minority of those truly at risk and have a significant false-positive rate of 60–80% (Yung et al., 2009). However, interventions at this stage do appear to have a significant impact on reducing the risk of progressing to an acute psychotic episode (see section on staged interventions)

The third EIS component: core clinical interventions in first-episode psychosis

These are divided into inpatient and community evidence-based clinical interventions.

Early psychosis inpatient services

Dedicated first-episode units are rare but there are a few notable examples include the EPPIC unit (originally opened in 1984 and now part of Orygen Youth Health), the LEO unit in south London, UK (opened in 2001), and the Early Psychosis Unit in Toronto, Canada, to name a few (Craig & Power, 2010). It is surprising that there are not more, given that most first-episode patients require hospitalization (Ajnakina et al., 2020; Fusar-Poli et al., 2020b) and these units are generally no more expensive to operate than generic acute wards. What is particularly concerning is that general adult wards are likely to fall well short in meeting the needs of young people presenting for the first time with psychosis and that accommodating them in these wards can be very traumatizing in itself (Jackson et al., 2004). Even if it is not possible to develop a specific EIP unit, it may prove possible to set aside a number of inpatients for FEP and promote a culture of EIP within the unit (e.g. as in one east London borough).

Inpatient EIP services should mirror what is provided by the community components of the EIS with the same ethos, assessments, treatment protocols, access to therapies, programmes, family support, and finally staff training and expertise. This is particularly relevant as FEP patients spend over a 100 days on average in hospital during their follow-up (average 7 years) and the majority will be detained for some of that period under mental health legislation (Ajnakina et al., 2020; Fusar-Poli et al., 2020a). So units should be closely integrated with community-based EIP teams with capacity for in-reach and continuity of care throughout the hospitalization process and post discharge.

EIP community services/teams

These MDT teams are the core component of all EIP services. They operate as assertive outreach community-based mental health teams with a capacity for home-based treatment and crisis intervention. Their role is to engage and provide timely EIP interventions through the course of the first episode of psychosis, recovery, and any relapses during the follow-up period. A keyworker/case manager (one of the clinicians in the MDT) and a doctor is appointed to each patient for the duration of the time with the EIP service. Keyworkers coordinate individual care plans, engagement with other interventions, monitor progress, respond to crises, liaise with outside agencies, and, depending on their skill set, provide EIP therapies and interventions. Online services and e-therapies have become an increasingly acceptable medium and may be a far more efficient way of delivering outreach services particularly for the younger population.

The fourth EIS component: staffing, training, supervision, management, and governance

All EIP MDT members should have comprehensive training and supervision in EIP as part of their induction and ongoing professional development. Local and national training schemes and workshops are very popular. Accredited courses (e.g. MSc course at Kings College London, UK) and training manuals are available online (www.orygen.org.au/Training/Resources/). Formal clinical academic and professional supervision structures need to be particularly transparent given close working relationships EIS clinicians, researchers, and peer support staff.

The fifth EIS component: funding and resources

An 'invest to save' approach to staffing and resources is essential. EISs require initial investment in order to be established. Savings are downstream, mainly through the reduction in inpatient bed usage and may not be directed back to EIS budgets. Initial funding is often piecemeal, dependent on grants, and takes several years to be incorporated into mainstream health budgets making it difficult to recruit enough staff initially. However, caseloads take 2–3 years to build up to capacity, allowing time to recruit and train in an incremental fashion. Similarly, it takes time for teams to accumulate and develop resources such as health promotion material—fortunately, there is a wealth of resources already online.

The sixth EIS component: service evaluation, development, and research

Continuous EIS evaluation is critical to ensure high-quality standards and fidelity to the early intervention model. This includes setting national targets, such as DUP, wait times, etc. Services should be audited annually using tools such as the Royal College of Psychiatrists' quality standards for EIP services (Chandra et al., 2018). User/carer participation and local agencies are essential partners in service evaluations and planning. EISs often have close partnerships with research bodies. This brings with it considerable benefits and may be the source of initial investment in the service. Local and national service and research networks provide considerable opportunities for mutual support, collaboration, and standardization (Table 13.2).

The future challenges for early intervention psychosis services

EIP services are now an integral part of many national mental health strategies even in countries where resources are traditionally very limited. EIP has proven its worth in the short term despite its critics. It has captured the imagination and sustained enthusiasm of health service managers, clinicians, academics, and community agencies. It is well received by young people, their families, and referrers.

There is now clear evidence of better outcomes with EIP and that it is more cost-effective than generic care. EIP has successfully driven reform and extra investment in mental health care. There is no legitimate premise to support 'late intervention' with older models of care. However, as with any new emerging model, EIP is a work in progress and there are a number of challenges to be faced. This includes putting more emphasis on strategies to reduce DUP (Malla, 2022), overcoming the obstacles of providing EIP to older adults (Reay et al., 2010), determining whether EISs are better placed within a youth mental health system (Malla et al., 2016), whether EIS should sustained for longer (e.g. 5 years), and the extent to which services should use e-health and online systems for clinical interventions. In the area of early detection, there is the prospect in the near future of discovering biomarkers and refining clinical measures to better identify for each individual what their risk of progression and treatment responses might be for different stages of psychosis, for example, the recently formed research network, Accelerated Medicines Partnership (AMP) Schizophrenia (SCZ) programme (https://nda.nih.gov/ampscz). This would better inform treatment recommendations (e.g. duration of treatment or early use of clozapine).

The principles of early intervention have already extended beyond the realm of psychosis into other areas of mental health (Insel, 2007), such as borderline personality disorder (Chanen et al., 2017). Early intervention is almost certainly applicable to most disorders that develop gradually and become persistent and disabling. Its vision of providing *personalized*, *participatory*, *pre-emptive*, and *predictive* care echoes developments in other fields of medicine. It is the premise for new models of youth mental health that have rapidly established themselves in a number of countries (Australia, Ireland, Canada, Denmark, and England) (Malla et al., 2016). It provides an exciting new challenge to mental health care and, given the extent of morbidity, one to which a response is long overdue. Meeting these challenges will be a test of the capacity of mental health reform and EIP in particular in the years to come.

Table 13.2 Useful sources of further information

Type	Source
Associations	International Early Psychosis Association (www.iepa.org.au/)
UK early intervention networks	IRIS (www.iris-initiative.co.uk) Early Intervention in Psychosis Network (EIPN) (www.rcpsych.ac.uk) Pan-London Network (PNP) for psychosis prevention
Fact sheets	www.mentalhealthfirstaid.csip.org.uk/~earlydetection/factsheets/ www.orygen.org.au
Patient booklets	Compton, M. & Broussard, B. (2009). *The First Episode of Psychosis: A Guide for Patients and Their Families*. Oxford: Oxford University Press
Textbooks	Edwards, J. & McGorry, P. (2002). *Implementing Early Intervention in Psychosis: A Guide to Establishing Early Intervention Services*. London: Martin Dunitz. Jackson, H. & McGorry, P. (Eds.) (2009). *The Recognition and Management of Early Psychosis: A Preventative Approach* (2nd ed.). Cambridge: Cambridge University Press. French, P., Smith, J., Shiers, D., Reed, M., & Rayne, M. (Eds.) (2010). *Promoting Recovery in Early Psychosis: A Practice Manual*. Oxford: Blackwell Publishing
Journals	*Early Intervention in Psychiatry*

REFERENCES

Aceituno, D., Vera, N., Prina, A., & McCrone, P. (2019). Cost-effectiveness of early intervention in psychosis: systematic review. *British Journal of Psychiatry*, **215**, 388–394.

Ajnakina, O., Stubbs, B., Francis, E., Gaughran, F., David, A. S., Murray, R. M., & Lally, J. (2020). Hospitalisation and length of hospital stay following first-episode psychosis: systematic review and meta-analysis of longitudinal studies. *Psychological Medicine*, **50**, 991–1001.

Allison, S., Bastiampillai, T., Malhi, G. S., & Castle, D. (2019). Does early intervention prevent chronic psychosis? A question for the Victorian Royal Commission into Mental Health. *Australian & New Zealand Journal of Psychiatry*, **53**, 943–945.

Alvarez-Jimenez, M., Priede, A., Hetrick, S. E., Bendall, S., Killackey, E., Parker, A. G., et al. (2012). Risk factors for relapse following treatment for first episode psychosis: a systematic review and meta-analysis of longitudinal studies. *Schizophrenia Research*, **139**, 116–128.

Alvarez-Jimenez. M., Bendall, S., Koval, P., Rice, S., Cagliarini, D., Valentine, L., et al. (2019). HORYZONS trial: protocol for a randomised controlled trial of a moderated online social therapy to maintain treatment effects from first-episode psychosis services. *BMJ Open*, **9**, e024104.

Amminger, G. P., Lin, A., Kerr, M., Weller, A., Spark, J., Pugh, C., et al. (2021). Cannabidiol for at risk for psychosis youth: a randomized controlled trial. *Early Intervention in Psychiatry*, **16**, 419–432.

Arranz, M. J., Salazar, J., & Hernández, M. H. (2021). Pharmacogenetics of antipsychotics: clinical utility and implementation. *Behavioural Brain Research*, **401**, 113058.

Barnett, J. & Jones, P. (2008). Genes and the social environment. In: Morgan, C., McKenzie, K., & Fearon, P. (Eds.), *Society and Psychosis* (pp. 58–74). Cambridge: Cambridge University Press.

Barnes, T. R. (2011). Evidence-based guidelines for the pharmacological treatment of schizophrenia: recommendations from the British Association for Psychopharmacology. *Journal of Psychopharmacology*, **25**, 567–620.

Behan, C., Masterson, S., & Clarke, M. (2017). Systematic review of the evidence for service models delivering early intervention in psychosis outside the stand-alone centre. *Early Intervention in Psychiatry*, **11**, 3–13.

Bertelsen, M., Jeppesen, P., Petersen, L., Thorup, A., Øhlenschlaeger, J., le Quach, P., et al (2008). Five-year follow-up of a randomized multicenter trial of intensive early intervention vs standard treatment for patients with a first episode of psychotic illness: the OPUS trial. *Archives of General Psychiatry*, **65**, 762–771.

Bertolote, J. & McGorry, P. (2005). Early intervention and recovery for young people with early psychosis: consensus statement. *British Journal of Psychiatry*, **187** (Suppl. 48), s116–s119.

Birchwood, M., Todd, P., & Jackson, C. (1998). Early intervention in psychosis. The critical period hypothesis. *British Journal of Psychiatry*, **172** (Suppl 33), s53–s59.

Bozzatello, P., Bellino, S., & Rocca, P. (2019). Predictive factors of treatment resistance in first episode of psychosis: a systematic review. *Frontiers in Psychiatry*, **10**, 67.

Breitborde, N. J. K., Srihari, V. H., & Wood, S. W. (2009). Review of the operational definition for first-episode psychosis. *Early Intervention in Psychiatry*, **3**, 259–265.

Brown, E., Gao, C. X., Staveley, H., Williams, G., Farrelly, S., Rickwood, D., et al. (2021a). The clinical and functional outcomes of a large naturalistic cohort of young people accessing national early psychosis services. *Australian and New Zealand Journal of Psychiatry*, **56**, 1265–1276.

Brown, E., Shrestha, M., & Gray, R. (2021b). The safety and efficacy of acceptance and commitment therapy against psychotic symptomatology: a systematic review and meta-analysis. *Revista Brasileira de Psiquiatria*, **43**, 324–336.

Camacho-Gomez, M. & Castellvi, P. (2020). Effectiveness of family intervention for preventing relapse in first-episode psychosis until 24 months of follow-up: a systematic review with meta-analysis of randomized controlled trials. *Schizophrenia Bulletin*, **46**, 98–109.

Cardno, A. (2014). Genetics and psychosis. *Advances in Psychiatric Treatment*, **20**, 69–70.

Carney, R., Cotter, J., Firth, J., Bradshaw, T., Yung, A.R. (2017). Cannabis use and symptom severity in individuals at ultra high risk for psychosis: a meta-analysis. *Acta Psychiatrica Scandinavia*, **136**, 5–15.

Carpenter, W. T. (2009). Anticipating DSM-V: should psychosis risk become a diagnostic class? *Schizophrenia Bulletin*, **35**, 841–843.

Catalan, A., Richter, A., Salazar de Pablo, G., Vaquerizo-Serrano, J., Mancebo, G., Pedruzo, B., et al. (2021). Proportion and predictors of remission and recovery in first-episode psychosis: systematic review and meta-analysis. *European Psychiatry*, **64**, e69.

Chan, S. K., So, H. C., Hui, C. L., Chang, W. C., Lee, E. H., Chung, D. W., et al. (2015). 10-year outcome study of an early intervention program for psychosis compared with standard care service. *Psychological Medicine*, **45**, 1181–1193.

Chandra, A., Patterson, E., & Hodge, S. (Eds.) (2018). *Standards for Early Intervention in Psychosis Services—1st Edition* (Publication number: CCQ1285). London: The Early Intervention in Psychosis Network & Royal College of Psychiatrists.

Chanen, A., Sharp, C., Hoffman, P., & Global Alliance for Prevention and Early Intervention for Borderline Personality Disorder (2017). Prevention and early intervention for borderline personality disorder: a novel public health priority. *World Psychiatry*, **16**, 215–216.

Chan, S., Chan, H., Devlin, J., Bastiampillai, T., Mohan, T., Hui, C. L. M., et al. (2019). A systematic review of long-term outcomes of patients with psychosis who received early intervention services. *International Review of Psychiatry*, **31**, 425–440.

Charlson, F. J., Ferrari, A. J., Santomauro, D. F., Diminic, S., Stockings, E., Scott, J. G., et al. (2018). Global epidemiology and burden of schizophrenia: findings from the Global Burden of Disease Study 2016. *Schizophrenia Bulletin*, **44**, 1195–1203.

Cheng, C., Dewa, C.S., Langill, G., Fata, M., & Loong, D. (2014). Rural and remote early psychosis intervention services: the Gordian knot of early intervention. *Early Intervention in Psychiatry*, **8**, 396–405.

Chen, Y. H., Hui, L. M., Lam, M., Law, C. W., Chiu, P. Y., Chung, W. S., et al. (2008). A double-blind randomized placebo-controlled relapse prevention study in remitted first-episode psychosis patients following one year of maintenance therapy. *European Psychiatry*, **23**, S107–S108.

Conus, P. (2016). Nonpharmacological substances for early intervention. In: Riecher-Rössler, A. & McGorry, P. D. (Eds.), *Early Detection and Intervention in Psychosis: State of the Art and Future Perspectives* (pp. 159–167). Basel: Karger.

Cooper, J., Mancuso, S. G., Borland, R., Slade, T., Galletly, C., & Castle, D. (2012). Tobacco smoking among people living with a psychotic illness: the second Australian Survey of Psychosis. *Australian and New Zealand Journal of Psychiatry*, **46**, 851–863.

Correll, C. U., Galling, B., Pawar, A., Krivko, A., Bonetto, C., Ruggeri, M., et al. (2018). Comparison of early intervention services vs treatment as usual for early-phase psychosis: a systematic review, meta-analysis, and meta-regression. *JAMA Psychiatry*, **75**, 555–565.

Correll, C. U., Fusar-Poli, P., Leucht, S., Karow, A., Maric, N., Moreno, C., et al. (2022). Treatment approaches for first episode and early-phase schizophrenia in adolescents and young adults: a Delphi consensus report from Europe. *Neuropsychiatric Disease and Treatment*, **18**, 201–219.

Craig, T. K., Garety, P., Power, P., Rahaman, N., Colbert, S., Fornells-Ambrojo, M., & Dunn, G. (2004). The Lambeth Early Onset (LEO) Team: randomised controlled trial of the effectiveness of specialised care for early psychosis. *British Medical Journal*, **329**, 1067–1070.

Craig, T. K. & Power, P. (2010). Inpatient provision in early psychosis. In: French, P., Smith, J., Shiers, D., Reed, M., & Rayne, M. (Eds.), *Promoting Early Intervention in Psychosis* (pp. 17–26). Oxford: Wiley Blackwell Press.

Douglas, K. S., Hart, S. D., Webster, C. D., & Belfrage, H. (2013). *HCR-20V3: Assessing Risk of Violence—User Guide*. Burnaby, Canada: Mental Health, Law, and Policy Institute, Simon Fraser University.

Drake, R. J., Husain, N., Marshall, M., Lewis, S. W., Tomenson, B., Chaudhry, I. B., et al. (2020). Effect of delaying treatment of first-episode psychosis on symptoms and social outcomes: a longitudinal analysis and modelling study, *Lancet Psychiatry*, **7**, 602–610.

Edwards, J., Cocks, J., Burnett, P., Maud, D., Wong, L., Yuen, H. P., et al. (2011). Randomized controlled trial of clozapine and CBT for first-episode psychosis with enduring positive symptoms: a pilot study. *Schizophrenia Research and Treatment*, **2011**, 394896.

Edwards, J., Maude, D., McGorry, P., Harrigan, S., & Cocks, J. (1998). Prolonged recovery in first-episode psychosis. *British Journal of Psychiatry*, **172** (Suppl. 33), 107–116.

ENSP Medical Management Writing Group (2014). *Medical Management in Early Psychosis: A Guide for Medical Practitioners*. Parkville: Orygen Youth Health Research Centre.

Faridi, K., Pawliuk, N., King, S., Joober, R., & Malla, A. K. (2009). Prevalence of psychotic and non-psychotic disorders in relatives of patients with a first episode psychosis. *Schizophrenia Research*, **114**, 57–63.

Fleischhacker, W.W., Oehl, M.A., & Hummer, M. (2003). Factors influencing compliance in schizophrenia patients. *Journal of Clinical Psychiatry*, **64** (Suppl. 16), 10–13.

Fowler, D., Hodgekins, J., Howells, L., Millward, M., Ivins, A., Taylor, G., et al. (2009). Can targeted early intervention improve functional recovery in psychosis? A historical control evaluation of the effectiveness of different models of early intervention service provision in Norfolk 1998–2007. *Early Intervention in Psychiatry*, **3**, 282–288.

Francey, S. M., O'Donoghue, B., Nelson, B., Graham, J., Baldwin, L., Yuen, H. P., et al. (2020). Psychosocial intervention with or without antipsychotic medication for first-episode psychosis: a randomized noninferiority clinical trial. *Schizophrenia Bulletin Open*, **1**, sgaa015.

Freudenreich, O., Schulz, S. C., & Goff, D. C. (2009). Initial medical work-up of first-episode psychosis: a conceptual review. *Early Intervention in Psychiatry*, **3**, 10–18.

Fusar-Poli P, Cappucciati M, Rutigliano G, et al. At risk or not at risk? A meta-analysis of the prognostic accuracy of psychometric interviews for psychosis prediction. World Psychiatry 2015; 14(3): 322-32.

Fusar-Poli, P., Davies, C., Solmi, M., Brondino, N., De Micheli, A., Kotlicka-Antczak, M., et al. (2019a). Preventive treatments for psychosis: umbrella review (just the evidence). *Frontiers in Psychiatry*, **10**, 764.

Fusar-Poli, P., Estradé, A., Spencer, T. J., Gupta, S., Murguia-Asensio, S., Eranti, S., et al. (2019b). Pan-London Network for Psychosis-Prevention (PNP). *Frontiers in Psychiatry*, **10**, 707.

Fusar-Poli, P., Salazar de Pablo, G., Correll, C. U., Meyer-Lindenberg, A., Millan, M. J., Borgwardt, S., et al. (2020a). Prevention of psychosis: advances in detection, prognosis, and intervention. *JAMA Psychiatry*, **77**, 755–765.

Fusar-Poli, P., Lai, S., Di Forti, M., Iacoponi, E., Thornicroft, G., McGuire, P., & Jauhar, S. (2020b). Early intervention services for first episode of psychosis in South London and the Maudsley (SLaM): 20 years of care and research for young people. *Frontiers in Psychiatry*, **11**, 577110.

Fusar-Poli, P., McGorry, P. D., & Kane, J. M. (2017). Improving outcomes of first-episode psychosis: an overview. *World Psychiatry*, **16**, 251–265.

Gaebel, W., Kerst, A., & Stricker, J. (2020). Classification and diagnosis of schizophrenia or other primary psychotic disorders: changes from ICD-10 to ICD-11 and implementation in clinical practice. *Psychiatria Danubina*, **32**, 320–324.

Gafoor, R., Craig, T., Garety, P., Power, P., & McGuire, P. (2010). Effect of early intervention on 5 year outcome in non-affective psychosis. *British Journal of Psychiatry*, **196**, 372–376.

Girgis, R. R., Diwadkar, V. A., Nutche, J. J., Sweeney, J. A., Keshavan, M. S., and Hardan, A. Y. (2006). Risperidone in first-episode psychosis: a longitudinal, exploratory voxel-based morphometric study. *Schizophrenia Research*, **82**, 89–94.

Gleeson, J. F., Cotton, S. M., Alvarez-Jimenez, M., Wade, D., Gee, D., Crisp, K., et al. (2013). A randomized controlled trial of relapse prevention therapy for first-episode psychosis patients: outcome at 30-month follow-up. *Schizophrenia Bulletin*, **39**, 436–448.

Gleeson, J., Linszen, D., & Wiersma, D. (2009). Relapse prevention in early psychosis. In: Jackson, H. & McGorry, P. D. (Eds.), *The Recognition and Management of Early Psychosis: A Preventative Approach* (pp. 349–364). Cambridge: Cambridge University Press.

Greenfield, P., Joshi, S., Christian, S., Lekkos, P., Gregorowicz, A., Fisher, H. L., & Johnson, S. (2018). First episode psychosis in the over 35s: is there a role for early intervention? *Early Intervention in Psychiatry*, **12**, 348–354.

Gross, G. (1989). The 'basic' symptoms of schizophrenia. *British Journal of Psychiatry*, **155** (Suppl. 7), 21–25.

Health Service Executive (2019). National clinical programme for early intervention for psychosis: model of care. https://www.hse.ie/eng/about/who/cspd/ncps/mental-health/psychosis/resources/hse-early-intervention-in-psychosis-model-of-care-executive-summary-june-2019.pdf

Hindocha, C., Quattrone, D., Freeman, T. P., Murray, R. M., Mondelli, V., Breen, G., et al. (2020). Do AKT1, COMT and FAAH influence reports of acute cannabis intoxication experiences in patients with first episode psychosis, controls and young adult cannabis users? *Translational Psychiatry*, **10**, 143.

Hjorthøj, C., Stürup, A. E., McGrath, J. J., & Nordentoft, M. (2017). Years of potential life lost and life expectancy in schizophrenia: a systematic review and meta-analysis. *Lancet Psychiatry*, **4**, 295–301.

Howes, O. D., Whitehurst, T., Shatalina, E., Townsend, L., Onwordi, E. C., Mak, T. L. A., et al. (2021). The clinical significance of duration of untreated psychosis: an umbrella review and random-effects meta-analysis. *World Psychiatry*, **20**, 75–95.

Huber, C. G. & Lambert, M. (2009). Treatment resistance in first-episode psychosis. In: Jackson, H. & McGorry, P. D. (Eds.), *The Recognition and Management of Early Psychosis: A Preventative Approach* (pp. 365–381). Cambridge, Cambridge University Press.

Hunt, G. E., Large, M. M., Cleary, M., Lai, H., & Saunders, J. B. (2018). Prevalence of comorbid substance use in schizophrenia spectrum disorders in community and clinical settings, 1990–2017: systematic review and meta-analysis. *Drug and Alcohol Dependence*, **191**, 234–258.

Insel, T. R. (2007). The arrival of pre-emptive psychiatry. *Early Intervention in Psychiatry*, **1**, 5–6.

International Early Psychosis Association Writing Group (2005). International clinical practice guidelines for early psychosis. *British Journal of Psychiatry*, **187** (Suppl. 48), s120–s124.

Jackson, C., Knott, C., Skeate, A., & Birchwood, M. (2004). The trauma of first episode psychosis: the role of cognitive mediation. *Australian & New Zealand Journal of Psychiatry*, **38**, 327–333.

Jackson, H. J, McGorry, P. D., Killackey, E., Bendall, S., Allott, K., Dudgeon, P., et al. (2008). Acute-phase and 1-year follow-up results of a randomized controlled trial of CBT versus befriending for first-episode psychosis: the ACE project. *Psychological Medicine*, **38**, 725–735.

James, A. C. & Broome, M. R. (2017). Antipsychotics in adolescent-onset psychosis: a work in progress. *Lancet Psychiatry*, **4**, e16–e17.

Jansen, J. E., Gleeson, J., Bendall, S., Rice, S., & Alvarez-Jimenez, M. (2020). Acceptance- and mindfulness-based interventions for persons with psychosis: a systematic review and meta-analysis. *Schizophrenia Research*, **215**, 25–37.

Johannessen, J. O., Larsen, T. K., Joa, I., Melle, I., Friis, S., Opjordsmoen, S., et al. (2005). Pathways to care for first-episode psychosis in an early detection healthcare sector: part of the Scandinavian TIPS study. *British Journal of Psychiatry*, **187**(Suppl. 48), s24–28.

Jongsma, H. E., Turner, C., Kirkbride, J. B., & Jones, P. B. (2019). International incidence of psychotic disorders, 2002–17: a systematic review and meta-analysis. *Lancet Public Health*, **4**, e229–e244.

Kahn, R. S., Fleischhacker, W. W., Boter, H., Davidson, M., Vergouwe, Y., Keet, I. P., et al. (2008). Effectiveness of antipsychotic drugs in first-episode schizophrenia and schizophreniform disorder: an open randomised clinical trial. *Lancet*, **371**, 1085–1097.

Kelleher, I., Connor, D., Clarke, M. C., Devlin, N., Harley, M., & Cannon, M. (2012). Prevalence of psychotic symptoms in childhood and adolescence: a systematic review and meta-analysis of population-based studies. *Psychological Medicine*, **42**, 1857–1863.

Kelleher, I. & DeVylder, J. E. (2017). Hallucinations in borderline personality disorder and common mental disorders. *British Journal of Psychiatry*, **210**, 230–231.

Kessing, L. V., Vradi, E., & Andersen, P. K. (2015). Life expectancy in bipolar disorder. *Bipolar Disorders*, **17**, 543–548.

Kessler, R. C., Berglund, P., Demler, O., Jin, R., Merikangas, K. R., & Walters, E. E. (2005). Lifetime prevalence and age-of-onset distributions of DSM-IV disorders in the National Comorbidity Survey Replication. *Archives of General Psychiatry*, **62**, 593–602.

Killackey, E., Allott, K., Jackson, H. J., Scutella, R., Tseng, Y. P., Borland, J., et al. (2019). Individual placement and support for vocational recovery in first-episode psychosis: randomised controlled trial. *British Journal of Psychiatry*, **214**, 76–82.

Kirkbride, J. B., Morgan, C., Fearon, P., Dazzan, P., Murray, R. M., & Jones, P. B. (2007). Neighbourhood-level effects on psychoses: re-examining the role of context. *Psycholological Medicine*, **37**, 1413–1425.

Krabbendam, L., Myin-Germeys, I., Bak, M., & van Os, J. (2005). Explaining transitions over the hypothesized psychosis continuum. *Australian & New Zealand Journal of Psychiatry*, **39**, 180–186.

Kurihara, T., Kato, M., Reverger, R., Tirta, I. G. R., & Kashima, H. (2005). Never-treated patients with schizophrenia in the developing country of Bali. *Schizophrenia Research*, **79**, 307–313.

Lally, J., Ajnakina, O., Stubbs, B., Cullinane, M., Murphy, K. C., Gaughran, F., & Murray, R. M. (2017). Remission and recovery from first-episode psychosis in adults: systematic review and meta-analysis of long-term outcome studies. *British Journal of Psychiatry*, **211**, 350–358.

Lappin, J. M., Heslin, M., Jones, P. B., Doody, G. A., Reininghaus, U. A., Demjaha, A., et al. (2016). Outcomes following first-episode psychosis—why we should intervene early in all ages, not only in youth. *Australian & New Zealand Journal of Psychiatry*, **50**, 1055–1063.

Leighton, S. P., Upthegrove, R., Krishnadas, R., Benros, M. E., Broome, M. R., Gkoutos, G. V., et al. (2019). Development and validation of multivariable prediction models of remission, recovery, and quality of life outcomes in people with first episode psychosis: a machine learning approach. *Lancet Digital Health*, **1**, e261–e270.

Lieberman, J. A., Tollefson, G. D., Charles, C., Zipursky, R., Sharma, T., Kahn, R. S., et al. (2005). Antipsychotic drug effects on brain morphology in first-episode psychosis. *Archives General Psychiatry*, **62**, 361–370.

Malla, A. (2022). Reducing duration of untreated psychosis: the neglected dimension of early intervention services. *American Journal of Psychiatry*, **179**, 259–261.

Malla, A., Iyer, S., McGorry, P., Cannon, M., Coughlan, H., Singh, S., et al. (2016). From early intervention in psychosis to youth mental health reform: a review of the evolution and transformation of mental health services for young people. *Social Psychiatry & Psychiatric Epidemiology*, **51**, 319–326.

Marshall, M., Harrigan, S. M., & Lewis, S. (2009). Duration of untreated psychosis: definition, measurement and association with outcome. In: Jackson, H. & McGorry, P. D. (Eds.), *The Recognition and Management of Early Psychosis: A Preventative Approach* (pp. 125–145). Cambridge: Cambridge University Press.

Mbewe, E., Haworth, A., Welham, J., Mubanga, D., Chazulwa, R., Zulu, M. M., et al. (2006). Clinical and demographic features of treated first-episode psychotic disorders: a Zambian study. *Schizophrenia Research*, **86**, 202–207.

McCrone, P., Dhanasiri, S., Patel, A., Knapp, M., & Lawton-Smith, S. (2008). *Paying the Price: The Cost of Mental Health Care in England to 2026*. London: The King's Fund.

McGlashan, T. H. (2006). Is active psychosis neurotoxic? *Schizophrenia Bulletin*, **32**, 609–613.

McGorry, P. D., Cocks, J., Power, P., Burnett, P., Harrigan, S., & Lambert, T. (2011). Very low-dose risperidone in first-episode psychosis: a safe and effective way to initiate treatment. *Schizophrenia Research and Treatment*, **2011**, 631690.

McGorry, P. D. & Hickie, I. B. (Eds.) (2019). *Clinical Staging in Psychiatry*. Cambridge: Cambridge University Press.

McGorry, P. D., Hickie, I. B., Yung, A. R., Pantelis, C., & Jackson, H. J. (2006). Clinical staging of psychiatric disorders: a heuristic framework for choosing earlier, safer and more effective interventions. *Australian & New Zealand Journal of Psychiatry*, **40**, 616–622.

McGorry, P., Johanessen, J. O., Lewis, S., Birchwood, M., Malla, A., Nordentoft, M., et al. (2010). Early intervention in psychosis: keeping faith with evidence-based health care. *Psychological Medicine*, **40**, 399–404.

McGrath, J. J., Saha, S., Al-Hamzawi, A., Alonso, J., Bromet, E. J., Bruffaerts, R., et al. (2015). Psychotic experiences in the general population: a cross-national analysis based on 31,261 respondents from 18 countries. *JAMA Psychiatry*, **72**, 697–705.

McHugo, M., Armstrong, K., Roeske, M. J., Woodward, N. D., Blackford, J. U., & Heckers, S. (2020). Hippocampal volume in early psychosis: a 2-year longitudinal study. *Translational Psychiatry*, **10**, 303.

McNab, C. & Linszen, D. (2009). Family intervention in early psychosis. In: Jackson, H. & McGorry, P. (Eds.), *The Recognition and Management of Early Psychosis: A Preventative Approach* (pp. 305–329). Cambridge: Cambridge University Press.

Mei, C., van der Gaag, M., Nelson, B., Smit, F., Yuen, H. P., Berger, M., et al. (2021). Preventive interventions for individuals at ultra high risk for psychosis: an updated and extended meta-analysis. *Clinical Psychology Review*, **86**, 102005.

Melle, I., Larsen, T. K., Haahr, U., Friis, S., Johannessen, J. O., Opjordsmoen, S., et al. (2004). Reducing the duration of untreated first-episode psychosis: effects on clinical presentation. *Archives of General Psychiatry*, **61**, 143–150.

Merlo, M. C., Hofer, H., Gekle, W, Berger, G., Ventura, J., Panhuber, I., et al. (2002). Risperidone, 2 mg/day vs. 4 mg/day, in first-episode, acutely psychotic patients: treatment efficacy and effects on fine motor functioning. *Journal of Clinical Psychiatry*, **63**, 885–891.

Miller, T. J., McGlashan, T. H., Rosen, J. L., Cadenhead, K., Cannon, T., Ventura, J., et al. (2003). Prodromal assessment with the structured interview for prodromal syndromes and the scale of prodromal symptoms: predictive validity, interrater reliability, and training to reliability. *Schizophrenia Bulletin*, **29**, 703–715.

Mitchell, A. J., Vancampfort, D., Sweers, K., van Winkel, R., Yu, W., & De Hert, M. (2013). Prevalence of metabolic syndrome and metabolic abnormalities in schizophrenia and related disorders—a systematic review and meta-analysis. *Schizophrenia Bulletin*, **39**, 306–318.

Morgan, C., Gayer-Anderson, C., Beards, S., Hubbard, K., Mondelli, V., Di Forti, M., et al. (2020). Threat, hostility and violence in childhood and later psychotic disorder: population-based case-control study. *British Journal of Psychiatry*, **217**, 575–582.

Naismith, S. L., Glozier, N., Carter, P. E., Scott, E., & Hickie, I. B. (2009). Early intervention or cognitive decline: is there a role for multiple behavioural interventions? *Early Intervention in Psychiatry*, **3**, 19–27.

National Institute for Health and Care Excellence (2013). Psychosis and schizophrenia in children and young people: recognition and management. Clinical guideline [CG155]. www.nice.org.uk/Guidance/CG155

National Institute for Health and Care Excellence (2014). Psychosis and schizophrenia in adults: prevention and management. Clinical guideline [CG178]. www.nice.org.uk/guidance/cg178

Nelson, B., Amminger, G. P., & McGorry, P. D. (2018). Recent meta-analyses in the clinical high risk for psychosis population: clinical interpretation of findings and suggestions for future research. *Frontiers in Psychiatry*, **9**, 502.

Neilssen, O. & Large, M. (2010). Rates of homicide during first episode of psychosis and after treatment: a systematic review and meta-analysis. *Schizophrenia Bulletin*, **36**, 702–712.

NHS England (2016). Implementing the early intervention in psychosis and waiting time standard: guidance (NHS England Publications Gateway Reference 04294). https://www.england.nhs.uk/wp-content/uploads/2023/03/B1954-implementing-the-early-intervention-in-psychosis-access-and-waiting-time-standard.pdf

O'Keeffe, D., Kinsella, A., Waddington, J. L., & Clarke, M. (2022). 20-Year prospective, sequential follow-up study of heterogeneity in associations of duration of untreated psychosis with symptoms, functioning, and quality of life following first-episode psychosis. *American Journal of Psychiatry*, **179**, 288–297.

Parellada, E. & Gassó, P. (2021). Glutamate and microglia activation as a driver of dendritic apoptosis: a core pathophysiological mechanism to understand schizophrenia. *Translational Psychiatry*, **11**, 271.

Patel, R., Reiss, P., Shetty, H., Broadbent, M., Stewart, R., McGuire, P., & Taylor, M. (2015). Do antidepressants increase the risk of mania and bipolar disorder in people with depression? A retrospective electronic case register cohort study. *BMJ Open*, **5**, e008341.

Pelizza, L., Pellegrini, C., Quattrone, E., Azzali, S., Landi, G., Pellegrini, P., & Leuci, E. (2020). Suicidal ideation in patients experiencing a first-episode psychosis: findings from the 2-year follow-up of the 'Parma Early Psychosis' program. *Suicide & Life-Threatening Behavior*, **50**, 838–855.

Pelosi, A. (2009). Is early intervention in the major psychiatric disorders justified? No. *BMJ*, **337**, a710.

Perkins, D. O., Gu, H., Boteva, K., & Lieberman, J. A. (2005). Relationship between duration of untreated psychosis and outcome in first-episode schizophrenia: a critical review and meta-analysis. *American Journal of Psychiatry*, **162**, 1785–1804.

Pharoah, F., Mari, J. J., Rathbone, J., & Wong, W. (2010). Family intervention for schizophrenia. *Cochrane Database of Systematic Reviews*, **12**, CD000088.

Pinfold, V., Smith, J., & Shiers, D. (2007). Audit of early intervention service development in England in 2005. *Psychiatric Bulletin*, **31**, 7–10.

Power, P., Iacoponi, E., Reynolds, N., Fisher, H., Russell, M., Garety, P., et al. (2007). The Lambeth Early Onset Crisis Assessment Team Study: general practitioner education and access to an early detection team in first-episode psychosis. *British Journal of Psychiatry*, **191**(Suppl. 51), s133–s139.

Power, P. & McGowan, S. (2011). Suicide risk management in early intervention. National Mental Health Development Unit. https://easacommunity.org/files/IRIS%20suicide-risk-management-in-the-first-epsiode-of-psychosis.pdf

Power, P., McGuire, P., Iacoponi, E., Garety, P., Morris, E., Valmaggia, L., et al. (2007). Lambeth Early Onset and Outreach and support in South London services. *Early Intervention in Psychiatry*, **1**, 97–103.

Power, P. & Robinson, J. (2009). Suicide prevention in first-episode psychosis. In: Jackson, H. & McGorry, P. (Eds.), *The Recognition and Management of Early Psychosis: A Preventative Approach* (pp. 257–282). Cambridge: Cambridge University Press.

Puntis, S., Minichino, A., De Crescenzo, F., Cipriani, A., Lennox, B., & Harrison, R. (2020). Specialised early intervention teams (extended time) for recent-onset psychosis. *Cochrane Database of Systematic Reviews*, **11**, CD013287.

Reay, R., Mitford, E., McCabe, K., Paxton, R., & Turkington, D. (2010). Incidence and diagnostic diversity in first-episode psychosis. *Acta Psychiatrica Scandinavica*, **121**, 315–319.

Reeves, S., Stewart, R., & Howard, R. (2002). Service contact and psychopathology in very-late-onset schizophrenia-like psychosis: the effects of gender and ethnicity. *International Journal Geriatric Psychiatry*, **17**, 473–479.

Reimann, H. & Hafner, H. (1973). Mental disorders of the elderly in Mannheim: an investigation of incidence rate. *Social Psychiatry*, **7**, 53–69.

Robinson, D., Woerner, M. G., Alvir, J. M., Bilder, R., Goldman, R., Geisler, S., et al. (1999). Predictors of relapse following response from a first episode of schizophrenia or schizoaffective disorder. *Archives of General Psychiatry*, **56**, 241–247.

Salazar de Pablo G, Radua J, Pereira J, et al. Probability of Transition to Psychosis in Individuals at Clinical High Risk: An Updated Meta-analysis. JAMA Psychiatry 2021; 78(9): 970-8.

Shiers, D., Jones, P. B., & Field, S. (2009). Early intervention in psychosis: keeping the body in mind. *British Journal of General Practice*, **59**, 395–396.

Schmidt, S. J., Schultze-Lutter, F., Schimmelmann, B. G., Maric, N. P., Salokangas, R. K., Riecher-Rössler, A., et al. (2015). EPA guidance on the early intervention in clinical high risk states of psychoses. *European Psychiatry*, **30**, 388–404.

Schoeler, T., Petros, N., Di Forti, M., Pingault, J. B., Klamerus, E., Foglia, E., et al. (2016). Association between continued cannabis use and risk of relapse in first-episode psychosis: a quasi-experimental investigation within an observational study. *JAMA Psychiatry*, **73**, 1173–1179.

Schooler, N., Rabinowitz, J., Davidson, M., Emsley, R., Harvey, P. D., Kopala, L., et al. (2005). Risperidone and haloperidol in first-episode psychosis: a long-term randomized trial. *American Journal of Psychiatry*, **162**, 947–953

Singh, S., Wright, C. T., Joyce, E., Barnes, T., & Burns, T. (2003). Developing early intervention services in the NHS: a survey to guide workforce and training needs. *Psychiatric Bulletin*, **27**, 254–258

Skikic, M. & Arriola, J. A. (2020). First episode psychosis medical workup: evidence-informed recommendations and introduction to a clinically guided approach. *Child and Adolescent Psychiatric Clinics of North America*, **29**, 15–28.

Somaiya, J., Thompson, A., O'Donoghue, B., & Brown, E. (2022). Delivery of an online psychosocial recovery program during COVID-19: a survey of young people attending a youth mental health service. *Early Intervention in Psychiatry*, **16**, 1259–1266.

Sunwoo, M., O'Connell, J., Brown, E., Lin, A., Wood, S. J., McGorry, P., & O'Donoghue, B. (2020). Prevalence and outcomes of young people with concurrent autism spectrum disorder and first episode of psychosis. *Schizophrenia Research*, **216**, 310–315.

Susai, S. R., Sabherwal, S., Mongan, D., Föcking, M., & Cotter, D. R. (2022). Omega-3 fatty acid in ultra-high-risk psychosis: a systematic review based on functional outcome. *Early Intervention in Psychiatry*, **16**, 3–16.

Taipale, H., Tanskanen, A., Correll, C. U., & Tiihonen, J. (2022). Real-world effectiveness of antipsychotic doses for relapse prevention in patients with first-episode schizophrenia in Finland: a nationwide, register-based cohort study. *Lancet Psychiatry*, **9**, 271–279.

Thien, K., Bowtell, M., Eaton, S., Bardell-Williams, M., Downey, L., Ratheesh, A., et al. (2018). Clozapine use in early psychosis. *Schizophrenia Research*, **199**, 374–379.

Thien, K. & O'Donoghue, B. (2019). Delays and barriers to the commencement of clozapine in eligible people with a psychotic disorder: a literature review. *Early Intervention in Psychiatry*, **13**, 18–23

Thornicroft, G. (2007). Most people with mental illness are not treated. *Lancet*, **370**, 807–808.

Trubetskoy, V., Pardiñas, A. F., Qi, T., Panagiotaropoulou, G., Panagiotaropoulou, G., Awasthi, S., Bigdeli, T. B., et al. (2022). Mapping genomic loci implicates genes and synaptic biology in schizophrenia. *Nature*, **604**, 502–508.

Vahia, I. V., Palmer, B. W., Depp, C., Fellows, I., Golshan, S., Kraemer, H. C., & Jeste, D. V. (2010). Is late-onset schizophrenia a subtype of schizophrenia? *Acta Psychiatrica Scandinavica*, **122**, 414–426.

Valmaggia, L. R., Byrne, M., Day, F., Broome, M. R., Johns, L., Howes, O., et al. (2015). Duration of untreated psychosis and need for admission in patients who engage with mental health services in the prodromal phase. *British Journal of Psychiatry*, **207**, 130–134.

van Os, J., Hanssen, M., Bijl, R. V., & Vollebergh, W. (2001). Prevalence of psychotic disorder and community level of psychotic symptoms: an urban-rural comparison. *Archives of General Psychiatry*, **58**, 663–668.

van Os, J. & Poulton, R. (2009). Environmental vulnerability and genetic-environmental interactions. In: Jackson, H. & McGorry, P. (Eds.), *The Recognition and Management of Early Psychosis: A Preventative Approach* (pp. 47–59). Cambridge: Cambridge University Press.

Velakoulis, D., Wood, S. J., Wong, M. T., McGorry, P. D., Yung, A., Phillips, L., et al. (2006). Hippocampal and amygdala volumes according to psychosis stage and diagnosis: a magnetic resonance imaging study of chronic schizophrenia, first-episode psychosis, and ultra-high-risk individuals. *Archives of General Psychiatry*, **63**, 139–149.

Vita, A. & Barlati, S. (2018). Recovery from schizophrenia: is it possible? *Current Opinion in Psychiatry*, **31**, 246–255.

Wießner, I., Falchi, M., Palhano-Fontes, F., Feilding, A., Ribeiro, S., & Tófoli, L. F. (2021). LSD, madness and healing: mystical experiences as possible link between psychosis model and therapy model. *Psychological Medicine*, **53**, 1151–1165.

Weinberger, D. & Berger, G. (2009). Genetic vulnerability. In: Jackson, H. & McGorry, P. (Eds.), *The Recognition and Management of Early Psychosis: A Preventative Approach* (pp. 32–46). Cambridge: Cambridge University Press.

Wilson, R. S., Yung, A. R., & Morrison, A. P. (2020). Comorbidity rates of depression and anxiety in first episode psychosis: a systematic review and meta-analysis. *Schizophrenia Research*, **216**, 322–329.

Wunderink, L., Nienhuis, F. J., Sytema, S., Slooff, C. J., Knegtering, R., & Wiersma, D. (2007). Guided discontinuation versus maintenance treatment in remitted first-episode psychosis: relapse rates and functional outcome. *Journal of Clinical Psychiatry*, **68**, 654–661.

Young, A. H., Ferrier, I. N., & Michalak, E. E. (Eds.) (2010). *Practical Management of Bipolar Disorder*. Cambridge: Cambridge University Press.

Yung, A. R., Klosterkotter, J., Cornblatt, B., & Schultze-Lutter, F. (2009). At-risk mental state and prediction. In: Jackson, H. & McGorry, P. (Eds.), *The Recognition and Management of Early Psychosis: A Preventative Approach* (pp. 83–105). Cambridge: Cambridge University Press.

Yung, A. R., Yuen, H. P., McGorry, P. D., Phillips, L. J., Kelly, D., Dell'Olio, M., et al. (2005). Mapping the onset of psychosis: the Comprehensive Assessment of At-Risk Mental States. *Australian & New Zealand Journal of Psychiatry*, **39**, 964–971.

Zalpuri, I. & Singh, M. K. (2017). Treatment of psychiatric symptoms among offspring of parents with bipolar disorder. *Current Treatment Options in Psychiatry*, **4**, 341–356.

Zhang, J. P., Gallego, J. A., Robinson, D. G., Malhotra, A. K., Kane, J. M., & Correll, C. U. (2013). Efficacy and safety of individual second-generation vs. first-generation antipsychotics in first-episode psychosis: a systematic review and meta-analysis. *International Journal of Neuropsychopharmacology*, **16**, 1205–1218.

Zipursky, R. B., Menezes, N. M., & Streiner, D. L. (2014). Risk of symptom recurrence with medication discontinuation in first-episode psychosis: a systematic review. *Schizophrenia Research*, **152**, 408–414.

14

Case management and assertive community treatment

Helen Killaspy and Alan Rosen

Introduction

Recent decades have seen the relocation of psychiatric care from hospital-based settings to community-based services in many countries. The initial phases of deinstitutionalization led to a replication of the general hospital outpatient clinic model for review of community patients by psychiatrists, but gradually services began to expand the support available to people with more severe mental health problems. Over time, the addition of nurses, psychologists, occupational therapists, and social workers led to the establishment of community mental health teams (CMHTs). As community health and social care provision expanded, it became an increasingly complex system to navigate. Case management was developed to address this by assigning individual staff to assess service users' needs and coordinate their treatment and care. Contemporary mental health services use a variety of models of case management of which assertive community treatment (ACT) is the most intensive and clearly defined form. Assertive outreach is another term for ACT used in the UK. In some countries, case managers are referred to as 'care coordinators'. This chapter explores these models of community mental health care, the evidence for them, and the possible explanations for the discrepancies in their effectiveness reported in the international literature.

Types of case management

Case management is the process of drawing together and ensuring coordinated delivery of all the services and interventions required to address service users' needs (e.g. medication, psychological and social interventions, appropriate accommodation, access to welfare benefits, assistance with day-to-day activities, budgeting and paying bills, and support to engage with education, employment, or other community-based activities). Various models of case management have been described and categorized according to the main focus and expected outcomes of the work (e.g. clinical, social networks, strengths, rehabilitation) or the type of support offered (e.g. passive response/brokerage or active response models) (Table 14.1) (see Rosen & Teeson, 2001). Case management has also been developed for specific groups of mental health service users (e.g. those receiving care from forensic services, older people, younger people, and those in the first episode of psychosis) as well as for people with other complex conditions (such as brain injury or neurological disorders). The brokerage model historically comprised of an administrative approach from relatively junior and generic, office-based staff that involved little more than referring service users to appropriate resources. Over time it has become increasingly clinically orientated, with assessments and interventions being led by more highly qualified and experienced mental health professionals working together in CMHTs and holding individual caseloads. The approach in many countries has also become more proactive and many contacts are made in the client's home. The main aims are to improve clinical and social outcomes and to intervene to avoid relapse and hospital admission wherever possible.

All mental health services are encouraged to use a 'recovery' orientation that engages clients in a collaborative 'doing with' partnership rather than a didactic 'doing to' approach (Roberts & Wolfson, 2004), regardless of the model of case management used. The analogy of evolution from a 'travel agent' to a 'travel companion' to a 'travel guide' has also been used to describe the proactive, supportive, collaborative, outreaching, and expert role of the case manager (Rosen & Teesson, 2001). More recently, the role of the case manager has been augmented and complemented by support workers, who are often individuals with lived experience of mental health problems or people with a family member with a mental health problem (often referred to as 'peer support workers'). A systematic review of studies of case management conducted in 2016 highlights the increasingly complex nature of the role of the case manager; 22 definitions and five models were identified, encompassing 69 different activities and 17 types of intervention (Lukersmith et al., 2016).

Evidence for case management

A systematic review of randomized controlled trials of case management (excluding ACT) found that it was efficacious at maintaining contact with service users but not at improving clinical outcomes

Table 14.1 Models of case management

Case management model	(A) Clinical (Stein and Test) (Harris and Bergman) (Lamb) (Kantor)	(B) Networking (Harris and Bergman) (Bachrach) (Drake)	(C) Strengths (Rapp)	(D) Rehabilitation (Anthony & Farkas)
1. Focus	INDIVIDUAL PERSPECTIVE i.e. dyad • Intensive outreach	SOCIAL SYSTEMS • Enhance impoverished networks	OPTIMISM • Empowerment • Mastery • Collaboration	EDUCATION/TRAINING • Brokerage • Skills • Support
2. Aims	1. To support the client to develop their: • functioning • sense of self • relationships • interests	1. To increase the capacity of the client's natural or devised social networks to provide: • emotional support • tangible aid • advice • information • companionship	1. To help client to become more competent and confident in managing various life skills (Midwest US Utopian Strain)	1. To broker or negotiate for all the services the client needs or wants
	2. Outreach into community	2. To enhance impoverished networks (e.g. of homeless clients) and to increase client's social margin	2. Achievements and opportunities more important than failures and limitations	2. To develop the client's skills and supports and improve their satisfaction with care
	3. Intensive (high frequency) contact at times of crisis		3. To foster collaboration	3. To develop client's autonomy and independence
3. Initial motivation required	Requires LOW initial engagement/cooperation/motivation		Requires HIGH initial engagement/education/cooperation/motivation	
4. Case manager role	Therapist or clinician (as well as securing resources)	Facilitator, Conductor, Network member	Collaborator and Companion	Manager, Broker of resources, Teacher guide
5. Training	Clinical professional background	Professional or para-professional group or system training	Graduate-level lay person (doesn't require extensive clinical knowledge)	Graduate with technical training in rehabilitation
6. Who benefits?	Clients who are difficult to engage Clients with a potential for insight	Clients with large, unhelpful networks (e.g. drug culture) or no networks (e.g. homeless)	Clients who are able to engage (not more marginalized groups, e.g. homeless, substance misuse)	Educated and goal-driven individuals

Adapted from Rosen, A. and Teesson, M. (2001). Does case management work? The evidence and the abuse of evidence based medicine. *Australian and New Zealand Journal of Psychiatry*, 35, 731–746.

including quality of life, symptoms, and social functioning (Marshall et al., 1998). Although a subsequent national study in Australia showed that case management reduced the chances of hospital admission for people with serious mental health problems threefold (Morgan et al., 2006), a systematic review of studies of various designs (not just randomized trials) found case management to be only moderately effective for service users with the most severe and complex mental health needs, especially when caseloads were high (Mueser et al., 1998). More intensive models with lower caseloads were developed to try to address this. Intensive case management has been defined as case management where the ratio of service users to staff is less than 20:1, and ACT is considered the most intensive form of case management (Burns et al., 2007) with ratios of around 10:1.

Development of ACT

One of the first models of community-based treatment was Stein and Test's (1980) 'Training in Community Living', an alternative approach to admission to psychiatric hospital in Madison, Wisconsin that involved moving ward staff out of the hospital to work with service users in their own homes. The model was tested in a randomized controlled trial and found to be able to prevent admissions (Stein & Test, 1980). It was successfully replicated in Sydney, Australia where substantially better outcomes for the subsample with schizophrenia were found (Hoult, 1986; Hoult et al., 1984) and it gradually evolved into two specific home treatment models: ACT and 24-hour mobile crisis resolution teams. Crisis resolution aims to treat people at home during a period of acute mental health crisis and avoid the need for hospital admission. It is an intensive, time-limited (usually to a few weeks or months) approach used for service users with any type of mental health problem. This model proved inadequate to keep individuals with severe and persistent disability from recurrent admissions to hospital and ACT was therefore developed with a specific focus on those with longer-term mental health problems such as schizophrenia, schizoaffective disorder, and bipolar affective disorder who have particularly complex problems (including functional and cognitive impairment and comorbidities such as substance misuse), social needs (such as homelessness and social isolation), and difficulties in engaging with standard community mental health services. This category of service users, historically, was often referred to as the 'revolving door' group due to their recurrent cycle of relapse in the community, readmission (often involuntarily), treatment, improvement in symptoms and functioning, discharge from hospital, failure to engage with community services, discontinuation of medication, relapse, and readmission. The ACT approach aims to address the needs of service users with more severe, persistent, or recurrent and complex problems for whom standard case management is inadequate. Leonard Stein, one of the co-founders of the ACT model, described it as a completely new class of intervention to case management, emphasizing critical differences in practice. In many countries, ACT is considered the 'gold standard' of case management (Rosen & Teeson, 2001; Rosen et al., 2007) that has gradually evolved into an internationally accepted model (McGrew et al., 1994) and that attempts to intervene in the 'revolving door' cycle to prevent readmission by maintaining therapeutic engagement and improving functioning through supporting adherence to treatment and care and facilitating successful community rehabilitation. The fidelity of ACT teams to this model can be assessed using the Dartmouth ACT Scale (DACTS; Teague et al., 1998). The model has further evolved with advances in evidence and practice to include other features (such as the adoption of a recovery-oriented approach, promotion of physical health, and family involvement), assessed using the Tool for Measurement of Assertive Community Treatment (TMACT; Monroe-DeVita et al., 2011).

Differences between standard case management and ACT

A number of books and guidelines have detailed ACT staffing and practice (Allness & Knoedler, 1998; Department of Health, 2001; Stein & Santos, 1998). Differences in ACT and standard case management by community mental health services are summarized in Table 14.2. The ACT team takes full responsibility for its clients when in the community and in hospital. ACT teams should be staffed with a full complement of the different mental health professional disciplines (psychiatry, nursing, occupational therapy, psychology, social work) and non-professional staff should also be represented such as support workers. Some staff should be service users in recovery, operating as peer support workers (Rosen et al., 2007) and there should be at least one vocational rehabilitation expert, a physical health care coordinator, and one co-occuring or 'dual' disorder expert (for service users with coexisting alcohol and other substance misuse and mental health problems) within the team. The team should have their own inpatient beds and be responsible for their own clients' admissions and discharges.

ACT staff work with smaller service user to staff ratios (maximum 10–12:1) than standard community mental health services (around 30–35 per worker) and the maximum total number of service users for an ACT team is around 100 (compared to around 350 for a standard CMHT). They also share their person-to-person work with other team members, so that over time all staff get to know all the team's clients. This is facilitated by working shifts to provide an extended hours service (usually around 12 hours per day including weekends) and by having daily team meetings where clients are discussed and the work for each day is planned. This sharing of cases is known as 'the team approach' or 'team case management'. Although some ACT teams use only team case management, there is no evidence to suggest that clients should not also have an individual case manager to coordinate their care by other team members and to coach and advocate for them (Rosen et al., 2007). In the standard case management model, there may be very little sharing of work between team members (other than covering each other's caseloads when a team member is away), with the exception of the psychiatrist and junior doctor who are likely to work alongside case managers with all the team's clients.

The small caseloads mean that ACT teams can provide a more intensive service, with around three times the number of face-to-face contacts of standard services (Killaspy et al., 2006). The bulk of these take place in the service user's home or elsewhere in the community whereas in standard case management, the majority of appointments are arranged at the team's office. Seeing service users at home or in another community location away from the office is known as '*in vivo*' work. The ACT teams prioritize assisting the individual with social needs as much as other aspects of treatment and support (such as medication), providing practical assistance with housing to support service users to maintain their tenancy, support with finances (such as assistance with banking and ensuring the client is

Table 14.2 Differences between ACT and standard community mental health services

ACT team	Standard community mental health team
Total team client number: 80–100	Total team client numbers: 300–350
Extended hours (0800–2100 every day)	Office hours only (0900–1700 Mon–Fri)
'In vivo' work, i.e. meet client at home or in café, park, etc.	Office-based appointments and home visits
Assertive engagement: multiple attempts, flexible and various approaches, e.g. befriending, offering practical support	Offer appointments at office and/or home visits
'No drop-out' policy, i.e. commitment to continue to try to engage over the long term	Discharge if unable to make or maintain contact
Maximum individual staff caseload: staff:client ratio = 1:12	Maximum individual staff caseload: staff:client ratio = 1:35
Team based approach, i.e. all team members work with all clients	Case management—very little sharing of work with individual clients between team members
Frequent (daily) team meetings to discuss clients and daily plans	Weekly team meetings
Use skills of team rather than outside agencies as much as possible	'Brokerage', i.e. referral to outside agencies for advice and services on, e.g. social security benefits, housing, employment, substance misuse

Data from Killaspy, H., Bebbington, P., Blizard, R., Johnson, S., Nolan, F., Pilling, S., & King, M. (2006). REACT: a Randomised Evaluation of Assertive Community Treatment in North London. *BMJ*, 332, 815–819.

receiving the welfare benefits they are entitled to), and support with everyday living tasks (such as personal hygiene, socializing, family contact, shopping, cooking, and cleaning). They use a collaborative approach to facilitate engagement and try to provide as much support as they can from the expertise of the ACT team members, rather than brokering out to other services.

Both standard case management and ACT provide individual and family/carer support, psychological interventions, and other evidence-based interventions including support with medication, but ACT teams have the flexibility, because of their smaller caseloads and extended hours, to provide more support including delivering and administering prescribed medications where necessary. This also means that if a service user is relapsing, the ACT team can increase their level of support, recalibrate medication rapidly, and hopefully avoid the need for admission, where standard services would need to make a referral to the crisis resolution service (where it exists) for more intensive home-based support. The ACT teams can also ensure that service users attend welfare, medical, and other health care appointments and complete required investigations and interventions to improve and maintain their general health. If the service user has difficulties organizing themselves to attend these appointments, the ACT team can also attend these appointments with them. The support and education that ACT can provide to families and informal carers is also more intensive than standard case management as they are more likely to meet due to the higher frequency of home visits and their ability to visit out of office hours (Killaspy et al., 2009a). This has been shown to result in greater client and family satisfaction with services than standard case management (Hoult et al., 1984).

Evidence for ACT

The ACT model is one of the most extensively evaluated mental health interventions and there is good evidence for its efficacy (Bond et al., 2001; Mueser et al., 1998). A Cochrane review published in 1998 identified 75 randomized controlled trials comparing ACT to some form of standard care such as an outpatient clinic or community mental health service. It included 17 of these in a meta-analysis that concluded that when targeted at high users of inpatient services, ACT reduced the costs of care by decreasing the frequency and length of admissions. Other positive outcomes included increased engagement with services, more stability in accommodation, and improved satisfaction for patients and their carers (Marshall & Lockwood, 1998). Its cost-effectiveness was further established in a subsequent review (Latimer, 1999). However, studies evaluating ACT in England and other European countries with well-developed community mental health services have not replicated these positive findings (Burns et al., 2002), possibly due to inadequate implementation of the ACT model and greater access to inpatient services. These issues are further explored later in this chapter.

The original Cochrane meta-analysis (Marshall & Lockwood, 1998) included only two European trials (Aberg-Wistedt, 1995; Audini et al., 1994), the rest being from the US or Canada. A randomized controlled trial of intensive case management/ACT in Australia showed modest advantage over standard case management for participants in social functioning but not in inpatient service use (Issakidis et al., 1999). Although this study was not funded to assess outcomes beyond 12-month follow-up and so further potential gains from longer-term ACT could not be reported, a number of randomized controlled trials of intensive case management for people with severe and enduring mental health problems in the UK also showed somewhat less impressive gains from ACT than the US trials (Burns et al., 1999; Harrison-Read et al., 2002; Holloway & Carson, 1998; Thornicroft et al., 1998). However, it is important to note that none of these studies were designed specifically to investigate the ACT model (McGrew et al., 1994). They were heavily criticized for their methodological limitations (Marshall et al., 1999) and their conclusions that ACT showed no advantage over standard care when the experimental intervention bore only limited resemblance to ACT (Rosen & Teesson, 2001). Recognizing the need for more evidence about the effectiveness of ACT in the UK, the Cochrane review recommended that a robust trial should be carried out (Marshall & Lockwood, 1998).

ACT in England and the REACT study

Despite the underwhelming findings of the UK studies, the strength of the international evidence in favour of ACT led to it being incorporated into the National Service Framework for Mental Health in England (Department of Health, 1999), a major policy initiative that provided guidance and funding for new community mental health services. By 2004, 263 ACT teams had been set up across the country (Department of Health, 2005). This provided an opportunity for a definitive randomized controlled trial to compare clinical outcomes and cost effectiveness of ACT with standard treatment from CMHTs for clients identified as difficult to engage and who were high users of inpatient care. Evaluating the effectiveness of ACT as teams developed had the advantage that professionals were enthusiastic and prepared for scrutiny of their work and there was less ethical concern about randomization to a service that was not available previously.

The Randomised Evaluation of Assertive Community Treatment in North London (REACT) study (Killaspy et al., 2006) involved 251 patients with a diagnosis of a severe and enduring mental health problem (such as schizophrenia, schizoaffective disorder, or bipolar affective disorder) who had high use of inpatient services in the previous 2 years and were identified by CMHTs as difficult to engage. They were randomly allocated to receive ACT from one of two local teams or to continue with their CMHT. All the teams were independently assessed for their model fidelity: one of the ACT teams was assessed as high fidelity and the other as 'ACT-like' (Wright et al., 2003) and all the CMHTs scored as having low ACT model fidelity. The features of the model that were missing for the two ACT teams were not having a substance misuse worker, not employing service users, and not offering a 24-hour service (although both operated in the evenings and weekends). These components were commonly missing across ACT teams in London at the time (Wright et al., 2003). The primary outcome was inpatient service use assessed 18 months after randomization and secondary outcomes included patient satisfaction, engagement, social functioning, symptoms, needs, attitudes towards medication, adverse events, substance misuse, and quality of life.

At follow-up there were no differences in any measure of inpatient service use, clinical functioning, or social functioning between ACT clients and those receiving standard case management from a CMHT (Killaspy et al., 2006). This finding had not changed at 36 months (Killaspy et al., 2009b) or at 10-year follow-up when inpatient service use, social outcomes, and adverse events were investigated (Killaspy et al., 2014). However, ACT clients were better engaged, less likely to drop out of contact with services, and more satisfied with their treatment and support from mental health services than those receiving standard care (Killaspy et al., 2006). The REACT study did not find that ACT was more cost-effective than standard case management, mainly because the bulk of health care costs are in inpatient service use (McCrone et al., 2009). Latimer (1999) found that higher-fidelity ACT reduced inpatient service use by nearly one-quarter more than lower-fidelity programmes but cautioned that, as service systems become less dependent on inpatient units, the cost advantages of ACT would become harder to achieve.

Possible reasons for international differences in effectiveness of ACT

The reasons why ACT does not appear to be as effective in the UK as the US, Australia, and Canada are summarized in Table 14.3. Possible explanations fall into three main categories: similarities between the ACT and comparison service, higher use of inpatient services in the local population, and inadequate implementation of the ACT model.

Similarities in ACT and comparison services

One possible explanation for the lack of effectiveness of ACT in the UK is that the services against which ACT has been compared were more community based than those in the earlier American trials and may have shared some aspects of the ACT approach. There is some evidence for this since although home treatment teams in the US (and Australia) have been reported to make more '*in vivo*' contacts than UK teams, CMHTs in the UK at the time of the REACT trial made more '*in vivo*' contacts than standard care comparison teams in the US (Burns et al., 2002). However, there does not appear to be evidence for a similar discrepancy in the use of home visiting in experimental and standard care approaches between Australia and the UK (Rosen & Teesson, 2001). Since '*in vivo*' work has been found to be one of the most effective components of home treatment (Catty et al., 2002) this difference may therefore be of some relevance in understanding the international research findings.

Morse and McKasson (2005) noted that outcomes from studies investigating the effectiveness of ACT were influenced by the degree to which comparison services offered ACT features. In the REACT study (Killaspy et al., 2006), although ACT model fidelity was low for the comparison community mental health services, they shared with the ACT teams four of seven features subsequently identified as important for the success of intensive case management: primary clinical responsibility, based in the community, team leader doing clinical work, and time-unlimited service (Burns et al., 2007). The other three 'critical ingredients' were that the team meets daily, shares responsibility for caseloads, and is available 24 hours.

High use of inpatient services in the local population

Another possible explanation for the different research findings is that inpatient mental health services in inner cities in the UK operate at a very high admission threshold and interventions aimed at reducing admissions are therefore unlikely to succeed (Burns, 2007). Although the focus on inpatient service use as the main outcome for assessing efficacy and effectiveness of ACT has been criticized as outdated (Rosen et al., 2008a), nevertheless, the participants in the REACT study who received ACT made no greater gains in *any* of the measures of clinical or social function than those receiving standard care. This suggests that CMHTs in the UK at the time of the REACT trial were providing a service which, with fewer face-to-face contacts and higher caseloads, was able to support clients and prevent admissions as effectively as a well-resourced ACT team (Killaspy et al., 2006, 2009b).

Inadequate ACT fidelity

Another possible explanation is that although studies of ACT services in the UK have consistently shown that they can successfully engage with 'hard-to-reach' clients, they were not operating with adequate ACT model fidelity to build on this to deliver the evidence-based interventions likely to improve clinical outcomes. A 2003 survey of ACT teams operating in England found that only 12% of the 222 teams who participated scored as having high model fidelity on the DACTS (Teague et al., 1998). Many did not provide an extended hours service, few had dedicated inpatient beds and few were adequately staffed to provide appropriate medical and psychosocial interventions: only half had a psychiatrist, only one-fifth had a psychologist, and very few had a substance misuse or vocational rehabilitation specialist. A postal survey of 187 ACT teams (of whom 104 responded) conducted a few years later showed little improvement in this situation: 36% had no psychiatrist, 34% had no occupational therapist, 52% had no psychologist, and 82% had no dedicated

Table 14.3 Factors that may influence the effectiveness of ACT

Factor	Description
Evolution and variability of treatment as usual	Services that ACT has been compared with vary. 'Standard' community mental health care has evolved and may replicate key aspects of the ACT model such as '*in vivo*' working and shared caseloads
Evolution of the ACT model	ACT often incorporates specific evidence-based interventions, expertise, and services (such as supported employment) but the delivery of these varies from team to team
Variability of the ACT model	Incorporation of ACT into other specialist mental health services (e.g. homeless services, early intervention services, forensic services, dual diagnosis services, etc.) may have introduced further variation in the approach
Failure to specify some aspects of the approach	Some aspects of ACT have not been clearly specified (the use or avoidance of coercion is an example) and may be of particular relevance in terms of effectiveness
Variability of social and economic context	In many areas, low-income housing and hospital-based care are severely restricted such that people with severe mental health problems are vulnerable to homelessness, incarceration, and other negative outcomes, but not high rates of hospitalization. Conversely, where there is an 'oversupply' of inpatient beds, studies of ACT are more likely to report a reduction in admissions
Variability in quality of ACT	The quality of ACT teams varies, fidelity assessment only captures some of the variance, and some teams are poorly implemented, supervised, and monitored for outcomes

inpatient beds. Almost all of these teams reported that their main aim was client engagement, suggesting that delivery of evidence-based interventions was not prioritized (Ghosh & Killaspy, 2010). A study that compared ACT in London and Melbourne, Australia also found important differences in staffing and model fidelity: London teams had around one-quarter the amount of input from a psychiatrist compared to Melbourne teams (0.6 full time equivalents per team caseload of 100, compared to 1.9 full-time equivalents); only half the London teams operated outside of office hours whereas all the Melbourne teams did so; the majority of Melbourne teams made the bulk of their client contacts 'in vivo' whereas this was the case for only a third of the London teams' contacts; the Melbourne teams scored higher for use of the team approach (Harvey et al., 2011).

A subsequent Cochrane review of trials of intensive case management, including ACT, has provided further corroboration of these possible explanations for the differences in effectiveness of ACT reported in the international literature (Dieterich et al., 2017). This review included 40 trials with a maximum follow-up period of 36 months. The studies were conducted in a larger range of countries than Marshall and Lockwood's (1998) original Cochrane review. Of the 40 trials, 26 compared intensive case management (i.e. case managers with a caseload maximum of 20 clients) with standard care comprising mainly outpatient clinic appointments, and the remaining 14 trials compared intensive case management with standard case management from a community-based team (with a caseload greater than 20 clients). In comparison with outpatient care, intensive case management was associated with slightly reduced inpatient service use and participants were less likely to drop-out of the trial. In comparison with standard case management, intensive case management was only found to be associated with being less likely to drop out of the trial. A meta-regression conducted as part of the review identified two factors associated with reduced inpatient service use: greater fidelity to the ACT model and a higher level of inpatient service use in the local population.

Active engagement or coercion in ACT

A consistent finding in the international literature is that ACT is more acceptable to 'hard-to-engage' clients than standard case management (Dietrich et al., 2017; Killaspy et al., 2006; Marsall & Lockwood, 1998; Mueser et al., 1998). This appears to be related to the particular style of the ACT approach that engages clients as partners in agreeing their care plans rather than directing them to accept treatment and support (Killaspy et al., 2009a). Although, conversely, it has been postulated that ACT is a coercive, intrusive, and paternalistic approach (Gomory, 2001), the co-founders of ACT have clearly stated that coercion is not part of the model (Test & Stein, 2001). A qualitative study of staff contacts with 45 clients of one ACT in Madison, Wisconsin found very few instances of coercive interactions and a wide range of collaborative approaches to increase clients' engagement (Angell et al., 2006). Similarly, Davidson and Campbell (2007) found that fewer coercive strategies were used by ACT staff in Northern Ireland than other community mental health service staff. In the REACT study (Killaspy et al., 2006), ACT clients' ratings of intrusiveness of the service were lower than CMHT clients, despite having three times the number of contacts, most of which were in their own homes. A qualitative study of clients of an ACT in the US identified various aspects of the approach that were in keeping with recovery orientated practice, such as flexibility, focusing on individuals' strengths, addressing concerns about medication, and building rapport through helping with practical and emotional support (Gandy-Guedes et al., 2018). This collaborative approach has also been reported to 'buffer' client and families' experiences of stigma and discrimination in the community (O'Reilly et al., 2019; Ye et al., 2016).

Specialist and adapted ACT

As the evidence base has evolved, many services have begun to offer variations on the traditional ACT or intensive case management approach, based on the 'critical ingredients', and sometimes targeting specific client groups. For example, specialist community services that work with people experiencing a first episode of psychosis were developed initially in Melbourne, Australia and have spread around the globe. These early intervention for psychosis services include many features of ACT (including smaller caseloads, more 'in vivo' work, and a greater focus on social outcomes such as engagement in education or employment) than standard community teams (Brewer et al., 2015).

Mental health rehabilitation services traditionally focus on those with longer-term, severe, and more complex mental health problems. Many community mental health rehabilitation teams were 're-badged' as Assertive Outreach Teams during the implementation of the National Service Framework for Mental Health in England in the early 2000s (Department of Health, 1999). Due to the lack of clear evidence for the effectiveness of ACT in England, however, there followed a period of disinvestment and there are now only a handful of Assertive Outreach Teams still in existence. However, in the last few years, there has been renewed interest in community rehabilitation teams which are now recommended by the National Institute for Health and Care Excellence (NICE) as a critical component of local mental health rehabilitation services for people with complex psychosis (NICE, 2020). These teams usually work with a shared team caseload, provide a more intensive approach than standard CMHTs, and make most of their contacts with clients 'in vivo'. These cycles of investment and disinvestment in different specialist teams for this client group are challenging, disrupt continuity of care, and are wasteful of resources. It is encouraging though that around two-thirds of NHS mental health trusts in England now have a community mental health rehabilitation team, suggesting that the specialist needs of this group are finally been recognized (Killaspy et al., 2013; Rosen et al., 2013).

Other examples of specialist ACT include teams that target homeless people with severe mental illness (Aubry et al., 2019; Coldwell, 2007), and teams that target those with comorbid substance misuse or alcohol dependence (Drummond et al., 2017; Petterson et al., 2014). There is also encouraging trial evidence from the US for the effectiveness of 'forensic ACT' for people with severe mental health problems who have had contact with the criminal justice system in terms of reduced markers of criminality and reduced inpatient service use (Lamberti et al., 2017). It is noteworthy that a large observational study of ACT teams in the Netherlands also reported reduced contact with the criminal justice system over time (van Vungt et al., 2016).

Evidence for ACT from elsewhere in Europe

Elsewhere in Europe the research on ACT has shown a similar picture to the UK. In the Netherlands, a randomized trial of ACT for clients with longer-term mental health problems and high levels of clinical need failed to find any clinical advantage for ACT over standard community care, although engagement and satisfaction were greater for ACT clients (Sytema et al., 2007). This finding is particularly interesting since the authors noted that there was no shortage of inpatient beds in the rural area where the study was carried out and therefore it might have been expected, given that ACT shows most impact on inpatient service use in areas with higher availability of inpatient beds (Burns et al., 2007; Dietrich et al., 2017), that it would have been associated with a reduction in inpatient days. On the other hand, one could argue that perhaps the easy availability of inpatient beds may have reduced the impetus on the ACT teams to reduce admissions.

In Denmark, a randomized controlled trial of ACT enhanced by family intervention and social skills training for patients experiencing their first episode of psychosis was associated with marginally greater improvements in positive and negative psychotic symptoms than patients who received standard CMHT care, but no difference in inpatient service use (Peterson et al., 2005). It is important to note, however, that the ACT service was office based and rarely carried out home visits and therefore its classification as ACT is questionable.

The implementation of ACT in Norway has also been evaluated, albeit not though not through a randomized trial, but positive findings in terms of reduced inpatient service have been reported (Clausen et al., 2016). Qualitative evaluation also highlighted its ability to improve the support available to and links with family members (Weimand et al., 2018).

Flexible ACT

Potentially more promising results have been found for 'Flexible ACT' (FACT), a Dutch hybrid or diluted variation on ACT which combines within the same team the delivery of ACT or intensive case management and standard care for patients requiring differing levels of support (van Veldhuizen, 2007). The model has been taken up in many Scandinavian countries and, to a smaller extent, in Germany and the UK.

A case–control study by Drukker et al. (2008) that used propensity score matching to compare outcomes for 240 recipients of FACT in one region of the Netherlands with clients receiving standard community care reported beneficial effects with regard to remission among those who were assessed at baseline as having unmet needs related to psychosis. This effect was stronger for those who had no comorbid alcohol problem. Similarly, Nugter et al. (2016) reported that more clients experienced remission and there were statistically significant improvements in compliance, unmet needs, and quality of life over the first 2 years of implementation of three new FACT teams in the Netherlands.

Firn et al. (2013) conducted an evaluation of the impact of a change in function of two ACT teams in south London to FACT teams. They used a 'mirror image' design whereby clients acted as their own controls, with data on service use and social outcomes compared between the 12 months before and after the service change. They found that the switch from ACT to FACT was associated with a reduction in inpatient service use, despite fewer face-to-face contacts, with no adverse effect on social outcomes such as housing stability or employment and no greater use of alternatives to admission such as home treatment teams. There were also considerable cost savings associated with the change in service model. Over each of the subsequent 3 years, clients had fewer admissions and inpatient days compared to the 12 months prior to the switch to FACT, but missed appointments increased. However, there was no increase in the use of crisis services (Firn et al., 2018).

Similarly positive results have also been reported elsewhere in the UK in a non-controlled evaluation of the amalgamation of an ACT team with CMHTs to form FACT teams (Sood et al., 2018). A retrospective before and after study evaluating FACT in Berlin, Germany also reported reductions in inpatient service use and involuntary admissions (Wullschleger et al., 2018). The implementation of FACT teams is also being evaluated in Norway where qualitative findings suggest they are welcomed by staff (Odden et al., 2019) and helping to build bridges between different components of the mental health system (Trane et al., 2021).

The most robust evaluation of FACT to date is that carried out by Munch Nielsen et al. (2021) who conducted a matched case–control study to evaluate the implementation of five FACT teams in Denmark. For clients who had previously been receiving care from CMHTs and those who had previously been receiving ACT, moving to the FACT model was associated with fewer psychiatric admissions but no significant difference in total psychiatric bed days was found for either group when compared to matched CMHT or ACT controls. Rather surprisingly, those who moved from ACT to FACT had more staff contacts than ACT controls, albeit most were office based rather than *in vivo*. The transition to FACT was not associated with more adverse events than controls for either group.

While these studies all provide positive findings for the benefits of FACT it is important to note that, to date, there have been no randomized trials comparing FACT with standard care or with ACT. However, as FACT becomes more widely implemented, it seems increasingly unlikely that such trials will be conducted. As Bond and Drake (2015) posit, ACT has made a monumental contribution to the way in which community mental health services are delivered and the key principles (outreach, delivery of services in the community, holistic and integrated services, and continuity of care) have been incorporated into many community mental health services and remain highly relevant for clients with more complex needs, while the flexibility of the approach enables it to adapt in response to different contexts and research. However, there is a nagging concern that hybrid teams that attempt to incorporate the assertive capability into a standard model of care, rather than implementing stand-alone ACT teams, may experience increasing dilution of the key ACT components over time due to pressure to attend to acute crises arising from new presentations or from routine case management, and/or due to gradual erosion of staffing levels. The assertive care component of FACT may have been sustained in the Netherlands by a powerful tool built into the model by its founder, Dr Remmers van Veldhuizen, which may not be available to FACT teams elsewhere; regular, robust external inspection and monitoring to ensure ongoing fidelity to the flexible assertive care function.

The impact of Covid-19 on case management

The Covid-19 pandemic has seen a huge shift in the way mental health services are delivered, with much greater use of technology and fewer face-to-face contacts. For those with less severe problems, this shift may be welcome in being more convenient than attending an appointment in person. However, for those with more severe or complex needs, telemedicine may not be appropriate due to lack of access or familiarity with the necessary technology (Moreno et al., 2020; Rosen, 2021). Remote methods of communication can also limit therapeutic rapport and reduce the opportunity for the assessment of non-verbal cues. This is particularly relevant for people with more severe mental disorders who may struggle with verbal communication. In addition, if staff are not visiting the person 'in vivo', they cannot assess their environment which can be a useful indicator of their current mental health and needs.

Some services are starting to employ a hybrid approach, using a mix of traditional face-to-face outreach together with telemedicine. There is some pre-pandemic evidence to support this. For example, Blankers et al. (2016) conducted a non-randomized pilot study comparing a blended version of FACT plus videoconferencing with standard FACT. They found both approaches were equally acceptable to service users, and quality of life and confidence were slightly greater for those receiving the blended approach. More research is needed to guide future developments in this area, but it is plausible that providing an adjustable mix of face-to-face and digital services, tailored to the service user's needs, may prove to be both clinically and cost-effective.

For people whose mental health problems are less severe or more stable, some countries have developed services that work at the interface of primary and secondary care. In Australia, shared care workers intervene at times of crisis to provide more intensive support to avoid admission to hospital where possible, as well as providing assessment and advice for new referrals from primary care to secondary mental health care services (Meadows, 1998). In the UK and many other countries, primary care liaison services offer a similar approach and many of these services have been able to shift to remote working through telemedicine without obvious negative consequences so far. However, for those with more severe mental health problems in the UK, although closer liaison between primary care and community mental health services is recommended to ensure access to physical health screening and treatment (NICE, 2020), case management remains in secondary care until the person has reached a level of stability that can be safely managed by their GP or through a primary care liaison service.

Summary

Case management systems may be employed effectively at different levels of intensity to meet the individual needs of different service users. At the lower end of intensity, support needs may simply involve regular medication review and general supportive counselling or coaching. This level of case management is increasingly devolved to primary care or primary care liaison services working across primary and secondary care. Service users with higher levels of need and more complex mental health problems require more intensive support from mobile CMHTs able to provide flexible and proactive response at times of crisis. For those with more severe and persistent problems, ACT has been shown to be the most effective mode of service delivery, but the results of trials of ACT are strongly influenced by the context of the health service within which it is operating and the degree to which model fidelity is achieved. Increasingly, hybrid models that offer greater flexibility of support, such as FACT, are gaining traction, particularly in Scandinavia with encouraging results from quasi-experimental evaluations. However, the lack of randomized controlled trial evaluation and longer-term sustainability studies of hybrid models is concerning and is in sharp contrast to the wealth of evidence for the effectiveness of high-fidelity ACT. The Covid-19 pandemic has accelerated the use of telepsychiatry as an alternative to face-to-face contacts. This appears appropriate for those with less severe mental health problems but an optimal mix of face-to-face and digital services, tailored to the individual's needs may prove to be clinically and cost-effective for those with more severe problems (Rosen, 2021; Rosen et al., 2020).

REFERENCES

Aberg-Wistedt, A., Cressell, T., Lidberg, Y., Liljenberg, B., & Osby, U. (1995). Two-year outcome of team-based intensive case management for patients with schizophrenia. *Psychiatric Services*, **46**, 1263–1266.

Allness, D. J. & Knoedler, W. H. (1998). *The PACT Model of Community-Based Treatment for Persons with Severe and Persistent Mental Illness. A Manual for PACT Start-Up*. Arlington, VA: National Alliance for the Mentally Ill.

Angell, B., Mahoney, C. A., & Martinez, N. I. (2006). Promoting treatment adherence in assertive community treatment. *Social Service Review*, **80**, 485–526.

Aubry, T., Bourque, J., Goering, P., Crouse, S., Veldhuizen, S., leBlanc, S., et al. (2019). A randomised controlled trial of the effectiveness of Housing First in a small Canadian city. *BMC Public Health*, **19**, 1154.

Audini, B., Marks, I. M., Lawrence, R. E., Connolly, J., & Watts, V. (1994). Home-based versus out-patient/in-patient care for people with serious mental illness. Phase II of a controlled study. *British Journal of Psychiatry*, **165**, 204–210.

Blankers, M., van Emmerik, A., Richters, B., & Dekker, J. (2016). Blended internet care for patients with severe mental illnesses: an open label prospective controlled cohort pilot study. *Internet Interventions*, **5**, 51–55.

Bond, G. R. & Drake, R. E. (2015). The critical ingredients of assertive community treatment. *World Psychiatry*, **14**, 240–242.

Bond, G. R., Drake, R. E., Mueser, K. T., & Latimer, E. (2001). Assertive community treatment for people with severe mental illness: critical ingredients and impact on patients. *Disease Management and Health Outcomes*, **9**, 141–159.

Brewer, W. J., Lambert, T. J., Witt, K., Dileo, J., Duff, C., Crlenjak, C., et al. (2015). Intensive case management for high-risk patients with first-episode psychosis: service model and outcomes. *Lancet Psychiatry*, **2**, 29–37.

Burns, T., Catty, J., Watt, H., Wright, C., Knapp, M., & Henderson, J. (2002). International differences in home treatment for mental health problems: results of a systematic review. *British Journal of Psychiatry*, **181**, 375–382.

Burns, T., Catty, J., Dash, M., Roberts, C., Lockwood A., & Marshall, M. (2007). Use of intensive case management to reduce time in hospital in people with severe mental illness: systematic review and meta-regression. *BMJ*, **335**, 336.

Burns, T., Creed, F., Fahy, T., Thompson, S., Tyrer, P., & White, I. (1999). Intensive versus standard case management for severe psychotic illness: a randomised trial. *Lancet*, **353**, 2185–2189.

Catty, J., Burns, T., Knapp, M., Watt, H., Wright, C., Henderson, J., et al. (2002). Home treatment for mental health problems: a systematic review. *Psychological Medicine*, **32**, 383–401.

Clausen, H., Ruud, T., Odden, S., Šaltytė Benth, J., Heiervang, K., Sverdvik, S., et al. (2016). Hospitalisation of severely mentally ill patients with and without problematic substance use before and during assertive community treatment: a naturalistic observational study. *BMC Psychiatry*, **16**, 125.

Coldwell, C. M. & Bender, W. S. (2007). The effectiveness of assertive community treatment for homeless populations with severe mental illness: a meta-analysis. *American Journal of Psychiatry*, **164**, 393–399.

Davidson, G. & Campbell, J. (2007). An examination of the use of coercion by assertive outreach and community mental health teams in Northern Ireland. *British Journal of Social Work*, **37**, 537–555.

Department of Health (1999). *The National Service Framework for Mental Health*. London: Department of Health.

Department of Health (2001). *Policy Implementation Guide: Assertive Community Treatment Teams*. London: Department of Health.

Department of Health (2005). *National Service Framework for Mental Health: Five Years On*. London: Department of Health.

Dieterich, M., Irving, C. B., Bergman, H., Khokhar, M. A., Park, B., & Marshall, M. (2017). Intensive case management for severe mental illness. *Cochrane Database of Systematic Reviews*, **1**, CD007906.

Drukker, M., Maarschalkerweerd, M., Bak, M., Driessen, G., à Campo, J., de Bie, A., et al. (2008). A real-life observational study of the effectiveness of FACT in a Dutch mental health region. *BMC Psychiatry*, **8**, 93.

Drummond, C., Gilburt, H., Burns, T., Copello, A., Crawford, M., Day, E., et al. (2017). Assertive community treatment for people with alcohol dependence: a pilot randomised controlled trial. *Alcohol and Alcoholism*, **52**, 234–241.

Firn, M., Hindhaugh, K., Hubbeling, D., Davies, G., Jones, B., & White, S. J. (2013). A dismantling study of assertive outreach services: comparing activity and outcomes following replacement with the FACT model. *Social Psychiatry and Psychiatric Epidemiology*, **48**, 997–1003.

Firn, M., White, S. J., Hubbeling, D., & Jones, B. (2018). The replacement of assertive outreach services by reinforcing local community teams: a four-year observational study. *Journal of Mental Health*, **27**, 4–9.

Gandy-Guedes, M., Manuel, J., George, M., McCray, S., & Negatu, D. (2018). Understanding engagement in the Program of Assertive Community Treatment (PACT) from the perspectives of individuals receiving treatment. *Social Work in Mental Health*, **16**, 400–418.

Ghosh, R. & Killaspy, H. (2010). A national survey of assertive community treatment services in England. *Journal of Mental Health*, **1**, 1–9.

Gomory, T. (2001). A critique of the effectiveness of assertive community treatment. *Psychiatric Services*, **52**, 1394–1395.

Harrison-Read, P., Lucas, B., Tyrer, P., Ray, J., Shipley, K., Simmonds, S., et al. (2002). Heavy users of acute psychiatric beds: randomised controlled trial of enhanced community management in outer London. *Psychological Medicine*, **32**, 403–416.

Harvey, C., Killaspy, H., Martino, S., White, S., Priebe, S., Wright, C., et al. (2011). A comparison of the implementation of assertive community treatment in Melbourne, Australia and London, England. *Epidemiology and Psychiatric Sciences*, **20**, 151–161.

Holloway, F. & Carson, J. (1998). Intensive case management for the severely mentally ill. *British Journal of Psychiatry*, **172**, 19–22.

Hoult, J., Rosen, A., & Reynolds, I. (1984). Community orientated treatment compared to hospital orientated treatment. *Social Science and Medicine*, **18**, 1005–1010.

Hoult, J. (1986). Community care of the acutely mentally ill. *British Journal of Psychiatry*, **149**, 337–344.

Issakidis, C., Sanderson, K., Teesson, M., Johnston, S., & Bulrich, N. (1999). Intensive case management in Australia: a randomised controlled trial. *Acta Psychiatrica Scandinavica*, **99**, 360–367.

Killaspy, H., Bebbington, P., Blizard, R., Johnson, S., Nolan, F., Pilling, S., & King, M. (2006). REACT: a Randomised Evaluation of Assertive Community Treatment in North London. *British Medical Journal*, **332**, 815–819.

Killaspy, H., Johnson, S., Pierce, B., Bebbington, P., Pilling, S., Nolan, F., et al. (2009a). A mixed methods analysis of interventions delivered by assertive community treatment and community mental health teams in the REACT trial. *Social Psychiatry and Psychiatric Epidemiology*, **44**, 532–540.

Killaspy, H., Kingett, S., Bebbington, P., Blizard, R., Johnson, S., Nolan, F., et al. (2009b). Three year outcomes of participants in the REACT (Randomised Evaluation of Assertive Community Treatment in North London) study. *British Journal of Psychiatry*, **195**, 82–83.

Killaspy, H., Marston, L., Omar, R., Green, N., Harrison, I., Lean, M., et al. (2013). Service quality and clinical outcomes: an example from mental health rehabilitation services in England. *British Journal of Psychiatry*, **202**, 28–34.

Killaspy, H., Mas-Exposito, L., Marston, L., & King, M. (2014). Ten year outcomes of participants in the REACT (Randomised Evaluation of Assertive Community Treatment in North London) study. *BMC Psychiatry*, **14**, 296.

Lamberti, J., Weisman, R., Cerulli, C., Williams, G., Jacobowitz, D., Mueser, K. et al. (2017). A randomized controlled trial of the Rochester forensic assertive community treatment model. *Psychiatric Services*, **68**, 1016–1024.

Latimer, E. (1999). Economic impacts of assertive community Treatment: a review of the literature. *Canadian Journal of Psychiatry*, **44**, 443–454.

Lukersmith, S., Millington, M., & Calvador-Carulla, L. (2016). What is case management? A scoping and mapping review. *International Journal of Integrated Care*, **16**, 1–13.

Marshall, M., Bond, G., Stein, L., Shepherd, G., McGrew, J., Hoult, J., et al. (1999). PRiSM Psychosis Study: design limitations, questionable conclusions. *British Journal of Psychiatry*, **175**, 501–503.

Marshall, M., Gray, A., Lockwood, A., & Green, R. (1998). Case management for people with severe mental disorders. *Cochrane Database of Systematic Reviews*, **2**, CD000050.

Marshall, M. & Lockwood, A. (1998). Assertive community treatment for people with severe mental disorders. *Cochrane Database of Systematic Reviews*, **4**, CD001089.

McCrone, P., Killaspy, H., Bebbington, P., Johnson, S., Nolan, F., Pilling, S. et al. (2009). The REACT study: cost-effectiveness of assertive community treatment in north London. *Psychiatric Services*, **60**, 908–913.

McGrew, J. H., Bond, G. R., Dietzen, L., & Salyers, M. (1994). Measuring the fidelity of implementation of a mental health program model. *Journal of Consulting and Clinical Psychology*, **62**, 670–678.

Meadows, G. (1998). Establishing a collaborative service model for primary mental health care. *Medical Journal of Australia*, **168**, 162–165.

Moreno, C., Wykes, T., Galderisi, S., Nordentoft, M., Crossley, N., Jones, N., et al. (2020). How mental health care should change as a consequence of the COVID-19 pandemic. *Lancet Psychiatry*, **7**, 813–824.

Monroe-DeVita, M., Teague, G. B., & Moser, L. L. (2011). The TMACT: a new tool for measuring fidelity to assertive community treatment. *Journal of the American Psychiatric Nurses Association*, **17**, 17–29.

Morgan, V., Korten, A., & Jablensky, A. (2006). Modifiable risk factors for hospitalization among people with psychosis: evidence from the National Study of Low Prevalence (Psychotic) Disorders. *Australia and New Zealand Journal of Psychiatry*, **40**, 683–690.

Morse, G. & McKasson, M. (2005). Assertive community treatment. In: Drake, R. E., Merrens, M. R., & Lynde, D. W. (Eds.), *Evidence Based Mental Health Practice: A Textbook* (pp. 317–47). New York: Norton.

Mueser, K. T., Bond, G. R., Drake, R. E., & Resnick, S. G. (1998). Models of community care for severe mental illness: a review of research on case management. *Schizophrenia Bulletin*, **24**, 37–74.

Munch Nielsen, C., Hjorthøj, C., Killaspy, H., & Nordentoft, M. (2021). The effect of flexible assertive community treatment in Denmark: a quasi-experimental controlled study. *Lancet Psychiatry*, **8**, 27–35.

National Institute for Health and Care Excellence (2020). Rehabilitation for adults with complex psychosis. NICE guideline [NG181]. https://www.nice.org.uk/guidance/ng181

Nugter, M. A., Engelsbel, F., Bähler, M., Keet, R., & van Veldhuizen, R. (2016). Outcomes of flexible assertive community treatment (FACT) implementation: a prospective real life study. *Community Mental Health Journal*, **52**, 898–907.

Odden, S., Landheim, A., Clausen, H., Stuen, H. K., Heiervang, K. S., & Ruud, T. (2019). Model fidelity and team members' experiences of assertive community treatment in Norway: a sequential mixed-methods study. *International Journal of Mental Health Systems*, **13**, 65.

O'Reilly, C. L., Paul, D., McCahon, R., Shankar, S., Rosen, A., & Ramzy, T. (2019). Stigma and discrimination in individuals with severe and persistent mental illness in an assertive community treatment team: perceptions of families and healthcare professionals. *International Journal of Social Psychiatry*, **65**, 570–579.

Petersen, L., Jeppesen, P., Thorup, A., Maj-Britt A., Øhlenschlæger, J., Torben Østergaard, C., et al. (2005). A randomised multicentre trial of integrated versus standard treatment for patients with a first episode psychotic illness. *BMJ*, **331**, 602.

Pettersen, H., Ruud, T., Ravndal, E., Havnes, I., & Landheim, A. (2014). Engagement in assertive community treatment as experienced by recovering clients with severe mental illness and concurrent substance use. *International Journal of Mental Health Systems*, **8**, 40.

Roberts, G. & Wolfson, P. (2004). The rediscovery of recovery: open to all. *Journal of Mental Health*, **10**, 37–49.

Rosen, A. (2021). We need to find right balance between telehealth, in-person care. Psychiatric News, 28 September. American Psychiatric Association. https://doi.org/10.1176/appi.pn.2021.10.8

Rosen, A., Bond, G. R., & Teesson, M. (2008a). Review: intensive case management for severe mental illness reduces rehospitalisation when previous hospital use has been high. *BMJ Mental Health*, **11**, 2.

Rosen, A., Clenaghan, P., Emerton, F., & Richards, S. (2008b). Integration of the crisis resolution function within community mental health teams. In: Johnson, S., Needle, J., Bindeman, J. P., & Thornicroft, G. (Eds), *Crisis Resolution and Home Treatment in Mental Health* (pp. 235–250). Cambridge: Cambridge University Press.

Rosen, A., Gill, N. S., & Salvador-Carulla, L. (2020). The future of community psychiatry and community mental health services. *Current Opinion in Psychiatry*, **33**, 375–390.

Rosen, A., Killaspy, H., & Harvey, C. (2013). Specialisation and marginalisation: how the assertive community treatment debate impacts on individuals with complex mental health needs. *The Psychiatrist*, **37**, 345–348.

Rosen, A., Mueser, K., & Teesson, M. (2007). Assertive community treatment—issues from scientific and clinical literature with implications for practice. *Journal of Rehabilitation Research and Development*, **44**, 1–13.

Rosen, A. & Teesson, M. (2001). Does case management work? The evidence and the abuse of evidence based medicine. *Australian and New Zealand Journal of Psychiatry*, **35**, 731–746.

Sood, L., Owne, A., Onvon, R., Sharma, A., Nigriello, J., Markham, D., et al. (2018). Flexible assertive community treatment (FACT) model in specialist psychosis teams: an evaluation. *British Journal of Psychiatry Bulletin*, **41**, 192–196.

Stein, L. I. & Santos, A. B. (1998). *Assertive Community Treatment of Persons with Severe Mental Illness*. New York: Norton.

Stein, L. I. & Test, M. A. (1980). Alternatives to mental hospital treatment. *Archives of General Psychiatry*, **37**, 392–397.

Sytema, S., Wunderink, L., Bloemers, W., Roorda, L., & Wiersma, D. (2007). Assertive community treatment in the Netherlands: a randomized controlled trial. *Acta Psychiatrica Scandinavica*, **116**, 105–112.

Teague, G. B., Bond, G. R., & Drake, R. E. (1998). Program fidelity in assertive community treatment: development and use of a measure. *American Journal of Orthopsychiatry*, **68**, 216–232.

Test, M. & Stein, L. (2001). Critique of the effectiveness of assertive community treatment. *Psychiatric Services*, **52**, 1396–1397.

Thornicroft, G., Wykes, T., Holloway, F., Johnson, S., & Smuzkler, G. (1998). From efficacy to effectiveness in community mental health services. PRiSM Psychosis Study 10. *British Journal of Psychiatry*, **173**, 423–427.

Trane, K., Aasbrenn, K., Rønningen, M., Odden, S., Lexén, A., & Landheim, A. (2021). Flexible assertive community treatment teams can change complex and fragmented service systems: experiences of service providers. *International Journal of Mental Health Systems*, **15**, 38.

van Veldhuizen, J. R. (2007). FACT: a Dutch version of ACT. *Community Mental Health Journal*, **43**, 421–433.

van Vugt, M. D., Kroon, H., Delespaul, P. A., & Mulder, C. L. (2016). Assertive community treatment and associations with delinquency. *International Journal of Law & Psychiatry*, **49**, 93–97.

Weimand, B., Israel, P., & Ewertzon, M. (2018). Families in assertive community treatment (ACT) teams in Norway: a cross-sectional study on relatives' experiences of involvement and alienation. *Community Mental Health Journal*, **54**, 686–697.

Wright, C., Burns, T., James, P., Billings, J., Johnson, S., Muijen, M., et al. (2003). Assertive outreach teams in London: models of operation. Pan London Assertive Outreach Study Part 1. *British Journal of Psychiatry*, **183**, 132–138.

Wullschleger, A., Berg, J., Bermpohl, F., & Montag, C. (2018). Can 'model projects of need-adapted care' reduce involuntary hospital treatment and the use of coercive measures? *Frontiers in Psychiatry*, **9**, 168.

Ye, J., Chen, T. F., Paul, D., McMahon, R., Shankar, S., Rosen, A., et al. (2016). Stigma and discrimination experienced by people living with severe and persistent mental illness in assertive community treatment settings. *International Journal of Social Psychiatry*, **62**, 532–541.

15

Principles and standards for medication management of individuals with serious mental illness

Thomas E. Smith and Delia C. Hendrick

Introduction

Psychotropic medications effectively treat a wide range of mood, psychotic, and anxiety disorders. Several large practical trials have demonstrated their effectiveness in 'real-world' populations and settings using clinically relevant outcomes such as all-cause medication discontinuation. Examples include clinical trials of antipsychotic (Jones et al., 2006; Kahn et al., 2008; Lieberman et al., 2005), antidepressant (S. Lewis et al., 2010; Rush et al., 2006; Sachs et al., 2007), and anxiolytic (Piacentini et al., 2014) medications. Recent meta-analyses have yielded additional important information for prescribers regarding the relative effectiveness and differential side effect profiles for classes of medications (Cipriani et al., 2018; Correll et al., 2021; Leucht et al., 2017, 2020; McDonagh et al., 2017; Zhou et al., 2020).

Medical societies, researchers, and expert panels have drawn upon this large body of evidence to create numerous medication management guidelines for prescribers working in community mental health settings. Examples include the American Psychiatric Association Clinical Practice Guidelines (American Psychiatric Association, n.d.), the National Institute for Health and Care Excellence (NICE) guidelines for mental health and behavioural conditions (NICE, 2021), the British Association for Psychopharmacology (BAP) Consensus Guidelines (BAP, 2021), the Cochrane Library Mental Health Reviews (Cochrane Library, n.d.), the World Federation of Societies of Biological Psychiatry (WFSBP) treatment guidelines (WFSBP, 2021), the Substance Abuse and Mental Health Services Administration (SAMHSA) Evidence-Based Practices Resource Center (SAMHSA, 2021), and the PORT Psychopharmacology Treatment Recommendations (Buchanan et al., 2010). These practice guidelines offer detailed support for clinical decision-making by presenting systematically developed medication management strategies in a standardized format.

Despite this large body of evidence supporting the effectiveness of psychotropic medication treatments, however, many patients with health conditions continue to receive no or inadequate treatment. The US National Comorbidity Survey indicated that up to 50% of individuals with a serious mental illness received no mental health treatment in the prior year (Wang et al., 2005). Only 16.5% of individuals with a major depressive disorder receive minimally adequate treatment in the prior year (Thornicroft et al., 2017) and only 46% of individuals with bipolar disorder receive any treatment in the prior 12 months (Blanco et al., 2017). Members of ethnoracially disadvantaged groups and low-income patients have even lower mental health service use compared with members of advantaged groups (Alegria et al., 2018).

When considering the complex interactions between social factors, comorbid conditions, side effect concerns, and patient preferences and attitudes regarding psychotropic medications, these high rates of inadequate treatment with psychotropic medication are not surprising. This chapter will therefore focus on strategies for maximizing patient engagement in medication management decisions and adherence to recommendations. We will focus on the initial assessment and engagement period as well as follow-up strategies and approaches. We will review shared decision-making (SDM) strategies known to improve adherence and identify key best practices as well as common avoidable practices for community mental health prescribers. Finally, we will describe and emphasize the importance of care management and collaboration both within multidisciplinary treatment teams as well as with outside providers and key support persons.

Psychopharmacology assessment

The initial psychopharmacology assessment is critical to development of an effective treatment plan.

Initial psychiatric evaluation

Prior to initiation of psychotropic medication treatment, the prescriber should complete and document a full psychiatric evaluation. The record should include documentation of the history of present illness, past psychiatric history including psychotropic medication history, and mental status examination. The initial evaluation should also include a summary of the patient's medical history and current medical conditions as well as pertinent family history (e.g. history of diabetes or heart disease), a review of systems, review of risk of harm to self or others, and a summary of active medical problems as well as current non-psychiatric medications (American Psychiatric Association, 2016).

The psychiatric evaluation also allows an opportunity to establish a therapeutic relationship with the patient and provides information necessary for SDM about treatment (see below) and for educating patients and family members (American Psychiatric Association, 2021). The assessment should consider the patient's ability to communicate, degree of cooperation, illness severity, and ability to recall historical details (American Psychiatric Association, 2016). Special attention should be paid to cultural factors that influence patients' perceptions of mental illness and symptoms as well as attitudes towards treatment. Some patients may benefit from a structured assessment of cultural factors (Lewis-Fernández et al., 2020).

Testing, diagnosis, and target symptoms

Some medication treatments require review of laboratory findings prior to initiation of treatment. Examples include documentation of renal functions prior to initiating lithium, review of electrocardiogram prior to initiating antidepressant or lithium treatment in patients with existing cardiovascular disease, and review of liver function tests in individuals with substance use disorders (SUDs) prior to initiating medications metabolized by the liver. Prior to prescribing a psychotropic medication, the prescriber should establish a primary psychiatric diagnosis or diagnoses. Target symptoms and/or behaviours should be defined for monitoring over time to determine response to the prescribed medication treatment, and at least one symptom or behaviour must be identified as the primary target for each medication prescribed.

There is growing interest in pharmacogenetic testing to identify genetic variants that predict treatment response to specific psychotropic medications. Combinatorial pharmacogenetic decision support tools have been developed which use algorithms to integrate information about multiple genetic variants into an easily interpretable report to guide medication prescribing. Currently, however, the expert consensus is that there are insufficient data to support widespread endorsement of these tools (American Academy of Child & Adolescent Psychiatry, 2020; Ontario Health (Quality), 2021; Zeier et al., 2018). Pharmacogenetic testing may nevertheless be helpful in certain circumstances, for example, to confirm whether a patient is a rapid or slow metabolizer of a specific medication when the patient's medication response or experience of side effects suggests an atypical metabolic profile. Another example involves determining whether a patient is at heightened risk of developing Stevens–Johnson syndrome/toxic epidermal necrolysis following initiation of anticonvulsant mood stabilizers, which is more likely among patients with human leucocyte antigen (HLA)-B*15:02 and HLA-A*31:01.

Measurement-based care

Measurement-based care involves the systematic administration of symptom rating scales and use of the results to drive medication management decisions (Fortney et al., 2017). Validated screens are available to assess and measure severity of depression, anxiety, trauma, attention deficit hyperactivity disorder, and substance use. Depression and anxiety symptom rating scales can also be used for sequential monitoring and documenting response to medication treatment. Numerous controlled trials have demonstrated that frequent and timely feedback of patient-reported symptoms to the prescriber improves medication management outcomes (Fortney et al., 2017). Nearly all medication management guidelines recommend systematic symptom assessments and experts have endorsed use of both patient-reported and clinician-administered symptom rating tools (Fortney et al., 2017; Rush, 2015).

Despite its demonstrated effectiveness, it has been estimated that fewer than 20% of behavioural health practitioners use measurement-based care in their practice (C. C. Lewis et al., 2019). Multiple barriers to implementation have been identified including concerns about patient confidentiality, practitioner beliefs that general clinical judgement is equally accurate, as well as concerns about time and resources necessary to support measurement-based care (C. C. Lewis et al., 2019). Prescribers and community mental health programme directors should be aware of and attempt to address these obstacles and support measurement-based approaches medication management.

Shared decision-making

In a 2015 survey, approximately half of mental health service users in England reported that they were not involved in treatment decisions to the extent they preferred (Care Quality Commission, 2015). Informed and engaged patients are more likely to adhere to treatment recommendations and receive care that best matches their needs and preferences. SDM is a communication model that aims to improve patients' knowledge about their conditions and treatment options and facilitate treatment decision-making by using a variety of decision aids and related approaches (Charles et al., 1997; Drake et al., 2009; Stacey et al., 2017; Thomas et al., 2021).

Effective medication management in community mental health settings involves prescribers working to understand patients' goals and preferences, reviewing pros and cons of potential medication options, and jointly deciding on a course of action. SDM promotes treatment decisions that are needed, wanted, and more likely to be implemented (Barry & Edgman-Levitan, 2012; Stiggelbout et al., 2012).

Goals and preferences

Prior to discussing specific treatment options, prescribers and patients should initiate a conversation about the patient's goals and preferences related to psychiatric medications. This conversation will be ongoing and should not delay initiation of medication treatment. Patients' goals and preferences evolve over time, however, and it is important for prescribers to reflect and review with patients their perceptions and attitudes regarding medication treatment in an ongoing manner (Coulter, 2017). It is critical, however, to frame initial discussions and decisions about medication treatment within the context of the patient's stated goals and preferences.

Initial discussions should explore the patient's decision-making preferences. For example, some patients prefer full autonomy and the ability to make all final decisions regarding treatment. Other patients, however, prefer to rely primarily (or exclusively) on the expert prescriber's judgement to make decisions regarding mediation treatment. Establishing goals and preferences will often require discussion with other members of the treatment team and key support persons including family members. This is especially important for patients with serious mental illness who may have cognitive difficulties that impact their judgement, memory, and decision-making abilities. Patient goals and preferences should be clearly documented in the medical record, as they will inform interventions offered by other members of the multidisciplinary team.

Prescribers can promote SDM by using structured decision aid tools (Alston et al., 2014; Wieringa et al., 2018). Decision aid tools elicit patient preferences and values, provide patient communication skills training, and engage the patient in participation in goal setting. These tools include brief text or diagrams but can be extensive and include booklets, websites, and videos (Alston et al., 2014; Elwyn et al., 2012; Weiringa et al., 2019). Patients are engaged and empowered when they recognize that they can choose among different treatment options.

Information regarding medication options

Additional key elements of SDM include choice awareness, option clarification, and discussion of harms and benefits (Weiringa et al., 2019). Prescribers should elicit what patients already know, attempt to address misinformation, and use decision aid tools to present new information about the effectiveness and side effect profiles of specific psychotropic medications. As noted above, there is clear evidence of significant variability in effectiveness and side effect profiles within classes of antidepressant, antipsychotic, and anxiolytic medications. Important examples include consideration of anticipated metabolic side effects associated with psychotropic medications and need for careful weight monitoring and management. Prescribers should provide information and tailor efforts to educate based upon the patient's cognitive capacities and preferences related to decision-making.

Informed patients will then transition from 'choice talk' to 'option talk', in which knowledge regarding options is reviewed in the context of their goals and preferences for treatment (Elwyn et al., 2012). In these discussions, prescribers can use additional SDM approaches including decision coaching and motivational and self-management strategies (Stacey et al., 2013; Zisman-Ilani, 2017).

Joint decision

Through this interactive process of reflection and discussion, the prescriber and patient reach a mutual decision about the subsequent choice of psychotropic medication and monitoring plan. It is critical to note that SDM discussions do not cease following decisions regarding the initial treatment plan. It should be an ongoing process that reviews the patient's response to the medication trial, any side effects experienced, and the patient's evolving goals and preferences related to treatment. SDM is best considered as an overall approach to engaging and empowering patients in their care.

SDM approaches have been proven effective in supporting treatment of individuals with mental illness. Decision support tools have been shown to impact perceived involvement in care, treatment engagement and adherence, and patient satisfaction in a range of patients with mental illness (Aljumah et al., 2015; Barr et al., 2019; Dixon et al., 2014; Finnerty et al., 2018; Hamann et al., 2007; LeBlanc et al., 2015; Loh et al., 2007; Raue et al., 2019; Robinson et al., 2018; Thomas et al., 2021; Treichler et al., 2020) and should be considered as a foundational approach for prescribers working in community mental health settings.

CommonGround model

The CommonGround program (Deegan et al., 2010) uses an SDM approach to support management of medication for patients with serious mental illnesses. CommonGround helps patients organize their health information into a particular format and outline decision points related to medication treatment. When CommonGround is fully implemented, the clinic waiting area is converted into a decision support centre with peer staff present to support and assist patients. Prior to seeing the prescriber, the patient logs in to a CommonGround secure website and creates a one-page health report to bring to the appointment with the prescriber. The health report notes the patient's goals for treatment and summarizes how the patient is currently using medications as well as questions/concerns about medications.

The CommonGround application includes additional SDM aids such as short videos of patients describing their recovery from illness as well as information about specific medications, and coping and recovery strategies. Following the appointment, the prescriber can summarize decisions made about medication treatment in the CommonGround application and the patient can authorize other individuals to access the program to support follow-up.

CommonGround is among the most studied SDM interventions (Thomas et al., 2021) with published reports documenting its positive impact on patient communication skills (Deegan et al., 2017), involvement in decision-making (Salyers et al., 2017), treatment engagement and adherence (Finnerty et al., 2018), symptoms (Salyers et al., 2017), and both patients' and providers' attitudes related to SDM (Deegan et al., 2008; Goscha & Rapp, 2015).

Initiation and ongoing medication management

Dose and duration of treatment

Prescribers should refer to established guidelines for information on usual starting doses and tapering strategies. Escalation of doses should be tailored to the patient's needs and circumstances, for example, doses are typically increased more frequently in inpatient settings when patients are experiencing more severe symptoms and/or the patient is having thoughts about harming themselves or others. At all times, however, the prescriber should aim to use the minimum effective dose of psychotropic medication.

Medication management guidelines typically include parameters for minimum dose and duration of psychotropic medications that would constitute an effective trial. Prescribers should attempt to continue trials to meet these standards before switching to another medication and distinguish between failed trials due to lack of efficacy versus lack of tolerance (e.g. the inability to achieve a minimum dose or duration of treatment due to side effects). When a patient requires a higher than recommended dose to achieve adequate response, the prescriber should clearly document the rationale and justification in the health record.

Deprescribing

Prescribers working in community mental health clinics will encounter several forms of polypharmacy. One involves patients taking high numbers of different types of medications, which is increasingly common as patients present with multiple comorbid conditions. A common example is the patient taking a psychotropic medication for a mental illness and taking additional medications to manage side effects from the psychotropic medication as well as common metabolic conditions including hypertension, dyslipidaemia, and type 2 diabetes mellitus. In survey data from 2015 to 2018, 21.5% of US adults reported taking at least three prescription medications and 11.2% were taking five or more prescription medications (National Center for Health Statistics, 2019).

Another common scenario involves psychotropic polypharmacy. Mojtabai and Olfson (2010) found that 59.8% of patients presenting for care in outpatient psychiatric settings were prescribed two or more and 33.2% were prescribed three or more psychotropic medications. A more recent report found that 86.1% of patients with schizoaffective disorder and 70.1% with schizophrenia were treated with two or more different classes of psychotropic medications (Stroup et al., 2018). Additionally, increasing numbers of patients are taking two or more medications from the same class to treat a specific condition: up to 30% of patients with schizophrenia have been prescribed two or more antipsychotic agents concurrently (Gallego et al., 2012; Horvitz-Lennon et al., 2022; Lung et al., 2018; Sneider et al., 2015) despite the lack of evidence that combining antipsychotic medications improves clinical response (Ortiz-Orendain et al., 2017). Nearly 60% of adult patients receiving treatment for depression are prescribed two or more psychotropic medications, including 22.7% who are prescribed at least two antidepressant medications from the same class (Rhee & Rosenheck, 2019). Psychotropic polypharmacy also has increased significantly in youth and young adults (Lagerberg et al., 2019); an estimated 300,000 US youth received medications from three or more psychotropic classes concomitantly in 2011–2016 (Zhang et al., 2021).

There are several reasons for high rates of psychotropic polypharmacy in community mental health settings including the increased number of medications available to treat common conditions, more patients presenting with multiple comorbid conditions, and the often-inadequate response rates to single agents. While there is no evidence base to support combining two or more antipsychotic medications for treatment of psychosis, psychotropic polypharmacy may be indicated for depressed adults for augmentation treatment or considerations of psychiatric multimorbidity (Rhee & Rosenheck, 2019). However, the concurrent administration of multiple drugs increases the risk of drug interactions and adverse effects including morbidity and mortality. Psychiatric polypharmacy is also associated with cumulative toxicity, poor medication adherence and treatment non-compliance (Sarkar, 2017).

Prescribers should avoid antipsychotic polypharmacy unless clearly indicated and should be adept at deprescribing when patients present with significant unjustified psychotropic polypharmacy.

Reeve et al. (2015) define deprescribing as: 'the process of withdrawal of an inappropriate medication, supervised by a health care professional with the goal of managing polypharmacy and improving outcomes' (p. 1254). Community mental health clinic prescribers should be able to recognize unnecessary polypharmacy and deprescribe as indicated. Resources that support deprescribing include staff and family education, tools for systematic review of medication regimens, and pharmacist consultation (Elbeddini et al., 2021). Examples of quality improvement programmes exist for deprescribing anticholinergic (Gannon et al., 2021) and antipsychotic medications (Hanson et al., 2021).

Timely follow-up

Prescribers or other members of the community mental health treatment team should check in with patients soon (ideally within 7–10 days) after starting a new psychotropic medication to evaluate adherence, review tolerability, and review any questions the patient may have. Subsequent follow-up visits should be scheduled as indicated based upon severity of symptoms, side effect and tolerability issues, and assessed risk for adverse outcomes.

During medication management visits the prescriber should assess the severity of target symptoms/behaviours and adjust medications accordingly. The prescriber should review whether psychotropic medication doses and trial durations are consistent with guidelines for the target condition(s), document the impact of prescribed medications on target symptoms/behaviours, and identify a clear rationale for either adjusting or maintaining doses. At each visit the prescriber also should assess for psychotropic medication side effects (including severity, with or without standardized scales) and adjust the medication regimen accordingly. Side effects can be managed by adjusting the dose or discontinuing the medication believed to be causing or contributing to the side effect, initiating a new medication to treat the side effect, or educating the patient regarding non-medication strategies for managing the side effect.

The prescriber should note when the patient has responded adequately to a medication trial and should review and inform the patient regarding strategies for maintenance treatment. The prescriber should review maintenance medication options with the patient including recommended duration of maintenance treatment, possible dosage adjustments for maintenance treatment, risk of recurrence with and without maintenance medication treatment, and approaches for monitoring early warning signs of recurrence.

Assessing adherence

Among those who do initiate treatment for a mental illness, it is estimated that 33–46% of clients routinely discontinue care (Kreyenbuhl et al., 2009; O'Brien et al., 2009). Community mental health providers also often treat patients with multiple complex comorbid conditions including personality and SUDs, who are much more difficult to engage in care (Chalker et al., 2015; Koekkoek et al., 2006; Ljungberg at al., 2016). Many patients experience social conditions such as chronic poverty, unemployment, unstable housing, and legal issues (Milfort et al., 2015), which impact their ability to adhere to treatment recommendations. Non-adherence rates among individuals with serious mental illness in community mental health settings are estimated to be greater than 80% (Schulze et al., 2019; Semahegn et al., 2018; Stentzel et al., 2018).

The patient's capacity and willingness to adhere to prescribed psychotropic medications should be assessed at the onset of treatment and during follow-up visits. If the patient is not responding to a prescribed medication, the prescriber should specifically inquire about adherence and address accordingly. Self-report and prescriber report are the most common methods used to assess adherence in clinical settings but are often inaccurate and may underestimate non-adherence (Velligan et al., 2009). Prescribers should also use more objective measures (e.g. pill counts, pharmacy records, and, when appropriate, serum levels). Family and other key support persons can also assist prescriber and patient efforts to understand and address low adherence.

Low adherence is often related to undesired side effects which can be easily addressed as noted above. Long-acting injectable antipsychotic medications are a useful option for many patients who have difficulty taking oral antipsychotic medications and have been shown to significantly lower rates of relapse and hospitalization (Kishimoto et al., 2021; Pacciarotti et al., 2019). In many instances, poor adherence is due to several complicated factors related to the patient's personal circumstances and experience of care. It is critical for prescribers to use a SDM approach when discussing adherence with patients. Whether managing side effects, addressing ambivalence about treatment, or managing other circumstances impacting on the patient's ability to take medications as prescribed, it will be important to frame the discussion in the context of the patient's goals and expectations and to engage other support persons as indicated.

Underutilized evidence-based psychopharmacological practices

Medication-assisted treatment for substance use disorders

SUDs are widespread and have high morbidity, mortality, and economical burdens. Interventions addressing SUDs involve screening and brief interventions (Steele et al., 2020) as well as psychosocial treatments such as contingency management, motivational enhancement, 'stages of change'-based treatments, and cognitive behavioural therapy-based interventions (Ray et al., 2020). Individuals with SUDs also benefit from interventions that provide integrated care for SUD comorbid mental illnesses (Mueser, 2001) and efforts to improve social capital and connectedness and offer employment opportunities (Klevan et al., 2021). Below we review pharmacotherapeutic interventions that prescribers working in community mental health settings should be able to offer.

Medication-assisted treatment (MAT) has emerged as an important evidence-based practice in treating opioid and alcohol use disorders (Table 15.1). In opioid-use disorders (OUDs), MAT decreases opioid overdose deaths, opioid use, and infectious disease transmission, and increases social functioning and retention in treatment (Ma et al., 2019; Mattick et al., 2014; Schwartz, 2013). MAT is approved for the treatment of OUDs and alcohol use disorders in the UK (NICE, 2022a, 2022b) and the US (SAMHSA, 2022).

Even in the US, where the opioid deaths have reached epidemic proportions and where numerous guidelines recommend it, MAT for OUDs is vastly underutilized (Knudsen et al., 2011). Limiting factors for providing MAT include prescriber availability, prescriber lack of comfort and support with diagnosing and treating addiction outside addiction clinics (Hawkins et al., 2021), and financial and public policy factors. Programmes that provide multidisciplinary, integrated, and coordinated care increase availability of MAT beyond specialty clinics (Lagisetty et al., 2017).

Three medications have been approved for the treatment of opioid dependence: methadone, buprenorphine/naloxone combination, and naltrexone. Methadone is a strong opioid agonist that carries risks of respiratory depression and QTc prolongation. Methadone also has many cytochrome P450-based interactions, subjecting individuals to plasma level variations and increased risk of side effects as well as risk of decreased efficacy. However, it remains a highly effective option in the treatment of OUD, a potentially fatal disease. In many countries, use of methadone for OUD is restricted to outpatient methadone clinics and daily staff-supervised administration.

The introduction of buprenorphine, a mixed opioid agonist/antagonist with an improved safety profile over methadone (lower risk of respiratory depression although still a risk in overdose or when mixed with alcohol or benzodiazepines), expands OUD MAT treatment to office-based individual prescribers. Several requirements and limitations to the use of methadone and buprenorphine/naloxone were temporarily lifted during the Covid-19 pandemic in recognition of the ongoing OUD pandemic in the US and in order to increase availability of MAT treatment. The third MAT option, naltrexone, is an opioid antagonist with a good safety profile that has been shown to be as effective as buprenorphine/naloxone for long-term treatment of OUDs. However, initiation of naltrexone in active opioid users is difficult due to the need for achieving detoxification first to avoid precipitated withdrawal. Naltrexone has also been used

Table 15.1 MAT options for opioid and alcohol use disorders

	Indication	Medication(s)	Actions
MAT for OUDs	Opioid dependence treatment	Methadone, buprenorphine/naloxone	Opioid agonists: suppress opioid withdrawal symptoms and attenuate the effects of opioids
	Opioid dependence treatment	Naltrexone	Opioid antagonist: blocks the effects of opioid agonists
	Opioid withdrawal treatment	Clonidine, lofexidine	Alpha-2 agonists: treat sympathomimetic signs of opioid withdrawal
	Opioid overdose treatment	Naloxone	Opioid antagonist: reverses opioid overdose
MAT for alcohol use disorders	Alcohol dependence treatment	Naltrexone	Opioid antagonist: decreases cravings
	Maintaining alcohol abstinence	Disulfiram	Inhibits aldehyde dehydrogenase: creates negative conditioning
	Maintenance treatment of alcohol dependence	Acamprosate	GABA agonist and partial glutamate (N-methyl-D-aspartate) antagonist; decreases dysphoria

to effectively treat alcohol use disorders since the 1970s, and despite a robust evidence base, remains vastly underutilized (Qeadan et al., 2021).

The three medications for OUDs each offer specific advantages and disadvantages but are considered equivalent in their overall effectiveness, and the choice of treatment should be based on the individual circumstances and preferences. Prescribers should use a SDM approach to ensure the choice of medication best matches the individual's needs, goals, and preferences. Prescribers and community mental health centre staff working with individuals with OUD should also be trained to administer naloxone to reverse acute opioid overdose. Many states in the US have allowed sales of naloxone kits for treating opioid overdose without a prescription and have started 'take-home naloxone' programmes, targeting opioid users, their family, and their friends, in an effort to curb opioid overdose death.

Nicotine cessation treatment

People with mental illness have high prevalence of nicotine use disorder, use more nicotine than smokers without mental illness (Ferron, et al., 2011; Ziedonis et al., 2008), and are less likely to quit and stay quit (Cook et al., 2014). Mental health and SUD treatment settings have lagged behind the medical facilities in enacting smoking bans and have been more likely to accept nicotine use disorder or even see it as necessary for people to maintain while in treatment for other conditions. Nicotine appears to provide cognitive enhancement (Heishman et al., 2010) and is viewed as an important coping tool by patients and many psychiatric care providers. Contrary to widespread beliefs, however, quitting smoking leads to improved mood, anxiety, and quality of life (Taylor et al., 2021). People with mental illness can quit and reverse the significant toll of smoking on their physical health (Banham & Gilbody, 2010). Side effects of medications and symptoms of mental illness can be treated appropriately without the use of tobacco.

Nicotine use disorder treatment involves agonist therapy (nicotine replacement therapy), medications to decrease cravings, and behavioural interventions, such as motivational enhancement techniques, cessation education, and skills training. There is evidence that people with serious mental illness benefit and tolerate strategies used in the general population, including medications such as bupropion and varenicline (Peckham et al., 2017). Psychiatric care providers need to be routinely assessing for nicotine use and utilize stage-of change- appropriate interventions. MAT is an important part of the treatment.

Identifying and managing metabolic conditions

People with any mental illness have higher risks for comorbid medical conditions. Chronic metabolic diseases are particularly prevalent in people with schizophrenia, bipolar disorders, and in people with depressive disorders. There are many contributing factors, but side effects of psychotropic medications play an important role. Antipsychotics, mood stabilizers, and antidepressants all can produce weight gain, and antipsychotics can also produce hypercholesterolaemia and diabetes, even independently of the weight gain.

Multiple organizations have issued guidelines for routine monitoring of metabolic, endocrine, and cardiac side effects (American Diabetes Association et al., 2004; Cohn & Sernyak, 2006; Cordes et al., 2008; Marder et al., 2004). Monitoring metabolic side effects of psychiatric medications is a relatively new task for psychiatrists and many may feel unprepared to take on the responsibility. Similarly, primary care providers have been less aware of these recommendations and less comfortable monitoring these parameters in patients with serious mental illness, further contributing to low uptake of these guidelines.

It is of utmost importance that prescribers working in community mental health centres are adept at screening for common medical conditions and counselling patients to reduce preventable cardiometabolic risk factors. In addition to awareness, system modifications allowing for routine laboratory referral and integration of the results in electronic health records, reminders, alerts, and patient registries are necessary to increase implementation of guidelines. System modifications facilitating communication between providers are needed to bridge fragmentation of care.

Psychiatric care providers need to be aware of medical care being delivered by other providers and communicate with them regularly and as needed to ensure patients are receiving necessary care. Stigma faced by patients with mental illness makes advocacy work necessary and important. Advocacy within the system can be effectively exerted by psychiatric care providers or by their delegates, such as nurse care coordinators embedded in mental health care management teams (Bury et al., 2022). Psychiatric care providers can play a key role in identifying and intervening when most appropriate, based on their identified competencies, local resources, and patient preferences for care. Co-management of common medical conditions when clinically necessary should be recognized as a potential component of the overall care of patients with mental illnesses; and systems changes, technology facilitation, and appropriate reimbursement mechanisms should be in place.

Care coordination and management to support medication management

Care management for patients with serious mental illness

Community-based support programmes have long been integral elements of comprehensive plans of care for patients with serious mental illness (Lim et al., 2022). More intensive care management programmes such as assertive community treatment and intensive care management have been repeatedly shown to reduce hospitalizations and improve engagement in care (Dieterich et al., 2017). Less has been published regarding non-intensive or routine care management for patients with serious mental illness treated in community mental health clinics. This is despite the many recent healthcare reforms that identify care management as the backbone of integrated public health programmes (Smith et al., 2021).

Patients with serious mental illness have unique care management needs related to the often-multiple functional deficits they experience in employment, self-care, and independent living, as well as cognitive deficits common to these illnesses including reality distortions, impulsivity, and impaired problem-solving and social skills. Stigma and lack of training among healthcare professionals further reinforce these needs. These patients need care management that is flexible and persistent—they are less likely to respond to cold telephone calls or mail offers of support typical of medical case management programmes. Care managers should be familiar with the local behavioural health system of care; patients with serious mental illness who frequently disengage with care are more likely to connect with mental health rather than primary care providers. Care managers must be experienced and comfortable working with patients with serious mental illness and should have basic training in using motivational interviewing, de-escalation, and reality testing techniques. Care managers must be able to advocate on behalf of the patient when the patient is not able to do so and must also be adept at mobilizing family and other key individuals to provide supports as indicated (Smith et al., 2021).

Coordination with other providers

Multidisciplinary team-based models are commonly used in community mental health settings. Team-based approaches take advantage of the diversity and breadth of provider skills and increase access to psychosocial rehabilitation practices proven to be effective for individuals with serious mental illness. Working within a team allows for coordination of medication management and psychiatric care with psychosocial rehabilitation, care management, and related efforts to address social determinants of health.

Multidisciplinary teams can provide care that is acceptable, accessible, and available (Smith et al., 2013). Team members can be trained to provide care that will enhance adherence and engagement using principles of trauma-informed care (Harris & Fallot, 2001), person-centred planning (Roca, 2020), SDM (Deegan et al., 2008), motivational interviewing (Frost et al., 2018), and harm reduction (Huhn & Gipson, 2021). Although many community mental health clinic sites struggle to provide adequate access to prescribers, it is nonetheless important to ensure opportunities for prescribers to collaborate with treatment team members. Innovative approaches to ensuring team collaboration include shared access to electronic mental health records and digital-based supervision of clinical staff (digital platforms can easily be leveraged to support supervision and collaboration).

Prescribers also should attempt to coordinate care with primary care providers and other specialists managing their patients' active medical conditions. Although time constraints and confidentiality concerns present common barriers to collaboration, communication and coordination with non-behavioural health providers will improve adherence, limit adverse medication events, and improve outcomes.

Coordination with family and key support persons

The prescriber should work with multidisciplinary team members to identify which family members or other persons are most likely to support psychotropic medication regimens as well as manage crises. Engagement of family and support persons greatly increases the likelihood of good outcomes. Depending on the patient's preferences, prescribers can communicate directly with family/support persons regarding the psychotropic medication regimen or can provide information to another member of the treatment team who will be the primary contact for the family/support person. Family and other key support persons can play a critical role assisting in monitoring response to medication treatments as well as adherence and side effects. Family and support persons also play critical roles helping patients manage crises and/or high-risk symptoms/behaviours (e.g. active suicidal ideation, potential medication diversion/abuse, marked symptom exacerbation, or acute trauma/loss).

REFERENCES

Alegria, M., Nakash, O., & NeMoyer, A. (2018). Increasing equity in access to mental health care: a critical first step in improving service quality. *World Psychiatry*, **17**, 43–44.

Aljumah, K. & Hassali, M. A. (2015). Impact of pharmacist intervention on adherence and measurable patient outcomes among depressed patients: a randomised controlled study. *BMC Psychiatry*, **15**, 219.

Alston, C. Z., Berger, S., Brownlee, G., Elwyn, F. J., Fowler, L. K., Hall, V. M., et al. (2014). *Shared Decision-Making Strategies for Best Care: Patient Decision Aids* (National Academy of Medicine Perspectives. Discussion paper). Washington, DC: National Academy of Medicine. https://nam.edu/perspectives-2014-shared-decision-making-strategies-for-best-care-patient-decision-aids/

American Academy of Child & Adolescent Psychiatry (2020). Policy statement: clinical use of pharmacogenetic tests in prescribing psychotropic medications for children and adolescents. https://www.aacap.org/aacap/Policy_Statements/2020/Clinical-Use-Pharmacogenetic-Tests-Prescribing-Psychotropic-Medications-for-Children-Adolescents.aspx

American Diabetes Association, American Psychiatric Association, American Association of Clinical Endocrinologists, & North American Association for the Study of Obesity (2004). Consensus development conference on antipsychotic drugs and obesity and diabetes *Diabetes Care*, **27**, 596–601.

American Psychiatric Association (2016). *Practice Guidelines for the Psychiatric Treatment of Adults* (3rd ed.). Washington, DC: American Psychiatric Association. https://psychiatryonline.org/doi/book/10.1176/appi.books.9780890426760

American Psychiatric Association (2021). *Practice Guidelines for the Treatment of Patients with Schizophrenia* (3rd ed.). Washington, DC: American Psychiatric Association. https://psychiatryonline.org/doi/book/10.1176/appi.books.9780890424841

American Psychiatric Association (n.d.). Clinical practice guidelines. https://www.psychiatry.org/psychiatrists/practice/clinical-practice-guidelines

Banham, L. & Gilbody, S. (2010). Smoking cessation in severe mental illness: what works? *Addiction*, **105**, 1176–1189.

Barr, P. J., Forcino, R. C., Dannenberg, M. D., Mishra, M., Turner, E., & Zisman-Ilani, Y. (2019). Healthcare Options for People Experiencing Depression (HOPE_D): the development and pilot testing of an encounter-based decision aid for use in primary care. *British Medical Journal Open*, **9**, e025375.

Barry, M. J. & Edgman-Levitan, S. (2012). Shared decision making—the pinnacle of patient-centered care. *New England Journal of Medicine*, **366**, 780–781.

Blanco, C., Compton, W. M., Saha, T. D., Goldstein, B. I., Ruan, W. J., Huang, B., et al. (2017). Epidemiology of DSM-5 bipolar I disorder: results from the National Epidemiologic Survey on Alcohol and Related Conditions—III. *Journal of Psychiatric Research*, **84**, 310–317.

British Association for Psychopharmacology (2021). BAP consensus guidelines. https://www.bap.org.uk/guidelines

Buchanan, R. W., Kreyenbuhl, J., Kelly, D. L., Noel, J. M., Boggs, D. L., & Fischer, B. A. (2010). The 2009 schizophrenia PORT psychopharmacological treatment recommendations and summary statements. *Schizophrenia Bulletin*, **36**, 71–93.

Bury, D., Hendrick, D., Smith, T. E., Metcalf, J., & Drake, R. E. (2022). The psychiatric nurse care coordinator on a multi-disciplinary, community mental health treatment team. *Community Mental Health Journal*, 58, 1354–1360.

Care Quality Commission (2015). *2015 Community Mental Health Survey. Statistical Release*. London: Care Quality Commission. https://www.cqc.org.uk/sites/default/files/20151020_mh15_statistical_release.pdf

Chalker, S. A., Carmel, A., Atkins, D. C., Landes, S. J., Kerbrat, A. H., & Comtois, K. A. (2015). Examining challenging behaviors of clients with borderline personality disorder. *Behavior Research and Therapy*, 75, 11–19.

Charles, C., Gafni, A., & Whelan, T. (1997). Shared decision-making in the medical encounter: what does it mean? (or it takes at least two to tango). *Social Science & Medicine*, 44, 681–692.

Cipriani, A., Furukawa, T. A., Salanti, G., Chaimani, A., Atkinson, L. Z., Ogawa, Y., et al. (2018). Comparative efficacy and acceptability of 21 antidepressant drugs for the acute treatment of adults with major depressive disorder: a systematic review and network meta-analysis. *Lancet*, 391, 1357–1366.

Cochrane Library (n.d.). Mental health reviews. https://www.cochranelibrary.com/cdsr/reviews/topics

Cohn, T. A. & Sernyak, M. J. (2006). Metabolic monitoring for patients treated with antipsychotic medications. *Canadian Journal of Psychiatry*, 51, 492–501.

Cook, B. L., Wayne, G. F., Kafali, E. N., Liu, Z., Shu, C., & Flores, M. (2014). Trends in smoking among adults with mental illness and association between mental health treatment and smoking cessation. *JAMA*, 311, 172–182.

Cordes, J., Sinha-Röder, A., Kahl, K. G., Malevani, J., Thuenker, J., Lange-Asschenfeldt, C., et al. (2008). Therapeutic options for weight management in schizophrenic patients treated with atypical antipsychotics. *Fortschritte der Neurologie-Psychiatrie*, 76, 703–714.

Correll, C. U., Kim, E. Sliwa, J. K., Hamm, M., Gopal, S., Mathews, M., et al. (2021). Pharmacokinetic characteristics of long-acting injectable antipsychotics for schizophrenia: an overview. *CNS Drugs*, 35, 39–59.

Coulter, A. (2017). Shared decision making: everyone wants it, so why isn't it happening? *World Psychiatry*, 16, 117–118.

Deegan, P. E. (2010). A web application to support recovery and shared decision making in psychiatric medication clinics. *Psychiatric Rehabilitation Journal*, 34, 23–28.

Deegan P. E., Carpenter-Song, E., Drake, R. E., Naslund, J. A., Luciano, A., & Hutchison, S. L. (2017). Enhancing clients' communication regarding goals for using psychiatric medications. *Psychiatric Services*, 68, 771–775.

Deegan, P. E., Rapp, C., Holter M., & Riefer, M. (2008). A program to support shared decision making in an outpatient psychiatric medication clinic. *Psychiatric Services*, 59, 603–605.

Dieterich, M., Irving, C. B., Bergman, H., Khokhar, M. A., Park, B., & Marshall, M. (2017). Intensive case management for severe mental illness. *Cochrane Database of Systematic Reviews*, 1, CD007906.

Dixon, L. B., Glynn, S. M., Cohen, A. N., Drapalski, A. L., Medoff, D., & Fang, L. J. (2014). Outcomes of a brief program, REORDER, to promote consumer recovery and family involvement in care. *Psychiatric Services*, 65, 116–120.

Drake, R. E., Cimpean, D., & Torrey, W. C. (2009). Shared decision making in mental health: prospects for personalized medicine. *Dialogues in Clinical Neuroscience*, 11, 455–463.

Elbeddini, A., Sawhney, M., Tayefehchamani, Y., Yilmaz, Z., Elshahawi, A., Josh Villegas, J., & Dela Cruz, J. (2021). Deprescribing for all: a narrative review identifying inappropriate polypharmacy for all ages in hospital settings. *BMJ Open Quality*, 10, e001509.

Elwyn, G., Frosch, D., Thomson, R., Joseph-Williams, N., Lloyd, A., Kinnersley, P., et al. (2012). Shared decision making: a model for clinical practice. *Journal of General Internal Medicine*, 27, 1361–1367.

Ferron, J. C., Brunette, M. F., He, X., Xie, H., McHugo, G. J., & Drake, R. E. (2011). Course of smoking and quit attempts among clients with co-occurring severe mental illness and substance use disorders. *Psychiatric Services*, 62, 353–359.

Finnerty, M. T., Layman, D. M., Chen, Q., Leckman-Westin, E., Bermeo, N., & Ng-Mak, D. S. (2018). Use of a web-based shared decision-making program: impact on ongoing treatment engagement and antipsychotic adherence. *Psychiatric Services*, 69, 1215–1221.

Fortney, J. C., Unützer, J., Wrenn, G., Pyne, J. M., Smith, G. R., Schoenbaum, M., et al. (2017). A tipping point for measurement-based care. *Psychiatric Services*, 68, 179–188.

Frost, H., Campbell, P., Maxwell, M., O'Carroll, R. E., Dombrowski, S. U., Williams, B., et al. (2018). Effectiveness of motivational interviewing on adult behaviour change in health and social care settings: a systematic review of reviews. *PLoS One*, 13, e0204890.

Gallego, J. A., Bonetti, J., Zhang, J., Kane, J. M., & Correll, C. U. (2012). Prevalence and correlates of antipsychotic polypharmacy: a systematic review and meta-regression of global and regional trends from the 1970s to 2009. *Schizophrenia Research*, 138, 18–28.

Gannon, J. M., Lupu, A., Brar, J., Brandt, M., Zawacki, S., John, S., et al. (2021). Deprescribing anticholinergic medication in the community mental health setting: a quality improvement initiative. *Research in Social and Administrative Pharmacy*, 17, 1841–1846.

Goscha, R. & Rapp, C. (2015). Exploring the experiences of client involvement in medication decisions using a shared decision making model: results of a qualitative study. *Community Mental Health Journal*, 51, 267–274.

Hamann, J., Cohen, R., Leucht, S., Busch, R. & Kissling, W. (2007). Shared decision making and long-term outcome in schizophrenia treatment. *Journal of Clinical Psychiatry*, 68, 992–997.

Hanson, H. M., Léveillé, T., Cole, M., Soril, L. J., Clement, F., Wagg, A., et al. (2021). Effect of a multimethod quality improvement intervention on antipsychotic medication use among residents of long-term care. *BMJ Open Quality*, 10, e001211.

Harris, M. E. & Fallot, R. D. (2001). *Using Trauma Theory to Design Service Systems*. San Francisco, CA: Jossey-Bass.

Hawkins, E. J., Danner, A. N., Malte, C. A., Blanchard, B. E., Williams, E. C., Hagedorn, H. J., et al. (2021). Clinical leaders and providers' perspectives on delivering medications for the treatment of opioid use disorder in Veteran Affairs' facilities. *Addiction Science & Clinical Practice*, 16, 55.

Heishman, S. J., Kleykamp, B. A., & Singleton, E. G. (2010). Meta-analysis of the acute effects of nicotine and smoking on human performance. *Psychopharmacology (Berlin)*, 210, 453–469.

Horvitz-Lennon, M., Volya, R., Zelevinsky, K., Shen, M., Donohue, J. M., Mulcahy, A., et al. (2022). Significance and factors associated with antipsychotic polypharmacy utilization among publicly insured US adults. *Administration and Policy in Mental Health and Mental Health Services Research*, 49, 59–70.

Huhn, A. S. & Gipson, C. D. (2021). Promoting harm reduction as a treatment outcome in substance use disorders. *Experimental and Clinical Psychopharmacology*, 29, 217–218.

Jones, P. B., Barnes, T. R., Davies, L., Dunn, G., Lloyd, H., Hayhurst, K. P., et al. (2006). Randomized controlled trial of the effect on quality of life of second- vs first-generation antipsychotic drugs in schizophrenia: Cost Utility of the Latest Antipsychotic Drugs in

Schizophrenia Study (CUtLASS 1). *Archives of General Psychiatry*, **63**, 1079–1087.

Kahn, R. S., Fleischhacker, W. W., & Boter, H. (2008). Effectiveness of antipsychotic drugs in first-episode schizophrenia and schizophreniform disorder: an open randomised clinical trial. *Lancet*, **371**, 1085–1097.

Kishimoto, T., Hagi, K., Kurokawa, S., Kane, J. M., & Correll, C. U. (2021). Long-acting injectable versus oral antipsychotics for the maintenance treatment of schizophrenia: a systematic review and comparative meta-analysis of randomised, cohort, and pre-post studies. *Lancet Psychiatry*, **8**, 387–404.

Klevan, T., Sommer, M., Borg, M., Karlsson, B., Sundet, R., & Kim, H. S. (2021). Part III: recovery-oriented practices in community mental health and substance abuse services: a meta-synthesis. *International Journal of Environmental Research and Public Health*, **18**, 13180.

Knudsen, H. K., Abraham, A. J., & Roman, P. M. (2011). Adoption and implementation of medications in addiction treatment programs. *Journal of Addiction Medicine*, **5**, 21–27.

Koekkoek, B., van Meijel, B., & Hutschemaekers, G. (2006). 'Difficult patients' in mental health care: a review. *Psychiatric Services*, **57**, 795–802.

Kreyenbuhl, J., Nossel, I. R., & Dixon, L. B. (2009). Disengagement from mental health treatment among individuals with schizophrenia and strategies for facilitating connections to care: a review of the literature. *Schizophrenia Bulletin*, **35**, 696–703.

Lagerberg, T., Molero, Y., D'Onofrio, B. M., Fernandez de la Cruz, L., Lichtenstein, P., Mataix-Cols, D., et al. (2019). Antidepressant prescription patterns and CNS polypharmacy with antidepressants among children, adolescents, and young adults: a population-based study in Sweden. *European Child and Adolescent Psychiatry*, **28**, 1137–1145.

Lagisetty, P., Klasa, K., Bush, C., Heisler, M., Chopra, V., & Bohnert, A. (2017). Primary care models for treating opioid use disorders: what actually works? A systematic review. *PLoS One*, **12**, e0186315.

LeBlanc, A., Herrin, J., Williams, M. D., Inselman, J. W., Branda, M. E., Shah, N. D., et al. (2015). Shared decision making for antidepressants in primary care: a cluster randomized trial. *JAMA Internal Medicine*, **175**, 1761–1770.

Leucht, S., Crippa, A., Siafis, S., Patel, M. X., Orsini, N., & Davis, J. M. (2020). Dose-response meta-analysis of antipsychotic drugs for acute schizophrenia. *American Journal of Psychiatry*, **177**, 342–353.

Leucht, S., Leucht, C., Huhn, M., Chaimani, S., Mavridis, D., Helfer, B., et al. (2017). Sixty years of placebo-controlled antipsychotic drug trials in acute schizophrenia: systematic review, Bayesian meta-analysis, and meta-regression of efficacy predictors. *American Journal of Psychiatry*, **174**, 927–942.

Lewis, C. C., Boyd, M., Puspitasari, A., Navarro, E., Howard, J., Kassab, H., et al. (2019). Implementing measurement-based care in behavioral health: a review. *JAMA Psychiatry*, **76**, 324–335.

Lewis, S., Geddes, J.R., Goodwin, G., Morriss, R., Rendell, J., Geddes, J. R., et al. (2010). Lithium plus valproate combination therapy versus monotherapy for relapse prevention in bipolar I disorder (BALANCE): a randomised open-label trial. *Lancet*, **375**, 385–395.

Lewis-Fernández, R., Aggarwal, N. K., & Kirmayer, L. J. (2020). The cultural formulation interview: progress to date and future directions. *Transcultural Psychiatry*, **57**, 487–496.

Lieberman, J. A., Stroup, T. S., McEvoy, J. P., Swartz, M. S., Rosenheck, R. A., Perkins, D. O., et al. (2005). Effectiveness of antipsychotic drugs in patients with chronic schizophrenia. *New England Journal of Medicine*, **353**, 1209–1223.

Lim, C. T., Caan, M. P., Kim, C. H., Chow, C. M., Leff, H. S., & Tepper, M. C. (2022). Care management for serious mental illness: a systematic review and meta-analysis. *Psychiatric Services*, **73**, 180–187.

Ljungberg, A., Denhov, A., & Topor, A. (2016). Non-helpful relationships with professionals—a literature review of the perspective of persons with severe mental illness. *Journal of Mental Health*, **25**, 267–277.

Loh, A., Simon, D., Wills, C. E., Kriston, L., Niebling, W., & Harter, M. (2007). The effects of a shared decision-making intervention in primary care of depression: a cluster randomized controlled trial. *Patient Education and Counseling*, **67**, 324–332.

Lung, S. L. M., Lee, H. M. E., Chen, Y. H. E., Chan, K. W. S., Chang, W. C., & Hui, L. M. C. (2018). Prevalence and correlates of antipsychotic polypharmacy in Hong Kong. *Asian Journal of Psychiatry*, **33**, 113–120.

Ma, J., Bao, Y. P., Wang, R. J., Su, M. F., Liu, M. X., Li, J. Q., et al. (2019). Effects of medication-assisted treatment on mortality among opioids users: a systematic review and meta-analysis. *Molecular Psychiatry*, **24**, 1868–1883.

Marder, S. R., Essock, S. M., Miller, A. L., Buchanan, R. W., Casey, D. E., Davis, J. M., et al. (2004). Physical health monitoring of patients with schizophrenia. *American Journal of Psychiatry*, **161**, 1334–1349.

Mattick, R. P., Breen, C., Kimber, J., & Davoli, M. (2014). Buprenorphine maintenance versus placebo or methadone maintenance for opioid dependence. *Cochrane Database Systematic Review*, **6**, CD002207.

McDonagh, M. S., Dana, T., Selph, S., Devine, E. B., Cantor, A., & Bougatsos, C. (2017). *Treatments for Schizophrenia in Adults: A Systematic Review* (Comparative Effectiveness Review No. 198). Rockville, MD: Agency for Healthcare Research and Quality.

Milfort, R., Bond, G. R., McGurk, S. R., & Drake, R. E. (2015). Barriers to employment among social security disability insurance beneficiaries in the Mental Health Treatment Study. *Psychiatric Services*, **66**, 1350–1352.

Mojtabai, R. & Olfson, M. (2010). National trends in psychotropic medication polypharmacy in office-based psychiatry. *Archives of General Psychiatry*, **67**, 26–36.

Mueser, K. T., Noordsy, D. L., Drake, R. E., & Fox, L. (2001). Integrated treatment for severe mental illness and substance abuse: effective components of programs for persons with co-occurring disorders. *Sante Mentale au Quebec*, **26**, 22–46.

National Center for Health Statistics (2019). Health, United States, 2019—data finder. https://www.cdc.gov/nchs/data/hus/2019/039-508.pdf

National Institute for Health and Care Excellence (2021). NICE guidelines for mental health and behavioral conditions. https://www.nice.org.uk/guidance/conditions-and-diseases/mental-health-and-behavioural-conditions

National Institute for Health and Care Excellence (2022a). Methadone and buprenorphine for the management of opioid dependence. https://www.nice.org.uk/guidance/ta114/chapter/1-Guidance

National Institute for Health and Care Excellence (2022b). Alcohol-use disorders: diagnosis, assessment and management of harmful drinking (high-risk drinking) and alcohol dependence. https://www.nice.org.uk/guidance/cg115/chapter/1-Guidance

O'Brien, A., Fahmy, R., & Singh, S. P. (2009). Disengagement from mental health services. *Social Psychiatry and Psychiatric Epidemiology*, **44**, 558–568.

Ontario Health (Quality) (2021). Multi-gene pharmacogenomic testing that includes decision-support tools to guide medication selection for major depression: a health technology assessment. *Ontario Health Technology Assessment Series*, **21**, 1–214.

Ortiz-Orendain, J., Castiello-de Obeso, S., Colunga-Lozano, L. E., Hu, Y., Maayan, N., & Adams, C. E. (2017). Antipsychotic combinations for schizophrenia. *Cochrane Database Systematic Review*, **28**, CD009005.

Pacchiarotti, I., Tiihonen, J., Kotzalidis, G. D., Verdolini, N., Murru, A., Goikolea, J. M., et al. (2019). Long-acting injectable antipsychotics (LAIs) for maintenance treatment of bipolar and schizoaffective disorders: a systematic review. *European Neuropsychopharmacology*, **29**, 457–470.

Peckham, E., Brabyn, S., Cook, L., Tew, G., & Gilbody, S. (2017). Smoking cessation in severe mental ill health: what works? An updated systematic review and meta-analysis. *BMC Psychiatry*, **14**, 252.

Piacentini, J., Bennett, S., Compton, S. N., Kendall, P. C., Birmahar, B., Albano, A. M., et al. (2014). 24- and 36-week outcomes for the child/adolescent anxiety multimodal study (CAMS). *Journal of the American Academy of Child & Adolescent Psychiatry*, **53**, 297–310.

Qeadan, F., Mensah, N. A., Gu, L. Y., Madden, E. F., Venner, K. L., & English, K. (2021). Trends in the use of naltrexone for addiction treatment among alcohol use disorder admissions in U.S. substance use treatment facilities. *International Journal of Environmental Research and Public Health*, **18**, 8884.

Raue, P. J., Schulberg, H. C., Bruce, M. L., Banerjee, S., Artis, A., Espejo, M., et al. (2019). Effectiveness of shared decision-making for elderly depressed minority primary care patients. *American Journal of Geriatric Psychiatry*, **27**, 883–893.

Ray, L. A., Meredith, L. R., Kiluk, B. D., Walthers, J., Carroll, K. M., & Magill, M. (2020). Combined pharmacotherapy and cognitive behavioral therapy for adults with alcohol or substance use disorders: a systematic review and meta-analysis. *JAMA Open Network*, **3**, e208279.

Reeve, E., Gnjidic, D., Long, J., & Hilmer, S. (2015). A systematic review of the emerging definition of 'deprescribing' with network analysis: implications for future research and clinical practice. *British Journal of Clinical Pharmacology*, **80**, 1254–1268.

Rhee, T. G. & Rosenheck, R. A. (2019). Psychotropic polypharmacy reconsidered: between-class polypharmacy in the context of multimorbidity in the treatment of depressive disorders. *Journal of Affective Disorders*, **252**, 450–457.

Robinson, D. G., Schooler, N. R., Correll, C. U., John, M., Kurian, B., Marcy, P., et al. (2018). Psychopharmacological treatment in the RAISE-ETP study: outcomes of a manual and computer decision support system based intervention. *American Journal of Psychiatry*, **175**, 169–179.

Roca, R. P. (2020). High-value mental health care and the person in the room. *Psychiatric Services*, **71**, 110–111.

Rush, A. J., Trivedi, M. H., Wisniewski, S. R., Nierenberg, A. A., Stewart, J. W., Warden, D., et al. (2006). Acute and longer-term outcomes in depressed outpatients requiring one or several treatment steps: a STAR*D report. *American Journal of Psychiatry*, **163**, 1905–1917.

Rush, A. J. (2015). Isn't it about time to employ measurement-based care in practice? *American Journal of Psychiatry*, **172**, 934–936.

Sachs, G. S., Nierenberg, A. A., Calabrese, J. R., Marangell, L. B., Wisniewski, S. R., Gyulai, L., et al. (2007). Effectiveness of adjunctive antidepressant treatment for bipolar depression. *New England Journal of Medicine*, **356**, 1711–1722.

Salyers, M. P., Fukui, S., Bonfils, K. A., Firmin, R. L., Luther, L., Goscha, R., et al. (2017). Consumer outcomes after implementing CommonGround as an approach to shared decision making. *Psychiatric Services*, **68**, 299–302.

Sarkar, S. (2017). Psychiatric polypharmacy, etiology and potential consequences. *Current Psychopharmacology*, **6**, 12–26.

Schulze, L. N., Stentzel, U., Leipert, J., Schulte, J., Langosch, J., Freyberger, H. J., et al. (2019). Improving medication adherence with telemedicine for adults with severe mental illness. *Psychiatric Services*, **70**, 225–228.

Schwartz, R. P., Gryczynski, J., O'Grady, K. E., Sharfstein, J. M., Warren, G., Olsen, Y., et al. (2013). Opioid agonist treatments and heroin overdose deaths in Baltimore, Maryland, 1995–2009. *American Journal of Public Health*, **103**, 917–922.

Semahegn, A., Torpey, K., Manu, A., Assefa, N., Tesfaye, G., & Ankomah, A. (2018). Psychotropic medication non-adherence and associated factors among adult patients with major psychiatric disorders: a protocol for a systematic review. *Systematic Reviews*, **7**, 1–5.

Smith, T. E., Easter, A., Pollock, M., Pope, L. G., & Wisdom, J. P. (2013). Disengagement from care: perspectives of individuals with serious mental illness and service providers. *Psychiatric Services*, **64**, 770–775.

Smith, T. E., Sullivan, A. T., & Druss, B. G. (2021). Redesigning public mental health systems post-COVID-19. *Psychiatric Services*, **72**, 602–605.

Sneider, B., Pristed, S. G., Correll, C. U., & Nielsen, J. (2015). Frequency and correlates of antipsychotic polypharmacy among patients with schizophrenia in Denmark: a nation-wide pharmacoepidemiological study. *European Neuropsychopharmacology*, **10**, 1669–1676.

Stacey, D., Kryworuchko, J., Belkora, J., Davison, B. J., Durand, M., & Eden, K. B. (2013). Coaching and guidance with patient decision aids: a review of theoretical and empirical evidence. BMC Medical *Informatics and Decision Making*, **13**(Suppl. 2), S11.

Stacey, D., Legare, F., Lewis, K., Barry, M. J., Bennett, C. L., Eden, K. B., et al. (2017). Decision aids for people facing health treatment or screening decisions. *Cochrane Database Systematic Review*, **4**, CD001431.

Steele, D. W., Becker, S. J., Danko, K. J., Balk, E. M., Adam, G. P., Saldanha, I. J., et al. (2020). Brief behavioral interventions for substance use in adolescents: a meta-analysis. *Pediatrics*, **146**, e20200351.

Stentzel, U., van den Berg, N., Schulze, L. N., Schwaneberg, T., Radicke, F., Langosch, J. M., et al. (2018). Predictors of medication adherence among patients with severe psychiatric disorders: findings from the baseline assessment of a randomized controlled trial (Tecla). *BMC Psychiatry*, **18**, 1–8.

Stiggelbout, A. M., van der Weijden, T., de Wit, M. P., Frosch, D., Légaré, F., Montori, V. M., et al. (2012). Shared decision making: really putting patients at the centre of healthcare. *British Medical Journal*, **344**, e256.

Stroup, T. S., Gerhard, T., Crystal, S., Huang, C., Tan, Z., Wall, M. M., et al. (2018). Psychotropic medication use among adults with schizophrenia and schizoaffective disorder in the United States. *Psychiatric Services*, **69**, 605–608.

Substance Abuse and Mental Health Services Administration (2021). Evidence-Based Practices Resource Center. https://www.samhsa.gov/resource-search/ebp

Substance Abuse and Mental Health Services Administration (2022). Medication assisted treatment. https://www.samhsa.gov/medication-assisted-treatmen

Taylor, G. M., Lindson, N., Farley, A., Leinberger-Jabari, A., Sawyer, K., Te Water Naudé, R., et al. (2021). Smoking cessation for improving mental health. *Cochrane Database of Systematic Reviews*, **3**, CD013522.

Thomas, E. C., Ben-David, S., Treichler, E., Roth, S., Dixon, L. B., Salzer, M., et al. (2021). A systematic review of shared decision-making interventions for service users with serious mental illnesses:

state of the science and future directions. *Psychiatric Services*, **72**, 1288–1300.

Thornicroft, G., Chatterji, S., Evans-Lacko, S., Gruber, M., Sampson, N., Aguilar-Gaxiola, S., et al. (2017). Undertreatment of people with major depressive disorder in 21 countries. *British Journal of Psychiatry*, **210**, 119–124.

Treichler, E. B. H., Avila, A., Evans, E. A., & Spaulding, W. D. (2020). Collaborative decision skills training: feasibility and preliminary outcomes of a novel intervention. *Psychological Services*, **17**, 54–64.

Velligan, D. I., Weiden, P. J., Sajatovic, M., Scott, J., Carpenter, D., Ross, R., et al. (2009). The expert consensus guideline series: adherence problems in patients with serious and persistent mental illness. *Journal of Clinical Psychiatry*, **70**(Suppl. 4), 1–46.

Wang, P. S., Lane, M., Olfson, M., Pincus, H. A., Wells, K. B., & Kessler, R. C. (2005). Twelve-month use of mental health services in the United States: results from the National Comorbidity Survey Replication. *Archives of General Psychiatry*, **62**, 629–640.

World Federation of Societies of Biological Psychiatry (2021). WFSBP treatment guidelines and consensus papers. https://www.wfsbp.org/educational-activities/wfsbp-treatment-guidelines-and-consensus-papers/

Wieringa, T. H., Rodriguez-Gutierrez, R., Spencer-Bonilla, G., de Wit, M., Ponce, O. J., Sanchez-Herrera, M. F., et al. (2019). Decision aids that facilitate elements of shared decision making in chronic illnesses: a systematic review. *Systematic Reviews*, **8**, 121.

Zhou, X., Teng, T., Zhang, Y., Del Giovane, C., Furukawa, T. A., Weisz, J. R., et al. (2020). Comparative efficacy and acceptability of antidepressants, psychotherapies, and their combination for acute treatment of children and adolescents with depressive disorder: a systematic review and network meta-analysis. *Lancet Psychiatry*, **7**, 581–601.

Zeier, Z., Carpenter, L. L., Kalin, N. H., Rodriguez, C. I., McDonald, W. M., Widge, A. S., et al. (2018). Clinical implementation of pharmacogenetic decision support tools for antidepressant drug prescribing. *American Journal of Psychiatry*, **175**, 873–886.

Zhang, C., Spence, O., Reeves, G., & dosReis, S. (2021). Characteristics of youths treated with psychotropic polypharmacy in the United States, 1999 to 2015. *JAMA Pediatrics*, **175**, 196–198.

Ziedonis, D., Hitsman, B., Beckham, J. C., Zvolensky, M., Adler, L. E., Audrain-McGovern, J., et al. (2008). Tobacco use and cessation in psychiatric disorders: National Institute of Mental Health report. *Nicotine and Tobacco Research*, **10**, 1691–1715.

Zisman-Ilani, Y., Barnett, E., Harik, J., Pavlo, A., & O'Connell, M. (2017). Expanding the concept of shared decision making for mental health: systematic search and scoping review of interventions. *Mental Health Review Journal*, **22**, 191–213.

16 Psychiatric outpatient clinics

Markus Koesters, Carolin Schneider, and Thomas Becker

Introduction

Specialist psychiatric outpatient services have not, in recent decades, been a priority for either the conceptual development or the study of community mental health care. General (or psychiatric) hospitals and community mental health team bases, at all of which outpatient clinics are held, can be considered community based as they are all located 'in the community'. However, there may have been an implicit assumption that services should be considered community based only if conceptually they have moved away from hospitals or other institutions. Also, the outpatient clinic model, in its traditional form, has been 'single-handed', with patients seeing a single practitioner at a time. Outpatient clinics therefore usually lack multidisciplinary input.

A review of the community-based UK mental health care system suggests that outpatient clinics are reported at more than two-thirds of so-called local implementation sites (Glover, 2007). There may also be a recent trend towards specialized clinics for subgroups of patients (e.g. people with affective disorders, mentally disordered offenders, young adults, new mothers, or patients with eating disorders). Also, there may be a degree of under-reporting of outpatient clinics in surveys of local mental health services (Glover, 2007). Historically, these services have been a core element in the provision of psychiatric treatment, and it is likely that outpatient care continues to be a service element meeting important clinical needs in a large number of people with mental disorders.

History of outpatient care

In Europe, outpatient care started in the second half of the nineteenth century with charitable organizations that aimed to implement post-discharge care in a period when mental health care was dominated by large asylums (Shorter, 2007). In the twentieth century, outpatient care was a key element in the mental health care reform movement that occurred in England between the 1930s through the 1960s (Freeman & Bennett, 1991). After the era of de-institutionalization, the developments in mental health care systems aimed at achieving a system of 'balanced care' (Thornicroft & Tansella, 1999), where outpatient treatment, more and more specialized and provided by multiprofessional teams, still plays a major role, supplemented by alternative community services and programmes (Becker & Vazquez-Barquero, 2001).

Functions of outpatient clinics

In this chapter, we review the literature on outpatient clinics. A systematic literature search including EMBASE, Medline, PsycInfo, and the Cochrane databases of controlled trials (CCTR) and systematic reviews (CDSR) was conducted, with the terms 'outpatient clinics' and 'mental health' or 'psychiatry' combined with comprehensive search strategies for controlled trials (The Cochrane Collaboration, 2009) and systematic reviews (Shojania & Bero, 2001). Although the search was intentionally broad with a high false-positive rate, about 1100 references were identified and only 62 publications remained for detailed evaluation after title and abstract screening. For further improvement of the literature search, a backward citation search of relevant key papers was also conducted.

The term *psychiatric outpatient clinics*, as used in this text, refers to facilities providing office-based support and therapy for people with mental disorders. It is important to bear in mind that the conceptual boundaries with other ambulatory settings such as (crisis intervention and) home treatment, day hospital care, case management, or assertive community treatment that are covered in other chapters of this book are sometimes blurred. Furthermore, there is substantial variety between outpatient clinics both across and within countries. While in Italy outpatient services are delivered mainly by outpatient clinics organized in mental health care centres, most having a multidisciplinary team (de Girolamo et al., 2007), psychiatrists ('Nervenärzte'), psychologists, and general practitioners in office practice, the majority of whom are single-handed, provide most of outpatient care services in Germany (Salize et al., 2007). Similarly, most outpatient clinics in England are staffed by doctors alone (Glover, 2007), whereas in France the availability and organization of the health service heavily depends on the region (Verdoux, 2007). Furthermore, outpatient clinics vary with respect to (Thornicroft & Tansella, 2004):

- referral (self-referral vs referral by primary care)
- appointment times (fixed appointment times vs open access)
- clinical contact (doctors alone or other disciplines)

- payment
- methods to enhance attendance rates
- response to non-attenders
- frequency and duration of appointments.

Evaluation of outpatient services

Outpatient treatment compared to other settings

Despite outpatient treatment being a standard component in most mental health care systems, there is only little evidence on the effectiveness of outpatient treatment as an element of the health care system as compared with other service components. However, the vast majority of treatment trials have been conducted within outpatient settings, and their results suggest that this setting is able to deliver effective treatment.

Outpatient compared to day hospital treatment

A Cochrane review summarized the evidence of day hospital versus outpatient care for people with schizophrenia (Shek et al., 2009). The review included only four randomized controlled trials that were conducted between 1966 and 1986 and concluded that there is insufficient evidence to draw a definite conclusion as to whether day hospital treatment (with higher treatment intensity) has an advantage over outpatient care. An older version of that review (Marshall et al. 2001a, 2001b) included an additional group of four studies of people with depression, anxiety, personality disorders, and neurotic disorders, and it drew similar conclusions. Two trials in this latter review suggested that day treatment might be superior to outpatient care in patients 'refractory to outpatient treatments', but data of these trials could not be combined due to differences in the reporting of data. On the basis of these reviews and all other studies reviewed, the conclusion was that it was insufficient to draw further conclusions regarding differential effects of the two treatment modalities (Marshall et al. 2001b).

Another study compared the efficacy of short-term day hospital with outpatient psychotherapy after 8 (Arnevik et al., 2009), 18 (Arnevik et al., 2010) and 36 months (Gullestad et al., 2012) as well as after 3 and 6 years (Antonsen, 2014) in patients with personality disorders. Results revealed that both groups improved in efficacy, but no statistical differences between the groups were found, with the exception of the 36-month follow-up, where outpatients achieved lower symptom scores than patients in the day hospital group. In contrast, a South Korean study (Kong, 2005) found advantages for a day treatment programme compared to the usual outpatient clinic care. In this study, 50 adult patients with eating disorders were randomized to a day treatment or standard outpatient care. There was significantly more improvement in most outcome measurements in people who were treated in the day treatment condition.

Outpatient compared to inpatient treatment

One fairly old and rather small trial compared specialized outpatient treatment as an alternative to full-time hospitalization. A sample of 20 patients with acute schizophrenia were randomly assigned to the two groups. There were no significant differences between the two groups in terms of treatment efficacy, but 'cost per remission' was about six times higher ($3330 vs $565) in the hospital group, although patients in the outpatient treatment group were given daily appointments and a regimen of pharmacotherapy, psychotherapy, and family counselling. In a pilot study, patients were randomized to home treatment or hospital-based outpatient treatment (Dewa et al., 2009). Both treatment modalities were part of a first-episode psychosis programme and provided care through a multidisciplinary team. The primary difference between both treatment modalities was the setting where care was delivered (home vs hospital setting). In both treatment groups, patients showed significant clinical improvement, but there was no difference in improvement rates between the groups. However, the results are based on a small sample of 29 completers.

Gowers et al. (2007) compared clinical effectiveness of three treatment settings for anorexia nervosa in adolescents. They randomized 170 adolescents to inpatient, specialist outpatient treatment, or treatment as usual in the general community. The clinical outcomes of the three treatment groups did not differ significantly at 1- and 2-year follow-up. Another study compared the effectiveness of outpatient, day hospital, and inpatient treatment in patients with cluster B personality disorder and found the inpatient group to show the largest improvements (Bartak, 2011). Similar results revealed the working group in a study with patients with cluster C personality disorder (Bartak, 2010). In this study, short-term inpatient treatment showed overall better improvements compared to short- and long-term outpatient, day hospital, or long-term inpatient treatment.

Outpatient compared to community mental health teams

Tyrer et al. (1998) randomized 155 patients to community multi-disciplinary teams or hospital-based outpatient care. The authors compared clinical outcomes and cost of care 1 year after discharge from inpatient care. Clinical outcomes were similar between the two groups, but readmission to hospital was more likely in the hospital-based care programme.

Limitations of the identified studies

Most of the studies mentioned above failed to show a significant difference in clinical efficacy between mental health care components. However, in a randomized controlled trial Sellwood et al. (1999) showed that, as compared with outpatient treatment alone, an additional home-based rehabilitation intervention significantly improved interpersonal functioning and social behaviour although there were no differences in positive or negative symptoms of psychosis. Given that there are effective pharmacological treatment options for most of the conditions studied, differences in the efficacy between service components might be negligible. However, there may be differences in other patient relevant outcomes beyond clinical efficacy (e.g. patient/user and carer satisfaction). Furthermore, there is a lack of evidence regarding the issue of what contributes to an effective outpatient clinic. Our literature search failed to reveal any trials comparing types of outpatient clinic with respect to clinical outcomes.

Costs of outpatient care

There is a general consensus that outpatient and community care are generally cheaper than care in hospital settings. There are, in fact, trials indicating that community treatment is also more cost-effective (Goldberg, 1991), but there are only few randomized controlled trials comparing cost-effectiveness of outpatient clinics compared to other service components. Byford (2007) published the economic evaluation of a trial comparing inpatient psychiatric treatment, specialist outpatient treatment, and general outpatient treatment (Gowers et al., 2007, see above). In terms of a broad service provision perspective, specialist outpatient treatment was the cheapest, whereas the general outpatient group was the most expensive treatment option, although the difference in costs between the three groups was not statistically significant. In cost-effectiveness analyses, specialist outpatient treatment had the highest probability of being cost-effective and combined outpatient treatments (specialist and general) also showed a greater probability of being more cost-effective than inpatient services.

The Cochrane review (Shek et al., 2009, see above) that compared day treatment with outpatient care concludes that the suggestion of day hospitals being more expensive than outpatient treatment is offset by the suggestion of savings in inpatient care. Another study compared costs of day hospital treatment versus outpatient psychotherapy at a specialist practice in people with personality disorder (Kvarstein et al., 2013). Kvarstein et al. (2013) report that cost-effectiveness differed between types of personality disorders and only in patients with avoidant personality disorder, day hospital treatment is more cost-effective due to the higher adjuvant health services in the outpatient setting.

Thus, it has remained unclear whether day hospitals are cost-effective as compared with outpatient treatment. Tyrer et al. (1998) concluded, that in their trial the hospital-based outpatient treatment was more expensive than community care, mainly because of the lower readmission rate in the latter group.

Conclusion

It is fair to conclude that the evidence on efficacy and effectiveness of psychiatric outpatient clinics, in comparison with other treatment settings, is insufficient. There is a lack of clarity as to whether 'packages of care' (outpatient clinic, community mental health team) are distinct with clearly defined, 'unique' borders delineating one from the other. Also, the body of evidence on distinct treatment modules (e.g. psychotropic drug treatment and psychotherapeutic interventions) applies to mental health care provision irrespective of the locus of care, and many treatment studies have found clinical improvement in pre–post, placebo, or head-to-head comparisons of patients, many or most of whom were seen in outpatient and community settings. It is likely that outpatient clinic work is 'hidden' in the comparator condition of 'treatment as usual' in many studies of non-hospital-based psychiatric treatment. There is a clinical consensus in many countries that such clinics are an efficient way of organizing assessment and treatment of people with mental disorders, provided that clinic sites are accessible to local populations. Nevertheless, outpatient clinics are simply methods of arranging clinical contact between staff and patients. The key issue is the content of the clinical interventions and the evidence of their efficacy (Thornicroft & Tansella, 2004). Outpatient clinics can be considered one valuable element of mental health care systems but settings of outpatient care may vary.

REFERENCES

Antonsen, B. T., Klungsøyr, O., Kamps, A., Hummelen, B., Johansen, M. S., Pedersen, G., et al. (2014). Step-down versus outpatient psychotherapeutic treatment for personality disorders: 6-year follow-up of the Ullevål personality project. *BMC Psychiatry*, **14**, 1–12.

Arnevik, E., Wilberg, T., Urnes, O., Johansen, M., Monsen, J. T., & Karterud, S. (2009). Psychotherapy for personality disorders: short-term day hospital psychotherapy versus outpatient individual therapy—a randomized controlled study. *European Psychiatry*, **24**, 71–78.

Arnevik, E., Wilberg, T., Urnes, Ø., Johansen, M., Monsen, J. T., & Karterud, S. (2010). Psychotherapy for personality disorders: 18 months' follow-up of the Ullevål Personality Project. *Journal of Personality Disorders*, **24**, 188–203.

Bartak, A., Andrea, H., Spreeuwenberg, M. D., Ziegler, U. M., Dekker, J., Rossum, B. V., et al. (2011). Effectiveness of outpatient, day hospital, and inpatient psychotherapeutic treatment for patients with cluster B personality disorders. *Psychotherapy and Psychosomatics*, **80**, 28–38.

Bartak, A., Spreeuwenberg, M. D., Andrea, H., Holleman, L., Rijnierse, P., Rossum, B. V., et al. (2010). Effectiveness of different modalities of psychotherapeutic treatment for patients with cluster C personality disorders: results of a large prospective multicentre study. *Psychotherapy and Psychosomatics*, **79**, 20–30.

Becker, T. & Vazquez-Barquero, J. L. (2001). The European perspective of psychiatric reform. *Acta Psychiatrica Scandinavica, Supplementum*, **104**, 8–14.

Byford, S., Barrett, B., Roberts, C., Clark, A., Edwards, V., Harrington, R., et al. (2007). Economic evaluation of a randomised controlled trial for anorexia nervosa in adolescents. *British Journal of Psychiatry*, **191**, 436–440.

de Girolamo, G., Bassi, M., Neri, G., Ruggeri, M., Santone, G., & Picardi, A. (2007). The current state of mental health care in Italy: problems, perspectives, and lessons to learn. *European Archives of Psychiatry and Clinical Neuroscience*, **257**, 83–91.

Dewa, C. S., Zipursky, R. B., Chau, N., Furimsky, I., Collins, A., Agid, O., et al. (2009). Specialized home treatment versus hospital-based outpatient treatment for first-episode psychosis: a randomized clinical trial. *Early Intervention in Psychiatry*, **3**, 304–311.

Freeman, H. L. & Bennett, D. H. (1991). Origins and development. In: Freeman, H. L. & Bennett, D. H. (Eds.), *Community Psychiatry* (pp. 40–70). Edinburgh: Churchill Livingstone.

Glover, G. (2007). Adult mental health care in England. *European Archives of Psychiatry and Clinical Neuroscience*, **257**, 71–82.

Goldberg, D. (1991). Cost-effectiveness studies in the treatment of schizophrenia: a review. *Social Psychiatry and Psychiatric Epidemiology*, **26**, 139–142.

Gowers, S. G., Clark, A., Roberts, C., Griffiths, A., Edwards, V., Bryan, C., et al. (2007). Clinical effectiveness of treatments for anorexia nervosa in adolescents: randomised controlled trial. *British Journal of Psychiatry*, **191**, 427–435.

Gullestad, F. S., Wilberg, T., Klungsøyr, O., Johansen, M. S., Urnes, Ø., & Karterud, S. (2012). Is treatment in a day hospital step-down program superior to outpatient individual psychotherapy for patients with personality disorders? 36 months follow-up of a randomized clinical trial comparing different treatment modalities. *Psychotherapy Research*, **22**, 426–441.

Kong, S. (2005). Day treatment programme for patients with eating disorders: randomized controlled trial. *Journal of Advanced Nursing*, **51**, 5–14.

Kvarstein, E. H., Arnevik, E., Halsteinli, V., Rø, F. G., Karterud, S., & Wilberg, T. (2013). Health service costs and clinical gains of psychotherapy for personality disorders: a randomized controlled trial of day-hospital-based step-down treatment versus outpatient treatment at a specialist practice. *BMC Psychiatry*, **13**, 1–13.

Marshall, M., Crowther, R., Almaraz-Serrano, A., Creed, F., Sledge, W., & Kluiter, H. (2001a). Systematic reviews of the effectiveness of day care for people with severe mental disorders: (1) acute day hospital versus admission; (2) vocational rehabilitation; (3) day hospital versus outpatient care. *Health Technology Assessment*, **5**, 1–75.

Marshall, M., Crowther, R., Almaraz-Serrano, A., & Tyrer, P. (2001b). Day hospital versus out-patient care for psychiatric disorders. *Cochrane Database of Systematic Reviews*, **2**, CD003240.

Salize, H. J., Rossler, W., & Becker, T. (2007). Mental health care in Germany: current state and trends. *European Archives of Psychiatry and Clinical Neuroscience*, **257**, 92–103.

Sellwood, W., Thomas, C. S., Tarrier, N., Jones, S., Clewes, J., James, A., et al. (1999). A randomised controlled trial of home-based rehabilitation versus outpatient-based rehabilitation for patients suffering from chronic schizophrenia. *Social Psychiatry and Psychiatric Epidemiology*, **34**, 250–253.

Shek, E., Stein, A. T., Shansis, F. M., Marshall, M., Crowther, R., & Tyrer, P. (2009). Day hospital versus outpatient care for people with schizophrenia. *Cochrane Database of Systematic Reviews*, **4**, CD003240.

Shojania, K. G. & Bero, L. A. (2001). Taking advantage of the explosion of systematic reviews: an efficient MEDLINE search strategy. *Effective Clinical Practice*, **4**, 157–162.

Shorter, E. (2007) The historical development of mental health services in Europe. In: Knapp, M., McDaid, D., Mossialos, E., & Thornicroft, G. (Eds.), *European Observatory on Health Systems and Policies Series: Mental Health Policy and Practice* across Europe (pp. 15–33). Milton Keynes: McGraw-Hill/Open University.

The Cochrane Collaboration (2009). Cochrane handbook for systematic reviews of interventions, version 5.0.2. www.cochrane-handbook.org

Thornicroft, G. & Tansella, M. (1999). *The Mental Health Matrix: A Manual to Improve Services*. Cambridge: Cambridge University Press.

Thornicroft, G. & Tansella, M. (2004). Components of a modern mental health service: a pragmatic balance of community and hospital care: overview of systematic evidence. *British Journal of Psychiatry*, **185**, 283–290.

Tyrer, P., Evans, K., Gandhi, N., Lamont, A., Harrison-Read, P., & Johnson, T. (1998). Randomised controlled trial of two models of care for discharged psychiatric patients. *BMJ*, **316**, 106–109.

Verdoux, H. (2007). The current state of adult mental health care in France. *European Archives of Psychiatry and Clinical Neuroscience*, **257**, 64–70.

17

Day hospital and partial hospitalization programmes

Aart H. Schene

Introduction

Partial hospitalization (PH) as a treatment modality for psychiatric disorders has evolved over more than 70 years now. PH fills the wide gap between inpatient or full-time hospitalization (FTH) on the one hand and outpatient or community mental health care on the other. For patients, carers, and professional staff PH has the potential to offer more than low-frequency outpatient visits while at the same time it prevents the disadvantages of a hospital admission.

In this chapter I discuss some of the main issues regarding the current status and the future development of PH: history, development, conceptual issues and definition, different types of PH programmes, (cost-)effectiveness of PH in comparison with FTH and outpatient treatment, selection criteria, treatment models, and therapeutic factors. In the last paragraph, I review the place of this component in the total of psychiatric services.

History

The history of PH goes back to the 1930s. Shortage of money urged Dzagharov (1937) to open a hospital without beds in Moscow in 1932. Next, Adams House started in Boston (1935) and Lady Chichester Hospital in Hove was the first in the UK in 1938. After these pre-war pioneers, the post-war period saw at first a slow further development: Marlborough Day Hospital in London (1946), Allan Memorial Institute in Montreal (1946), Yale University Clinic (1948), Menninger Clinic (1949), Bristol Day Hospital (1951), Massachusetts Mental Health Center (1952), and the Maudsley Day Hospital (1953).

Two post-war PH pioneers, Bierer and Cameron, deserve mention. Bierer (1951) initiated a Social Psychotherapy Centre (later Marlborough Day Hospital) in London in 1946. In his view, the day hospital was the predecessor of the era of social psychiatry. Later, he described the day hospital as a treatment centre independent of the hospital, with preventive, outpatient, and temporary inpatient services, and based on the principles of the therapeutic community (Bierer, 1961). The main focus was to keep patients in contact with their normal living environment.

Cameron (1947) introduced the term 'day hospital' in 1946 when he opened such a service as part of the Allan Memorial Institute of Psychiatry being part of a large general hospital. Cameron described it as an extension and addition to FTH. In comparison with Bierer, whose ideas very much resemble the later philosophy of the US community mental health centres, Cameron had a more medical view on psychiatry. Without knowing it, these two pioneers represented two distinct visions on the later development of PH: the day hospital and day treatment.

Further development of PH differed much between different countries. For the UK, Farndale (1961) described the rapid increase of day hospital settings in the late 1950s as a 'day hospital movement'. Between 1959 and 1979, the number of day hospitals increased from 58 to 303 (Brocklehurst, 1979). 'Better Services for the Mentally Ill' (1975) had mentioned a ratio of day hospital places of 30 per 100,000 and of day centre places of 60 per 100,000. Between 1974 and 1982, day hospital places rose from 9400 to 15,300. For day care centres the rise in that period was from 3600 to 5000 places. The US saw the growth of PH in the 1960s mainly as a result of the 1963 Community Mental Health Center Construction Act, while countries such as the Netherlands and Germany started to develop PH as late as the 1970s and 1980s (Bosch & Veltin 1983; Schene, 1985; Schene et al., 1986).

Development and further growth

During its first decades, the development of PH was initiated and stimulated by different motives. Firstly, the post-war period saw a growing optimism about the possibilities of treating mental disorders. Not only by biological methods but also by individual and group psychotherapeutic techniques as well as occupational, family, and social psychiatric methods. Secondly, PH pioneers saw the hospital setting with its strong boundaries towards the outside world as a less adequate structure to use these new type of treatments. Thirdly, the 1960s showed that PH could have an important and specific role in the run-down of large mental hospitals and in the further development of community-oriented psychiatry. Finally, effectiveness studies like those of Kris (1960), Zwerling and Wilder (1962),

Meltzhoff and Blumenthal (1966), and Herz et al. (1971) contributed to a scientific support of this new type of treatment and gradually decreased the prejudices of hospital-oriented clinicians and other staff.

Also related to the process of deinstitutionalization was the rise in day care centres. When patients with long-term psychiatric disabilities have to live in the community, staff and services once located within the hospital should be redistributed within the community. Day hospitals fulfilled the acute service while day care centres started as maintenance programmes and in many places developed into psychosocial rehabilitation centres.

Comparison with inpatient and outpatient services

To understand its inherent qualities, we compare PH with inpatient and outpatient services. In comparison with the former, PH has the advantages that the disruption to life's normal routine (finances, housemaking, social contacts, hobbies, etc.) is less pronounced. Scapegoating the patient is less severe, as is the rejection by family members and other relatives. Contact with children and partner can be continued. Daily interaction with the outside world gives the patient good opportunities to develop skills and to generalize those from the therapeutic environment to the normal living situation (Dibella et al., 1982; Schene, 1985).

There also is a constant interplay in the way in which the patient and family or support system interact with each other. Because patients have to travel each day, they expect to get an active treatment and not just to 'hang around on the ward'. The change from inpatient to PH to outpatient can be more gradual. PH is accepted more easily by patient and carers, providing the opportunity to intervene in an earlier stage of the illness or decompensation. The therapeutic climate gives less opportunities for regression, stimulates healthy behaviour, and produces less loss of self-esteem (Davidson et al., 1996). Stigmatization of patients might be lower as well as costs.

The disadvantages of PH, in comparison with FTH, for patients, are the daily travelling, the fact that they get less structure, support, and care, and mostly have no 24-hour availability of staff. They do not have the opportunity to be free of family or network contacts for a period of time, which in certain cases can be healing. For professionals, the control of aggression and other disturbing behaviours is less easy and therefore more distressing. They have to decide each day anew if patients can go home. Involuntary admissions are not possible.

In comparison with outpatient treatment, PH has the advantage to give more intensive, more differentiated, and mostly multidisciplinary treatment. Medical diagnostics, assessments, observations, and certain therapeutics are more easily given. PH also provides more structure, more support, and more contact and learning opportunities with other patients. The disadvantages of PH in comparison with outpatient treatment are more stigmatization, more opportunity for regression, and more travelling.

Definition of partial hospitalization

A Task Force on Partial Hospitalization of the American Psychiatric Association (Casarino et al., 1982) was first to define PH as an ambulatory treatment programme that includes the major diagnostic, medical, psychiatric, psychosocial, and prevocational treatment modalities, designed for patients with serious mental disorders, who require coordinated intensive, comprehensive, and multidisciplinary treatment not provided in an outpatient setting.

DiBella et al. (1982) defined psychiatric PH more quantitatively as a psychiatric treatment programme of eight or more waking hours per week, designed for improvement of a group of six or more ambulatory patients, provided by two or more multidisciplinary clinical staff, and consisting of carefully coordinated, multimodality interconnected therapies within a therapeutic milieu. Patients participate regularly in the entire programme, which occurs almost always during at least 2 days per week for at least 3 weeks, with most of the treatment periods of at least 3 hours but less than 24 hours.

Later Block and Lefkovitz (1991) restricted the definition of PH to a time-limited, ambulatory, active treatment programme that offers therapeutically intensive, coordinated, and structured clinical services within a stable therapeutic milieu. Programmes are designed to serve individuals with significant impairment resulting from a psychiatric, emotional, or behavioural disorder.

In summary, PH means multidisciplinary, multimodality, and comprehensive programmes, available to several or groups of patients with severe mental illness, with regular opening hours and patient participation of at least 2 days per week, with most of the participation periods of at least 3 hours but less than 12 hours. It may be an acute (admission within 48–72 hours) or non-acute service; patients can participate somewhere in the range between low (two half-days per week) and high intensity (4–5 days per week) and the length of participation can be a few weeks to indefinite.

Typology of partial hospitalization

In the field of PH, an amalgam of terms and terminology is being used including day services, day hospital, partial hospital, day treatment, day centre, and day care. In different countries these terms may have different meanings. This confusion has to do with the wish to categorize and characterize PH services for which many criteria could be used: target population, type of treatment, duration of treatment or care, staff composition, organizational structure, and connection with other mental health services, etc.

Looking at specific target populations (Farndale, 1961), we can distinguish age groups (young children, adolescents, adults, old people), diagnostic categories (Bystritsky et al., 1996; Gerlinghoff et al., 1998; Lussier et al., 1997; Rosie et al., 1995) or combinations like elderly and infirm old people, mentally defective patients, disabled persons, young patients with schizophrenia, and others.

Considering the connection with the mother institution, we find services that are freestanding and organizationally independent, freestanding but organizationally connected with other mental health services, freestanding on the terrain of a psychiatric or general hospital, units where patients use the same facilities as inpatients, and PH integrated on a psychiatric unit, which also contains inpatient and outpatient services.

Considering the part of the day, a distinction in day treatment, evening treatment, evening and night treatment, and weekend treatment can be made (De Hert et al., 1996; DiBella et al., 1982; Schene, 1985). With regard to programmes, we can distinguish short-term, medium-term, and long-term services. The therapeutic orientation can be medical psychiatric, psychotherapeutic, or more rehabilitative. PH has to be distinguished from psychosocial rehabilitation programmes (self-help houses, Fountain House, therapeutic social clubs, and lounge programmes).

Four functions of partial hospitalization

In the UK, a distinction is made between day hospitals and day centres. Day hospitals offer (1) active treatment, including medication and a range of professional interventions (psychological, social, occupational), aimed at people who need more intensive treatment than could be given on an outpatient basis; or (2) rehabilitation for those for whom day treatment is a step in the transition process from inpatient treatment towards the community (Shepherd, 1991). Day centres, on the other hand, meet clients' long-term needs for support and social contact, assisting them in adjusting or re-adjusting to the demands of work and trying to relieve the strain on the family.

In the US, a distinction is made between day hospital, day treatment, and day care (Rosie, 1987) as well as between the intensive care model, rehabilitation model, and chronic care model (Klar et al., 1982). The day hospital/intensive care model provides diagnostic and treatment services for acutely ill patients who would otherwise be treated on traditional psychiatric inpatient units. The typical length of stay is between 4 and 8 weeks.

The day treatment programme/rehabilitation model provides an alternative to outpatient care for patients who have severe impairments in vocational or social performance. These programmes strive for symptom reduction and improved functioning and have a length of stay between 3 and 12 months.

The day care centre/chronic care model is indicated for patients who would otherwise require custodial care, for patients who might deteriorate in the community, and for patients who require regular treatment but cannot tolerate a more active treatment programme. It has modest expectations of patient improvement, high symptom tolerance, and a supportive, practical treatment approach. It offers maintenance care and social programming for individuals who require daily structure and supervision to prevent relapse. The length of stay is more than 1 year (Catty et al., 2007; Holloway, 1991).

To summarize and integrate these different classifications Schene et al. (1988) described PH in terms of the distinct functions it could fulfil in the total mental health care system and distinguished four types:

1. Alternative to acute inpatient: a medically oriented staff with high staff/patient ratio offers PH in or close to a general hospital for patients with acute illnesses who would otherwise be treated as inpatients
2. Continuation of acute inpatient: transition to outpatient care can be organized on or close to the inpatient unit; staff, patients, and treatment resemble those of the first function
3. Extension to outpatient care: either for specialized intensive treatment or rehabilitation for patients who do not require inpatient care but who benefit from more intensive care than is possible on an outpatient basis
4. Day care or rehabilitation: long-term maintenance or rehabilitation of patients with chronic, debilitating mental disorders.

Evaluative research

The main questions researchers have tried to answer considered the (cost-)effectiveness of PH in comparison with FTH as well as with outpatient treatment. The evaluative research on PH has been reviewed extensively, first in non-systematic reviews (Di Bella et al., 1982; Creed et al., 1989a; Herz, 1982; Mason et al., 1982; Parker & Knoll, 1990; Rosie, 1987; Schene, 2004; Schene & Gersons, 1986) but more recent systematic ones have been published as well (Catty et al., 2007; Horvitz-Lennon, 2001; Marshall et al., 2003, 2011). However, the underlying questions of all reviews are comparable:

1. For what percentage of patients otherwise hospitalized is PH a good alternative?
2. What is the (cost-)effectiveness of PH in comparison with FTH?
3. What is the (cost-)effectiveness of PH in comparison with outpatient treatment or day care?

Effectiveness of partial versus full-time hospitalization

Acute day hospital treatment as an alternative for inpatient treatment has been studied in randomized controlled trials (RCTs) in the US (Herz et al., 1971; Sledge et al., 1996; Washburn et al., 1976; Zwerling & Wilder 1962, 1964), the UK (Creed et al., 1989b, 1990, 1997; Dick et al., 1985a, 1985b; Priebe et al., 2006), and the Netherlands (Kluiter et al., 1992; Schene et al., 1993). Three non-RCTs give some additional information (Fink et al., 1978; Michaux et al., 1972; Penk et al., 1978).

The aim of most studies was to randomize the patient population admitted to acute psychiatric wards towards FTH or PH in order to find how many patients could be treated by PH just as well as by FTH. However, in most studies not all admitted patients could actually be randomized. Only Zwerling and Kluiter did a randomized study on an unselected group of patients referred to FTH. All other studies suffered from design violation between admission and randomization, mostly because patients were 'too ill' to be randomized. This pre-randomization attrition influences the percentage of the population randomized to PH that after randomization had to be admitted to FTH: the smaller the selection before randomization, the higher the percentage of patients who failed in PH and had to be admitted to FTH. Zwerling, for instance, randomized 100% of admitted patients but had to admit 34% of those randomized to PH. For the other studies these percentages were respectively: 100% and 39.2% (Kluiter), 55% and 12% (Creed), 42% and 12% (Schene), 22% and 0% (Herz), 22% and 0% (Dick), and 15% and 0% (Washburn).

Earlier studies were less stringent and sophisticated in their methodology. Later studies had more differentiated outcome measures, made better descriptions of their patient selection, also measured family burden, costs, and satisfaction with services, and calculated the use of medication. In their Cochrane review, Marshall et al. (2003) concluded that for between 18.4% and 39.1% of otherwise FTH patients PH is a feasible alternative. Both PH and FTH are just as effective (on social functioning, burden on carers, deaths (suicide, homicide, all causes), number unemployed at follow-up, and readmission) but PH has three main advantages: a more rapid improvement in mental state, a higher satisfaction with services, and lower costs. This group updated their Cochrane systematic review in 2011 (Marshall et al., 2011) and then reported the following main findings from ten trials, which included 2685 people. There is moderate evidence that the duration of index admission is longer for patients in day hospital care than inpatient care. There is no difference between day hospital care and inpatient care for being readmitted to inpatient/day patient care after discharge. It is likely that there is no difference between day hospital care and inpatient care for being unemployed at the end of the study, for quality of life, or for treatment satisfaction. The authors concluded that caring for people in acute day hospitals is as effective as inpatient care in treating acutely ill psychiatric patients.

More recently, Heekeren et al. (2020) conducted a comparison of FTH and PH in among 44 patients in Switzerland and found no significant differences between the two settings in terms of external assessment of symptoms, subjective symptom burden, functional level, quality of life, treatment satisfaction, and number of treatment days. Treatment in the day hospital was about 45% cheaper compared to inpatient treatment. The conclusions of this study were that acutely ill psychiatric patients of different symptom severity can be treated just as well in an acute day hospital instead of being admitted to the hospital. In addition, when direct treatment costs are considered, there are clear cost advantages for day hospital treatment (Heekeren et al., 2020). A somewhat larger comparison was carried among over 300 patients at an acute psychiatric day care unit in Spain, and found that improvement was greater among patients with bipolar disorder than among those with psychosis or depressive disorder. Longer length of stay in the day hospital, and greater baseline symptom severity were identified as predictors of good clinical response. The authors interpreted the findings to show that intensive care in an acute psychiatric day hospital is feasible and effective for patients suffering from an acute mental disorder, with important differences in effectiveness between diagnostic groups (Vazquez-Bourgon et al., 2021).

The overall conclusion must be that PH can be a good alternative for about 20–40% of patients in need of acute psychiatric admission. For that population there are no differences between PH and FTH in the reduction of symptoms while there is some tendency that social functioning has a better outcome in PH, although this difference has disappeared 2 years later. This finding from earlier studies, was not replicated in some later studies (Creed et al., 1990; Kluiter et al., 1992; Schene et al., 1993), but more recently Kallert et al. (2007) did. From their multicentre RCT they concluded that day hospital care was as effective as conventional inpatient care with respect to psychopathological symptoms and quality of life, but more effective on social functioning (at discharge and 3- and 12-month follow-up). Because of its sample size (n = 1117), this study has 'more than doubled the existing evidence base' for the day hospital being a 'viable and clinically effective alternative to inpatient admission for approximately one fifth of all acute admissions'.

All RCTs together tell us something about contraindications for PH: patients who could harm themselves or others, who fail to care for themselves, who given their symptomatology have no support systems, who are homeless, who also suffer from a severe addiction disorder, patients with organic disorders, and those in need of somatic treatment or nursing care. In all those cases, patients have to be admitted to inpatient services first.

Other outcome measures showed that satisfaction with services is equal or somewhat better in PH (Priebe et al., 2006; Schene et al., 1997). Also, family members are more satisfied, while almost all studies have shown no difference in family or caregiver burden. Only Creed et al. (1997) found day hospital patients were less of a burden to their carers at 1 year post admission. Schene et al. (1993), Wiersma et al. (1995), Sledge et al. (1996a), and Priebe et al. (2006) found no difference in readmissions, while Creed et al. (1990) found more readmissions for those treated in FTH.

Apart from Kris (1965), Herz et al. (1971), and Sledge et al. (1996a), all RCTs found PH to have a longer treatment duration than FTH. This might be related to greater acceptance of PH by patients, more satisfaction, and more compliance with services. However, a relation with the time needed to reach treatment effectiveness as well as Hawthorne effects, are other explanations. Schene et al. (1993) mentioned the interaction of treatment length and treatment intensity as a possible causative factor: PH combines a lower intensity with a longer duration of treatment, while FTH has a higher intensity combined with a shorter duration.

Cost-effectiveness of partial versus full-time hospitalization

Four RCTs have also considered costs. Wiersma et al. (1995) found over a 2-year period direct costs (number of inpatient and day patients days and outpatient contacts) for PH and FTH were more or less the same. In this study, costs per day for PH and FTH were the same as well as the number of staff needed to run the service. Because patients' compliance and satisfaction with services both for patient and families was better in PH, they concluded that day treatment can be considered a cost-effective alternative to inpatient treatment.

Sledge et al. (1996b) compared FTH with a day hospital/crisis respite programme. Over a 10-month period, the experimental condition was $7100 (20%) cheaper than FTH. In particular, the index admission was 43% less expensive due to operating costs which were twice as high in FTH. Personal costs were equal in both conditions as well as effectiveness. Therefore, Sledge concluded that in his study PH was less expensive for two reasons: the length of stay during index admission was 7 days less in PH and operating costs were lower.

Creed et al. (1997) assessed costs over 12 months after the date of admission. They found that overall day hospital treatment was £1994 less expensive than FTH for the 30–40% of potential admissions that can be treated in this way. Although day hospital patients were less of a burden to their carers, the latter may bear additional costs.

Priebe et al. (2006) found the costs of the day hospital patients to be higher than the inpatients. Reasons for this were the longer treatment time in the day hospital, the fact that half of the day hospital group also received inpatient care, and the cost per day at the day hospital, which was around 70% of the cost of a day on the inpatient wards, so relatively high.

Acute day hospital care

The percentages of an admissions cohort eligible for PH is, of course, dependent on other patient, network or support, and service characteristics. If, for instance, patients are well integrated into community support systems, this percentage will rise. If the threshold for psychiatric admissions is high, because of a shortage of beds in a certain region, it will be lower because patients will be more severe. Residents and junior staff (Kluiter et al., 1992; Platt et al., 1980; Washburn et al., 1976) also seem to lower this percentage. Acute day hospital care seems to have better opportunities with a well-trained and skilled staff with an attitude favouring PH (Herz et al., 1971; Schene, 1992). The service has to be closely connected to inpatient services, having available all diagnostic and treatment facilities necessary for acutely ill psychiatric patients.

Practical issues such as transport from home to service and, if needed, overnight accommodation or a backup bed (Gudeman et al., 1983) are also important prerequisites. Additional support at home by, for instance, a community psychiatric nurse, a 24-hour crisis telephone service, and the opportunity for outreach to patients in crisis can help to make PH a success for a higher percentage of the admitted patient group.

Partial hospitalization and beds

In a day hospital functioning as an alternative to inpatient hospitalization, Turner and Hoge (1991) studied the use of an overnight hospitalization or backup bed. Twenty per cent of patients admitted to the day hospital used the backup bed (47% for 1 night, 19% for 2 nights, and 34% for 3 nights). The main reasons were psychotic symptoms (44% of backup admissions), dangerousness (81%), and extreme agitation (5%). Of all episodes, 73% returned to the day hospital and 27% resulted in FTH. Only 50% of the backup bed users were able to complete their day hospitalization, the other 50% received a standard FTH.

To really understand the relation between the use of FTH, PH, and outpatient services we first consider for a specific catchment area the total number of days that acutely ill patients should spend in a hospital setting because that setting is more effective or protective than outpatient care. Second, we consider the percentage of the total amount of days which could be spent just as safely and effectively in an acute day hospital. Of all patients referred for FTH, k% will spend their whole admission in FTH, l% will have a combination of x days in FTH and y days in PH (the percentage x/x + y will vary between 1 and 99) and m% will spend their total time in PH (Schene, 1992).

Effectiveness of partial hospitalization versus outpatient treatment

Comparisons between PH and outpatient treatment suffer from quite diverse populations and settings and so even more complicated methodologies (Schene, 2004). A distinction should be made between (1) day hospitals or day treatment programmes, emphasizing treatment and run by medical services with the psychotic patient as target group; (2) the same as (1) but with the non-psychotic patient as target group; and (3) facilities or day care centres run by non-medical services (e.g. social services) and providing long-term care.

Regarding the first category (long-term mostly psychotic patients as target population), only three trials comparing day care medical services with outpatient services were performed in the US before 1980. Meltzhoff and Blumenthal (1966) found better results for PH for patient with chronic schizophrenia: fewer admissions days, more work, and greater independence. Day treatment changed the deterioration of those patients. Guy et al. (1969) reported that medication and PH for patients with schizoaffective disorder has advantages in terms of reduction of symptoms. Linn et al. (1979) studied 122 male patients with schizophrenia and found a better outcome on symptoms at the end of the 2-year study period and better social functioning during the whole 2-year period. There were no differences in readmissions. Also Weldon et al. (1979) showed better functioning and significant more work or training after 3 months. The quality of these studies was insufficient to show evidence that day hospital care had substantial advantages over outpatient care. Authors of a Cochrane review (Shed et al., 2009), however, concluded that they had 'the impression' that day hospital does reduce time in inpatient care. Data to support the idea that day hospital or outpatient care helps avoid admission was not strong. Because all trials were undertaken over decades ago, results are difficult to apply in the context of modern outpatient services. It seems that meanwhile this type of PH has been superseded by case management approaches and vocational rehabilitation programmes.

Regarding the second category of comparison of outpatient and PH (treatment refractory non-psychotic patients as target population) the Cochrane review of Marshall et al. (2003) could include only four studies, with the following target populations: borderline personality disorders (Bateman & Fonaghy, 1999), affective disorders and personality disorders (Piper et al., 1993, 1996), persistent anxiety or depression (Dick et al., 1991), and anxiety or depressive neurosis (Tyrer et al., 1987). Because of the quite different settings and heterogeneous populations definite conclusions could not be drawn. However, considering the total picture, the authors concluded tentatively that day treatment might be superior to continued outpatient treatment in terms of improving symptoms and social functioning. Differences in necessary inpatient admissions were not found, patient satisfaction results were equivocal, while participation rates might be lower in day treatment compared to outpatient treatment.

Regarding the third category (facilities or day care centres run by non-medical services) Catty et al. (2007) designed a Cochrane review to determine the effects of non-medical day centre care for people with severe mental illness, but the 12 studies they found were all on medical and not on non-medical day centres. There is a clear need for RCTs of day centre care compared to other forms of day care.

Therapeutic factors

Hoge et al. (1988) studied therapeutic factors in a day hospital functioning as an alternative to FTH. Patients and staff mentioned the following therapeutic factors in declining frequency: structure, interpersonal contact, medication, altruism, catharsis, learning, mobilization of family support, connection to community, universality, patient autonomy, successful completion, and security. He concluded that it was striking that PH in this setting provides security and structure while simultaneously promoting patient responsibility and autonomy.

Schreer (1988) did a comparable study in a private, non-for-profit, short-term psychiatric partial hospital with more affective and less psychotic disorders than Hoge et al. She found interpersonal contact just as important, but feedback on behaviour, universality, and learning to be more important, while structure, medication, and security were less important.

Davidson et al. (1996) studied the social environment of a conventional psychiatric inpatient setting with that of a combined day hospital and crisis respite programme. The day hospital programme had higher expectations for patient functioning, a lower tolerance for deviance, more patient choice, and allowing for more continuation of patients' ongoing community involvement. The programme had a more stimulating and attractive physical environment and social milieu. It promoted higher levels of patient functioning and activity, increased help with daily living skills and social and recreational resources, and more integration of patients into the community outside the facility.

Discussion and conclusions

PH has become an important, highly differentiated sector of mental health services, representing a spectrum which overlaps with FTH on the one end and outpatient services on the other. There is enough evidence to consider PH to be a good alternative for about one-fifth to one-third of acute patients in need of FTH. Operating costs might be lower, but personal costs are about equal. For this reason, integrated admission units which offer FTH and PH in a flexible way seem to be the most practical and need-based way of working. Patients treated on those units start to sleep at home as soon as their clinical condition allows them to do so. The number of nights at home per week can be increased according to their condition. In our own Programme for Mood Disorders, all admitted patients are screened for PH at admission. If possible, they start PH immediately; if not, they start FTH. Some are treated in FTH for the whole length of their admission. For most patients, however, a combination of FTH and PH is made during their 8–16-week stay.

Not only the clinical condition of patients determines the utilization of PH. Staff attitudes and skills, hospital policy, staff-to patient ratios, structured programming, resources for managing clinical emergencies, distance from home to PH service, attitudes of family members, payment of service, and others certainly also have their influence. Choosing for PH in an early phase and not only when patients' decompensation is so severe that only FTH is still possible makes PH an important function in a comprehensive system of care. For such a short-term PH to be an alternative to FTH, Hoge et al. (1987) described five functions: reduction of acute symptoms (first 2 weeks), decrease of demoralization (weeks 3 and 4), facilitating community re-entry (weeks 1–4), education and skill building (weeks 3–4), and connection to community (week 4).

Looking at PH as an extension to outpatient care, the conclusions are less clear. For patients with severe psychopathology who do not respond to regular outpatient treatment, PH seems to have some advantages for those with psychosis. For those with personality disorders, PH might be an effective alternative for continued outpatient treatment. For both types of patients, cost-effectiveness studies are lacking.

Hoge et al. (1992) had the opinion that this type of PH should be changed into assertive community treatment. Rosie et al. (1995) described that this view may be correct for patients with psychotic disorders, but does not hold for patients with personality disorders or severe neurosis. For them, a time-limited 4-month programme had good outcome if it had a close relationship to a highly active outpatient clinic. What the future will bring in this field is not clear. Further research with RCTs comparing PH and intensive outpatient treatment with a long-term follow-up is needed.

Finally, the fourth function of PH, rehabilitation or day centre care, is rarely discussed in research terms. It is one of the cornerstones of community support systems, with a strong emphasis on training, support, and continuity of care. However, it lends itself to careful evaluation in the future. Trials comparing day care centres with intermittent day treatment programmes or with intensive forms of outpatient care are certainly lacking.

Acknowledgements

Professor Aart Schene died during the preparation of the second edition of this textbook, and this chapter has been updated by Graham Thornicroft. The editors would like to pay tribute to the outstanding contributions made to the field of mental health by Professor Schene.

REFERENCES

Bateman, A. & Fonaghy, P. (1999). Effectiveness of partial hospitalization in the treatment of borderline personality disorder: a randomized controlled trial. *American Journal of Psychiatry*, **156**, 1563–1569.

Bierer, J. (1951). *The Day Hospital: An Experiment in Social Psychiatry and Syntho-Analytic Psychotherapy*. London: H. K. Lewis and Co.

Bierer, J. (1961). Day hospitals, further developments. *International Journal of Social Psychiatry*, **7**, 148–151.

Block, B. M. & Lefkovitz, P. M. (1991). *Standards and Guidelines for Partial Hospitalization*. Alexandria, VA: American Association for Partial Hospitalization.

Bosch, G. & Veltin, A. (1983). *Die Tagesklinik als teil der psychiatrischen Versorgung*. Köln: Rheinland-Verlag GmbH.

Brocklehurst, J. (1979). The development and present status of day hospitals. *Age and Ageing*, **8**, 76–79.

Bystritsky, A., Muford, P. R., Rosen, R. M., Martin, K. M., Vapnik, T., Borbis, E. E., & Wolson, R. C. (1996). A preliminary study of partial hospital management of severe obsessive-compulsive disorder. *Psychiatric Services*, **47**, 170–174.

Cameron, D. E. (1947). The day hospital: an experimental form of hospitalization for psychiatric patients. *Modern Hospital*, **69**, 60–62.

Casarino, J. P., Wilner, M., & Maxey, J. T. (1982). American Association for Partial Hospitalization (AAHP) standards and guideline for partial hospitalization. *International Journal of Partial Hospitalization*, **1**, 15–21.

Catty, J. S., Burns, T., Comas, A., & Poole, Z. (2007). Day centres for severe mental illness. *Cochrane Database of Systematic Reviews*, **1**, CD001710.

Creed, F., Anthony, P., Godbert, K., & Huxley, P. (1989b). Treatment of severe psychiatric illness in a day hospital. *British Journal of Psychiatry*, **154**, 341–347.

Creed, F., Black, D., & Anthony, P. (1989a). Day-hospital and community treatment for acute psychiatric illness; a critical appraisal. *British Journal of Psychiatry*, **154**, 300–310.

Creed, F., Black, D., Anthony, P., Osborn, M., Thomas, P., & Tomenson, B. (1990). Randomized controlled trial of day versus inpatient psychiatric treatment. *British Medical Journal*, **300**, 1033–1037.

Creed, F., Mbaya, P., Lancashire, S., Tomenson, B., Williams, B., & Holme, S. (1997). Cost-effectiveness of day and inpatient psychiatric treatment. *BMJ*, **314**, 1381–1385.

Davidson, L., Kraemer Tebes, J., Rakfeldt, J., & Sledge, W. H. (1996). Differences in social environment between inpatient and day hospital-crisis respite settings. *Psychiatric Services*, **47**, 714–720.

De Hert, M., Thys, E., Vercruyssen, V., & Peuskens, J. (1996). Partial hospitalization at night: the Brussels Nighthospital. *Psychiatric Services*, **47**, 527–528.

DiBella, G., Weitz, G. W., Pogntes Bergen, D., & Yurmark, J. L. (Eds.) (1982). *Handbook of Partial Hospitalization*. New York: Brunner/Mazel.

Dick, P. H., Cameron, L., Cohen, D., Barlow, M., & Ince, A. (1985b). Day and full time psychiatric treatment: a controlled comparison. *British Journal of Psychiatry*, **147**, 246–250.

Dick, P. H., Ince, A., & Barlow, M. (1985a). Day treatment: suitability and referral procedure. *British Journal of Psychiatry*, **142**, 250–253.

Dick, P. H., Sweeney, M. L., & Crombie, I. K. (1991). Controlled comparison of day-patient and out-patient treatment for persistent anxiety and depression. *British Journal of Psychiatry*, **158**, 24–27.

Dzagharov, M. A. (1937). Experience in organizing a day hospital for mental patients. *Neuropathologi Psikhiatri*, **6**, 137–146.

Farndale, J. (1961). *The Day Hospital Movement in Great Britain*. London: Pergamon Press.

Gerlinghoff, M., Backmund, H., & Franzen, U. (1998). Evaluation of a day treatment programme for eating disorders. *European Eating Disorders Review*, **6**, 96–106.

Gudeman, J. E., Shore, M. F., & Dickey, B. (1983). Day hospitalization and an inn instead of inpatient care for psychiatric patients. *New England Journal of Medicine*, **308**, 749–753.

Guy, W., Gross, M., Hogarty, G. E., & Dennis, H. (1969). A controlled evaluation of day hospital effectiveness. *Archives of General Psychiatry*, **201**, 329–338.

Heekeren, K., Antoniadis, S., Habermeyer, B., Obermann, C., Kirschner, M., Seifritz, E., et al. (2020). Psychiatric acute day hospital as an alternative to inpatient treatment. *Frontiers in Psychiatry*, **11**, 471.

Herz, M. I. (1982). Research overview in day treatment. *International Journal of Partial Hospitalization*, **1**, 33–45.

Herz, M. I., Endicott, J., Spitzer, R. L., & Mesnikoff, A. (1971). Day versus inpatient hospitalization: a controlled study. *American Journal of Psychiatry*, **127**, 1371–1381.

Hoge, M. A., Farrell, S. P., Munchnel, M. E., & Strauss, J. S. (1988). Therapeutic factors in partial hospitalization. *Psychiatry*, **51**, 199–210.

Hoge, M. A., Farrell, S. P., Strauss, J. S., & Munchnel Posner, M. (1987). Functions of short-term partial hospitalization in a comprehensive system of care. *International Journal of Partial Hospitalization*, **4**, 177–188.

Hoge, M. A., Davidson, L., Leonard Hill, W., Turner, V. E., & Ameli, R. (1992). The promise of partial hospitalization: a reassessment. *Hospital and Community Psychiatry*, **43**, 345–354.

Holloway, F. (1991). Day care in an inner city I. Characteristics of the attenders. *British Journal of Psychiatry*, **158**, 805–810.

Horvitz-Lennon, M., Normand, S. L., Gaccione, P., & Frank, R. G. (2001). Partial versus full hospitalization for adults in psychiatric distress: a systematic review of the published literature (1957–1997). *American Journal of Psychiatry*, **158**, 676–685.

Kallert, T. W., Priebe, S., McCabe, R., Kiejna, A., Rymaszewska, J., Nawka, P., et al. (2007). Are day hospitals effective for acutely ill psychiatric patients? A European multicenter randomized controlled trial. *Journal of Clinical Psychiatry*, **68**, 278–287.

Klar, H., Francis, A., & Clarkin, H. (1982). Selection criteria for partial hospitalization. *Hospital and Community Psychiatry*, **33**, 929–933.

Kluiter, H., Giel, R., Nienhuis, F. J., Rüphan, M., & Wiersma, D. (1992). Predicting feasibility of day treatment for unselected patients referred for inpatient psychiatric treatment: results of a randomized trial. *American Journal of Psychiatry*, **149**, 1199–1205.

Kris, E. B. (1960). Intensive short-term treatment in a day care facility for the prevention of rehospitalization of patients in the community showing recurrence of psychotic symptoms. *Psychiatric Quarterly*, **34**, 83–88.

Kris, E. B. (1965). Day hospitals. *Current Therapeutic Research*, **7**, 1331–1340.

Linn, M. W., Caffey, E. M., Klett, C. J., Hogarty, G. E., & Lamb, H. R. (1979). Day treatment and psychotropic drugs in the aftercare of schizophrenic patients. *Archives of General Psychiatry*, **36**, 1055–1066.

Lussier, R. G., Steiner, J., Grey, A., & Hansen, C. (1997). Prevalence of dissociative disorders in an acute care day hospital population. *Psychiatric Services*, **48**, 244–246.

Marshall, M., Crowther, R., Almaraz-Serrano, A.M., Creed, F., Sledge, W.H., Kluiter, H, et al. (2003). Day hospital versus admission for acute psychiatric disorders. *Cochrane Database of Systematic Reviews*, **1**, CD004026.

Marshall, M., Crowther, R., Sledge, W. H., Rathbone, J., & Soares-Weiser, K. (2011). Day hospital versus admission for acute psychiatric disorders. *Cochrane Database of Systematic Reviews*, **12**, CD004026.

Mason, J., Louks, J., Burmer, G., & Scher, M. (1982). The efficacy of partial hospitalization: a review of recent literature. *International Journal of Partial Hospitalization*, **1**, 251–269.

Mbaya, P., Creed, F., & Tomenson, B. (1998). The different uses of day hospitals. *Acta Psychiatrica Scandinavica*, **98**, 283–287.

Meltzhoff, J. & Blumenthal, R. (1966). *The Day Treatment Center: Principles, Application and Evaluation*. Springfield IL: Charles C. Thomas.

Michaux, M. H., Chelst, M. R., Foster, S. A., Prium, R. J., & Dasinger, E. M. (1972). Day- and full-time treatment, a controlled comparison. *Current Therapeutic Research*, **14**, 279–292.

Parker, S. P. & Knoll, J. L., 3rd. (1990). Partial hospitalization: an update. *American Journal of Psychiatry*, **147**, 156–160.

Penk, W. E., Charles, H. L., & Van Hoose, T. A. (1978). Comparative effectiveness of day hospital and inpatient psychiatric treatment. *Journal of Consulting & Clinical Psychology*, **46**, 94–101.

Piper, W. E., Rosie, J. S., Azim, H. F. A., & Joyce, A. S. (1993). A randomized trial of psychiatric day treatment for patients with affective and personality disorders. *Hospital and Community Psychiatry*, **44**, 757–763.

Piper, W. E., Rosie, J. S., Joyce, A. S., & Azim, H. F. A. (1996). *Time-Limited Day Treatment for Personality Disorders*. Washington, DC: American Psychological Association.

Platt, S. D., Knights, A. C., & Hirsch, S. R. (1980). Caution and conservatism in the use of a psychiatric day hospital; evidence from a research project that failed. *Psychiatric Research*, **3**, 123–132.

Priebe, S., Jones, G., McCabe, R., Briscoe, J., Wright, D., Sleed, M., & Beecham, J. (2006). Effectiveness and costs of acute day hospital treatment compared with conventional in-patient care: randomised controlled trial. *British Journal of Psychiatry*, **188**, 243–249.

Rosie, J. S. (1987). Partial hospitalization: a review of recent literature. *Hospital and Community Psychiatry*, **38**, 1291–1299.

Rosie, J. S., Azim, H. F. A., Piper, W. E., & Joyce, A. S. (1995). Effective psychiatric day treatment: historical lessons. *Psychiatric Services*, **46**, 1019–1026.

Schene, A. H. (1985). *Psychiatric Partial Hospitalization: An Overview* (in Dutch). Utrecht: Netherlands Center of Mental Health.

Schene, A. H. & Gersons, B. P. R. (1986). Effectiveness and application of partial hospitalization. *Acta Psychiatrica Scandinavica*, **74**, 335–340.

Schene, A. H., van Lieshout, P., & Mastboom, J. (1986). Development and current status of partial hospitalization in the Netherlands. *International Journal of Partial Hospitalization*, **3**, 237–246.

Schene, A. H., van Lieshout, P., & Mastboom, J. (1988). Different types of partial hospitalization programs: results from a nationwide study. *Acta Psychiatrica Scandinavica*, **75**, 515–520.

Schene, A. H. (1992). *Psychiatric Partial and Full-Time Hospitalization: A Comparative Study* (Dissertation (in Dutch)). Utrecht: University of Utrecht.

Schene, A. H., van Wijngaarden, B., & Gersons, B. P. R. (1997). Partial or full-time hospitalization: patients' preferences. In: M. Tansella (Ed.), *Making Rational Mental Health Services* (pp. 145–54). Roma: Il Pensiero Scientifico Editore.

Schene, A. H., van Wijngaarden, B., Poelijoe, N. W., & Gersons, B. P. R. (1993). The Utrecht comparative study on psychiatric day treatment and inpatient treatment. *Acta Psychiatrica Scandinavica*, **87**, 427–436.

Schreer, H. (1988). Therapeutic factors in psychiatric day hospital treatment. *International Journal of Partial Hospitalization*, **4**, 307–319.

Shek, E., Stein, A.T., Shansis, F.M., Marshall, M., Crowther, R., & Tyrer, P. (2009). Day hospital versus outpatient care for people with schizophrenia. *Cochrane Database of Systematic Reviews*, **4**, CD003240.

Shepherd, G. (1991). Day treatment and care. In: Bennett, D. H. & Freeman, H. L. (Eds.), *Community Psychiatry* (pp. 396–414). London: Churchill Livingstone.

Sledge, W. H., Tebes, J., Rakfeldt, J., Davidson, L., Lyons, L., & Druss, B. (1996a). Day hospital/crisis respite care versus inpatient care, part I: clinical outcomes. *American Journal of Psychiatry*, **153**, 1065–1073.

Sledge, W. H., Tebes, J., Wolff, N., & Helminiak, T. W. (1996b). Day hospital/crisis respite care versus in-patient care, part II: service utilization and costs. *American Journal of Psychiatry*, **153**, 1074–1083.

Turner, V. E. & Hoge, M. A. (1991). Overnight hospitalization of acutely ill day hospital patients. *International Journal of Partial Hospitalization*, **7**, 23–36.

Tyrer, P., Remington, M., & Alexander, J. (1987). The outcome of neurotic disorders after out-patient and day hospital care. *British Journal of Psychiatry*, **151**, 57–62.

Vazquez-Bourgon, J., Gomez Ruiz, E., Hoyuela Zaton, F., Salvador Carulla, L., Ayesa Arriola, R., Tordesillas Gutierrez, D., et al. (2021). Differences between psychiatric disorders in the clinical and functional effectiveness of an acute psychiatric day hospital, for acutely ill psychiatric patients. *Revista de Psiquiatria y Salud Mental*, **14**, 40–49.

Washburn, S., Vannicelli, R., Longabaugh, R., & Scheff, B. J. (1976). A controlled comparison of psychiatric daytreatment and inpatient hospitalization. *Journal of Consulting & Clinical Psychology*, **44**, 665–675.

Weldon, E., Clarkin, J.E., Hennessy, J. J., & Frances, A. (1979). Day hospital versus outpatient treatment. A controlled study. *Psychiatric Quarterly*, **51**, 144–150.

Wiersma, D., Kluiter, H., Nienhuis, F. J., Ruphan, M., & Giel, R. (1995). Costs and benefits of hospital and day treatment with community care of affective and schizophrenic disorders. *British Journal of Psychiatry*, **27**, 52–59.

Zwerling, I. & Wilder, J. F. (1962). Day hospital treatment for acutely psychotic patients. *Current Psychiatric Therapies*, **2**, 200–210.

Zwerling, I. & Wilder, J. F. (1964). An evaluation of the applicability of the day hospital in treatment for acutely disturbed patients. *Israel Annals of Psychiatry and Related Disciplines*, **2**, 162–185.

18

Inpatient treatment

Frank Holloway and Derek Tracy

Introduction

This chapter seeks to describe the role of inpatient care within contemporary community-oriented mental health services. We put current provision within a historical context. Inpatient services are here defined as hospitals: 24-hour residential settings that, at a minimum, provide nursing and medical care and within which people can be detained against their will. This is what we mean when we employ the term 'beds', a physical location where people stay for a period of time.

At the outset we have to acknowledge that effective psychological, social, and physical treatments for mental disorders can be provided in other settings, including, in some instances, forms of residential accommodation not meeting the aforementioned criteria. Inpatient admission happens as a result of a complex interaction between an individual's mental health problems, the availability and feasibility of alternative social and therapeutic supports, and frequently also a perceived necessity for compulsory treatment. Nowadays admission is generally a result of assessed serious risk to self or others and often follows an episode of disturbed behaviour or significant self-harm.

We outline the history of inpatient mental health care, review the international literature on trends in inpatient provision, and set out the contemporary range of inpatient services. We go on to review the limited literature on the quality of inpatient care and discuss what constitutes best practice. Throughout, we emphasize that inpatient care should function as a component of a comprehensive and local mental health system.

The authors both work in England and this chapter inevitably reflects this perspective (health care policy is devolved to the four component countries of the UK). Since 1948, mental health services have been funded through the NHS and care is free at the point of access, although the precise details of the funding, commissioning, and provision of services has evolved over time. Social care is means-tested and often requires a contribution from the recipient, though not for people who have been detained under longer-term provisions of the Mental Health Act. The UK reports lower than average bed numbers for a high-income country and has a relatively advanced system of community care.

Early times

Family care of people with mental disability has been the norm throughout history and across cultures, with the possibility of additional support from religious institutions and charitable foundations. The earliest recognizable examples of what we would now call psychiatric inpatient units are within the Bimaristans that were founded in the major cities of the Islamic world. Bimaristans were multifunctional hospitals, often with dedicated inpatient psychiatric provision. Drawing on Islamic models, facilities for the care of the insane were gradually developed across Europe from the late Middle Ages.

In medieval and early modern times there was only one dedicated facility for the reception of 'lunatics' in England—the Bethlem in London, which has been much referenced in art, literature, and popular culture from the sixteenth century onwards (Arnold, 2008). Later 'mad doctors' (a descriptive term that had no particular stigma attached to it) could earn a good living in offering treatment to the insane in private 'madhouses', although there was no particular medical monopoly in the trade in lunacy (Porter, 1990). Throughout the eighteenth century an increasing number of madhouses opened, many of which supplemented the Bethlem in providing care for people without means—so-called pauper lunatics.

People could move between the madhouse and informal care. The eighteenth-century poet and hymnist William Cowper spent some time in a madhouse run by Dr Nathaniel Cotton, where he was mechanically restrained from killing himself. On recovery he spent the rest of his life in a very caring religious family household, where he was supported through further episodes of 'madness' (Cecil, 1933). Cowper's later experience was a particularly productive example of the phenomenon of 'boarding out' someone with a mental illness, an early and effective form of community care.

We know that conditions in the eighteenth- and early nineteenth-century madhouse could be degrading (Porter, 1990; Scull, 1983), although Cowper was in retrospect very positive about his experience at Dr Cotton's asylum. We also know from the report of a House of Commons committee considering regulation of madhouses that people left hospital: in 1799, the Bethlem admitted 201 patients and reported having 'cured and discharged' 179 patients and buried 20. Of the 243 residents on 31 December 1799, 130 were described as 'under cure' and 113 as 'incurable'(Sharpe, 1815, p. 388). These data come from a time when the Bethlem's reputation was at a particularly low point.

Moral treatment and the asylum movement

Moral treatment

The York Retreat was founded in 1796 by the Quaker tea merchant William Tuke. It followed the death of Hannah Mills, a member of the local Quaker community, shortly after her admission to York Asylum, where conditions were poor. The early years of the Retreat were documented by William Tuke's grandson Samuel in his *Description of the Retreat* (Tuke, 1815). Samuel Tuke devoted a chapter of his book to 'moral treatment'. He used terminology popularized in Revolutionary France by Phillipe Pinel, who described 'traitement moral' as a new approach to care in the asylum. This involved sympathy and kindness and freedom from restraint.

The Retreat offered a positive environment, where patients were treated with respect and encouraged to be involved in a daily routine of activity and leisure specific to their previous life and interests. Patients were talked to as human beings 'in a kind, and somewhat low tone of voice' and encouraged to develop self-restraint. The use of chains and corporal punishment, common in the eighteenth century madhouse, was forbidden. (A chapter in Tuke's book recounts the empirical work of the first physician to the asylum exploring the ineffective medical treatments then available—other than warm baths for women with melancholia.)

The rise of the asylum

By the early nineteenth century, reformers in Europe and the US were clear that what was required were purpose-built asylums organized on the therapeutic principles of moral treatment (Scull, 1983). Care in asylums that took people in at an early stage in their illness would lead to cure and discharge. Conditions in asylums improved and non-restraint was introduced into the growing system of public asylums, instigated in the UK by John Conolly at the Hanwell Insane Asylum. A high proportion of patients admitted to early nineteenth-century asylums were discharged either 'cured' or 'relieved'.

During the latter part of the nineteenth century and the first half of the twentieth century, English and American asylums entered what has been described as a 'long sleep'. Therapeutic optimism declined in parallel with the rise of a 'degeneracy' model of mental disorder. By 1890, more people each year were dying in hospital than being discharged 'cured' (Scull, 1983). Asylums grew in size and new asylums were built, often on the periphery of conurbations or the principal town of a county.

Even during these bleak years there was evidence of interest in supporting people who left the asylum. In 1879, the Reverend Henry Hawkins, chaplain to Colney Hatch Asylum, founded the Mental Aftercare Association 'to facilitate the readmission of the poor friendless female convalescent from Lunatic Asylums into social life'.

From the asylum to community care

Reform and discontent

The system of public asylums in England and Wales expanded during the first half of the twentieth century. Community care has, perhaps surprisingly, been public policy since the 1930 Mental Treatment Act.[1] This encouraged local authorities, then responsible for the asylum system, to set up systems of aftercare. The Act for the first time allowed for informal admission to a public mental hospital (the new term for asylums). Progress towards community care was delayed by the Great Depression and the Second World War. Postwar, the mental hospital system was incorporated into the NHS. The 1950s and 1960s saw a range of innovations in community care including outpatient clinics, day hospitals, community psychiatric nursing, the rise of psychiatric social work, and increasing residential provision for aftercare. As the mental hospitals shrank, acute inpatient care was commonly provided in district general hospital psychiatric units, although 'chronic' patients would end up in the mental hospital.

Professional attitudes towards mental illness changed during the period after the Second World War, partly due to an influx of doctors who had worked with the psychiatric casualties of the war and had more optimistic views about mental illness. The 'open door' movement involved both literally and metaphorically unlocking the ward doors within the mental hospitals. Hospitals became more permeable institutions. Admission rates increased but discharges increased faster. Innovators introduced novel approaches that David Clark described in his short book *Social Therapy in Psychiatry* (1974, p. 11) as 'help[ing] people change to a state more tolerable to themselves and others'. These approaches included industrial therapy, which is now largely forgotten, and the much-diminished therapeutic community movement.[2] Clark was passionate about psychiatric treatment being a joint enterprise between 'the client' and a range of other people not only from established professional backgrounds but including administrators and maintenance staff.

However, despite significant reform of how mental hospitals worked, there was a growing suspicion of institutions and institutional care (Jones & Fowles, 1984). The sociologist Erving Goffman described the 'total institution' and its deadening effects on its inmates (Goffman, 1961) (Clark knew and admired Goffman's work). Russell Barton, a psychiatrist, coined the term 'institutional neurosis', characterized as a syndrome of apathy, lack of initiative, and loss of interest in the outside world seen in mental hospital patients that in his view was caused by institutional life (Barton, 1959). In the Three Hospitals Study, Wing and Brown (1970) identified a 'clinical poverty' syndrome of blunted affect, poverty of speech, and social withdrawal. They demonstrated that the functioning and attitudes towards discharge of patients with schizophrenia were related to the social

---

[1] The history of mental health care can be followed in evolving mental health legislation. England and Wales share their mental health law. Northern Ireland and Scotland each has a different legal framework.
[2] One of us spent a memorable day as a student on an acute ward at Fulborn that was run on Therapeutic Community lines.

conditions of the particular hospital they were resident in. A series of scandals about the conditions in learning disability, elderly care, and mental hospitals that emerged in the 1960s and 1970s had a powerful effect on professional and public attitudes in reinforcing the view that care in institutions was a bad thing (Martin, 1984).

Deinstitutionalization

The first large English mental hospital closure, Banstead Hospital, took place in 1986. The TAPS study monitored the closure of Friern Barnet Hospital in North London (previously Colney Hatch and at its peak the largest mental hospital in Europe). The majority of patients were discharged from inpatient care, usually to high support settings, and their clinical and social outcomes were good (Leff & Treiman, 2000). A smaller group of hard-to-discharge patients moved to new specialist inpatient facilities and again did well over the following years (Treiman & Leff, 2002). The vast majority of the traditional asylums closed in the subsequent 15 years (The Time Chamber, 2020). Mental hospital sites were repurposed in many different ways. Bansted became a prison and Friern Barnet a high-end gated residential development. Warlingham Park which was a pioneer of the 'open door' movement and community psychiatric nursing, is now a desirable suburban housing estate. Other sites have been redeveloped as district general hospitals, often with attached psychiatric units.

Hospital closure, when carried out well, was successful for the patients caught up in the process. It came at the cost of very severe pressure on the reduced remaining inpatient services with high bed occupancy, increasing 'acuity' on wards, raised thresholds for admission, and a long-term trend of increasing use of compulsory admission. Community care, albeit supported by an evolving range of inpatient provision, became the dominant paradigm (Killaspy, 2006).

In the 1990s, adult mental health services typically consisted of a community mental health team that related to a geographical catchment area and the local general practitioner practices and a local acute inpatient ward. Medical staff would work across the inpatient/community divide. There was limited access to specialist care. Subsequently, in the 2000s, policy mandated the development of a range of specialist community teams. The link between a particular inpatient ward and the locality team, previously a strength of UK mental health services, was broken. This was due to pressing policy concerns, for example, a requirement to develop single-sex accommodation. Increasingly the medical workforce was divided between inpatient and community work, although inpatient psychiatry is not a recognized speciality in the UK. The inpatient/community split has been heavily debated, usually with more heat than light: see Burns and Baggaley (2018).

Bed numbers in England, despite significant population growth, declined steadily from the early 1950s from a peak of over 150,000 in 1954/1955 to a reported 18,000 NHS mental illness and learning disability beds in 2021. NHS provision has for many years been supplemented by private and independent sector beds, the vast majority of which are funded by the NHS. Laing and Buisson, a market intelligence organization, reported that these beds represented 30% of the total in 2017, which would suggest the total mental illness bed provision in England in 2021 was in the region of 26,000 (45 beds per 100,000 total population).[3] Cost undoubtedly plays a major role in current discussions on 'appropriate bed numbers', with up to 50% of secondary care mental health budgets spent on a resource that provides for less than 3% of patients at any given time.

International trends in inpatient services

Bed reductions across the world

The trend in England for a decline from a peak in inpatient beds has been seen across the world, although the size and date of the peak varies between countries. Among high-income countries the earliest peak was in New Zealand in 1950 (500/100,000 total population) and the latest Japan in 1990 (290/100,000) (Table 18.1). The process of bed reduction, which is commonly described as 'deinstitutionalization', has had unique trajectories in different jurisdictions. The US and the UK started to reduce beds at the same time and from very similar rates of inpatient beds and are now at roughly the same level but the changes were much more rapid in the US, following a slew of court judgments mandating hospital closure. Some countries have seen very marked decreases—notably Italy, which aggressively closed mental hospitals following implementation from 1978 of Law 180. By 2019, Italy reported 8/100,000 beds, down from a peak of 224/100,000 in 1963. Japan is an interesting outlier at the other end of the spectrum because the decline in bed numbers started very late and has been very modest. Japan now has by far the highest rate of inpatient beds per head in the world—at the time of writing 259/100,000 population. The discrepancy between Italy, reporting '40 years without a mental hospital' (Barbui et al., 2018), and Japan, which has scarcely begun the deinstitutionalization process (Kanata, 2016), cannot be explained by differences in the prevalence of mental disorder or the effectiveness or otherwise of community care. It must be the result of powerful sociocultural and administrative processes that lie beyond the scope of this chapter.

The World Health Organization, the European Union, and the OECD collate and report information on mental health care including data on psychiatric beds. This shows how variable the number of beds is, as is seen by the OECD data described above and in Table 18.1. There is additionally systematic variation in beds (and all other mental health resources) between groupings of countries according to World Bank income group (World Health Organization, 2018). Low-income countries report an average of 29 times fewer beds than high-income countries (Table 18.2).

Problems with the data

Bed data that are reported in national and international statistics cannot be read uncritically. The bed numbers in the UK reported by the OECD, which is scrupulous about data sources, specifically excludes private and independent sector provision (OECD, 2021), estimated to represent 30% of the bed total in England. The most

---

[3] At the time of writing, NHS-funded activity in the private and independent sector is captured by NHS Digital but is not publicly available. The most recent comprehensive bed data for England were produced in 2010 in a report by the Care Quality Commission that was quoted in the previous edition of this book.

SECTION 4 Treatment and service components

Table 18.1 Psychiatric inpatient beds in selected high-income countries: changes over time

Country	Beds per 100,000 total population	Peak year and beds	Ratio of beds maximum:contemporary
Australia (2016)	42	1965 271/100,000	6.9:1
Canada (2019)	36	1965 400/100,000	11.4:1
France (2019)	82	1974 250/100,000	3.1:1
Germany (2019)	131	1965 177/100,000	1.3:1
Ireland (2019)	33	1958 500/100,000	15.1:1
Italy (2019)	8	1963 224/100,000	28.0:1
Japan (2019)	259	1990 290/100,00	1.1:1
Netherlands (2019)	80	1955 260/100,000	3.2:1
New Zealand (2019)	32	1949 ~500/100,00	15.6:1
Spain (2019)	36	1974 130/1000,000	3.6:1
UK (2020)	33	1955 350/100,000	10.6:1
US (2018)	25	1955 339/100,000	13.7:1

Source: for current beds: OECD (2022). Hospital beds (indicator). doi: 10.1787/0191328e-en (accessed 10 January 2022). Peak year from multiple publications.

recently published comprehensive survey of inpatient provision in the US, which provides data from 2014, describes a highly fragmented system of inpatient provision with multiple providers funded through complex arrangements that work at national, state, and local levels with a significant contribution from work-based insurance. The study reports 31.9 beds per 100,000 population (National Association of State Mental Health Program Directors, 2017). This compares with 21 beds per 100,000 for that year in OECD figures. A census of inpatients in Ireland undertaken in 2019 identified 2308 occupied beds, representing 46.8 inpatients per 100,000 compared with the OECD reported figure of 33 per 100,000 (Daly & Craig, 2019). A study of the discrepancy between Italy and Canada, which has experienced severe bed shortage despite a much higher number of beds and relatively advanced community services, suggested that a very large element of the apparent discrepancy between the countries was definitional since 'rehabilitation' units in Italy that look and feel like longer-term inpatient provision are not defined as 'inpatient beds' (which is in fact accurate in terms of our initial definition because these units by law cannot not take detained patients) (O'Reilly & Shum, 2017).

Transinstitutionalization

Sceptical voices have also identified a process of 'transinstitutionalization', in which the hospital bed reductions seen in wealthy countries were matched by an increase in people living in other forms of restricted setting (Priebe et al., 2005). There is certainly striking evidence that as hospitals closed, the prison population increased, although these phenomena may well be unrelated. More persuasively, across the world and for a range of care groups, mini-institutions (e.g. hostels, care homes, nursing homes, secure homes for children, and specialist provision for people with learning disability) have sprung up to replace now-closed large institutions.

Inpatient care into the twenty-first century

The traditional UK mental hospital contained wards with differing functions ranging from acute wards for the reception of newly admitted patients, through wards offering rehabilitation and resettlement, to 'back wards' for patients who were not expected to be discharged. Elderly, frail patients would be separately accommodated. The large and quite separate system of hospitals that catered for people with 'mental handicap' was replaced by a network of small specialist inpatient units for people with intellectual disability and/or autism either as a primary problem or an important comorbidity.

Contemporary UK mental health services are almost entirely funded by the state but provision is through a mixed economy of NHS, not-for-profit, and private sector providers. Providers work within an ever-changing commissioning framework. The competitive advantage of NHS providers lies largely in their close links with a geographical locality and local commissioners and the potential ability to work effectively across the inpatient/community divide. The independent sector's competitive advantage is flexibility, with an ability to offer services targeted at underserved highly specialist care groups and acute and psychiatric intensive care unit overspill beds when local NHS capacity is exhausted, as it was in the 1990s and has been in the 2010s and 2020s. Some NHS providers can also use academic links to offer highly specialist inpatient care, for example, for people with severe affective disorder or treatment-resistant psychosis.

Acute care

In the UK today, acute inpatient care is most commonly provided in relatively small free-standing acute units serving a local catchment area (approximately 250,000 population). Acute wards work within NHS health trusts, which have large (approximately 1 million population) catchment areas and are subject to bed management processes that place a patient in any available bed. Most acute wards are now single sex. Where in-trust beds are not available, acute private sector care is purchased.

Table 18.2 Total adult inpatient care indicators (mental hospital, forensic inpatient units, psychiatric wards, community residential facilities) by World Bank income group

	Beds per 100,000 population (median)	Admissions per 100,000 population (median)
Low income	1.9	17.5
Lower-middle	6.3	43.8
Upper-middle	24.3	117.2
High	54.6	334.1

Source: World Health Organization (2018). Mental Health Atlas 2017. Geneva: World Health Organization (p. 36).

Across a wider geographical area, acute wards are supplemented by psychiatric intensive care units that manage patients who present with severe agitation and aggression that cannot be safely managed in an acute ward (Rule, 2019). In some services there may be a specialized short-term assessment or 'triage' ward, although evaluation has not shown systematic benefits of the triage system (Williams et al., 2014). A recent development in England is the 'provider collaborative' where several organizations come together, usually within 'integrated care systems' (Tracy et al., 2023). These allow delivery of specialist inpatient services that no single NHS trust might have the need or ability to provide, for example, female psychiatric intensive care units, acute provision for children and young persons (Child and Adolescent Mental Health Services (CAMHS)), and mother-and-baby units. This also allows a 'shared bed capacity' to reduce usage of the private sector. However, acute care is only one component of a much broader system of inpatient care (Smith et al., 2015, pp. 12–15).

Forensic inpatient services

Historically, UK mental hospitals have been complemented by four 'high secure' hospitals, which admit offender patients who are recognized as presenting a particularly serious threat to others or have committed a serious offence. An expanding network of 'medium secure' provision was developed from 1980 onwards, partly to allow downsizing of the high secure estate and partly to expand total 'forensic' provision. The initial expectation was that patients would spend a maximum of 2 years before discharge from medium security, but this proved illusory. Medium secure provision now includes rehabilitation and longer-term care services. There is also now a further class of 'low secure' provision that in England operates as part of the 'forensic' system. In contrast to other high-income countries a significant proportion of the forensic estate is in the independent sector. Commissioning arrangements for forensic provision in England are separate from the commissioning of other inpatient services and at the time of writing are led by NHS-led provider collaboratives operating at a regional level.

Rehabilitation

Closing the mental hospitals failed to end the need for longer-term inpatient care for people whose severe mental health problems did not resolve rapidly in acute wards and who could not be supported in community-based living settings. As a result, there has been continuing need for a spectrum of inpatient psychiatric rehabilitation services. These include community rehabilitation units that emphasize enhancing living skills and seek to optimize medication management; high-dependency units that take in people with severe refractory symptoms of their illness, comorbidities, and potentially challenging behaviours; longer-term facilities supporting people with complex care needs; 'locked' rehabilitation units that manage people presenting significant risk: and a range of units that offer highly specialist care for people with very specific needs such as acquired brain damage, severe personality disorder, and comorbid autism (Davies & Killaspy, 2015). A 2019 survey of rehabilitation services in England undertaken by the Care Quality Commission (CQC, 2019a) identified 3622 individuals in a designated rehabilitation bed, with a majority of beds being provided by the independent sector. Patients placed in rehabilitation services were often 'out of area', with obvious impacts on the care pathway.

Inpatient rehabilitation is only one component of a wider rehabilitation pathway that is, in the words of a recent National Institute for Health and Care Excellence (NICE) guideline on rehabilitation for adults with complex psychosis, 'embedded in a local comprehensive mental healthcare service' (NICE, 2020).

Complex care

The landscape of inpatient provision now includes units with varying levels of security offering treatment for people with a personality disorder diagnosis (commonly providing trauma-focused work); CAMHS services that manage young persons who present with severe self-harming behaviours; services offering inpatient treatment for people with eating disorders; specialist services for people with acquired brain injury and neurodegenerative disorders; specialist services for people with diagnoses of learning disability and autism; and some continuing care of people suffering from dementia associated with severe behavioural problems. The importance of private and independent sector provision, which is largely invisible to community-based practitioners, cannot be overestimated. The pathway for an individual out of highly specialist care can be very challenging but is much eased if there is a local community team that has relevant expertise working towards discharge.

Inpatient services in the US

The US has both a complex pattern of funding health care and a very mixed economy of providers which include state mental hospitals, community hospitals, academic centres, and non-profit and for-profit hospitals, and a separate system for veterans. Although there is legislation and regulation at the federal level, each state has its own mental health legislation and policy. Funding streams include money from the federal government, state and local government, insurance, and direct payments from the patient. Reimbursement systems are very complex for the provider to negotiate and there are enormous transaction costs in the US health care system.

Tertiary care state hospitals in the US focus especially on people with psychotic illness that is not responsive to acute care, often characterized by danger to self or others; some units are further specialized for violence or personality disorders (especially borderline personality) with self-harm, or individuals with psychosis and significant cognitive impairments. Admissions to the state hospitals serve as the safety net for patients who are uninsured or do not respond to acute care. In recent years there is an increasing presence of patients committed with forensic histories or on court order for restoration of competence or NGRI (not guilty for reason of insanity): these patients can be very difficult to discharge (National Association of State Mental Health Program Directors, 2014). A few private, not-for-profit, hospitals are centres of excellence and sites for highly specialized inpatient treatment (e.g. McLean Hospital, Cornell-Westchester, Menninger, and Sheppard Pratt), although the number of these tertiary centres has declined.

Concerns about inpatient care

There is an overriding concern over access to timely and effective treatment for mental illness. Many countries report significant bed shortages, particularly Anglophone countries that have aggressively deinstitutionalized, and rising thresholds for admission.

Coercion and control

In England, compulsory admissions increased from the late 1980s onwards, with the exception of small declines in the years 2002–2009 (CQC, 2019b), which was a time of unprecedented investment in community services. Few inpatient units now lack a lock on their front door that prevents free movement. Whether the locked door works is a matter for debate. Data from over 15 years of admissions to hospitals in Germany, which has far higher bed numbers than England, found that those with an open door policy had fewer suicide attempts, absconsions, and suicides than locked wards (Huber et al., 2016).

Involuntary admission in England is commoner among people from an ethnic minority background and internationally is associated with socioeconomic deprivation, a diagnosis of psychosis, and previous involuntary admission (Walker et al., 2019). The troubling fact that the majority of people who remain in hospital for prolonged periods are there against their will—which must colour the interaction between staff and patient—was a major driver behind current proposals to reform the Mental Health Act (Independent Review of the Mental Health Act 1983, 2018).

One area of significant concern is the use of restraint, prolonged seclusion, and long-term segregation, particularly of children and young people, and autistic people and/or with a learning disability. A study found that diagnosed or suspected autism was by far the most common clinical diagnosis associated with the use of long-term segregation outside forensic settings, although psychosis and personality disorder also featured (CQC, 2018). Anyone familiar with psychiatric hospital environments will be aware how disturbing they can be for autistic people, though some wards are working towards providing 'autism friendly' environments. The quite small but important group of individuals with learning disability or autism in long-term segregation are now subject to Independent Care (Education) and Treatment Reviews (CQC, 2021).

Inpatient staff have routinely to balance a range of highly complex legal, ethical, and practical issues. Mental health legislation gives staff wide-ranging powers over someone who is detained. Patients may be under observation regimes, have medication administered against their wishes, be physically restrained, and be allowed leave only at staff discretion. These powers come with legal and ethical duties that include working in a way that is compatible with human rights legislation while at the same time following required procedures that maintain the individual's safety and promote their recovery. All professions have codes of conduct governing their behaviour but in reality how people negotiate these complex issues will be determined by the training they receive, their own moral compass, and the culture they work in. There is some international evidence that staff training is effective in reducing coercive practices (Barbui et al., 2021).

Failures of care

The reports into the hospital scandals of the 1960s and 1970s described in graphic detail how things could go wrong in the culture of inpatient services (Martin, 1984). More recently in the UK, evidence emerged in a BBC TV documentary that aired in May 2011 about serious abuse of patients at Winterbourne View, a small hospital for people with learning disability. Detailed reviews were held about what went wrong, which identified criminal behaviour by staff and failures of governance and regulatory oversight (Department of Health, 2012).

The policy response was the 'Transforming Care' programme, which envisaged that rigorous review of inpatients with learning disability and/or autistic and with challenging behaviour would result in most patients being discharged to bespoke community-based settings. Progress has been slow and by the end of 2021, 2085 adults and children with learning disability and/or autistic remained in specialist inpatient units, with an average length of stay of 5.4 years (CQC, 2019b). This represents almost 10% of the total mental health inpatient provision.

Evidence of unacceptable treatment of such patients within learning disability/autism inpatient units has continued to emerge, the most notable example being revelations in another BBC documentary of abuse at Whorlton Hall that aired in 2019. At the time of writing, no similar systemic examples of the dramatic collapse of the quality of care has recently been identified in other forms of inpatient provision. However, it is quite common for units to experience criticism for specific failures that have, for example, led to patient suicide or other serious adverse outcomes.

Out of sight, out of mind?

An additional issue has been the use of 'out-of-area' beds both for acute overspill and the longer-term care of people requiring more specialist care. It is not uncommon for people to be transferred, usually by a secure ambulance, from one end of England to another in order to be placed in an 'appropriate' bed, with inevitable effects on continuity of care and the ability of carers to offer support.

Information flows across the inpatient/community divide are often poor even when a person well known to the local mental health services is admitted to a local bed. Existing electronic patient record systems are often poorly structured and are seldom interoperable between services. Problems are clearly exacerbated when someone is placed out of area. Discontinuities of care due to moves between hospitals for clinical or bed management reasons can add further distress and make the metaphorical patient journey feel like a game of snakes and ladders. As an example, someone moving down from medium to low security can paradoxically experience more restrictions on their liberty as the new team gets to know them. There are simple and effective measures that services can take to reduce the use of out-of-area inpatient treatment, of which the most obvious is making sure local services and commissioners are aware of the problem and try to address it in a systematic fashion (Bennett et al., 2011).

The journey for a person with complex needs out of hospital can be very difficult, may involve a great deal of negotiation between agencies, and requires significant expertise to manage.

The built environment

Internationally, there are marked differences in the quality of inpatient environments. Many units in the UK are located in old buildings that are not fit for purpose and are dismal and poorly maintained. Many new buildings are similarly cramped, noisy, depressing, and with poor standards of fittings. There may be a lack of space and equipment for rehabilitative activities.

What do inpatient services do and how do they do it?

In 2005, the then Department of Health for England (now Department of Health and Social Care) stated that:

> The purpose of an adult acute psychiatric inpatient service is to provide a high standard of humane treatment and care in a safe and therapeutic setting for service users in the most acute and vulnerable stage of their illness. It should be for the benefit of those service users whose circumstances or acute care needs are such that they cannot at that time be treated and supported appropriately at home or in an alternative, less restrictive setting. (Department of Health, 2005, p. 5)

This view, which can essentially be summed up as admission being an always undesirable last resort when all else has failed, is replicated in the current literature, which largely focuses on demonstrating the efficacy of alternatives to inpatient admission. It also reflects the practice in contemporary inpatient psychiatry to focus on short-term symptomatic or behavioural stabilization and as rapid a discharge as possible, often without a great deal of curiosity about locating the acute problem in a longer-term context. The managerial metric is overwhelmingly on avoiding admission and reducing length of stay if admission occurs, a perspective that is reflected in the benchmarking criteria that are used to assess NHS providers. People who absolutely cannot be discharged will eventually be transferred into longer-term settings without much optimism from decision-makers about the outcome. This narrative ignores the potential benefits of treatment in a well-run, therapeutically oriented inpatient service.

Treatment and care are delivered by the staff team. The typical ward team will include psychiatrists, nurses and support workers, occupational therapists, clinical pharmacists, and, increasingly, psychologists. Different settings may also include other core staff members. An eating disorder ward requires specialist dietetic input; CAMHS units will tend to include family therapists and teachers; and old age services will draw on physiotherapists and speech-and-language therapists. Some organizations have been trialling novel roles aimed to bridge the traditional patient–staff hierarchy, with positions such as peer support workers. Ideally the inpatient team works closely with community-based colleagues including social workers and housing officers. In the integrated care systems currently being introduced in England that aim to cross traditional boundaries between physical and mental health, there is an emerging growth in the utilization of relevant professionals, such as physiotherapists and diabetes nurses (Tracy et al., 2023).

Inpatient care pathways

There has been great enthusiasm for the mental health care pathway. This is understood as a quasi-algorithmic process that describes who does what during the metaphorical patient journey following admission, with prescribed timescales for the provision of NICE-compliant interventions and a set of expected outcomes. The concept was imported from the management of elective surgical interventions such as a hip replacement, where there are clearly expected outcomes within a predictable time-frame and people who fall off the pathway can be readily identified. In principle, discharge planning should begin at the point of admission with close liaison occurring between the inpatient service and an identified community team, potentially augmented by short-term support from the local crisis response/home treatment team.

What actually happens is a much less smooth and predictable process described by the nursing academic Len Bowers and colleagues (Bowers et al., 2009). This starts with the presence of a mental illness/problem that might prompt the need for admission and the unavailability or unfeasibility of alternative options such as family or mental health service support, then a decision to admit which will be made by multiple actors and results in a rather wide-ranging set of activities that occur in hospital that (one hopes) will result in resolution of the clinical and social issues that led to admission, and indeed address additional issues (such as previously undertreated physical health problems).

The inpatient experience

What actually goes on during an admission is surprisingly poorly described. The literature that exists suggests that service users in acute units report limited interaction with staff, poor information about treatments, a lack of activities on the ward, and boredom (Wykes et al., 2018), with staff spending about 50% of their time interacting with patients (Sharac et al., 2010). One early study noted, depressingly, that leave from the ward was the most valued aspect of inpatient stays (McIntyre et al., 1989). That said, patients do consistently report valuing the quality of the nursing care they receive, particularly the empathy, warmth, and respect that they experience. These positives are balanced by negatives when patients experience apparently arbitrary behaviour by nurses, coercion and punishment, and a tendency for staff to congregate in the office to the exclusion of attention to the patients (Quirk & Lelliott, 2004). Too often the inpatient unit experience is of a place to stay while receiving drug treatments in a controlled environment during ever-shorter stays (Markowitz, 2008). At the extreme, some patients report being traumatized by their experiences of treatment in hospital as a result of coercive physical interventions (Prytherch et al., 2020).

What happens on an inpatient ward?

Initial assessment and information gathering is crucial for good quality care, although the elaboration of a thorough biopsychosocial formulation is quite rare. Staff working in inpatient settings need to develop a relationship with the patient—a skill captured in the forensic psychiatry literature as 'relational security'. There are also very basic issues that may need to be addressed such as hygiene and personal care, adequate food and fluid intake, and management of physical health problems. Inpatient services will of course deploy management and treatment strategies that seek to deal with the problems that resulted in admission. In an ideal world, discharge planning eases the process of return to community living and should include a review of the person's living conditions, current social supports, and ability to function. One vital resource is the patient's social network and an effective service will go out of its way to engage with family and carers. Care packages can be developed to enable safe discharge. This will inevitably require close contact with community services and interagency working. As a result of the Covid-19 pandemic services have learnt to facilitate digital meetings with carers and staff (Dave et al., 2021).

Inpatient services are proficient at offering evidence-based physical treatments such as medication and electroconvulsive therapy. Occupational therapists have particular skills in the assessment of functioning, engagement of a patient in meaningful activities, and planning, with the person, for future needs after discharge. In some acute units, short-term psychological assessments are now available: these can help determine suitability for longer-term psychological treatment in the community, provide brief on-site interventions, and develop a formulation of an individual's background and difficulties to assist the person and team's understanding and management of their difficulties on the ward. Group therapy and peer support activities are perhaps understudied in terms of the potential gains from sharing experiences with others in crises, though they have an evidence base. There is an emerging literature on inpatient-specific interventions, for example, cognitive behavioural therapy modified for psychosis (Wood et al., 2020). More specialist services should be able to deploy a much wider range of interventions, for example, trauma-focused work in personality disorder units and detailed behavioural analysis in intellectual disability services that feed into an effective positive behaviour support plan.

Aggression and violence are a fact of life in many acute inpatient services (Bowers, 2014). Core principles in the NICE guideline on the short-term management of violence and aggression include improving service user experience and the training of staff in recognizing risk factors and de-escalation (NICE, 2015). Coercive interventions, such as rapid tranquillization, restraint, and seclusion, will occur but can be carried out with sensitivity and professionalism. Understanding the processes that underlie the existence of conflict and the requirement for containment in psychiatric wards lies at the heart of the Safewards initiative (https://www.safewards.net/) and reducing restrictive practice collaborative (Royal College of Psychiatrists, 2021) and can form the basis of a wide set of interventions aimed at improving patient and staff experience (Bowers et al., 2015).

Developing a positive ward culture

One factor associated with the abuse identified at Whorlton Hall was the hospital's closed culture, an issue that has long been recognized as a risk factor for poor care (Martin, 1984). A healthy ward culture seems to lie at the heart of effective inpatient services. David Clark, writing 50 years ago, summarized three elements of a positive hospital environment: activity—keeping people engaged as much as possible in things they find meaningful; freedom—as far as possible limiting restrictions on a person's ability to move, choose, and act as they wish; and responsibility—maximizing choice and personal autonomy (Clark, 1974). This view, written during the era of the mental hospital, is both fully in line with current thinking about human rights and in enormous tension with the protocolized, risk-averse culture that dominates contemporary mental health services. Helping frontline staff deal with this tension is a key skill for service leaders. Managers and leaders at all levels in contemporary practice have responsibility to value, facilitate, and reward the growth of best care.

Regulation, quality assurance, and quality improvement

Regulation in England

The CQC is the regulator for all health and social care in England. It registers all providers then goes on to assess the quality of care of a service against five generic standards: is the service safe? Is it effective? Is it caring? Is it responsive? Is it well led? Each standard is ranked on a scale from 'outstanding', through 'good' and 'requires improvement', to 'inadequate'. The inspectors come to an overall assessment of the service in these domains. Where practice is rated as inadequate, the CQC takes enforcement action. Inspectors of mental health services have expertise in the field and will review issues such as the availability of staff and the quality of their training, systems of risk management and medication management, the use of restrictive interventions, care planning, staff interactions with patients, the ward environment, and the quality of leadership in the service. Inspection reports are publicly available documents. There is also a parallel regime within the CQC that monitors the use of mental health legislation, which feeds into the overall inspection framework.

The CQC has, itself, been criticized over failure to identify settings where there has been a collapse in quality of care: Whorlton Hall was repeatedly assessed as 'Good' in inspections before revelations of abuse. Two independent reports were commissioned to review inspection and regulation activities at Whorlton Hall, which made wide-ranging recommendations for improving the inspection process including encouraging inspectors to identify a closed culture (Murphy, 2020a, 2020b).

There is a requirement for all organizations in the UK to have policies and procedures that safeguard children and vulnerable adults in protecting them from harm (financial, emotional, physical and sexual, and neglect). Safeguarding concerns when they arise must be conveyed to the local social services authority as the lead agency. Inpatient units have a duty to convey concerns about harms experienced by patients to a designated safeguarding team.

Serious adverse outcomes are routinely monitored across the UK. The National Confidential Inquiry into Suicide and Safety in Mental Health (NCISH) has for many years reviewed aggregate data on suicide and homicide associated with mental health problems and developed the 'Safer Services' toolkit to reduce the incidence of suicide in wards and other clinical environments (NCISH, 2022). Inpatient suicides decreased markedly over the decade from 2008, as did to a lesser extent homicide by people known to mental health services (NCISH, 2021).

Quality assurance and quality improvement

The Centre for Quality Improvement (CCQI) at the Royal College of Psychiatrists runs a number of quality networks, including networks for working age, older adult and CAMHS inpatient services and forensic services (https://www.rcpsych.ac.uk/improving-care/ccqi/what-we-do). There are also networks for other specialist inpatient services including mother and baby, eating disorder, rehabilitation, and psychiatric intensive care units. These networks offer learning events and conferences, networking opportunities including email groups, and accreditation to subscribing units in a developmental process that involves self-assessment then peer review against defined standards. The networks build up libraries and evidence of best practice, counter-balancing the largely numbers-driven national datasets with clinical examples and standards of good care.

Over the years the standards evolve—the working age inpatient standards are currently in their seventh edition (Penfold et al., 2019). The working age standards cover admission and assessment, care planning and treatment, referral, discharge and transfer, patient and carer experience, staffing and training, environment and facilities, and governance. There is some cross-sectional evidence of improvement over time in the quality of care provided in participating acute services (Chaplin et al., 2018). A cluster randomized controlled trial comparing low secure services that were or were not participating in a peer review network failed to find significant differences in ward-level and patient-level outcomes. Interestingly, staff in participating units reported feeling safer but experienced more burn-out (Aimola et al., 2018).

Although the CCQI accreditation process is similar across service types the content of standards differs: for example, for obvious reasons issues of security (physical, procedural, and relational) are prominent in the forensic standards (Townsend et al., 2021). At this point, CCQI accreditation is optional for services; however, there is a general consensus that commissioners of services will increasingly not accept or pay for those that do not have the relevant approval.

Another element of quality improvement is participation in audit. A good example is another CCQI initiative—the Prescribing Observatory for Mental Health (POMH-UK), which carries out large-scale audits of prescribing practices against contemporary clinical guidelines. Audit results are fed back to participating provider organizations, which fund the work through membership fees. POMH-UK has recently reported on 15 years of work (Barnes & Paton, 2020) and can provide evidence of change in clinical practice.

Licensing, regulation, and monitoring of services in the US

Health care in the US is essentially a marketplace with providers competing for customers and resources. Providers are licensed at the state level according to local regulations, which vary markedly between states (Shields et al., 2018). Some states prescribe minimum staffing levels, provision of particular forms of care, systematic monitoring of adverse events, and specific environmental issues, such as access to outdoor spaces, though most do not. Hospitals need to be accredited in order to receive funding through Medicare and Medicaid. Accreditation also attracts patients and insurers and therefore offers a competitive advantage to providers.

More than 80% of inpatient facilities are accredited through the Joint Commission (Sheilds et al., 2018), which is a long-established non-profit body that according to its website evaluates 'more than 22,000 health care organizations and programs in the United States'. The process for accreditation is somewhat similar to that adopted by CQC and CCQI with external review of the organization backed by submission of data that includes (1) screening on admission for violence risk, substance use, psychological trauma and patient strengths; (2) hours of physical restraint use; (3) hours of seclusion use; and (4) patients discharged on multiple antipsychotic medication with appropriate justification (Joint Commission, 2021, pp. 33–68). The reviewer methodology is firmly behind a paywall. However, there is no systematic mechanism for ensuring that organizations learn from mistakes and no national system for learning from seriously adverse outcomes as exists in the UK.

Conclusion

The scientific literature on inpatient care is notable in two regards: its paucity and the general focus on poor practice or process markers (Tracy & Phillips, 2022). There are ethical and methodological complexities in researching inpatient care, but it can be done (Wykes et al., 2018). Without such work we are unlikely to identify and disseminate effective elements of care. One systemic problem is the failure to adopt standardized outcome measures in routine practice. The clinical reality is that most people come into hospital with very severe problems and leave significantly improved.

The issues facing inpatient services are profound: from financial and staffing resources to questions about the model of (and evidence for) the care provided. Just maintaining the current system is challenging. Recruitment and retention are under huge pressure and the emphasis is often on maintaining minimum staffing levels that can ensure safety. Professional time is considerably eaten into by administrative tasks.

Key questions surrounding inpatient care include the following: what should happen within wards? What constitutes best practice? And how can this be disseminated? Alternatives to acute wards are being developed. 'Crisis houses' are a noteworthy example (Butt et al., 2019) and include services targeted at women who have suffered trauma, and for whom standard inpatient care was found to exacerbate symptomatology (Prytherch et al., 2020).

Inpatient treatment remains an essential component of a comprehensive mental health service. People who become inpatients nowadays have on average more complex needs than in the past. Effective inpatient services need to have good links with competent community services to ensure effective discharge planning.

REFERENCES

Aimola, L., Jasim, S., Bassett, P., Bassett, P., Quirk, A., Worrall, A., et al. (2018). Impact of a peer-review network on the quality of inpatient low secure mental health services: cluster randomised controlled trial. *BMC Health Services Research*, **18**, 994–1004.

Arnold, C. (2008). *Bedlam*. London: Pocket Books.

Barbui, C., Papola, D., & Saraceno, B. (2018). Forty years without a mental hospital. *International Journal of Mental Health Systems*, **12**, 43.

Barbui, C., Purgato, M., Abdulmalik, J., Caldas-de-Almeida, J. M., Eaton, J., Gureje, O., et al (2021). Efficacy of interventions to reduce coercive treatment in mental health services: umbrella review of randomised evidence. *British Journal of Psychiatry*, **218**, 185–195.

Barnes, T. R. E. & Paton, C. (2020). *The Prescribing Observatory for Mental Health 15-Year Report College*. London: Royal College of Psychiatrists Centre for Quality Improvement.

Barton, R. (1959). *Institutional Neurosis*. Bristol: John Wright.

Bennett, A., Killaspy, H., Ryan, T., Davies, G., & Meier, R. (2011). *In Sight and in Mind: A Toolkit to Reduce the Use of Out of Area Mental Health Services*. London: Royal College of Psychiatrists. https://mentalhealthpartnerships.com/resource/in-sight-and-in-mind-a-toolkit-to-reduce-the-use-of-out-of-area-mental-health-services/

Bowers, L. (2014). Safewards: a new model of conflict and containment on psychiatric wards. *Journal of Psychiatric and Mental Health Nursing*, **21**, 499–508.

Bowers, L., Chaplin, R., Quirk, A., & Lelliott, P. (2009). A conceptual model of the aims and functions of acute inpatient psychiatry. *Journal of Mental Health*, **18**, 316–325.

Bowers, L., James, K., Quirk, A., Simpson, A., SUGAR, Stewart, D., & Hodsoll, J. (2015). Reducing conflict and containment rates on acute psychiatric wards: the Safewards cluster randomized controlled trial. *International Journal of Nursing Studies*, **52**, 1412–1422.

Burns, T. & Baggaley, M. (2018). Splitting in-patient and out-patient responsibility does not improve patient care. *British Journal of Psychiatry*, **210**, 6–9.

Butt, M. F., Walls, D., & Bhattacharya, R. (2019). Do patients get better? A review of outcomes from a crisis house and home treatment team partnership. *BJPsych Bulletin*, **43**, 106–111.

Care Quality Commission (2018). *Out of Sight—Who Cares? A Review of Restraint, Seclusion and Segregation for Autistic People, and People with a Learning Disability and/or Mental Health Condition*. Newcastle upon Tyne: Care Quality Commission.

Care Quality Commission (2019a). *Mental Health Rehabilitation Inpatient Services: Results from the 2019 Information Request*. Newcastle upon Tyne: Care Quality Commission.

Care Quality Commission (2019b). Mental Health Act: The *Rise* in the *Use* of the MHA to *Detain People* in England. Newcastle upon Tyne: Care Quality Commission. https://www.cqc.org.uk/publications/themed-work/mental-health-act-rise-mha-detain-england

Care Quality Commission (2021). Restraint, segregation and seclusion review: progress report. https://www.cqc.org.uk/publications/themes-care/restraint-segregation-seclusion-review-progress-report-december-2021

Cecil, D. (1933). *The Stricken Deer*. London: Constable and Company.

Chaplin, R., Raphael, H., & Beavon, M. (2018). The impact of accreditation for 10 years on inpatient units for adults of working age in the United Kingdom *Psychiatric Services*, **69**, 1053–1055.

Clark, D. H. (1974). *Social Therapy in Psychiatry*. Harmondsworth: Penguin.

Daly, A. & Craig, S. (2019). *Irish Psychiatric Units and Hospitals Census 2019 Main Findings*. Dublin: Health Research Board.

Dave, S., Abraham, S., Ramkisson, R., Matheiken, S., Pillai, A. S., Reza, H., et al. (2021). Digital psychiatry and COVID-19: the big bang effect for the NHS? *BJPsych Bulletin*, **45**, 259–263.

Davies, S. & Killaspy, H. (2015). Rehabilitation in hospital settings. In: Holloway, F., Kalidindi, S., Killaspy, H., & Roberts, G. (Eds.), *Enabling Recovery: The Principles and Practice of Rehabilitation Psychiatry* (pp. 262–278). London: RCPsych Publications.

Department of Health (2005). *Mental Health Policy Implementation Guide: Adult Acute Inpatient Care Provision*. London: Department of Health.

Department of Health (2012). *Transforming Care: A National Response to Winterbourne View Hospital*. London: Department of Health.

Goffman, E. (1961). *Asylums*. New York: Doubleday.

Huber, C. G., Schneeberger, A. R., Kowalinski, E., Frohlich, D., von Felten, S., Walter, M., et al. (2016). Suicide risk and absconding in psychiatric hospitals with and without open door policies: a 15 year, observational study. *Lancet Psychiatry*, **3**, 842–849.

Independent Review of the Mental Health Act 1983 (2018). Modernising the Mental Health Act. Increasing *Choice, Reducing Compulsion*. Final Report of the Independent Review of the Mental Health Act 1983. London: Department of Health and Social Care.

Joint Commission (2021). Specifications manual for Joint Commission National Quality Measures. Version 2021B2. https://manual.jointcommission.org/Home/WebHome

Jones, K. & Fowles, A. J. (1984). *Ideas on Institutions*. London: Routledge and Kegan Paul.

Kanata, T. (2016). Japanese mental health care in historical context. Why did Japan become a country with so many psychiatric care beds? *Social Work/Maatskaplike Werk*, **52**, 471–489.

Killaspy, H. (2006). From asylum to community care: learning from experience. *British Medical Bulletin*, **79–80**, 245–258.

Leff, J. & Trieman, N. (2000). Long stay patients discharged from psychiatric hospitals. Social and clinical outcomes after five years in the community. TAPS Project 46. *British Journal of Psychiatry*, **176**, 217–223.

McIntyre, K., Farrell, M., & David, A. S. (1989). What do psychiatric in-patients really want? *BMJ*, **298**, 159–160.

Markowitz, J. C. (2008). A letter from America: rescuing inpatient psychiatry *Evidence Based Mental Health*, **11**, 68–69.

Martin, J. P. (1984). *Hospitals in Trouble*. Oxford: Basil Blackwell.

Murphy, G. (2020a). CQC inspections and regulation of Whorlton Hall 2015–2019: an independent review. Care Quality Commission. https://www.cqc.org.uk/news/stories/cqc-publishes-independent-review-its-regulation-whorlton-hall-between-2015-2019

Murphy, G. (2020b). CQC inspections and regulation of Whorlton Hall 2015–2019 second independent report. Care Quality Commission. https://www.cqc.org.uk/news/stories/cqc-publishes-second-part-independent-review-its-regulation-whorlton-hall

National Association of State Mental Health Program Directors (2014). *The Vital Role of State Psychiatric Hospitals*. Arlington, VA: National Association of State Mental Health Program Directors.

National Association of State Mental Health Program Directors (2017). *Trend in Psychiatric Inpatient Capacity, United States and Each State 1970 to 2014*. Arlington, VA: National Association of State Mental Health Program Directors.

National Confidential Inquiry into Suicide and Safety in Mental Health (2021). *Annual Report: England, Northern Ireland, Scotland and Wales 2021*. Manchester: University of Manchester.

National Confidential Inquiry into Suicide and Safety in Mental Health (2022). *Safer Services: A Toolkit for Specialist Mental Health Services and Primary Care*. Manchester: University of Manchester. https://documents.manchester.ac.uk/display.aspx?DocID=40697

National Institute for Health and Care Excellence (2015). Violence and aggression: short-term management in mental health, health and community settings (NICE Guideline NG10). https://www.nice.org.uk/guidance/ng10

National Institute for Health and Care Excellence (2020). Rehabilitation for adults with complex psychosis (NICE guideline NG181). www.nice.org.uk/guidance/ng181

OECD (2021). Health statistics. Definitions, sources and methods. All psychiatric care beds in hospital. http://www.oecd.org/health/health-data.htm

O'Reilly, R. & Shum, J. Y.-H. (2017). Pitfalls of comparing psychiatric bed numbers across jurisdictions: lessons from Canada and Italy. *Research Insights*, **14**, 2–8.

Penfold, N., Nugent, A., Clarke, H., & Colwill, A. (2019). *Standards for Acute Inpatient Services for Working Age Adults*. London: Royal College of Psychiatrists College Centre for Quality Improvement.

Porter, R. (1990). *Mind-Forg'd Manacles*. Harmondsworth: Penguin.

Priebe, S., Badesconyi, A., Fioritti, A., et al. (2005). Reinstitutionalisation in mental health care: comparison of data on service provision from six European countries. *British Medical Journal*, **330**, 123–126.

Prytherch, H., Cooke, A., & Marsh, I. (2020). Coercion or collaboration: service-user experiences of risk management in hospital and a trauma-informed crisis house. *Psychosis*, **13**, 93–104.

Quirk, A. & Lelliott, P. (2004). Users' experience of in-patient services. In: Campling, P., Davies, S., & Farquharson, G. (Eds.), *From Toxic Institutions to Therapeutic Environments: Residential Settings in Mental Health Services* (pp. 45–54). London: Gaskell.

Royal College of Psychiatrists (2021). MH-SIP—reducing restrictive practice (RRP): scale up and spread. https://www.rcpsych.ac.uk/improving-care/nccmh/quality-improvement-programmes/MHSIP-reducing-restrictive-practice

Rule, A. (2019). Psychiatric intensive care. In: Barrera, A., Attard, C., & Chaplin, R. (Eds.), *Oxford Textbook of Inpatient Psychiatry* (pp. 305–311). Oxford: Oxford University Press.

Scull, A. T. (1983). Museums of Madness. Harmondsworth: Penguin.

Sharac, J., McCrone, P., Sabes-Figuera, R., Csipke, E., Wood, A., & Wykes, T. (2010). Nurse and patient activities and interaction on psychiatric inpatients wards: a literature review. *International Journal of Nursing Studies*, **47**, 909–917.

Sharpe, J. B. (1815). *Report, Together with the Minutes of Evidence, and an Appendix of Papers from the Committee Appointed to Consider of Provision Being Made for the Better Regulation of Madhouses in England*. London: Baldwin Craddock and Joy and R Hunter. https://wellcomecollection.org/works/aw92nswj/items?canvas=7

Shields, M. C., Stewart, M. T., & Delaney, K. R. (2018). Patient safety in inpatient psychiatry: a remaining frontier for health policy. *Health Affairs*, **37**, 1853–1861.

Smith, G., Nicholson, K., Fitch, C., & Mynors-Wallis, L. (2015). *The Commission to Review the Provision of Acute Inpatient Psychiatric Care for Adults in England, Wales and Northern Ireland*. Background Briefing Paper. London: The Commission on Acute Adult Psychiatric Care.

The Time Chamber (2020). The asylums list. https://www.thetimechamber.co.uk/beta/sites/asylums/asylum-history/the-asylums-list

Townsend, K., Rodriguez, K., & Deacon, J. (2021). *Standards for Forensic Mental Health Services: Low and Medium Secure Care—Fourth Edition*. London: Royal College of Psychiatrists, College Centre for Quality Improvement

Tracy, D. K., Holloway, F., Hanson, K., Kananai, N., Trainer, M., Dimond, I., et al. (2023). Why care about integrated care 2. Integrated care systems: an irresistible force changing mental health services. *BJPsych Advances*, **29**, 19–30.

Tracy, D. K. & Phillips, D. (2022). What is good acute psychiatric care (and how would you know)? *World Psychiatry*, **21**, 166–167.

Treiman, N. & Leff, J. (2002). Long-term outcome of long-stay psychiatric inpatients considered unsuitable to live in the community. TAPS Project 44. *British Journal of Psychiatry*, **181**, 428–432.

Tuke, S. (1815). *Description of the Retreat, An Institution Near York for Insane Persons*. York: W. Alexander.

Walker, S., Mackay, E., Barnett, P., Sheridan Rains, L., Leverton, M., Dalton-Locke, C., et al. (2019). Clinical and social factors associated with increased risk for involuntary psychiatric hospitalisation: a systematic review, meta-analysis, and narrative synthesis. *Lancet Psychiatry*, **6**, 1039–1053.

Williams, P., Csipke, E., Rose, D., Koeser, L., McCrone, P., Tulloch, A. D., et al (2014). Efficacy of a triage system to reduce length of hospital stay. *British Journal of Psychiatry*, **204**, 480–485.

Wing, J. K. & Brown, G. W. (1970). *Institutionalism and Schizophrenia*. Cambridge: Cambridge University Press.

Wood, L., Williams, C., Billings, J., & Johnson, S. (2020). A systematic review and meta-analysis of cognitive behavioural informed psychological interventions for psychiatric inpatients with psychosis. *Schizophrenia Research*, **222**, 133–144.

World Health Organization (2018). *Mental Health Atlas 2017*. Geneva: World Health Organization. https://apps.who.int/iris/handle/10665/272735

Wykes, T., Csipke, E., Rose, D., Craig, T., McCrone, P., Williams, P., et al. (2018). Patient involvement in improving the evidence base on mental health inpatient care: the PERCEIVE programme. *Programme Grants Applied Research*, **6**, 7.

19

Residential care

Geoff Shepherd and Rob Macpherson

Introduction

We all need somewhere to live where we feel safe and comfortable. Given this simple fact, it is unfortunate that for far too long, housing has been seen as at the periphery of the concerns of most mental health professionals, service providers, and researchers. While the importance of adequate housing may be recognized in principle, little research has been done to identify staffing and management practices associated with high-quality care, or to improve outcomes. Meanwhile, people with severe mental health problems continue to live in substandard accommodation and struggle to gain access to decent and affordable housing (Kirby & Keon, 2006).

This chapter explores these issues. We will describe the historical and policy background, review current issues, and bring together the available research to make practical, evidence-based suggestions for improving the quality of residential care. The context is the 'mixed economy' of care that now characterizes housing provision for people with mental health problems in the UK and in most of northern Europe, Australasia, and North America. This has grown up as we have moved away from long-term care in hospital. The 'total institution' has thus disappeared, but we now have many smaller 'institutions', with different management authorities, cultures, and values. How have we arrived at this point?

Historical and policy background

In England, the central theme in the development of residential care for people with mental health problems over the last 60 years has been the move from NHS-funded hospital care to a multiplicity of independent 'for-profit' and 'not-for-profit' community service providers. Similar developments have taken place in most other developed countries. Thus, long-stay hospital beds in England and Wales reduced from 155,000 in 1955 to fewer than 3000 half a century later (O'Brien, 2010). The policy background that drove this dramatic change was signalled in the NHS 'Hospital Plan' over 60 years ago (Ministry of Health, 1962), which announced an intention to move towards a more community-based system of care. *Care in the Community* (Department of Health and Social Security, 1981) then shifted the responsibility for managing residential care from regional health authorities towards local authorities (local government) and in 1990 the National Health Service and Community Care Act (Department of Health, 1990) enabled agencies other than the NHS and local authorities to become involved in providing these facilities. Subsequently *Partnership in Action* (Department of Health, 1998a) emphasized the importance of joint working between statutory and independent sector agencies and then the 'Supporting People' strategy (Office of the Deputy Prime Minister, 2002) set out explicitly to coordinate all housing support for vulnerable people, including those with mental health problems.

During these changes, a tension has emerged between the aims of 'community care' for most people and the needs of a relatively small group of highly disabled patients who require some kind of specialist, 'institutional' provision—albeit resembling community-based and home-like facilities as much as possible. Despite the successes of community care, patients continue to present to services with multiple and complex needs of such severity that care in non-specialist facilities does not seem feasible. Up to now, their needs have also been included in policy. For example, the *National Service Framework for Mental Health* (Department of Health, 1999) recommended a small number of intensive, high dependency places in specialist residential facilities which would provide high-quality medical and nursing care for the most disabled. These were called '24-hour nursed care' or 'hospital hostels' (Shepherd, 1995). In 2009, a new mental health policy document to replace the NSF was published (*New Horizons*; Department of Health, 2009). Its vision was for improved prevention of mental health problems, through early intervention and 'social inclusion' and the successful challenging of inequality and stigma. But, it says little about those with the greatest and most complex needs. There is therefore a danger that the needs of this group will be overlooked as policy moves towards more 'preventative' and 'public health' models (Mountain et al., 2009).

Another important policy theme which has emerged as the hospitals have been reduced in number and size, has been the most appropriate mechanisms for regulation and quality inspection in a new, multiple provider, environment. In England and Wales a range of monitoring frameworks have been established by different bodies to set standards and attempt to shape practice (e.g. Department of Health, 2003, 2007; Office of the Deputy Prime Minister, 2005; Royal College of Psychiatrists, 2010). There has also been a succession of regulatory bodies (in England three in the last 20 years) to oversee arrangements for the inspection of standards. The latest, the Care Quality Commission (CQC), was set up in 2009 to regulate all adult health and social care services. It uses a system of registration, together with a familiar combination of standards, self-assessment, and emergency inspections (much as its predecessors the Commission for Health Improvement and the Healthcare Commission). The threat to 'deregister' individual providers for conspicuously poor standards of care suggests that it may have more impact than previous regulatory bodies; whether it will be any more effective in raising *general* standards waits to be seen. Previous experience suggests not (Walshe, 2003). Improving the quality of local care is essentially a local matter and this has not changed in the last 200 years.

Another area of policy development that continues to impact mental health services, including residential care, is that associated with the principles of 'recovery' (Shepherd et al., 2008; Slade, 2009a, 2009b). These aim to make services more supportive of individuals' recovery 'journeys', recognizing the centrality of life goals as opposed to symptom management, the importance of a sense of being 'in control' rather than continually directed by others, and of personal hopes and ambitions as opposed to the often reduced expectations of professionals. These ideas now underpin public mental health policy in several countries and we will examine their specific implications for residential care later. Before doing that, let us try to clarify terms.

Defining terms

The range of residential alternatives is notoriously difficult to classify. However, Lelliott et al. (1996) produced a typology some years ago which is still useful. This is shown in **Table 19.1**.

This classificatory scheme suggests that the different forms of supported accommodation can be arranged on a dimension of staffing levels from acute inpatient wards with constant staffing and relatively high numbers of staff; through high staffed hostels, low staffed hostels; staffed care homes with sleeping night staff; and group homes without staff on the premises, but regular visiting.

The problem of this kind of classification for modern residential services is that the changes in the pattern of care over the past 60 years towards a more mixed model of providers have also been associated with a move towards more 'supported housing', where the care is delivered to the person in their home by peripatetic staff teams, rather than by fixed staffing associated with a single facility (hence, these options need to be added). This means that levels of care are much more flexible and the person can live as independently as possible most of the time. It also reflects the consistent research findings that service users generally favour more autonomy and wish to avoid shared housing options that seem too like the institutions they were set up to replace (see 'Quality of care and quality of life'). At the same time, it opens up the possibility of using a much greater range of 'ordinary housing' options in a more cost-efficient way and accords with current thinking on the importance of 'social inclusion'.

Estimating needs

One of the major practical reasons for wishing to develop agreed and consistent definitions of sheltered and supported housing is so that these can be used to inform planning for the range of different kinds of accommodation required to meet the needs of a specific, local population. For the reasons given above, this has become increasingly difficult as planning has come to depend more and more on the simple availability of general housing stock. Nevertheless, there are some interesting examples in the literature of attempts to do this and these are summarized in **Table 19.2**.

Despite these kinds of studies, there is still no generally agreed system of local needs assessment for residential care and no recognized instrument to assess housing need at an individual level (Strathdee & Jenkins, 1996). In practice, the development of local provisions appears to be largely determined by history and factors such as demography, transport, unemployment, ethnic composition, funding priorities, attitudes of primary care, and effectiveness of specialist mental health services. Some of these can be partially taken into account by sophisticated quantitative modelling (e.g. Glover, 1996), but at the heart of such algorithms remain guesses, albeit sensible and well-informed guesses, about what numbers of different kinds of provisions a given pattern of local morbidity implies.

Table 19.1 The spectrum of residential care

Facility type	Usual number of places	Night cover	Day cover	Ratio of staff:residents	% of staff with care qualification
Forensic unit	>6	Waking	Constant	1.3	62
Acute ward	>6	Waking	Constant	1.3	63
Long-stay ward	>6	Waking	Constant	0.9	49
High-staffed hostel	>6	Waking	Constant	0.7	15
Mid-staffed hostel	>6	Sleep-in	Constant	0.4	14
Low-staffed hostel	>6	On call/none	Regular	0.2	15
Group home	<6	On call/none	Visited	0.2	33
Staffed care home	>6	Sleep-in	Constant	1.0	7
Dedicated supported housing schemes	Individual flats/small houses up to 4 places	No	Available in complex	0.5 (average)	Unknown
Outreach support in individual tenancy	Usually individual flats	Rarely	Intermittent	0.5 up to 3	Unknown

Modified from Lelliott et al. (1996).

Table 19.2 Estimates of local housing needs through survey methods

Authors	Country	Method	Main findings
Shepherd et al. (1997)	UK	Census of acute bed usage in a nationally representative sample	Highlighted the need for specialist rehabilitation placements or 24-hour, 'nursed care' units
Fitz and Evenson (1999)	US	Large-scale, systematic assessment of local needs	Community living skills, social skills, and problem behaviour were the primary characteristics affecting adjustment to residential settings
Durbin et al. (2001)	Canada	Survey of inpatients	Five levels of care developed, only 10% of current inpatients needed to remain in hospital, 60% could live independently in the community with appropriate support
Bartlett et al. (2001)	UK	Analysis of 730 acute admissions	Many patients might have benefited from alternative, community-based services. A quarter could have been supported effectively in the community in specialist accommodation if available
Freeman et al. (2004)	Australia	Survey of all state and non-governmental high support housing services	State and non-government services useful, but significant numbers of unmet social and psychological needs in residents
Commander and Rooprai, (2008)	UK	Survey of acute in-patients	Almost 20% of acute beds occupied by patients for more than 6 months. 'By far the majority' required 24-hour nursed care, need to improve access to this provision
Cowman and Whitty (2016)	Ireland	Accommodation needs assessed among acute psychiatric inpatients	On average 38% of acute inpatients had accommodation related needs

The problem of accurately estimating demand is further complicated by the fact that one kind of housing or accommodation can often 'substitute' for another. Thus, high support hostels may substitute for inpatient beds; flexible community teams may substitute for sheltered housing (or hospital beds); family care with intensive professional support may substitute for professional support or specialist housing; and so on. Housing needs assessments therefore cannot be separated from the functioning and dynamics of the total service 'system' and the confidence limits surrounding any estimates of need for different kinds of accommodation remain large (Johnson et al., 1996).

For all these reasons, it is probably more sensible to begin a local planning process by conducting a simple inventory of local housing availability to see who is currently accommodated (i.e. survey of levels of disability and case mix in existing provision). If one then adds in information on who is currently excluded (e.g. estimates of the number of homeless mentally ill people) and these figures are combined with local information about the availability of general housing stock, then this should give a starting point in terms of development priorities. On the basis of national information, shortages in high dependency housing and flexible, intensive community support are likely to be the areas of greatest deficiencies (Audit Commission, 1998; Department of Health, 1998b).

The impact of service developments

In England, the *National Service Framework for Mental Health* (Department of Health, 1999) prompted the development of a range of new specialist community-based teams, focusing on patients with specific needs (crisis and home treatment, assertive outreach, and early intervention). This new pattern of services led, in turn, to a significant reappraisal of traditional concepts of the limits of 'community care'. Thus, it is now clear that many service users who would previously have been in hospital for long periods, or in the 'revolving door' of repeated admissions, can now be successfully supported in the community with well-functioning, specialist teams. However, the success of these specialist teams has resulted in a further reduction in acute beds and this has put pressure on the community teams in terms of their ability to support people with severe and complex problems living in facilities that are run by largely non-statutory providers.

Whether this constitutes a process of 're-institutionalization' depends on what you count as an 'institution'. In England, the majority of the residential alternatives that have been developed in the community show few of the common features of institutional care (large size, impersonal routines, lack of contact with the community). Indeed, it is their lack of 'institutionalization' that seems to account for the higher rates of satisfaction reported by patients resettled from the large hospitals (Leff et al., 1994; Thornicroft et al., 2005). Of course, this is not necessarily the same in countries where larger, more 'institutional' units are common.

In all cases, tensions have emerged around the problems of 'partnership working' between mental health services and housing providers in the new system. For example, there is often a perception on the part of clinical teams that housing providers can choose who they will accept and, not surprisingly, tend to choose the apparently 'easier' clients. Conversely, many independent sector providers believe that statutory services simply want to 'dump' difficult problems on to them and then fail to give adequate support and follow-up. Both views reflect stereotypes, but both also contain a degree of truth. These attitudes underline the need for statutory and non-statutory agencies to work closely together (e.g. through joint training). But, given its importance as an everyday, practical problem, the problems of improving joint working have received surprisingly little attention as a research topic.

In England the process of 'deinstitutionalization' is now effectively complete and there are only a few remaining long-stay in-patient units, providing mainly medium stay (i.e. 1–2 years), 24-hour nursed care for 'new' long-stay patients (Killaspy et al., 2005). A study of changes in services across nine European countries by Priebe et al. (2008) showed a similar picture.

In addition to the increase in placements in sheltered and supported housing, what other changes in services have occurred?

There has certainly been a growth in forensic beds and prison places which cannot be explained by changes in prevalence or patterns of morbidity among patients with severe mental illness (Priebe et al., 2008). For example, between 1994 and 2003 the number of NHS secure beds rose from 1080 to 2560 and detained admissions increased from 600 to 1400/year (of which one in five were treated in private or independent sector facilities). Similarly, in England and Wales the number of prison places increased by 32,500 (66%) from 1995 to 2009 (Ministry of Justice, 2009). However, when one considers the case mix of residents in these different facilities it is clear that while there is some overlap between patients in secure and semi-secure beds and those who might have been in 'mainstream' hospitals, the diagnostic profile of those with mental illness in the prison system is quite different—less than 10% with psychosis, high rates of personality disorder, low levels of literacy and frequent drug and alcohol abuse (Singleton et al., 1998; Brunette et al, 2004). Thus, while it is possible that there may have been some 're-institutionalization' of people with mental health problems from 'open' hospitals to secure and semi-secure provisions, it is unlikely that there has been much 're-institutionalization' back to prison.

Perhaps more importantly, there have been changes in public perceptions regarding the risks posed by people with mental illness in the community. These were exacerbated, in the early days of the run-down of the mental hospitals in England, by cases like that of Christopher Clunis, a man with schizophrenia who was well known to local services, but who had fallen out of follow-up and eventually murdered a member of the public in an Underground station in London (Coid, 1994). Not surprisingly, these kinds of events attracted substantial media attention and, despite the lack of evidence of any *actual* increase in homicides committed by people with mental illness (Shaw et al., 1999), they contributed to a shift in attitudes—public and professional—towards the need for greater use of secure provisions.

Changes in the pattern of residential provisions have also been driven directly by an increasing emphasis on a 'market philosophy', where private providers are encouraged to try to increase their 'market share' in competition with traditional state provisions. This has also happened across Europe (Priebe et al., 2005) and, as indicated, has been 'successful' in that new providers have been encouraged into the 'market'. However, it has led to concerns regarding the costs and quality of care provided. Secure services are often remote from the geographical area where the patient originated and this makes it difficult to maintain contact with local community services. It can also lead to difficulties in monitoring progress and unnecessarily protracted lengths of stay. The separation of vulnerable patients from their families and friends then makes successful resettlement more difficult (Ryan et al., 2006). Finally, physical and organizational isolation has repeatedly been shown to be a common factor in hospital abuse scandals (Martin, 1984) and these same factors can operate within residential units if they become similarly isolated. It is therefore welcome that the regulator in England (CQC) includes private and independent sector provisions within its remit.

Staffing and staff training

As indicated above, one of the biggest challenges resulting from the growth of non-statutory providers is that many more staff are now involved who do not have formal mental health training or qualifications (Phelan & Strathdee, 1994). In some ways this is an advantage since they are less likely to have traditional, 'institutional' attitudes but, as we noted earlier, staff untrained to deal with difficult clinical problems are more likely to be reluctant to accept such individuals into their care. In terms of the development and evaluation of training programmes for residential care staff, the evidence is limited and mixed. It is summarized in Table 19.3.

Part of the reason for the failure to develop and evaluate training programmes for residential care staff is that it has not been clear exactly what skills they require. The application of 'expressed emotion' (EE) models from the research with family carers (Ball et al., 1992) is one model that seems intuitively plausible. Regarding recruitment and selection of staff, while it is recognized that staff characteristics are important, almost no attention has been given to developing more reliable and valid selection criteria. Again, the 'low

Table 19.3 Training and quality of care

Authors	Country	Method	Main findings
Sorensen-Snyder et al. (1994)	Sweden	Survey of staff in 15 residential care homes	Association between staff critical comments and resident subjective quality of life. Staff high EE associated with illness severity, suggesting a complex interaction between attitudes and levels of morbidity
Peterson and Barland (1995)	US	State hospital staff trained workers in community care facilities caring for people with severe mental illness	After a 17-week programme, community staff reported high satisfaction and the overall quality of the service was reported to improve, with reduced staff turnover
Shepherd et al. (1996)	UK	Survey of residential care	Patients with the highest levels of disability tended to receive the least interaction and more negative interactions when they did occur
Senn et al. (1997)	UK	Survey as part of the TAPS study	Almost a quarter of reprovision schemes offered no training at all, not even in the management of violence or risk
Raskin et al. (1998)	US	Psychoeducational programme for staff in community residences	Staff liked the networking and mental health component. Service users also became more active and had fewer admissions
Gabrielian et al. (2024)	US	Assessment of impact of implementing a training programme for service providers for homeless people	The pilot programme was feasible and acceptable

TAPS, Team for the Assessment of Psychiatric Services.

EE' model may have applicability as a framework for staff selection (e.g. select staff who are low on blame and criticism) but has not been empirically tested. The involvement of service users (consumers) as part of the selection process also appears to be widely used but, to our knowledge, has not been formally evaluated.

The qualities of effective leaders in residential care teams and how best to develop and support them have also received little specific attention. In other areas of teamwork, successful leaders seem to able to combine good 'task' skills (analysing problems, setting clear goals, agreeing responsibilities) with good 'socioemotional' skills (involving colleagues, recognizing their strengths, inviting collaborative decision-making), see Alimo-Metcalfe and Alban-Metcalf (2006). There is no reason why this same mix of positive qualities should not apply to leaders in residential staff teams but, again, this has not been investigated within an evaluative framework.

'Quality of care' and 'quality of life'

Before discussing more of the research literature, we should clarify what we mean by the terms '*quality of care*' and '*quality of life*'. 'Quality of care' implies evaluation from an external perspective (e.g. as reflected in positive changes in functioning) whereas 'quality of life' refers to subjective satisfaction by residents with the care delivered and the physical environment.

In terms of quality of care, the most important factor appears to be the effectiveness of individually centred, targeted programmes of care. The strongest evidence for this comes from studies of 'hospital hostels' where there is 24-hour professional care (Fakhoury et al., 2005). Service users going through these units tend to show positive improvements in functioning—including some reductions in violence—compared with controls and this seems to be associated with the delivery of highly individualized, 'user-centred' programmes (Shepherd et al., 1996; Trieman & Leff, 1996). Such programmes combine structure and support, in the context of frequent, high quality ('low EE') staff-resident interactions.

The quality of the physical environment may also affect quality of care. For example, Baker and Douglas (1990) studied the effect of the quality of the housing environment on community adjustment over a 9-month period in a large sample (n = 729) of clients in community support programmes in upstate New York. Clients who were resident in housing rated 'good' or 'fair' showed significant improvements in functioning and no increases in maladaptive behaviour compared with those in housing rated as 'poor'. In a large-scale systematic review of the quality of institutional care for people with longer term mental health problems, Taylor et al. (2009) found eight domains of institutional care that were key to recovery: living conditions, interventions for schizophrenia, physical health, restraint and seclusion, staff training and support, therapeutic relationships, autonomy, and service user involvement. Evidence was strongest for specific interventions for schizophrenia, but this may have been due to the mixed quality of the available research evidence.

Among the most important factors in determining *quality of life* as perceived by the service user are choice (including choice over which setting in which to live) and the absence of unnecessary rules and restrictions (Owen et al., 1996). In relation to choice, as indicated earlier, it is a consistent finding that service users tend to express a preference for more independent living, in ordinary housing, with flexible, domiciliary support, rather than living with staff (Hogberg et al., 2006; Owen et al., 1996; Tanzman, 1993). In addition, if these choices are followed then there is good evidence that satisfaction will increase (Keck, 1990; Nelson et al., 2007a; Srebnick et al., 1995).

However, the literature also contains several examples where staff or family perceptions conflict with service users' preferences. Minsky et al. (1995) found that the choice of 80 long-term inpatients was overwhelmingly to live alone, with family, or chosen room mate, with only 4% preferring options with live-in staff. By contrast, 61% of staff felt this to be the best option. Massey and Wu (1993) surveyed service users in a Florida mental health centre and found similarly that service users prioritized personal choice, location, and (interestingly) proximity to mental health services more often than staff. A Canadian study by Piat et al. (2008) found that mental health case managers tended to prefer supported accommodation with structure (i.e. staffing) 'built-in' to the accommodation, whereas service users preferred their own apartments, and the importance of case managers was also reported by Nelson et al. (2007b). Friedrichs et al. (1999) found that for service users living independently, they and their families reported isolation to be a significant problem and family members tended to prefer housing which provided support and structure. The research therefore suggests that staff—and family members—tend to opt for more 'safe' housing options, with staff on site; while service users value independence and privacy.

Regarding the importance of minimizing '*unnecessary rules and restrictions*', in the Team for the Assessment of Psychiatric Services (TAPS) study (see 'Outcomes') it is striking how much change there was in measures of 'restrictiveness' when patients moved from hospital to community settings (Leff, 1997). These changes were often small (e.g. being able to access the kitchen at 9.00 pm and make a cup of tea; having the choice over what to eat and who to eat with) but these small choices made a big difference to the quality of peoples' lives (Borge et al., 1999). The increased satisfaction ('quality of life') consistently associated with the move from hospital to community seems to be largely a direct reflection of the value of these small increments in perceived autonomy (Shepherd et al., 1996).

Stigma

Another important consequence of moving care from hospital to community is that it becomes necessary to deal directly with public attitudes, specifically stigma. In England, public attitudes towards people with mental health problems living in the community have generally softened in recent years. For example, in 2010, 66% agreed with the statement, 'Residents have nothing to fear from people coming into their neighbourhoods to obtain mental health services', this compares with 62% in 2009 (TNS UK, 2010). However, while the public may have become generally less fearful, they are still likely to have specific fears about actual developments in their neighbourhood. Hence, the study by Wolff et al. (1996) is still important. They evaluated the effectiveness of a community education programme aimed at preparing a local neighbourhood for a new supported housing scheme. They targeted approximately 150 people, providing information sheets, a video, a public meeting with a 'question-and-answer' session, a barbecue, and other social events. Common stereotypes of dangerousness were addressed and the public were reassured that residents would not be simply 'dumped' and left to fend for themselves. The study found a small increase in knowledge concerning mental illness, but a significant reduction in fearful and rejecting attitudes. This confirms several different anti-stigma programmes and shows that they *can* make a difference providing they are clearly targeted and involve direct contact, in controlled conditions, between those holding the prejudice and those who are the object of it (Thornicroft et al., 2007). More recently public attitudes to people with mental health problems have improved in England at the time when the nationwide Time to Change anti-stigma programme was active (Thornicroft et al., 2022).

Recovery

As indicated earlier, there continues to be considerable interest in the concept of 'recovery' in residential care (e.g. Dinniss et al., 2007). However, there is also still confusion concerning the meaning of 'recovery' and what evidence is available to support the approach (Shepherd et al., 2008; Warner, 2009). In residential care, recovery is mainly about the style and quality of care, in particular the extent to which attempts are made to empower the person to take their own decisions and pursue their own priorities, rather than those of professionals. Hence, it relates closely to the key dimensions of 'choice' and 'control' mentioned above. A method of improving the quality of recovery-oriented services has been proposed by Shepherd et al. (2010).

In England, the move towards a 'recovery-orientation' has been encouraged by attempts to increase the '*personalization*' of care (Department of Health, 2008). This has included attempts to provide patients with individual 'budgets', where they are given direct funding and helped to make their own choices about residential (and day care) options. This approach is still controversial and uptake has been slow (Social Care Institute for Excellence, 2009). The central problem is providing appropriate help and support to individuals who find it difficult to express their views and difficult to manage their own care. There are also obvious dangers of exploitation and abuse. Nevertheless, this approach is becoming more common in relation to residential options for people over 65 and, with increasing pressures on budgets, it is likely to become more widely used for adults of all ages in the future.

Outcomes

In relation to outcomes, due to ethical, logistical, and conceptual problems, the evaluation of different forms of residential care is not an area where there are many randomized controlled trials. However, there are many other ways of assessing outcomes and we will consider attempts to assess housing initiatives at the whole service level, individual housing schemes, and also narrative approaches, which give rich, qualitative information from an individual perspective.

The research on 'deinstitutionalization' has consistently demonstrated that the functioning of long-stay patients resettled in the community is generally improved and they are more satisfied compared with those remaining in hospital. The TAPS study examined the progress of more than 700 patients leaving Friern and Claybury hospitals in north London over a period of more than 5 years (Leff, 1997). Following resettlement, service users showed reduced negative symptoms, increased social networks and functioning, and reported higher levels of satisfaction with their living situation compared with the matched controls. There were no differences regarding the severity of positive symptoms or the rates of suicide or crime. Forty per cent of the 72 patients who were initially 'difficult to place' went on to be resettled from hospital over the next 5 years, suggesting that even the most disabled people could manage in less institutional settings, providing appropriate support is available. There were some concerns regarding fragmentation and the possible inadequacy of community services, but overall the results are generally viewed as demonstrating that properly funded, planned resettlement of long-stay patients from asylums results in significant social benefits and increased quality of life without any increased risk of harmful outcomes. If all costs were taken into account, care was slightly less expensive for the community group, but increased with increasing levels of disability (Beecham et al., 1997).

Uncontrolled, prospective follow-up studies of community resettlement in several different countries show a very similar picture. Studies in Australia (Andrews et al., 1990), California (Segal & Kotler, 1993), Northern Ireland (Donnelly et al., 1996), Norway (Borge et al., 1999), and Italy (Barbato et al., 2004) have all generally found improved satisfaction for people moving to the community, stable levels of symptomatology (no increase or decrease), and relatively few subsequent long-term readmissions.

Turning now to specific types of residential care, the one which has probably been most studied is '24-hour nursed care' ('hospital hostels'). The outcome evidence for these kinds of units was reviewed by Macpherson and Jerrom (1999). The data from one randomized controlled trial and a number of matched controlled trials and uncontrolled follow-up studies suggest that they are effective in improving the functioning of up to 40% of residents sufficiently for them to be resettled into the community after an average of 2–3 years. Residents generally made more progress than controls regarding their social functioning; they showed increased contact with the community; and higher levels of satisfaction. Overall, costs were generally less than acute beds.

The outcome evidence for other forms of accommodation is very limited. In their review, Fakhoury et al. (2002) found 28 largely descriptive studies from the US, Canada, and Europe. They noted that the research was of variable quality and problems of definition, design, and methodology made it difficult to draw firm conclusions regarding the clinical and cost-effectiveness of differing forms of supported accommodation. Similarly, Chilvers et al. (2002) attempted a Cochrane review of studies of supported flats within designated housing schemes (staffed 'core and cluster' facilities) compared with dispersed, 'ordinary housing', outreach support. They found no randomized controlled studies and highlighted the need for more—and better—research. Kyle and Dunn (2008) systematically reviewed 29 studies, using a method to allocate levels of evidence according to the robustness of the research method. They found good evidence that housing interventions have a positive impact on hospital use in the homeless, but weak evidence for similar effects with people with severe mental illness who were not homeless. There was generally weak, or very weak, evidence of a beneficial effect of supported housing on psychiatric symptoms and, at best, medium evidence of an association between housing and quality of life. These reviews illustrate the wide variety of study methods used and the complex, and at times conflicting, results of studies in this area. A selection of studies that are informative are summarized in **Table 19.4**.

Table 19.4 Quality outcome studies

Authors	Country	Method	Main findings
Hodgkins et al. (1990)	Canada	Comparison of 61 inpatients in Montreal placed into designated supported apartments with 51 individuals on the waiting list	No differences in service use after 2 years, but control group showed significantly more thought disorder from 12 months attributed to the stress of living closely with other mentally ill individuals in a poorly supervised setting
Nelson et al. (1998)	Canada	Study of the quality of care provided in a variety of care settings	Number of living companions, housing concerns, and having a private room predicted 'community adaptation' (measured by scales rating emotional well-being and personal empowerment)
Seidman et al. (2003)	US	Randomized controlled trial, followed up homeless people with severe mental illness for 18 months after random allocation to independent apartments or to group homes	Neuropsychological functioning improved significantly for both groups, but executive functioning decreased significantly for the group living in independent apartments. Authors suggest that living alone may result in a lack of social interaction leading to deleterious effects on cognitive functioning
Tsemberis et al. (2004)	US	Random allocation of 208 participants with severe mental illness and substance misuse to a housing programme which offered immediate housing without expectation of psychiatric treatment compliance or abstinence from substance use, compared with transitional housing which required compliance and sobriety	No differences in psychiatric symptoms or substance abuse. Results challenge the common practice of linking access to housing with a requirement to accept treatment and sobriety
O'Connell et al. (2023)	US	Randomised controlled trial-5 year follow up data	Access to housing contributed 4% to the improvement in quality of life in supported housing settings

Turning now to the qualitative studies, Chesters et al. (2005) reported on the narratives of 15 residents of supported housing programme in Australia. These highlighted the importance of supported housing as an integral part of recovery-focused services. The participants reported that people with mental health problems found it difficult to get effective care and treatment (other than education) in the community. The authors concluded that people need the benefits of decent public housing *and* ongoing support. They also warned that not all communities are welcoming and that friendships can be even less easy to secure than housing and support. In a study using interviews with supported housing residents in Ontario, Canada, Walker and Seasons (2002) found that four themes emerged: loneliness, poor quality of housing, a desire for greater understanding, and social inclusion. Forchuk et al. (2006), again working in Canada, used a focus group methodology to study the housing experiences of people with severe mental illness living in the community. They likened the devastating impact of loss through mental illness to the effects of a tornado, with periods of losing ground, struggling to survive, and then eventually gaining stability. From a professional perspective, Hogberg et al. (2006) carried out a qualitative analysis of interviews with nine nurses in Sweden. They noted a central theme of respect for the service user's self-determination, but also saw a key role for the professional in providing a link between the service user and their local neighbourhood.

These qualitative studies give insights into the lives of people living with serious mental illness in the community. However, they are most useful when it is possible to relate people's subjective experience to quantitative data regarding 'quality of care'—staffing levels, quality of interaction, leadership, management regimes, etc. Thus, it is not just the case that 'more research' would be useful, but more 'mixed method' research is most likely to help us improve the quality of resident's experience.

Over the last decade there has been a renewed research interest in the provision of residential care in the mental health sector. A particular field of growth has the 'Home Chez Soi' or 'Housing First' model from Canada (Aubry et al., 2015) who describe this as a 'paradigm shift in the delivery of community mental health services'. In this model, people with severe mental illness who are homeless are supported through assertive community treatment or intensive case management to move into regular housing. This report of a demonstration project reported that Housing First is a promising approach, yielding superior outcomes in helping people to rapidly exit homelessness and establish stable housing. People receiving Housing First achieved superior housing outcomes and showed more rapid improvements in community functioning and quality of life than those receiving treatment as usual. Housing First has also been studied in relation to the impact on criminal justice outcomes. Leclair et al. (2019) systematically reviewed this literature and found five studies were included with a total of 7128 participants. The results suggested that on average Housing First has little impact on criminal justice involvement.

Richter and Hoffmann (2017a) have contributed an overview of independent housing and support for people with severe mental illness. They identified 24 papers from studies with homeless people and eight from studies with non-homeless people. Overall, results from independent housing and support settings are not inferior to results from institutionalized settings. They went on to identify the priorities of residents (Richter & Hoffmann, 2017b). This second review and meta-analysis included eight studies with 3134 consumers, of whom 84% expressed a preference for independent living over living institutionalized settings.

A more recent overview has been published by Parker et al. (2019) who differentiated two types of residential care: community-based residential care, which emerged in the context of deinstitutionalization, and the more recent transitional residential rehabilitation approach. The authors concluded that while there is qualitative evidence to suggest consumers value the support provided by community rehabilitation units, there is an absence of methodologically sound quantitative research about the consumer outcomes achieved by these services.

Summary

1. In terms of *planning and estimating needs*, any definitions of residential alternatives must be multidimensional and should include a consideration of the whole system of supported accommodation, including all the available private, charitable, and statutory services. They should also reflect the established value and attraction to service users of flexible, 'supported housing' models, rather than traditional group homes and hostels with fixed staffing. Local planning should be built on locally collected information about *who* the housing network is serving (and who it is not). It should not rely on 'norms'. Any planning process must not neglect the needs of those requiring the highest levels of support and a range of models of specialist residential provision, including '24-hour nursed care' should be available in each locality.

2. In terms of *housing developments*, new projects are increasingly likely to be managed by independent sector providers. To improve 'partnership working' between statutory and non-statutory agencies there needs to be a mutual respect and understanding regarding their respective roles and responsibilities. Support for providers through education and joint working with community mental health teams is necessary and should be seen as an integral part of the work of both agencies.

3. In terms of *user preferences*, new housing developments should try to take into account, as far as possible, the expressed preferences of service users regarding their living arrangements, even if these are different from professionals and family carers. Apart from expressed preferences, there is little evidence to assist in the judgement as to which service users will fare well in which different kinds of accommodation. Resident satisfaction should also be regularly assessed as it may show significant changes over time. Loneliness and isolation may be problems for some people, but so can stress caused by close proximity to others who show disturbed and distressing behaviour. Staff in housing services should consider carefully whether there is any justification for excluding service users with a history of substance abuse or 'challenging behaviour'. Every attempt should be made to manage these kinds of problems as part of the ongoing support provided.

4. In terms of *staffing and interventions*, more attention needs to be given to the development and evaluation of joint training initiatives, aimed at improving the knowledge and skills of residential care workers. Attention should also be given to staff selection processes in order to identify those who will be most effective in their interactions with residents. Particularly careful consideration should be given to the desirable attributes of project leaders and to mechanisms for supporting and helping them develop their leadership skills. Housing regimes which maximize choice and independence are likely to be most highly valued by residents.

5. The adoption of a 'recovery orientation' in mental health services will challenge those working in residential care to provide good-quality accommodation of the type service users want and maintain a focus on the individual and the importance of choice and control. This may conflict with aspects of a 'business' model where there is an emphasis on 'throughput' and cost efficiency.

6. In terms of *outcomes*, in general those resettled from long-stay hospitals show few advantages in terms of clinical symptoms but function better socially, are happier, and cost less than their counterparts remaining in hospital. The evidence in favour of transitional 24-hour nursed care for the 'new' long stay is generally positive; however, it may be unattractive to some service users. Other 'high-support' options may therefore need to be developed. Regarding the differential effectiveness of other types of provision, the evidence is limited and, once again, user preferences should probably predominate as these are most reliably associated with good outcomes.

7. There is a need for better quality, carefully designed, *quantitative research* which investigates the relationship between 'quality of care' variables and objective improvements in clinical and/or social functioning. There is also a need for better quality, carefully designed, *qualitative research* which explores the experience of service users and staff in residential care settings and investigates the relationship between 'quality of care' variables and 'quality of life' (satisfaction). Both methods should be combined for maximum effect.

8. There is clearly emerging evidence that the Housing First/Chez Soi model may confer benefits for community residential care in high-income settings, especially for people who have been homeless.

Conclusion

Housing should be at the centre of community mental health. In order to achieve meaningful improvements in housing provision, we need to adopt a whole-systems, multiagency, collaborative approach. Services have evolved rapidly since the closure of the psychiatric institutions and further changes in response to various ideological and policy developments are inevitable. The challenges for professionals working with people who need supported accommodation are as much to do with promoting social inclusion and challenging stigma and discrimination, as they are about providing the right clinical support and treatment. Residential care is certainly an area where 'more research is needed', but we would also be able to make considerable progress *now* if we were simply to implement what we already know.

REFERENCES

Alimo-Metcalf, B. & Alban-Metcalf, J. (2006). More good leaders for the public sector. *International Journal of Public Sector Management*, 19, 293–315.

Andrews, G., Teesson, M., Stewart, G., & Hoult, J. (1990). Follow-up of community placement of the chronic mentally ill in New South Wales. *Hospital and Community Psychiatry*, 41, 184–188.

Aubry, T., Nelson, G., & Tsemberis, S. (2015). Housing First for people with severe mental illness who are homeless: a review of the research and findings from the At Home-Chez Soi demonstration project. *Canadian Journal of Psychiatry*, 60, 467–474.

Audit Commission (1998). *Home Alone*. London: Audit Commission.

Baker, F. & Douglas, C. (1990). Housing environments and community adjustments of severely mentally ill patients. *Community Mental Health Journal*, 26, 497–505.

Ball, R. A., Moore, E., & Kuipers, L. (1992). Expressed emotion in community care staff. A comparison of patient outcomes in a nine month follow-up of two hostels. *Social Psychiatry and Psychiatric Epidemiology*, 27, 35–39.

Barbato, A., D'Avanzo, B., Rocca, G., Amatulli, A., & Lampugnani, D. (2004). A study of long-stay patients resettled in the community after closure of a psychiatric hospital in Italy. *Psychiatric Services*, 55, 67–70.

Bartlett, C., Holloway, J., Evans, M., Owens, J., & Harrison, G. (2001). Alternatives to psychiatric in-patient care: a case-by-case survey of clinician judgements. *Journal of Mental Health*, 10, 535–546.

Beecham, J., Hallam, A., Knapp, M., Baines, B., Fenyo, A., & Asbury, M. (1997). Costing care in hospital and in the community. In: Leff, J. (Ed.), *Care in the Community: Illusion or Reality?* (pp. 93–108). Chichester: John Wiley & Sons.

Borge, L., Martinsen, E. W., Ruud, T., Watne, O., & Friis, S. (1999). Quality of life, loneliness and social contact among long-term psychiatric patients. *Psychiatric Services*, 50, 81–84.

Brunette, M. F., Mueser, K. T., & Drake, R. E. (2004). A review of research on residential programs for people with severe mental illness and co-occurring substance use disorders. *Drug and Alcohol Review*, 23, 471–481.

Chesters, J., Fletcher, M., & Jones, R. (2005). Mental illness, recovery and place. *Australian e-Journal for the Advancement of Mental Health*, 4, 89–97.

Chilvers, R., MacDonald, G. M., & Hayes, A. A. (2002). Supported housing for people with severe mental disorders. *Cochrane Database of Systematic Reviews*, 4, CD000453.

Coid, J. (1994). The Christopher Clunis enquiry. *Psychiatric Bulletin*, 18, 449–452.

Commander, M. & Rooprai, D (2008). Survey of long-stay patients on acute psychiatric wards. *The Psychiatrist*, 32, 380–383.

Cowman, J. & Whitty, P. (2016). Prevalence of housing needs among inpatients: a 1 year audit of housing needs in the acute mental health unit in Tallaght Hospital. *Irish Journal of Psychological Medicine*, 33(3), 159–164. doi:10.1017/ipm.2015.74 [published Online First: 2016/09/01].

Department of Health (1990). *NHS and Community Care Act*. London: HMSO.

Department of Health (1996). *The Spectrum of Care: Local Services for People with Mental Health Problems*. London: HMSO.

Department of Health (1998a). *Partnership in Action: New Opportunities for Joint Working between Health and Social Services: A Discussion Document*. London: HMSO.

Department of Health (1998b). *Modernising Mental Health Services: Safe, Sound and Supportive*. London: HMSO.

Department of Health (1999). *National Service Framework for Mental Health: Modern Standards and Service Models*. London: Department of Health.

Department of Health (2003). *Care Homes for Adults (18–65) and Supplementary Standards for Care Homes Accommodating Young People Aged 16 and 17: National Minimum Standards*. London: TSO.

Department of Health (2007). *Essence of Care: Benchmarks for the Care Environment*. London: Department of Health.

Department of Health (2008). *An Introduction to Personalisation*. London: Department of Health.

Department of Health (2009). *New Horizons: A Shared Vision for Mental Health*. London: Mental Health Division, Department of Health.

Department of Health and Social Security (1981). *Care in the Community: A Consultative Document on Moving Resources for Care in England*. London: HMSO.

Dinniss, S., Roberts, G., Hubbard, C., Hounsell, J., & Webb, R. (2007). User-led assessment of a recovery service using DREEM. *Psychiatric Bulletin*, 31, 124–127.

Donnelly, M., McGilloway, S., Mays, N., Knapp, M., Kavanagh, S., Beecham, J., & Fenyo, A. (1996). Leaving hospital: one and two-year outcomes of long-stay psychiatric patients discharged to the community. *Journal of Mental Health*, 5, 245–255.

Durbin, J., Cochrane, J., Goering, P., & Macfarlane, D. (2001). Needs-based planning: evaluation of a level of care planning model. *Journal of Behavioural Health Services and Research*, 28, 67–80.

Fakhoury, W. K. H., Murray, A., Shepherd, G., & Priebe, S. (2002). Research in supported housing. *Social Psychiatry and Psychiatric Epidemiology*, 37, 301–315.

Fakhoury, W. K. H., Priebe, S., & Quraishi, M. (2005). Goals of new long stay patients in supported housing a UK study. *International Journal of Social Psychiatry*, 51, 45–54.

Fitz, D. & Evenson, R. C. (1999). Recommending client residence: a comparison of the St Louis Inventory of Community Living Skills and global assessment. *Psychiatric Rehabilitation Journal*, 23, 107–112.

Forchuk, C., Ward-Griffin, C., Csiernik, R., & Turner, C. (2006). Surviving the tornado of mental illness: psychiatric survivors' experiences of getting, losing and keeping housing. *Psychiatric Services*, 57, 558–562.

Freeman, A., Malone, J., & Hunt, G. E. (2004). A statewide survey of high support services for people with chronic mental illness: assessment of needs for care, level of functioning and satisfaction. *Australian and New Zealand Journal of Psychiatry*, 38, 811–819.

Friedrich, R., Hollingsworth, B., Hradeck, E., & Culp, K. R. (1999). Family and client perspectives on alternative residential settings for persons with severe mental illness. *Psychiatric Services*, 50, 509–514.

Gabrielian, S., Hamilton, A. B., Gelberg, L., et al. (2024). Testing an implementation package in a housing skills training pilot for homeless-experienced persons with serious mental illness. *Implementation Research and Practice*, 5, 26334895241236679. doi:10.1177/26334895241236679 [published Online First: 2024/03/07].

Glover, G. (1996). The Mental Illness Needs Index (MINI). In: Thornicroft, G. & Strathdee, G. (Eds.), *Commissioning Mental Health Services* (pp. 53–58). London: HMSO.

Hodgkins, S., Cyr, M., & Gaston, L. (1990). Impact of supervised apartments on the functioning of mentally disordered adults. *Community Mental Health Journal*, 26, 507–515.

Hogberg, T., Magnusson, H. T., & Lutzen, K. (2006). Living by themselves? Psychiatric nurses' views on supported housing for persons with severe and persistent mental illness. *Journal of Psychiatric and Mental Health Nursing*, 13, 735–741.

Johnson, S., Thornicroft, G., & Strathdee, G. (1996). Assessing population needs. In: Thornicroft, G. & Strathdee, G. (Eds.), *Commissioning Mental Health Services* (pp. 37–52). London: HMSO.

Keck, J. (1990). Responding to consumer housing preferences: the Toledo experience. *Psychosocial Rehabilitation Journal*, 13, 51–58.

Killaspy, H., Harden C., Holloway, F., & King, M. (2005). What do mental health rehabilitation services do and what are they for? A national survey in England. *Journal of Mental Health*, 14, 157–165.

Kirby, M. & Keon, W. J. (2006). Voices of people living with mental illness. In: *Out of the Shadows at Last: Transforming Mental Health, Mental Illness and Addiction Services in Canada* (pp. 1–20). Ottawa: Standing Senate Committee on Social Affairs, Science and Technology.

Kyle, T. & Dunn, J. R. (2008). Effects of housing circumstances on health, quality of life and healthcare use for people with severe mental illness: a review. *Health and Social Care in the Community*, 16, 1–15.

Leclair, M. C., Deveaux, F., Roy, L., Goulet, M. H., Latimer, E. A., & Crocker, A. G. (2019). The impact of housing first on criminal justice outcomes among homeless people with mental illness: a systematic review. *Canadian Journal of Psychiatry*, **64**, 525–530.

Leff, J., Thornicroft, G., Coxhead, N., & Crawford, C. (1994). A five year follow up of long stay patients discharged to the community. *British Journal of Psychiatry*, **165**(Suppl. 25), 13–17.

Leff, J. (1997). *Care in the Community: Illusion or Reality?* London: Wiley.

Lelliott, P., Audini, B., Knapp, M., & Chisholm, D. (1996). The mental health residential care study: classification of facilities and descriptions of residents. *British Journal of Psychiatry*, **169**, 39–47.

Macpherson, R. & Jerrom, W. (1999). Review of twenty-four hour nursed care. *Advances in Psychiatric Treatment*, **5**, 146–153.

Martin, J. P. (1984). *Hospitals in Trouble*. Oxford: Basil Blackwell.

Massey, O. T. & Wu, L. (1993). Important characteristics of independent housing for people with severe mental illness: perspectives of case managers and consumers. *Psychosocial Rehabilitation Journal*, **17**, 81–92.

Ministry of Health (1962). *The Hospital Plan for England and Wales* (Cmnd, 1604). London: HMSO.

Ministry of Justice (2009). *Story of the Prison Population 1995–2009 England and Wales* (Statistics bulletin). London: Ministry of Justice.

Minsky, S., Riesser, G. G., & Duffy, M. (1995). The eye of the beholder: housing preferences of inpatients and treatment teams. *Psychiatric Services*, **46**, 173–176.

Mountain, D., Killaspy, H., & Holloway, F. (2009). Mental health rehabilitation services in the UK in 2007. *The Psychiatrist*, **33**, 215–218.

Nelson, G., Aubry, T., & Lafrance, A. (2007b). A review of the literature on the effectiveness of housing and support, assertive community treatment, and intensive case management interventions for persons with mental illness who have been homeless. *American Journal of Orthopsychiatry*, **77**, 350–361.

Nelson, G., Brent Hall, G., & Walsh-Bowers, R. (1998). The relationship between housing characteristics, emotional well-being and the personal empowerment of psychiatric consumer/survivors. *Community Mental Health Journal*, **34**, 57–69.

Nelson, G., Sylvestre, J., & Aubry, T. (2007a). Housing choice and control, housing quality, and control over professional support as contributors to the subjective quality of life and community adaptation of people with severe mental illness. *Administration and Policy in Mental Health and Mental Health Services Research*, **34**, 89–100.

O'Brien, M. (2010). Written answer, 5 February 2010. https://www.theyworkforyou.com/wrans/?id=2010-02-05a.315539.h&s=O%27Brien+Mike#g315539.r0

O'Connell, M., Tsai, J., & Rosenheck, R. (2023). Beyond supported housing: correlates of improvements in quality of life among homeless adults with mental illness. *Psychiatric Quarterly*, **94**(1), 49–59. doi:10.1007/s11126-022-10010-x [published Online First: 2022/12/21].

Office of the Deputy Prime Minister (2002). *The NHS and the Supporting People Strategy: Building the Links*. London: Office of the Deputy Prime Minister.

Office of the Deputy Prime Minister (2005). *Using the Quality Assessment Framework*. London: Office of the Deputy Prime Minister.

Owen, C., Rutherford, V., Jones, M., Wright, C., Tennant, C., & Smallman, A. (1996). Housing accommodation preferences of people with psychiatric disabilities. *Psychiatric Services*, **47**, 628–632.

Parker, S., Hopkins, G., Siskind, D., Harris, M., McKeon, G., Dark, F., & Whiteford, H. (2019). A systematic review of service models and evidence relating to the clinically operated community-based residential mental health rehabilitation for adults with severe and persisting mental illness in Australia. *BMC Psychiatry*, **19**, 55.

Peterson, P. & Borland, A. (1995). Use of state hospital staff to provide training for staff of community residential facilities. *Psychiatric Services*, **46**, 506–508.

Phelan, M. & Strathdee, G. (1994). Living in the community: training house officers in mental health. *Journal of Mental Health*, **3**, 229–233.

Piat, M., Lesage, A., Boyer, R., Dorvil, H., Couture, A., Grenier, G., & Bloom, D. (2008). Housing for persons with serious mental illness: consumer and service provider preferences. *Psychiatric Services*, **59**, 1011–1017.

Priebe, S., Badesconyi, A., Fioritti, A., Hansson, L., Kilian, R., Torres-Gonzales, F., et al. (2005). Reinstitutionalisation in mental health care: comparison of data on service provision from six European countries. *BMJ*, **330**, 123–126.

Priebe, S., Frottier, P., Gaddini, A., Killian, R., Lauber, C., Martinez-Leal, R., et al. (2008). Mental health care institutions in nine European countries, 2002 to 2006. *Psychiatric Services*, **59**, 570–573.

Raskin, A., Mghir, R., Peszke, M., & York, D. (1998). A psychoeducational program for caregivers of the chronic mentally ill residing in community residences. *Community Mental Health Journal*, **34**, 393–402.

Richter, D. & Hoffmann, H. (2017a). Independent housing and support for people with severe mental illness: systematic review. *Acta Psychiatria Scandinavica*, **136**, 269–279.

Richter, D. & Hoffmann, H. (2017b). Preference for independent housing of persons with mental disorders: systematic review and meta-analysis. *Administration and Policy in Mental Health*, **44**, 817–823.

Royal College of Psychiatrists (2010). *Accreditation for Inpatient Mental Health Services (AIMS)*. London: Royal College of Psychiatrists.

Ryan, T., Pearsall, A., Hatfield, B., & Poole, R. (2006). Long term care for serious mental illness outside the NHS. A study of out of area placements. *Journal of Mental Health*, **13**, 425–429.

Segal, S. P. & Kotler, P. L. (1993). Sheltered care residence: ten-year personal outcomes. *American Journal of Orthopsychiatry*, **63**, 80–83.

Seidman, L. J., Schutt, R. K., Caplan, B. C., Tolomiczenko, G. S., Turner, W. M., & Goldfinger, S. M. (2003). The effect of housing interventions on neuropsychological functioning among homeless people with mental illness. *Psychiatric Services*, **54**, 905–908.

Senn, V., Kendal, R., & Trieman, N. (1997). The TAPS project 38: level of training and its availability to carers within group homes in a London district. *Social Psychiatry & Psychiatric Epidemiology*, **32**, 317–322.

Shaw, J., Appleby, L., Amos, T., McDonnell, R., Harris, C., McCann, K., et al. (1999). Homicide, mental disorder and clinical care in people convicted of homicide: national clinical survey. *BMJ*, **318**, 1240–1244.

Shepherd, G. (1995). The ward in a house: residential care for the severely disabled. *Journal of Mental Health*, **31**, 53–69.

Shepherd, G., Beadsmoore, A., Moore, C., Hardy, P., & Muijen, M. (1997). Relation between bed use, social deprivation, and overall bed availability in acute psychiatric units and alternative residential options: a cross sectional survey, one day census data and staff interviews. *BMJ*, **314**, 262–266.

Shepherd, G., Boardman, J., & Burns, M. (2010). *Making Recovery a Reality* (Briefing paper). London: Sainsbury Centre for Mental Health.

Shepherd, G., Boardman, J., & Slade, M. (2008). *Implementing Recovery: A Methodology for Organisational Change* (Policy paper). London: Sainsbury Centre for Mental Health.

Shepherd, G., Muijen, M., Dean, R., & Cooney, M. (1996). Residential care in hospital and in the community—quality of care and quality of life. *British Journal of Psychiatry*, **168**, 448–456.

Singleton, N., Meltzer, H., & Gatward, R. (1998). *Psychiatric Morbidity among Prisoners in England and Wales*. London: Office for National Statistics.

Slade, M. (2009a). *Personal Recovery and Mental Illness: A Guide for Mental Health Professionals*. Cambridge: Cambridge University Press.

Slade, M. (2009b). *100 Ways to Support Recovery*. London: Rethink.

Social Care Institute for Excellence (2009). Research briefing 20: the implementation of individual budget schemes in adult social care. http://www.scie.org.uk/publications/briefings/briefing20/index.asp

Sorensen-Snyder, K., Wallace, C., Moe, K., & Liberman, R. (1994). Expressed emotion by residential care operators and residents' symptoms and quality of life. *Hospital and Community Psychiatry*, **45**, 1141–1143.

Srebnik, D., Livingstone, J., Gordon, L., & King, D. (1995). Housing choice and community success for individuals with serious and persistent mantal illness. *Community Mental Health Journal*, **31**, 139–152.

Strathdee, G. & Jenkins, R. (1996). Purchasing mental health care for primary care. In: Thornicroft, G. & Strathdee, G. (Eds.), *Commissioning Mental Health Services* (pp. 71–83). London: HMSO.

Tanzman, B. (1993). An overview of surveys of mental health consumers' preferences for housing and support services. *Hospital & Community Psychiatry*, **44**, 450–455.

Taylor, T. L., Killaspy, H., Wright, C., Turton, P., White, S., Kallert, T. W., et al. (2009). A systematic review of the international published literature relating to quality of institutional care for people with longer term mental health problems. *Biomed Central Psychiatry*, **9**, 55–73.

Thornicroft, G., Bebbington, P., & Leff, J. (2005). Outcomes for long-term patients one year after discharge from a psychiatric hospital. *Psychiatric Services*, **56**, 1416–1422.

Thornicroft, G., Diana, R., Kassam, A., & Sartorius, N. (2007). Stigma: ignorance, prejudice or discrimination? *British Journal of Psychiatry*, **190**, 192–193.

Thornicroft, G., Sunkel, C., Alikhon Aliev, A., et al. (2022). The Lancet Commission on ending stigma and discrimination in mental health. *Lancet*, **400**(10361), 1438–1480. doi:10.1016/S0140-6736(22)01470-2 [published Online First: 2022/10/13].

TNS UK (2010). Attitudes to mental illness 2010 research report. https://webarchive.nationalarchives.gov.uk/ukgwa/20130107215027/http://www.dh.gov.uk/en/Publicationsandstatistics/Publications/PublicationsStatistics/DH_114795

Trieman, N. & Leff, J. (1996). The TAPS Project. 36: the most difficult to place long-stay psychiatric in-patients outcome one year after relocation. *British Journal of Psychiatry*, **169**, 289–292.

Tsemberis, S., Gulcur, L., & Nakae, M. (2004). Housing First, consumer choice and harm reduction for homeless individuals with a dual diagnosis. *Research and Practice*, **94**, 651–656.

Walker, R. & Seasons, M. (2002). Supported housing for people with serious mental illness: resident perspectives on housing. *Canadian Journal of Community Mental Health*, **21**, 137–151.

Walshe, K. (2003). *Regulating Healthcare*. Maidenhead: Open University Press.

Warner, R. (2009). Recovery from schizophrenia and the recovery model. *Current Opinion in Psychiatry*, **22**, 374–380.

Wolff, G., Pathare, S., Craig, T., & Leff, J. (1996). Public education for community care: a new approach. *British Journal of Psychiatry*, **168**, 441–447.

20

Individual placement and support
The evidence-based practice of supported employment

Deborah R. Becker, Gary R. Bond, and Robert E. Drake

Introduction

In most societies, employment is a major avenue to social inclusion (Grove et al., 2005). The benefits of working include increasing one's financial resources, being productive and contributing to society, utilizing one's skills and talents, enhancing self-esteem, improving self-image, meeting other people, and structuring one's time. People with severe mental illness benefit from employment in these same ways. In addition, work enables many to recover from the disabling effects of mental illness.

Expectations for people with severe mental illness have changed drastically in the last three decades. Clients who once were relegated to day treatment and sheltered employment are now working competitively. The most successful employment practice to assist people develop a working life is a form of supported employment called individual placement and support (IPS). IPS has been standardized, tested, and implemented in several countries, especially the US.

Principles and practice of IPS supported employment

Created in the 1980s for people with developmental disabilities, supported employment assists people with disabilities to work competitively alongside others who are not disabled. Supported employment transforms 'train-place' approaches (preparation and prevocational training precede any job search) to 'place-train' efforts (training occurs after starting a job) (Wehman & Moon, 1988). Modified for people with severe mental illness, IPS supported employment focuses on helping clients find regular part-time or full-time jobs.

The eight guiding principles of IPS supported employment and how they contrast with traditional vocational services are listed in **Table 20.1**.

- First, IPS integrates behavioural health and vocational services through multidisciplinary teams. The IPS specialist can join one or two multidisciplinary treatment teams and meets at least weekly with each team to review clients, coordinate services, and update plans.
- Second, the only eligibility requirement for services is a desire to work a competitive job. People are not screened for work readiness or other prerequisites.
- Third, people are assisted in obtaining comprehensive benefits counselling to learn about work incentive programmes and how work may affect their benefits. Many people with mental illness receive health, disability, welfare, or other benefits (primarily from Social Security, Medicaid, and Medicare in the US). They are hesitant to return to work because they fear losing these benefits, and accurate information can help them make good decisions.
- Fourth, the goal is competitive employment. IPS specialists, sometimes called employment specialists, help people to find jobs that pay at least minimum wage and provide the benefits that others receive in the same position. The jobs are not set aside for people with disabilities, such as sheltered work or time-limited positions that are negotiated by a rehabilitation facility or mental health agency.
- Fifth, IPS specialists assist individuals to seek competitive jobs directly, without requiring lengthy prevocational assessments, trainings, sheltered work, or work adjustment activities. While the length of the job search varies, most individuals contact potential employers within 1 month and obtain a desired job within about 3 or 4 months.
- Sixth, IPS specialists make frequent contacts with employers, systematically building relationships with them to learn about their business needs before suggesting possible work candidates.
- Seventh, client preferences determine the type of job, the work environment, decisions about disclosure of disability to the employer, and type of job supports. IPS specialists assist clients to find jobs that are consistent with their preferences, skills, and previous experiences.
- Eighth, IPS specialists provide supports to the client after obtaining employment for as long as they want. Although clients differ in their desire and need for support, the general guideline for IPS

Table 20.1 IPS supported employment compared to traditional approaches.

IPS supported employment	Traditional vocational approaches
Integration of mental health, substance abuse, and employment services is important. IPS specialists are usually employed by the mental health agency. They attend weekly meetings with clinicians to discuss clients and their goals. State vocational rehabilitation also collaborates closely with supported employment programmes	Services are often brokered, meaning that clients receive mental health services, substance abuse services, and vocational services at separate agencies
All clients who want to work are eligible. Motivation to work is an important predictor of success. Clients are not screened out due to substance abuse, symptoms, hospitalization history, treatment non-adherence, or other factors	Traditional vocational programmes often attempt to assess which clients are 'ready' for employment and to screen out those who appear to have the most significant barriers, including substance abuse, to employment
Clients are encouraged to meet with a person trained in benefits (e.g. a certified work incentive counsellor) to learn how benefits would be affected by part- or full-time employment	Many traditional programmes also offer referrals to benefit specialists
Competitive employment is the goal. These are regular jobs in the community that pay at least minimum wage, not jobs that are set aside for people with disabilities	Some programmes focus on competitive jobs, while others focus on sheltered jobs such as workshops or enclave groups of clients working under the supervision of staff
The job search is rapid. Clients are not asked to participate in vocational evaluation or work adjustment programmes, as these 'pre-vocational, activities' are not related to better employment outcomes	Clients are frequently required to complete vocational testing, vocational adjustment programmes, or other pre-vocational groups before searching for a community job
IPS specialists systematically build relationships with employers to learn about their business needs before suggesting a possible work candidate. IPS specialists make multiple in-person visits with hiring managers to build trust and then introduce a qualified work candidate based on the skills and positions that the employer has described	Job developers identify available jobs through public job listings, such as on websites and job centres
Client preferences are important. Client preferences may refer to type of work, job location, number of hours worked each week, work shift, disclosure of disability to employer, etc.	Some traditional programmes offer only limited choices. This causes problems because, just like anyone else, clients tend to stay employed longer at jobs that meet their preferences
IPS specialists provide supports to working people as needed and desired. The supported employment team may provide long-term supports (typically for at least 1 year). Mental health practitioners sometimes provide supports to people who have been working successfully for more than a year	Follow-along supports are typically offered on a time-limited basis, often for 90 days

programmes is to provide regular support for 1 year after a client is working steadily. Afterward, the client transitions off the IPS supported employment caseload, and their primary mental health practitioner asks about the job during their regular sessions.

Review of the research

Systematic reviews and meta-analyses of the IPS literature have found that IPS is effective in improving competitive employment outcomes for people with serious mental illness (Brinchmann et al., 2020; Frederick & VanderWeele, 2019; Kinoshita et al., 2013; Marshall et al., 2014; Metcalfe et al., 2018; Modini et al., 2016; Suijkerbuijk et al., 2017). The practice has been well described (Becker & Drake, 2003; Swanson & Becker, 2013) and a fidelity scale outlines its critical components (Becker et al., 2019; Bond et al., 2012b).

Day treatment conversions: quasi-experimental studies

Starting in the late 1980s in the US, there were several evaluations of day treatment programmes that converted their rehabilitation services to supported employment. Drake and colleagues (1994) compared employment outcomes for people attending day treatment to those people who participated in a former day treatment programme that converted to IPS supported employment. In the conversion site, day treatment counsellor positions were changed to IPS specialist positions. Clients continued to receive mental health services (i.e. medication management, case management, etc.) but were encouraged to consider obtaining a competitive job with the support of an IPS specialist and the rest of the mental health team.

Employment outcomes significantly increased for those people receiving IPS employment services. Clients, family members, and staff were interviewed 1 year later and reported positively about the changes. The expressed concern about social activities was met by peer support services (Torrey et al., 1995). The finding of increased employment outcomes was replicated in four additional studies (Bailey et al., 1998; Becker et al., 2001; Drake et al., 1996a; M. Gold & Marrone, 1998). Clark (1998) demonstrated that replacing day treatment with IPS supported employment led to cost savings.

Randomized controlled trials

Twenty-eight randomized controlled trials (RCTs) of high-fidelity IPS supported employment for people with serious mental illness demonstrated consistently favourable employment outcomes as compared to traditional stepwise employment services (Bond et al., 2020; Drake et al., 2016). Across these studies, the competitive employment rate was 55% for people who received IPS supported employment as compared to 25% for people who received traditional vocational services. A meta-analysis found that, compared to control participants, IPS participants gained employment on average 2 months sooner, maintained employment four times longer during follow-up, earned three times the amount from employment, and were three times as likely to work 20 hours or more per week (Bond et al., 2012a). IPS studies conducted in the US included rural (P. B. Gold et al., 2006) and urban (Bond et al., 2007; Drake et al., 1999; Lehman et al., 2002; Mueser et al., 2004) communities, diverse populations including African Americans (Bond et al., 2007; Drake et al., 1999, Lehman et al., 2002), Latinos (Mueser et al., 2004), and older adults (Twamley et al., 2008). These studies compared IPS supported employment to leading vocational approaches of the day, including skills training (Drake et al., 1996b) and psychosocial rehabilitation (Bond et al., 2007). Internationally, RCTs conducted in four continents have all found favourable outcomes for IPS (North America, Europe, Asia, and Australia) (Drake et al., 2019).

Long-term trajectories

The goal of vocational services is, of course, long-term careers rather than short-term jobs. Findings from two longitudinal, mixed-methods (quantitative and qualitative) studies indicate that many people who receive IPS supported employment continue to work in satisfying jobs that they consider careers over time. An initial 10-year follow-up of participants in an IPS supported employment study found that 47% were working (Salyers et al., 2004). A second follow-up study of two cohorts of clients from the same mental health centre interviewed 8 and 12 years after participating in IPS supported employment studies found that 71% were currently working and 71% had worked more than half of the follow-up period (Becker et al., 2007). Clients reported that medication adjustments, working part time, and continued supports were important factors. Despite consistent employment, neither study found that clients on disability benefits had stopped receiving them completely. More recently, two IPS RCTs also found long-term employment outcomes favouring IPS. A Swiss study found that, at 5-year follow-up, 44% of IPS participants compared to 11% of participants receiving traditional vocational rehabilitation group were steady workers (i.e. competitively employed at least 30 months of the 60-month follow-up) (Hoffmann et al., 2014). A follow-up study of a multisite RCT of IPS for disability beneficiaries conducted examining outcomes over a 5-year period starting 3 years after the study had ended found significantly higher annual employment earnings for IPS (Baller et al., 2020).

Cost studies

A 2004 study estimated the costs of IPS employment services in seven IPS programmes throughout the US (Latimer et al., 2004). Although estimates varied according to local salaries and caseload sizes, a comprehensive cost analysis completed in 2013 estimated an annual per-client cost in the $3500–$5000 range for an IPS specialist maintaining a caseload of 18 (Salkever, 2013).

Two large European studies have found IPS to be less costly as well as more effective than standard vocational services in consideration of all programme costs, including mental health treatment (Christensen et al., 2020; Knapp et al., 2013). In both studies, the lower cost of psychiatric inpatient care for IPS participants was a major cost savings. In the US, day treatment programmes converting to IPS have resulted in substantial savings (Clark, 1998). A recently completed cost-effectiveness analysis of IPS for US veterans with post-traumatic stress disorder found that the annual per-client costs of all vocational and health services were $4000 greater for IPS clients than clients enrolled in a transitional work programme, but IPS was significantly more effective (Stroupe et al., 2022).

Cognitive studies

Several studies have investigated enhancing supported employment with cognitive remediation.

Several researchers are testing approaches to improve problems with memory, concentration, speed, and other cognitive areas in relation to work (McGurk & Wykes, 2008). A restorative approach, for example, includes computerized practice of cognitive functioning. Compensatory approaches may include job-specific coping strategies and job accommodations designed to help clients circumvent cognitive difficulties. Several controlled trials involving supported employment have found higher employment rates for clients receiving a cognitive intervention (e.g. McGurk, Mueser, Feldman, et al., 2007; McGurk, Mueser, Welsh, et al., 2015), but others have not replicated success (Christensen et al., 2019).

First psychotic episode and work and school

As part of early intervention, recent studies have focused on work and school for people with first-episode psychosis.

In the past decade, clinical research has emphasized early interventions for people with a first psychotic episode. One strategy involves return to daily life activities like work and school through IPS supported employment. Nuechterlein and colleagues (2020) reported that 92% of the young adults receiving both school and work support through IPS supported employment obtained either a competitive job and/or enrolled in school. Three other RCTs of IPS for young adults with early psychosis have also found significantly better employment outcomes for IPS participants (Erickson et al., 2021; Killackey et al., 2008, 2019).

Implementation and fidelity

IPS supported employment has been implemented in routine settings in most states in the US (Pogue et al., 2022). Many jurisdictions and local sites utilize the IPS Fidelity Scale (Becker et al., 2019) as a guide to implementation. High-fidelity implementation typically requires initial training, supervision, and fidelity assessment over 6–12 months (Becker et al., 2008). The 25-item IPS Fidelity Scale outlines the critical components of the practice with benchmarks, like a roadmap or a compass. It has been validated and revised based on research and recommendations from expert IPS trainers (Becker et al., 2019). A large and growing body of research has demonstrated IPS fidelity is significantly correlated with employment outcomes (Lockett et al., 2016).

Dissemination

IPS supported employment was developed in the US, and adoption has occurred widely there, including more than 80% of state mental health systems and all Veterans Health Administration centres (Pogue et al., 2022). More than 1000 IPS teams in the US serve over 60,000 clients with serious mental illness per year. The 27 states in the IPS learning community (Becker et al., 2014) have been expanding IPS services more rapidly than other states, perhaps because they provide interagency collaboration, training and technical assistance, reviews of fidelity and data, and funding (Pogue et al., 2022). The IPS Employment Center and IPS Learning Community provide online training, technical assistance, data analysis, fidelity monitoring, and regular communication through newsletters, bimonthly calls, and an in-person annual meeting. Although the economy and local unemployment affect IPS outcomes (Cook et al., 2006), quarterly employment outcomes in IPS Learning Community states have remained above 40%, even during the great recession and the Covid-19 pandemic (IPSworks.org).

The lack of a simple funding system continues to limit IPS expansion in the US. Because states and programmes need to combine, or braid, funding from multiple sources, funding remains the primary barrier to more widespread implementation (Bazelon Center for Mental Health Law, 2018; Drake et al., 2016).

IPS supported employment is also spreading in more than 20 other countries (Drake, 2020). RCTs in several countries (reviewed earlier in this chapter) have spurred this development over the past 15 years. The increasing numbers of adults on disability due to psychiatric illnesses is stressing democracies with free enterprise systems throughout the world (OECD, 2009). Countries of course vary considerably in terms of economic, workforce, health care, and disability regulations (Burns et al., 2007). Nevertheless, most high-income countries and some middle-income countries have adopted IPS because they recognize that employment is a central component of recovery for many people with serious mental illness and that IPS is a highly effective intervention.

Conclusion

IPS embodies disability rights and human rights. People with severe mental illnesses want to work, not only to improve their economic status but also as part of the process of recovery. Employment enhances one's self-image, self-esteem, relationships, and many other aspects of quality of life; it also helps people to manage symptoms and illnesses. The IPS supported employment model has demonstrated robust success in improving rates of competitive employment in many countries. Barriers nevertheless remain, including bureaucratic resistance within the mental health and vocational rehabilitation systems, failures to align funding with evidence-based practices in general, antiquated disability regulations in many countries, and the economic downturn of recent years. Widespread uptake will require further efforts.

REFERENCES

Bailey, E. L., Ricketts, S. K., Becker, D. R., Xie, H., & Drake, R. E. (1998). Do long-term day treatment clients benefit from supported employment? *Psychiatric Rehabilitation Journal*, **22**, 24–29.

Baller, J., Blyler, C., Bronnikov, S., Xie, H., Bond, G. R., Filion, K., & Hale, T. (2020). Long-term follow-up of a randomized trial of supported employment for social security disability beneficiaries with mental illness. *Psychiatric Services*, **71**, 243–249.

Bazelon Center for Mental Health Law (2018). *Advances in Employment Policy for Individuals with Serious Mental Illness*. Washington, DC: Bazelon Center for Mental Health Law.

Becker, D. R., Bond, G. R., McCarthy, D., Thompson, D., Xie, H., McHugo, G. J., & Drake, R. E. (2001). Converting day treatment centers to supported employment programs in Rhode Island. *Psychiatric Services*, **52**, 351–357.

Becker, D. R. & Drake, R. E. (2003). *A Working Life for People with Severe Mental Illness*. New York: Oxford University Press.

Becker, D. R., Drake, R. E., & Bond, G. R. (2014). The IPS supported employment learning collaborative. *Psychiatric Rehabilitation Journal*, **37**, 79–85.

Becker, D. R., Lynde, D., & Swanson, S. J. (2008). Strategies for statewide implementation of supported employment: The Johnson & Johnson–Dartmouth Community Mental Health Program. *Psychiatric Rehabilitation Journal*, **31**, 296–299.

Becker, D. R., Swanson, S., Reese, S. L., Bond, G. R., & McLeman, B. M. (2019). *Supported Employment Fidelity Review Manual* (4th ed.). Lebanon, NH: IPS Employment Center.

Becker, D. R., Whitley, R., Bailey, E. L., & Drake, R. E. (2007). Long-term employment trajectories among participants with severe mental illness in supported employment. *Psychiatric Services*, **58**, 922–928.

Bond, G. R., Campbell, K., & Drake, R. E. (2012a). Standardizing measures in four domains of employment outcome for individual placement and support. *Psychiatric Services*, **63**, 751–757.

Bond, G. R., Drake, R. E., & Becker, D. R. (2020). An update on individual placement and support. *World Psychiatry*, **19**, 390–391.

Bond, G. R., Peterson, A. E., Becker, D. R., & Drake, R. E. (2012b). Validation of the revised Individual Placement and Support Fidelity Scale (IPS-25). *Psychiatric Services*, **63**, 758–763.

Bond, G. R., Salyers, M. P., Dincin, J., Drake, R. E., Becker, D. R., Fraser, V. V., & Haines, M. (2007). A randomized controlled trial comparing two vocational models for persons with severe mental illness. *Journal of Consulting and Clinical Psychology*, **75**, 968–982.

Brinchmann, B., Widding-Havneraas, T., Modini, M., Rinaldi, M., Moe, C. F., McDaid, D., et al. (2020). A meta-regression of the impact of policy on the efficacy of individual placement and support. *Acta Psychiatrica Scandinavica*, **141**, 206–220.

Burns, T., Catty, J., Becker, T., Drake, R. E., Fioritti, A., Knapp, M., et al. (2007). The effectiveness of supported employment for people with severe mental illness: a randomised controlled trial. *Lancet*, **370**, 1146–1152.

Christensen, T. N., Kruse, M., Hellström, L., & Eplov, L. F. (2020). Cost-utility and cost-effectiveness of individual placement support and cognitive remediation in people with severe mental illness: results from a randomised clinical trial. *European Psychiatry*, **64**, e3.

Christensen, T. N., Wallstrøm, I. G., Stenager, E., Bojesen, A. B., Gluud, C., Nordentoft, M., & Eplov, L. F. (2019). Effects of individual placement and support supplemented with cognitive remediation and work-focused social skills training for people with severe mental illness: a randomized clinical trial. *JAMA Psychiatry*, **76**, 1232–1240.

Clark, R. E. (1998). Supported employment and managed care: can they coexist? *Psychiatric Rehabilitation Journal*, **22**, 62–68.

Cook, J. A., Mulkern, G., Grey, D. D., Burke-Miller, J., Blyler, C. R., Razzano, L. A., et al. (2006). Effects of local unemployment rate on vocational outcomes in a randomized trial of supported employment for individuals with psychiatric disabilities. *Journal of Vocational Rehabilitation*, **25**, 71–84.

Drake, R. E. (2020). Special issue: international implementation of individual placement and support. *Psychiatric Rehabilitation Journal*, **43**, 1–82.

Drake, R. E., Becker, D. R., Biesanz, J. C., Torrey, W. C., McHugo, G. J., & Wyzik, P. F. (1994). Rehabilitation day treatment vs. supported employment: I. Vocational outcomes. *Community Mental Health Journal*, **30**, 519–532.

Drake, R. E., Becker, D. R., Biesanz, J. C., Wyzik, P. F., & Torrey, W. C. (1996a). Day treatment versus supported employment for persons with severe mental illness: a replication study. *Psychiatric Services*, 47, 1125–1127.

Drake, R. E., Becker, D. R., & Bond, G. R. (2019). Introducing individual placement and support (IPS) supported employment in Japan. *Psychiatry and Clinical Neurosciences*, 73, 47–49.

Drake, R. E., Bond, G. R., Goldman, H. H., Hogan, M. F., & Karakus, M. (2016). Individual placement and support services boost employment for people with serious mental illness, but funding is lacking. *Health Affairs*, 35, 1098–1105.

Drake, R. E., McHugo, G. J., Bebout, R. R., Becker, D. R., Harris, M., Bond, G. R., & Quimby, E. (1999). A randomized clinical trial of supported employment for inner-city patients with severe mental illness. *Archives of General Psychiatry*, 56, 627–633.

Drake, R. E., McHugo, G. J., Becker, D. R., Anthony, W. A., & Clark, R. E. (1996b). The New Hampshire study of supported employment for people with severe mental illness: vocational outcomes. *Journal of Consulting and Clinical Psychology*, 64, 391–399.

Erickson, D. H., Roes, M. H., Digiacomo, A., & Burns, A. (2021). Individual placement and support boosts employment for early psychosis clients, even when baseline rates are high. *Early Intervention in Psychiatry*, 15, 662–668.

Frederick, D. E. & VanderWeele, T. J. (2019). Supported employment: meta-analysis and review of randomized controlled trials of individual placement and support. *PLoS One*, 14, e0212208.

Gold, M. & Marrone, J. (1998). Mass Bay Employment Services (a service of Bay Cove Human Services, Inc.): a story of leadership, vision, and action resulting in employment for people with mental illness. *Roses and Thorns from the Grassroots: A Series Highlighting Organizational Change in Massachusetts*, **Spring**, 1–4. https://files.eric.ed.gov/fulltext/ED460446.pdf

Gold, P. B., Meisler, N., Santos, A. B., Carnemolla, M. A., Williams, O. H., & Kelleher, J. (2006). Randomized trial of supported employment integrated with assertive community treatment for rural adults with severe mental illness. *Schizophrenia Bulletin*, 32, 378–395.

Grove, B., Secker, J., & Seebohm, P. (Eds.) (2005). *New Thinking about Mental Health and Employment*. Abingdon: Radcliffe Publishing.

Hoffmann, H., Jäckel, D., Glauser, S., Mueser, K. T., & Kupper, Z. (2014). Long-term effectiveness of supported employment: five-year follow-up of a randomized controlled trial. *American Journal of Psychiatry*, 171, 1183–1190.

Killackey, E. J., Allott, K., Jackson, H. J., Scutella, R., Tseng, Y., Borland, J., et al. (2019). Individual placement and support for vocational recovery in first-episode psychosis: randomised controlled trial. *British Journal of Psychiatry*, 214, 76–82.

Killackey, E. J., Jackson, H. J., & McGorry, P. D. (2008). Vocational intervention in first-episode psychosis: individual placement and support v. treatment as usual. *British Journal of Psychiatry*, 193, 114–120.

Kinoshita, Y., Furukawa, T. A., Omori, I. M., Marshall, M., Bond, G. R., Huxley, P., & Kingdon, D. (2013). Supported employment for adults with severe mental illness. *Cochrane Database of Systematic Reviews* 2010, CD008297.

Knapp, M., Patel, A., Curran, C., Latimer, E., Catty, J., Becker, T., et al. (2013). Supported employment: cost-effectiveness across six European sites. *World Psychiatry*, 12, 60–68.

Latimer, E., Bush, P., Becker, D. R., Drake, R. E., & Bond, G. R. (2004). How much does supported employment for the severely mentally ill cost? An exploratory survey of high-fidelity programs. *Psychiatric Services*, 55, 401–406.

Lehman, A. F., Goldberg, R. W., Dixon, L. B., McNary, S., Postrado, L., Hackman, A., & McDonnell, K. (2002). Improving employment outcomes for persons with severe mental illness. *Archives of General Psychiatry*, 59, 165–172.

Lockett, H., Waghorn, G., Kydd, R., & Chant, D. (2016). Predictive validity of evidence-based practices in supported employment: a systematic review and meta-analysis. *Mental Health Review Journal*, 21, 261–281.

Marshall, T., Goldberg, R. W., Braude, L., Dougherty, R. H., Daniels, A. S., Ghose, S. S., et al. (2014). Supported employment: assessing the evidence. *Psychiatric Services*, 65, 16–23.

McGurk, S. R., Mueser, K. T., Feldman, K., Wolfe, R., & Pascaris, A. (2007). Cognitive training for supported employment: 2–3 year outcomes of a randomized controlled trial. *American Journal of Psychiatry*, 164, 437–441.

McGurk, S., Mueser, K. T., Welsh, J., Drake, R. E., Becker, D. R., McHugo, G., & Xie, H. (2015). A randomized controlled trial of cognitive enhancement treatment for people with severe mental illness who do not respond to supported employment. *American Journal of Psychiatry*, 172, 852–861.

McGurk, S. R. & Wykes, T. (2008). Cognitive remediation and vocational rehabilitation. *Psychiatric Rehabilitation Journal*, 31, 350–359.

Metcalfe, J. D., Drake, R. E., & Bond, G. R. (2018). Economic, labor, and regulatory moderators of the effect of individual placement and support among people with severe mental illness: a systematic review and meta-analysis. *Schizophrenia Bulletin*, 44, 22–31.

Modini, M., Tan, L., Brinchmann, B., Wang, M., Killackey, E., Glozier, N., et al. (2016). Supported employment for people with severe mental illness: a systematic review and meta-analysis of the international evidence. *British Journal of Psychiatry*, 209, 14–22.

Mueser, K. T., Clark, R. E., Haines, M., Drake, R. E., McHugo, G. J., Bond, G. R., et al. (2004). The Hartford study of supported employment for persons with severe mental illness. *Journal of Consulting and Clinical Psychology*, 72, 479–490.

Nuechterlein, K. H., Subotnik, K. L., Ventura, J., Turner, L. R., Gitlin, M. J., Gretchen-Doorly, D., et al. (2020). Enhancing return to work or school after a first episode of schizophrenia: the UCLA RCT of individual placement and support and workplace fundamentals module training. *Psychological Medicine*, 50, 20–28.

OECD (2009). Pathways onto (and off) disability benefits: assessing the role of policy and individual circumstances. http://www.oecd.org/officialdocuments/publicdisplaydocumentpdf/?cote=DELSA/ELSA/WP5(2009)5anddocLanguage=En

Pogue, J. A., Bond, G. R., Drake, R. E., Becker, D. R., & Logsdon, S. (2022). Growth of IPS supported employment programs in the US: an update. *Psychiatric Services*, 73, 533–538.

Salkever, D. S. (2013). Social costs of expanding access to evidence-based supported employment: concepts and interpretive review of evidence. *Psychiatric Services*, 64, 111–119.

Salyers, M. P., Becker, D. R., Drake, R. E., Torrey, W. C., & Wyzik, P. F. (2004). Ten-year follow-up of clients in a supported employment program. *Psychiatric Services*, 55, 302–308.

Stroupe, K. T., Jordan, N., Richman, J., Cao, L., Burt, J., Kertesz, S., et al. (2022). Cost effectiveness of individual placement and support compared to transitional work program for veterans with post-traumatic stress disorder. *Administration and Policy in Mental Health and Mental Health Services Research*, 49, 429–439.

Suijkerbuijk, Y. B., Schaafsma, F. G., van Mechelen, J. C., Ojajärvi, A., Corbière, M., & Anema, J. R. (2017). Interventions for obtaining and maintaining employment in adults with severe mental illness, a network meta-analysis. *Cochrane Database of Systematic Reviews*, **9**, CD011867.

Swanson, S. J. & Becker, D. R. (2013). *IPS Supported Employment: A Practical Guide*. Lebanon, NH: Dartmouth Psychiatric Research Center.

Torrey, W. C., Becker, D. R., & Drake, R. E. (1995). Rehabilitative day treatment versus supported employment: II. Consumer, family and staff reactions to a program change. *Psychosocial Rehabilitation Journal*, **18**, 67–75.

Twamley, E. W., Narvaez, J. M., Becker, D. R., Bartels, S. J., & Jeste, D. V. (2008). Supported employment for middle-aged and older people with schizophrenia. *American Journal of Psychiatric Rehabilitation*, **11**, 76–89.

Wehman, P. & Moon, M. S. (Eds.) (1988). *Vocational Rehabilitation and Supported Employment*. Baltimore, MD: Paul Brookes.

21
Programmes to support family members and caregivers

Samantha Jankowski, Amy L. Drapalski, and Lisa B. Dixon

Introduction

Most individuals with schizophrenia or other serious mental illnesses have regular contact with family members, and these family members often provide substantial support and assistance to their ill relative (Chien et al., 2006; Hackman & Dixon, 2008; Resnick et al., 2005). Although providing support to a relative with mental illness is often rewarding on many levels, caring for a relative with a mental illness can also be extremely demanding and lead to feeling overwhelmed, frustrated, worried, and depressed. Limited knowledge of mental illness, mental health treatments, and the mental health service system, coupled with the increased demands associated with taking on a caregiver role, can contribute to significant family stress, distress, and burden. In turn, this increased burden may impede a family's ability to maintain the support and assistance that their ill relative may need to manage an illness and achieve recovery goals. Several programmes have been developed to address the varying needs and preferences of family members and caregivers of individuals with serious mental illness. This chapter aims to discuss the potential impact of mental illness on the family and its relationship to family needs, the basic tenets or principles of effective family programmes delivered in clinical and community settings, several prominent family interventions, the evidence for their effectiveness, and barriers to programme use.

The impact of mental illness on the family

Many aspects of providing support for an individual with a serious mental illness can be rewarding. However, observing mental illness in a family member and experiencing its effects can be traumatic for families. Moreover, the time and effort required to provide this support can create additional burden for family members. Family members are often the first to notice emerging signs or symptoms of an illness. However, due to limited prior experience with mental illness, these behaviours are rarely recognized as such and, even when they are, can be distressing and disturbing for family members. Consequently, families may alternate between periods of denial or avoidance of emerging issues or problems and feeling overwhelmed or overcome by the illness and its effect on the family functioning (Lucksted et al., 2012). These changes may lead family members to experience additional burden—often described in terms of objective and subjective burden. Objective burden typically refers to clear, observable disruptions in the family unit or family roles that stem from the added responsibilities associated with caring for a relative with an illness (Hackman & Dixon, 2008). These can include financial strain or hardship created by the need to financially support a relative, loss of social support or social disengagement due to active efforts to avoid others and minimize rejection, limited time to engage in social activities as a result of the time constraints created by additional caregiver responsibilities, and disruption in daily routines and family relationships and roles.

Subjective burden refers to the psychological impact of the illness on the family, often manifested in the form of psychological distress, particularly depression, anxiety, and anger (Lefley, 1989). Factors associated with greater distress include caregiver health problems, limited social support, negative appraisals of caregiving, providing frequent assistance, and needing to monitor medication (Lerner et al., 2018). Family members often worry about the health and welfare of their ill relative, the potential for future relapses and hospitalizations, and their ability to help their family member successfully cope with an illness (Drapalski et al., 2009). Depression is also common and may result from feelings of grief and loss as family members attempt to come to terms with the potential need to change their own expectations concerning their relative's future functioning and goals. Moreover, depression, frustration, and anger may also occur in reaction to the added responsibility associated with supporting a relative, the challenges family members may face in their attempts to support their relative, and the potential changes family members may need to make in their own lives or in terms of their own future plans as a result of their relative's illness (Drapalski et al., 2009).

Not surprisingly, greater objective and subjective burden may produce a family environment that is stressful for both the family and the individual with the illness. However, providing family members with information to help them better understand a relative's illness and ways to help them cope with their illness, assistance with developing more effective communication and problem-solving skills, and support in helping family members better manage the difficulties and struggles that may come with supporting a relative with an illness, can all serve to minimize family burden (Dixon et al., 2001b; Falloon & Pederson, 1985; Hazel et al., 2004). Results of several studies assessing the perceived needs of family members of individuals with serious mental illness echo this sentiment, with family members expressing the need for information on mental illness and its treatment, coping strategies and problem-solving skills, the structure and function of the mental health system and the different roles of mental health treatment providers, community resources (e.g. housing, employment, social/recreational programmes), and future planning (Drapalski et al., 2008; Hatfield, 1978; Lefley, 1989; Smith, 2003; Winefield & Harvey, 1994).

Importantly, working with family members is a dynamic process with multiple phases and changing needs and preferences over time, since family members often go through a recovery process (Spaniol & Nelson, 2015). Spaniol and Nelson (2015) suggest that certain types of family interventions may be better suited for particular phases of recovery. For example, psychoeducation may help families with recognition and acceptance, while peer-led programmes may be helpful for coping or personal advocacy.

Basic principles and goals of family programmes

Over the past 40 years, many family programmes have been developed in an attempt to meet the needs of individuals with serious mental illness and their families. These programmes define family broadly to include any individual who serves as a support to the individual with the illness. As such, 'family' may include parents, siblings, spouses or significant others, or children; extended family such as cousins, aunts, or uncles; or persons outside the family such as close friends or peers. Programmes can generally be characterized as clinic-based, that is, delivered by a member of the clinical team, generally by a clinician, and those that are delivered in the community (peer-delivered). Programmes delivered within the clinician setting generally require consent of the consumer for the family to participate and include family psychoeducation (FPE) and brief family education and consultation. Peer-delivered programmes provide opportunities for families to receive support on their own behalf and include National Alliance on Mental Illness (NAMI) Family-to-Family and NAMI Homefront programmes.

Although these programmes can differ in terms of their content, structure, and format, effective, evidence-based family treatments all tend to adhere to several core principles and incorporate several critical features (Dixon et al., 2001b). These core elements, outlined by a panel of international experts convened by the World Schizophrenia Fellowship (1998), are viewed as central in helping providers to work collaboratively with individuals with serious mental illness and their families to best promote positive outcomes for both the individual with the illness and their family (Dixon et al., 2001b). These features include the following:

- Establishing and maintaining a collaborative and supportive relationship with the consumer with illness and family
- Attention to the needs of the consumer and the family
- Treating family as equal partners in treatment planning and delivery
- Exploration and clarification of the consumer's and family's treatment expectations
- Assessment and evaluation of family strengths and weaknesses as they pertain to their ability to support their ill relative
- Address feelings of loss
- Sensitivity to the family distress and conflict
- Provision of relevant information/education when needed
- Development of crisis management and response plan
- Communication and problem-solving skill development
- Assisting families in the expansion of social support networks (e.g. NAMI)
- Awareness of potential differences in the needs of families and flexibility in meeting those needs.

Connecting the family with other professionals once the family work has been completed: programmes to support family members and caregivers

As noted previously, many family programmes have been developed in an effort to address the needs of individuals with serious mental illness and their families. Although these programmes vary substantially in terms of their structure, content, and focus, all share several common features including developing a supportive, collaborative relationship with the consumer and family member, providing education and information on mental illness and its treatment, and helping families develop more effective skills for coping with some of the effects of the illness (often including communication and problem-solving skills) (Murray-Swank et al., 2007; Pfammatter et al., 2006). Moreover, each programme has demonstrated benefits for both consumers and family members. Thus, the availability of a variety of programmes allows providers to work with consumers and family members to decide which programme best meets their individual needs and preferences concerning involvement. We first describe clinician-led services delivered in a clinical context and then community-delivered, peer-led services.

Family psychoeducation (FPE)

FPE programmes initially developed with the goal of improving consumer outcomes by reducing or minimizing the level of expressed emotion exhibited by family members of individuals with schizophrenia and other serious mental illnesses. Expressed emotion refers to the extent of criticism or emotional overinvolvement directed towards an individual with mental illness by another individual (typically a family member) (Bebbington & Kuipers, 1994). High levels of expressed emotion among family members has been associated with greater relapse rates in individuals with both schizophrenia (Bebbington & Kuipers, 1994) and bipolar disorder (Miklowitz et al., 1988).

For example, in a study of individuals with schizophrenia, Bebbington and Kuipers (1994) found that individuals with families evaluated as being high in expressed emotion evidenced more than double the relapse rate (50%) compared to families evaluated as being low in expressed emotion (21%). Research on FPE over the past several decades suggests that are a number of benefits to participation in FPE programmes extend to all families, regardless of the level of expressed emotion (Bebbington & Kuipers, 1994; Murray-Swank & Dixon, 2005). Notably, much of this research focused on individuals who had recently been or were currently hospitalized.

Although specific FPE programmes may vary somewhat in terms of content, structure, and format, most FPE programmes include several core features: (1) provision of psychoeducation, (2) skill building (particularly communication and problem-solving), and (3) increased opportunities for receiving support (Murray-Swank et al., 2007). However, as noted earlier, the way in which these components are delivered can vary depending on the specific programme. For example, some FPE programmes are designed to be conducted with an individual family (Anderson et al., 1986; Falloon et al., 1984; Mueser & Glynn, 1999), while others are conducted in a group setting with several families participating at one time (McFarlane, 2002).

While many programmes have been developed primarily with families of individuals with schizophrenia in mind, in the family-focused treatment (FFT) programme the content and focus of the sessions has been modified to better address the specific needs of families of individuals with bipolar disorder (Miklowitz & Goldstein, 1997). Finally, some programmes such as behavioural family treatment (Falloon et al., 1984; Mueser & Glynn, 1999) and multifamily group therapy (McFarlane, 2002, 2016) include both the family and the individual with mental illness in sessions, while others involve only the family. Importantly in these programme subtypes, consumer outcomes are primary and consumer consent is required for families to participate.

Regardless of the differences in the content, structure, and format of the programme, the effectiveness of FPE for individuals with serious mental illness has been clearly established. Results from several meta-analyses of FPE programmes have demonstrated the effectiveness of FPE for individuals with schizophrenia, particularly with regard to relapse and rehospitalization rates (Baucom et al., 1998; Pfammater, et al., 2006; Pharoah et al., 2010; Pitschel-Walz et al., 2001). In an analysis of 53 studies, Pharoah et al. (2010) found that family intervention decreased relapse rates (definitions varied by study and included recurrence or deterioration of symptoms or hospitalization) and hospital admissions, increased medication compliance, and improved social impairment and levels of expressed emotions in families.

Another meta-analysis by Pitschel-Walz and colleagues (2001) found that better outcomes were associated with length in treatment with greater benefits evidenced in those that participated in programmes for more than 3 months. Results from other meta-analyses are even more pronounced. Baucom and colleagues (1998) found that participation in an FPE programme lasting at least 9 months can reduce relapse and rehospitalization rates by approximately 50%. Other studies have found that participation in FPE was associated with a number of positive outcomes including better rates of employment (McFarlane et al., 1996, 2000), social functioning (Montero et al., 2001), life satisfaction (Resnick et al., 2004), and reduced negative symptoms (Dyck et al., 2000).

While most studies on FPE have included families of individuals with schizophrenia, studies examining the effects for families of individuals with other diagnoses such as bipolar disorder and major depression suggest similar positive effects. Modelled after behavioural family treatment programmes for schizophrenia (Falloon et al., 1984), FFT is a psychoeducation programme that includes the same core components found in FPE programmes for individuals with schizophrenia (e.g. illness education, communication skills development, and problem-solving training), but these elements are modified or tailored to address the specific needs of individuals with bipolar disorder and their families (Miklowitz & Goldstein, 1997). In a randomized clinical trial comparing FFT to usual care, Miklowitz and colleagues (2003) found that participation in FFT was associated with significantly lower relapse rates (34% vs 54%), more extended periods of time between periods of symptom exacerbation (53.2 days vs 73.2 days), better medication adherence, and less depression 2 years after completing the programme (Miklowitz et al., 2003).

Similarly, Rea and colleagues (2003) compared the effects of using FFT as an adjunct to medication management to individual treatment and medication management (Rea et al., 2003). Results were even more pronounced with individuals receiving FFT being less likely to relapse (28% vs 60%) or be rehospitalized (12% vs 60%) 1 year after hospital discharge than those who received individual therapy as an adjunct to medication. Other studies have demonstrated benefits of participation in psychoeducational programmes for couples for individuals with depression (Emanuels-Zuurveen & Emmelkamp, 1997; Leff et al., 2000). Although these findings suggest that FPE may be equally beneficial for individuals with other serious mental illnesses and their families, particularly when programmes are tailored to meet the specific needs and experiences of those individuals and families, additional studies are needed.

The benefits associated with participation in FPE programmes appear to be sustained well after the completion of the programme. Pitschel-Walz and colleagues (2006) examined relapse rates and days of hospitalization over a 7-year period following discharge. They found that individuals with schizophrenia whose families participated in FPE during the index hospitalization were significantly less likely to relapse (54%) during the 7 years post-hospitalization than those who did not (88%). In addition, individuals who families received FPE spent significantly fewer days in the hospital (75 days) than those whose families did not receive FPE (225 days), suggesting that the benefits of FPE programmes may be maintained and possibly enhanced over time (Pitschel-Walz et al., 2006). Additional studies are needed to determine the long-term impact of FPE on consumer outcomes including relapse and rehospitalization rates as well as family outcomes.

Participation in FPE can also impact family outcomes. A meta-analysis reviewing outcomes of FPE across numerous settings found that participation was associated with a significant decrease in the objective and subjective burden, negative feelings towards the family member with the illness, and family conflict experienced by family members (Cuijpers, 1999). Other studies have found that participation in FPE was associated with improved well-being (Falloon et al., 1985) and better overall family functioning (Cuipers, 1999).

Similarly, Lyman et al. (2014) found that multifamily psychoeducation groups were associated with improved problem-solving ability and reduced family burden. Thus, given the overwhelming evidence of the positive effects of FPE, particularly in terms of relapse and rehospitalization rates, numerous groups such as the American Psychiatric Association, the Schizophrenia Patient Outcomes Research Team (PORT), and others have recommended that FPE programmes be offered to the families of individuals with serious mental illness. In fact, in the most recent iteration of the

Schizophrenia PORT recommendations indicated that all individuals with schizophrenia be offered FPE that includes illness education, coping and crisis management skills training, and support that lasts at least 6 months (Dixon et al., 2010).

Brief education and family consultation

Similar to FPE, briefer educational programmes and family consultation were developed with the goals of increasing knowledge, reducing burden, and minimizing distress in families of individuals with serious mental illness. These programmes may serve as alternative or complementary programmes to FPE, particularly in cases where participation in FPE may not be feasible, practical, or perceived as needed (Cohen et al., 2008). In these cases, shorter, more targeted programmes or services, such as brief family education or family consultation, may be beneficial.

Brief family education

Brief education programmes are time-limited and focused, often lasting from 6 to 12 weeks or more. Sessions are usually led by a mental health professional and often focus on specific educational and/or skills training goals such as providing families with education on mental illness, its aetiology, and its treatment; helping families develop effective communication and problem-solving skills; improving self-care and coping skills; crisis management and relapse prevention; and increasing the opportunity for mutual support. For example, Posner and colleagues (1992) had family members attend eight, 90-minute sessions that focused on educating family members concerning schizophrenia, its aetiology, and illness treatment; the effects of mental illness on the family; and available community resources. Another programme developed and evaluated by Magliano and colleagues (2006) had families participating in educational sessions for 6 months that proceeded in stages starting with an assessment of family needs, then informational/educational sessions, communication skills training, and finally problem-solving.

Although the benefits of briefer family intervention programmes may be somewhat diminished in comparison to longer programmes, participation in these programmes has been shown to lead to many positive outcomes for individuals with schizophrenia. These benefits appear to differ from study to study and have included fewer symptoms (Merinder et al., 1999), better self-care (Magliano et al., 2006; Xiong et al., 1994), and better treatment adherence (Pitschel-Walz et al., 2006; Xiong et al., 1994) in individuals with illness and greater knowledge of the illness (Posner et al., 1992) and less perceived burden and distress among family members (Cuijpers, 1999). However, the impact on relapse and rehospitalization rates is less clear. While results from some studies have suggested that participation in brief educational programmes may be associated with longer periods of time between relapses (Merinder et al., 1999), fewer hospitalizations (Chien & Lee, 2010), and shorter hospitalizations (Chien & Lee, 2010), other have not (Posner et al., 1992). Despite the variability in outcomes, the apparent benefits of brief family education programme led to the Schizophrenia PORT recommendation that individuals with schizophrenia and their families be offered brief educational programmes in cases where participation in longer FPE programmes are not possible or not of interest to family members (Dixon et al., 2010). Few studies have examined the use of brief psychoeducational programmes for families of individuals with other serious mental illnesses.

Family consultation

Family consultation offers another alternative to working with families of individuals with mental illness. Similar to the psychoeducational programmes previously discussed, family consultation involves providing families with information and education on mental illness and its treatment and helps families to develop better coping skills. However, in contrast, family consultation typically involves a provider meeting with an individual family (rather than several families at a time) to target the individual needs of the family. The consultation can vary in length depending on the needs and goals of the family. Family consultation may be particularly useful in situations where the family can identify a specific problem or need that can be addressed in a relatively short period of time. In addition, since family consultation can be conducted in the absence of the person with the illness, it can be useful in situations where the individual with the illness is unwilling or unable to participate.

Most family consultations begin with an assessment with the client and/or the family to determine the focus or primary goal of the consultation effort. After identifying a particular problem or goal to be addressed, potential options for addressing the problem are discussed and a joint decision concerning how best to address that goal is reached. This may include providing families with additional education on relevant topics, helping families identify and access community resources, working with families to help them develop more effective communication, problem-solving, and other coping skills, or engaging the family in problem-solving around a particular issue (Family Institute for Education, Practice and Research & New York State Office of Mental Health, 2007). As such, the consultation length is often dependent on both the problem and the method by which the family has chosen to attempt to address the problem.

Only a few studies have systematically evaluated the effectiveness of family consultation; however, these studies suggest potential benefits to participation in these programmes. In one such study, Solomon and colleagues (1997) compared a brief psychoeducational programme to a family consultation programme. Participants included individuals with schizophrenia spectrum disorders, bipolar disorder, or major depression. The brief educational programme included ten 2-hour sessions that involved both education on mental illness and its treatment and assistance in developing coping skills. In contrast, family consultation involved the family engaging in individual consultation with a mental health provider. Consultation sessions were conducted either in person or over the telephone and were provided on an as-needed basis up to a maximum of 15 hours of consultation over 3-months. They found that participation in both brief family education and family consultation led to improved self-efficacy concerning the family's ability to successfully manage and cope with their relative's mental illness (Solomon et al., 1996, 1997). Participation did not, however, lead to greater family contact with the mental health services system, suggesting the need to help family members connect with the relative's treatment providers (Solomon et al., 1998).

Spiegel and Wissler (1987) evaluated a family consultation programme in which a consultation team came to the family's home for 4–6 weeks following discharge from an inpatient setting to provide them with education, problem-solving, and crisis intervention skills development. Although conducted with only a small number of families, results show that those whose family received the consultation had fewer days in the hospital, greater use of outpatient services, and better self-reported adjustment than those who did not receive consultation. Although additional research on the impact of family consultation is clearly needed, these studies suggest that family consultation could be useful for some families, particularly in situations where an identified a problem or goal can be addressed in a short period of time.

Shared decision-making and family involvement

Although prior programmes have shown positive outcomes, underutilization of these programmes is common and may arise from a mismatch between consumer and family preferences. One programme that was created to address this issue and to recognize the heterogeneity of consumer preferences is the Recovery-Oriented Decisions for Relatives' Support (REORDER) programme, which utilizes shared decision-making principles to promote recovery and encourage consumers to consider and express preferences for family involvement in care (Dixon et al., 2014). REORDER includes three consumer 50-minute sessions where clients define their recovery goals and consider family involvement, and three family educational sessions where families are provided with support and education to help promote the consumer's recovery goals. In a study conducted by Dixon et al. (2014), 85% of REORDER participants attended at least one consumer session and of those, 59% had at least one family session. At 6 months, participants had reduced paranoid ideation and improvements in ability to ask for help when needed and taking risks to enhance recovery.

Informal family involvement

Although research on the impact of more informal family involvement is limited, more informal family–provider contact may allow for the needs to the family to be addressed in a similar, albeit somewhat diminished or diluted, way to more structured programmes. This involvement may include intermittent telephone contacts with family members, a family member's attendance for part of an individual's treatment session, participation in treatment planning, period family meeting with a provider, or written information or handouts sent or brought home for family members (Drapalski et al., 2009). More informal contact with family members may create opportunities for educating family members on mental illness, its aetiology and its treatment, correcting any misconceptions family members may have regarding the illness, and working collaboratively with family members to identify strategies and develop skills for helping the ill relative cope with the illness, all of which may serve to improve the family relationship and reduce family burden.

Peer-led programmes

In addition to family programmes offered by mental health providers in the clinical context, several peer-led, community-based programmes have also been developed to address the needs of families. Based on theories of stress, coping, and adaptation, the primary goal of these programmes is to improve family outcomes, and, as such, these programmes differ in several ways from the family programmes mentioned earlier (Dixon et al., 2001a). The central feature of peer-led family education programmes, such as the NAMI Family-to-Family education programme and NAMI Homefront, is that they are led by trained family members of individuals with mental illness who have previously completed the programme rather than by clinicians involved in the psychiatric care of the consumer. These programmes tend to be shorter in length (ranging from 6 to 12 weeks), attended by several families at one time, and held in the community (rather than a treatment facility). They aim to provide family members with education on mental illness, mental health treatments, and the mental health services system; to help the family develop skills to help their relative better cope with their illness and the family better cope with stressors that may be associated with their caregiver role; and to offer opportunities for mutual support. Importantly, these programmes provide opportunities for family members to receive support even if a consumer does not provide consent for family services available in the clinical setting or if a consumer is not receiving treatment.

Several studies have evaluated the effectiveness of these community-based, peer-led programmes. Participants in these studies have typically included family members of individuals with a range of serious mental illnesses, such as schizophrenia spectrum disorders, bipolar disorder, and major depression. Participation in peer-led lead family education programmes has been associated with many positive client and family outcomes. Results from seminal uncontrolled and waitlist-control trials of the NAMI Family-to-Family 12 week programme showed a greater sense of empowerment in families (Dixon et al., 2001a, 2004), less displeasure or worry associated with their relative (Dixon et al., 2001a, 2004), more knowledge of mental illness and the mental health care system (Dixon et al., 2004), and improved self-care (Dixon et al., 2004). These effects were sustained at 6-month follow-up (Dixon et al., 2001a, 2004). RCT results also showed significant improvements in empowerment, knowledge, and emotion-focused coping as defined by increased acceptance and problem-solving and reduced distress (Dixon et al., 2011). In addition, a recent study conducted in New York City in a naturalistic setting by Mercado et al. (2016) replicated these results and found additional gains in positive reframing and emotional support.

In response to the effectiveness of these programmes and a need to help military families after the terrorist attacks on 11 September 2001, the NAMI Homefront programme was created for military and veteran families as a six-session programme based on NAMI Family-to-Family that focuses on topics relevant to these individuals, such as post-traumatic stress disorder, traumatic brain injury, anxiety, and depression. It provides an online option in order to increase access for rural and active-duty military families (Haselden et al., 2019). Similar to other Family-to-Family programmes, participants receive information about mental illness and learn coping mechanisms including communication skills and problem-solving, self-care, and crisis planning. Results suggested positive effects on empowerment, distress, family functioning, coping, knowledge of mental illness, and experiences of caregiving that persist 6 weeks after programme completion (Haselden et al., 2019). These effects did not differ by online or in-person modality.

Results from these programmes underscore the importance of peer-led interventions. Some suggest that the impact of these programmes may be due in part to the fact that the information and support is provided by an individual with similar lived experiences (Solomon, 2004). Thus, through shared experience, group leaders may be able to offer families a different and more authentic perspective on the family relationship and caregiver role and provide examples of effective strategies for helping their relative better manage their illness, which may be received more positively by participants and lead to increased confidence in the participants' own ability to successfully cope with a relative's illness (Pickett-Schenk et al., 2006a, 2008; Solomon, 2004). In addition, many mental health education and advocacy organizations such as NAMI (US), Depression and Related Affective Disorders (DRADA; UK), and the National Schizophrenia Fellowship (UK), sponsor or provide information on support groups available to family members. Family support groups often afford family members the opportunity to obtain mutual support and understanding from others who share common experiences. Thus, these groups may be useful for family members who need additional emotional support.

Integrated community models for family involvement

Another approach that has been developed to include family members in clinical care and take patient preferences into consideration is the open dialogue (OD) approach, which is both an integrative therapeutic intervention and way of organizing services for individuals with psychosis (Seikkula et al., 2001). This approach originated in Finland and has been more recently adapted in other European countries, the US, and Australia. OD encourages families to participate in the treatment process immediately after referral to psychiatric services and throughout treatment, preferably in the consumer's home (Freeman et al., 2019; Seikkula et al., 2001). The intervention focuses on fostering dialogue with consumers and social network members rather than on symptom reduction. A review conducted by Lakeman (2014) has suggested that in small cohorts of individuals in Western Lapland, Finland, participation in OD has resulted in reduced duration of untreated psychosis, functional recovery with minimal use of antipsychotics, few residual symptoms, and lack of use of disability benefits.

Another observational study comparing OD participants with first-episode psychosis to a control group consisting of Finnish individuals with first-episode psychosis found no difference between annual incidence of first-episode psychosis, diagnosis, and suicide rates over a 19-year period (Bergström et al., 2018). However, hospitalization duration, disability usage, and need for antipsychotic medications was significantly lower for the OD group (Bergström et al., 2018). A feasibility study conducted with individuals with first-episode psychosis in the US found that OD was successfully integrated into clinical services with good client engagement, high client satisfaction and perceptions of shared decision-making, and improvements in symptoms and functioning (Gordon et al., 2016). Although these results have been promising, a recent review by Freeman et al. (2019) suggested that quantitative and qualitative studies have lacked methodological rigour and have a high risk of bias. Therefore, there is a need for more randomized control trials in this area.

Addressing barriers to family involvement

Although many programmes have been developed for families, as little as 8–15% of families participate in formal family programmes (Dixon et al., 1999; Magliano et al., 2006; Resnick et al., 2005). A number of system/provider, consumer, and family-related barriers may prevent family members from participation in these programmes and make participation impractical or impossible (Luckstead et al., 2012). Additionally, a mismatch between consumer and family preferences could contribute to underutilization of family programmes or a consumer may not provide consent for families to participate in clinical services. In a Veterans Affairs Family Forum, several factors to improve family involvement were identified including leadership support, training in FPE for clinical staff, adequate resources to implement psychoeducation including flexible work hours and funding for implementation, and complementary strategies to involve family members in care for whom FPE may not be appropriate (Cohen et al., 2008). Efforts have been made to address these problems including development of REORDER, peer-led programmes, and programmes that offer a more flexible online format to reach a wider array of families such as NAMI Homefront; however, more implementation research is needed. Additionally, more research is needed regarding engagement factors across different ethnic groups, age, and socioeconomic status (Luckstead et al., 2012).

Conclusion

Families often require considerable information, education, skills, and support to minimize the additional burden that may come with caring for an individual with serious mental illness and help them support their relative in their mental illness recovery. Several programmes aimed at providing family members and caregivers of individuals with serious mental illness with the information and education, skills, and support they need to support an ill relative have been developed. While research suggests that longer FPE programmes may produce the best outcomes, briefer programmes such as brief family education and family consultation as well as family involvement in ongoing care or treatment have also proven beneficial and may be preferable for some families. By helping consumers and family members to consider ways to involve family in treatment and explore options concerning family programmes, mental health providers can better determine which of these programmes would best address the needs and potentially produce the most positive outcomes for each family.

REFERENCES

Anderson, C. M., Reiss, D. J., & Hogarty, G. E. (1986). *Schizophrenia and the Family*. New York: Guilford Press.

Baucom, D. H., Shoham, V., Mueser, K. T., Daiuto, A. D., & Stickle, T. R. (1998). Empirically supported couple and family interventions for marital distress and adult mental health problems. *Journal of Consulting and Clinical Psychology*, **66**, 53–58.

Bebbington, P. & Kuipers, L. (1994). The clinical utility of expressed emotion in schizophrenia. *Acta Psychiatrica Scandinavica*, **382**, 46–53.

Bergström, T., Seikkula, J., Alakare, B., Mäki, P., Köngäs-Saviaro, P., Taskila, J. J., et al. (2018). The family-oriented open dialogue approach in the treatment of first-episode psychosis: nineteen-year outcomes. *Psychiatry Research*, **270**, 168–175.

Chien, W. T., Chan, S. W. C., Thompson, D. R. (2006). Effects of a mutual support group for families of Chinese people with schizophrenia: 18 month follow-up. *British Journal of Psychiatry*, **189**, 41–49.

Chien, W. T. & Lee, I. Y. L. (2010). The schizophrenia care management program for family caregivers of Chinese patient with schizophrenia. *Psychiatric Services*, 61, 317–320.

Cohen, A. N., Glynn, S. M., Murray-Swank, A., Barrio, C., Fischer, E. P. McCutcheon, S. I., et al. (2008). The family forum: directions for the implementation of family psychoeducation for severe mental illness. *Psychiatric Services*, 59, 40–48.

Cuijpers, P. (1999). The effects of family intervention on relatives' burden: a meta-analysis. *Journal of Mental Health*, 8, 275–285.

Dixon, L. B., Dickerson, F., Bellack, A. S., Bennett, M., Dickinson, D., Goldberg, R. W., et al. (2010). The 2009 Schizophrenia PORT psychosocial treatment recommendations and summary statements. *Schizophrenia Bulletin*, 36, 48–70.

Dixon, L. B., Glynn, S. M., Cohen, A. N., Drapalski, A. L., Medoff, D., Fang, L. J., et al. (2014). Outcomes of a brief program, REORDER, to promote consumer recovery and family involvement in care. *Psychiatric Services*, 65, 116–120.

Dixon, L. B., Lucksted, A., Medoff, D. R., Burland, J., Stewart, B., Lehman, A. F., et al. (2011). Outcomes of a randomized study of a peer-taught family-to-family education program for mental illness. *Psychiatric Services*, 62, 591–597.

Dixon, L., Lucksted, A., Stewart, B., Burland, J., Brown, C. H., Postrado, L., et al. (2004). Outcomes of the peer-taught 12-week family-to-family education program for severe mental illness. *Acta Psychiatrica Scandinavica*, 109, 207–215.

Dixon, L., Lyles, A., Scott, J., Lehman, A., Postrado, L., Goldman, H., et al. (1999). Services to families of adults with schizophrenia: from treatment recommendations to dissemination. *Psychiatric Services*, 50, 233–238.

Dixon, L., McFarlane, W. R., Lefley, H., Lucksted, A., Cohen, M., Falloon, I., et al. (2001b). Evidence-based practices for services to families of people with psychiatric disabilities. *Psychiatric Services*, 52, 903–910.

Dixon, L., Stewart, B., Burland, J., Delahanty, J., Lucksted, A., & Hoffman, M. (2001a). Pilot study of the effectiveness of the family-to-family education program. *Psychiatric Services*, 52, 965–967.

Drapalski, A. L., Marshall, T., Seybolt, D., Medoff, D., Peer, J., Leith, J., et al. (2008). The unmet needs of families of adults with mental illness and preferences regarding family services. *Psychiatric Services*, 59, 655–662.

Drapalski, A. L., Leith, J., & Dixon, L. (2009). Involving families in the care of persons with schizophrenia and other serious mental illnesses: history, evidence, and recommendations. *Clinical Schizophrenia and Related Psychosis*, 3, 39–49.

Dyck, D., Short, R., Hendryx, M., Norell, D., Myers, M., Patterson, T., et al. (2000). Management of negative symptoms among patients with schizophrenia attending multiple-family groups. *Psychiatric Services*, 51, 513–519.

Emanuaels-Zuurveen, L. & Emmelkamp, P. M. G. (1997). Spouse-aided therapy with depressed patients. *Behavior Modification*, 21, 62–77.

Falloon, I. R. H., Boyd, J., & McGill, C. (1984). *Family Care of Schizophrenia*. New York: Guilford Press.

Falloon, I. R., Boyd, J. L., McGill, C. W. Williamson, M., Razani, J., Moss, H. B., et al. (1985). Family management in the prevention of morbidity of schizophrenia: clinical outcome of a two-year longitudinal study. *Archives of General Psychiatry*, 42, 887–896.

Falloon, I. R. & Pederson, J. (1985). Family management in the prevention of morbidity of schizophrenia: the adjustment of the family unit. *British Journal of Psychiatry*, 147, 156–163.

Family Institute for Education, Practice and Research & New York State Office of Mental Health (2007). Competency training in consumer centered family consultation (Unpublished manuscript). Department of Psychiatry, University of Rochester, Rochester, NY.

Freeman, A. M., Tribe, R. H., Stott, J. C., & Pilling, S. (2019). Open dialogue: a review of the evidence. *Psychiatric Services*, 70, 46–59.

Gordon, C., Gidugu, V., Rogers, E. S., DeRonck, J., & Ziedonis, D. (2016). Adapting open dialogue for early-onset psychosis into the US health care environment: a feasibility study. *Psychiatric Services*, 67, 1166–1168.

Hackman, A. & Dixon, L. (2008). Issues in family services for persons with schizophrenia. *Psychiatric Times*, 25, 1–2.

Haselden, M., Brister, T., Robinson, S., Covell, N., Pauselli, L., & Dixon, L. (2019). Effectiveness of the NAMI Homefront program for military and veteran families: in-person and online benefits. *Psychiatric Services*, 70, 935–939.

Hatfield A. B. (1978). Psychological costs of schizophrenia to the family. *Social Work*, 23, 355–359.

Hazel, N. A., McDonell, M. G., Short, R. A., Berry, C. M. Voss, W. D., Rodgers, M. I., et al. (2004). Impact of multiple-family groups for outpatients with schizophrenia on caregiver's distress and resources. *Psychiatric Services*, 55, 34–41.

Lakeman, R. (2014). The Finnish open dialogue approach to crisis intervention in psychosis: a review. *Psychotherapy in Australia*, 20, 28–35.

Leff, J., Vearnals, S., Brewin, C. R., Wolff, G., Alexander, B., Asen, E., et al. (2000). Randomized controlled trial of antidepressants v. couple therapy in the treatment and maintenance of people with depression living with a partner: clinical outcome and costs. *British Journal of Psychiatry*, 177, 95–100.

Lefley, H. P. (1989). Family burden and family stigma in major mental illness. *American Psychologist*, 44, 556–560.

Lerner, D., Chang, H., Rogers, W. H., Benson, C., Lyson, M. C., & Dixon, L. B. (2018). Psychological distress among caregivers of individuals with a diagnosis of schizophrenia or schizoaffective disorder. *Psychiatric Services*, 69, 169–178.

Lucksted, A., McFarlane, W., Downing, D., & Dixon, L. (2012). Recent developments in family psychoeducation as an evidence-based practice. *Journal of Marital and Family Therapy*, 38, 101–121.

Lyman, D. R., Braude, L., George, P., Dougherty, R. H., Daniels, A. S., Ghose, S. S., & Delphin-Rittmon, M. E. (2014). Consumer and family psychoeducation: assessing the evidence. *Psychiatric Services*, 65, 416–428.

Magliano, L., Fiorillo, A., Malangone, C., De Rosa, C., & Maj, M. (2006). Patient functioning and family burden in a controlled, real-world trial of family psychoeducation for schizophrenia. *Psychiatric Services*, 57, 1784–1791.

McFarlane, W. R. (2002). *Multifamily Groups in the Treatment of Severe Psychiatric Disorders*. New York: Guilford Press.

McFarlane, W. R. (2016). Family interventions for schizophrenia and the psychoses: a review. *Family Process*, 55, 460–482.

McFarlane, W. R., Dixon, L., Lukens, E., & Lucksted, A. (2003). Family psychoeducation and schizophrenia: a review of the literature. *Journal of Marital Therapy*, 29, 223–245.

McFarlane, W. R., Dushay, R. A., Stastny, P., Deakins, S. M., & Link, B. (1996). A comparison of two levels of family-aided assertive community treatment. *Psychiatric Services*, 47, 744–750.

McFarlane W. R., Dushay, R. A., Deakins, S. M., Stastny, P., Lukens, E. P., Toran, J., et al. (2000). Employment outcomes in family-aided assertive community treatment. *American Journal of Orthopsychiatry*, 70, 203–214.

Mercado, M., Fuss, A. A., Sawano, N., Gensemer, A., Brennan, W., McManus, K., et al. (2016). Generalizability of the NAMI family-to-family education program: evidence from an efficacy study. *Psychiatric Services*, **67**, 591–593.

Merinder, L. B., Viuff, A. G., Laugensen, H. D., Clemmensen, K., Misfelt, S., & Espensen, B. (1999). Patient and relative education in community psychiatry: a randomized controlled trial regarding its effectiveness. *Social Psychiatry and Psychiatric Epidemiology*, **34**, 287–294.

Miklowitz, D. J., George, E. L., Richards, J. A., Simoneau, T. L., & Suddath, R. L. (2003). A randomized study of family-focused psychoeducation and pharmacotherapy in the outpatient management of bipolar disorder. *Archives of General Psychiatry*, **60**, 904–912.

Miklowitz, D. J. & Goldstein, M. J. (1997). *A Family-Focused Treatment Approach*. New York: Guilford Press.

Miklowitz, D. J., Goldstein, M. J., Nuechterlein, K. H., Snyder, K. S., & Mintz, J. (1988). Family factors and the course of bipolar affective disorder. *Archives of General Psychiatry*, **45**, 225–231.

Montero, I., Asencio, A., Hernandez, I., Masanet, M. S. J., Lacruz, M., Bellver, F., et al. (2001). Two strategies for family intervention in schizophrenia: a randomized trial in a mediterranean environment. *Schizophrenia Bulletin*, **27**, 661–670.

Mueser, K. T. & Glynn, S. M. (1999). *Behavioral Family Therapy for Psychiatric Disorders* (2nd ed.). Oakland, CA: New Harbinger Publications.

Murray-Swank, A. & Dixon, L. (2005). Evidence based practices for working with families of individuals with serious mental illness. In: Drake, R., Merrens, M., & Lynde, D. (Eds.), *Evidence-Based Mental Health Practice: A Textbook* (pp. 424–52). New York: W. W. Norton and Company.

Murray-Swank, A., Glynn, S., Cohen, A. N., Sherman, M., Medoff, D. P., Fang, L. J., et al. (2007). Family contact, experience of family relationships, and views about family involvement in treatment among VA consumers with serious mental illness. *Journal of Rehabilitation Research and Development*, **44**, 801–812.

Pfammatter, M., Junghan, U. M., & Brenner, H. D. (2006). Efficacy of psychological therapy in schizophrenia: conclusions from meta-analyses. *Schizophrenia Bulletin*, **32**(Suppl. 1), S64–S80.

Pharoah, F., Mari, J. J., Rathbone, J., & Wong, W. (2010). Family intervention for schizophrenia. *Cochrane Database of Systematic Reviews*, **12**, CD000088.

Pickett-Schenk, S. A., Bennett, C., Cook, J. A., Steigman, P., Lippincott, R., Villagracia, I., et al. (2006b). Changes in caregiving satisfaction and information needs among relatives of adults with mental illness: results of a randomized evaluation of a family-led education intervention. *American Journal of Orthopsychiatry*, **76**, 545–553.

Pickett-Schenk, S. A., Cook, J. A., Steigman, P., Lippencott, R., Bennett, C., & Grey, D. D. (2006a). Psychological well-being and relationship outcomes in a randomized study of family-led education. *Archives of General Psychiatry*, **63**, 1043–1050.

Pickett-Schenk, S. A., Lippincott, R. C., Bennett, C., & Steigman, P. J. (2008). Improving knowledge about mental illness through family-led education: the journey of hope. *Psychiatric Services*, **59**, 49–56.

Pitschel-Walz, G., Bauml, J., Bender, W., Engel, R. R., Wagner, M., & Kissling, W. (2006). Psychoeducation and compliance in the treatment of schizophrenia: results of the Munich Psychosis Information Project Study. *Journal of Clinical Psychiatry*, **67**, 443–452.

Pitschel-Walz, G., Leucht, S., Bauml, J., Kissling, W., & Engel, R. R. (2001). The effect of family interventions on relapse and rehospitalization in schizophrenia-a meta-analysis. *Schizophrenia Bulletin*, **21**, 73–92.

Posner, C. M., Wilson, K. G., Kral, M. J., Lander, S., & McIlwraith, R. D. (1992). Family psychoeducational support groups in schizophrenia. *American Journal of Orthopsychiatry*, **62**, 206–218.

Rea, M. M., Tompson, M. C., Miklowitz, D. J., Goldstein, M. J., Hwang, S., & Mintz, J. (2003). Family-focused treatment versus individual treatment for bipolar disorder: results of a randomized clinical trial. *Journal of Consulting and Clinical Psychology*, **71**, 482–492.

Resnick, S. G., Rosenheck, R. A., Dixon, L., & Lehman, A. F. (2005). Correlates of family contact with the mental health system: allocation of a scarce resource. *Mental Health Services Research*, **7**, 113–121.

Resnick, S. G., Rosenheck, R. A., & Lehman, A. F. (2004). An exploratory analysis of correlates of recovery. *Psychiatric Services*, **55**, 540–547.

Seikkula, J., Alakare, B., & Aaltonen, J. (2001). Open dialogue in psychosis I: an introduction and case illustration. *Journal of Constructivist Psychology*, **14**, 247–265.

Smith, G. C. (2003). Patterns and predictors of service use and unmet needs among aging families of adults with severe mental illness. *Psychiatric Services*, **4**, 871–877.

Solomon, P. (2004). Peer support/peer provided services underlying processes, benefits, and critical ingredients. *Psychiatric Rehabilitation Journal*, **25**, 281–288.

Solomon, P., Draine, J., Mannion, E., & Meisel, M. (1996). Impact of brief family psychoeducation on self-efficacy. *Schizophrenia Bulletin*, **22**, 41–50.

Solomon, P., Draine, J., Mannion, E., & Meisel, M. (1997). Effectiveness of two models of brief family education: retention of gains by family members of adults with serious mental illness. *American Journal of Orthopsychiatry*, **67**, 177–186.

Solomon, P., Draine, J., Mannion, E., & Meisel, M. (1998). Increased contact with community mental health resources as a potential benefit of family education. *Psychiatric Services*, **49**, 333–339.

Spaniol, L. & Nelson, A. (2015). Family recovery. *Community Mental Health Journal*, **51**, 761–767.

Spiegel, D. & Wissler, T. (1987). Using family consultation as psychiatric aftercare for schizophrenic patients. *Hospital and Community Psychiatry*, **38**, 1096–1099.

Winefield, H. & Harvey, E. (1994). Needs of family caregivers in chronic schizophrenia. *Schizophrenia Bulletin*, **20**, 557–566.

World Schizophrenia Fellowship (1998). *Families as Partners in Care: A Document Developed to Launch a Strategy for the Implementation of Family Education, Training, and Support*. Toronto: World Schizophrenia Fellowship.

Xiong, W., Phillips, M. R., Hu, X., Wang, R., Dai, Q., Kleinman, J., & Kleinman, A. (1994). Family-based intervention for schizophrenic patients in China: a randomized controlled trial. *British Journal of Psychiatry*, **165**, 239–247.

22

Managing co-occurring physical disorders in mental health care

Delia C. Hendrick and Robert E. Drake

Introduction

Over centuries, ancient philosophers, historians, and physicians recognized that the health of the mind and body were intimately connected. However, Western medicine development led to an artificial separation of the two, attempting to isolate, name, and understand conditions and find specific, evidence-based treatments. The success of this effort in Western medicine also meant that physical and mental health increasingly represented separate entities, studied and addressed in separate systems of care, competing for attention at the level of the system, individual, and provider. Today, the drive to reunify them confronts many barriers at the level of the society and the individual.

Individuals with any mental illness have increased rates of medical comorbidity, especially, people with serious mental illness (SMI)—which refers to schizophrenia, bipolar disorder, severe depression, and any other severe and disabling psychiatric illness. The increased medical comorbidity refers both to increased odds of using acute medical services (Himelhoch et al., 2004) and increased rates of chronic medical illnesses. In fact, many common chronic medical conditions have elevated prevalence and may develop at a younger age in people with mental illness; certain conditions are particularly prevalent (Table 22.1).

Bidirectional relationships exist between specific conditions, such as between depression and coronary heart disease (Fang et al., 2020; DeHert et al., 2018; Y. Wang et al., 2018; Wium-Andersen et al., 2020), between depression and diabetes (Sherwood et al., 2011), and between anxiety disorders and asthma or heart disease (Emdin et al., 2016; Tully et al., 2015).

Physical disorders account for high morbidity, high mortality, and earlier death for people with *psychosis*, compared to the general population (Chang et al., 2011; Heiberg et al., 2018; Hjorthøj et al., 2017; Kilbourne et al., 2009; Lawrence et al., 2013; Nordentoft et al., 2013; Ösby et al., 2016; Saha et al., 2007). A major part of this increased morbidity and mortality is due to cardiovascular and metabolic disorders, including heart disease, diabetes, hyperlipidaemia, and obesity (Correll et al., 2014; Foguet-Boreu et al., 2016; Lieberman et al., 2005; Meyer et al., 2005; Stubbs et al., 2015; Vancampfort et al., 2016). Compared to the general population, people with schizophrenia have significantly higher rates of respiratory disorders, probably due to the large prevalence of smoking as well as the vulnerability to pneumonia imparted by antipsychotics and premature aging (Suetani et al., 2021). In addition to metabolic, cardiovascular, and respiratory disorders, people with *bipolar*

Table 22.1 Common medical comorbidities in specific mental illnesses

Mental illness	Medical comorbidity
Schizophrenia/psychosis/bipolar disorders	Metabolic diseases (obesity, diabetes) Cardiovascular disease Chronic respiratory disorders (e.g. chronic obstructive pulmonary disease) Gastrointestinal disorders HIV infection Hepatitis C infection
Depression	Metabolic diseases (diabetes, hyperlipidaemia) Pain conditions Neurological disorders
Anxiety disorders	Asthma Cardiovascular disease
Tobacco use disorder	Cancer Chronic respiratory illnesses Cardiovascular disease
Alcohol use disorder	Cardiovascular disease (cardiomyopathy, atrial fibrillation) neurological disorders (neuropathy, Wernicke–Korsakoff encephalopathy) Liver disease Pancreatitis Cancer (digestive, lung, and breast cancers)
Cannabis use disorder	Cardiovascular disease Stroke
Intravenous drug use (opioids/stimulants)	HIV infection Hepatitis C infection Acute infectious syndromes (subacute bacterial endocarditis, abscesses) Acute cardiovascular disease (strokes, myocardial infarction, sudden death) overdose deaths

disorder are at high risk also for migraine headache, thyroid disease, and osteoarthritis (Forty et al., 2014).

People with *unipolar depressive disorders* may also have elevated metabolic risk, as well as higher risk for pain conditions and for neurological disorders (Amiri et al., 2019; Cai et al., 2019; Kim et al., 2018; Stubbs et al., 2017b; S. Wang et al., 2018), while people with *anxiety disorders* have increased prevalence of asthma and cardiovascular disease (Batelaan et al., 2014; Vogelzangs et al., 2010). People with *substance use disorders* (SUDs) have increased rates of medical pathology specific to the substance and modality of use, with the most severe complications, including overdose deaths, associated with intravenous drug use. Chronic pain is common among people with drug use disorders, sometimes triggering a drug use disorder or developing as a comorbidity.

Tobacco smoking remains the leading cause of preventable death in the general population in the US. People with any mental illness are more likely to use nicotine than those in the general population, and people with schizophrenia are likely to smoke more cigarettes a day and are less likely to quit and stay quit (Cook et al., 2014; Ziedonis et al., 2008). One-third of all cancer deaths, and many chronic respiratory illnesses, cardiovascular illnesses, and deaths are attributable to smoking (Centers for Disease Control and Prevention, n.d.).

Alcohol use disorders, which are more prevalent in people with depressive disorders, anxiety disorders, or schizophrenia, represent an additional risk factor for suicide (McHugh et al., 2019) and are also associated with many types of physical illnesses in a dose-dependent manner (Table 22.1).

As legal *cannabis* has been increasingly available, cannabis use has increased (Compton et al., 2019), and emerging data suggest an associated increase in cardiovascular disease (especially haemorrhagic strokes in women) (Auger et al., 2020). The association with respiratory diseases is controversial.

As consequences of high rates of medical comorbidity, people with mental illness, especially those with comorbid SUDs, may experience reduced physical functioning, early institutionalization in nursing homes, worse mental health outcomes, lower quality of life, and early mortality, especially cardiovascular mortality. In particular, people with SMI, compared to people of the same age without mental illness, have 10–15-year shorter life spans (Crump et al., 2013; Lawrence et al., 2013; Walker et al., 2015). Morbidity, disability, and early mortality in people with SMI resemble the health of people much older in the general population.

Reasons for medical morbidity and early mortality

Poor medical health and early mortality among individuals with mental illness are due to several factors, summarized in Table 22.2 and described in detail below.

Genetic risks

Studies of early psychosis in schizophrenia patients show that these individuals have a higher likelihood of having diabetes mellitus and metabolic abnormalities at the time of their first presentation and prior to treatment (De Hert et al., 2006; Lang et al., 2021; Verma et al., 2009). This finding may indicate a common genetic vulnerability and may also explain the observed increased risk of people with schizophrenia to develop cardiovascular disease. Some genetic studies have provided additional support for a potential common genetic predisposition for schizophrenia and diabetes mellitus (Postolache et al., 2019*)*, but large data from genome-wide analysis have not found evidence of shared genetics between schizophrenia and cardiovascular disease (Veeneman et al., 2021). Other genome-wide studies have found that genetic vulnerability to depression was associated with higher coronary artery disease and myocardial infarction risks, partly mediated by type 2 diabetes mellitus and smoking (Lu et al., 2021).

Genetic factors implicated in elevated risk for mental illness are also associated with elevated risk of SUDs, which explains in part the high comorbidity observed between the two conditions. For example, the 5HTTLPR polymorphism in the serotonin transporter gene was associated with higher risk for both major depressive disorder and alcohol dependence (Oo et al., 2016).

Social determinants of health

Chronic, pervasive, socioeconomic stress has been associated in other populations with premature ageing, likely due to increased allostatic load as measured by several cardiovascular, metabolic, and inflammatory biomarkers (Bird et al., 2010; Geronimus et al., 2006). Links between stress, shortened telomeres, and psychopathology potentially run across generations (Epel et al., 2018). People with SMI experience pervasive stress, such as poverty, isolation, unemployment, homelessness, incarceration, and overt or subtle chronic stigma and discrimination, in addition to the suffering of being unwell mentally and physically. In the US, one aspect of chronic stress involves criminal justice system involvement. Many people with SMI have been sent to jail or prison for minor crimes during the US era of mass incarceration, and about 50% of patients in community mental health centres now have justice-system involvement (Anderson et al., 2015; Robertson et al., 2014). In the US, people of colour, those from ethnic minorities, and other stigmatized groups have suffered disproportionately (Hinton et al., 2018; Mahaffey et al., 2018). Structural racism, embedded in the economic

Table 22.2 Causes of medical morbidity and early mortality

Genetic or epigenetic	Genetic or illness-related vulnerabilities
Societal harm/social determinants of health	Poverty Stigma and discrimination Unemployment Homelessness
Health care behaviours	Unhealthy diet Reduced physical activity Alcohol, nicotine, and drug toxicity
Medication side effects	Endocrine and metabolic (obesity, diabetes mellitus, hyperlipidaemia, hyperprolactinaemia, osteoporosis) Cardiovascular (coronary artery disease, stroke, sudden death) Neurological (extrapyramidal symptoms, tardive dyskinesia)
Inadequate medical care	Reduced access to health care Reduced quality of health care Inattention to physical health Misattribution of symptoms
Violent premature death	Suicide Accidents, violence, overdoses

system as well as in cultural and societal norms in the US, reinforces discriminatory beliefs, values, and distribution of resources, affecting all aspects of health care (Bailey et al., 2017, 2021).

Over the course of a lifetime, these factors converge to produce premature ageing, high medical burden, and early mortality. These vulnerabilities underline the importance of addressing social determinants of health, primary and secondary prevention health improvement programmes, early mental illness screening, and treatment adhering to the standard of care for chronic illness management for people with SMI.

Health care behaviours

People with mental illness, in particular SMI, tend to have sedentary lifestyles and diets with higher calorie and sodium intake (Teasdale et al., 2019), which are risk factors for obesity, hyperlipidaemia, diabetes mellitus, and cardiovascular disease. Contributors to inactivity and unhealthy diets are features of specific mental illnesses (such as negative symptoms of schizophrenia, avoidance behaviours of anxiety, and low motivation of depressive disorders), side effects of treatment (such as sedation), in addition to restricted access to healthy diets and exercise due to poverty, social isolation, and unemployment.

The elevated rates of comorbid drug use in people with any mental illness, including high rates of nicotine, alcohol, and other drug use, represent other critical risk factors for high morbidity and early mortality. In the US, people with all disabilities have high rates of what are called 'deaths of despair': deaths due to alcohol and drug toxicity and suicide (Olfson et al., 2021).

Health care behaviours are difficult to address in the general population and in people with mental illness, but effective interventions promoting physical activity and healthy diets can be integrated into comprehensive and concomitant treatments addressing comorbidities, including SUDs (Bartels et al., 2018).

Medication side effects

Psychiatric medications, although an important part of treatment, can contribute to medical morbidity and mortality.

Most second-generation antipsychotics can produce hypercholesterolaemia, hypertriglyceridaemia, diabetes, and significant weight gain (Barton et al., 2020), but metabolic complications can occur even in the absence of weight gain. Different antipsychotics have different metabolic profiles, and people respond differently to individual medications. These effects can be magnified during concomitant treatment with other medications that have similar side effects, such as lithium, valproate, or depot progesterone.

Occasionally, the onset of marked increases in lipids and/or blood sugar after the start of an antipsychotic has led to life-threatening complications such as acute pancreatitis due to severe hypertriglyceridaemia (risk high with triglyceride level >1000 mg/dL) or diabetic ketoacidosis (Jin et al., 2002; Koller et al., 2003; Wilson et al., 2003). In addition to producing metabolic conditions and increasing the risk for coronary artery disease and cardiovascular events, antipsychotics have been implicated in an increase in cardiac sudden death of unclear aetiology, possibly related to QTc prolongation (Ray et al., 2009).

Mood stabilizers are effective treatments for stabilization of acute depression and mania episodes as well as for episode prevention. They are associated with specific well-known medical complications and require screening, monitoring, and awareness of multiple medication interactions. Lithium is associated with numerous potential side effects such as diarrhoea, polyuria, increased thirst, and enuresis, whereas valproate is associated with increased sedation and infection. Both can be associated with weight gain (Cipriani et al., 2013; Macritchie et al., 2013).

Many side effects of medications, particularly sexual side effects, weight gain, extrapyramidal symptoms, drowsiness and fatigue, hair loss, or acne, decrease medication adherence (Ashoorian et al., 2015; Dibonaventura et al., 2012; Mercke et al., 2000; Perkins, 2002). Some side effects—such as sedation, gastrointestinal side effects, dizziness, etc.—contribute to low function, unemployment, and lower quality of life (Keefe et al., 2020). These non-life-threatening side effects tend to be ignored by medical professionals, and people who experience such side effects may feel that the medical professional ignores them and may resort to discontinuing the medications to eliminate the interference with things that are important to them (Deegan, 2005).

Psychiatric providers must actively manage side effects of medications by choosing the medication carefully to start with, by systematically using a process of shared decision-making (SDM), by maintaining a prescribing style that minimizes type of medication used, doses and interactions, systematic deprescribing, awareness and monitoring of individual response, systematic screening for, and treating the side effects, following guidelines, and providing and advocating for quality care.

Inadequate medical care

Although 50% of psychiatric patients have known medical problems and another 35% suffer from previously unidentified medical problems, people with SMI tend to receive inadequate medical care. Regardless of access to care, people with SMI have a decreased likelihood of receiving preventive care, treatment for the conditions they have, and needed specialized medical procedures (Druss et al., 2000; Roberts et al., 2007).

In the US, the CATIE trials identified rates of non-treatment of 30% for diabetes, 60% for hypertension, and almost 90% for dyslipidaemia in people with schizophrenia (Nasrallah, 2006). A large meta-analysis of studies across the world looking at cardiovascular disease screening and treatment in people with mental disorders found significant disparities for screening, any intervention, and treatment with specific medications for cardiovascular disorders across all mental disorders (except for cardiovascular medications in mood disorders). Disparities were largest for schizophrenia, although they differed across countries (Solmi et al., 2021).

An abundance of guidelines addressing metabolic comorbidity and monitoring parameters exists, but the uptake in routine clinical practice has been slow (American Diabetes Association et al., 2004; Cohn & Sernyak, 2006; Yatham et al., 2018). Taking responsibility for the treatment of metabolic conditions is one barrier. Many psychiatrists are uncomfortable treating physical conditions, while many general medical providers are uncomfortable interacting with SMI patients and using antipsychotic medications.

While stigma and a tendency to explain the clinical picture with one diagnosis only (Jones et al., 2008) (usually mental illness or SUD in the case of comorbidity) are important additional deterrents, health care system factors such as lack of access and fragmentation present additional barriers to care. Individuals with co-occurring conditions often experience uncoordinated care resulting in lower quality of care, poor health outcomes, and higher health care costs (Frandsen et al., 2015; Walker et al., 2015). In the US, for example, the medical and psychiatric systems of care are generally separated through training, geographical/physical setting, medical records systems, and insurance coverage. The subsequent communication and coordination difficulties are significant barriers to care, especially for people with comorbid psychiatric and medical illness. While best methods to integrate care are still debated, co-ordinated and integrated medical and psychiatric care is better care; achieving it should be an important goal in every system.

Violent premature death

The common problems of suicides, accidents, violence, and overdoses related to substance abuse are discussed in another chapter.

Intervention approaches

In this section, we review interventions to improve physical health and decrease the risk of early mortality in people with mental illness. All such interventions emphasize prevention. Because people with mental illness are at increased risk for developing a variety of medical conditions, effective treatment starts with primary prevention (intervening before the medical condition appears) by addressing smoking, diet, sedentarism, substance use, oral health, vaccinations, and age-appropriate and common medical conditions screening, immediately upon recognition of mental illness. When a medical condition appears, secondary prevention includes evidence-based practices to identify the medical condition in the earliest stages and prevent its progression: for example, patient and provider education, medication change, lifestyle improvements, and treating SUDs (including nicotine use disorders). Tertiary prevention (meant to help people live with the comorbidity, prevent exacerbations, and limit the negative consequences) addresses self-management of chronic disorders, social supports, and lifestyle issues to prevent disability (Drake & Bond, 2021).

These interventions, all aimed to improve care of people with mental illness by preventing and treating medical comorbidity, can be grouped by their focus on patients, providers, or systems (Table 22.3). We detail several interventions below.

Shared decision-making

One important goal is helping people become more knowledgeable and more active in choosing and monitoring their own medications or other treatment interventions, termed SDM (Deegan & Drake, 2006). People with mental illness should be involved in the process of SDM in all aspects of care. SDM increases the quality of decisions (knowledge, participation, and congruence with values) (Beebe et al., 2005; Drake & Deegan, 2009; Malm et al., 2003; Priebe et al., 2007) and perhaps medication adherence because people may tolerate some side effects when they have a choice through SDM. Specific SDM interventions addressing paired clinician and patient teams improve SDM and patient-perceived quality of care (Alegria et al., 2018).

Metabolic screening

Many organizations have issued guidelines for routine monitoring of metabolic, endocrinological, and cardiac side effects (American

Table 22.3 Recommendations to improve physical health and longevity

1. Patient-centred interventions	SDM for choosing psychiatric treatment, according to individual goals and side effects tolerance
	Access to evidence-based, most effective treatments
	Health improvement interventions to focus on diet and exercise
	Smoking cessation programmes[a]
	Integrated dual diagnosis interventions[a]
2. Provider-centred interventions	Provider education and support: • Increase awareness of metabolic and other medical risk • Guidelines for monitoring and screening • Establishing standards of care for people with mental illness • Increase psychiatric providers comfort with treating metabolic conditions and using psychotropic medications according to the SDM process, and ongoing risk evaluation
	Supporting metabolic monitoring (systems of reminders, access to labs and lab results, etc.)
	Advocating for treatment of known medical conditions according to standards of care in the general population
3. System-centred interventions	Ensure access to prevention, primary care, and specialty care
	Connect medical care and mental health care (using appropriate staff and technology)
	Integrate social care and medical/mental health care
	Address social determinants of health with evidence-based practices, such as supported employment

[a] These interventions are addressed in other chapters in this textbook.

Diabetes Association et al., 2004; Cohn & Sernyak, 2006; Cordes et al., 2008; Marder et al., 2002). Metabolic monitoring includes monitoring of weight, body mass index, waist circumference, fasting glucose, haemoglobin A1c, and lipids. Most measures should begin at baseline and repeat at variable intervals: from 4 to 12 weeks to at least once a year after initiation or change in antipsychotic treatment, often with increasing frequency of monitoring if patients are at higher risk. Providers should maintain awareness of the need for monitoring, from the very first few weeks of a new antipsychotic treatment and for the duration of the antipsychotic treatment. System improvements, such as registries, automated reminders of screening measures, and leadership support, can support screening (Melamed et al., 2019).

Weight management interventions

Obesity and metabolic diseases have become widespread in developed countries in the general population, and they disproportionately affect people with mental illness. Interventions for weight management in the general population have focused on diet, exercise, pharmacology, and bariatric surgery. All interventions have in common modest, short-term, highly variable results in the general population (Ward et al., 2015), and they are less studied in people with mental illness. Importantly, attaining a normal weight is unnecessary to reduce metabolic risk: a 5% reduction in weight has benefits on blood sugar and lipid levels and can therefore ameliorate cardiovascular risk (Franz et al., 2015).

Poor diet and sedentarism are well-recognized risk factors, and nutritious diet and regular exercise have benefits to health well beyond weight loss (Jerome et al., 2017; Posadzki et al., 2020), including in people with mental illness, even in prevention and treatment of various psychopathologies (Ashdown-Franks et al., 2020; Morres et al., 2019; Stubbs et al., 2017a). Diet interventions may be associated with weight loss, and in people with SMI appear to be more effective when closer to antipsychotic initiation (Teasdale et al., 2017). For people with mental illness, interventions focused on diet and exercise reduce or prevent weight gain in the short-term (Faulkner & Cohn, 2006; Faulkner et al., 2007; Loh et al., 2006). Maintenance of results in the long term has not been assessed in people with mental illness, but likelihood of maintaining the weight loss in the long term is low in the general population. Some degree of weight loss and increase in physical activity achieved during intensive interventions appear to maintain 6 years later (Fothergill et al., 2016).

To implement a habit involving regular physical activity in people with mental illness, interventions have used geographic planning, cognitive behavioural therapy focused on changing behaviours, addressing motivation, and pairing exercise with incentives and socialization (Alvarez-Jimenez et al., 2008; Bartels et al., 2015; Naslund et al., 2017; Romain et al., 2020).

Pharmacological interventions for weight management in people with SMI have focused on changing antipsychotics, switching from polypharmacy to monotherapy, and adding specific medications to promote weight loss or prevent weight gain. Changing antipsychotics can alleviate metabolic risk. Switching from a high metabolic risk to a low metabolic risk antipsychotic has correlated with improved prevalence of metabolic syndrome, weight maintenance or loss, and cardiovascular risk decrease of 13–33% (Meyer, 2002; Meyer et al., 2005; Ried et al., 2003, 2006; Rosenheck et al., 2009; Sisking et al., 2021). The American Diabetes Association recommends switching antipsychotics when weight gain exceeds 5% during the first few months of starting an antipsychotic (American Diabetes Association et al., 2004). Switching from polypharmacy (at least two antipsychotics) to monotherapy also resulted in weight loss, although about a third of participants discontinued treatment altogether after switching (Essock et al., 2011).

Pharmacological interventions for weight management in people on antipsychotics provide modest benefits (Faulkner et al., 2007). Metformin is a well-tolerated, inexpensive, and commonly used medication in the general population for prevention and initial treatment of diabetes type 2. Large randomized controlled trials and subsequent reviews showed that, when added to an antipsychotic likely to produce weight gain, metformin significantly moderates the weight gain, with minimal side effects (DeSilva et al., 2016; Wu et al., 2008a, 2008b). Recent studies suggest that using samidorphan (an opioid antagonist), or GLP1 agonists may also reduce weight in people taking psychotropics (Correll et al., 2020; Larsen et al., 2017).

Bariatric surgery procedures have been shown in randomized controlled trials to be much more effective than lifestyle interventions in the short term, and, in observational studies, to be associated with improvement in weight, metabolic parameters, cardiovascular events, and mortality at 10–20 years of follow-up (Arterburn & Courcoulas, 2014). In a multicentre cohort study, people who had mental illness prior to surgery achieved the same weight loss after bariatric surgery as people without mental illness, but needed more acute medical care postoperatively (Fisher et al., 2017). Small retrospective studies have indicated the possibility of psychiatric symptom exacerbation in those with SMI (Shelby et al., 2015) and possible onset of SUDs, including alcohol and illicit drug use disorders, postoperatively in all (King et al., 2017). Thus, bariatric surgery should be an option in the SDM process for treatment of obesity and metabolic conditions for people with mental illness.

Substance use disorder treatment

SUDs are significant and frequent comorbidities in people with mental illness, greatly increasing the risks to health and mortality (Baghaie et al., 2017; Dickey et al., 2002; Onyeka et al., 2019). Although people with mental illness are at high risk for developing a SUD, no studies of preventing SUDs in this population exist. Evidence does exist on prevention of tobacco use, alcohol use, and illicit drug use in the general adolescent population by using early, school-based interventions (MacArthur et al., 2018). Once established, SUDs can be treated effectively with evidence-based interventions such as medication-assisted treatments, peer support interventions, contingency management, motivational interventions, cognitive behavioural therapy interventions, and comprehensive residential treatments (Drake et al., 2008), in the context of integrated, concurrent treatment of SUDs and mental illness. Nicotine use disorder, which is highly prevalent in people with mental illness, especially in people with SMI (Ziedonis et al., 2008), was historically an accepted comorbidity in mental health and substance use treatment fields, but the toll on physical health is heavy. The evidence shows that quitting smoking leads to improved mood, anxiety, and quality of life (Taylor et al., 2021). People with SMI benefit from the same strategies used in the general population, including medication-assisted treatments for nicotine cessation (Peckham et al., 2017) (see Chapter 24).

Integrating medical and psychiatric care

Like others in society, people with mental illness need routine primary medical care and specialized care for serious or chronic conditions. The literature on medical care for people with SMI assumes that greater coordination or integration of medical and mental health care can improve each area. Different approaches have been suggested: dually trained physicians, increasing the role of the psychiatrist in providing primary care, introducing public health nurses in community mental health centres, using case managers or nurses as care coordinators to help link people with SMI with medical providers, enhancing primary care by establishing specialized medical clinics focused entirely on health of people with SMI, or co-locating the medical care team and the mental health team in the same setting (Bartels et al., 2018; Cimpean & Drake, 2011; Thornicroft et al., 2019; Whiteman et al., 2016).

In the UK, integrated care relies heavily on general practitioners, primary care case registers and incentives, and explicit guidelines for cooperation between primary and secondary care (England & Lester, 2005; National Collaborating Centre for Mental Health, 2009). In the US, no consensus exists regarding a specific approach to connecting mental health care and medical care for people with SMI. Current efforts to develop integrated care include the development of the certified community behavioural health clinic model (https://www.thenationalcouncil.org/ccbhc-success-center/ccbhcta-overview), which provides access to physical and behavioural health care, and the federally qualified health centres (https://www.hrsa.gov/opa/eligibility-and-registration/health-centers/fqhc/

index.html), which are adding behavioural health to physical health care. These approaches have proven successful in limited locations and are being expanded with federal funding. Successful integration will likely require guidelines accessible during the episode of care, making physical health a close priority (Ruud et al., 2020), access to vital signs measurements, laboratory analysis, electrocardiograms, training of behavioural health providers to support self-management of chronic medical illness, integrating assertive community treatment and primary care (Vanderlip et al., 2017), and employing nurses to support care, advocacy, and collaborative efforts with medical care providers (Bury et al., 2022).

Information technology could enhance all approaches to integrating psychiatric and medical care. Computerized reminders, effective in primary medical clinics, might be used to improve the rates of adherence with guidelines for basic medical services in mental health as well. Computerized clinical decision support systems can improve outcomes if they exchange data within an electronic medical record, generate reports of measures, and provide feedback and computerized prompts to providers (Dorr et al., 2007). Numerous smartphone apps have been developed to support self-management. Finally, the introduction of patient portals in the US, supporting direct access of patients to their electronic health record, might support better communication between patients and their providers and ultimately, a patient-centred, self-managed approach to integration (Lyles et al., 2020).

Summary and conclusions

Physical health comorbidity and threats to normal longevity are ubiquitous issues for people with mental illness, who are vulnerable to poor medical health, considerable morbidity, and early mortality. To improve outcomes, interventions should address primary, secondary, and tertiary prevention, always centring on the patient, the provider, and the system of care. Interventions must address the following issues: (1) improving health care behaviours, such as diet, exercise, and smoking cessation, adherence, and follow-up; (2) enhancing the monitoring and management of side effects related to psychiatric medications; and (3) ensuring preventive health care, routine medical care, and specialty referrals.

Physical health is inextricably linked with mental health, functional performance, and quality of life. Effective psychiatric rehabilitation requires accessible, holistic, integrated care.

REFERENCES

Alegria, M., Nakash, O., Johnson, K., Ault-Brutus, A., Carson, N., Fillbrunn, M., et al. (2018). Effectiveness of the DECIDE interventions on shared decision making and perceived quality of care in behavioral health with multicultural patients: a randomized clinical trial. *JAMA Psychiatry*, **75**, 325–335.

Alvarez-Jimenez, M., Hetrick, S. E., Gonzalez-Blanch, C., Gleeson, J. F., & McGorry, P. D. (2008). Non-pharmacological management of antipsychotic-induced weight gain: systematic review and meta-analysis of randomised controlled trials. *British Journal of Psychiatry*, **193**, 101–107.

American Diabetes Association, American Psychiatric Association, American Association of Clinical Endocrinologists, & North American Association for the Study of Obesity (2004). Consensus development conference on antipsychotic drugs and obesity and diabetes. *Diabetes Care*, **27**, 596–601.

Amiri, S., Behnezhad, S., & Azad, E. (2019). Migraine headache and depression in adults: a systematic review and meta-analysis. *Neuropsychiatry*, **33**, 131–140.

Anderson, A., von Esenwein, S., Spaulding, A., & Druss, B. (2015). Involvement in the criminal justice system among attendees of an urban mental health center. *Health and Justice*, **3**, 4.

Arterburn, D. E. & Courcoulas, A. P. (2014). Bariatric surgery for obesity and metabolic conditions in adults. *BMJ*, **349**, g3961.

Ashdown-Franks, G., Firth, J., Carney, R., Carvalho, A. F., Hallgren, M., Koyanagi, A., et al. (2020). Exercise as medicine for mental and substance use disorders: a meta-review of the benefits for neuropsychiatric and cognitive outcomes. *Sports Medicine*, **50**, 151–170.

Ashoorian, D., Davidson, R., Rock, D., Dragovic, M., & Clifford, R. (2015). A clinical communication tool for the assessment of psychotropic medication side effects. *Psychiatry Research*, **230**, 643–657.

Auger, N., Paradis, G., Low, N., Ayoub, A., He, S., & Potter, B. J. (2020). Cannabis use disorder and the future risk of cardiovascular disease in parous women: a longitudinal cohort study. *BMC Medicine*, **18**, 328.

Baghaie, H., Kisely, S., Forbes, M., Sawyer, E., & Siskind, D. J. (2017). A systematic review and meta-analysis of the association between poor oral health and substance abuse. *Addiction*, **112**, 765–779.

Bailey, Z., Feldman, J., & Bassett, M. (2021). How structural racism works—racist policies as a root cause of U.S. racial health inequities. *New England Journal of Medicine*, **384**, 768–773.

Bailey, Z. D., Krieger, N., Agénor, M., Graves, J., Linos, N., & Bassett, M. T. (2017). Structural racism and health inequities in the USA: evidence and interventions. *Lancet*, **389**, 1453–1463.

Bartels, S. J., DiMilia, P. R., Fortuna, K. L., & Naslund, J. A. (2018). Integrated care for older adults with serious mental illness and medical comorbidity: evidence-based models and future research directions. *Psychiatric Clinics of North America*, **41**, 153–164.

Bartels, S. J., Pratt, S. I., Aschbrenner, K. A., Barre, L. K., Naslund, J. A., Wolfe, R., et al. (2015). Pragmatic replication trial of health promotion coaching for obesity in serious mental illness and maintenance of outcomes. *American Journal of Psychiatry*, **172**, 344–352.

Barton, B. B., Segger, F., Fischer, K., Obermeier, M., & Musil, R. (2020). Update on weight-gain caused by antipsychotics: a systematic review and meta-analysis. *Expert Opinion on Drug Safety*, **19**, 295–314.

Batelaan, N. M., ten Have, M., van Balkom, A. J., Tuithof, M., & de Graaf, R. (2014). Anxiety disorders and onset of cardiovascular disease: the differential impact of panic, phobias and worry. *Journal of Anxiety Disorders*, **28**, 252–258.

Beebe, L. H., Tian, L., Morris, N., Goodwin, A., Allen, S. S., & Kuldau, J. (2005). Effects of exercise on mental and physical health parameters of persons with schizophrenia. *Issues in Mental Health Nursing*, **26**, 661–676.

Bird, C. E., Seeman, T. E., Escarce, J. J., Basurto-Dávila, R., Finch, B. K., Dubowitz, T., et al. (2010). Neighborhood socioeconomic status and biological 'wear & tear' in a nationally representative sample of U.S. adults. *Journal of Epidemioliogy and Community Health*, **64**, 860–865.

Bury, D., Hendrick, D., Smith, T., Metcalfe, J., & Drake, R. (2022). The psychiatric nurse care coordinator on a multi-disciplinary, community mental health treatment team. *Community Mental Health Journal*, **58**, 1354–1360.

Cai, W., Mueller, C., Li, Y. J., Shen, W. D., & Stewart, R. (2019). Post stroke depression and risk of stroke recurrence and mortality: a systematic review and meta-analysis. *Ageing Research Reviews*, **50**, 102–109.

Centers for Disease Control and Prevention (n.d.). Fast facts and fact sheets: smoking and cigarettes. https://www.cdc.gov/tobacco/data_statistics/fact_sheets/fast_facts/index.htm

Chang, C. K., Hayes, R. D., Perera, G., Broadbent, M. T., Fernandes, A. C., Lee, W. E., et al. (2011). Life expectancy at birth for people with serious mental illness and other major disorders from a secondary mental health care case register in London. *PLoS One*, **6**, e19590.

Cimpean, D. & Drake, R. E. (2011). Treating co-morbid chronic medical conditions and anxiety/depression. *Epidemiology and Psychiatric Sciences*, **20**, 141–150.

Cipriani, A., Reid, K., Young, A. H., Macritchie, K., & Geddes, J. (2013). Valproic acid, valproate and divalproex in the maintenance treatment of bipolar disorder. *Cochrane Database of Systematic Reviews*, **10**, CD003196.

Cohn, T. A. & Sernyak, M. J. (2006). Metabolic monitoring for patients treated with antipsychotic medications. *Canadian Journal of Psychiatry/Revue Canadienne de Psychiatrie* **51**, 492–501.

Compton, W. M., Han, B., Jones, C. M., & Blanco, C. (2019). Cannabis use disorders among adults in the United States during a time of increasing use of cannabis. *Drug and Alcohol Dependence*, **204**, 107468.

Cook, B. L., Wayne, G. F., Kafali, E. N., Liu, Z., Shu, C., & Flores, M. (2014). Trends in smoking among adults with mental illness and association between mental health treatment and smoking cessation. *JAMA*, **311**, 172–182.

Cordes, J., Sinha-Roder, A., Kahl, K. G., Malevani, J., Thuenker, J., Lange-Asschenfeldt, C., et al. (2008). Therapeutic options for weight management in schizophrenic patients treated with atypical antipsychotics. *Fortschritte der Neurologie-Psychiatrie*, **76**, 703–714.

Correll, C. U., Robinson, D. G., Schooler, N. R., Brunette, M. F., Mueser, K. T., Rosenheck, R. A., et al. (2014). Cardiometabolic risk in patients with first-episode schizophrenia spectrum disorders: baseline results from the RAISE-ETP study. *JAMA Psychiatry*, **71**, 1350–1363.

Correll, C. U., Newcomer, J. W., Silverman, B., DiPetrillo, L., Graham, C., Jiang, Y., et al. (2020). Effects of olanzapine combined with samidorphan on weight gain in schizophrenia: a 24-week phase 3 study. *American Journal of Psychiatry*, **177**, 1168–1178.

Crump, C., Winkleby, M. A., Sundquist, K., & Sundquist, J. (2013). Comorbidities and mortality in persons with schizophrenia: a Swedish National Cohort Study. *American Journal of Psychiatry*, **170**, 324–333.

Deegan, P. E. (2005). The importance of personal medicine: a qualitative study of resilience in people with psychiatric disabilities. *Scandinavian Journal of Public Health Supplement*, **66**, 29–35.

Deegan, P. E., & Drake, R. E. (2006). Shared decision making and medication management in the recovery process. *Psychiatric Services*, **57**, 1636–1639.

De Hert, M., Detraux, J., & Vancampfort, D. (2018). The intriguing relationship between coronary heart disease and mental disorders. *Dialogues in Clinical Neuroscience*, **20**, 31–40.

De Hert, M., van Winkel, R., Van Eyck, D., Hanssens, L., Wampers, M., Scheen, A., & Peuskens, J. (2006). Prevalence of diabetes, metabolic syndrome and metabolic abnormalities in schizophrenia over the course of the illness: a cross-sectional study. *Clinical Practice and Epidemiology in Mental Health*, **2**, 14.

De Silva, V. A., Suraweera, C., Ratnatunga, S. S., Dayabandara, M., Wanniarachchi, N., & Hanwella, R. (2016). Metformin in prevention and treatment of antipsychotic induced weight gain: a systematic review and meta-analysis. *BMC Psychiatry*, **16**, 341.

Dibonaventura, M., Gabriel, S., Dupclay, L., Gupta, S., & Kim, E. (2012). A patient perspective of the impact of medication side effects on adherence: results of a cross-sectional nationwide survey of patients with schizophrenia. *BMC Psychiatry*, **12**, 20.

Dickey, B., Normand, S. L., Weiss, R. D., Drake, R. E., & Azeni, H. (2002). Medical morbidity, mental illness, and substance use disorders. *Psychiatric Services*, **53**, 861–867.

Dorr, D., Bonner, L. M., Cohen, A. N., Shoai, R. S., Perrin, R., Chaney, E., & Young, A. S. (2007). Informatics systems to promote improved care for chronic illness: a literature review. *Journal of the American Medical Informatics Association*, **14**, 156–163.

Drake, R. E. & Bond, G. R. (2021). Psychiatric crisis care and the more is less paradox. *Community Mental Health Journal*, **57**, 1230–1236.

Drake, R. E. & Deegan, P. E. (2009). Shared decision making is an ethical imperative. *Psychiatric Services*, **60**, 1007.

Drake, R. E., O'Neal, E. L., & Wallach, M. A. (2008). A systematic review of psychosocial interventions for people with co-occurring substance use and severe mental disorders. *Journal of Substance Abuse Treatment*, **34**, 123–138.

Druss, B. G., Bradford, D. W., Rosenheck, R. A., Radford, M. J., & Krumholz, H. M. (2000). Mental disorders and use of cardiovascular procedures after myocardial infarction. *JAMA*, **283**, 506–511.

Emdin, C. A., Odutayo, A., Wong, C. X., Tran, J., Hsiao, A. J., & Hunn, B. H. (2016). Meta-analysis of anxiety as a risk factor for cardiovascular disease. *American Journal of Cardiology*, **118**, 511–519.

England, E. & H. Lester. (2005). Integrated mental health services in England: a policy paradox. *International Journal of Integrated Care*, **5**, e24.

Epel, E. S. & Prather, A. A. (2018). Stress, telomeres, and psychopathology: toward a deeper understanding of a triad of early aging. *Annual Review of Clinical Psychology*, **14**, 371–397.

Essock, S. M., Schooler, N. R., Stroup, T. S., McEvoy, J. P., Rojas, I., Jackson, C., & Covell, N. H. (2011). Schizophrenia Trials Network. Effectiveness of switching from antipsychotic polypharmacy to monotherapy. *American Journal of Psychiatry*, **168**, 702–708.

Fang, Y., Qin, T., Liu, W., Ran, L., Yang, Y., Huang, H., et al. (2020). Cerebral small-vessel disease and risk of incidence of depression: a meta-analysis of longitudinal cohort studies. *Journal of the American Heart Association*, **9**, e016512.

Faulkner, G. & Cohn, T. A. (2006). Pharmacologic and nonpharmacologic strategies for weight gain and metabolic disturbance in patients treated with antipsychotic medications. *Canadian Journal of Psychiatry/Revue Canadienne de Psychiatrie*, **51**, 502–511.

Faulkner, G., Cohn, T., & Remington, G. (2007). Interventions to reduce weight gain in schizophrenia. *Cochrane Database of Systematic Reviews*, **1**, CD005148.

Fisher, D., Coleman, K. J., Arterburn, D. E., Fischer, H., Yamamoto, A., Young, D. R., et al. (2017). Mental illness in bariatric surgery: a cohort study from the PORTAL network. *Obesity (Silver Spring)*, **25**, 850–856.

Foguet-Boreu, Q., Fernandez San Martin, M. I., Flores Mateo, G., Zabaleta Del Olmo, E., Ayerbe García-Morzon, L., Perez-Piñar López, M., et al. (2016). Cardiovascular risk assessment in patients with a severe mental illness: a systematic review and meta-analysis. *BMC Psychiatry*, **16**, 141.

Forty, L., Ulanova, A., Jones, L., Jones, I., Gordon-Smith, K., Fraser, C., et al. (2014). Comorbid medical illness in bipolar disorder. *British Journal of Psychiatry*, **205**, 465–472.

Fothergill, E., Guo, J., Howard, L., Kerns, J. C., Knuth, N. D., Brychta, R., et al. (2016). Persistent metabolic adaptation 6 years after 'The Biggest Loser' competition. *Obesity (Silver Spring)*, **24**, 1612–1619.

Frandsen, B. R., Joynt, K. E., Rebitzer, J. B., & Jha, A. K. (2015). Care fragmentation, quality, and costs among chronically ill patients. *American Journal of Managed Care*, **21**, 355–362.

Franz, M. J., Boucher, J. L., Rutten-Ramos, S., & VanWormer, J. J. (2015). Lifestyle weight-loss intervention outcomes in overweight and obese adults with type 2 diabetes: a systematic review and meta-analysis of randomized clinical trials. *Journal of the Academy of Nutrition and Dietetics*, **115**, 1447–1163.

Geronimus, A. T., Hicken, M., Keene, D., & Bound, J. (2006). 'Weathering' and age patterns of allostatic load scores among blacks and whites in the United States. *American Journal of Public Health*, **96**, 826–833.

Heiberg, I. H., Jacobsen, B. K., Nesvåg, R., Bramness, J. G., Reichborn-Kjennerud, T., Næss, Ø., et al. (2018). Total and cause-specific standardized mortality ratios in patients with schizophrenia and/or substance use disorder. *PLoS One*, **13**, e0202028.

Himelhoch, S., Weller, W., Wu, A. W., Anderson, G. F., & Cooper, L. A. (2004). Chronic medical illness, depression, and use of acute medical services among Medicare beneficiaries. *Medical Care*, **42**, 512–521.

Hinton, E., Henderson, L., & Reed, C. (2018). *An Unjust Burden: The Disparate Treatment of Black Americans in the Criminal Justice System*. New York: Vera Institute of Justice.

Hjorthøj, C., Stürup, A. E., McGrath, J. J., & Nordentoft, M. (2017). Years of potential life lost and life expectancy in schizophrenia: a systematic review and meta-analysis. *Lancet Psychiatry*, **4**, 295–301.

Jerome, G. J., Young, D. R., Dalcin, A. T., Wang, N. Y., Gennusa, J., 3rd, Goldsholl, S., et al. (2017). Cardiorespiratory benefits of group exercise among adults with serious mental illness. *Psychiatry Research*, **256**, 85–87.

Jin, H., Meyer, J. M., & Jeste, D. V. (2002). Phenomenology of and risk factors for new-onset diabetes mellitus and diabetic ketoacidosis associated with atypical antipsychotics: an analysis of 45 published cases. *Annals of Clinical Psychiatry*, **14**, 59–64.

Jones, S., Howard, L., & Thornicroft, G. (2008). 'Diagnostic overshadowing': worse physical health care for people with mental illness. *Acta Psychiatrica Scandinavica*, **118**, 169–171.

Keefe, K., Styron, T., O'Connell, M., Mattias, K., Davidson, L., & Costa, M. (2020). Understanding family perspectives on supported employment. *International Journal of the Society of Psychiatry*, **66**, 76–83.

Kilbourne, A. M., Morden, N. E., Austin, K., Ilgen, M., McCarthy, J. F., Dalack, G., & Blow, F. C. (2009). Excess heart-disease-related mortality in a national study of patients with mental disorders: identifying modifiable risk factors. *General Hospital Psychiatry*, **31**, 555–563.

Kim, M., Kim, Y. S., Kim, D. H., Yang, T. W., & Kwon, O. Y. (2018). Major depressive disorder in epilepsy clinics: a meta-analysis. *Epilepsy & Behavior*, **84**, 56–69.

King, W. C., Chen, J. Y., Courcoulas, A. P., Dakin, G. F., Engel, S. G., Flum, D. R., et al. (2017). Alcohol and other substance use after bariatric surgery: prospective evidence from a U.S. multicenter cohort study. *Surgery for Obesity and Related Diseases*, **13**, 1392–1402.

Koller, E. A., Cross, J. T., Doraiswamy, P. M., & Malozowski, S. N. (2003). Pancreatitis associated with atypical antipsychotics: from the Food and Drug Administration's MedWatch surveillance system and published reports. *Pharmacotherapy*, **23**, 1123–1130.

Lang, X., Liu, Q., Fang, H., Zhou, Y., Forster, M. T., et al. (2021). The prevalence and clinical correlates of metabolic syndrome and cardiometabolic alterations in 430 drug-naive patients in their first episode of schizophrenia. *Psychopharmacology*, **238**, 3643–3652.

Larsen, J. R., Vedtofte, L., Jakobsen, M. S. L., Jespersen, H. R., Jakobsen, M. I., Svensson, C. K., et al. (2017). Effect of liraglutide treatment on prediabetes and overweight or obesity in clozapine- or olanzapine-treated patients with schizophrenia spectrum disorder: a randomized clinical trial. *JAMA Psychiatry*, **74**, 719–728.

Lawrence, D., Hancock, K. J., & Kisely, S. (2013). The gap in life expectancy from preventable physical illness in psychiatric patients in Western Australia: retrospective analysis of population based registers. *BMJ*, **346**, f2539.

Lieberman, J. A., Stroup, T. S., McEvoy, J. P., Swartz, M. S., Rosenheck, R. A., Perkins, D. O., et al. (2005). Effectiveness of antipsychotic drugs in patients with chronic schizophrenia. *New England Journal of Medicine*, **353**, 1209–1223.

Loh, C., Meyer, J. M., & Leckband, S. G. (2006). A comprehensive review of behavioral interventions for weight management in schizophrenia. *Annals of Clinical Psychiatry*, **18**, 23–31.

Lu, Y., Wang, Z., Georgakis, M. K., Lin, H., & Zheng, L. (2021). Genetic liability to depression and risk of coronary artery disease, myocardial infarction, and other cardiovascular outcomes. *Journal of the American Heart Association*, **10**, e017986.

Lyles, C. R., Nelson, E. C., Frampton, S., Dykes, P. C., Cemballi, A. G., & Sarkar, U. (2020). Using electronic health record portals to improve patient engagement: research priorities and best practices. *Annals of Internal Medicine*, **172**(Suppl. 11), S123–S129.

MacArthur, G., Caldwell, D. M., Redmore, J., Watkins, S. H., Kipping, R., White, J., et al. (2018). Individual-, family-, and school-level interventions targeting multiple risk behaviours in young people. *Cochrane Database of Systematic Reviews*, **10**, CD009927.

Macritchie, K. A., Geddes, J. R., Scott, J., Haslam, D. R., & Goodwin, G. M. (2013). Valproic acid, valproate and divalproex in the maintenance treatment of bipolar disorder. *Cochrane Database of Systematic Reviews*, **10**, CD003196.

Mahaffey, C., Stevens-Watkins, D., & Leukefeld, C. (2018). Life after: examining the relationship between socio-behavioral factors and mental health among African American ex-offenders. *International Journal of Offender Therapy and Comparative Criminology*, **62**, 3873–3889.

Malm, U., Ivarsson, B., Allebeck, P., & Falloon, I. R. (2003). Integrated care in schizophrenia: a 2-year randomized controlled study of two community-based treatment programs. *Acta Psychiatrica Scandinavica*, **107**, 415–423.

Marder, S. R., Essock, S. M., Miller, A. L., Buchanan, R. W., Davis, J. M., Kane, J. M., et al. (2002). The Mount Sinai conference on the pharmacotherapy of schizophrenia. *Schizophrenia Bulletin*, **28**, 5–16.

McEvoy, J. P., Meyer, J. M., Goff, D. C., Nasrallah, H. A., Davis, S. M., Sullivan, L., et al. (2005). Prevalence of the metabolic syndrome in patients with schizophrenia: baseline results from the Clinical Antipsychotic Trials of Intervention Effectiveness (CATIE) schizophrenia trial and comparison with national estimates from NHANES III. *Schizophrenia Research*, **80**, 19–32.

McHugh, R. K. & Weiss, R. D. (2019). Alcohol use disorder and depressive disorders. *Alcohol Research: Current Reviews*, **40**, arcr.v40.1.01.

Melamed, O. C., Wong, E. N., LaChance, L. R., Kanji, S., & Taylor, V. H. (2019). Interventions to improve metabolic risk screening among adult patients taking antipsychotic medication: a systematic review. *Psychiatric Services*, **70**, 1138–1156.

Mercke, Y., Sheng, H., Khan, T., & Lippmann, S. (2000). Hair loss in psychopharmacology. *Annals of Clinical Psychiatry*, **12**, 35–42.

Meyer, J. M. (2002). A retrospective comparison of weight, lipid, and glucose changes between risperidone- and olanzapine-treated inpatients: metabolic outcomes after 1 year. *Journal of Clinical Psychiatry*, **63**, 425–433.

Meyer, J. M., Nasrallah, H. A., McEvoy, J. P., et al. (2005). The Clinical Antipsychotic Trials of Intervention Effectiveness (CATIE)

Schizophrenia Trial: clinical comparison of subgroups with and without the metabolic syndrome. *Schizophrenia Research*, **80**, 9–18.

Morres, I. D., Hatzigeorgiadis, A., Stathi, A., Comoutos, N., Arpin-Cribbie, C., Krommidas, C., & Theodorakis, Y. (2019). Aerobic exercise for adult patients with major depressive disorder in mental health services: a systematic review and meta-analysis. *Depression and Anxiety*, **36**, 39–53.

Mueser, K. T., Drake, R. E., & Wallach, M. A. (1998). Dual diagnosis: a review of etiological theories. *Addictive Behaviors*, **23**, 717–734.

Naslund, J. A., Whiteman, K. L., McHugo, G. J., Aschbrenner, K. A., Marsch, L. A., & Bartels, S. J. (2017). Lifestyle interventions for weight loss among overweight and obese adults with serious mental illness: a systematic review and meta-analysis. *General Hospital Psychiatry*, **47**, 83–102.

Nasrallah, H. A. (2006). Metabolic findings from the CATIE trial and their relation to tolerability. *CNS Spectrums*, **11**(7 Suppl. 7), 32–39.

National Collaborating Centre for Mental Health (2009). *Core Interventions in the Treatment and Management of Schizophrenia in Primary and Secondary Care (Update)* (National Clinical Practice Guideline Number 82). London: National Institute for Health and Clinical Excellence.

Nordentoft, M., Wahlbeck, K., Hällgren, J., Westman, J., Osby, U., Alinaghizadeh, H., et al. (2013). Excess mortality, causes of death and life expectancy in 270,770 patients with recent onset of mental disorders in Denmark, Finland and Sweden. *PLoS One*, **8**, e55176.

Olfson, M., Cosgrove, C., Altekruse, S. F., Wall, M. M., & Blanco, C. (2021). Deaths of despair: adults at high risk for death by suicide, poisoning, or chronic liver disease in the U.S. *Health Affairs*, **40**, 505–512.

Onyeka, I. N., Collier Høegh, M., Nåheim Eien, E. M., Nwaru, B. I., & Melle, I. (2019). Comorbidity of physical disorders among patients with severe mental illness with and without substance use disorders: a systematic review and meta-analysis. *Journal of Dual Diagnosis*, **15**, 192–206.

Oo, K. Z., Aung, Y. K., Jenkins, M. A., & Win, A. K. (2016). Associations of 5HTTLPR polymorphism with major depressive disorder and alcohol dependence: a systematic review and meta-analysis. *Australian and New Zealand Journal of Psychiatry*, **50**, 842–857.

Ösby, U., Westman, J., Hällgren, J., & Gissler, M. (2016). Mortality trends in cardiovascular causes in schizophrenia, bipolar and unipolar mood disorder in Sweden 1987–2010. *European Journal of Public Health*, **26**, 867–871.

Peckham, E., Brabyn, S., Cook, L., Tew, G., & Gilbody, S. (2017). Smoking cessation in severe mental ill health: what works? An updated systematic review and meta-analysis. *BMC Psychiatry*, **17**, 252.

Perkins, D. O. (2002). Predictors of noncompliance in patients with schizophrenia. *Journal of Clinical Psychiatry*, **63**, 1121–1128.

Posadzki, P., Pieper, D., Bajpai, R., Makaruk, H., Könsgen, N., Neuhaus, A. L., & Semwal, M. (2020). Exercise/physical activity and health outcomes: an overview of Cochrane systematic reviews. *BMC Public Health*, **20**, 1724.

Postolache, T. T., Del Bosque-Plata, L., Jabbour, S., Vergare, M., Wu, R., & Gragnoli, C. (2019). Co-shared genetics and possible risk gene pathway partially explain the comorbidity of schizophrenia, major depressive disorder, type 2 diabetes, and metabolic syndrome. *American Journal of Medical Genetics. Part B, Neuropsychiatric Genetics*, **180**, 186–203.

Priebe, S., McCabe, R., Bullenkamp, J., Hansson, L., Lauber, C., Martinez-Leal, R., et al. (2007). Structured patient-clinician communication and 1-year outcome in community mental healthcare: cluster randomised controlled trial. *British Journal of Psychiatry*, **191**, 420–426.

Ray, W. A., Chung, C. P., Murray, K. T., Hall, K., & Stein, C. M. (2009). Atypical antipsychotic drugs and the risk of sudden cardiac death. *New England Journal of Medicine*, **360**, 225–235.

Ried, L. D., Renner, B. T., Bengtson, M. A., Wilcox, B. M., & Acholonu, W. W., Jr. (2003). Weight change after an atypical antipsychotic switch. *Annals of Pharmacotherapy*, **37**, 1381–1386.

Ried, L. D., Renner, B. T., McConkey, J. R., Bengtson, M. A., & Lopez, L. M. (2006). Increased cardiovascular risk with second-generation antipsychotic agent switches. *Journal of the American Pharmacists Association: JAPhA*, **46**, 491–498.

Roberts, L., Roalfe, A., Wilson, S., & Lester, H. (2007). Physical health care of patients with schizophrenia in primary care: a comparative study. *Family Practice*, **24**, 34–40.

Robertson, A. G., Swanson, J. W., Frisman, L. K., Lin, H., & Swartz, M. S. (2014). Patterns of justice involvement among adults with schizophrenia and bipolar disorder: key risk factors. *Psychiatric Services*, **65**, 931–938.

Romain, A. J., Bernard, P., Akrass, Z., St-Amour, S., Lachance, J. P., Hains-Monfette, G., et al. (2020). Motivational theory-based interventions on health of people with several mental illness: a systematic review and meta-analysis. *Schizophrenia Research*, **222**, 31–41.

Rosenheck, R. A., Davis, S., Covell, N., Essock, S., Swartz, M., Stroup, S., et al. (2009). Does switching to a new antipsychotic improve outcomes? Data from the CATIE Trial. *Schizophrenia Research*, **107**, 22–29.

Ruud, T., Høifødt, T. S., Hendrick, D. C., Drake, R. E., Høye, A., Landers, M., et al. (2020). The Physical Health Care Fidelity Scale: psychometric properties. *Administration and Policy in Mental Health*, **47**, 901–910.

Saha, S., Chant, D., & McGrath, J. (2007). A systematic review of mortality in schizophrenia: is the differential mortality gap worsening over time? *Archives of General Psychiatry*, **64**, 1123–1131.

Shelby, S. R., Labott, S., & Stout, R. A. (2015). Bariatric surgery: a viable treatment option for patients with severe mental illness. *Surgery for Obesity and Related Diseases*, **11**, 1342–1348.

Sherwood, A., Blumenthal, J. A., Hinderliter, A. L., Koch, G. G., Adams, K. F., Jr, Dupree, C. S., et al. (2011). Worsening depressive symptoms are associated with adverse clinical outcomes in patients with heart failure. *Journal of the American College of Cardiology*, **57**, 418–423.

Siskind, D., Gallagher, E., Winckel, K., Hollingworth, S., Kisely, S., Firth, J., et al. (2021). Does switching antipsychotics ameliorate weight gain in patients with severe mental illness? A systematic review and meta-analysis. *Schizophrenia Bulletin*, **47**, 948–958.

Solmi, M., Fiedorowicz, J., Poddighe, L., Delogu, M., Miola, A., Høye, A., et al. (2021). Disparities in screening and treatment of cardiovascular diseases in patients with mental disorders across the world: systematic review and meta-analysis of 47 observational studies. *American Journal of Psychiatry*, **178**, 793–803.

Stubbs, B., Vancampfort, D., De Hert, M., & Mitchell, A. J. (2015). The prevalence and predictors of type two diabetes mellitus in people with schizophrenia: a systematic review and comparative meta-analysis. *Acta Psychiatrica Scandinavica*, **132**, 144–157.

Stubbs, B., Vancampfort, D., Rosenbaum, S., Firth, J., Cosco, T., Veronese, N., et al. (2017). An examination of the anxiolytic effects of exercise for people with anxiety and stress-related disorders: a meta-analysis. *Psychiatry Research*, **249**, 102–108.

Stubbs, B., Vancampfort, D., Veronese, N., Thompson, T., Fornaro, M., Schofield, P., et al. (2017). Depression and pain: primary data and meta-analysis among 237 952 people across 47 low- and middle-income countries. *Psychological Medicine*, **47**, 2906–2917.

Suetani, S., Honarparvar, F., Siskind, D., Hindley, G., Veronese, N., Vancampfort, D., et al. (2021). Increased rates of respiratory disease in schizophrenia: a systematic review and meta-analysis including 619,214 individuals with schizophrenia and 52,159,551 controls. *Schizophrenia Research*, **237**, 131–140.

Taylor, G. M., Lindson, N., Farley, A., Leinberger-Jabari, A., Sawyer, K., te Water Naudé, R., et al. (2021). Smoking cessation for improving mental health. *Cochrane Database Systematic Review*, **3**, CD013522.

Teasdale, S. B., Ward, P. B., Rosenbaum, S., Samaras, K., & Stubbs, B. (2017). Solving a weighty problem: systematic review and meta-analysis of nutrition interventions in severe mental illness. *British Journal of Psychiatry*, **210**, 110–118.

Teasdale, S. B., Ward, P. B., Samaras, K., Firth, J., Stubbs, B., Tripodi, E., & Burrows, T. L. (2019). Dietary intake of people with severe mental illness: systematic review and meta-analysis. *British Journal of Psychiatry*, **214**, 251–259.

Thornicroft, G., Ahuja, S., Barber, S., Chisholm, D., Collins, P. Y., Docrat, S., et al. (2019). Integrated care for people with long-term mental and physical health conditions in low-income and middle-income countries. *Lancet Psychiatry*, **6**, 174–186.

Tully, P. J., Turnbull, D. A., Beltrame, J., Horowitz, J., Cosh, S., Baumeister, H., Wittert, G. A. (2015). Panic disorder and incident coronary heart disease: a systematic review and meta-regression in 1131612 persons and 58111 cardiac events. *Psychological Medicine*, **45**, 2909–2920.

Vancampfort, D., Correll, C. U., Galling, B., Probst, M., De Hert, M., Ward, P. B., et al. (2016). Diabetes mellitus in people with schizophrenia, bipolar disorder and major depressive disorder: a systematic review and large scale meta-analysis. *World Psychiatry*, **15**, 166–174.

Vanderlip, E. R., Henwood, B. F., Hrouda, D. R., Meyer, P. S., Monroe-DeVita, M., Studer, L. M., et al. (2017). Systematic literature review of general health care interventions within programs of assertive community treatment. *Psychiatric Services*, **68**, 218–224.

Veeneman, R. R., Vermeulen, J. M., Abdellaoui, A., Sanderson, E., Wootton, R. E., Tadros, R., et al. (2021). Exploring the relationship between schizophrenia and cardiovascular disease: a genetic correlation and multivariable Mendelian randomization study. *Schizophrenia Bulletin*, **48**, 463–473.

Verma, S. K., Subramaniam, M., Liew, A., & Poon, L. Y. (2009). Metabolic risk factors in drug-naive patients with first-episode psychosis. *Journal of Clinical Psychiatry*, **70**, 997–1000.

Vogelzangs, N., Seldenrijk, A., Beekman, A. T., van Hout, H. P., de Jonge, P., & Penninx, B. W. (2010). Cardiovascular disease in persons with depressive and anxiety disorders. *Journal of Affective Disorders*, **125**, 241–248.

Walker, E. R., McGee, R. E., & Druss, B. G. (2015). Mortality in mental disorders and global disease burden implications: a systematic review and meta-analysis. *JAMA Psychiatry*, **72**, 334–341.

Wang, S., Mao, S., Xiang, D., & Fang, C. (2018). Association between depression and the subsequent risk of Parkinson's disease: a meta-analysis. *Progress in Neuro-Psychopharmacology & Biological Psychiatry*, **86**, 186–192.

Wang, Y., Yang, H., Nolan, M., Burgess, J., Negishi, K., & Marwick, T. H. (2018). Association of depression with evolution of heart failure in patients with type 2 diabetes mellitus. *Cardiovascular Diabetology*, **17**, 19.

Ward, M. C., White, D. T., & Druss, B. G. (2015). A meta-review of lifestyle interventions for cardiovascular risk factors in the general medical population: lessons for individuals with serious mental illness. *Journal of Clinical Psychiatry*, **76**, e477–e486.

Whiteman, K. L., Naslund, J. A., DiNapoli, E. A., Bruce, M. L., & Bartels, S. J. (2016). Systematic review of integrated general medical and psychiatric self-management interventions for adults with serious mental illness. *Psychiatric Services*, **67**, 1213–1225.

Wilson, D. R., D'Souza, L., Sarkar, N., Newton, M., & Hammond, C. (2003). New-onset diabetes and ketoacidosis with atypical antipsychotics. *Schizophrenia Research*, **59**, 1–6.

Wium-Andersen, M. K., Wium-Andersen, I. K., Prescott, E. I. B., Overvad, K., Jørgensen, M. B., & Osler, M. (2020). An attempt to explain the bidirectional association between ischaemic heart disease, stroke and depression: a cohort and meta-analytic approach. *British Journal of Psychiatry*, **217**, 434–441.

Wu, R. R., Zhao, J. P., Guo, X. F., He, Y. Q., Fang, M. S., Guo, W. B., et al. (2008a). Metformin addition attenuates olanzapine-induced weight gain in drug-naive first-episode schizophrenia patients: a double-blind, placebo-controlled study. *American Journal of Psychiatry*, **165**, 352–358.

Wu, R. R., Zhao, J. P., Jin, H., Shao, P., Fang, M. S., Guo, X. F., et al. (2008b). Lifestyle intervention and metformin for treatment of antipsychotic-induced weight gain: a randomized controlled trial. *JAMA*, **299**, 185–193.

Yatham, L. N., Kennedy, S. H., Parikh, S. V., Schaffer, A., Bond, D. J., Frey, B. N., Sharma, V., et al. (2018). Canadian Network for Mood and Anxiety Treatments (CANMAT) and International Society for Bipolar Disorders (ISBD) 2018 guidelines for the management of patients with bipolar disorder. *Bipolar Disorder*, **20**, 97–170.

Ziedonis, D., Hitsman, B., Beckham, J. C., Zvolensky, M., Adler, L. E., Audrain-McGovern, J., et al. (2008). Tobacco use and cessation in psychiatric disorders: National Institute of Mental Health report. *Nicotine & Tobacco Research*, **10**, 1691–1715.

Illness self-management programmes

Kim T. Mueser and Susan Gingerich

Introduction

In recent years there has been a growth in programmes aimed at teaching illness self-management skills to individuals with a major mental illness. This trend reflects a broader trend in modern medicine towards adopting a more collaborative approach that includes the patient and family members in the management of chronic medical disorders. Education about psychiatric disorders and teaching of illness self-management strategies is now a common practice in the mental health field, and a growing number of programmes have been developed with standard curriculum and teaching methods designed to achieve this. While the goal of these programmes is to improve illness self-management through better adherence to treatment recommendations and improved skills for coping with persistent symptoms and impairments, the management of psychiatric disorders in these programmes is generally viewed as a collaborative process that involves the client, treatment team, and family members or friends.

We begin this chapter with a review of factors that led to the development and growth of illness self-management programmes. We then discuss the goals of illness self-management programmes, followed by a review of different approaches to teaching illness self-management. We then address research supporting illness self-management, and briefly describe several programmes. We conclude with a brief summary of illness self-management for people with serious psychiatric disorders.

Historical factors in the development of self-management programmes for mental illness

The notion that people with a serious psychiatric disorder are capable of helping themselves is not a new one. Over 160 years ago the Alleged Lunatics' Friend Society was founded in England for the purposes of helping people with a serious psychiatric disorder cope with their illness (Frese & Davis, 1997). In the 1940s, former state hospital patients began to meet together to provide support for one another in New York City, which eventually gave rise to Fountain House, and the development of psychosocial clubhouses designed for individuals with a serious mental illness to support one another in moving forward in their lives (Beard et al., 1982). Over the past several decades, a confluence of factors has led to the development of illness self-management programmes for psychiatric disorders. Two important factors merit particular attention, including the rise of the consumer and recovery movement, and the shift towards shared decision-making in general medicine. These factors are briefly described below.

The consumer and recovery movement

The consumer and recovery movement evolved over the past five decades, spurred on by changes in attitudes and beliefs about serious mental illness and its treatment, and research on the long-term course of these disorders. In the wake of deinstitutionalization, and following changes in laws that prohibited people from being hospitalized in the absence of evidence that they presented a grave danger to themselves or others, increasing numbers of people with serious psychiatric disorders began to express dissatisfaction with their treatment in the mental health system, and were afforded the opportunity of meeting and supporting each other in voicing their objections (Chamberlin, 1978). These individuals often objected to the word 'patient' as suggesting a passive role in treatment, with those in the US opting for the term *consumer* (of mental health services), and those in Great Britain opting for the term *service user*.

Consumers expressed their dissatisfaction with several different aspects of the mental health system. First, they objected to the presumed chronicity of serious mental illnesses such as schizophrenia, and to mental health professionals who sought to explain to them that their psychiatric disorders were lifelong and they should accept this and either modify their hopes and dreams accordingly, or give up on them altogether (Deegan, 1990). Bolstered by a growing body of research demonstrating that the long-term outcome of schizophrenia was in fact much better than previously thought, and that significant numbers of persons demonstrated improvement and even remission of their disorder over the long-term (Harrison et al., 2001; Salzer et al., 2018), consumers argued for a broader definition of recovery that was based not on remission of psychopathology, but rather on the personally meaningful process that involves living and growing beyond or in spite of having a mental illness (Anthony, 1993; Davidson, 2003; Deegan, 1988; Roe & Chopra, 2003). Although the concept of recovery continues to generate debate (Bellack, 2006), and many different definitions have been offered (National Academies of Sciences, Engineering, and Medicine, 2016; Ralph & Corrigan, 2005), the shift away from defining recovery in medical terms and towards defining it in more personal terms drew attention to the importance of engaging individuals in identifying their own treatment goals, rather than narrowly focusing on the reduction of symptoms and impairments.

Second, consumers objected to the traditional, hierarchical and often coercive decision-making process that dominated psychiatric treatment (Blaska, 1990; Campbell, 1997; Carling, 1995). They complained that their concerns were frequently ignored by treatment providers, and that rather than providing them with the help and care they needed, they were often further traumatized by the very system that was supposed to serve them (Fisher, 1992; Jennings, 1994). Consumers argued that they needed to be the ones to set the goals of treatment, and demanded respect and collaboration from treatment providers (Segal et al., 1993).

Third, as part of the rise of the self-help movement in the 1970s (Gartner & Riessman, 1977; L. Kurtz, 1988), consumers began to look to their peers as critical to their own empowerment and recovery (Freese, 2008). A growing body of writings by consumers testified to the importance of illness self-management strategies to helping individuals get on with their lives (Copeland, 1994; Leete, 1989). As the desire for illness self-management strategies grew, so did curriculum, groups, and settings that responded to this need.

Shared decision-making

Parallel to the rise of the consumer and recovery movement, the modern practice of medicine was undergoing a similar radical shift. While traditional medical practice was hierarchical in nature, with the doctor instructing the patient on what needed to be done to treat the disorder, two trends emerged that led to a reappraisal and change of this practice. First, the problem of poor adherence to doctors' treatment recommendations became increasingly clear. Although effective treatments for many diseases existed, patients often failed to follow their doctor's recommendations, leading to worse than expected outcomes (Blackwell, 1976). Second, as the variety of treatment options for different diseases grew, so did the risks and benefits, and the task of medical decision-making became more complex. The best or optimal treatment for a given disease was often less clear. Patient preferences in treatment decisions became an important consideration, as patients naturally differed in the outcomes they most valued and the side effects they least wanted, resulting in different treatment decisions for the same disease.

Shared decision-making was developed in order to engage and invest patients in making decisions about the treatment and management of an illness, based on the outcomes they desired (Wennberg, 1988). Shared decision-making involves teaching the person about the nature of their disease, discussing the advantages and disadvantages of different treatment options, and then involving the person in making treatment decisions based on a consideration of the likely outcomes (Charles et al., 1997, 1999). As shared decision-making required that individuals be educated about the nature of their diseases and the different treatment options, teaching them this information became standard medical practice, which extended to psychiatry (Deegan et al., 2008; Dixon et al., 2016).

The goals of illness self-management programmes

Psychiatric illness self-management programmes are aimed at teaching clients how to manage their psychiatric disorders in collaboration with others. Although a range of different programmes have been developed, most share a common set of goals, including to:

- instil hope for a better quality of life and a more favourable course of illness by improving illness self-management skills
- foster the development of a collaborative approach between clients and treatment providers in establishing treatment goals and choosing treatment options
- provide information about the nature of the individual's psychiatric illness and options for treating it
- teach strategies for monitoring the course of the illness and for preventing or minimizing symptom relapses and hospitalizations
- improve social support for illness self-management
- teach effective strategies for coping with persistent symptoms and illness-related impairments
- teach strategies for reducing the negative effects of stress
- assist clients in making lifestyle changes in order to facilitate the management of the psychiatric illness.

Methods for improving illness self-management

A wide range of methods have been developed to achieve the goals of illness self-management. Some of these methods are nearly universal across different programmes, such as psychoeducation, whereas others vary from one programme to another, such as peer support and skills training. In addition to the methods used across programmes, they also differ with respect to the teaching modality (e.g. individual or group) and the provider (e.g. peer, professional). Eight different strategies for teaching illness self-management are briefly described below: psychoeducation, medication adherence strategies, relapse prevention training, coping strategies for persistent symptoms, stress management, social skills training, peer support, and family psychoeducation.

Psychoeducation

Psychoeducation refers to teaching information about a psychiatric disorder in an interactive fashion that engages the client's interest in the information and its perceived relevance to their lives and goals (Ascher-Svanum & Krause, 1991; Swezey & Swezey, 1976). Psychoeducation includes a combination of didactic teaching strategies with frequent questions and prompts to help individuals relate the information to their own personal experiences and circumstances. A variety of materials may be used to teach information about a psychiatric disorder, including handouts, DVDs, posters, and other media. A summary of the topic areas frequently addressed in psychoeducation programmes for serious mental disorders is provided in **Box 23.1**.

Medication adherence strategies

Non-adherence to prescribed medications is an important predictor of relapses and hospitalizations for persons whose psychiatric disorders have been previously stabilized with medication (Miner et

> **Box 23.1** Outline of curriculum for psychoeducation about psychiatric disorders
>
> - Name of psychiatric disorder and how a diagnosis is established
> - Prevalence, onset, and possible courses of the disorder
> - Characteristic symptoms and related problems
> - Theories about the aetiology of the disorder and factors affecting its course (e.g. stress-vulnerability model)
> - Reducing negative attitudes and beliefs about mental illness
> - Pharmacological treatment:
>   - Names and types of medication
>   - Clinical effects
>   - Side effects
> - Psychosocial treatment:
>   - Psychotherapy and counselling (e.g. cognitive behavioural therapy)
>   - Illness self-management programmes
>   - Family psychoeducation
>   - Psychiatric rehabilitation (e.g. social skills training, cognitive remediation, supported employment)
> - Family and other social supports
> - Self-help/peer support.

Table 23.1 Strategies for helping clients increase their adherence to prescribed medications

Strategy	Description
Psychoeducation	Provide information about medications, their effects and side effects
Behavioural tailoring	Help client incorporate taking medication into their daily routine
Pill boxes or organizers	Facilitate client taking medication by using pill boxes or organizers
Alarms and other prompts	Teach client how to use alarms (e.g. on one's mobile phone) and other electronic prompts to take medication
Simplify medication regimen	In collaboration with prescriber, reduce number of different medications and number of times per day medication is taken
Motivational interviewing	Explore with client how taking medication can help them achieve personal goals
Social skills training	Teach client skills for interacting with and expressing concerns to medication prescriber
Depot medications	Explore with client potential benefits of taking depot antipsychotic medications over oral medication
Enlisting assistance of family members or other supporters	Explore with client how family members or other supporters could help them set up a system for taking medications and/or provide prompts for taking them

al., 1997). There are many different reasons why people do not take their prescribed medications (Roe et al., 2009; Weiden et al., 1995), as described below.

Some clients do not take their medication regularly because they do not fully understand the purpose of the medication, or may have misconceptions about the effects of medication. For example, many clients believe that if they are not experiencing symptoms, they do not need to keep taking their medication; they do not know that medication also prevents symptom relapses. Some people do not take medication because they believe it is addictive, or they are afraid of interactions between the medication and alcohol and/or street drugs. Another common reason for non-adherence is that people simply forget to take their medication at the appropriate times. Medication side effects, such as weight gain, sexual difficulties, restlessness, or sedation are other factors that can precipitate medication discontinuation. Lack of accurate information about the effects of medications and their side effects may also lead to medication discontinuation when clients do not feel confident, comfortable, and socially skilled at discussing their concerns with their prescriber. Last, individuals may not take their medication because they do not see how it can improve their lives or help them achieve their goals. Individuals with serious psychiatric disorders vary in their insight into their symptoms, and even those who are aware of their symptoms may not place a high priority on reducing symptoms or reducing symptom relapses.

A wide range of interventions have been developed to increase adherence to prescribed medication. Programmes that target medication adherence typically teach a number of different strategies, tailored to the individual needs of the client. Commonly used strategies for increasing medication adherence are summarized in Table 23.1.

Relapse prevention training

For many individuals, serious psychiatric disorders are episodic, with the severity of symptoms fluctuating over time, occasionally requiring psychiatric hospitalization when the person poses a threat to self or others. A relapse is defined as either the re-emergence of symptoms (in a client whose symptoms were previously in remission) or the worsening of symptoms (in a client with persistent symptoms), accompanied by a deterioration in functioning, such as increased problems at work or school, social difficulties, or reduction in self-care. Relapses tend to occur gradually, over several weeks, and are often preceded by subtle changes or *early warning signs* that are unique to the individual, such as a mild increase in depression, social withdrawal, or difficulties with concentration. Whether or not early warning signs precede the re-emergence or worsening of psychiatric symptoms, there is usually a window of opportunity for rapid intervention during the early stages of a relapse that can prevent a deterioration in functioning and full-blown relapse from occurring (Herz, 1984). The most common type of rapid intervention that can stave off a relapse if detected early enough is an increase in the individual's medication (Herz et al., 2000).

Relapse prevention training involves teaching the client about the nature of relapse, helping the individual identify their early warning signs or first symptoms of relapse, developing a plan for monitoring signs and symptoms, and taking rapid action at the first indication of a possible relapse. Relapse prevention plans should be regarded as a 'living document' that can be changed and improved over time to make it more effective. The steps of developing a relapse prevention plan are summarized in Box 23.2.

Coping strategies for persistent symptoms

Many individuals with serious mental disorders experience persistent symptoms, even when they are adherent to their prescribed medications. For example, hallucinations, paranoia, delusions of reference, depression, anxiety, sleep problems, or cognitive difficulties may persist and lead to distress and interference with everyday functioning and the enjoyment of life. Phenomenological studies

> **Box 23.2** Steps of developing a relapse prevention plan
>
> 1. If possible, in addition to working with the patient to develop the plan, try to involve a family member or friend who is close to the client.
> 2. Identify triggers of previous relapses, such as specific stressful situations.
> 3. Identify two or three specific early warning signs of relapse based on a discussion of the past one or two relapses.
> 4. Develop a system for monitoring the early warning signs of relapse.
> 5. Determine an action plan for responding to early warning signs of relapse, including who should be contacted.
> 6. Write down the plan, including the specific early warning signs that are being monitored and the telephone numbers of any important contact people.
> 7. Rehearse the plan in a role-play, post the plan in a prominent location, and give copies to anyone with an assigned role in the plan.
> 8. If a relapse occurs, after the client is safe and the situation has been stabilized, convene a meeting with the client and others who are involved in the plan, praise everyone for implementing those parts of the plan that went well, and then modify the plan to make it more effective.

and personal accounts of individuals with serious mental disorders have shown that many people develop coping strategies for reducing the distress and interference caused by persistent symptoms (Breier & Strauss, 1983; Leete, 1989).

While many individuals with serious mental disorders spontaneously develop strategies for coping with persistent symptoms, many others do not. However, effective coping strategies can be systematically taught using cognitive behavioural teaching principles (Tarrier, 1992). Coping skills can be taught using the following steps:

1. Focus on symptoms that either cause distress or interfere with an area of functioning that the client wants to improve.
2. Explore with the client the situations in which the symptom is most and least problematic.
3. Identify coping strategies that the client currently uses to deal with the target symptom and the effectiveness of those strategies.
4. If the client reports using effective strategies to cope with the symptom, but these strategies are infrequently utilized, make a plan with the client to increase their use of those skills on a regular basis.
5. After increasing the utilization of coping skills that the client already uses, review and describe other possible strategies for coping with the symptom.
6. Help the client select another coping strategy to learn.
7. Model (demonstrate) the new coping skill in a role-play for the client.
8. Engage the client in practising the new coping strategy in a role-play.
9. Praise the client for trying the new strategy, make adaptations to the strategy if necessary, and engage the client in additional role-plays to practise it as needed.
10. Develop a plan with the client to practise the new coping strategy outside of the session, focusing first on easier and more manageable situations.
11. Follow-up on the plan and make modifications to the coping strategy and practise it as needed.
12. Help the client develop at least two or three coping strategies for each symptom, as coping self-efficacy is related to the number of strategies people report using.

A wide range of different coping strategies has been developed to help individuals manage persistent symptoms and impairments more effectively. In addition to individual or group-based teaching of coping strategies using the principles of cognitive behavioural therapy, a growing number of digital tools have been developed to teach such skills, such as smartphone apps (Ben-Zeev et al., 2018) and online platforms (Gottlieb et al., 2017). Table 23.2 summarizes some coping strategies for the most common symptoms.

Stress management

Stress is a well-established precipitant of symptom exacerbations (Zubin & Spring, 1977). While the minimization of unnecessary stress can be a valuable illness management strategy, stress is an inherent part of life, and many of the goals that clients have involve stress, such as working in an interesting job, pursuing an educational degree, having a loving relationship, or being a parent. Therefore, teaching stress management skills is another common component of illness self-management programmes.

Illness self-management programmes use a variety of different strategies to improve coping with stress, with most strategies drawn from or adapted from stress management techniques developed for the general population (Davis et al., 2008; Woolfolk et al., 2008). Commonly used stress management techniques include relaxed breathing, using positive imagery, and muscular relaxation (Gingerich & Mueser, 2011).

Social skills training

Social support and social contact are strong predictors of the course of serious mental disorders, including relapses and rehospitalizations (Erickson et al., 1989; Strauss & Carpenter, 1977). Therefore, improving social support and the quality of social relationships has the potential to facilitate the management and outcome of these disorders. Social skills training, which involves systematically teaching more effective interpersonal skills by breaking complex skills into their constituent elements and then teaching these elements through a combination of modelling, role-play rehearsal, positive and corrective feedback, and home assignments to practise skills, is a widely used approach to improving the quality of social relationships for people with serious mental disorders (Mueser et al., 2024). Examples of commonly taught social skills include starting conversations, expressing positive feelings, making a request, and finding common interests.

Peer support

Individuals with a serious mental disorder who are coping effectively and moving ahead with their lives can serve as important peer supports and role models for others who are struggling with their disorder (Clay et al., 2005; Davidson et al., 2012). People who are successfully managing their psychiatric disorder, and who have rewarding lives in areas such as work, school, social relationships, leisure time, and living situation, can provide credible and realistic hope to others who may be discouraged about their lives and their future. Instilling hope for a better life can provide the impetus for learning illness self-management.

Table 23.2 Examples of coping strategies for persistent symptoms

Depression	Anxiety
• Schedule pleasant events • Use positive self-talk • Challenge negative, self-defeating thoughts • Increase activity level	• Learn relaxation strategies • Gradually expose oneself to feared but safe situations • Use positive self-talk • Challenge negative, self-defeating thoughts
Hallucinations	**Cognitive difficulties**
• Shift attention (e.g. listen to music) • Use positive self-talk • Accept that voices will not go away but need not be a major focus of your attention • Increase contact with others	• Remove distractions to improve attention • Over-practise to improve psychomotor speed • Use memory aids (e.g. pocket calendar) to reduce forgetting • Learn step-by-step problem-solving to address problems
Sleep problems	**Negative symptoms**
• Choose a standard time to go to bed and get up each day • Avoid napping even if you don't get enough sleep the previous night • Avoid caffeine after 5 p.m. • Develop a relaxing bedtime routine • If you have trouble sleeping for 30 minutes, get out of bed for 10–15 minutes and then return to bed	• Break down big goals into smaller goals and steps • Schedule regular pleasant activities to engage in • Focus on the future not the past • Praise yourself for your efforts and accomplishing small steps

Family psychoeducation

Family stress does not cause serious mental disorders, but can be a precipitant of relapse in some individuals (Butzlaff & Hooley, 1998). Family stress may be due in part to the significant challenges of helping a relative deal with a severe mental disorder (Hatfield & Lefley, 1993), but can also be due to a lack of understanding about the nature of the disorder and its treatment (Barrowclough & Hooley, 2003). Many families have not been given information about their relative's psychiatric disorder and its treatment, making it difficult for them to support their relative's adherence to treatment recommendations and work towards personal goals. Families may also not have a working relationship with their relative's treatment team, preventing them from getting timely help when their relative's illness worsens. These families often have significant amounts of contact with their relative, and are in an ideal position to work collaboratively with the treatment team if they are provided with the information and skills they need to help their relative learn how to better manage their disorder.

Family psychoeducation programmes have been developed in order to reduce stress in the family, increase the knowledge of family members (including the client) about the mental disorder and its treatment, to improve family support for the client's adherence to the recommended treatments, to monitor the course of the psychiatric disorder, and to work with the client to achieve their personal recovery goals. A variety of family programmes have been developed for people with a mental disorder using either single-family or multiple-family group treatment modalities, which include the client in family sessions (Lefley, 2009). Many of the strategies for improving illness self-management previously described are incorporated into family programmes, such as psychoeducation, developing a relapse prevention plan, implementing strategies for reducing stress in the family, and training in communication and problem-solving skills to reduce stress and improve social support (Anderson et al., 1986; Barrowclough & Tarrier, 1992; Falloon et al., 1984; Kuipers et al., 2002; Mueser & Glynn, 1999; Weissman de Mamani et al., 2021). Multifamily group formats incorporate these strategies and also provide peer support to clients and their relatives (McFarlane, 2002).

Research on illness self-management

Numerous studies have been conducted to evaluate the effectiveness of different approaches to teaching illness self-management to people with serious mental disorders. In a review of 40 randomized controlled trials evaluating different approaches to illness self-management training, Mueser et al. (2002) concluded that there is evidence supporting four major methods for teaching illness self-management: psychoeducation, medication adherence strategies, relapse prevention training, and coping skills training. More recent reviews of research on illness self-management reached similar conclusions (Bighelli et al., 2021; Lean et al., 2019; Morin & Franck, 2017).

Some amount of psychoeducation is a necessary part of illness self-management programmes in order to facilitate client involvement in shared decision-making about treatment. Early research suggested that although psychoeducation programmes alone led to significant improvements in knowledge about mental illness and its treatment, they did not reduce symptoms or relapses (Mueser et al., 2002), suggesting that psychoeducation was necessary but not sufficient to equip clients with the skills they need to manage their psychiatric disorder effectively. However, a more review of research on psychoeducation have concluded that it does in fact improve the course of psychiatric illness (Xia et al., 2011; Zhao et al., 2015).

Although Mueser et al. (2002) reviewed research on a wide range of different strategies for improving medication adherence, they found that only one strategy enjoyed consistent support in controlled trials: behavioural tailoring. *Behavioural tailoring* involves helping the client incorporate the taking of medication into their daily routine so that the person is reminded to take medication at the appropriate times (e.g. having the client place his medication next to his toothbrush so that he is reminded to take his medication when he brushes his teeth in the morning and evening).

There is also strong support for the effectiveness of training in the prevention of relapses and hospitalizations (Bighelli et al., 2021; Lean et al., 2019; Mueser et al., 2002). Similarly, controlled studies of teaching coping strategies for persistent symptoms also demonstrated significant reductions in symptom severity and distress related to symptoms. Teaching coping strategies is routinely incorporated into cognitive behavioural therapy for psychosis, which has been found to reduce the severity of psychotic and negative symptoms in schizophrenia (Turner et al., 2018, 2020).

The research literature on social skills training has steadily accumulated over the past three decades, with growing evidence supporting its effectiveness (M. M. Kurtz & Mueser, 2008). The most recent meta-analysis of controlled research on social skills training for schizophrenia reported moderate effect sizes for the impact of skills training on improving both social functioning and negative symptoms (Turner et al., 2018). Thus, social skills training has support for improving illness self-management skills in persons with serious psychiatric disorders.

There is also a strong evidence base supporting the effectiveness of professionally led family psychoeducation programmes for serious psychiatric disorders (Camacho-Gomez & Castellvi, 2020; Pharoah et al., 2010; Reinares et al., 2014). The most effective family programmes are those that are relatively long term (minimum 9 months), develop a collaborative relationship between the treatment team and family members, involve educating the family about mental illness and its treatment, help the family develop a relapse prevention plan, and reduce family burden and stress (Harvey, 2018). Both single- and multifamily group formats have been found to be effective at improving the management of serious psychiatric disorders.

Only a limited amount of research has evaluated the benefits of peer support programmes for improving illness self-management (Barber et al., 2008; Chinman et al., 2014). The results of the research conducted thus far is inconclusive, although the study of peer support programmes involves methodological challenges for researchers since those programmes are often embedded within larger self-help programmes that are difficult to randomly assign individuals to. More research is needed on this important approach to illness self-management.

Standardized illness self-management programmes

A number of illness self-management programmes have been standardized and are widely available to people with a serious mental disorder. We briefly describe several of those programmes below.

Illness Management and Recovery programme

The Illness Management and Recovery (IMR) is a programme in which clients set personal recovery goals at the beginning of the programme, break those goals down into smaller goals and steps which they work towards over the course of the programme, and then learn illness self-management information and skills in order to help them achieve their personal goals (Gingerich & Mueser, 2005, 2010, 2011). The curriculum is divided into 11 topic areas or modules, each requiring three to seven sessions to complete. It takes an average of 5–10 months of either twice-weekly or weekly sessions to complete the overall programme, although persons with more severe symptoms may take longer. The module topics include the following:

1. Recovery strategies
2. Practical facts about schizophrenia/bipolar disorder/depression
3. Stress-vulnerability model and strategies for treatment
4. Building social support
5. Using medications effectively
6. Drug and alcohol use
7. Reducing relapses
8. Coping with stress
9. Coping with problems and persistent symptoms
10. Getting your needs met in the mental health system
11. Healthy lifestyles.

Each module includes a handout for the client and teaching guidelines for the clinician. The guidelines for each module provide recommendations for using psychoeducational, cognitive behavioural, and motivational enhancement teaching strategies. Home assignments are collaboratively developed at the end of each session, and clients are encouraged to involve family members and other supporters in helping them practise their illness management skills and work on their personal goals. The IMR programme can be implemented in either an individual or group modality.

The IMR programme was developed following a comprehensive review of research on illness self-management (Mueser et al., 2002), and was designed to include the core effective elements described in the previous section on research (psychoeducation, behavioural tailoring for medication adherence, relapse prevention training, coping skills training, and social skills training). Since the development of the IMR programme, it has been translated into over 19 languages and multiple controlled studies have been conducted in six different countries. While there are some inconsistencies in findings across studies, most have reporting beneficial effects of IMR on illness self-management and related outcomes when compared to usual services (McGuire et al., 2014).

In addition, one study evaluated whether the IMR programme could be implemented with high fidelity to the treatment model in routine treatment settings serving people with serious mental illness in the US (McHugo, et al., 2007). Based on a standardized training and consultation model, the IMR programme was implemented at 12 community mental health centres throughout the US, with fidelity assessments conducted at baseline and every 6 months for 2 years. The results indicated that good levels of fidelity could be achieved 6 months after the initial training, with modest improvements at 1 year that were maintained at the 2-year fidelity assessment. This study supported the feasibility of implementing the IMR programme in routine treatment settings serving people with serious psychiatric disorders.

The IMR programme has also been adapted to meet the special needs of specific groups of individuals with serious mental illness, as well as for individuals from different cultures. For example, the Integrated IMR programme combines teaching psychiatric and physical illness self-management to people with serious mental illness and common comorbid disorders such as diabetes and cardiovascular disease (Bartels et al., 2014), while guidelines have been developed for providing IMR to individuals with very severe psychiatric impairment receiving treatment on Assertive Community Treatment teams (Monroe-DeVita et al., 2018). IMR has been adapted and implemented successfully in a diverse range of different non-Western cultures, including in Japan (Fujita et al., 2010), Tanzania (Johnson et al., 2009), and Arab-Israelis (Daass-Iraqi et al., 2020).

Social and Independent Living Skills programme

The Medication Management and Symptom Management modules are two of eight different skills training modules that form the Social and Independent Living Skills (SILS) programme (Kopelowicz & Liberman, 1994). These modules were developed for persons with schizophrenia spectrum disorders with the aim of providing them with information about pharmacological and psychosocial treatments, developing a relapse prevention plan, and teaching strategies for coping with persistent symptoms. Other modules in the SILS programme include Basic Conversational Skills, Recreation for Leisure, Community Reentry (for inpatients anticipating discharge into the community), Substance Abuse Management, Workplace Fundamentals, and Friendship and Intimacy.

All of the modules in this programme are taught using the principles of social skills training, based on video demonstrations of topic areas and skills. Modules are designed to be taught in a group format, although they can also be taught individually. Each module includes a core set of materials, including an instructor's manual, participants' workbooks, a demonstration video, and fidelity and outcome measures. For the Medication Management module, teaching is organized around four topic areas: the benefits of medication, self-administration and self-monitoring of medication effects, coping with side effects, and negotiating medication issues with health providers. The Symptom Management module is organized around four skill areas: identifying early warning signs of relapse and seeking early intervention, devising a relapse prevention plan, coping with persistent symptoms, and avoiding substance abuse. The duration of time needed to complete each module depends on the frequency of sessions and level of functioning of participants, with 3–6 months of twice-weekly sessions required to teach a module to outpatients.

A significant amount of research has been conducted on the Medication Management and Symptom Management modules, which are often provided in the context of skills training in other areas (Liberman, 2007). Controlled research shows that clients participating in these modules acquire and retain targeted information and skills over 1 year, as compared with other non-skills training interventions (Eckman et al., 1992; Wirshing et al., 1992). Research on the dissemination of modules in the SILS programme indicates that clinicians can implement the module with high fidelity to the programme (Liberman, 2007).

Wellness Recovery Action Plan

The Wellness Recovery Action Plan (WRAP) was developed as a general, standardized programme for helping individuals with recurring health and emotional problems to develop healthier and more rewarding lives (Copeland, 1997; Copeland & Mead, 2004). WRAP is a structured programme in which an individual or group of persons is guided through developing a written plan for managing or reducing distressing symptoms and making other desired changes in their lives. WRAP is aimed at helping people with a variety of mental health problems regain control and balance in their life, and it therefore does not provide information about specific disorders or treatments. The WRAP programme is divided into seven different components, each one including written plans that the client maintains in a workbook:

1. Creating a daily maintenance plan
2. Identifying triggers, early warning signs, and signs of potential crisis
3. Developing a crisis plan
4. Establishing a nurturing lifestyle (e.g. more healthy living)
5. Setting up a support system and self-advocating
6. Increasing self-esteem
7. Relieving tension and stress.

Teaching is typically done through a combination of lecture and discussion, with time taken to complete the plan and receive advice and support. WRAP is usually provided by trained consumers, who use their own experiences to inspire others to realize that they can recover their wellness.

Although limited research has evaluated the WRAP programme, a number of controlled trials have been conducted in recent years (e.g. Cook et al., 2012; Jonikas et al., 2013). A recent meta-analysis that included the results of five controlled trials reported that WRAP was more effective at improving self-perceived recovery outcomes, but not for improving clinical symptoms (Canacott et al., 2019). However, research on this programme is still at a relatively early stage, and definitive conclusions about its effectiveness cannot be reached.

Dialectical behaviour therapy

Dialectical behaviour therapy (DBT) is a comprehensive psychotherapeutic approach that was originally developed with a primary focus on reducing self-injurious and suicidal behaviour, but now is more broadly applied to persons with borderline personality disorder (Linehan, 1993, 2014). *Dialectic* or *dialectics* refers to the process of resolving conflict between two apparently contradictory ideas or forces through a synthesis of the two or establishing truths on both sides, rather than attempting to prove one right and the other wrong. In DBT, dialectics are employed at the level of the therapeutic relationship by the clinician's combined use of validation and acceptance of the client as they are, with the strategies aimed at changing behaviour and achieving a better balance in the client's functioning. Dialectics are also used to help clients strike a balance between the *reasonable mind* and the *emotional mind* in striving to develop a *wise mind* that combines the two and an integrated fashion.

In practice, DBT involves a wide array of cognitive behavioural techniques to improve interpersonal skills (e.g. social skills training), self-management of negative emotions (e.g. cognitive restructuring), and practical problem-solving. These are combined with mindfulness-based approaches (e.g. focusing on the present, taking a non-judgemental stance) aimed at promoting acceptance and tolerance of the person as they are, including any unpleasant feelings and thoughts. DBT is usually provided using a combination of weekly individual psychotherapy and group skills training sessions, with the clinicians providing DBT also participating in weekly case consultation meetings among themselves. Specific guidelines are provided for establishing a clear treatment contract between the client and clinician before the beginning of the programme, and to specify in advance the nature of additional contacts and rules concerning these contacts (e.g. telephone calls regarding thoughts of self-injury).

Following the development of DBT, a body of controlled research has gradually emerged supporting the effectiveness of the approach (e.g. Bohus et al., 2004; Verheul et al., 2003). Research on DBT has reported several positive effects, including significant reductions in suicidal behaviour and improvement in common emotional problems such as depression, hopelessness, and anger. A recent meta-analysis of 18 controlled studies of DBT found the intervention had a significantly greater impact on reducing self-harming behaviour and psychiatric emergency service utilization (DeCou et al., 2019).

Summary and conclusions

It is now widely accepted that people with serious psychiatric disorders are highly capable of being active partners with professionals, family members, and other supporters in the treatment of their disorder and that the provision of optimal mental health treatment requires this kind of partnership. Illness self-management programmes are aimed at developing a collaborative relationship between clients and treatment providers, engaging clients in establishing treatment goals, educating them about the nature of their disorder so that they can make informed decisions about their treatment, teaching them strategies for monitoring their disorder and preventing relapses, teaching them strategies for coping with persistent symptoms or disorder-related impairments, instilling hope for a better future, and increasing social support for improved illness self-management and making progress towards goals. A number of standardized programmes have been developed to teach clients illness self-management information and skills.

Research on approaches to illness self-management provides empirical support for both comprehensive illness self-management programmes as well as specific treatment strategies. Evidence-based illness self-management strategies include psychoeducation about the disorder and its treatment, behavioural tailoring to help the client incorporate taking medication into their daily routines, relapse prevention training, teaching coping skills for persistent symptoms, social skills training to improve social support, and family psychoeducation to develop a collaborative relationship between treatment providers and the family and to teach families (including the client) the principles of illness management. The adoption of more collaboratively based treatment approaches for serious psychiatric disorders that recognize the importance of involving the client and significant others in decision-making, combined with the growth in empirically supported strategies and programmes for teaching illness self-management, brings the ultimate goal of recovery within reach of many more people with these disorders.

REFERENCES

Anderson, C. M., Reiss, D. J., & Hogarty, G. E. (1986). *Schizophrenia and the Family*. New York: Guilford Press.

Anthony, W. A. (1993). Recovery from mental illness: the guiding vision of the mental health service system in the 1990s. *Psychosocial Rehabilitation Journal*, **16**, 11–23.

Ascher-Svanum, H. & Krause, A. A. (1991). *Psychoeducational Groups for Patients with Schizophrenia: A Guide for Practitioners*. Gaithersburg, MD: Aspen.

Barber, J., Rosenheck, R., Armstrong, M., & Resnick, S. G. (2008). Monitoring the dissemination of peer support in the VA healthcare system. *Community Mental Health Journal*, **44**, 433–441.

Barrowclough, C. & Hooley, J. M. (2003). Attributions and expressed emotion: a review. *Clinical Psychology Review*, **23**, 849–880.

Barrowclough, C. & Tarrier, N. (1992). *Families of Schizophrenic Patients: Cognitive Behavioural Intervention*. London: Chapman and Hall.

Bartels, S. J., Pratt, S. I., Mueser, K. T., Wolfe, R., Santos, M. M., Naslund, J. A., Xie, H., & Riera, E. G. (2014). Integrated psychiatric and medical illness self-management for adults with serious mental illness: a randomized clinical trial. *Psychiatric Services*, **65**, 330–337.

Beard, J. H., Propst, R. N., & Malamud, T. J. (1982). The Fountain House model of rehabilitation. *Psychosocial Rehabilitation Journal*, **5**, 47–53.

Bellack, A. S. (2006). Scientific and consumer models of recovery in schizophrenia: concordance, contrasts, and implications. *Schizophrenia Bulletin*, **32**, 432–442.

Ben-Zeev, D., Brian, R. M., Jonathan, G., Razzano, L. A., Pashka, N., Carpenter-Song, E., et al. (2018). Mobile health (mhealth) versus clinic-based group intervention for people with serious mental illness: a randomized controlled trial. *Psychiatric Services*, **69**, 978–985.

Bighelli, I., Rodolico, A., García-Mieres, H., Pitschel-Walz, G., Hansen, W. P., Schneider-Thoma, J., et al. (2021). Psychosocial and psychological interventions for relapse prevention in schizophrenia: a systematic review and network meta-analysis. *Lancet Psychiatry*, **8**, 969–980.

Blackwell, B. (1976). Treatment adherence. *British Journal of Psychiatry*, **129**, 513–531.

Blaska, B. (1990). The myriad medication mistakes in psychiatry: a consumer's view. *Hospital and Community Psychiatry*, **41**, 993–997.

Bohus, M., Haaf, B., Simms, T., Limberger, M. F., Schmahl, C., Unckel, C., et al. (2004). Effectiveness of inpatient dialectical behavioral therapy for borderline personality disorder: a controlled trial. *Behaviour Research and Therapy*, **42**, 487–499.

Breier, A. M. & Strauss, J. S. (1983). Self-control of psychotic behavior. *Archives of General Psychiatry*, **40**, 1141–1145.

Butzlaff, R. L. & Hooley, J. M. (1998). Expressed emotion and psychiatric relapse. *Archives of General Psychiatry*, **55**, 547–552.

Camacho-Gomez, M. & Castellvi, P. (2020). Effectiveness of family intervention for preventing relapse in first-episode psychosis until 24 months of follow-up: a systematic review with meta-analysis of randomized controlled trials. *Schizophrenia Bulletin*, **46**, 98–109.

Campbell, J. (1997). How consumers/survivors are evaluating the quality of psychiatric care. *Evaluation Review*, **21**, 357–363.

Canacott, L., Moghaddam, N., & Tickle, A. (2019). Is the Wellness Recovery Action Plan (WRAP) efficacious for improving personal and clinical recovery outcomes? A systematic review and meta-analysis. *Psychiatric Rehabilitation Journal*, **42**, 372–381.

Carling, P. J. (1995). *Return to Community: Building Support Systems for People with Psychiatric Disabilities*. New York: Guilford Press.

Chamberlin, J. (1978). *On Our Own: Patient-Controlled Alternatives to the Mental Health System*. New York: Hawthorne.

Charles, C., Gafni, A., & Whelan, T. (1997). Shared decision-making in the medical encounter: what does it mean? (or it takes at least two to tango). *Social Science and Medicine*, **44**, 681–692.

Charles, C., Gafni, A., & Whelan, T. (1999). Decision-making in the physician-patient encounter: revisiting the shared treatment decision-making model. *Social Science and Medicine*, **49**, 651–661.

Chinman, M., George, P., Dougherty, R. H., Daniels, A. S., Ghose, S. S., Swift, A., et al. (2014). Peer support services for individuals with serious mental illnesses: assessing the evidence. *Psychiatric Services*, **65**, 429–441.

Clay, S., Schell, B., Corrigan, P., & Ralph, R. (Eds.) (2005). *On Our Own, Together: Peer Programs for People with Mental Illness*. Nashville, TN: Vanderbilt University Press.

Cook, J. A., Copeland, M. E., Jonikas, J. A., Hamilton, M. M., Razzano, L. A., Grey, D. D., et al. (2012). Results of a randomized controlled trial of mental illness self-management using Wellness Recovery Action Planning. *Schizophrenia Bulletin*, **38**, 881–891.

Copeland, M. E. (1994). *Living Without Depression and Manic Depression*. Oakland, CA: New Harbinger.

Copeland, M. E. (1997). *Wellness Recovery Action Plan*. Brattleboro, VT: Peach Press.

Copeland, M. E. & Mead, S. (2004). *Wellness Recovery Action Plan and Peer Support: Personal, Group and Program Development*. Dummerston, VT: Peach Press.

Daass-Iraqi, S., Mashiach-Eizenberg, M., Garber-Epstein, P., & Roe, D. (2020). Impact of a culturally adapted version of illness management and recovery on Israeli Arabs with serious mental illness. *Psychiatric Services*, **71**, 951–954.

Davidson, L. (2003). *Living Outside Mental Illness: Qualitative Studies of Recovery in Schizophrenia*. New York: New York University Press.

Davidson, L., Bellamy, C., Guy, K., & Miller, R. (2012). Peer support among persons with severe mental illnesses: a review of evidence and experience. *World Psychiatry*, **11**, 123–128.

Davis, M., Eshelman, E. R., McKay, M., & Fanning, P. (2008). *The Relaxation and Stress Reduction Workbook* (6th ed.). Oakland, CA: New Harbinger Publications.

DeCou, C. R., Comtois, K. A., & Landes, S. J. (2019). Dialectical behavior therapy is effective for the treatment of suicidal behavior: a meta-analysis. *Behavior Therapy*, **50**, 60–72.

Deegan, P. E. (1988). Recovery: the lived experience of rehabilitation. *Psychosocial Rehabilitation Journal*, **11**, 11–19.

Deegan, P. E. (1990). Spirit breaking: when the helping professionals hurt. *The Humanistic Psychologist*, **18**, 301–313.

Deegan, P. E., Rapp, C. A., Holter, M., & Riefer, M. (2008). Best practices: a program to support shared decision making in an outpatient psychiatric medication clinic. *Psychiatric Services*, **59**, 603–605.

Dixon, L. B., Holoshitz, Y., & Nossel, I. (2016). Treatment engagement of individuals experiencing mental illness: review and update. *World Psychiatry*, **15**, 13–20.

Eckman, T. A., Wirshing, W. C., Marder, S. R., Liberman, R. P., Johnston-Cronk, K., Zimmermann, K., et al. (1992). Technique for training schizophrenic patients in illness self-management: a controlled trial. *American Journal of Psychiatry*, **149**, 1549–1555.

Erickson, D. H., Beiser, M., Iacono, W. G., Fleming, J. A. E., & Lin, T. (1989). The role of social relationships in the course of first-episode schizophrenia and affective psychosis. *American Journal of Psychiatry*, **146**, 1456–1461.

Falloon, I. R. H., Boyd, J. L., & McGill, C. W. (1984). *Family Care of Schizophrenia: A Problem-Solving Approach to the Treatment of Mental Illness*. New York: Guilford Press.

Fisher, D. B. (1992). Humanizing the recovery process. *Resources*, **4**, 5–6.

Frese, F. J. I. (2008). Self-help activities. In: K. T. Mueser & D. V. Jeste (Eds.), *Clinical Handbook of Schizophrenia* (pp. 298–305). New York: Guilford Press.

Frese, F. J. I. & Davis, W. W. (1997). The consumer-survivor movement, recovery, and consumer professionals. *Professional Psychology: Research and Practice*, **28**, 243–245.

Fujita, E., Kato, D., Kuno, E., Suzuki, Y., Uchiyama, S., Watanabe, A., et al. (2010). Implementing the illness management and recovery program in Japan. *Psychiatric Services*, **61**, 1157–1161.

Gartner, A. & Riessman, F. (1977). *Self-Help in the Human Services*. San Francisco, CA: Jossey-Bass Publishers.

Gingerich, S. & Mueser, K. T. (2005). Illness management and recovery. In: Drake, R. E., Merrens, M. R., & Lynde, D. W. (Eds.), *Evidence-Based Mental Health Practice: A Textbook* (pp. 395–424). New York: Norton.

Gingerich, S. & Mueser, K. T. (2010). *Illness Management and Recovery Implementation Resource Kit* (rev. ed.). Rockville, MD: Center for Mental Health Services, Substance Abuse and Mental Health Services Administration. http://mentalhealth.samhsa.gov/cmhs/CommunitySupport/toolkits/illness/

Gingerich, S. & Mueser, K. T. (2011). *Illness Management and Recovery: Personalized Skills and Strategies for Those with Mental Illness* (3rd ed.). Center City, MN: Hazelden.

Gottlieb, J. D., Gidugu, V., Maru, M., Tepper, M., Davis, M. J., Greenwold, J., et al. (2017). Randomized controlled trial of an internet cognitive behavioral skills-based program for auditory hallucinations in persons with psychosis. *Psychiatric Rehabilitation Journal*, **40**, 283–292.

Harrison, G., Hopper, K., Craig, T., Laska, E., Siegel, C., Wanderling, J., et al. (2001). Recovery from psychotic illness: a 15- and 25-year international follow-up study. *British Journal of Psychiatry*, **178**, 506–517.

Harvey, P. D., McGurk, S. R., Mahncke, H., & Wykes, T. (2018). Controversies in computerized cognitive training. *Biological Psychiatry: Cognitive Neuroscience and Neuroimaging*, **3**, 907–915.

Hatfield, A. B. & Lefley, H. P. (1993). *Surviving Mental Illness: Stress, Coping, and Adaptation*. New York: Guilford Press.

Herz, M. I. (1984). Recognizing and preventing relapse in patients with schizophrenia. *Hospital and Community Psychiatry*, **35**, 344–349.

Herz, M. I., Lamberti, J. S., Mintz, J., Scott, R., O'Dell, S. P., McCartan, L., et al. (2000). A program for relapse prevention in schizophrenia: a controlled study. *Archives of General Psychiatry*, **57**, 277–283.

Jennings, A. F. (1994). On being invisible in the mental health system. *Journal of Mental Health Administration*, **21**, 374–387.

Johnson, D. P., Ringo, E. J., Lyimo, A., Nolan, J., & Whetten, K. (2009). Implementation of group psychoeducation for severe mental illness in East Africa: lessons learned in Tanzania. *International Psychology Bulletin*, **12**, 17–19.

Jonikas, J. A., Grey, D. D., Copeland, M. E., Razzano, L. A., Hamilton, M. M., Floyd, C. B., et al. (2013). Improving propensity for patient self-advocacy through wellness recovery action planning: results of a randomized controlled trial. *Community Mental Health Journal*, **49**, 260–269.

Kopelowicz, A. & Liberman, R. P. (1994). Self-management approaches for seriously mentally ill persons. *Directions in Psychiatry*, **14**, 1–7.

Kuipers, L., Leff, J., & Lam, D. (2002). *Family Work for Schizophrenia: A Practical Guide* (2nd ed.). London: Gaskell.

Kurtz, L. (1988). Mutual aid for affective disorders: the manic depressive and depressive association. *American Journal of Orthopsychiatric Association, Inc.*, **58**, 152–155.

Kurtz, M. M. & Mueser, K. T. (2008). A meta-analysis of controlled research on social skills training for schizophrenia. *Journal of Consulting and Clinical Psychology*, **76**, 491–504.

Lean, M., Fornells-Ambrojo, M., Milton, A., Lloyd-Evans, B., Harrison-Stewart, B., Yesufu-Udechuku, A., et al. (2019). Self-management interventions for people with severe mental illness: systematic review and meta-analysis. *British Journal of Psychiatry*, **214**, 260–268.

Leete, E. (1989). How I perceive and manage my illness. *Schizophrenia Bulletin*, **15**, 197–200.

Lefley, H. (2009). *Family Psychoeducation in Serious Mental Illness: Models, Outcomes, Applications*. New York: Oxford University Press.

Liberman, R. P. (2007). Dissemination and adoption of social skills training: social validation of an evidence-based treatment for the mentally disabled. *Journal of Mental Health*, **16**, 595–623.

Linehan, M. M. (1993). *Cognitive-Behavioral Treatment of Borderline Personality Disorder*. New York: Guilford Press.

Linehan, M. M. (2014). *DBT Skills Training Manual* (2nd ed.). New York: Guilford.

McFarlane, W. R. (2002). *Multifamily Groups in the Treatment of Severe Psychiatric Disorders*. New York: Guilford Press.

McGuire, A. B., Kukla, M., Green, A. K., Mueser, K. T., & Salyers, M. P. (2014). Illness management and recovery: a review of the literature. *Psychiatric Services*, **65**, 171–179.

McHugo, G. J., Drake, R. E., Whitley, R., Bond, G. R., Campbell, K., Rapp, C., et al. (2007). Fidelity outcomes in the national implementing evidence-based project. *Psychiatric Services*, **58**, 1279–1284.

Miner, C. R., Rosenthal, R. N., Hellerstein, D. J., & Muenz, L. R. (1997). Prediction of compliance with outpatient referral in patients with schizophrenia and psychoactive substance use disorders. *Archives of General Psychiatry*, **54**, 706–712.

Monroe-DeVita, M., Morse, G., Mueser, K. T., McHugo, G. J., Xie, H., Hallgren, K. A., et al. (2018). Implementing illness management and recovery within assertive community treatment: a pilot trial of feasibility and effectiveness. *Psychiatric Services*, **69**, 562–571.

Morin, L. & Franck, N. (2017). Rehabilitation interventions to promote recovery from schizophrenia: a systematic review. *Frontiers in Psychiatry*, **8**, 100.

Mueser, K. T., Bellack, A. S., Gingerich, S., Agresta, J., & Fulford, D. (2024). *Social Skills Training for Schizophrenia: A Step-by-Step Guide* (Third ed.). Guilford Press.

Mueser, K. T., Corrigan, P. W., Hilton, D., Tanzman, B., Schaub, A., Gingerich, S., et al. (2002). Illness management and recovery for severe mental illness: a review of the research. *Psychiatric Services*, **53**, 1272–1284.

Mueser, K. T. & Glynn, S. M. (1999). *Behavioral Family Therapy for Psychiatric Disorders* (2nd ed.). Oakland, CA: New Harbinger.

National Academies of Sciences, Engineering, and Medicine (2016). *Measuring Recovery from Substance Use or Mental Disorders: Workshop Summary*. Washington, DC: National Academies Press.

Pharoah, F., Mari, J., Rathbone, J., & Wong, W. (2010). Family intervention for schizophrenia. *Cochrane Database of Systematic Reviews*, **12**, CD000088.

Ralph, R. O. & Corrigan, P. W. (Eds.) (2005). *Recovery in Mental Illness: Broadening Our Understanding of Wellness*. Washington, DC: American Psychological Association.

Reinares, M., Sánchez-Moreno, J., & Fountoulakis, K. N. (2014). Psychosocial interventions in bipolar disorder: what, for whom, and when. *Journal of Affective Disorders*, **156**, 46–55.

Roe, D. & Chopra, M. (2003). Beyond coping with mental illness: toward personal growth. *American Journal of Orthopsychiatry*, **73**, 334–344.

Roe, D., Goldblatt, H., Baloush-Klienman, V., Swarbrick, M., & Davidson, L. (2009). Why and how people decide to stop taking prescribed psychiatric medication: exploring the subjective process of choice. *Psychiatric Rehabilitation Journal*, **33**, 38–46.

Salzer, M. S., Brusilovskiy, E., & Townley, G. (2018). National estimates of recovery-remission from serious mental illness. *Psychiatric Services*, **69**, 523–528.

Segal, S. P., Silverman, C., & Temkin, T. (1993). Empowerment and self-help agency practice for people with mental disabilities. *Social Work*, **38**, 705–712.

Strauss, J. S. & Carpenter, W. T. (1977). Prediction of outcome in schizophrenia III. Five-year outcome and its predictors. *Archives of General Psychiatry*, **34**, 159–163.

Swezey, R. L. & Swezey, A. M. (1976). Educational theory as a basis for patient education. *Journal of Chronic Diseases*, **29**, 417–422.

Tarrier, N. (1992). Management and modification of residual positive psychotic symptoms. In: Birchwood, M. & Tarrier, N. (Eds.), *Innovations in the Psychological Management of Schizophrenia* (pp. 147–169). Chichester: John Wiley and Sons.

Turner, D. T., McGlanaghy, E., Cuijpers, P., van der Gaag, M., Karyotaki, E., & MacBeth, A. (2018). A meta-analysis of social skills training and related interventions for psychosis. *Schizophrenia Bulletin*, **44**, 475–491.

Turner, D. T., Reijnders, M., van der Gaag, M., Karyotaki, E., Valmaggia, L. R., Moritz, S., et al. (2020). Efficacy and moderators of cognitive behavioural therapy for psychosis versus other psychological interventions: an individual-participant data meta-analysis. *Frontiers in Psychiatry*, **11**, 402.

Verheul, R., Van Den Bosch, L. M. C., Koetter, M. W. J., De Ridder, M. A. J., Stijnen, T., & Van Den Brink, W. (2003). Dialectical behaviour therapy for women with borderline personality disorder: 12-month, randomised clinical trial in the Netherlands. *British Journal of Psychiatry*, **182**, 135–140.

Weiden, P. J., Mott, T., & Curcio, N. (1995). Recognition and management of neuroleptic noncompliance. In: Shriqui, C. L. & Nasrallah, H. A. (Eds.), *Contemporary Issues in the Treatment of Schizophrenia* (pp. 411–433). Washington, DC: American Psychiatric Press.

Weisman de Mamani, A., McLaughlin, M., Altamirano, O., Lopez, D., & Ahmad, S. S. (2021). *Culturally Informed Therapy for Schizophrenia: A Family-Focused Cognitive Behavioral Approach*, Clinician Guide. New York: Oxford University Press.

Wennberg, J. E. (1988). Improving the medical decision-making process. *Health Affairs*, **7**, 99–105.

Wirshing, W. C., Marder, S. R., Eckman, T., Liberman, R. P., & Mintz, J. (1992). Acquisition and retention of skills training methods in chronic schizophrenic outpatients. *Psychopharmacology Bulletin*, **28**, 241–245.

Woolfolk, R. L., Sime, W. E., & Barlow, D. H. (2008). *Principles and Practice of Stress Management* (3rd ed.). New York: Guilford Press.

Xia, J., Merinder, L. B., & Belgamwar, M. R. (2011). Psychoeducation for schizophrenia. *Cochrane Database of Systematic Reviews*, **15**(6).

Zhao, S., Sampson, S., Xia, J., & Jayaram, M. B. (2015). Psychoeducation (brief) for people with serious mental illness. *Cochrane Database of Systematic Reviews*, **4**(CD010823).

Zubin, J. & Spring, B. (1977). Vulnerability: a new view of schizophrenia. *Journal of Abnormal Psychology*, **86**, 103–126.

24

Co-occurring substance use disorders

Robert E. Drake, Kim T. Mueser, and Delia C. Hendrick

Introduction

Substance use disorders are common comorbidities among people with all types of mental health conditions, often worsening the course of mental illness and personal suffering, family distress, societal problems, and health costs. In this chapter we first review the generic characteristics of people with co-occurring substance use disorders, including prevalence, complications, and need for integrated treatment. We then describe integrated treatment and some of the effective interventions, including the need for approaches that are tailored for some of the common target groups and the individuals within those groups. Finally, we discuss the challenges of implementing integrated treatment within typical community mental health programmes.

Prevalence

People with serious mental illness (SMI) have greatly increased rates of co-occurring alcohol and drug use disorders (COD) compared to the general population. For example, while the lifetime rate of substance use disorder in the general population is about 16%, approximately 50% of individuals with SMI have lifetime COD (Kessler et al., 1997; Mueser et al., 2000; Regier et al., 1990). People with common mental health disorders other than SMI, including anxiety, depression, and post-traumatic stress disorder, also have substantially increased rates of COD, approximately 25–30% (Kessler et al., 1997). More recent data from the annual National Survey of Drug Use and Health in the US show lower past-year rates: for example, only 25–30% of people with SMI report symptoms of COD in the past year (NIDA, 2020). However, these surveys come from households and therefore miss people who are homeless, transient, incarcerated, or living in other institutions such as group homes, rehabilitation centres, or hospitals (Substance Abuse and Mental Health Services Administration, 2020)—locations with high rates of SMI and COD.

The reasons for such high prevalence are complex. Three broad categories encompass plausible explanations: common underlying third factors, mental illness leading to substance use disorder, and substance use disorder leading to mental illness (Mueser et al., 1998; Noordsy et al., 2013). Regarding underlying factors, genetic research shows that many of the genes that increase vulnerability for SMI also increase vulnerability for substance use disorders (Andersen et al., 2017; Hartz et al., 2018; Khokhar et al., 2018). In addition, psychosocial risk factors such as adverse childhood events, stress, and trauma can also predispose to both types of disorders (National Institute on Drug Abuse, 2020). Interactions also occur between genetic and environmental factors. For example, stress, trauma, or drug use can cause epigenetic changes that influence gene expression (Cheah et al., 2014; Peña et al., 2014).

Causality can sometimes be more unidirectional. Specific mental disorders, such as attention deficit hyperactivity disorder and anxiety disorders, are definite risk factors for COD (Grant et al., 2016; Wu et al., 2011). People affected by mental illness often attempt to use alcohol and other drugs to alleviate symptoms of mental illness, but evidence shows that even minimal use of alcohol, other drugs, or prescribed medications can worsen symptoms and lead to substance use disorders over time (Brunette et al., 2003; Drake & Wallach, 1993; Post & Kalivas, 2013). Substance use may also lead to brain changes associated with mental illness and that predispose to mental illness (Ross & Peselow, 2012). Common examples include heavy marijuana use precipitating psychosis and sometimes schizophrenia (Henquet et al., 2005; Manrique-Garcia et al., 2012) and heavy alcohol use leading to depression (Connor et al., 2009; Powell et al., 1987). In summary, multiple pathways can account for the high comorbidity between mental illness and substance use disorder.

Complications related to co-occurring alcohol and drug use disorders

Regardless of the causes, COD adds to the stress of living with a mental illness. Complications for affected individuals include diagnostic uncertainty (Caton et al., 2005), relapses (Linszen et al., 1994), hospitalizations (Haywood et al., 1995), family conflict (Niv et al., 2007) and loss of family support (Dixon et al., 1995), unemployment (Poremski et al., 2014), suicide (Ostergaard et al., 2017), victimization (Goodman et al., 2001), homelessness (Caton et al., 1994), non-compliance with medications and other treatments (Owen et al., 1996), justice system involvement and incarceration (Abram &

Teplin, 1991), traumatic brain injury (McHugo et al., 2017), serious infectious diseases such as HIV and hepatitis C (Rosenberg et al., 2001), and violence (Swartz et al., 1998). For example, the Macarthur Violence Risk Assessment Study, which included extensive follow-up information on over 1000 people with SMI, showed that the rate of violence among those with a major mental disorder who did not misuse substances was indistinguishable from their non-substance-misusing neighbourhood controls, but COD doubled the risk of violence (Steadman et al., 1998). In another study of inner-city patients with SMI, over three-quarters screened positive for at least one traumatic brain injury, and these episodes were associated with arrests, incarcerations, and homelessness (McHugo et al., 2017). As a simple rule, COD correlates with nearly all adverse effects, at a rate many times higher than for those with mental illness alone.

COD also creates problems for families, communities, and treatment systems. In addition to experiencing family disruptions, family members are the most likely targets of violence, which typically occurs in the home (Stuart, 2003). COD affects communities in various ways, including public nuisance crimes, homelessness, and interference with business. Treatment systems experience higher costs because patients with COD are prone to missed appointments, emergency department visits, and hospitalizations (Bartels et al., 1993; Dickey & Azeni, 1996).

These myriad effects of COD on adverse behaviour, family support, and community problems have suggested a poor prognosis for individuals with COD, reinforced by numerous short-term studies. For example, one study found virtually no 6-month improvements in COD among patients with the highest level of psychiatric severity (McLellan et al., 1983).

Course of co-occurring alcohol and drug use disorders

Although symptoms, social function, and disruptive behaviour among people with SMI and COD indicate serious problems at presentation, many people with early psychosis stop substance use quickly to avoid further relapses (Wisdom et al., 2011). For those with persistent COD, several (but not all) studies demonstrate diminishing problems and high rates of recovery over longer time intervals. These studies include a two-year naturalistic follow-up of patients with early psychosis and COD (Drake et al., 2011) as well as several follow-ups of patients in studies of assertive community treatment (Bartels et al., 1995; Drake et al., 2006, 2016, 2020; Essock et al., 2006; Morse et al., 2006). In the 2-year naturalistic follow-up of early psychosis patients with concurrent substance use, alcohol dependence, drug dependence, positive and negative symptoms of psychosis, family relationships, and friendships improved significantly, despite low rates of any specific interventions. In the assertive community treatment studies, all of which incorporated some types of COD interventions (discussed below), follow-ups ranging from four to 16 years indicated steady improvement trends in substance use, psychiatric symptoms, and social function. These trajectories were similar in rural and urban areas (Mueser et al., 2001).

Recovery may occur rapidly, slowly, or not at all for individuals within studies (Xie et al., 2009). The differences have to do with client characteristics, intervention characteristics, and environmental context (Alverson et al., 2000, 2001; Frisman et al., 2009; Mueser et al., 1997). For example, earlier intervention, before people have lost family and other supports, is always preferable. One recent cohort study showed very high rates of recovery for young men with SMI and COD in intensive treatment over 1 year (Acquilano et al., 2020). Participants in this study had several advantages, including 3–6 months of residential stabilization followed by intensive and assertive community treatment, both of which are evidence-based practices. By contrast, an inner-city study of chronically ill patients with SMI and COD found little recovery over two years, perhaps due to the older ages of participants, their location in impoverished, high-crime neighbourhoods, and lack of residential stabilization and assertive community treatment (McHugo et al., 2021). Another study, a longitudinal ethnography, identified several contextual factors that correlated with recovery: (1) regular engagement in an enjoyable activity; (2) decent, stable housing; (3) a loving relationship with someone sober who accepted the participant's mental illness; and (4) a positive, valued relationship with a mental health professional (Alverson et al., 2000).

Treatment

Historically, interventions for COD in people with SMI relied on either parallel or sequential treatment approaches. In the parallel approach, different clinicians, usually working for different agencies, provided separate treatments for mental illness and COD. In the sequential approach, clinicians first treated one disorder, followed by the second disorder. Both approaches are considered ineffective for most individuals with SMI (Polcin, 1992; Ridgely et al., 1990).

In contrast to parallel and sequential treatments, integrated treatment is a widely recommended, evidence-based approach in which the same clinician or team of clinicians takes responsibility for combining interventions for the two (and usually more) disorders and provides mental health and substance use services concurrently (Hendrickson, 2006; McGovern et al., 2008; Mueser et al., 2003a; Weiss & Connery, 2011). Integrated treatment combines and modifies multiple interventions in a coherent treatment plan (Mueser & Drake, 2007).

Principles of integrated treatment

Functional analysis

To conduct a functional analysis, the clinician gathers detailed information about the nature of the substance use, the client's activities, and possible reasons for using substances. The goal is to gain an understanding of the client's functioning across different life domains, such as relationships, family support or conflict, self-care, involvement in work or school activities, leisure activities, and symptoms. Details about the client's pattern of using substances include the types of substances used, situations in which they are used, motives for use, frequency and intensity of use, and the perceived positive and negative effects of using. The functional analysis leads to an understanding of how substance use fits into the client's life, including factors that maintain ongoing substance use and present a barrier to sobriety. Rather than assuming that substance use is an irrational behaviour that clients are compelled to engage in despite its negative consequences, a functional analysis assumes that substance use is maintained by the positive effects of using substances and the negative effects of not using, recognizing that the positive effects are often short-lived compared to the long-term negative effects.

Substance use is usually associated with at least one of four common motives: *reduction of distress* (e.g. coping with hallucinations, depression, or anxiety); *leisure and recreation* (e.g. because substances produce pleasure); *social facilitation* (e.g. something to do with friends, a way to meet people, peer pressure); and *structure and a sense of purpose* (e.g. something to look forward to) (Carey & Carey, 1995; Dixon et al., 1991; Mueser et al., 1995). Understanding the perceived reasons for using substances creates empathy and informs treatment planning. Clients are more successful in achieving sobriety if they are helped to develop alternative ways of getting their needs met.

Stages of treatment

Individuals with COD typically go through several stages in treatment (Mueser et al., 2003a; Osher & Kofoed, 1989). At the *engagement stage*, the goal is to establish a therapeutic relationship before making efforts to persuade the client to work on substance use problems. Outreach to connect with clients in the community, helping clients resolve a crisis or pressing problem, and providing practical assistance are common ways of establishing this relationship. In the *persuasion stage*, clients who have a working relationship may still not be motivated to develop a sober lifestyle. The goal is therefore to help them develop motivation to reduce substance use and achieve sobriety. Motivational interviewing and shared decision-making are common strategies. The *active treatment stage* focuses on helping the client reduce and give up substance use. Strategies include psychiatric rehabilitation to develop new skills for getting needs met in less destructive ways, developing a relapse prevention plan, practising skills for dealing with high-risk situations (e.g. being offered substances by friends), supported employment, and participation in a self-help group. When the client achieves sobriety, the *relapse prevention stage* focuses on maintaining new habits and supports for recovery, such as work and social relationships, and managing relapses. Interventions are most effective when they align with the client's stage of treatment. For example, when a therapeutic relationship has been established but there is no evidence that the client is motivated to develop a sober lifestyle, treatment should focus on instilling motivation rather than achieving sobriety.

Comprehensive, longitudinal involvement

People typically recover from COD over months and years rather than after one episode of treatment (Drake et al., 2016; 2020). Living a satisfying life without alcohol and drugs typically requires new ways of dealing with anxiety and depression, new habits, new friends, new relationships, new values, new jobs, and new leisure activities. Changing all these areas takes time. During the recovery process, a constant, accepting, hopeful relationship can help people through difficult times, including relapses and failures. A competent provider or team helps clients in many areas: not just avoiding alcohol and drugs but also finding new areas of satisfaction, establishing social relationships with people who support sobriety, developing new skills, and acquiring self-confidence.

Shared decision-making

No single intervention or path to recovery works for all people with COD. At each stage of treatment, clinicians and clients should discuss multiple options and try different strategies. For example, does the individual in active treatment want to use cognitive behaviour therapy, a COD treatment group, faith-based support, a self-help group, a medication, a new job, or some combination of these? Shared decision-making means that the clinician provides information on all options, helps the individual to make choices, and travels with the client during setbacks and successes, always instilling hope and encouragement.

Specific interventions

Several effective interventions for COD exist, including individual, group, and family therapies, contingency management, residential, employment, and medication approaches. Details on these interventions are available in in several books (McGovern et al., 2008; Mueser et al., 2003a). One fundamental feature of COD interventions is that they are individually tailored to address at least two disorders. For example, skills training may focus on developing new relationships, finding a job, mending family relationships, or rejecting harmful relationships with drug dealers. Family therapy must teach families to understand and help their relatives with SMI and COD, including the interactions between mental illness and misused substances. Medication management must address psychiatric symptoms and substance use disorders, while carefully avoiding medications that are prone to misuse.

Psychotherapy

Motivational interviewing, cognitive behaviour therapy, and relapse prevention training are the core individual psychotherapies for COD (Barrowclough et al., 2001; Graham et al., 2004). They focus on motivating clients to develop a sober lifestyle, helping them acquire the skills for illness self-management, and relapse prevention (Gingerich et al., 2018). These therapeutic strategies are essential for every COD provider.

Group intervention

Group intervention is an evidence-based practice for COD (Drake et al., 2008). Specific interventions have demonstrated excellent reductions of substance use (Bellack et al., 2006; Weiss et al., 2000, 2007). Numerous groups have been developed and manualized group interventions for people with COD (Bellack et al., 2007; Gingerich et al., 2018; Gråwe et al., 2007; McGovern et al., 2010; Mueser et al., 2003a; Mueser et al., 2004; Weiss & Connery, 2011).

Peer support and 12-step groups for people with COD are also common, including Alcoholics Anonymous, Narcotics Anonymous, and Dual Diagnosis Anonymous. All these groups can be modified for specific profiles: For example, common groups exist for young mothers with trauma histories and opioid addiction, physicians with anxiety/depression and stimulant use, homeless people with chronic alcoholism, and young African American men with COD who are returning to their communities after incarceration. The great advantage of group interventions is that people recognize that their lives are similar and help themselves by helping their peers. A further advantage of peer support groups is that they are free and available every day in most communities. Peer support groups have some specific advantages. In Oregon, professionally led groups have been difficult to sustain due to workforce and financing issues, but Dual Diagnosis Anonymous groups have proliferated around the state (Monica et al., 2010).

Family therapy

Family therapy is an evidence-based practice for people with substance use disorders of all variations (O'Farrell & Fals-Stewart, 2006). Families need education, support, and skills training, even more so when their relatives have SMI and COD. Specific family interventions address families with a relative experiencing SMI and COD (Barrowclough et al., 2001; Mueser et al., 2013). Multiple family groups combine supports from professionals and peers.

Case management

Case management interventions for COD are intensive, team-based, multidisciplinary, outreach-oriented, and clinically coordinated; they usually involve the assertive community treatment (ACT) model (Stein & Test, 1980). Studies of ACT have produced inconsistent results on substance use outcomes, but they have shown consistent positive outcomes on other domains, such as increasing engagement, decreasing hospital use, increasing community tenure, and improving quality of life (Drake et al., 1998; Essock et al., 2006; Morse et al., 2006). The beneficial effects of ACT may have specific advantages for subgroups of clients with COD. For example, one secondary analysis reported that COD clients with antisocial personality disorder who received integrated treatment on ACT teams improved significantly more in number of days drinking and spent fewer days in jail than similar clients who received integrated treatment on standard case management teams, whereas there was no difference in the effectiveness of ACT and standard case management for dual disorder clients without antisocial personality (Frisman et al., 2009).

Residential interventions

Residential interventions are an effective treatment for patients with COD (Brunette et al., 2004; Drake et al., 2008). Approaches vary considerably, and longer-term residential treatment (6 months or more) tends to be more effective. Residential interventions are important for high-risk populations, such as those who have been homeless, incarcerated, or unresponsive to less intensive outpatient interventions.

Contingency management

Contingency management, another evidence-based intervention for COD, involves carefully scheduled rewards, often monetary payments, to reinforce abstinence (Higgins et al., 2008). The strategy is effective, even for people with very chronic histories of COD (Destoop et al., 2021; Sigmon & Higgins, 2006). However, in the US at least, paying people for not using drugs has never been politically feasible.

Medications

Medications that help people decrease or stop substance use are now available for several substance use disorders, including opioids, alcohol, and nicotine. These interventions can be effective for clients with COD (Mueser et al., 2003b; Petrakis et al., 2004, 2006; Robertson et al., 2018). Chapter 15 in this volume on medication management by Smith and Hendrick describes these medications and strategies for their use. Some studies indicate that clozapine can be effective in patients with SMI and COD (Brunette et al., 2011; Drake et al., 2000).

Social determinants

Recovery often requires addressing social determinants—safe housing, employment, income above the poverty level, family and peer support, health insurance, and overcoming stigma (Jeste & Pender, 2022). These supports are difficult to arrange, and clinicians often fail to recognize that social determinants are more powerful than treatment and may consider them secondary or ancillary (Hood et al., 2016). Nevertheless, interventions directed at social determinants should be integrated with mental health, substance use, and COD services. For example, several studies show that integrating supported employment with mental health and COD services is a central part of the recovery process for many patients (Drake et al., 2012). Studies also show that COD is not an impediment to competitive employment; in fact, mental health clients with COD benefit as much as those without COD (Campbell et al., 2011; Mueser et al., 2011). Similarly, supportive housing is more effective when closely integrated with mental health care (McHugo et al., 2004).

Co-occurring alcohol and drug use disorder programmes

As above, several effective COD interventions are available, including counselling, peer support, medications, supported employment, and others. Integrated treatment programmes vary considerably, but all combine and tailor interventions for specific features of the target group as well as for the individuals within each group. For example, programmes for long-term homeless clients typically combine supportive housing, group counselling, self-help groups, and medications, but individuals within these programmes receive specific interventions according to needs and preferences. Programmes for young mothers with PTSD and substance use disorder often combine cognitive behaviour or exposure-based PTSD treatments with parenting interventions, childcare, safe housing, and medications. Early psychosis programmes typically incorporate supported education and employment, family psychoeducation, illness management counselling, and medications. Programmes for young men leaving incarceration may include help obtaining benefits, education, supported employment, counselling for antisocial cognitions and impulsive behaviours, self-help groups, and medications. Each target group has relevant needs, and individuals within these group have specific goals and preferences for interventions.

Implementing co-occurring alcohol and drug use disorder interventions

Although evidence-based interventions exist, implementing COD programmes presents extensive challenges (Drake et al., 2001). Although the US federal government has been advocating integrated services for over three decades (Ridgely et al., 1990), minimal progress has been made in creating integrated services for people with SMI and COD (McGovern et al., 2004, 2006, 2007, 2010). The barriers to integration are extensive: the fields of mental health care and addiction treatment have developed independently; government regulations and oversight, provider organizations, and funding mechanisms are fragmented; the workforces and training programmes differ; stigma remains pervasive; and philosophies of recovery often conflict.

Integrated treatments that implement evidence-based principles with fidelity can achieve significant outcomes (McHugo et al., 1999), but implementations are often unsuccessful or erode over time. Involving all major participants (service users, family members, clinicians, programme leaders, and mental health policymakers) in the planning process, incorporating training and fidelity reviews in the implementation, and reviewing quality continuously may enhance success (Torrey et al., 2002). Clinicians from different backgrounds, working together with the same clients, usually learn from each other and appreciate the benefits of multimodal treatment.

Research

The research literature on integrated treatment of dual disorders has been periodically reviewed over the past several years as research has grown (Chow et al., 2013; Donald et al., 2005; Drake et al., 2008; Kavanagh & Mueser, 2007; Ley, 2003). One comprehensive review identified 45 unique studies of psychosocial treatment, including 22 randomized controlled trials and 23 quasi-experimental studies (Drake et al., 2008). Although the literature supports integrated treatment in general and several specific interventions, few studies have examined how to combine interventions for specific groups.

One important research finding is that a successful programme produces a range of positive clinical and functional outcomes. For example, clients should be managing mental health and substance use conditions, should be achieving educational and/or employment goals, should have an adequate income and safe housing, and should have positive relationships with social network members who support their recovery (Acquilano et al., 2020). Nevertheless, few programmes have the administrative and financial support, the multidisciplinary staff, the expert supervision, and the quality monitoring to address these standards.

Conclusion

A large proportion of people with mental disorders experience COD. For people with SMI, the rate of COD is about 50%; for those with other common mental disorders, such as anxiety or depression, the rates are still high, approximately 25–30%. Although the natural course of COD tends towards improvements in several domains of illness management and social functioning over time, recovery may take many years, and not everyone will recover. Treatment should aim to enhance the process and shorten the time for recovery.

Integrated treatment, which denotes one clinician or team of clinicians who combine mental health and substance use interventions, has developed an extensive evidence base over the last 30 years. Several specific interventions have proven effective, but interventions should vary by clinical population and by individual needs. Few clinical studies have addressed the heterogeneity and complexity of the population.

Administrating, funding, training, supervising, and implementing high-quality, effective, persisting programmes that provide integrated treatment, even for specific groups, has been extremely challenging. Considerable work remains to be done in nearly all behavioural health systems.

REFERENCES

Abram, K. & Teplin, L. (1991). Co-occurring disorders among mentally ill jail detainees: implications for public policy. *The American Psychologist*, **46**, 1036–1044.

Acquilano, S. C., Noel, V., Gamache, J., Hendrick, D. C., & Drake, R. E. (2020). Outcomes of a community-based, co-occurring disorders treatment program. *International Mental Health and Addiction*, **19**, 1615–1624.

Alverson, H., Alverson, M., & Drake, R. E. (2000). An ethnographic study of the longitudinal course of substance abuse among people with severe mental illness. *Community Mental Health Journal*, **36**, 557–569.

Alverson, H., Alverson, M., & Drake, R. E. (2001). Social patterns of substance use among people with dual diagnoses. *Mental Health Services Research*, **3**, 3–14.

Andersen, A. M., Pietrzak, R. H., Kranzler, H. R., Ma, L., Zhou, H., Liu, X., et al. (2017). Polygenic scores for major depressive disorder and risk of alcohol dependence. *JAMA Psychiatry*, **74**, 1153–1160.

Balyakina, E., Mann, C., Ellison, M., Sivernell, R., Fulda, K. G., Sarai, S. K., & Cardarelli, R. (2014). Risk of future offense among probationers with co-occurring substance use and mental health disorders. *Community Mental Health Journal*, **50**, 288–295.

Barrowclough, C., Haddock, G., Tarrier, N., Lewis, S., Moring, J., O'Brien, R., et al. (2001). Randomized controlled trial of motivational interviewing, cognitive behavior therapy, and family intervention for patients with comorbid schizophrenia and substance use disorders. *American Journal of Psychiatry*, **158**, 1706–1713.

Bartels, S. J., Drake, R. E., & Wallach, M. A. (1995). Long-term course of substance use disorders among persons with severe mental disorders. *Psychiatric Services*, **46**, 248–251.

Bartels, S. J., Teague, G. B., Drake, R. E., Clark, R. E., Bush, P. W., & Noordsy, D. L. (1993). Substance abuse in schizophrenia: service utilization and costs. *Journal of Nervous and Mental Disease*, **181**, 227–232.

Bellack, A. S., Bennett, M. E., & Gearon, J. S. (2007). Behavioral Treatment for Substance Abuse in People with Serious and Persistent Mental Illness: A Handbook for Mental Health Professionals. New York: Taylor and Francis.

Bellack, A. S., Bennet, M. E., Gearon, J. S., Brown, C. H., & Yang, Y. (2006). A randomized clinical trial of a new behavioral treatment for drug abuse in people with severe and persistent mental illness. *Archives of General Psychiatry*, **63**, 426–432.

Brunette, M. F., Dawson, R., O'Keefe, C. D., Narasimhan, M., Noordsy, D. L., Wojcik, J., & Green, A. I. (2011). A randomized trial of clozapine versus other antipsychotics for cannabis use disorder in patients with schizophrenia. *Journal of Dual Diagnosis*, **7**, 50–63.

Brunette, M. F., Mueser, K. T., & Drake, R. E. (2004). A review of research on residential programs for people with severe mental illness and co-occurring substance use disorders. *Drug and Alcohol Review*, **23**, 471–481.

Brunette, M. F., Noordsy, D. L., Xie, H., & Drake, R. E. (2003). Benzodiazepine use and abuse among patients with severe mental illness and co-occurring substance use disorder. *Psychiatric Services*, **54**, 1395–1401.

Campbell, K., Bond, G. R., & Drake, R. E. (2011). Who benefits from supported employment? *Schizophrenia Bulletin*, **37**, 370–380.

Carey, K. B. & Carey, M. P. (1995). Reasons for drinking among psychiatric outpatients: relationship to drinking patterns. *Psychology of Addictive Behaviors*, **9**, 251–257.

Caton, C. L. M., Drake, R. E., Hasin, D., Dominguez, B., Shrout, P. E., Samet, S., & Schanzer, B. (2005). Differences between early phase primary psychotic disorders with concurrent substance use and substance-induced psychoses. *Archives of General Psychiatry* **62**, 137–145.

Caton, C., Shrout, P., Eagle, P., Opler, L. A., Felix, A., & Dominguez, B. (1994). Risk factors for homelessness among schizophrenic men: a case-control study. *American Journal of Public Health*, **84**, 265–270.

Cheah, S. Y., Lawford, B. R., Young, R. M., Connor, J. P., Phillip Morris, C., & Voisey, J. (2014). BDNF SNPs are implicated in comorbid alcohol dependence in schizophrenia but not in alcohol-dependent patients without schizophrenia. *Alcohol and Alcoholism*, **49**, 491–497.

Chow, C. M., Wieman, D., Cichocki, B., Qvicklund, H., & Hiersteiner, D. (2013). Mission impossible: treating serious mental illness and substance use co-occurring disorder with integrated treatment: a meta-analysis. *Mental Health and Substance Use*, **6**, 150–168.

Conner, K. R., Pinquart, M., & Gamble, S. A. (2009). Meta-analysis of depression and substance use among individuals with alcohol use disorders. *Journal of Substance Abuse Treatment*, **37**, 127–137.

Destoop, M., Docx, L., Morrens, M., & Dom, G. (2021). Meta-analysis on the effect of contingency management for patients with both psychotic and substance use disorders. *Journal of Clinical Medicine*, **10**, 616.

Dickey, B. & Azeni, H. (1996). Persons with dual diagnoses of substance abuse and major mental illness: their excess costs of psychiatric care. *American Journal of Public Health*, **86**, 973–977.

Dixon, L., Haas, G., Weiden, P. J., Sweeney, J., & Frances, A. J. (1991). Drug abuse in schizophrenic patients: clinical correlates and reasons for use. *American Journal of Psychiatry*, **148**, 224–230.

Dixon, L., McNary, S., & Lehman, A. (1995). Substance abuse and family relationships of persons with severe mental illness. *American Journal of Psychiatry*, **152**, 456–458.

Donald, M., Dower, J., & Kavanagh, D. J. (2005). Integrated versus non-integrated management and care for clients with co-occurring mental health and substance use disorders: a qualitative systematic review of randomised controlled trials. *Social Science & Medicine*, **60**, 1371–1383.

Drake, R. E., Bond, G. R., & Becker, D. R. (2012). *Individual Placement and Support: An Evidence-based Approach to Supported Employment*. New York: Oxford University Press.

Drake, R. E., Caton, C., Xie, H., Gorroochurn, P., Hsu, E., Samet, S., & Hasin, D. (2011). A prospective 2-year follow-up of emergency department admissions with primary psychoses or substance-induced psychoses. *American Journal of Psychiatry*, **168**, 742–748.

Drake, R. E., Essock, S. M., Shaner, A., Carey, K. B., Minkoff, K., Kola, L., et al. (2001). Implementing dual diagnosis services for clients with severe mental illness. *Psychiatric Services*, **52**, 469–476.

Drake, R. E., Luciano, A., Mueser, K. T., Covell, N. H., Essock, S. M., Xie, H., & McHugo, G. J. (2016). Longitudinal course of clients with co-occurring schizophrenia-spectrum and substance use disorders in urban mental health centers: a seven-year prospective study. *Schizophrenia Bulletin*, **42**, 202–211.

Drake, R. E., McHugo, G. J., Clark, R. E., Teague, G. B., Xie, H., Miles, K., & Ackerson, T. H. (1998). Assertive community treatment for patients with co-occurring severe mental illness and substance use disorder: a clinical trial. *American Journal of Orthopsychiatry*, **68**, 201–215.

Drake, R. E., McHugo, G. J., Xie, H., Fox, M., Packard, J., & Helmstetter, B. (2006). Ten-year recovery outcomes for clients with co-occurring schizophrenic and substance use disorders. *Schizophrenia Bulletin*, **32**, 464–473.

Drake, R. E., O'Neal, E. L., & Wallach, M. A. (2008). A systematic review of psychosocial interventions for people with co-occurring substance use and severe mental disorders. *Journal of Substance Abuse Treatment*, **34**, 123–138.

Drake, R. E. & Wallach, M. A. (1993). Moderate drinking among people with severe mental illness. *Hospital and Community Psychiatry*, **44**, 780–782.

Drake, R. E., Xie, H., & McHugo, G. J. (2020). A 16-year prospective study of community mental health patients with co-occurring serious mental illness and substance use disorder. *World Psychiatry*, **19**, 397–398.

Drake, R. E., Xie, H., McHugo, G. J., & Green, A. I. (2000). The effects of clozapine on alcohol and drug use disorders among schizophrenic patients. *Schizophrenia Bulletin*, **26**, 441–449.

Essock, S. M., Mueser, K. T., Drake, R. E., Covell, N. H., McHugo, G. J., Frisman, L. K., et al. (2006). Comparison of ACT and standard case management for delivering integrated treatment for co-occurring disorders. *Psychiatric Services*, **57**, 185–196.

Frisman, L. K., Mueser, K. T., Covell, N. H., Lin, H.-J., Crocker, A., Drake, R. E., & Essock, S. M. (2009). Use of integrated dual disorder treatment via assertive community treatment versus clinical case management for persons with co-occurring disorders and antisocial personality disorder. *Journal of Nervous and Mental Disease*, **197**, 822–828.

Gingerich, S., Mueser, K. T., Meyer-Kalos, P. S., Fox-Smith, M., & Freedland, T. (2018). *Enhanced Illness Management and Recovery E-IMR*. St. Paul, MN: Minnesota Center for Chemical and Mental Health, School of Social Work, College of Education and Human Development, University of Minnesota.

Goodman, L. A., Salyers, M. P., Mueser, K. T., Rosenberg, S. D., Swartz, M., Essock, S. M., et al. (2001). Recent victimization in women and men with severe mental illness: prevalence and correlates. *Journal of Traumatic Stress*, **14**, 615–632.

Graham, H. L., Copello, A., Birchwood, M. J., Mueser, K. T., Orford, J., McGovern, D., et al. (2004). *Cognitive-Behavioural Integrated Treatment (C-BIT): A Treatment Manual for Substance Misuse in People with Severe Mental Health Problems*. Chichester: John Wiley & Sons.

Grant, B. F., Saha, T. D., Ruan, W. J., Goldstein, R. B., Chou, S. P., Jung, J., et al. (2016). Epidemiology of DSM-5 drug use disorder: results from the National Epidemiologic Survey on alcohol and related conditions-III. *JAMA Psychiatry*, **73**, 39–47.

Gråwe, R. W., Hagen, R., Espeland, B., & Mueser, K. T. (2007). The Better Life Program: effects of group skills training for persons with severe mental illness and substance use disorders. *Journal of Mental Health*, **16**, 625–634.

Hartz, S. M., Horton, A. C., Oehlert, M., Carey, C. E., Agrawal, A., Bogdan, R., et al. (2018). Association between substance use disorder and polygenic liability to schizophrenia. *Biological Psychiatry*, **82**, 709–715.

Haywood, T. W., Kravitz, H. M., Grossman, L. S., Cavanaugh, J. L., Jr, Davis, J. M., & Lewis, D. A. (1995). Predicting the 'revolving door' phenomenon among patients with schizophrenic, schizoaffective, and affective disorders. *American Journal of Psychiatry*, **152**, 856–861.

Hendrickson, E. L. (2006). *Designing, Implementing, and Managing Treatment Services for Individuals with Co-Occurring Mental Health and Substance Use Disorders: Blueprints for Action.* New York: Haworth Press.

Henquet, C., Krabbendam, L., Spauwen, J., Kaplan, C., Lieb, R., Wittchen, H. U., & van Os, J. (2005). Prospective cohort study of cannabis use, predisposition for psychosis, and psychotic symptoms in young people. *British Medical Journal*, **330**, 11.

Higgins, S. T., Silverman, K., & Heil, S. H. (2008). *Contingency Management in Substance Abuse Treatment.* New York: Guilford Press.

Hood, C. M., Gennusp, K. P., Swain, G. R., & Catlin, B. B. (2016). County health rankings: relationships between determinant factors and health outcomes. *American Journal of Preventive Medicine*, **50**, 129–135.

Jeste, D. V. & Pender, V. B. (2022). Social determinants of mental health. Recommendations for research, training, practice, and policy. *JAMA Psychiatry*, **79**, 283–284.

Kavanagh, D. J. & Mueser, K. T. (2007). Current evidence on integrated treatment for serious mental disorder and substance misuse. *Journal of the Norwegian Psychological Association*, **5**, 618–637.

Kessler, R. C., Crum, R. M., Warner, L. A., Nelson, C. B., Schulenberg, J., & Anthony, J. C. (1997). Lifetime co-occurrence of DSM-III-R alcohol abuse and dependence with other psychiatric disorders in the National Comorbidity survey. *Archives of General Psychiatry*, **54**, 313–321.

Khokhar, J. Y., Dwiel, L. L., Henricks, A. M., Doucette, W. T., & Green, A. I. (2018). The link between schizophrenia and substance use disorder: a unifying hypothesis. *Schizophrenia Research*, **194**, 78–85.

Ley, A. J. (2003). Cochrane review of treatment outcome studies and its implications for future developments. In: Graham, H. L., Copello, A., Birchwood, M. J., & Mueser, K. T. (Eds.), *Substance Misuse in Psychosis: Approaches to Treatment and Service Delivery* (pp. 349–365). Chichester: John Wiley & Sons.

Linszen, D., Dingemans, P., & Lenior, M. (1994). Cannabis abuse and the course of recent-onset schizophrenic disorders. *Archives of General Psychiatry*, **51**, 273–279.

Manrique-Garcia, E., Zammit, S., Dalman, C., Hemmingsson, T., Andreasson, S., & Allebeck, P. (2012). Cannabis, schizophrenia and other non-affective psychoses: 35 years of follow-up of a population-based cohort. *Psychological Medicine*, **42**, 1321–1328.

McGovern, M. P., Drake, R. E., Merrens, M. R., Mueser, K. T., Brunette, M. B., & Hendrick, R. (2008). *Hazelden Co-occurring Disorders Program: Integrated Service for Substance Use and Mental Health Problems.* Center City, MN: Hazelden.

McGovern, M. P., Fox, T. S., Xie, H., & Drake, R. E. (2004). A survey of clinical practices and readiness to adopt evidence-based practices: dissemination research in an addiction treatment system. *Journal of Substance Abuse Treatment*, **26**, 305–312.

McGovern, M. P., Lambert-Harris, C., McHugo, G. J., Giard, J., & Mangrum, L. (2010). Improving the dual diagnosis capability of addiction and mental health treatment services: implementation factors associated with program level changes. *Journal of Dual Diagnosis*, **6**, 237–250.

McGovern, M. P., Matzkin, A. L., & Giard, J. (2007). Assessing the dual diagnosis capability of addiction treatment services: the Dual Diagnosis Capability in Addiction Treatment (DDCAT) Index. *Journal of Dual Diagnosis*, **3**, 111–123.

McGovern, M. P., Mueser, K. T., Hamblen, J. L., & Jankowski, M. K. (2010). *Cognitive-Behavioral Therapy for PTSD: A Program for Addiction Professionals.* Center City, MN: Hazelden.

McGovern, M. P., Xie, H., Segal, S. R., Siembab, L., & Drake, R. E. (2006). Addiction treatment services and co-occurring disorders: prevalence estimates, treatment practices, and barriers. *Journal of Substance Abuse Treatment*, **31**, 267–275.

McHugo, G. J., Bebout, R. R., Harris, M., Cleghorn, S., Herring, G., Xie, H., et al. (2004). A randomized controlled trial of integrated versus parallel housing services for homeless adults with severe mental illness. *Schizophrenia Bulletin*, **30**, 969–982.

McHugo, G. J., Drake, R. E., Haslett, W. R., Krassenbaum, S. R., Mueser, K. T., Sweeney, M. A., & Harris, M. (2021). Algorithm-driven substance use disorder treatment for inner-city clients with serious mental illness and multiple impairments. *Journal of Nervous and Mental Disease*, **209**, 92–99.

McHugo, G. J., Drake, R. E., Teague, G. B., Xie, H., & Sengupta, A. (1999). The relationship between model fidelity and client outcomes in the New Hampshire Dual Disorders Study. *Psychiatric Services*, **50**, 818–824.

McHugo, G. J., Krassenberg, S., Donley, S., Corrigan, J. D., Boggner, J., & Drake, R. E. (2017). The prevalence and correlates of traumatic brain injury among people with co-occurring serious mental illness and substance use disorders. *Journal of Head Trauma Rehabilitation*, **32**, E65–E74.

McLellan, A. T., Luborsky, L., Woody, G., O'Brien, C. P., & Druley, K. A. (1983). Predicting response to alcohol and drug abuse treatments. *Archives of General Psychiatry*, **40**, 620–625.

Monica, C., Nikkel, R. E., & Drake, R. E. (2010). Dual diagnosis anonymous in Oregon. *Psychiatric Services*, **61**, 738–740.

Morse, G. A., Calsyn, R. J., Klinkenberg, D. W., Helminiak, T. W., Wolff, N., Drake, R. E., et al. (2006). Treating homeless clients with severe mental illness and substance use disorders: costs and outcomes. *Community Mental Health Journal*, **42**, 377–404.

Mueser, K. T., Bellack, A. S., Gingerich, S., Agresta, J. & Fulford, D. (2004). Social skills training for schizophrenia: A step-by-step Guide(3rd ed). New York GuilFord Press.

Mueser, K. T., Bond, G. R., Drake, R. E., & Resnick, S. G. (1998). Models of community care for severe mental illness: a review of research on case management. *Schizophrenia Bulletin*, **24**, 37–74.

Mueser, K. T., Campbell, K., & Drake, R. E. (2011). The effectiveness of supported employment in people with dual disorders. *Journal of Dual Diagnosis*, **7**, 90–102.

Mueser, K. T. & Drake, R. E. (2007). Comorbidity: what have we learned and where have we gone? *Clinical Psychology: Science and Practice*, **14**, 64–69.

Mueser, K. T., Drake, R. E., & Miles, K. M. (1997). The course and treatment of substance use disorder in persons with severe mental illness. In: Onken, L. S., Blaine, J. D., Genser, S., & Horton, A. M. (Eds.), *National Institute of Drug Abuse (NIDA) Research Monograph Series, 172: Treatment of Drug-Dependent Individuals with Comorbid Mental disorders* (pp. 86–109). Rockville, MD: US Department of Health and Human Services.

Mueser, K. T., Drake, R. E., & Wallach, M. A. (1998). Dual diagnosis: a review of etiological theories. *Addictive Behaviors*, **23**, 717–734.

Mueser, K. T., Essock, S. M., Drake, R. E., Wolfe, R. S., & Frisman, L. K. (2001). Rural and urban differences in dually diagnosed patients: implications for service needs. *Schizophrenia Research*, **48**, 93–107.

Mueser, K. T., Glynn, S. M., Cather, C., Xie, H., Zarate, R., Smith, M. F., et al. (2013). A randomized controlled trial of family intervention for co-occurring substance use and severe psychiatric disorders. *Schizophrenia Bulletin*, **39**, 658–672.

Mueser, K. T., Nishith, P., Tracy, J. I., DeGirolamo, J., & Molinaro, M. (1995). Expectations and motives for substance use in schizophrenia. *Schizophrenia Bulletin*, **21**, 367–378.

Mueser, K. T., Noordsy, D. L., Drake, R. E., & Fox, L. (2003a). *Integrated Treatment for Dual Disorders: A Guide to Effective Practice.* New York: Guilford Press.

Mueser, K. T., Noordsy, D. L., Fox, L., & Wolfe, R. (2003b). Disulfiram treatment for alcoholism in severe mental illness. *American Journal on Addictions*, **12**, 242–252.

Mueser, K. T., Yarnold, P. R., Rosenberg, S. D., Swett, C., Miles, K. M., & Hill, D. (2000). Substance use disorder in hospitalized severely mentally ill psychiatric patients: prevalence, correlates, and subgroups. *Schizophrenia Bulletin*, **26**, 179–192.

National Institute on Drug Abuse (2020). Research report: common comorbidities with substance use disorders research report. https://nida.nih.gov/publications/research-reports/common-comorbidities-substance-use-disorders

Niv, N., Lopez, S. R., Glynn, S. M., & Mueser, K. T. (2007). The role of substance use in families, attributions and affective reactions to their relative with severe mental illness. *Journal Nervous and Mental Disease*, **195**, 307–314.

Noordsy, D. L., Mishra, M. K., & Mueser, K. T. (2013). Models of relationships between substance use and mental disorders. In P. Miller (Ed.), *Principles of Addiction: Comprehensive Addictive Behaviors and Disorders* (**Vol. 1**, pp. 489–495). Academic Press.

O'Farrell, T. J. & Fals-Stewart, W. (2006). *Behavioral Couples Therapy for Alcoholism and Drug Abuse*. New York: Guilford Press.

Osher, F. C. & Kofoed, L. L. (1989). Treatment of patients with psychiatric and psychoactive substance use disorders. *Hospital and Community Psychiatry*, **40**, 1025–1030.

Ostergaard, M. L. D., Nordentoft, M., & Hjorthoj, C. (2017). Associations between substance use disorders and suicides or suicide attempts in people with mental illness: a Danish nation-wide, prospective, registry-based study of patients diagnosed with schizophrenia, bipolar disorder, unipolar depression or personality disorder. *Addiction*, **112**, 1250–1259.

Owen, R. R., Fischer, E. P., Booth, B. M., & Cuffel, B. J. (1996). Medication noncompliance and substance abuse among patients with schizophrenia. *Psychiatric Services*, **47**, 853–858.

Peña, C. J., Bagot, R. C., Labonté, B., & Nestler, E. J. (2014). Epigenetic signaling in psychiatric disorders. *Journal of Molecular Biology*, **426**, 3389–3412.

Petrakis, I. L., Nich, C., & Ralevski, E. (2006). Psychotic spectrum disorders and alcohol abuse: a review of pharmacotherapeutic strategies and a report on the effectiveness of naltrexone and disulfiram. *Schizophrenia Bulletin*, **32**, 644–654.

Petrakis, I. L., O'Malley, S., Rounsaville, B., Poling, J., McHugh-Strong, C., Krystal, J. H. (2004). Naltrexone augmentation of neuroleptic treatment in alcohol-abusing patients with schizophrenia. *Psychopharmacology (Berlin)*, **172**, 291–297.

Polcin, D. L. (1992). Issues in the treatment of dual diagnosis clients who have chronic mental illness. *Professional Psychology: Research and Practice*, **23**, 30–37.

Poremski, D., Whitley, R., & Latimer, E. (2014). Barriers to obtaining employment for people with severe mental illness experiencing homelessness. *Journal of Mental Health*, **23**, 181–185.

Post, R. M. & Kalivas, P. (2013). Bipolar disorder and substance misuse: pathological and therapeutic implications of their comorbidity and cross-sensitisation. *British Journal of Psychiatry Journal of Mental Science*, **202**, 172–176.

Powell, B. J., Read, M. R., Penick, E. C., Miller, N. S., & Bingham, S. F. (1987). Primary and secondary depression in alcoholic men: an important distinction? *Journal of Clinical Psychiatry*, **48**, 98–101.

Regier, D. A., Farmer, M. E., Rae, D. S., Locke, B. Z., Keith, S. J., Judd, L. L., & Goodwin, F. K. (1990). Comorbidity of mental disorders with alcohol and other drug abuse: results from the Epidemiologic Catchment Area (ECA) study. *Journal of the American Medical Association*, **264**, 2511–2518.

Ridgely, M. S., Goldman, H. H., & Willenbring, M. (1990). Barriers to the care of persons with dual diagnoses: organizational and financing issues. *Schizophrenia Bulletin*, **16**, 123–132.

Robertson, A. G., Easter, M. M., Lin, H., Frisman, L. K., Swanson, J. W., & Swartz, M. S. (2018). Medication-assisted treatment for alcohol-dependent adults with serious mental illness and criminal justice involvement: effects on treatment utilization and outcomes. *American Journal of Psychiatry*, **175**, 665–673.

Rosenberg, S. D., Goodman, L. A., Osher, F. C., Swartz, M. S., Essock, S. M., Butterfield, M. I., et al. (2001). Prevalence of HIV, hepatitis B and hepatitis C in people with severe mental illness. *American Journal of Public Health*, **91**, 31–37.

Ross, S. & Peselow, E. (2012). Co-occurring psychotic and addictive disorders: neurobiology and diagnosis. *Clinical Neuropharmacology*, **35**, 235–243.

Sigmon, S. C. & Higgins, S. T. (2006). Voucher-based contingent reinforcement of marijuana abstinence among individuals with serious mental illness. *Journal of Substance Abuse Treatment*, **30**, 291–295.

Steadman, H. J., Mulvy, E. P., Monahan, J., Robbins, P. C., Appelbaum, P. S., Grisso, T., et al. (1998). Violence by people discharged from acute psychiatric inpatient facilities and by others in the same neighbourhoods. *Archives of General Psychiatry*, **55**, 393–404.

Stein, L. I. & Test, M. A. (1980). Alternatives to mental hospital treatment: conceptual, model, treatment program and clinical evaluation. *Archives of General Psychiatry*, **37**, 392–397.

Stuart, H. (2003). Violence and mental illness: an overview. *World Psychiatry*, **2**, 121–124.

Substance Abuse and Mental Health Services Administration (2006). *Results from the 2005 National Survey on Drug Use and Health: National Findings* (Office of Applied Studies, NSDUH Series H-30, DHHS Publication No. SMA 06-4194). Washington, DC: Department of Health and Human Services.

Substance Abuse and Mental Health Services Administration (2020). National Survey of Drug Use and Health tables, 2020. https://www.samhsa.gov/data/report/2020-nsduh-detailed-tables

Swartz, M. S., Swanson, J. W., Hiday, V., Borum, R., Wagner, H. R., & Burns, B. J. (1998). Violence and severe mental illness: the effects of substance abuse and non-adherence to medication. *American Journal of Psychiatry*, **155**, 226–231.

Torrey, W. C., Drake, R. E., Cohen, M., Lynde, D., Gorman, P., & Wyzik, P. (2002). The challenge of implementing integrated dual disorders treatment services. *Community Mental Health Journal*, **38**, 507–521.

Weiss, R. D. & Connery, H. S. (2011). *Integrated Group Therapy for Bipolar Disorder and Substance Abuse*. New York: Guilford Press.

Weiss, R. D., Griffin, M. L., Greenfield, S. F., Najavits, L. M., Wyner, D., Soto, J. A., & Hennen, J. A. (2000). Group therapy for patients with bipolar and substance dependence: results of a pilot study. *Journal of Clinical Psychiatry*, **61**, 361–367.

Weiss, R. D., Griffin, M. L., Kolodziej, M. E., Greenfield, S. F., Najavits, L. M., Daley, D. C., et al. (2007). A randomized trial of integrated group therapy versus group drug counseling for patients with bipolar disorder and substance dependence. *American Journal of Psychiatry*, **164**, 100–107.

Wisdom, J. P., Manuel, J. I., & Drake, R. E. (2011). Substance abuse in people with first-episode psychosis: a systematic review of course and treatment. *Psychiatric Services*, **62**, 1007–1012.

Wu, L.-T., Gersing, K., Burchett, B., Woody, G. E., & Blazer, D. G. (2011). Substance use disorders and comorbid axis I and II psychiatric disorders among young psychiatric patients: findings from a large electronic health records database. *Journal of Psychiatric Research*, **45**, 1453–1462.

Xie, H., Drake, R. E., & McHugo, G. J. (2009). The 10-year course of substance use disorder among patients with severe mental illness: an analysis of latent class trajectory groups. *Psychiatric Services*, **60**, 804–811.

25
Behavioural health technologies and telehealth

John Torous and Elizabeth Carpenter-Song

Introduction

Mental health problems are a significant and growing source of disability globally (World Health Organization (WHO), 2021a, 2021b). There are numerous barriers to accessing mental health care, including a lack of mental health providers in many global settings (WHO, 2021c), limited mental health literacy (Andrade et al., 2014), stigma (Dockery et al., 2015), and cost (Rowan et al., 2013). Digital technologies have great potential for helping to overcome barriers to access by offering timely, low-barrier, and potentially anonymous forms of support for mental health problems.

There has been growing recognition of the ways in which digital technologies can be used to support mental health (Ben-Zeev et al., 2020; Buck et al., 2020; Lecomte et al., 2020; Santarossa et al., 2018) reflected in the large volume of smartphone applications available (IQVIA Institute for Human Data Science, 2017) as well as investments in the development of digital health technologies (Shah & Berry, 2021). In addition, current evidence demonstrates high interest in and acceptability of mobile technology use by individuals living with mental illness (Carpenter-Song, 2020; Carpenter-Song et al., 2018; Firth et al., 2016; Jonathan et al., 2019; Noel et al., 2019; Roberts et al., 2018; Santarossa et al., 2018). Despite substantial interest, there had not been wide adoption and use of digital technologies in routine mental health care settings (Chiauzzi & Newell, 2019; Noel et al., 2019; Wisniewski & Torous, 2020), with implementation identified as a key challenge for the field (Mohr et al., 2017).

This situation is now rapidly changing in the context of the global COVID-19 pandemic. Leaders in the field of digital mental health note that the pandemic catalysed a 'paradigm shift' for digital health technologies (Torous et al., 2021) as public health restrictions necessitated the rapid transition away from in-person care delivery. As COVID-19 persists, mental health digital tools like smartphone apps and telehealth offer safe, evidence-based solutions to meet the rising need for care. The transition to digital care has been rapid—in one published case an entire clinic converted to 100% online care in 72 hours (Yellowlees et al., 2020)—and many services are expected to remain digital even after pandemic restrictions subside (Predmore et al., 2021). Policy changes, including the relaxation of privacy regulations to support non-traditional telehealth applications as well as changes to reimbursements for remote services, enabled this transformation in mental health care delivery (Kopelovich et al., 2021; Department of Health and Human Services, 2020). In this context, attitudes and practices regarding the use of digital technologies to augment mental health care appear to be changing. Evidence from a recent study in 17 countries indicates increased use of digital technologies in mental health settings and support for uptake during the pandemic (Kinoshita et al., 2020). Shifting perspectives on digital mental health reflect a growing awareness born out from pandemic experiences of the potential of technology to support scalable, affordable, and accessible mental health care (Torous et al., 2021). Rapid transformations of care in the context of COVID-19 are likely to endure beyond the pandemic (Bartels et al., 2020; Ben-Zeev, 2020; Goldman et al., 2020; Inkster et al., 2020; Torous et al., 2020a). Many leaders in the mental health field are advocating for expanding access to digital health care (Ben-Zeev, 2020; Inkster et al., 2020; Torous et al., 2020a).

In this chapter, we outline the range of approaches within digital mental health care; review recent evidence of the feasibility, acceptability, and effectiveness of technologies to support mental health; discuss strategies for evaluating the large volume of digital mental health technologies currently available; examine current challenges for the field; and offer perspectives on future directions and approaches to support meaningful and equitable outcomes through the use of digital mental health technologies. Given the scope of the space, we focus on mobile technology although do provide broad examples across many diverse digital tools.

What are digital mental health technologies?

While telepsychiatry has been in place for decades as a solution to meet mental health needs in settings with limited access to specialty providers, digital mental health technologies include a wider array of approaches to delivering care and supporting mental health. A recent review of digital health technologies focuses on developments in smartphone apps, virtual reality, social media, and chatbots (Torous et al., 2021). To this list, we would add mental health internet/web applications as well as recent innovations in telehealth.

Digital mental health tools have been designed to meet a range of needs. Some address symptoms to strengthen self-management of serious mental illnesses, including schizophrenia, bipolar disorder, and major depressive disorder (Ben-Zeev et al., 2018), post-traumatic stress disorder (Kuhn et al., 2014), as well as common mental disorders such as depression and anxiety (Firth et al., 2017a, 2017b). Other tools leverage the strengths of digital technology to link users to supportive peer communities (Fortuna et al., 2020). Others have been developed to support person-centred care and communication in psychiatric medication management (Deegan et al., 2008). Some tools leverage passive sensing features of modern smartphones such as step counts, voice analytics from phone calls, and text analytics from social media use to inform predictions of illness relapse or other outcomes such as social isolation. This approach is often referred to as 'digital phenotyping' and reflects efforts to individualize psychiatric care through real-time, patient-level data. Digital mental health technologies range from tools that are entirely self-guided to those that are human supported and integrated with traditional mental health care.

Digital mental health tools vary with respect to whether or not they were developed using rigorous research methods and evidence-based approaches. Many commercially available smartphone apps, for example, may claim to be 'evidence based', but have not been rigorously tested to evaluate their feasibility, acceptability, or effectiveness. A review of commercially available apps reported that less than 2% were supported by original research evidence (Baxter et al., 2020). Yet it is also the case that the few apps with strong evidence for use with serious mental illnesses are not yet publicly available (Kopelovich et al., 2021). This situation presents a challenge for those with mental illness and service providers to identify and access digital tools that are consistent with current evidence. This challenge will be discussed in more detail later in this chapter.

Overview of current evidence

The potential of digital technologies to address unmet mental health needs is reflected in the accumulating evidence indicating that some technology-delivered interventions may be as effective as in-person interactions (Ben-Zeev et al., 2018; Gire et al., 2017; Hubley et al., 2016; Lecomte et al., 2020; Santarossa et al., 2018; Wright et al., 2019). Telepsychiatry and digital mental health technologies show promise for mitigating long-standing disparities in access to care for people living in rural or other low-resource settings (Biagianti et al., 2017; Gire et al., 2017; Mahmoud et al., 2020; Torous et al., 2017). Technology-based approaches may also improve engagement and retention for high-risk patients (Ben-Zeev et al., 2016; Buck et al., 2020). Yet researchers have also noted that available evidence regarding the effectiveness of digital mental health interventions may be limited in important ways by small sample sizes, lack of control groups, and short follow-up periods (Carter et al., 2021; Neary & Schueller, 2018).

Context-specific evidence from global settings and diverse clinical and demographic populations is necessary to understand both the potential and limitations of digital mental health approaches as well as to identify gaps in knowledge in this area. In this section, we provide an overview of current evidence regarding digital mental health in low- and middle-income countries (LMICs) and for specific mental health conditions.

Digital mental health in low- and middle-income countries

Mental health conditions account for a large global burden of disease and are increasing globally (WHO, 2021a). The WHO reports that there has been a 13% increase in mental health conditions worldwide in the past decade (to 2017) (WHO, 2021a). Depression is a leading cause of disability and contributes to a high global burden of disease (WHO, 2021b). Yet the vast majority of people with mental disorders do not have access to adequate mental health treatment; more than 75% of people in LMICs receive no treatment (WHO, 2021b). In low-income countries there are fewer than two mental health workers per 100,000 population compared to over 60 per 100,000 in high-income countries (WHO, 2021c). Digital mental health approaches hold potential for mitigating the treatment gap in low-resource settings by offering low-barrier ways to access mental health supports. Evidence from large surveys demonstrates that most people have access to mobile devices even in low-resource settings (Silver et al., 2019), creating opportunities to leverage technology to support unmet mental health needs.

There is a growing body of research examining digital mental health approaches in LMICs. This work is being conducted in diverse global settings, with most studies in East Asia, South Asia, and Central or Latin America (Carter et al., 2021). Researchers have noted that certain regions, including Central and Southeast Asia, the Middle East, Eastern Europe, and Africa are less well represented in current literature (Carter et al., 2021), suggesting the need to expand efforts in these settings.

Several systematic reviews of digital mental health in LMICs provide evidence of the feasibility and acceptability of technology-based approaches in LMICs as measured through patient satisfaction and adherence (Carter et al., 2021; Jimenez-Molina et al., 2019; Kaonga & Morgan, 2019; Naslund et al., 2017). Recently, there have been increased efforts to examine the clinical effectiveness of digital mental health interventions in LMICs (Carter et al., 2021). One recent systematic review found that two-thirds of included studies (n = 23) reported improvements in mental health measures at follow-up and most studies evaluating digital interventions for common mental disorders (n = 20) reported significant findings (Carter et al., 2021). The latter finding aligns with evidence from a recent meta-analysis by Fu and colleagues (2020) that found that digital mental health interventions were moderately effective compared to control conditions.

Yet current research into the clinical effectiveness of digital approaches remains limited by small sample sizes and short follow-up periods (Carter et al., 2021; Fu et al., 2020) as well as few studies reporting standardized effect sizes (Carter et al., 2021). There is also a dearth of research on cultural adaptation of digital health interventions developed outside of LMICs but then applied to them. Applying ethnographic approaches may provide a practical means to customize a plethora of existing digital health tools to be more relevant and effective for LMICs and diverse populations (Kozelka et al., 2021; Rodriguez et al., 2020). Carter and colleagues (2021) also note that their review of 37 digital intervention studies in 13 LMICs yielded no studies that reported worsening of symptoms or negative acceptability or dissatisfaction, which may suggest publication bias. The limitations of current evidence of clinical effectiveness of digital interventions in LMICs points to the need for rigorous randomized controlled trials with larger sample sizes in these settings (Carter et al., 2021). The need to generate rigorous evidence regarding the effectiveness of digital mental health interventions in LMICs is especially pressing given their potential to offer accessible supports for mental health in settings with few mental health workers and treatment resources.

Digital mental health and specific mental health conditions

Evidence from specific mental health conditions supports broad feasibility, although evidence of efficacy and effectiveness remains nascent. Still, evidence is rapidly emerging across disorders such as depression, anxiety, and schizophrenia. As this evidence base grows, use is rapidly accelerating, and even before COVID-19 there was high interest among particular groups like youth (Cohen et al., 2021). Formal numbers remain unknown, but by all indicators uptake and demand has only increased around COVID-19 (Inkster, 2021).

Considering apps for depression, effect size sizes from symptom reduction have varied from negligent to large depending on the study. During the height of the COVID-19 pandemic, emerging evidence suggests people turned to mood apps at higher rates for emotional support (Inkster, 2021). Large health care systems have also begun to implement use of these apps in routine clinical care during this same time period (Mordecai et al., 2021). In larger reviews and meta-analysis, the effect of cognitive behavioural therapy (CBT) apps has generally been reported as negligent to small (Hrynyschyn & Dockweiler, 2021), although mediators such as human support have been shown to improve outcomes (Lungu et al., 2020; Mohr et al., 2019). The role of human support in driving engagement and engagement itself as it relates to outcomes in these apps remains an active area of research (Molloy & Anderson, 2021). In one larger study examining market research data from the general population, real-world engagement with a mood and anxiety-related app was suggested to be approximately 5% or lower after 10 days (Baumel et al., 2019). Recent research is also now focusing beyond the impact of any particular app but rather towards understanding mechanisms of action. For example, a recent review reported that apps may offer smaller effect towards reducing symptom and improving well-being, but a medium effect size (g = 0.49) for emotional regulation (Eisenstadt et al., 2021).

Much of the research on anxiety apps parallels that of depression apps. A 2020 systematic review of app interventions found that nearly 12% have focused on anxiety, and across all studies 80% utilize elements of CBT (Miralles et al., 2020). A 2019 systematic review and meta-analysis reported no overall effect for self-help related anxiety apps (Weisel et al., 2019), although, as noted above, the role of human support has since become a focus to address this challenge. A 2021 systematic review of anxiety and mood apps reported on the need for more persuasive design embedded in these apps to drive engagement and effectiveness (Wu et al., 2021). The review suggests four areas of importance for this design including facilitating the primary purpose of the app, promoting user–app interactions, leveraging social relationships, and increasing app credibility. While recent reviews of anxiety apps do suggest a positive effect size for generalized anxiety (g = 0.30) symptoms, stress levels (g = 0.35), and social anxiety symptoms (g = 0.58) (Linardon et al., 2019), these effects must be understood in the context of data from pilot studies that are subject to high rates of bias.

Apps for psychotic disorders also have strong preliminary evidence although the same limitations as noted above for depression and anxiety apps remain. Interest in those with these conditions is high. A 2021 study of those with first-episode psychosis reported that 95% are already using technology to better understand or cope with their condition, and 70% report using apps for health (Buck et al., 2021). Focusing on engagement challenges unique to apps for these conditions, a 2021 review noted four core factors including the direct impact of psychotic symptoms and illness: an individual's response to psychosis, the extent of prior and current day-to-day exposure, integration of technology, and intervention/technology aspects (Arnold et al., 2021). Still, many recent studies are working around these barriers through offering human support around the app use and outcomes around engagement and expectations have become important considerations for study (Allan et al., 2019).

Numerous small but interesting studies around psychosis have been published in recent years and draw frequently on CBT principles also utilized in depression and anxiety apps. The FOCUS smartphone app, which offers self-management and coping resources, has reported efficacy results in two studies (Ben-Zeev et al., 2014, 2018), and recently the authors reported that it may be more cost-effective than peer-led interventions. The Canadian App4Independence (A4i) (Kidd et al., 2019), which offers coping strategies and connects users to resources and a peer support community, also reported numerous clinical benefits. The UK Actissit app (Bucci et al., 2018), offering CBT strategies for coping, reported improvements in negative, general, and overall psychotic symptoms. Numerous other apps targeting schizophrenia like SAVVy (Bell et al., 2020), MACS (Moitra et al., 2021), SMARTapp (Hanssen et al., 2020), PRIME (Schlosser et al., 2018), ClinTouch (Lewis et al., 2020), WeCOPE (Steare et al., 2020), and MyJourney3 (Whelan et al., 2015) have each reported positive evidence of smartphone apps to improve clinical symptoms across four domains associated with relapse: mood, anxiety, negative symptoms, and positive symptoms. While exact estimates of effect sizes of these interventions are challenging given varied methodology and reporting of results, the above studies indicate at least a small effect across mood, anxiety, and psychotic symptoms.

Evaluation of digital apps for mental health

Evaluating digital applications is a key area of emerging work in the field of digital mental health. There is widespread availability of digital apps for health and wellness, with over 300,000 health apps currently available (IQVIA Institute for Human Data Science, 2017) and more than 400 million downloads of medical apps globally (Muoio, 2019). Unfortunately, despite their wide availability, the majority of commercially available mental health apps have not been rigorously evaluated (Neary & Schueller, 2018; Torous et al., 2019a; Weisel et al., 2019), and some researchers have raised concerns regarding the validity of evidence used to support claims of efficacy in mental health apps (Cosgrove et al., 2020). Adding to concern, some mental health apps contain information inconsistent with current practice guidelines (Nicholas et al., 2015), and some apps have been found to contain potentially harmful information (Larsen et al., 2016). Recent reviews of mental health apps currently available on the commercial app stores continue to support these concerns. For example, a 2021 review of these CBT apps reported that they represent a 'heterogeneous group offering a range of evidence-based and non-evidence-based CBT techniques' (Martinengo et al., 2021).

In the absence of rigorous evaluation and with few regulations in digital health (Torous & Haim, 2018), people experiencing mental illness and clinicians have been left to navigate this new and complex health landscape with few supports. Consequently, researchers have expressed concern that many people struggling with mental health challenges may be using unreviewed and unsupported mental health apps potentially in lieu of evidence-based treatments (Neary & Schueller, 2018; Weisel et al., 2019).

While randomized controlled trials represent the 'gold standard' for evaluating the effectiveness of mental health apps (Mohr et al., 2021a), the fast-paced development and dissemination of commercial mental health apps pose a substantial challenge for such evaluation given the time required to conduct and publish findings from a randomized controlled trial (Neary & Schueller, 2018). More nimble and pragmatic modes of evaluation are necessary for informing the safe use of mental health apps. Rating models and guidelines have been developed over the past several years to address this need such as the Mobile App Rating Scale (MARS) (Stoyanov et al., 2015), and the Enlight guidelines (Baumel et al., 2017) among at least 70 others (Lagan et al., 2021). Researchers have called for standards and principles for evaluating mental health apps that address key areas of concern, including data safety and privacy, effectiveness, user-experience/adherence, and data integration (Torous et al., 2019a). These principles have been brought together in the App Advisor Initiative and App Evaluation Model of the American Psychiatric Association (American Psychiatric Association, 2021; Torous et al., 2018). These principles also guide an interactive platform, the M-Health Index and Navigation Database (MIND) (Beth Israel Deaconess Medical Center, 2020; Lagan et al., 2020) that facilitates identification of mental health apps that have been rigorously vetted according to the American Psychiatric Association framework.

Challenges in digital mental health

User engagement

Despite the potential of digital mental health interventions to help overcome many barriers to mental health care, user engagement with digital technologies is a continuing challenge within the field. As noted previously in this chapter, many research studies are limited by short follow-up periods. As a result, there is limited knowledge regarding long-term use of digital technologies. Existing evidence suggests that although digital health apps are highly available and frequently downloaded, many people stop using health apps 2 weeks after download (Dorsey et al., 2017; Torous et al., 2019). Researchers have noted that barriers to sustained use may reflect problems with app usability; meaningful input from patients and clinicians is often missing in the design and development phases (Torous et al., 2019). Including those with lived experience of mental illness and clinicians in the process of identifying unmet needs and in the design of digital interventions may enhance long-term engagement by helping to ensure that tools developed provide intrinsic value for their intended users (Biagianti et al., 2017).

Many factors impact user engagement with digital mental health technologies. A recent systematic review found user, program, and technology/environment characteristics that either facilitated or impeded engagement (Borghouts et al., 2021). Specifically, the authors found that severity of mental health symptoms, technical problems, and lack of personalization were common barriers to engagement (Borghouts et al., 2021). This is not to suggest that engagement is impossible in any populations, and a recent paper exploring a depression/anxiety-related app noted even those with the highest levels of symptom burden can still engage and benefit (Mohr et al., 2021b). Common facilitators of engagement were digital interventions that cultivated social connectedness as well as increasing insight and feelings of control over one's health (Borghouts et al., 2021).

Access to digital mental health

Even in high-income countries like the US, digital health is not yet accessible to all. Issues of diversity, equity, and inclusion cannot be ignored. While nearly 90% of the US population has access to a smartphone in 2022, access is lower among those who are older, have less education, live in rural areas, or are from minority or disadvantaged communities. But in terms of accessing the internet, smartphones may actually be utilized more than computers by the most disadvantaged patients (Roberts et al., 2020) and are thus deserving of focus as the primary device for health care interactions. While limited internet access because of either poverty or rural locations cannot be ignored, substantial efforts like the new 2021 US Infrastructure bill are devoting considerable resources towards bridging this digital divide. Digital literacy is a second and equally pressing digital divide that must also be bridged to make digital mental health truly accessible.

Implementation in routine mental health care settings

Despite accumulating evidence of the feasibility, acceptability, and effectiveness of digital technologies within the context of research studies, this has not resulted in widespread adoption of technology-based approaches in routine mental health care settings (Chiauzzi & Newell, 2019; Mohr et al., 2017; Noel et al., 2019; Wisniewski & Torous, 2020). As attitudes towards technology and practices have changed during the COVID-19 pandemic, there is an opportunity to build on the rapid transition to telehealth to integrate other forms of technology-based mental health care.

Mohr and colleagues (2017) have identified several issues that have hindered adoption and implementation. In particular, they highlight insufficient attention to the context of mental health services and lack of input from stakeholders in the development and testing of digital mental health technologies (Mohr et al., 2017). Consequently, benefits found in highly controlled research studies are rarely successfully transferred to real-world practice settings. Drop-out and non-engagement in these real-world uses are often far higher than reported at baseline in clinical studies (Torous et al., 2020b). Mohr and colleagues (2017) advocate examining the 'ecosystem' around technology rather than a narrow focus on the digital 'product'; conducting studies in mental health service settings that simultaneously examine treatment effects and implementation; and involving patient, health care providers, administrators, and information technology specialists in the process of developing digital interventions through user-centred design (Mohr et al., 2017). Other researchers point to the role of qualitative and ethnographic methods in providing insight into the context and use of digital mental health technologies (Carpenter-Song et al., 2018; Kozelka et al., 2021). Engaging stakeholders and attending to contexts of mental health care delivery recognizes that digital mental health approaches are not 'one size fits all' and need to be co-constructed with the communities they are intended to serve to maximize their uptake and benefit (Kozelka et al., 2021). New research is also beginning to explore the numerous mediators around digital health outcomes (e.g. emotional, interpersonal, and cognitive) and promises more mechanism-driven and personalized approaches (Domhardt et al., 2021).

Innovations in digital mental health care delivery

Technology specialist

Leaders in digital mental health have identified the need to support mental health stakeholders in their use of technology as means to address engagement and implementation challenges (Ben-Zeev et al., 2015; Wisniewski & Torous, 2020). Mental health clients and clinicians face difficulty finding tools that are consistent with best practices, easy to use, and secure in a digital landscape with an overwhelming number of options (Lecomte et al., 2020). Many clients find digital tools challenging to use (Wisniewski & Torous, 2020). Clinicians are often unsure of how best to select and use mHealth tools (Waalen et al., 2019), and clinical workflows in busy mental health centres create challenges for implementing digital tools because effort to integrate technology may be seen as burdensome to clinicians (Gagnon et al., 2016).

Responding to the current lack of effective support to improve clinician and client adoption and meaningful use of digital tools (Waalen et al., 2019), the 'technology specialist' is a new role in mental health service delivery (Carpenter-Song, 2020; Carpenter-Song et al., 2022; Noel et al., 2019). The technology specialist works collaboratively with clients and clinicians to integrate digital tools in routine mental health care. Digital tools are selected to support clients' individualized recovery goals and are evaluated for evidence, usability, and privacy/security according to the App Evaluation Model of the American Psychiatric Association (American Psychiatric Association, 2021; Torous et al., 2018). The technology specialist provides ongoing support to clients and clinicians to encourage use of, and communication regarding, the digital tool in the person's mental health care. Preliminary evidence regarding feasibility, acceptability, and impact of the technology specialist is promising (Carpenter-Song et al., 2022).

Technology-enabled clinical care

As one example of integrating mobile technology directly into care, we present details on technology-enabled clinical care (TECC) as a novel means to offer agile, personalized, and scalable mental health care (Rauseo-Ricupero & Torous, 2021). TECC harnesses three key aspects of this potential to offer effective care: (1) smartphone apps, (2) technology specialists, and (3) traditional telehealth. Utilizing the free and open-source mindLAMP app created by the Division of Digital Psychiatry at the Beth Israel Deaconess Medical Center, Boston (Torous et al., 2019b), TECC uses the smartphone app for two purposes: (1) data collection outside of sessions and (2) practising skills and homework completion also outside of sessions. These data (e.g. mood symptoms, step count, sleep patterns, etc.) are used to provide clinical insights and predictions that can be discussed by the patient and clinician at telehealth visits. This enables the clinician and patient to focus less on history gathering and more on interpreting what occurred between sessions and working on new solutions and skills. mindLAMP can also offer app-based interventions like mindfulness, goal tracking, safety planning, and more—thus, it provides patients a resource and tool to use between sessions and extend the reach of care. At each clinical visit, the clinician can use the mindLAMP portal to customize the app to the unique needs of the patient (e.g., change surveys, schedule of mindfulness, etc.) for use between visits. To ensure app use and help patients around any technology challenges, the clinic employs a specific type of technology specialist, a digital navigator, to provide technical and motivational support both inside and outside of visits. The TECC model is designed to ensure that technology does not reduce the autonomy of either the clinician or patient as the technology is designed to serve the unique clinical needs of each case at each visit through customization as driven by care needs and assisted through the direct hands-on implementation of the technology specialist.

Concluding remarks

The potential of telehealth for mental health has been realized during the COVID-19 pandemic as utilization and interest increased. While this focus on synchronous telehealth has made care more available, potential of asynchronous telehealth technologies like smartphone apps that we have focused on in this chapter is even greater. Engagement and clinical integration remain two of the largest challenges today, but new research and approaches like the technology specialist offer a bright future.

REFERENCES

Allan, S., Bradstreet, S., Mcleod, H., Farhall, J., Lambrou, M., Gleeson, J., et al. (2019). Developing a hypothetical implementation framework of expectations for monitoring early signs of psychosis relapse using a mobile app: qualitative study. *Journal of Medical Internet Research*, **21**, e14366.

American Psychiatric Association (2021). App Advisor—an American Psychiatric Association initiative. App evaluation model. https://www.psychiatry.org/psychiatrists/practice/mental-health-apps/the-app-evaluation-model

Andrade, L. H., Alonso, J., Mneimneh, Z., Wells, J. E., Al-Hamzawi, A., Borges, G., et al. (2014). Barriers to mental health treatment: results from the WHO World Mental Health surveys. *Psychological Medicine*, **44**, 1303–1317.

Arnold, C., Farhall, J., Villagonzalo, K. A., Sharma, K., & Thomas, N. (2021). Engagement with online psychosocial interventions for psychosis: a review and synthesis of relevant factors. *Internet Interventions*, **25**, 100411.

Bartels, S. J., Baggett, T. P., Freudenreich, O., & Bird, B. L. (2020). COVID-19 emergency reforms in Massachusetts to support behavioral health care and reduce mortality of people with serious mental illness. *Psychiatric Services*, **71**, 1078–1081.

Baumel, A., Muench, F., Edan, S., & Kane, J. M. (2019). Objective user engagement with mental health apps: systematic search and panel-based usage analysis. *Journal of Medical Internet Research*, **21**, e14567.

Baumel, A., Faber, K., Mathur, N., Kane, J. M., & Muench, F. (2017). Enlight: a comprehensive quality and therapeutic potential evaluation tool for mobile and web-based eHealth interventions. *Journal of Medical Internet Research*, **19**, e82.

Baxter, C., Carroll, J. A., Keogh, B., & Vandelanotte, C. (2020). Assessment of mobile health apps using built-in smartphone sensors for diagnosis and treatment: systematic survey of apps listed in international curated health app libraries. *JMIR mHealth and uHealth*, **8**, e16741.

Bell, I. H., Rossell, S. L., Farhall, J., Hayward, M., Lim, M. H., Fielding-Smith, S. F., & Thomas, N. (2020). Pilot randomised controlled trial of a brief coping-focused intervention for hearing voices blended with smartphone-based ecological momentary assessment and intervention (SAVVy): feasibility, acceptability and preliminary clinical outcomes. *Schizophrenia Research*, **216**, 479–487.

Ben-Zeev, D. (2020). The digital mental health genie is out of the bottle. *Psychiatric Services*, **71**, 1212–1213.

Ben-Zeev, D., Brenner, C. J., Begale, M., Duffecy, J., Mohr, D. C., & Mueser, K. T. (2014). Feasibility, acceptability, and preliminary efficacy of a smartphone intervention for schizophrenia. *Schizophrenia Bulletin*, **40**, 1244–1253.

Ben-Zeev, D., Brian, R. M., Jonathan, G., Razzano, L., Pashka, N., Carpenter-Song, E., et al. (2018). Mobile health (mHealth) versus clinic-based group intervention for people with serious mental illness: a randomized controlled trial. *Psychiatric Services*, **69**, 978–985.

Ben-Zeev, D., Buck, B., Meller, S., Hudenko, W. J., & Hallgren, K. A. (2020). Augmenting evidence-based care with a texting mobile interventionist: a pilot randomized controlled trial. *Psychiatric Services*, **71**, 1218–1224.

Ben-Zeev, D., Drake, R., & Marsch, L. (2015). Clinical technology specialists. *BMJ*, **350**, h945.

Ben-Zeev, D., Scherer, E. A., Gottlieb, J. D., Rotondi, A. J., Brunette, M. F., Achtyes, E. D., et al. (2016). mHealth for schizophrenia: patient engagement with a mobile phone intervention following hospital discharge. *JMIR Mental Health*, **3**, e34.

Beth Israel Deaconess Medical Center (2020). M-Health Index and Navigation Database. https://mindapps.org/

Biagianti, B., Hidalgo-Mazzei, D., & Meyer, N. (2017). Developing digital interventions for people living with serious mental illness: perspectives from three mHealth studies. *Evidence-Based Mental Health*, **20**, 98–101.

Borghouts, J., Eikey, E., Mark, G., De Leon, C., Schueller, S. M., Schneider, M., et al. (2021). Barriers to and facilitators of user engagement with digital mental health interventions: systematic review. *Journal of Medical Internet Research*, **23**, e24387.

Bucci, S., Barrowclough, C., Ainsworth, J., Machin, M., Morris, R., Berry, K., et al. (2018). Actissist: proof-of-concept trial of a theory-driven digital intervention for psychosis. *Schizophrenia Bulletin*, **44**, 1070–1080.

Buck, B., Chander, A., & Ben-Zeev, D. (2020). Clinical and demographic predictors of engagement in mobile health vs. clinic-based interventions for serious mental illness. *Journal of Behavioral and Cognitive Therapy*, **30**, 3–11.

Buck, B., Chander, A., Tauscher, J., Nguyen, T., Monroe-DeVita, M., & Ben-Zeev, D. (2021). mHealth for young adults with early psychosis: user preferences and their relationship to attitudes about treatment-seeking. *Journal of Technology in Behavioral Science*, **6**, 667–676.

Carpenter-Song, E. (2020). Promoting meaningful recovery with digital mental health care. *Epidemiology and Psychiatric Sciences*, **29**, e105.

Carpenter-Song, E., Acquilano, S. C., Noel, V., Al-Abdulmunem, M., Torous, J., & Drake, R. E. (2022). Individualized intervention to support mental health recovery through implementation of digital tools into clinical care: feasibility study. *Community Mental Health Journal*, **58**, 99–110.

Carpenter-Song, E., Noel, V. A., Acquilano, S. C., & Drake, R. E. (2018). Real-world technology use among people with mental illnesses: qualitative study. *JMIR Mental Health*, **5**, e10652.

Carter, H., Araya, R., Anjur, K., Deng, D., & Naslund, J. A. (2021). The emergence of digital mental health in low-income and middle-income countries: a review of recent advances and implications for the treatment and prevention of mental disorders. *Journal of Psychiatric Research*, **133**, 223–246.

Chiauzzi, E. & Newell, A. (2019). Mental health apps in psychiatric treatment: a patient perspective on real world technology usage. *JMIR Mental Health*, **6**, e12292.

Cohen, K. A., Stiles-Shields, C., Winquist, N., & Lattie, E. G. (2021). Traditional and nontraditional mental healthcare services: usage and preferences among adolescents and younger adults. *Journal of Behavioral Health Services & Research*, **48**, 537–553.

Cosgrove, L., Karter, J. M., Morrill, Z., & McGinley, M. (2020). Psychology and surveillance capitalism: the risk of pushing mental health apps during the COVID-19 pandemic. *Journal of Humanistic Psychology*, **60**, 611–625.

Deegan, P. E., Rapp, C., Holter, M., & Riefer, M. (2008). Best practices: a program to support shared decision making in an outpatient psychiatric medication clinic. *Psychiatric Services*, **59**, 603–605.

Department of Health and Human Services (2020). OCR announces notification of enforcement discretion for telehealth remote communications during the COVID-19 nationwide public health emergency. https://www.hhs.gov/hipaa/for-professionals/special-topics/emergency-preparedness/notification-enforcement-discretion-telehealth/index.html

Dockery, L., Jeffery, D., Schauman, O., Williams, P., Farrelly, S., Bonnington, O., et al. (2015). Stigma- and non-stigma-related treatment barriers to mental healthcare reported by service users and caregivers. *Psychiatry Research*, **228**, 612–619.

Domhardt, M., Engler, S., Nowak, H., Lutsch, A., Baumel, A., & Baumeister, H. (2021). Mechanisms of change in digital health interventions for mental disorders in youth: systematic review. *Journal of Medical Internet Research*, **23**, e29742.

Dorsey, E. R., McConnell, M. V., Shaw, S. Y., Trister, A. D., & Friend, S. H. (2017). The use of smartphones for health research. *Academic Medicine*, **92**, 157–160.

Eisenstadt, M., Liverpool, S., Infanti, E., Ciuvat, R. M., & Carlsson, C. (2021). Mobile apps that promote emotion regulation, positive mental health, and well-being in the general population: systematic review and meta-analysis. *JMIR Mental Health*, **8**, e31170.

Firth, J., Cotter, J., Torous, J., Bucci, S., Firth, J. A., & Yung, A. R. (2016). Mobile phone ownership and endorsement of 'mhealth' among people with psychosis: a meta-analysis of cross-sectional studies. *Schizophrenia Bulletin*, **42**, 448–455.

Firth, J., Torous, J., Nicholas, J., Carney, R., Pratap, A., Rosenbaum, S., & Sarris, J. (2017a). The efficacy of smartphone-based mental health interventions for depressive symptoms: a meta-analysis of randomized controlled trials. *World Psychiatry*, **16**, 287–298.

Firth, J., Torous, J., Nicholas, J., Carney, R., Rosenbaum, S., & Sarris, J. (2017b). Can smartphone mental health interventions reduce symptoms of anxiety? A meta-analysis of randomized controlled trials. *Journal of Affective Disorders*, **218**, 15–22.

Fortuna, K. L., Naslund, J. A., LaCroix, J. M., Bianco, C. L., Brooks, J. M., Zisman-Ilani, Y., et al. (2020). Digital peer support mental health interventions for people with a lived experience of a serious mental illness: systematic review. *JMIR Mental Health*, **7**, e16460.

Fu, Z., Burger, H., Arjadi, R., & Bockting, C. L. (2020). Effectiveness of digital psychological interventions for mental health problems in low-income and middle-income countries: a systematic review and meta-analysis. *Lancet Psychiatry*, **7**, 851–864.

Gagnon, M.-P., Ngangue, P., Payne-Gagnon, J., & Desmartis, M. (2016). m-Health adoption by healthcare professionals: a systematic review. *Journal of the American Medical Informatics Association*, **23**, 212–220.

Gire, N., Farooq, S., Naeem, F., Duxbury, J., McKeown, M., Kundi, P. S., et al. (2017). mHealth based interventions for the assessment and treatment of psychotic disorders: a systematic review. *mHealth*, **3**, 33.

Goldman, M. L., Druss, B. G., Horvitz-Lennon, M., Norquist, G. S., Kroeger Ptakowski, K., Brinkley, A., et al. (2020). Mental health policy in the era of COVID-19. *Psychiatric Services*, **71**, 1158–1162.

Hanssen, E., Balvert, S., Oorschot, M., Borkelmans, K., van Os, J., Delespaul, P., & Fett, A. K. (2020). An ecological momentary intervention incorporating personalised feedback to improve symptoms and social functioning in schizophrenia spectrum disorders. *Psychiatry Research*, **284**, 112695.

Hrynyschyn, R., & Dockweiler, C. (2021). Effectiveness of smartphone-based cognitive behavioral therapy among patients with major depression: systematic review of health implications. *JMIR mHealth and uHealth*, **9**, e24703.

Hubley, S., Lynch, S. B., Schneck, C., Thomas, M., & Shore, J. (2016). Review of key telepsychiatry outcomes. *World Journal of Psychiatry*, **6**, 269–282.

Inkster, B. (2021). Early warning signs of a mental health tsunami: a coordinated response to gather initial data insights from multiple digital services providers. *Frontiers in Digital Health*, **2**, 64.

Inkster, B., O'Brien, R., Selby, E., Joshi, S., Subramanian, V., Kadaba, M., et al. (2020). Digital health management during and beyond the COVID-19 pandemic: opportunities, barriers, and recommendations. *JMIR Mental Health*, **7**, e19246.

IQVIA Institute for Human Data Science. (2017). *The Growing Value of Digital Health: Evidence and Impact on Human Health and the Healthcare System*. Parsippany, NJ: IQVIA Institute for Human Data Science.

Jiménez-Molina, Á., Franco, P., Martínez, V., Martínez, P., Rojas, G., & Araya, R. (2019). Internet-based interventions for the prevention and treatment of mental disorders in Latin America: a scoping review. *Frontiers in Psychiatry*, **10**, 664.

Jonathan, G., Carpenter-Song, E. A., Brian, R. M., & Ben-Zeev, D. (2019). Life with FOCUS: a qualitative evaluation of the impact of a smartphone intervention on people with serious mental illness. *Psychiatric Rehabilitation Journal*, **42**, 182–189.

Kaonga, N. N., & Morgan, J. (2019). Common themes and emerging trends for the use of technology to support mental health and psychosocial well-being in limited resource settings: a review of the literature. *Psychiatry Research*, **281**, 112594.

Kidd, S. A., Feldcamp, L., Adler, A., Kaleis, L., Wang, W., Vichnevetski, K., et al. (2019). Feasibility and outcomes of a multi-function mobile health approach for the schizophrenia spectrum: App4Independence (A4i). *PloS One*, **14**, e0219491.

Kinoshita, S., Cortright, K., Crawford, A., Mizuno, Y., Yoshida, K., Hilty, D., et al. (2020). Changes in telepsychiatry regulations during the COVID-19 pandemic: 17 countries and regions' approaches to an evolving healthcare landscape. *Psychological Medicine*, **52**, 2606–2613.

Kopelovich, S. L., Monroe-DeVita, M., Buck, B. E., Brenner, C., Moser, L., Jarskog, L. F., et al. (2021). Community mental health care delivery during the COVID-19 pandemic: practical strategies for improving care for people with serious mental illness. *Community Mental Health Journal*, **57**, 405–415.

Kozelka, E. E., Jenkins, J. H., & Carpenter-Song, E. (2021). Advancing health equity in digital mental health: lessons from medical anthropology for global mental health. *JMIR Mental Health*, **8**, e28555.

Kuhn, E., Greene, C., Hoffman, J., Nguyen, T., Wald, L., Schmidt, J., et al. (2014). Preliminary evaluation of PTSD Coach, a smartphone app for post-traumatic stress symptoms. *Military Medicine*, **179**, 12–18.

Lagan, S., Sandler, L., & Torous, J. (2021). Evaluating evaluation frameworks: a scoping review of frameworks for assessing health apps. *BMJ Open*, **11**, e047001.

Lagan, S., Aquino, P., Emerson, M. R., Fortuna, K., Walker, R., & Torous, J. (2020). Actionable health app evaluation: translating expert frameworks into objective metrics. *NPJ Digital Medicine*, **3**, 1–8.

Larsen, M. E., Nicholas, J., & Christensen, H. (2016). A systematic assessment of smartphone tools for suicide prevention. *PLoS One*, **11**, e0152285.

Lecomte, T., Potvin, S., Corbière, M., Guay, S., Samson, C., Cloutier, B., et al. (2020). Mobile apps for mental health issues: meta-review of meta-analyses. *JMIR mHealth uHealth*, **8**, e17458.

Lewis, S., Ainsworth, J., Sanders, C., Stockton-Powdrell, C., Machin, M., Whelan, P., et al. (2020). Smartphone-enhanced symptom management in psychosis: open, randomized controlled trial. *Journal of Medical Internet Research*, **22**, e17019.

Linardon, J., Cuijpers, P., Carlbring, P., Messer, M., & Fuller-Tyszkiewicz, M. (2019). The efficacy of app-supported smartphone interventions for mental health problems: a meta-analysis of randomized controlled trials. *World Psychiatry*, **18**, 325–336.

Lungu, A., Jun, J. J., Azarmanesh, O., Leykin, Y., Connie, E., & Chen, J. (2020). Blended care-cognitive behavioral therapy for depression and anxiety in real-world settings: pragmatic retrospective study. *Journal of Medical Internet Research*, **22**, e18723.

Mahmoud, H., Vogt, E. L., Dahdouh, R., & Raymond, M. L. (2020). Using continuous quality improvement to design and implement a telepsychiatry program in rural Illinois. *Psychiatric Services*, **71**, 860–863.

Martinengo, L., Stona, A. C., Griva, K., Dazzan, P., Pariante, C. M., von Wangenheim, F., & Car, J. (2021). Self-guided cognitive behavioral therapy apps for depression: systematic assessment of features, functionality, and congruence with evidence. *Journal of Medical Internet Research*, **23**, e27619.

Miralles, I., Granell, C., Díaz-Sanahuja, L., Van Woensel, W., Bretón-López, J., Mira, A., et al. (2020). Smartphone apps for the treatment of mental disorders: systematic review. *JMIR mHealth and uHealth*, **8**, e14897.

Mohr, D. C., Azocar, F., Bertagnolli, A., Choudhury, T., Chrisp, P., Frank, R., et al. (2021a). Banbury Forum consensus statement on the path forward for digital mental health treatment. *Psychiatric Services*, **72**, 677–683.

Mohr, D. C., Kwasny, M. J., Meyerhoff, J., Graham, A. K., & Lattie, E. G. (2021b). The effect of depression and anxiety symptom severity on clinical outcomes and app use in digital mental health treatments: meta-regression of three trials. *Behaviour Research and Therapy*, **147**, 103972.

Mohr, D. C., Schueller, S. M., Tomasino, K. N., Kaiser, S. M., Alam, N., Karr, C., et al. (2019). Comparison of the effects of coaching and receipt of app recommendations on depression, anxiety, and engagement in the IntelliCare platform: factorial randomized controlled trial. *Journal of Medical Internet Research*, 21, e13609.

Mohr, D. C., Weingardt, K. R., Reddy, M., & Schueller, S. M. (2017). Three problems with current digital mental health research … and three things we can do about them. *Psychiatric Services*, 68, 427–429.

Moitra, E., Park, H. S., & Gaudiano, B. A. (2021). Development and initial testing of an mhealth transitions of care intervention for adults with schizophrenia-spectrum disorders immediately following a psychiatric hospitalization. *Psychiatric Quarterly*, 92, 259–272.

Molloy, A. & Anderson, P. L. (2021). Engagement with mobile health interventions for depression: a systematic review. *Internet Interventions*, 26, 100454.

Mordecai, D., Histon, T., Neuwirth, E., Heisler, W. S., Kraft, A., Bang, Y., et al. (2021). How Kaiser Permanente created a mental health and wellness digital ecosystem. *NEJM Catalyst Innovations in Care Delivery*, 2, 1.

Muoio, D. (2019). Global mental health apps exceeded 400 M in 2018. *Mobi Health News*. https://www.mobihealthnews.com/content/global-medical-app-downloads-exceeded-400m-2018

Naslund, J. A., Aschbrenner, K. A., Araya, R., Marsch, L. A., Unützer, J., Patel, V., & Bartels, S. J. (2017). Digital technology for treating and preventing mental disorders in low-income and middle-income countries: a narrative review of the literature. *Lancet Psychiatry*, 4, 486–500.

Neary, M. & Schueller, S. M. (2018). State of the field of mental health apps. *Cognitive and Behavioral Practice*, 25, 531–537.

Nicholas, J., Larsen, M. E., Proudfoot, J., & Christensen, H. (2015). Mobile apps for bipolar disorder: a systematic review of features and content quality. *Journal of Medical Internet Research*, 17, e198.

Noel, V. A., Acquilano, S. C., Carpenter-Song, E., & Drake, R. E. (2019). Use of mobile and computer devices to support recovery in people with serious mental illness: survey study. *JMIR Mental Health*, 6, e12255.

Predmore, Z. S., Roth, E., Breslau, J., Fischer, S. H., & Uscher-Pines, L. (2021). Assessment of patient preferences for telehealth in post-COVID-19 pandemic health care. *JAMA Network Open*, 4, e2136405.

Rauseo-Ricupero, N., & Torous, J. (2021). Technology enabled clinical care (TECC): protocol for a prospective longitudinal cohort study of smartphone-augmented mental health treatment. *JMIR Research Protocols*, 10, e23771.

Roberts, L. W., Chan, S., & Torous, J. (2018). New tests, new tools: mobile and connected technologies in advancing psychiatric diagnosis. *NPJ Digital Medicine*, 1, 6.

Roberts, E. T., & Mehrotra, A. (2020). Assessment of disparities in digital access among Medicare beneficiaries and implications for telemedicine. *JAMA Internal Medicine*, 180, 1386–1389.

Rodriguez-Villa, E., Naslund, J., Keshavan, M., Patel, V., & Torous, J. (2020). Making mental health more accessible in light of COVID-19: scalable digital health with digital navigators in low and middle-income countries. *Asian Journal of Psychiatry*, 54, 102433.

Rowan, K., McAlpine, D. D., & Blewett, L. A. (2013). Access and cost barriers to mental health care, by insurance status, 1999–2010. *Health Affairs*, 32, 1723–1730.

Santarossa, S., Kane, D., Senn, Y. C., & Woodruff, J. S. (2018). Exploring the role of in-person components for online health behavior change interventions: can a digital person-to-person component suffice? *Journal of Medical Internet Research*, 20, e144.

Schlosser, D. A., Campellone, T. R., Truong, B., Etter, K., Vergani, S., Komaiko, K., & Vinogradov, S. (2018). Efficacy of PRIME, a mobile app intervention designed to improve motivation in young people with schizophrenia. *Schizophrenia bulletin*, 44, 1010–1020.

Shah, R. N. & Berry, O. O. (2021). The rise of venture capital investing in mental health. *JAMA Psychiatry*, 78, 351–352.

Silver, L., Smith, A., Johnson, C., Taylor, K., Jiang, J., Anderson, M., & Rainie, L. (2019). Mobile connectivity in emerging economies. *Pew Research Center*, 7 March. https://www.pewresearch.org/internet/2019/03/07/mobile-connectivity-in-emerging-economies/

Steare, T., O'Hanlon, P., Eskinazi, M., Osborn, D., Lloyd-Evans, B., Jones, R., et al. (2020). Smartphone-delivered self-management for first-episode psychosis: the ARIES feasibility randomised controlled trial. *BMJ Open*, 10, e034927.

Stoyanov, S. R., Hides, L., Kavanagh, D. J., Zelenko, O., Tjondronegoro, D., & Mani, M. (2015). Mobile app rating scale: a new tool for assessing the quality of health mobile apps. *JMIR mHealth and uHealth*, 3, e3422.

Torous, J., Andersson, G., Bertagnoli, A., Christensen, H., Cuijpers, P., Firth, J., et al. (2019a). Towards a consensus around standards for smartphone apps and digital mental health. *World Psychiatry*, 18, 97.

Torous, J., Bucci, S., Bell, I. H., Kessing, L. V., Faurholt-Jepsen, M., Whelan, P., et al. (2021). The growing field of digital psychiatry: current evidence and the future of apps, social media, chatbots, and virtual reality. *World Psychiatry*, 20, 318–335.

Torous, J. B., Chan, S. R., Gipson, S. Y. M. T., Kim, J. W., Nguyen, T. Q., Luo, J., & Wang, P. (2018). A hierarchical framework for evaluation and informed decision making regarding smartphone apps for clinical care. *Psychiatric Services*, 69, 498–500.

Torous, J., Firth, J., Mueller, N., Onnela, J. P., & Baker, J. T. (2017). Methodology and reporting of mobile health and smartphone application studies for schizophrenia. *Harvard Review of Psychiatry*, 25, 146–154.

Torous, J. & Haim, A. (2018). Dichotomies in the development and implementation of digital mental health tools. *Psychiatric Services*, 69, 1204–1206.

Torous, J., Jän Myrick, K., Rauseo-Ricupero, N., & Firth, J. (2020a). Digital mental health and COVID-19: using technology today to accelerate the curve on access and quality tomorrow. *JMIR Ment Health*, 7, e18848.

Torous, J., Lipschitz, J., Ng, M., & Firth, J. (2020b). Dropout rates in clinical trials of smartphone apps for depressive symptoms: a systematic review and meta-analysis. *Journal of Affective Disorders*, 263, 413–419.

Torous, J., Wisniewski, H., Bird, B., Carpenter, E., David, G., Elejalde, E., et al. (2019b). Creating a digital health smartphone app and digital phenotyping platform for mental health and diverse healthcare needs: an interdisciplinary and collaborative approach. *Journal of Technology in Behavioral Science*, 4, 73–85.

Waalen, J., Peters, M., Ranamukhaarachchi, D., Li, J., Ebner, G., Senkowsky, J., et al. (2019). Real world usage characteristics of a novel mobile health self-monitoring device: results from the Scanadu Consumer Health Outcomes (SCOUT) Study. *PLoS One*, 14, e0215468.

Weisel, K. K., Fuhrmann, L. M., Berking, M., Baumeister, H., Cuijpers, P., & Ebert, D. D. (2019). Standalone smartphone apps for mental health—a systematic review and meta-analysis. *NPJ Digital Medicine*, 2, 1–10.

Whelan, P., Machin, M., Lewis, S., Buchan, I., Sanders, C., Applegate, E., et al. (2015). Mobile early detection and connected intervention to coproduce better care in severe mental illness. *Studies in Health Technology and Informatics*, **216**, 123–126.

Wisniewski, H. & Torous, J. (2020). Digital navigators to implement smartphone and digital tools in care. *Acta Psychiatrica Scandinavica*, **141**, 350–355.

World Health Organization (2021a). Health topics: mental health-burden. https://www.who.int/health-topics/mental-health#tab=tab_2

World Health Organization (2021b). Fact sheets—depression. https://www.who.int/news-room/fact-sheets/detail/depression

World Health Organization (2021c). *Mental Health Atlas 2020*. Geneva: World Health Organization.

Wright, J. H., Mishkind, M., Eells, T. D., & Chan, S. R. (2019). Computer-assisted cognitive-behavior therapy and mobile apps for depression and anxiety. *Current Psychiatry Reports*, **21**, 62.

Wu, A., Scult, M. A., Barnes, E. D., Betancourt, J. A., Falk, A., & Gunning, F. M. (2021). Smartphone apps for depression and anxiety: a systematic review and meta-analysis of techniques to increase engagement. *NPJ Digital Medicine*, **4**, 1–9.

Yellowlees, P., Nakagawa, K., Pakyurek, M., Hanson, A., Elder, J., & Kales, H. C. (2020). Rapid conversion of an outpatient psychiatric clinic to a 100% virtual telepsychiatry clinic in response to COVID-19. *Psychiatric Services*, **71**, 749–752.

26

Forensic community mental health services

Lisa Wootton, Penelope Brown, and Alec Buchanan

Introduction

Mental health care, like other forms of health care, takes place in a social context. The context in which outpatient treatment is provided to people whose mental disorders are complicated by a history of criminal offending has changed substantially over the past half century. Other chapters in this volume describe the closures of large hospitals and the move to providing care in community settings. For many patients of mental health services with offending histories, this move has been associated with a change in goals and emphasis in the treatment they receive. Risk assessment and risk management are now at the centre of their care (see Mullen, 2002), whether the responsibility for providing them falls on general or specialist services. This chapter is about how this new emphasis has developed and what effect it has had on the treatment that patients receive.

Over the past 30 years community forensic psychiatric services have become widespread both in the US and in Europe. The treatment they provide differs according to the needs of different jurisdictions. In the US, forensic assertive community treatment teams based on the assertive community treatment model developed in response to evidence that people with mental illness who were in contact with the criminal justice system were not receiving adequate services and were ending up in prison as a result (Hoge et al., 2009). Outpatient civil commitment was introduced from the 1980s onwards in many states by advocates seeking to ensure that 'revolving door' patients received the treatment they needed, whether they sought that care or not. In the UK, most patients of forensic community services have been discharged from secure hospitals.

An unproductive discussion in the middle years of the twentieth century over whether people with mental disorders were 'dangerous' had been replaced by the 1990s with descriptions of risk assessment and risk management (Monahan, 1988; Mullen & Ogloff, 2009; Snowden, 1997). These descriptions amounted both to the identification of a problem and a way of addressing it, quantifying risk of violence and other adverse outcomes in non-binary and consistent ways that made planning treatment with the explicit aim of managing that risk more feasible. In the twenty-first century this practice has been integrated into routine care, in North America through the development of structured rating scales designed to help clinicians manage risk and more formally in the UK with the adoption of the Care Programme Approach.

Of course, notorious acts of violence by people with mental illnesses, always uncommon, have not ceased. But along with the responsibility to manage risk has come a perception that services are responsible for the consequences when violence occurs (see Szmukler, 2000). Sometimes those events are outside a psychiatrist's power to control. Irrespective, values such as confidentiality and the need to do no harm have been forced to yield to a new emphasis on collaborating with criminal justice agencies. Repeatedly reminded in the press and, for 30 years, by inquiries (see Ritchie et al., 1994) of the failures of treatment to prevent serious violence by people in contact with services, psychiatrists in the UK feel that they are not only, reasonably, expected to help their patients but also, less reasonably, to routinely collaborate in efforts to control them (see Holloway & Davies, 2017).

The social context

Diversion

Research suggests that between one-third to one-half of people in police custody have some form of mental disorder. Between one-fifth and one-half of defendants at court have also been estimated to have a mental disorder (Brown et al., 2022). Mood disorders, neurodevelopmental disorders, and substance abuse are particularly frequent (McKinnon et al., 2013; Payne-James et al., 2005; Young et al., 2013). The Bradley Report, published in 2009, began from the premise that many of these people should not be in the criminal justice system, at all:

> While public protection remains the priority, there is a growing consensus that prison may not always be an appropriate environment for those with severe mental illness and that custody can exacerbate mental ill health, heighten vulnerability and increase the risk of self-harm and suicide. (Bradley, 2009, p. 7)

The Report called for more diversion from criminal justice and into health services and more multi-agency collaboration between health service and criminal justice staff. This has led to the development of liaison and diversion services covering police stations and courts, which aim to identify vulnerable people entering the justice system at an early stage and direct them to appropriate care pathways (NHS Commissioning Board, 2013). Australia has seen similar initiatives (Davidson et al., 2016).

More controversially, the report argued that meeting the complex needs of mentally disordered offenders is part of the core business not only of forensic services but also of general psychiatry (Senior et al., 2017). In the US, also, the 2000s have seen greater collaboration between criminal justice and mental health agencies. Examples include mental health professionals training police crisis intervention teams in how to interact most appropriately with people with mental disorders and when to use alternatives to incarceration, in the continuing development of mental health courts where treatment can be offered in lieu of incarceration, and in pilot projects such as Ohio's 'Succeeding at Home' programme, which provides treatment for substance use disorder and mental health conditions to men released from jails and prisons (Ohio Ex-Offender Reentry Coalition, 2010).

Published frameworks and guidelines have gone some way towards addressing the wide variation in services in different jurisdictions in the US, although resource constraints have rendered their adoption patchy (see D'Amora et al., 2017). In the UK to date, the Bradley Report does not appear to have led to a flood of patients being referred to community mental health services (Her Majesty's Inspectorate of Probation, 2021; Holloway & Davies, 2017). It may be that this is at least in part because the need is being met, in contrast to what would be regarded as optimal elsewhere in twenty-first-century mental health, through the increased funding and use of inpatient care.

Community mental health input to prisons

The UK in the 2000s embarked on an attempt to integrate prison mental health care with community services. Research in the 1990s had suggested that between 7% of sentenced men and 14% of women suffered from psychosis (Singleton et al., 1998). In 2001, the UK departments responsible for health and prisons jointly published guidance whereby prison mental health care would be delivered by staff directly employed by the health service. One consequence was the development of 'in-reach' teams. Initially, these teams often faced staff retention and recruitment difficulties. Whether for this or other reasons, initial improvements were limited, with evidence of discharge planning at the time of prison release noted in barely over half of cases in one study and evidence of direct contact between the prison and the community mental health team in only 38% (Lennox et al., 2012). High levels of psychiatric morbidity in prisons internationally has led to a suggestion that all prisons should have systems in place for the identification of those with serious mental health problems, including case finding on arrival to prison and allocation to appropriate level of service, including pharmacological and psychological interventions, substance misuse services, and trauma-focused and sex/gender-specific interventions (Fazel et al., 2016).

Probation and public policy on offender management

Probation policy governing the supervision of mentally disordered offenders also changed in the 2000s. In the UK the Offender Rehabilitation Act 2014 (Ministry of Justice, 2014) introduced mandatory supervision for people released from prison part-way through a sentence of less than 12 months. The 35 individual Probation Trusts were replaced by a single National Probation Service. A review of community sentences permitted courts (with the consent of the offender) to add a 'Mental Health Treatment Requirement' (MHTR) lasting for up to 3 years. MHTRs have not been widely used and evidence for their effectiveness has been inconsistent. In 2012–2013, only 765 were made either as part of a Community Order (CO) or Suspended Sentence Order (SSO)—567 CO requirements and 198 SSOs. They accounted for fewer than 1% of all community orders (National Offender Management Service, 2014; see also Beswick & Gunn, 2017). Since 2018 there has been a renewed interest following the pilot of a new protocol which seeks to address the perceived barriers to their use (Molyneaux et al., 2021).

Multi-Agency Public Protection Arrangements (MAPPA) were introduced in England and Wales by the Criminal Justice and Court Services Act (2000). The act, designed as a public protection measure, created local multi-agency panels, managed by police and probation services, to coordinate risk management in high-risk offenders. In 2003 the legislation was amended to include the prison service and introduced a 'duty to cooperate' on nine other agencies, including health. The number of people who are MAPPA 'eligible' (see 'Information Sharing') continues to grow and in 2020–2021 it was 87,657 (Ministry of Justice, 2021). Clinicians have expressed concerns regarding the type and quantity of clinical information that is expected to be shared (Yakeley et al., 2012), and regarding the decision-making processes around disclosure of an offender's history to a third party (such as an employer or partner) without the offender's consent (Penny & Craissati, 2012). The challenges and controversies related to information sharing are addressed further below.

The growth in forensic inpatient provision

In 1990, Bluglass had noted: 'Forensic psychiatrists will … be anxious to resist being regarded as psychiatry's jailers in a reorganized health service; a risk which they may face as mental hospitals close down' (Bluglass, 1990, p. 8). The closure of large general psychiatric hospitals over the past 40 years has coincided with a substantial expansion of secure psychiatric provision. The number of people detained under mental health legislation in high and medium secure units in England and Wales has risen over that period (Rutherford & Duggan, 2008) and by 2011 secure psychiatric services cared for up to 8000 people, approximately 3500 of whom were in 'medium secure' units (Centre for Mental Health, 2011, p. 6).

Psychiatrists have indeed expressed concerns that this growth in secure provision has become immune to the usual constraints of funding and clinical necessity (Wilson et al., 2011). General psychiatric services had traditionally been wary of taking large numbers of offender patients and the expansion in forensic inpatient beds has been an important contributor to the development of specialist, forensic outpatient services. The bed numbers, however, also indicate the extent to which psychiatry now shares with the criminal justice system the task of detaining those deemed to pose a risk to others. The prison population in England and Wales at the end of 2021 was 80,000. As prison numbers remain relatively stable in the UK, so the proportion of all those detained who are under mental health care has grown. This is likely to be due to a combination of an increased recognition of mental disorder among those involved in the criminal justice system and increases in bed numbers which have allowed for the detention of people who may not have been detained in the past.

Unfairness and bias

There is now increasing evidence that criminal justice and mental health systems focus coercion disproportionately on Black and other ethnic minority patients. Psychiatry, with its background in medicine, its focus on the individual, and its obligation to do good has the opportunity, as well as the professional obligation, to ensure that where its patients are concerned, the need to protect the public is balanced against a proper respect for the people it treats. Rose has summarized the positive steps that psychiatrists working in the community can take to increase the chances of their overall contribution being to the benefit of their patients and others (Rose, 2017). They can remain aware of the limits on their abilities to assess risk in mentally disordered individuals; they can oppose measures that criminalize mental health problems or that would take advantage of the stigma associated with mental illness to demand that psychiatry itself become more carceral; and, finally, they can shift the focus from concerns about notorious, even demonized, individuals onto the damaging and pervasive effects of prisons and imprisonment on mental health.

The provision of care

The structure and goals of care

The statistical association between mental illness and risk of criminal recidivism is weak (Bonta et al., 2014) and the best predictors of re-arrest among people with mental illness are the same as those for the general population (Skeem et al., 2009). Although the methodological difficulties in investigating causation are substantial, research suggests that for most crimes by most people with mental illness, the crime is not accounted for by symptoms (Skeem et al., 2014) and it is unusual for risk management to focus on one symptom or set of symptoms. Instead, the treatment of people with mental illness involved with the criminal justice system has the same goals as the treatment of non-offender people: ameliorating symptoms, minimizing disability, maximizing community functioning and supporting individualized recovery (Rotter et al., 2017).

Those goals, however, will usually be developed in collaboration with the patient and informed by knowledge of the kinds of problems that are most strongly associated with the patient finding themselves back in prison. Many people with offending histories, including those with mental illness, have substance use problems and, statistically, this is the patient characteristic most strongly linked to re-incarceration (Wilson & Wood, 2014).

People who have been incarcerated or been detained for a long time in hospital may have lost both their accommodation and the networks that would previously have supported them. Providing family education and structure is difficult with broken families but it may still be possible to enhance a patient's level of community support (Jewell et al., 2012). People with mental illnesses who have been in prison are doubly stigmatized when looking for work; supported employment, particularly combined with the associated assessment, training, and placement services, is an effective intervention (Kane et al., 2015). Peer support often has an important role, both in maintaining abstinence and in problem-solving (Luciano et al., 2014). Enabling people with severe mental illness to find and retain employment is a key component of the NHS's Five Year Forward View for Mental Health (NHS England, 2016).

Treatment with medication

Many outpatients under forensic care suffer from psychosis. Research on community samples shows that people with psychosis have approximately four times the risk of engaging in violent behaviour compared with the general population (Fazel et al., 2009). The type of psychosis does not appear substantially to affect the risk and most of the increase appears to be the result of comorbid substance use. Treatment appears to mitigate, and in some studies abolish, this increased risk (Fazel et al., 2014; Keers et al., 2014; Swanson et al., 2008). The results are heterogeneous but some antipsychotics, and in particular clozapine, may be more effective than others (Sariaslan et al., 2021). However, treatment of psychosis in all settings is associated with high rates of discontinuation (Tracy & Gaughran, 2017). Hopes that the introduction of 'second-generation' antipsychotics would help address this problem have not been realized (Jones et al., 2006; Lieberman et al., 2005).

In the UK, for the treatment of psychosis the National Institute for Health and Care Excellence recommends initial treatment with oral antipsychotic medication in conjunction with psychological measures such as family therapy and individual cognitive behavioural therapy. Long-acting injectable medications are widely used in forensic practice in part because discontinuing medication is usually a risk factor for violence and this method of administration ensures a patient has received the prescribed dose. It is not yet clear whether long-acting injections of second-generation antipsychotics are associated with lower rates of non-compliance, although there are suggestions that these drugs cause less pain at the injection site and fewer 'break-through' extrapyramidal side effects on the day of injection (Jann et al., 1985). Smokers typically require a higher dose of clozapine to achieve therapeutic levels and those who resume their habit on leaving a 'smoke free' forensic hospital or prison may require monitoring of their clozapine blood levels.

Factors that have been shown by research to be associated with improved adherence are typically divided into those relating to the patient, to the type of medication, and to the environment, although patients have preferences that can trump research findings. Of patient characteristics, good illness insight and a positive attitude to medication are the only variables that have been consistently linked to treatment adherence (Tracy & Gaughran, 2017). Neither type of medication (whether first or second generation), mode of administration, or treatment side effects (Buchanan 1992, 1998) have been shown consistently to exert an effect. Environmental factors have been the subject of fewer studies. Predictably perhaps, having a good relationship with one's treating psychiatrist is usually said to improve compliance, along with paying patients to take their medication, though the latter is ethically contentious (Tracy & Gaughran, 2017; see Chapter 29, this volume).

Mood stabilizing medication is effective in reducing violent offending in those with a diagnosis of bipolar disorder but not other diagnoses (Fazel et al., 2014). Medication to treat attention deficit hyperactivity disorder also appears to be effective in reducing offending (Lichtenstein et al., 2012) and more specifically violent offending, as is medication to treat addictive disorders (Chang et al., 2016).

The treatment of people who have histories of sexual offending is usually conducted by specialist services. In addition to history and examination, evaluation typically includes a hormonal profile, a range of behavioural questionnaires and instruments, and an assessment of the risk of recidivism. Pharmacological treatment is often combined with psychological treatment. A task force report by the World Federation of Societies of Biological Psychiatry (Thibaut et al., 2010) reviews pharmacotherapy with selective serotonin reuptake inhibitors, antiandrogens, and gonadotropin-releasing hormone analogues. It also outlines an algorithm titrating that treatment against the effects on desire and sexual behaviour that are sought. The topic is reviewed in detail by Bradford et al. (2017).

Treatment with psychotherapy

Van Velsen and Norton (2017) summarized the psychotherapeutic objective:

> The main aim of treating out-patient mentally-disordered offenders is to improve their mental health or prevent its deterioration. This is to enable them to exercise, maximally, their potential for making healthier choices. Optimally, this helps them to refrain from criminal behaviour that is under their conscious control, albeit such behaviour is often driven by impulses that are irrational and unconscious, i.e., of which they are, by definition, unaware. Additionally, the aim is to promote their more creative engagement with life and so reduce the suffering of self and others. (p. 179)

Treatment often involves sharing information with a range of professionals and agencies. This is particularly the case where the welfare of children is involved and families have been victims. Many of those agencies and professional will have standards and approaches that differ from those of psychiatry, especially relating to confidentiality. Mechanisms for multidisciplinary working need to take account of this.

Psychotherapy with patients who have offending histories employs the same range of techniques as psychotherapy in other settings. Problems are frequently enacted interpersonally, rather than articulated (Gilligan, 1999) and patients, particularly those who feel they have been coerced into treatment, may perceive treatment more as part of their problem than its solution (Lockwood, 1992). Managing anxiety in patient, therapist, or both (Norton & McGauley, 1998) is a crucial part of the task, to the extent that some define one aim of treatment as being to improve the patient's capacity to contain anxiety and hence to inhibit its discharge through antisocial or criminal behaviour (Van Velsen & Norton, 2017).

Appropriate supervision of the therapist is important, particularly regarding the detection of boundary infringements and their management. Transference reactions are of central importance in understanding the therapeutic encounter, and have the potential to split otherwise cohesive therapeutic teams (Gabbard, 1986). Terminations of therapy should not usually coincide with change of external environment, such as moving to a community setting, because such moves can themselves be destabilizing. Lists of contraindications to psychotherapy in forensic patients have been published (Meloy & Yakeley, 2010). These include sadistic aggressive behaviour resulting in serious injury, the absence of any remorse for (or justification of) destructive behaviour, a history lacking in any meaningful attachments, and certain cases of learning disability. Practice is heterogeneous, however. Clarity as to the objective and the availability of experienced supervision seem key.

Practitioners specializing in providing psychotherapy for people with histories of sexual offending emphasize that what are often the most immediate and salient aspects of someone's clinical presentation—victim empathy, acknowledging rather than denying harmful behaviour, and offence-related attitudes and insight—are usually of little help in assessing risk (Craissati, 2004). They recommend a more actuarial and instrument-based approach, with important caveats: predictive statistics apply to populations, not individuals; low base rates mean than even instruments with good predictive validity will have high false positive or false negatives, or both; and instruments should only be used in populations in which they have been shown to be valid. Even where these caveats are acknowledged, it is important to bear in mind the limits of risk assessment. Craissati and Sindall (2009) examined 94 repeat offences committed by offenders on probation in London. Most of the men fell into the 'medium' risk range on actuarial assessments.

Risk assessment in community settings

Violence risk assessment in community settings differs in several respects from risk assessments conducted when a patient is in a hospital. The greater availability in community settings of weapons, illegal drugs, and potential victims are obvious reasons. But the low prevalence (base rate) of serious violence in most mental health samples means that even the best methods of assessment, whether instrument based or clinical, are seriously inaccurate when they are used to attempt to identify individuals who will act violently (Buchanan & Leese, 2001; Singh et al., 2014). Finally, the ability of clinicians to identify the people their patients will encounter and the circumstances in which they will encounter them are much more limited in the community than when the patient is in hospital.

Whatever the setting, one of the principal challenges for practitioners lies in integrating two very different approaches to violence risk assessment. One of these approaches involves identifying which known, evidence-based risk factors are present in the case at hand (a 'correlation-based' approach). The other is based on the traditional, clinical, assumption that violence occurs for reasons or motives and that the clinician's understanding of those reasons can be used to prevent future violence (a 'causation-based' approach). The correlation-based approach saw the development of a series of actuarial instruments in the late 1900s (Harris et al., 1993). Other structured instruments, developed later, sought to combine a structured approach to information gathering with the use of clinical understanding ('structured professional judgement'; see Webster et al., 1997). Some have suggested that clinicians can obtain some of the benefits of correlation- and cause-based approaches by first identifying risk factors and then interpreting those risk factors in the light of the patient's affect, beliefs, and intentions (Buchanan & Norko, 2011).

The methods of risk assessment in community settings and the risk factors for violence in those settings have been reviewed by Buchanan and Norko (2017). Whichever approach is adopted, assessments of risk in the community are often limited by a lack of information, not only about the patient's background and mental health history but also relating to environmental factors such as what a patient spends their days doing. Mitigating this problem by using multiple sources of information, ensuring good communication between members of a multidisciplinary team, and good record keeping is important, as is remembering that levels of risk fluctuate in individuals and focusing on the time interval until the patient is likely to be seen again. It is also important to acknowledge that there are times when risk cannot be managed while a patient remains in the community.

Tensions and controversies

Information sharing

Managing offenders with mental disorders, especially in community settings, requires the sharing of information. Information sharing between health and justice agencies can be fraught with ethical tensions. Patients have the right to confidential medical treatment, and clinicians must uphold both data protection laws and the duty of confidentiality to their patients. On the other hand, there are circumstances in which clinicians are required or permitted to disclose information, including when there is a risk of harm to the individual or someone else (including in cases relating to child protection, terrorism, fitness to drive, or certain infectious diseases), and when there is a legal requirement to disclose.

The police often request information from community mental health services concerning the mental state of people they have arrested. It is important that the needs of individuals with mental disorder be identified and managed as early as possible in the criminal justice system, including ensuring that essential treatment is made available. Data-sharing agreements are often lacking, however, and there is a need for caution when sharing medical information without consent whether or not the legal thresholds for doing so are clearly met. This includes the contentious issue of police requests for medical information used to inform charging decisions. Clinicians are often asked for both factual information as well as opinions on issues such as mental state at the time of the alleged offence, which may be beyond their expertise or role. Despite authoritative guidance that whether or not a defendant 'had capacity' at the time of an alleged offence should not be used to inform charging decisions because this term lacks legal precision (Crown Prosecution Service, 2019), police and prosecution in the UK continue to request medical opinions on this question. Treating clinicians should exercise particular caution when responding to requests likely to have an impact on the therapeutic relationship.

In the UK there is a duty on health services to cooperate with MAPPA. There are strict criteria in relation to who is 'MAPPA eligible' (National MAPPA Team & HM Prison and Probation Services Public Protection Group, 2021). The person needs to be actively serving a prison sentence longer than 12 months; on a section 37 or section 37/41; or on the sex offenders register for a specified violent, sexual or terrorism offence.[1] The purpose of MAPPA is for agencies to work collaboratively to assess and manage risk and, therefore, a key component of this is information sharing (National MAPPA Team & HM Prison and Probation Services Public Protection Group, 2021). Generally, this takes place within Multi-Agency Public Protection meetings.

The MAPPA Confidentiality and Equality Statement acknowledges professional duties of confidentiality but states that information is shared under an understanding that, 'it is felt that the risk presented by the offender is so great that issues of public or individual safety outweigh those rights of confidentiality' (National MAPPA Team & HM Prison and Probation Services Public Protection Group, 2016). This suggests that the threshold for sharing information described by the General Medical Council will usually be met: information is being disclosed as required or permitted by law[2] and in the public interest.[3] The General Medical Council also indicates 'you must' participate in procedures set up to protect the public from violent and sex offenders, such as MAPPA (General Medical Council, 2017, p. 36). However, there are guiding principles to be considered and the Royal College of Psychiatrists (2017) is clear: psychiatrists 'should be ready to defend a patient's rights in this context' (p. 9). Any information shared must be kept to a minimum and be absolutely relevant, necessary, and justified for the specific context in which it is shared, even where a clear information-sharing agreement is present.

Information sharing in the public interest is a highly complex area where the focus of the professional can be shifted away from patient care and protecting privacy. Importantly, it remains a case-by-case clinical decision whether information sharing is needed to prevent serious harm (Taylor & Yakeley, 2019). For UK practitioners, the General Medical Council (2017) states: 'If you are not sure how the law applies in a particular situation, you should consult a Caldicott or data guardian, a data protection officer, your defence body or professional association, or seek independent legal advice' (p. 11).

Community treatment under legal mandates

The last 30 years have seen the introduction of new ways of legally mandating psychiatric treatment for patients living in the community. One cause may be the reduction in psychiatric inpatient provision in many countries, a reduction which leaves policymakers and clinicians with fewer options when risk cannot be managed through voluntary treatment in the community. The language of legal mandates can be confusing. In the US, mandatory psychiatric treatment (but not medication) in the community was introduced as 'involuntary outpatient civil commitment' (Geller, 2006; King, 1995; Swartz & Swanson, 2002) but is now widely referred to as 'assisted outpatient treatment', arguably a euphemism. The legal mandate distinguishes assisted outpatient treatment from assertive community treatment, a widely used programme for treating mental illness in the US. Although most US states have involuntary outpatient

---

[1] These offences are specified in schedule 15 of the Criminal Justice Act 2003 (https://www.legislation.gov.uk/ukpga/2003/44/schedule/15). Rarely, cases can be brought outside these criteria as category 3 cases.

[2] From the GMC, 2017, p. 16: 'You should satisfy yourself that the disclosure is required by law and you should only disclose information that is relevant to the request. Wherever practicable, you should tell patients about such disclosures, unless that would undermine the purpose, for example by prejudicing the prevention, detection or prosecution of serious crime.'

[3] From the GMC, 2017, p. 33: 'there can be a public interest in disclosing information to protect individuals or society from risks of serious harm, such as from serious communicable diseases or serious crime'.

commitment laws, many make little use of them and only five states had more than 1000 people under outpatient commitment orders in 2010 (NRI, 2015).

The question of whether mandated community treatment improves clinical outcomes has been the subject of debate. Neither of two US randomized trials (Steadman et al., 2001; Swartz et al., 1999) showed a simple intent-to-treat difference between the outpatient commitment and control groups in terms of the number of admissions or hospital inpatient days. Analyses of subgroups, however, particularly those who were under a court order for longer periods, have suggested benefits to compulsion that warrant further investigation. Australian and UK studies examining broadly similar legislation to that in the US have failed to show the same benefits (Burns et al., 2013; Kisely et al., 2005). Comparing studies internationally is difficult. The services that patients receive in both the experimental and control groups inevitably vary. It is unlikely that the question of whether mandated community treatment improves clinical outcomes will be resolved without further, high-quality, randomized controlled trials. The issues were reviewed in detail by Buchanan et al. (2017).

Mentally disordered offenders and generic outpatient services

One consequence of the development of specialist services for mentally disordered offenders has been a perception that those services will be where most people with offending histories will receive their treatment (Wootton et al., 2017). The development of community mental health care across Europe coincided with the decline in the large psychiatric hospitals (Shorter, 2007). In the UK, a 'sectorized' or 'catchment area' model of services developed, based on multi-disciplinary community mental health teams (Burns, 2010). These sectorized services remain but are now often supplemented by 'functionally defined' teams in fields that include assertive outreach, crisis intervention and early intervention in psychosis, as well as community forensic services (Ozdural, 2006). Financial constraints have limited the introduction of specialized, functionally defined services and fostered something of a move back to community mental health teams, albeit sometimes with reduced funding. Crisis and early intervention services have usually been retained (Holloway & Davies, 2017). A perception that resources are short has probably contributed to the relative lack of movement of patients from forensic to generic community services.

Several characteristics of generic community mental health services limit their ability to manage risk. The proliferation of functionally defined teams inevitably increases the number of transitions between teams that a patient will make during their treatment. With the passage of time, for instance, their psychosis will move beyond the window for early intervention. Each transition requires a transfer of information and involves a loss of much of the personal knowledge gained by staff over the time they have treated the person. These difficulties are particularly relevant to the management of risk in patients who are ambivalent about treatment. Inquiries following individual homicides often mention a failure to understand the inner world of the patient (Petch & Bradley, 1997), a task made more difficult when care is transferred from one team to another.

Resource constraints can also contribute to inexperienced staff working without consistent supervision and a lack of communication between health and other agencies, two other factors that inquiries identify as contributory when risk management fails to prevent violence (Buchanan, 1999). Community mental health teams often identify tensions between their traditional clinical values and obligations to share information and participate in new clinical arrangements, such as assertive community treatment, that challenge previously accepted notions of a patient's right to refuse treatment or to be free from coercive interventions (Holloway & Davies, 2017).

Although consultation and joint working with forensic services have been seen as potentially mitigating some of these concerns, this is not always the case. The limits of their training can leave forensic psychiatrists unfamiliar with some of the realities, and resource limitations, of community mental health treatment. Risk assessment tools used by forensic psychiatrists in inpatient settings are often not applicable to non-institutionalized patients (Duggan, 1997). The research base is limited but to date has failed to demonstrate a benefit of adopting forensic models of working to community mental health care (Coid et al., 2007; Humber et al., 2011; Solomon & Draine, 1995). Since most forensic models place an emphasis on case management, this is consistent with earlier work showing no difference, in terms of violent outcomes, between intensive case management and standard services through a community mental health team (Walsh et al., 2001).

Integration and separate provision

As some of us have noted previously, no one has found a way of making a doctor or a service look after a patient whom they have deemed, disingenuously or otherwise, 'inappropriate' or 'in need of services which we are unable to provide'. In the UK at least, it may be that when long-standing anxieties of generic services about the appropriateness of some offender patients are combined with increasing resource constraints, the prospects for meaningful collaboration between forensic outpatient services and their generic colleagues are grim. What were once described as parallel service structures (Gunn, 1977), where patients with similar illnesses and similar clinical needs are provided with different services because of their history of contact with forensic inpatient services, may increasingly become the norm. The challenge then becomes one of ensuring that the same forces that led to the exclusion of many of these patients from services at previous points in their psychiatric careers do not lead to them receiving a more restrictive, and less recovery oriented, model of care (Simpson & Penney, 2011).

Conclusion

The first section of this chapter described the social and political context in which people with mental disorders and histories of offending receive mental health care in the UK and elsewhere. This context is critical also to whether the understandably cautious response of general psychiatric services to the prospect of offender patients becoming a greater part of their workload can be overcome. In many countries, resources are already stretched. Without adequate resources and the confidence that those resources will not be withdrawn over the short or medium term, it is difficult to see how any meaningful integration of forensic and generic services will take place.

A continued growth of predominantly parallel models of care would ultimately be to the disadvantage of patients of community forensic psychiatric services. Managing the range of clinical challenges over the long term requires a range of service elements, including emergency departments and acute admission wards, that community mental health teams make use of routinely but which are often less familiar to specialist staff. A lack of critical mass denies many forensic services the opportunity to develop their own specialist services, such as early intervention services, that are increasingly expected elsewhere. If mentally disordered offenders are consistently to receive the standards of community care expected elsewhere in psychiatry, it will require a sustained social and political commitment to overcoming these challenges.

REFERENCES

Beswick, J. & Gunn, M. (2017). The law in England and Wales on mental health treatment in the community. In: Buchanan, A. & Wootton L. (Eds.), *Care of the Mentally Disordered Offender in the Community* (2nd ed., pp. 61–76). Oxford: Oxford University Press.

Bluglass, R. (1990). The scope of forensic psychiatry. *Journal of Forensic Psychiatry*, **1**, 5–9.

Bonta, J., Blais, J., & Wilson, H. A. (2014). A theoretically informed meta-analysis of the risk for general and violent recidivism for mentally disordered offenders. *Aggression and Violent Behavior*, **19**, 278–287.

Bradford, J., de Amorim Levin, G., Ahmed, A., & Gulati, S. (2017). Sex offender treatment. In: Buchanan, A. & Wootton L. (Eds.), *Care of the Mentally Disordered Offender in the Community* (2nd ed., pp. 203–218). Oxford: Oxford University Press.

Bradley, K. (2009). *Lord Bradley's Review of People with Mental Health Problems or Learning Disabilities in the Criminal Justice System.* London: Department of Health.

Brown, P., Bakolis, I., Appiah-Kusi, E., Hallett, N., Hotopf, M., &Blackwood, N. (2022). Prevalence of mental disorders in defendants at criminal court. *BJPsych Open*, **8**, e92.

Buchanan, A. (1992). A two-year prospective study of treatment compliance in patients with schizophrenia. *Psychological Medicine*, **22**, 787–797.

Buchanan, A. (1998). Treatment compliance in schizophrenia. *Advances in Psychiatric Treatment*, **4**, 227–234.

Buchanan, A. (1999). Independent inquiries into homicide. *BMJ*, **318**, 1089–1090.

Buchanan, A., Kisely, S., Moseley, D., Rugkåsa, J., Swanson, J., & Swartz, M. (2017). Community psychiatric treatment under legal mandates: the international experience. In: Buchanan, A. & Wootton L. (Eds.), *Care of the Mentally Disordered Offender in the Community* (2nd ed., pp. 243–266). Oxford: Oxford University Press.

Buchanan, A. & Leese, M. (2001). Detention of people with dangerous severe personality disorders. *Lancet*, **358**, 1955–1959.

Buchanan, A. & Norko, M. (2011). Violence risk assessment. In: Buchanan, A. & Norko, M. (Eds.), *The Psychiatric Report* (pp. 224–239). Cambridge: Cambridge University Press.

Buchanan, A. & Norko, M. (2017). Violence risk in community settings. In: Buchanan, A. & Wootton L. (Eds.), *Care of the Mentally Disordered Offender in the Community* (2nd ed., pp. 219–239). Oxford: Oxford University Press.

Burns, T. (2010). The rise and fall of assertive community treatment? *International Review of Psychiatry*, **22**, 120–127.

Burns, T., Rugkåsa, J., Molodynksi, A., Dawson, J., Yeeles, K., Vazquez-Montes, M., et al. (2013). Community treatment orders for patients with psychosis: a randomised controlled trial (OCTET). *Lancet*, **381**, 1627–1633.

Centre for Mental Health (2011). *Pathways to Unlocking Secure Mental Health Care.* London: Centre for Mental Health.

Chang, Z., Lichtenstein, P., Långström, N., Larsson, H., & Fazel, S. (2016). Association between prescription of major psychotropic medications and violent reoffending after prison release. *Journal of the American Medical Association*, **316**, 1798–1807.

Coid, J. W., Hickey, N., & Yang, M. (2007). Comparison of outcomes following after-care from forensic and general adult psychiatric services. *British Journal of Psychiatry*, **190**, 509–514.

Craissati, J. (2004). *Managing high risk sex offenders in the community: A psychological approach.* Routledge.

Craissati, J. & Sindall, O. (2009). Serious further offences: an exploration of risk and typologies. *Probation Journal*, **56**, 9–27.

Crown Prosecution Service (2019). Mental health: suspects and defendants with mental health conditions or disorders. https://www.cps.gov.uk/legal-guidance/mental-health-suspects-and-defendants-mental-health-conditions-or-disorders

D'Amora, D., Tran, M., & Osher, F. (2017). Achieving positive outcomes for justice-involved people with behavioural health disorders. In: Buchanan, A. & Wootton L. (Eds.), *Care of the Mentally Disordered Offender in the Community* (2nd ed., pp. 77–96). Oxford: Oxford University Press.

Davidson, F., Heffernan, E., Greenberg, D., Butler, T., & Burgess, P. (2016). A critical review of Mental Health Court Liaison Services in Australia: a first national survey. *Psychiatry, Psychology and Law*, **23**, 908–921.

Duggan, C. (1997). Introduction. Assessing risk in the mentally disordered. *British Journal of Psychiatry*, **170**(Suppl. 32), 1–3.

Fazel, S., Gulati, G., Linsell, L., Geddes, J. R., & Grann, M. (2009). Schizophrenia and violence: systematic review and meta-analysis. *PLoS Medicine*, **6**, e1000120.

Fazel, S., Hayes, A., Bartellas, K., Clerici, M., & Tresteman, R. (2016). The mental health of prisoners: a review of prevalence, adverse outcomes and interventions. *Lancet Psychiatry*, **3**, 871–881.

Fazel, S., Zetterqvist, J., Larsson, H., Langstrom, N., & Lichtenstein, P. (2014). Antipsychotics, mood stabilisers, and risk of violent crime. *Lancet*, **384**, 1206–1214.

Gabbard, G. O. (1986). The special hospital patient. *International Review of Psychoanalysis*, **13**, 333–347.

Geller, J. L. (2006). The evolution of outpatient commitment in the USA: from conundrum to quagmire. *International Journal of Law and Psychiatry*, **29**, 234–248.

General Medical Council (2017). Confidentiality: good practice in handling patient information. https://www.gmc-uk.org/-/media/documents/gmc-guidance-for-doctors---confidentiality-good-practice-in-handling-patient-information----70080105.pdf

Gilligan, J. (1999). *Violence: Reflections on Our Deadliest Epidemic* (Forensic Focus 18). London: Jessica Kingsley Publishers.

Gunn, J. (1977). Management of the mentally abnormal offender: integrated or parallel. *Proceedings of the Royal Society of Medicine*, **70**, 877–880.

Harris, G., Rice, M., & Quinsey, V. (1993). Violent recidivism of mentally disordered offenders: the development of a statistical prediction instrument. *Criminal Justice and Behavior*, **20**, 315–335.

Her Majesty's Inspectorate of Probation (2021). *A Joint Thematic Inspection of the Criminal Justice Journey for Individuals with Mental Health Needs and Disorders.* Manchester: Her Majesty's Inspectorate of Probation.

Hoge, S. K., Buchanan, A. W., Kovasznay, B. M., & Roskes, E. J. (2009). Outpatient services for the mentally ill involved in the criminal justice system. *American Psychiatric Association Task Force Report:* Washington, DC, 1–15.

Holloway, F. & Davies, T. (2017). The community mental health team and the mentally disordered offender. In: Buchanan, A. & Wootton L. (Eds.), *Care of the Mentally Disordered Offender in the Community* (2nd ed., pp. 303–324). Oxford: Oxford University Press.

Humber, N., Hayes, A., Wright, S., & Fahy, T. (2011). A comparative study of forensic and community psychiatric patients with integrated and parallel models of care. *Journal of Forensic Psychiatry and Psychology*, **22**, 183–202.

Jann, M. W., Ereshefsky, L., & Saklad, S. R. (1985). Clinical pharmacokinetics of the depot antipsychotics. *Clinical Pharmacokinetics*, **10**, 315–333.

Jewell, T. C., Smith, A. M., Hoh, B., Ladd, S., Evinger, J., Lamberti, J. S., et al. (2012). Consumer centered family consultation: New York State's recent efforts to include families and consumers as partners in recovery. *American Journal of Psychiatric Rehabilitation*, **15**, 44–60.

Jones, P. B., Barnes, T. R., Davies, L., Dunn, G., Lloyd, H., Hayhurst, K. P., et al. (2006). Randomized controlled trial of the effect on quality of life of second- vs first-generation antipsychotic drugs in schizophrenia: Cost Utility of the Latest Antipsychotic Drugs in Schizophrenia Study (CUtLASS 1). *Archives of General Psychiatry*, **63**, 1079–1087.

Kane, J. M., Schooler, N. R., Marcy, P., Correll, C. U., Brunette, M. F., Mueser, K. T., et al. (2015). The RAISE early treatment program for first-episode psychosis: background, rationale, and study design. *Journal of Clinical Psychiatry*, **76**, 240–246.

Keers, R., Ullrich, S., Destavola, B. L., & Coid, J. W. (2014). Association of violence with emergence of persecutory delusions in untreated schizophrenia. *American Journal of Psychiatry*, **171**, 332–339.

King, E. F. (1995). Outpatient civil commitment in North Carolina: constitutional and policy concerns. *Law and Contemporary Problems*, **58**, 251–281.

Kisely, S., Smith, M., Preston, N. J., & Xiao, J. (2005). A comparison of health service use in two jurisdictions with and without compulsory community treatment. *Psychological Medicine*, **35**, 1357–1367.

Lennox, C., Senior, J., King, C., Hassan, L., Clayton, R., Thornicroft, G., & Shaw, J. (2012). The management of released prisoners with severe and enduring mental illness. *Journal of Forensic Psychiatry and Psychology*, **23**, 67–75.

Lichtenstein, P., Halldner, L., Zetterqvist, J., Sjolander, A., Serlachius, E., Fazel, S., et al. (2012). Medication for attention deficit-hyperactivity disorder and criminality. *New England Journal of Medicine*, **367**, 2006–2014.

Lieberman, J., Stroup, T., McEvoy, J., Swartz, M., Rosenheck, R., Perkins, D., et al. (2005). Effectiveness of antipsychotic drugs in patients with chronic schizophrenia. *New England Journal of Medicine*, **353**, 1209–1223.

Lockwood, G. (1992). Psychoanalysis and the cognitive therapy of personality disorders. *Journal of Cognitive Psychotherapy*, **6**, 25–42.

Luciano, A., Belstock, J., Malmberg, P., McHugo, G. J., Drake, R. E., Xie, H., et al. (2014). Predictors of incarceration among urban adults with co-occurring severe mental illness and a substance use disorder. *Psychiatric Services*, **65**, 1325–1331.

McKinnon, I., Srivastava, S., Kaler, G., & Grubin, D. (2013). Screening for psychiatric morbidity in police custody: results from the HELP-PC project. *The Psychiatrist*, **37**, 389–394.

Meloy, J. R. & Yakely, J. (2010). Psychodynamic treatment of antisocial personality disorder. In: Clarkin, J., Fonagy, P., & Gabbard, G. (Eds.), *Psychodynamic Treatment of Personality Disorders: A Clinical Handbook* (pp. 311–336). Arlington, VA: American Psychiatric Publishing Inc.

Ministry of Justice (2014). *Offender Rehabilitation Act 2014*. London: Ministry of Justice.

Ministry of Justice (2021). *Multi-Agency Public Protection Arrangements (MAPPA) Annual Report: 2020 to 2021*. London: Ministry of Justice.

Molyneaux, E., San Juan, N., Brown, P., Lloyd-Evans, B., & Oram, S. (2021). A pilot programme to facilitate the use of mental health treatment requirements: professional stakeholders' experiences. *British Journal of Social Work*, **51**, 1041–1059.

Monahan, J. (1988). Risk assessment of violence among the mentally disordered: generating useful knowledge. *International Journal of Law and Psychiatry*, **11**, 249–257.

Mullen, P. (2002). Introduction. In: Buchanan, A. & Wootton L. (Eds.), *Care of the Mentally Disordered Offender in the Community* (2nd ed., pp. xiii–xix). Oxford: Oxford University Press.

Mullen, P. & Ogloff, J. (2009). Assessing and managing the risk of violence towards others. In: Gelder, M. G., Andreasen, N. C., López-Ibor, J. J., & Geddes, J. R. (Eds.), *New Oxford Textbook of Psychiatry* (2nd ed., **Vol. 2**, pp. 1991–2002). Oxford: Oxford University Press.

National Health Service England (2016). *Implementing the Five Year Forward View for Mental Health*. Redditch: NHS England.

National MAPPA Team & HM Prison and Probation Services Public Protection Group (2021). MAPPA guidance. Gov.UK. https://www.gov.uk/government/publications/multi-agency-public-protection-arrangements-mappa-guidance

National MAPPA Team & HM Prison and Probation Services Public Protection Group (2016). MAPPA guidance: appendices and forms. Gov.UK. https://www.gov.uk/government/publications/multi-agency-public-protection-arrangements-mappa-guidance

National Offender Management Service Commissioning Group (2014). Supporting community order treatment requirements. https://assets.publishing.service.gov.uk/government/uploads/system/uploads/attachment_data/file/426676/Supporting_CO_Treatment_Reqs.pdf

NHS Commissioning Board (2013). Liaison and diversion operating model 2013/14. NHS England. https://www.england.nhs.uk/wp-content/uploads/2014/04/ld-op-mod-1314.pdf

Norton, K. R. W. & McGauley, G. (1998). *Counselling Difficult Clients*. London: Sage.

NRI (2015). State mental health agency data search. http://www.nri-incdata.org/

Ohio Ex-Offender Reentry Coalition (2010). *2010 Annual Report*. Columbus, OH: Ohio Ex-Offender Reentry Coalition.

Ozdural, S. (2006). The role of a community forensic mental health team. *Psychiatric Bulletin*, **30**, 36.

Payne-James, J. J., Wall I. J., & Bailey, C. (2005). Patterns of illicit drug use of prisoners in police custody in London, UK. *Journal of Clinical Forensic Medicine*, **12**, 196–198.

Penny, C. & Craissati, J. (2012). Decisions on disclosure to third parties made at MAPP meetings: opinions and practice. *The Psychiatrist*, **36**, 379–385.

Petch, E. & Bradley, C. (1997). Learning the lessons from homicide inquiries: adding insult to injury? *Journal of Forensic Psychiatry*, **8**, 161–184.

Ritchie, J. H., Dick, D., & Lingham, R. (1994). *The Report of the Inquiry into the Care and Treatment of Christopher Clunis*. London: HMSO.

Rose, N. (2017). Society, madness and control. In: Buchanan, A. & Wootton L. (Eds.), *Care of the Mentally Disordered Offender in the Community* (2nd ed., pp. 3–27). Oxford: Oxford University Press.

Rotter, M., Barber-Rioja, V., & Schombs, F. (2017). Recovery and recidivism reduction for offenders with mental illness. In: Buchanan, A. & Wootton L. (Eds.), *Care of the Mentally Disordered Offender in the Community* (2nd ed., pp. 117–128). Oxford: Oxford University Press.

Royal College of Psychiatrists (2017). Good psychiatric practice: confidentiality and information sharing (3rd ed.) (College Report CR209). https://www.rcpsych.ac.uk/docs/default-source/improving-care/better-mh-policy/college-reports/college-report-cr209.pdf?sfvrsn=23858153_2

Rutherford, M. & Duggan, S. (2008). Forensic mental health services: facts and figures on current provision. *British Journal of Forensic Practice*, **10**, 4–10.

Sariaslan, A., Leucht, S., Zetterqvist, J., Lichtenstein, P., & Fazel, S. (2021). Associations between individual antipsychotics and the risk of arrests and convictions of violent and other crime: a nationwide within-individual study of 74 925 persons. *Psychological Medicine*, **52**, 1–9.

Senior, J., Hayes, A., & Shaw, J. (2017). UK health policy in relation to mentally disordered offenders in the community. In: Buchanan, A. & Wootton L. (Eds.), *Care of the Mentally Disordered Offender in the Community* (2nd ed., pp. 29–46). Oxford: Oxford University Press.

Shorter, E. (2007). The historical development of mental health services in Europe. In: Knapp, M., McDaid, D., Mossialos, E., & Thornicroft, G. (Eds.), *Mental Health Policy and Practice across Europe* (pp. 15–33). Maidenhead: Open University Press.

Simpson, A. & Penney, S. (2011). The recovery paradigm in forensic mental health services. *Criminal Behaviour and Mental Health*, **21**, 299–306.

Singh, J., Fazel, S., Gueorguieva, R., & Buchanan, A. (2014). Rates of violence in patients classified as high risk by structured risk assessment instruments. *British Journal of Psychiatry*, **204**, 180–187.

Singleton, N., Meltzer, H., Gatward, R., Coid, J., & Deasy, D. (1998). *Survey of Psychiatric Morbidity among Prisoners in England and Wales*. London: Office for National Statistics.

Skeem, J. L., Manchak, S., Vidal, S., & Hart, E. (2009, March). *Probationers with Mental Disorder: What (Really) Works?* Paper presented at the American Psychology and Law Society (AP-LS) Annual Conference, San Antonio, TX.

Skeem, J. L., Winter, E., Kennealy, P. J., Eno Louden, J., & Tatar, J. R., II. (2014). Offenders with mental illness have criminogenic needs, too: toward recidivism reduction. *Law and Human Behavior*, **38**, 212–224.

Snowden, P. (1997). Practical aspects of clinical risk assessment and management. *British Journal of Psychiatry*, **170**(Suppl. 32), 32–34.

Solomon, P. & Draine, J. (1995). One-year outcomes of a randomised trial of case management with seriously mentally ill clients leaving jail. *Evaluation Review*, **19**, 256–273.

Steadman, H. J., Gounis, K., Dennis, D., Hopper, K., Roche, B., Swartz, M., & Robbins, P. C. (2001). Assessing the New York City involuntary outpatient commitment pilot program. *Psychiatric Services*, **52**, 330–336.

Swanson, J. W., Swartz, M. S., Van Dorn, R. A., Volavka, J., Monahan, J., Stroup, T. S., et al. (2008). Comparison of antipsychotic medication effects on reducing violence in people with schizophrenia. *British Journal of Psychiatry*, **193**, 37–43.

Swartz, M. S. & Swanson, J. W. (2002). Involuntary outpatient commitment in the United States: practice and controversy. In: Buchanan, A. (Ed.), *Care for the Mentally Disordered Offender in the Community* (pp. 199–221). Oxford: Oxford University Press.

Swartz, M. S., Swanson, J. W., Wagner, H. R., Burns, B. J., Hiday, V. A., & Borum, R. (1999). Can involuntary outpatient commitment reduce hospital recidivism?: findings from a randomized trial with severely mentally ill individuals. *American Journal of Psychiatry*, **156**, 1968–1975.

Szmukler, G. (2000). Homicide inquiries: what sense do they make? *Psychiatric Bulletin*, **24**, 6–10.

Taylor, R. & Yakeley, J. (2019). Working with MAPPA: ethics and pragmatics. *BJPsych Advances*, **25**, 157–165.

Thibaut, F., De La Barra, F., Gordon, H., Cosyns, P., & Bradford, J. M. (2010). The World Federation of Societies of Biological Psychiatry (WFSBP) Guidelines for the Biological Treatment of Paraphilias. *World Journal of Biological Psychiatry*, **11**, 604–655.

Tracy, D. & Gaughran, F. (2017). Treatment with medication. In: Buchanan, A. & Wootton L. (Eds.), *Care of the Mentally Disordered Offender in the Community* (2nd ed., pp. 149–177). Oxford: Oxford University Press.

Van Velsen, C. & Norton, K. (2017). Outpatient psychotherapeutic approaches with mentally disordered offenders. In: Buchanan, A. & Wootton L. (Eds.), *Care of the Mentally Disordered Offender in the Community* (2nd ed., pp. 179–202). Oxford: Oxford University Press.

Walsh, E., Gilvarry, C., Samele, C., Harvey, K., Manley, C., Tyrer, P., et al. (2001). Reducing violence in severe mental illness: randomised controlled trial of intensive case management compared with standard care. *BMJ*, **323**, 1093–1096.

Webster, C., Douglas, K., Eaves, D., & Hart, S. D. (1997). *HCR-20: Assessing Risk for Violence (Version 2)*. Vancouver: Simon Fraser University, Mental Health, Law, and Policy Institute.

Wilson, S., James, D., & Forrester, A. (2011). The medium-secure project and criminal justice mental health. *Lancet*, **378**, 110–111.

Wilson, J. A. & Wood, P. B. (2014). Dissecting the relationship between mental illness and return to incarceration. *Journal of Criminal Justice*, **42**, 527–537.

Wootton, L., Fahy, T., Wilson, S., & Buchanan, A. (2017). The interface of general psychiatric and forensic psychiatric services. In: Buchanan, A. & Wootton L. (Eds.), *Care of the Mentally Disordered Offender in the Community* (2nd ed., pp. 325–342). Oxford: Oxford University Press.

Yakeley, J., Taylor, R., & Cameron, A. (2012). MAPPA and mental health-10 years of controversy. *The Psychiatrist*, **36**, 201–204.

Young, S., Goodwin, E. J., Sedgwick, O., & Gudjonsson, G. H. (2013). The effectiveness of police custody assessments in identifying suspects with intellectual disabilities and attention deficit hyperactivity disorder. *BMC Medicine*, **11**, 1–11.

SECTION 5
Ethical and legal aspects

27. **Ethical framework for community mental health** 283
    Abraham Rudnick, Cheryl Forchuk, and George Szmukler

28. **International human rights and community mental health** 291
    Oliver Lewis and Peter Bartlett

29. **Treatment pressures, coercion, and compulsion** 301
    George Szmukler and Paul S. Appelbaum

27

Ethical framework for community mental health

Abraham Rudnick, Cheryl Forchuk, and George Szmukler

Introduction

Community mental health services have been developing in the last few decades. In the process a number of ethical issues have arisen. Some of these deserve attention as they are relatively distinct from ethical issues related to hospital mental health services. Application of established ethical approaches in the context of community mental health services has required revision of these approaches or alternatives to them. The aim of this chapter is to revisit key ethics concepts, to discuss ethical issues in community mental health services, and to provide an updated basis for an ethical framework for community mental health.

We will present definitions and central theories in ethics, an overview of bioethics, and ethical issues related to community mental health services, addressing generic as well as distinctive problems. We will consider conservative and radical approaches (the latter partly based on community psychology research and practice). We also discuss challenges arising from an ethics of community mental health services (such as the view that social justice as in 'social inclusion' goes beyond fair resource allocation), as well as emerging opportunities and threats (such as digital technology).

Definitions and central theories in ethics

Ethics addresses moral problems, sometimes termed ethical problems or dilemmas. In health care, ethical problems are commonly viewed as the tension between two or more morally defensible alternative actions, including inaction (Beauchamp & Childress, 2009). Ethical theories suggest various ways of addressing and resolving such ethical problems. The most veteran and well-established ethical theories are 'utilitarianism' (or more generally 'consequentialism'), which considers outcomes; 'deontology', which considers duties; and 'virtue ethics', which considers intentions. More novel ethical theories include 'rights-based theory' and 'care ethics' (Rudnick, 2001), among others.

Consequentialism and deontology are arguably the broadest in scope and the most influential ethical theories in contemporary health care and probably in contemporary life in general—at least in the Western world. For example, the notion of human rights, a mainstay of contemporary attitudes to life in the Western world, can be argued to derive from deontology, since duties to others entail rights of those others and vice versa, and as the notion of duties precedes the notion of rights, at least historically. Both consequentialism and deontology are also considered self-sufficient (unlike most other ethical theories such as virtue ethics). And both may have particular relevance to community mental health, especially in relation to consideration of populations as well as individuals.

Consequentialism is based on the argument that consequences or outcomes of actions (and of inactions) determine whether an action (or an inaction) with ethical implications is moral or immoral. In its simplest form, that of hedonistic-like utilitarianism, consequentialism considers pleasure or happiness and pain or suffering as the outcomes of importance, and determines the morality or immorality of an action (or inaction) based on whether it produces more pleasure or happiness than pain or suffering, either of an individual or counted over a number of individuals if more than one individual is affected by the action (or inaction). Two general types of utilitarianism have been described: act utilitarianism, which maintains that the morality of each action is to be determined in relation to the favourable or unfavourable consequences that emerge from that action, and rule utilitarianism, which maintains that a behavioural code or rule is morally right if the consequences of adopting that rule are more favourable than unfavourable to everyone (Dershowitz, 2004, p. 242). Arguably, rule utilitarianism is conceptually more similar to deontology than act utilitarianism is.

Deontology is based on the argument that moral duties or obligations determine whether an action (or an inaction) is moral or immoral. Deontology was first developed systematically by Kant in the eighteenth century (MacIntyre, 1998), and since then it has been further developed and diversified. In its simplest form, deontology considers universal obligations as the duties of importance, and determines the morality or immorality of an action (or inaction) based on whether it upholds a universal obligation; famously, Kant argued that there is a universal obligation to tell the truth, even if that means disclosing the location of a potential victim to a person known to plan that victim's murder. More generally, Kant formulated the 'categorical imperative', which is an impartiality—applicable to all people—condition, stating that an action (or inaction) is ethically acceptable if it holds for any person who could hypothetically be involved in the particular circumstances, including the person(s) conducting the action (or inaction) if he were to be at the receiving end of the action (or inaction). A neo-Kantian version of this requirement, developed by John Rawls, is that ethical decision-making should be conducted behind a 'veil of ignorance' (which can be formulated as not knowing whether the person will be the instigator or recipient of the action), which strips the ethical decision-maker of any personal considerations that may disrupt impartiality. A variant of Kant's formulation is that persons should be considered ends in themselves, rather than merely the means for other ends. The question who constitutes a 'person' is still open for discussion, and is particularly relevant in bioethics, for example, in relation to obligations towards malformed human fetuses and embryos, as mentioned below (Kant claimed that only rational beings are full-fledged persons, hence he declined full-fledged personhood to animals and to human children). Also subject to such considerations are human adults who lack decision-making capacity, for example, due to disruptive psychosis (Kant declined full-fledged personhood to such psychotic human adults too).

Overview of bioethics

Health care ethics, or bioethics (as it has been termed in recent decades), has a history of thousands of years, both in the Western world and elsewhere (Jonsen, 2000). Most well known in relation to ancient health care ethics is the Hippocratic oath. Although partly dated, for example, in its consideration of physician duties to slaves, it still retains universally applicable components—for example, its requirements to do no (intentional) harm and to maintain confidentiality (Lloyd, 1983). Admittedly, these Hippocratic requirements are not considered absolute now; sometimes harm may be necessary for benefit (e.g. in relation to chemotherapy for cancer) and sometimes confidentiality may have to be breached (e.g. in order to protect third parties who are at risk due to a patient's illness). However, they are still central considerations in health care ethics. Importantly, self-determination or autonomy, specifically patients' choice in relation to their health care, is not addressed in the Hippocratic oath; it is only since the advent of bioethics, a few decades ago, that it has been widely considered a key component of health care ethics, particularly in the Western world (Jonsen, 1998).

Contemporary bioethics includes various, sometimes conflicting, approaches. The most well known is 'principlism'. Four main moral principles that drive moral action are identified. These may come into conflict with each other (or conflict can occur within one principle), with such conflict resulting in a bioethical problem. These principles are (1) respect for autonomy or self-determination (sometimes termed respect for persons or their choices), (2) beneficence (i.e. benefiting the person(s) directly involved), (3) non-maleficence (i.e. doing no/least harm, which is sometimes combined with beneficence as a balance of most benefit and least harm), and (4) justice (fairness, particularly to third parties or others involved or affected, as in resource allocation) (Beauchamp & Childress, 2009). These principles are considered to ground key tenets of bioethics, such as confidentiality of personal health information. An example of an alternative approach to 'principlism' is 'care ethics', largely based on virtue ethics and casuistry (context-specific considerations) (Rudnick, 2001). Another example is 'dialogical bioethics', in which predetermined principles are replaced with reasoned communication (but which appears to require the principle of justice as fairness) (Rudnick, 2002, 2007). Note that contemporary bioethics addresses areas of health care beyond clinical practice, such as health-related research, administration and policy, as well as speculative health care such as cryogenic medicine (Rudnick, 2011).

Some of the major subjects for bioethics to date have included end-of-life situations, beginning-of-life situations, and risk/benefit-to-others situations. In these, a bioethical problem is evident, requiring reasoned resolution in order to decide on an acceptable health-related action (or inaction). End-of-life situations address euthanasia (mercy killing), physician-assisted death, withholding or withdrawing life support, and other potential and actual health care procedures that either shorten or do not prolong the life of a person who is terminally ill, irreversibly unconscious, or incurably suffering. Beginning-of-life situations address abortion, artificial insemination, and other potential and actual health care procedures that curtail or alternatively enable the continuation of life of a human fetus, embryo, or newborn.

Risk/benefit-to-others situations address the impact of health, ill health, and health care-related procedures involving one or more individuals on other people. A paradigmatic example of a benefit-to-others situation is that of health-related human research, where persons are invited to participate in health-related research which is not necessarily expected to benefit (and may indeed harm) them, but which is expected to benefit others such as future patients. The need to protect human research participants and to obtain and respect their voluntary informed consent (or refusal) to participate in research was highlighted by the exposure of the Nazi medical experiments in the Doctors' Trial at the Nuremberg Tribunal in 1947, and the resulting ten principles of human research known as the Nuremberg Code (Jonsen, 2000, pp. 100–102). A paradigmatic psychiatric example of a risk-to-others situation is that of the Tarasoff decisions, whereupon it was determined in the California court system in the mid-1970s that health care providers are obliged to warn and to protect third parties in relation to identified physical risk posed to these third parties by mentally ill individuals, where the risk is caused by their mental illness (L. W. Roberts & Dyer, 2004, p. 104). Such obligations may breach confidentiality of mentally ill individuals, which we discuss below.

The context of community mental health care and related ethical challenges

Community mental health care involves a change in locus of care (from hospital to community), funding arrangements, and treatment techniques. It establishes a network of services offering crisis intervention, continuing care, accommodation, occupation, and social support which together help people with mental health problems to retain or recover valued social roles (or to promote 'social inclusion'). Usually the focus of services has been on those with severe mental illness. To understand the context of community psychiatry it is important to consider both psychiatric care of *individuals* in the community and psychiatric care in relation to *community*. If the goal of treatment is 'social inclusion' then both aspects require careful consideration.

Mental health care of individuals in the community

To ensure that patients in the community receive the benefits of the range of services that they may require, widespread practice of 'case management' or its variants has been adopted. The aims are to ensure continuity of care, accessibility to often fragmented and independently managed services, accountability, and efficiency. A more intensive model of case management is commonly adopted for people with persistent symptoms who are difficult to engage in treatment—assertive community treatment. Assertive community treatment aims to prevent the service user from dropping out of treatment and brings treatment *to* the patient. If the patient defaults from treatment, the community team may actively seek out the patient to re-establish contact.

Patients with severe mental illness have a diverse range of needs that can often only be met by an array of services and agencies. Access to these may require a substantial flow of relevant personal information between care providers concerning the service user. The nature of the therapeutic relationships between staff and service user also changes in community-based treatment. The key worker or other members of the interdisciplinary team provide a broad range of interventions. As well as medication and standard psychological treatments, they may work with the patient in their ordinary community settings, including the home, to rehabilitate basic living skills. This special, personal relationship may be used to encourage the service user to adhere to treatment.

The role of the community itself is crucial to 'community care'. Public fears that care in the community for persons with mental illness are prone to failure are common. Responses to these fears by government, public agencies, and community members may greatly affect practice. 'Risk thinking' leads to attempts at its management, control, or surveillance through classifications of risky persons, registers, databases, regulatory mechanisms, and so on. Risk may become a professional responsibility with new forms of regulation and governance of professional judgement and actions (Rose, 1998). Thus clinical practice in some areas has moved in the direction of greater social control at the expense of autonomy (Holloway, 1996). At the same time, in many places, there has been a move towards more person-centred and recovery-oriented care that encourages the development and use of autonomy, such as in supported (rather than sheltered) programmes (G. Roberts et al., 2006).

Key dilemmas in clinical practice in the community

These can be grouped under four headings: privacy, confidentiality, coercion, and conflicts of duty.

Privacy

Assertive treatment programmes bring treatment to service users, often in their residence whether it be home, hostel, or boarding house. Visits, some uninvited, may be made by mental health professionals. Indeed, visits may continue even when the patient's explicit desire is that they cease.

Since much treatment occurs in the community, there is also an increased likelihood that it becomes visible to the public. The curiosity of neighbours may be aroused, particularly with repeated visits, and especially if attempts to gain entry are rebuffed by the patient. Neighbours may deduce that the person being visited is a service user.

Furthermore, as treatment becomes more visible to the public, new expectations may be generated that a community mental health team can be called to deal with a difficult person suspected to be a patient. Even if a public assessment is not carried out, an acknowledgement by the team that they may have a role may reveal to bystanders that the person is a psychiatric patient (if already so) or label them as one (if not).

If the patient assessed as representing a risk defaults from treatment, the team may be expected to make every effort to re-establish contact. The team may inform the police if the person could pose a significant risk of serious harm to self or others. The nature of the relationship between clinician and service user may shift from care to supervision. In some cases, assertive treatment, instead of ensuring that service users receive the care they need, may lead them to being labelled as 'dangerous' leading to exclusion from community services or amenities, including housing.

Confidentiality

In medicine, it is generally understood that information obtained from a patient will not be disclosed to others without the patient's consent. In community mental health services, where the patient is commonly treated by an interdisciplinary team, sharing of information is common. Service users may not know that this is to be expected. More complex is the sharing of information between agencies—health, social, voluntary, housing, and so on. Very needy patients' access to benefits and other goods may depend on information about them being revealed to those in a position to supply them. Since information may flow regularly, confidentiality may receive less emphasis. There may develop an attitude that 'the patient has less to lose by certain breaches of confidentiality than other kinds of patients do' (Diamond & Wikler, 1985).

Confidentiality may be breached ostensibly in the interests of the patient as above, or for the protection of others. The latter is considered below, including the interests of family and carers.

Treatment pressures and 'coercion'

A range of pressures may be exerted by community mental health teams to gain the patient's cooperation with treatment. These can be placed in a rough hierarchy—persuasion, interpersonal leverage, inducements (or offers), threats ('coercion' proper), and compulsion. These 'treatment pressures', so critical in the practice of psychiatry, are described in detail by Szmukler and Appelbaum (2008) and in Chapter 29 and will not be further discussed here.

Conflict of duty to patient versus others

Risk of harm to others

As previously discussed, the negative climate in which community mental health services may operate often provokes the question of the degree to which a mental health professional has a duty to protect others. If a specific risk of serious harm to an identified person is assessed, the clinician's duty to protect that person is usually reasonably clear. When the risk to others is general, judgements are more problematic.

Expectations of the public about what mental health services should do to control disturbed behaviour may change with a growing emphasis on community care. For example, the mental health team may be asked to intervene by neighbours or shopkeepers, when they are disturbed by a service user's behaviour. A further aspect may be the possibility that if the team does not act, prejudice against the service user will increase and their community tenure may be threatened. The balance between the duty of care to the patient and to the local community may be difficult to strike.

Mental health professionals are expected to be competent in assessing risk to others as well as to patients themselves. This often requires information from a range of informants, particularly concerning previous incidents of violence and risk factors such as substance abuse. On occasion, the mere seeking of information concerning the service user's past behaviour may reveal that the person is being treated by a mental health team. It may even raise unwarranted anxieties in their minds. The predictive accuracy of risk assessments, especially for serious harms—suicide or serious violence—is poor. Because such events are rare, false-positive predictions hugely outnumber true positives, even with the best risk assessment instruments. Important ethical issues thus arise (Szmukler & Rose, 2013).

Informal carers

Informal carers, usually family, are often central to effective community care. However, the extent to which carers' own needs should be met is often quite uncertain. Where there is a danger of serious physical harm to the carer, the clinician's responsibility is usually straightforward. Far more common are less grave threats to a carer's well-being which nevertheless have serious effects on well-being. Carers may experience difficulty in coping with burdensome behaviours, lack critical knowledge about their relative's illness, and may not know to whom to turn for support, or what support they might expect or be entitled to. The patient may prohibit any contact with the family. It may be unclear then to what extent the mental health team owes a duty of care to the family (Szmukler & Bloch, 1998).

Approaches to addressing the ethical challenges

Acting in the health interests of the service user

Szmukler and Appelbaum (2008) and elsewhere in this volume (see Chapter 29) discuss two approaches to ethical decision-making based on forms of 'paternalism'. These are a 'capacity/best interests' framework and a 'paternalism' framework. It is argued there that these frameworks can be applied to the full range of ethical dilemmas described above. Note that paternalism may not be fully independent from some principlist considerations, particularly from the consideration of beneficence. The reader is referred to the above-mentioned references for a fuller discussion of these approaches. An alternative approach is that of 'dialogical bioethics', where even non-capacitous service users are engaged in dialogue in order to enhance their participation in ethical decision-making as much as possible and to obtain their input and enrich it (as well as others'), including obtaining their assent (incapable agreement) or dissent (incapable disagreement), as the case may be. Even in situations where grave risk is expected for the person or for others, this approach may be sufficient, considering it involves dialogue and input from all stakeholders involved (although it may not be fully independent from some principlist considerations, particularly from the consideration of justice). For a fuller discussion of this approach, the reader is referred to previous publications by Rudnick (2002, 2007). This approach is arguably a key element of the recently developed 'open dialogue' approach to reducing coercion in mental health care (Olson et al., 2014), and is in keeping with the emphasis on 'supported decision-making' in the United Nations Convention on the Rights of Persons with Disabilities 2006 (see Chapter 28).

Preventing harm to others

Szmukler and Appelbaum (see Chapter 29) discuss the difficulties in deciding when to intervene in a 'coercive' manner for the protection of others. They argue that there is an important conceptual distinction between interventions serving the health interests of service users versus those for the protection of others. The latter may result—through the agency of mental health legislation—in 'preventive detention' or preventive coercive measures that discriminate against people with mental disorders since people not suffering from a mental disorder but who are equally risky cannot be dealt with in such a manner unless they have first committed an offence. Clinical ethical dilemmas in this area are important (see Chapter 29 for further discussion of this matter).

Psychiatric care in relation to community: the context

Individual patient goals of social inclusion and community integration imply the need for a receptive community. Considerations include issues of stigma and discrimination, organization of mental health services, and access to social determinants of health. These issues speak to justice, among other moral and ethical considerations.

Oppression, stigma, and discrimination are major issues that impede community integration of individuals with mental illness and perpetuate health disparities (Thornicroft, 2006). People with mental illnesses have been identified to be the most devalued of all people with disabilities (Lyons & Ziviani, 1995). They face negative attitudes and discriminating behaviours, frequently from family members, co-workers, the communities they live in (Schulze & Angermeyer, 2003), and even health care providers (Drake et al., 1999; Geller, 2001). Negative perceptions include beliefs that sufferers are incompetent, unpredictable, violent, hard to talk with, less intelligent, less trustworthy, and less likely to have valuable things to say (Crisp et al., 2000; Overton & Medina, 2008). Fear of this experience is sufficient to prevent some people from seeking help, and is a factor in premature treatment discontinuation (Sirey et al., 2001). Discrimination and stigma play a role in access to social determinants of health such as access to housing (Forchuk et al., 2006a, 2006b), employment (Baldwin & Marcus, 2006; Shied, 2005), and friends (Alexander & Link, 2003).

Other community factors also affect the potential for community integration. Availability and organization of mental health services is important. For example, people in rural areas may relocate to unfamiliar and undesired urban areas solely for accessing mental health services and at times with entire families (Forchuk et al., 2011). Unavailability of public transportation can also impede access to services (Forchuk et al., 2006a, 2011). These are but a few examples of community level issues that affect the individual.

Discrimination and stigma also play a role in relation to public policy and the priority given (or not given) to people diagnosed with a mental illness. Public policy can have a dramatic effect on the potential for social inclusion. Forchuk et al. (2007) described and analysed how the lack of connection between policy changes within the mental health field, housing, and income support created a situation which dramatically increased the number of people with mental illnesses who have become homeless. In contrast, using a strategy to explicitly reconnect and partner mental health services with providers of housing and of income support dramatically reduced the number of people discharged from psychiatric wards to homelessness (Forchuk et al., 2008).

When problems with social inclusion occur, one cannot assume that the problem lies with the individual patient. A conclusion that the underlying problem is either with the patient or the community will lead to very different responses and proposed interventions. Thus, community level issues have significant ethical implications.

Key dilemmas in community level psychiatry

A myriad of potential ethical issues exist at the community level. Some key dilemmas include (1) beneficence—doing good for whom?; (2) social justice and basic human rights; (3) the obligation to advocate or to 'whistle-blow'; and (4) understanding ethics within legal frameworks.

1. Beneficence–doing good for whom?

When working with individual patients, it is usually clear who the identified 'patient' is. However, with a community focus this may be unclear. With multiple vulnerable subgroups, prioritizing the needs of one may disadvantage another. For example, the common focus given to people with serious and persistent mental illnesses can mean that people with moderate mental health problems are unable to get services unless they deteriorate sufficiently to 'qualify'. In Ontario, Canada, a priority group for public housing has been people fleeing domestic violence. This group is almost always female and does often include people with mental illness. This seems to be a good policy and practice. However, with the current shortage of public housing, this has made it extremely difficult in many communities for others (such as men with mental illness, or intact families) to get public housing. As well, the policy is specific to intimate partners so even violence from a different family does not result in the same priority rating.

2. Social justice and basic human rights

Concerns about 'doing good for whom?' relate to resource allocation within a system with insufficient resources for all. This leads to issues concerning social justice and human rights. Social justice is based on the ideal of fair distribution (Morris, 2002). Essential questions to be addressed include 'Which inequalities matter most?' (Powers & Faden, 2006) and 'Is our society just?' (Davison et al., 2006). When people with mental illness are without adequate food and shelter, their basic human rights are arguably not being addressed (Forchuk et al., 2006b). Health care providers can contribute to this denial of basic human rights by ignoring the societal context of services. For example, discharging people from psychiatric wards to no fixed address has resulted in people, with no previous history of homelessness, being still homeless 6 months later or joining the sex trade to avoid homelessness (Forchuk et al., 2008).

3. The obligation to advocate or to whistle-blow

If health care professionals witness the denial of basic human rights or abuses, do obligations follow? In some cases, this will be a part of professional codes of ethics or standards. Some workplaces put restrictions on employees regarding taking information from the workplace to a public forum. To counter this, some jurisdictions have legislation protecting 'whistle blowers' who bring to light serious problems involving their workplace. Solutions in these situations often involve developing alliances with other groups and individuals to carry forward concerns to the political and public arenas. However, large community issues facing community psychiatric patients, such as homelessness, poverty, and lack of services, will take great efforts and time to overcome.

4. Understanding ethics within legal frameworks

Legal frameworks as well as ethical frameworks require consideration. Legal frameworks underpinning mental health acts, hospital acts, community treatment orders, health professional practices, and privacy can vary considerably, yet they form part of the context of community care. There can be tensions between legal and ethical frameworks which should be identified and addressed as best possible, including implementing legislative changes when possible and appropriate. Many people with mental illness are now entangled with the criminal justice system in myriad ways and are in the community under various conditions of parole, probation, conditional discharge, and so on. The legal system often requests various kinds of reports. Hence coercion, confidentiality and other ethical issues arise. The demands of the legal system should be weighed in relation to the patient's interests. When there is conflict between such demands and such interests, judicial demands may have to take precedence in the short term, but if deliberation reveals that these judicial demands are ethically unsound, advocacy for legislative and other legal change as well as for related cultural change may be required.

An example of the relation between ethics and law relates to sex offenders, who in many places are now discharged from prison and remanded to mental health care. Mental health care providers may feel unable to provide care for these patients, may fear for the safety of community members, and may be intimidated by the frequent media accounts of the horrific offences sometimes perpetrated by such patients, while recognizing their fiduciary duty to these patients. To address this set of challenges, mental health care providers and their administrators can champion wide stakeholder collaboration, such as with the police, to try to ensure public safety while keeping confidentiality breaches to the necessary minimum, and with health policy decision-makers and regulators, to try to secure and use adequate specialized resources to provide best care for these patients within legal constraints.

Digital technology

In the last decade or two, digital technology has often been used as part of mental health services. For example, electronic health records, telepsychiatry, internet-based psychotherapy, self-help mental wellness apps, and more have been introduced. Some of this has been accelerated by the Covid-19 pandemic, such as remotely delivered mental health care (Daigle & Rudnick, 2020). Such digital technology poses both opportunities and threats with prominent ethical aspects. For example, access to internet-based mental health services may be considered a human right (Reglitz & Rudnick, 2020), and as such its unavailability in some areas of the world (such as some parts of many low-income countries as well as some rural or remote parts of high-income countries) can be considered unethical. Similarly, people who are living in poverty or unhoused frequently do not have access to internet-based solutions. Solutions to remedy these situations may involve private sector industry, such as telecommunication and other corporations, which may raise further ethical questions (e.g. in relation to financial conflicts of interests and more); remediation may require applying universal design so that exploratory implementation prioritizes disadvantaged communities after which the general population could benefit from the exploratory results (as SpaceLink seems to be proceeding lately in remote areas of Canada for satellite access to broadband internet).

Conclusion

Ethics in relation to community mental health are important and often complex. Such ethics involve knowledge of general ethical approaches, such as the well-established consequentialism, deontology, and virtue ethics, as well as more novel approaches, such as care ethics. We argue that mental health professionals require basic skills in bioethics thinking, such as application of 'principlism', as well as awareness of other bioethical approaches, such as dialogical bioethics and—somewhat in contrast—benevolent paternalism. The ethical problems encountered in community mental health, which these approaches address, range from traditional problems, such as the use of coercion, to relatively novel problems, such as those of the community as a unit of ethical analysis and digital technology as a set of opportunities and threats. Further discussion and research are required in relation to these and other relevant ethical problems in order to address changing services and policies in relation to community mental health. Community mental health care providers, who may be regularly confronted with ethical problems such as those described here and who may want to seek ethical guidance in relation to these problems, can access written resources, as illustrated in the further reading and reference lists of this chapter, as well as engage in multidisciplinary team discussions and in consultations with ethicists and ethics committees that are available now in some community mental health settings. Further development of such consultation and capacity building resources in the area of community mental health may be in order.

Summary

1. In health care, ethical problems are commonly viewed as the tension between two or more morally defensible alternative actions, including inaction, and ethical theories, such as consequentialism/utilitarianism, deontology, and virtue ethics, suggest various ways of addressing and resolving such ethical problems.
2. Bioethics involves ethics of health-related matters, both clinical and other, such as in relation to health policy and research. 'Principlism', a widely used bioethical approach, comprises considerations of autonomy, beneficence, non-maleficence, and justice, in addition to context. Alternatives to principlism, such as 'dialogical bioethics' and—somewhat in contrast—benevolent paternalism, may be helpful in bioethical decision-making, although they may not be fully independent from some principlist considerations (such as justice and beneficence, respectively).
3. In community mental health, consideration needs to be given to both the individual person/patient as well as to the community as a unit of analysis. Issues of disability and community integration could be related to the person/patient and/or to the broader community as a whole.
4. Privacy, confidentiality, coercion, and conflicts of duty are key sets of dilemmas in the practice of mental health care in the community.
5. Community level considerations include (1) beneficence—doing good for whom?; (2) social justice and basic human rights; (3) the obligation to advocate or to 'whistle-blow'; and (4) understanding ethics within legal frameworks.
6. Digital technology involves opportunities and threats, such as in relation to improving access to mental health services while addressing conflicts of interests of private sector providers.

FURTHER READING

Akhtar, N., Forchuk, C., McKay, K. A., Fisman, S., & Rudnick A. (2020). *Handbook of Person-Centered Mental Health Care*. Boston, MA: Hogrefe.

Backlar, P. & Cutler, D. L. (Eds.) (2002). *Ethics in Community Mental Health Care: Commonplace Concerns*. New York: Kluwer/Plenum.

Blackburn, S. (2021). *Ethics: A Very Short Introduction* (2nd ed.). Oxford: Oxford University Press.

REFERENCES

Alexander, L. A. & Link, B. G. (2003). The impact of contact stigmatizing attitudes toward people with mental illness. *Journal of Mental Health*, **12**, 271–289.

Baldwin, M. L., & Marcus, S. C. (2006). Perceived and measured stigma among workers with serious mental illness. *Psychiatric Services*, **57**, 388–392.

Beauchamp, T. L. & Childress, J. F. (2009). *Principles of Biomedical Ethics* (6th ed.). New York: Oxford University Press.

Crisp, A. H., Gelder, M. G., Rix, S., Meltzer, H., & Rowlands, O. (2000). Stigmatisation of people with mental illnesses. *British Journal of Psychiatry*, **177**, 4–7.

Daigle, P. & Rudnick, A. (2020). Shifting to remotely delivered mental health care: quality improvement in the COVID-19 pandemic. *Psychiatry International*, **1**, 31–35.

Davison, C., Edwards, N., & Robinson, S. (2006). *Social Justice: A Means to an End, an End in Itself*. Ottawa: Canadian Nurses Association.

Dershowitz, A. (2004). *Rights from Wrongs: A Secular Theory of the Origins of Rights*. New York: Basic Books.

Diamond, R. J. & Wikler, D. (1985). Ethical problems in the community treatment of the chronically mentally ill. In: Stein, L. I. & Test, M. A. (Eds.), *Training in Community Living Model: A Decade of Experience* (pp. 169–196). San Francisco, CA: Josey-Bass.

Drake, R. E., McHugo, G. J., Bedout, R. R., Becker, D. R., Marris, M., Bond, G. R., et al. (1999). A randomized clinical trial of supported employment for inner-city patients with severe mental disorders. *Archives of General Psychiatry*, **56**, 62.

Forchuk, C., Joplin, L., Schofield, R., Csiernik, R., Gorlick, C., & Turner, K. (2007). Housing, income support and mental health: points of disconnection. *Health Research Policy Systems*, **5**, 14.

Forchuk, C., Macclure, S. K., Van Beers, M., Smith, C., Csiernik, R., Hoch, J., et al. (2008). Developing and testing an intervention to prevent homelessness among individuals discharged from psychiatric wards to shelters and 'no fixed address'. *Journal of Psychiatric and Mental Health Nursing*, **15**, 569–575.

Forchuk, C., Montgomery, P., Berman, H., Ward-Griffin, C., Csiernik, R., Gorlick, C., et al. (2011). Gaining ground, losing ground: the paradoxes of rural homelessness. In: Forchuk, C., Csiernik, R., & Jensen, E. (Ed.), *Homelessness, Housing and the Experiences of Mental Health Consumer-Survivors: Finding Truths—Creating Change* (pp. 328–344). Toronto: Canadian Scholars Press.

Forchuk, C., Nelson, G., & Hall, G. B. (2006a). 'It's important to be proud of the place you live in': housing problems and preferences of psychiatric survivors. *Perspectives in Psychiatric Care*, **42**, 42–52.

Forchuk, C., Russell, G., Kingston-Macclure, S., Turner, S., & Dill, S. (2006). From psychiatric ward to the streets and shelters. *Journal of Psychiatric and Mental Health Nursing*, **13**, 301–308.

Forchuk, C., Ward-Griffin, C., Csiernik, R., & Turner, K. (2006b). Surviving the tornado of mental illness: psychiatric survivors' experiences of getting, losing, and keeping housing. *Psychiatric Services*, **57**, 558–562.

Geller, J. L. (2001). Taking issue: ain't no such thing as a schizophrenic. *Psychiatric Services*, **52**, 715.

Holloway, F. (1996). Community psychiatric care: from libertarianism to coercion. Moral panic and mental health policy in Britain. *Health Care Analysis*, **4**, 235–243.

Jonsen, A. R. (1998). *The Birth of Bioethics*. New York: Oxford University Press.

Jonsen, A. R. (2000). *A Short History of Medical Ethics*. New York: Oxford University Press.

Lloyd, G. E. R. (Ed.) (1983). *Hippocratic Writings*. London: Penguin.

Lyons, M. & Ziviani, J. (1995). Stereotypes, stigma and mental illness: learning from fieldwork experiences. *American Journal of Occupational Therapy*, **49**, 1002–1008.

MacIntyre, A. A. (1998). *Short History of Ethics: A History of Moral Philosophy from the Homeric Age to the Twentieth Century* (2nd ed.). London: Routledge.

Morris, P. (2002). The capabilities perspective. A framework for social justice. *Families in Society*, **83**, 365–373.

Olson, M., Seikkula, J., & Ziedonis, D. (2014). *The Key Elements of Dialogic Practice in Open Dialogue*. Worcester, MA: University of Massachusetts Medical School. http://www.do-ge.ch/uploads/1/3/9/9/13993272/keyelementsv1.109022014.pdf

Overton, S. L. & Medina, S. L. (2008). The stigma of mental illness. *Journal of Counseling and Development*, **86**, 143–151.

Powers, M. & Faden, R. (2006). *Social Justice: The Moral Foundations of Public Health and Health Policy*. New York: Oxford University Press.

Reglitz, M. & Rudnick, A. (2020). Internet access as a right for realizing the human right to adequate mental (and other) health care. *International Journal of Mental Health*, **49**, 97–103.

Roberts, G., Davenport, S., Holloway, F., & Tattan, T. (Ed.) (2006). *Enabling Recovery: The Principles and Practice of Rehabilitation Psychiatry*. London: Gaskell.

Roberts, L. W. & Dyer, A. R. (2004). *Concise Guide to Ethics in Mental Health Care*. Washington, DC: American Psychiatric Publishing.

Rose, N. (1998). Governing risky individuals: the role of psychiatry in new regimes of control. *Psychiatry, Psychology and Law*, **5**, 177–195.

Rudnick, A. (2001). A meta-ethical critique of care ethics. *Theoretical Medicine*, **22**, 505–517.

Rudnick, A. (2002). The ground of dialogical bioethics. *Health Care Analysis*, **10**, 391–402.

Rudnick, A. (2007). Processes and pitfalls of dialogical bioethics. *Health Care Analysis*, **15**, 123–135.

Rudnick, A. (Ed.) (2011). *Bioethics in the 21st Century*. London: InTech.

Schulze, B. & Angermeyer, M. C. (2003). Subjective experiences of stigma. A focus group study of schizophrenic patients, their relatives and mental health professionals. *Social Science & Medicine*, **56**, 299–312.

Shied, T. L. (2005). Stigma as a barrier to employment: mental disability and the Americans with Disabilities Act. *International Journal of Law and Psychiatry*, **28**, 670–690.

Sirey, J. A., Bruce, M. L., Alexopoulos, G. S., Perlick, D. A., Raue, P., Friedman, S. J., et al. (2001). Perceived stigma as a predictor of treatment discontinuation in young and older outpatients with depression. *American Journal of Psychiatry*, **158**, 479–481.

Szmukler, G. & Appelbaum, P. (2008). Treatment pressures, leverage, coercion and compulsion in mental health care. *Journal of Mental Health*, **17**, 233–244.

Szmukler, G. & Bloch, S. (1998) Family involvement in the care of people with psychoses: an ethical argument. *British Journal of Psychiatry*, **171**, 401–405.

Szmukler, G. & Rose, N. (2013) Risk assessment in mental health care: values and costs. *Behavioral Science and the Law*, **31**, 125–140.

Thornicroft, G. (2006). *Shunned: Discrimination Against People with Mental Illness*. New York: Oxford University Press.

28

International human rights and community mental health

Oliver Lewis and Peter Bartlett

Introduction

This chapter concerns human rights relating to people with mental health issues living in the community. It seeks to explain how international human rights law can work in a variety of ways to foster a person's equal right to live independently and be included in the community on an equal basis, with choices equal to others.

Each individual country may have legislation and policy to underpin community living. These may include social security payments and personal budgets to help people live independently, accessible housing arrangements, provision of personal assistance and other mental health-related supports, community primary health services and specialist mental health services, as well as non-discrimination provisions relating to vocational training and employment, and more widely to the provision of all goods and services. Such legislation and policy are essential in setting and regulating standards of human rights within countries. These arrangements differ widely between countries, and for practical reasons a comparative legal analysis lies outside the scope of this chapter.

Instead, this chapter concerns the layers of international law and standards that sit above domestic law, directing and influencing domestic law and policy in order to bring about positive changes to the lived experiences of persons with mental health issues living in the community. The second section of the chapter ('International human rights law') is a primer on international human rights law: the treaties and other standards, how they apply to people with mental health issues living in the community, and how they are implemented and monitored. The third section ('The dawn of a new era?') introduces elements of the United Nations (UN) Convention on the Rights of Persons with Disabilities (hereinafter 'CRPD'),[1] and examines its philosophical underpinnings, the obligations on the State to implement it, and sets out its innovative features at the domestic level to coordinate policy action and to monitor implementation. It also outlines the Optional Protocol to the CRPD and the international mechanisms established to monitor State compliance.[2] The fourth section ('Human rights underpinning community mental health') explains some of the CRPD rights which impact community mental health, and the next three sections ('Right to health', 'Right to live in the community', and 'Right to legal capacity') provide an analysis of three of these rights in depth. The conclusion in the final section suggests actions which community mental health practitioners could take to ensure that the State respects, protects, and fulfils the rights of people with mental health issues in the community.

When the first edition of this book was published in 2011, there was little academic commentary on the CRPD, the treaty having been adopted in 2006. In the last 10 years or so, this paucity has turned into an embarrassment of riches—Google Scholar now numbers the books and articles referring to the CRPD in the tens of thousands, from legal, medical, social work and social care, philosophical, historical, anthropological, and other perspectives, written by academics, practitioners, and persons with disabilities. This is an introductory chapter, and cannot engage with that literature, but people wishing to pursue the themes in this chapter should be aware—there is lots out there to sink your teeth into.

International human rights law

International law flows from agreements ('treaties' or 'conventions') made between countries ('States' or 'States Parties' in the legal language) in intergovernmental organizations such as the Council of

---

[1] Convention on the Rights of Persons with Disabilities adopted by the UN General Assembly, New York, 13 December 2006, ref: Doc.A/61/611. A full text of the CRPD may be found at https://www.ohchr.org/EN/HRBodies/CRPD/Pages/ConventionRightsPersonsWithDisabilities.aspx (accessed 22 February 2022).

[2] Optional Protocol to the Convention on the Rights of Persons with Disabilities, adopted by the UN General Assembly, New York, 13 December 2006, ref: Doc.A/61/611.

Europe[3] and the UN. For present purposes, international law is not imposed on a State without its consent. That is to say, States negotiate and agree to the terms of agreements, and take part in formulating the standards and organize how the international monitoring of the implementation of those standards takes place. Quite how these various laws and standards work depends on the legal instrument in question. The most important laws are treaties which States have negotiated between themselves. Often, civil society organizations have participated in the negotiations.

Modifications or additions to human rights treaties may also be adopted and these are usually called 'protocols' or 'optional protocols'. A treaty (and any protocol attached to it) is binding on the State that 'ratifies'[4] it. The text of a treaty determines the obligations on States to implement it. Precisely how this is done will depend on the laws of the State, but certainly, the State will need to review the arrangements of laws, policies, and budgets, and will need to adopt a baseline report as to the practice in reality. A State will usually need to pass laws to bring its domestic arrangements into line with the treaty, and enforce those laws (e.g. through its criminal and civil domestic legislation, institutions, and procedures). This will have knock-on effects for public bodies, private entities, and individual people, since States have duties to respect, protect, and fulfil the rights set out in the treaty.

It is the State that will be held to account under international law, not any particular individual, local authority, or health care service. The mechanism of accountability will depend on the terms of the treaty. Often, there is a requirement that States report periodically (say, every 4 years) on implementation. Sometimes, there are international bodies that adjudicate complaints from people in the country who consider that their rights under the treaty have been violated.[5] While those bodies tend to rely on moral suasion on States in implementation of their decisions, the public visibility of State non-compliance can have some effect: it looks bad in diplomatic terms to be non-compliant. Further, the outcome document of a treaty monitoring body can be used by national human rights institutions, non-governmental organizations, political parties, and the media domestically to raise awareness and hold the government to account.

There is a considerable array of international law. People with mental health issues are meant to benefit from these provisions as much—or as little—as anyone else.[6] Thus, for example, a girl does not cease to benefit from the UN Convention on the Rights of the Child because she has a mental health problem.

A wide array of international law is relevant to people with mental health issues. Obvious examples include the 1966 International Covenant on Civil and Political Rights (ICCPR),[7] which sets out the right to life, to freedom from torture, to expression and association, to freedom from interference with private and family life, and to vote. The ICCPR's sister treaty is the International Covenant on Economic, Social and Cultural Rights,[8] which provides, among others, for the right to the enjoyment of the highest attainable standard of physical and mental health, the right to healthy working conditions, social insurance, adequate standard of living and adequacy of housing, education, and participation in cultural life. All of these rights are fundamental to enable people with mental health issues to live in the community. As will be laid out below, they are given further focus in the CRPD.

The treaties covering children,[9] girls and women,[10] people of racial and ethnic minorities,[11] and migrant workers[12] all apply to persons with mental health issues. So too does the treaty dealing with the prohibition of torture, cruel, inhuman, and degrading treatment or punishment, whose ambit covers the inappropriate use of psychiatric treatments, restraints, and seclusion.[13] A new UN convention on the rights of older people is in the works, but has not yet reached fruition—but watch this space.

Alongside the global UN mechanisms are regional mechanisms to protect human rights. These include the African system, the Inter-American system, and the European system. The European Convention on Human Rights and Fundamental Freedoms (hereinafter 'ECHR'), is particularly important, both because its

---

[3] The Council of Europe should not be confused with the European Union (EU). The EU has 26 Member States (no longer including the UK, although transitional arrangements following Brexit mean that considerable EU law has been adopted into UK law, at least for the time being). The Council of Europe has 46 Member States from across Europe, and includes a wide variety of countries not members of the EU (e.g. Turkey, the Caucasus, and the UK). Its remit is to promote and protect democracy, the rule of law, and human rights. Brexit had no effect on the UK's membership in or relationship with the Council of Europe.

[4] Essentially, this means agreeing fully to implement the contents of the treaty domestically. Processes for that will differ, depending on the country. They sometimes, for example, require approval from State legislatures, as well as agreement from the relevant government minister(s). Sometimes a state 'signs' a treaty, which is one step away from ratification and signals that the State has an intention to ratify the treaty in the future.

[5] In addition to the Optional Protocol to the CRPD, the Human Rights Committee may receive individual communications relating to States parties to the First Optional Protocol to the International Covenant on Civil and Political Rights; the Committee on the Elimination of Discrimination Against Women may receive individual complaints relating to States parties to the Optional Protocol to the Convention on the Elimination of Discrimination Against Women; the Committee against Torture may consider individual communications relating to States parties who have made the necessary declaration under Article 22 of the Convention Against Torture; the Committee for the Elimination of Racial Discrimination may consider individual communications relating to States parties who have made the necessary declaration under article 14 of the Convention on the Elimination of Racial Discrimination; and the Convention on Migrant Workers contains provision for allowing individual communications to be considered by the Committee on Migrant Workers and these provisions will become operative when ten States parties have made the necessary declaration under article 77.

[6] In this chapter, the term 'mental health problems' is taken to include anyone labelled with psychosocial disabilities, mental disorders, or mental illness.

[7] Adopted by General Assembly resolution 2200A (XXI) on 16 December 1966.

[8] International Covenant on Economic, Social and Cultural Rights, adopted by General Assembly resolution 2200A (XXI) on 16 December 1966.

[9] Convention on the Rights of the Child (adopted by General Assembly resolution 44/25 on 20 November 1989). See particularly Article 23 which sets out rights specifically for children with physical or mental disabilities and which obliges States to carry out a range of actions to promote the child's self-reliance and facilitate the child's active participation in the community.

[10] Convention on the Elimination of All Forms of Discrimination against Women (adopted by General Assembly resolution 34/180 on 18 December 1979).

[11] International Convention on the Elimination of All Forms of Racial Discrimination (adopted by General Assembly resolution 2106 (XX) on 21 December 1965).

[12] International Convention on the Protection of the Rights of All Migrant Workers and Members of Their Families (adopted by General Assembly resolution 45/158 on 18 December 1990).

[13] Convention against Torture and Other Cruel, Inhuman or Degrading Treatment or Punishment (adopted by General Assembly resolution 39/46 on 10 December 1984).

jurisprudence is more developed than other courts in the other regions, and because the ECHR can be invoked and is largely enforceable in domestic courts of the 46 Member States of the Council of Europe. This chapter does not discuss all potentially relevant international law, and readers concerned by specific client groups or human rights issues will need to become acquainted with the international law that relates to their specific concern. The jurisprudence of the ECHR to date has concerned primarily issues relating to detention rather than preventing it, and analyses have been dealt with elsewhere.[14]

Instead, the focus of this chapter is the CRPD. Unlike the ECHR which covers human rights broadly, the CRPD focuses specifically on the rights of persons with disabilities. Instead of defining disability, the CRPD defines 'persons with disabilities', to 'include those who have long-term physical, mental, intellectual or sensory impairments which in interaction with various barriers may hinder their full and effective participation in society on an equal basis with others'.[15] It is without doubt that persons with mental health issues fall within the ambit of the CRPD.

One of the reasons that the CRPD came into existence in 2006 was the global gap between rights rhetoric and lived reality. The CRPD itself points out that international human rights instruments have for many years 'proclaimed and agreed that everyone is entitled to all the rights and freedoms set forth therein, without distinction of any kind',[16] yet the international community was '[c]oncerned that, despite these various instruments and undertakings, persons with disabilities continue to face barriers in their participation as equal members of society and violations of their human rights in all parts of the world'.[17] Over a decade later, these statements are still likely to resonate with anyone working in mental health systems.

Two reasons for the implementation failure of pre-CRPD human rights treaties are inadequate coordination at the domestic policy level and inadequate independent monitoring of the implementation. The drafters of the CRPD were well aware of these policy failures and ensured that the new treaty binds States to establish implementation and monitoring mechanisms. These include a governmental coordinating body to facilitate activities relevant to the implementation of the Convention across different ministries and departments, and down into regions and localities.[18] The CRPD also places an obligation on States to establish or designate an independent mechanism (such as an ombudsman or a national human rights institution) to promote and protect the rights of persons with disabilities and to monitor the domestic implementation of the Convention.[19] States are required to ensure that persons with disabilities and their representative organizations have opportunities to be involved and participate in this monitoring process.[20]

People with mental health issues can play a part in monitoring the CRPD's implementation. The CRPD also makes it a treaty obligation to 'closely consult with and actively involve' people with disabilities (which includes people with mental health issues) '[i]n the development and implementation of legislation and policies to implement the [CRPD], and in other decision-making processes concerning issues relating to persons with disabilities'.[21] This provision echoes a statement in the CRPD's preamble, that 'persons with disabilities should have the opportunity to be actively involved in decision-making processes about policies and programmes, including those directly concerning them'.[22]

At the UN level, the CRPD establishes a treaty monitoring body, the 'Committee on the Rights of Persons with Disabilities' (hereafter the 'CRPD Committee').[23] The CRPD Committee publishes guidance ('General Comments') on its interpretation of the CRPD, and these are well worth a read as a way into the understanding of the detail of the Convention.[24] The General Comments are authoritative, but not formally binding: they are meant to provoke a 'productive dialogue' with States Parties and other actors.

In addition, the CRPD Committee considers national reports provided by governments and assesses overall compliance by the individual countries—a more traditional monitoring role.[25] These observations can be influenced by others in those countries—including by organizations of persons with mental health issues or advocacy groups—who may submit their own reports in advance of the Committee's deliberations. The CRPD Committee then has discussions (called 'constructive dialogues') with governmental representatives at its sessions in Geneva. The outcome document is the Committee's 'concluding observations', which are not legally binding, but are public documents which can be used to advocate politically for laws, policies, and practices to be changed. The Committee also adjudicates on individual complaints submitted to it, from people in States which have ratified the Optional Protocol to the CRPD. In this context, the Committee will behave in a fashion broadly analogous to a court, determining the admissibility and merits of the case before it.[26]

The dawn of a new era?

The CRPD was adopted by the UN General Assembly in December 2006, and it entered into force in May 2008. As of January 2022, it had been ratified by 182 'States', including the UK.[27] In 2008, the then UN

---

[14] For an extended discussion of the ECHR jurisprudence relating to people with mental health problems (and people with intellectual disabilities), see Bartlett et al. (2007) (also available on Google books).
[15] CRPD, Art. 1.
[16] CRPD, preambulatory paragraph (a).
[17] CRPD, preambulatory paragraph (k).
[18] CRPD, Art. 33(1).
[19] CRPD, Art. 33(2).
[20] CRPD, Art. 33(3).
[21] CRPD, Art. 4(3).
[22] CPRD, perambulatory para. (o).
[23] CRPD, Art. 34.
[24] As of February 2022, seven General Comments have been issued. These explore Equal Access to the Law (CRPD/C/GC/1, 2014), Accessibility (CRPD/C/GC/2, 2014), Women and Girls with Disability (CRPD/C/GC/3, 2016), Inclusive Education (CRPD/C/GC/4, 2016), Independent Living (CRPD/C/GC/5, 2017), Equality and Non-Discrimination (CRPD/C/GC/6, 2018), and Participation of Persons with Disabilities in Implementation and Monitoring of the Convention (CRPD/C/GC/7, 2018). All of these are available at https://www.ohchr.org/en/hrbodies/crpd/pages/gc.aspx (accessed 18 February 2022).
[25] CRPD, Arts. 35 and 36.
[26] Its case law is included in the UN database of jurisprudence, located at https://juris.ohchr.org/
[27] See https://www.ohchr.org/Documents/HRBodies/CRPD/OHCHR_Map_CRPD.pdfl (accessed 22 February 2022). An additional nine countries had signed, but not yet ratified. 97 countries, including the UK, had ratified the optional protocol, allowing complaints to the CRPD Committee from individual citizens: https://www.ohchr.org/Documents/HRBodies/CRPD/OHCHR_Map_CRPD-OP.pdf

Secretary General, Kofi Annan, described the adoption of the CRPD as, 'the dawn of a new era—an era in which disabled people will no longer have to endure the discriminatory practices and attitudes that have been permitted to prevail for all too long' (UN Press Release, 2006). The Convention signals an end to a paradigm where people with disabilities, including people with mental health issues, are treated as objects: objects of treatment, management, charity, pity, and fear. The new era brings with it a shift in thinking about disability and mental health, one in which people with mental health issues are viewed not as objects, but as subjects of human rights on an equal basis with others.

How far the Convention will be meaningful for people with disabilities still remains to be seen. Its success will be largely dependent on whether a variety of stakeholders—including community mental health practitioners—embrace its provisions. Its success will also be dependent on the effectiveness of governmental coordination and on independent monitoring, as noted earlier.

Whatever the future holds in store, the text marks a significant departure from previous human rights instruments for a variety of reasons. People with disabilities, including global and regional organizations comprising people with mental health issues, were themselves directly involved in the negotiations leading to the Convention.[28] UN Member States were the official negotiators of the CRPD, and they are the duty-bearers to ensure its implementation. That said, persons with disabilities, including people with mental health issues—including many people from the global south—were key to shaping the text in a way which was unprecedented at the UN. This involvement has resulted in a Convention with great specificity, relevance, and ownership by the disabilities movements.

The CRPD uses the language and approach of classic human rights expressly and unreservedly in a treaty relating to people with disabilities. Previously, treaties that adopted a clear human rights approach either included people with disabilities by implication, or excluded them specifically (provisions allowing detention of people with mental health issues are an obvious example).[29] There have been other international instruments—of a lower rank than treaties—that have focused on the rights of persons with disabilities. Although these documents used some human rights rhetoric, they pre-supposed that considerably greater control, regulation, and substituted decision-making was appropriate for people with mental health issues than for the population as a whole. The 1991 UN Mental Illness Principles serve as an example here.[30]

By comparison, the CRPD contains a set of guiding principles, including the 'freedom to make one's own choices' (and by implication the dignity of risk to make one's own mistakes on an equal basis with others),[31] '[r]espect for difference and acceptance of persons with disabilities as part of human diversity and humanity',[32] and the principle that people with disabilities have should enjoy '[f]ull and effective participation and inclusion in society'.[33] These philosophical underpinnings come from a human rights model and sit more comfortably with other UN human rights treaties than with the pre-existing specialist instruments which, as noted above, tended to assume that rights needed to be lowered downwards to justify the removal of rights—of autonomy, of liberty, of physical and mental integrity—for people with mental health issues.

In addition to principles, the CRPD articulates a list of general obligations on States in order to ensure compliance with the CRPD's provisions. These obligations include adopting appropriate legislation and taking other measures in order to implement the convention.[34] States must abolish laws that constitute discrimination,[35] and take '*all* appropriate measures to eliminate discrimination on the basis of disability by any person, organization or private enterprise'.[36] The CRPD contains a disability mainstreaming provision, so that States must 'to take into account the protection and promotion of the human rights of persons with disabilities in *all* policies and programmes' (emphasis added), not only in disability policies or mental health policies.[37] Of particular relevance to community mental health practitioners is the general obligation on training on CRPD rights for staff working with people with disabilities, 'so as to better provide the assistance and services guaranteed by those rights'.[38]

One of the top concerns of civil society organizations during the negotiations leading up to the Convention was institutionalization of people with mental health issues and people with other types of disabilities. Removing people from society and placing them in long-term closed institutions is closely connected with other human rights concerns, namely treatment without consent and sometimes by force, as well as the removal of a person's legal capacity rendering them powerless to make choices about their own lives. The gradual closure of residential institutions and establishing in parallel a variety of community-based services are the focus of this textbook as a whole, and are of prime importance in the CRPD. In the next sections we will outline how community mental health practitioners can use the CRPD to support independent living.

Human rights underpinning community mental health

This section lays out in general terms the rights contained in the CRPD. The following three sections address provisions which may be of particular relevance for the concerns of community mental health practitioners and their clients.

---

[28] These included the World Network of Users and Survivors of Psychiatry, which, in conjunction with many other non-governmental organizations acted in concert within the International Disability Caucus.

[29] See Article 5(1)(e) of the ECHR, which suspends the right to liberty for several groups including 'persons of unsound mind'. For more on the history of pre-CRPD provisions applied to persons with disabilities, see Lewis and Pathare (2020).

[30] 'Principles for the protection of persons with mental illness and the improvement of mental health care' (adopted by UN General Assembly resolution 46/119 of 17 December 1991).

[31] CRPD, Art. 3(a).

[32] CRPD, Art. 3(d).

[33] CRPD, Art. 3(c).

[34] CRPD, Art. 4(1)(a).

[35] CRPD, Art. 4(1)(b).

[36] CRPD, Art. 4(1)(e) (emphasis added).

[37] CRPD, Art. 4(1)(c). This means, for example, that the rights of persons with mental health problems need to be considered not merely in the context of mental health law or legal capacity law, but also in policy areas diverse as housing, travel, insurance, energy, defence, education, transport, and international development.

[38] CRPD, Art. 4(1)(i).

The CRPD contains a classic array of what have been termed 'civil and political rights' which exist in the ICCPR (see earlier 'International human rights law' section of the chapter), such as the right to liberty (Article 14 of the CRPD) and integrity of the person (Article 17), and the rights to freedom of expression (Article 21) and privacy (Article 22). The CRPD echoes the ICCPR and the UN Convention against Torture by containing an absolute prohibition on torture, cruel, inhuman, or degrading treatment or punishment (Article 15). In addition, it outlaws medical and scientific experimentation without consent (Article 15). It sets out rights to equal recognition before the law and to legal capacity (Article 12—a topic which we will address the section 'Right to legal capacity') and access to justice (Article 13). It provides the right to vote and participate in public affairs (Article 29). These are rights that already, at least to a considerable degree, apply to people with mental health issues, through pre-existing international laws. These civil and political rights generally date from eighteenth-century Western thought, and are generally rights to be free from State intervention. They are potentially significant for persons with mental health issues in the community. A reduction of the power of the State to detain an individual in a psychiatric hospital, for example, is in many ways a prerequisite for a person with a mental health problem to maintain their life in the community, and Article 14 of the CRPD provides a particularly strong statement framed as a right.

These are sometimes called 'negative rights'—that the State must stop, refrain from doing something, or prevent something from happening. Some scholars argue that civil and political rights do not cost much money. This assumption is tested by the CRPD. In order to protect people with disabilities against ill-treatment (disability hate crime, or violence in mental health settings, as examples) a State must actively ensure that there is an adequate criminal law, as well as fund and manage a police force and a justice system including prisons and probation services, as well as set standards for the treatment of people in mental health services, ensure staff undergo minimum training, and the like. The CRPD places much emphasis on preventing all forms of disability-based discrimination, including the failure to provide 'reasonable accommodation' to people with disabilities in order to equalize their rights upwards on an equal basis with others. All of this comes with a price tag.[39]

The CRPD further contains a variety of what have traditionally been labelled 'economic, social and cultural rights'. Some of these reflect earlier treaty rights (particularly in the International Covenant on Economic, Social and Cultural Rights, see earlier 'International human rights law' section). These include the right to an adequate standard of living and the right to health. However, a number of these rights go beyond previously articulated international law. The right to health and the right to live in the community will be discussed in greater detail in the following sections, but it is appropriate also to provide a brief overview of the broader range of rights, as they work in concert with the right to health and the right to community life to provide the legal structure for a new era of community mental health.

The CRPD protects the right to relationships, to sexual activity, and to family life (Article 23). While other international instruments protect these rights in general, the CRPD provides a detailed articulation of these rights, including the right to decide the number and spacing of one's children, the right to age-appropriate sexual education and information, the right to retain one's fertility, and the right to assistance from the State in the performance of child-rearing duties. While the State retains the right to remove a child from his or her family when it is in the best interests of the child, such removal may not be on the basis of the disability of the child or the parent(s).

The CRPD also contains the right to education, understood as inclusive education in the general school system, rather than segregated education in facilities only for children with disabilities.[40] It also contains a parallel right to individualized educational support in environments that maximize academic and social development.[41] There are provisions of particular importance for children labelled with mental health issues or behavioural problems, as well as those with intellectual or learning disabilities who are at risk of exclusion from mainstream educational settings.[42] The CRPD rejects 'special education' where children with disabilities are taught together using different curricula than regular schools and achieving lower educational outcomes. Instead, there needs to be 'a transformation in culture, policy and practice in all formal and informal educational environments to accommodate the differing requirements and identities of individual students, together with a commitment to removing the barriers that impede that possibility'.[43] The pivot towards an inclusive educational system for all echoes the preamble to the CRPD which talks about the existing and potential contributions which people with disabilities can make to the well-being and diversity of communities.[44] This is underpinned by one of the principles which should be read into each of the Convention's provisions, namely a '[r]espect for difference and acceptance of persons with disabilities as part of human diversity and humanity'.[45]

In addition to the right to education, the CRPD includes the right to work and employment, in which there are specific requirements that non-discrimination programmes be introduced to cover 'conditions of recruitment, hiring and employment, continuance of employment, career advancement and safe and healthy working conditions',[46] that reasonable accommodation be made of the different needs of employees that flow from their disabilities,[47] and that people with disabilities be employed in the public sector.[48]

---

[39] CRPD, Art. 2.

[40] For more detail on the right to education under the CRPD, see General Comment 4 of the CRPD on the Right to Inclusive Education (2016), available at https://www.ohchr.org/en/hrbodies/crpd/pages/gc.aspx

[41] CRPD, Art. 24.

[42] For an application of the right to education for children with disabilities, see *Mental Disability Advocacy Center v. Bulgaria*, decided under the European Social Charter by the European Committee on Social Rights, October 2008. For a report which sets out the right for children with disabilities to inclusive education, see Inclusion International, 'Better Education for All When We're Included Too', 2009 (https://inclusion-international.org/resource/better-education-for-all-a-global-report/); and for an overview of how the right to education applies to children with disabilities, see CRPD Committee, 'General comment No. 4 on Article 24—the right to inclusive education', 25 November 2016.

[43] CRPD Committee, 'General comment No. 4 on Article 24—the right to inclusive education', 25 November 2016, para. 9, and for an analysis of the law, see de Beco et al. (2019).

[44] CRPD, perambulatory paragraph (m).

[45] CRPD, Art. 3(d).

[46] Art. 27(1)(a).

[47] Art. 27(1)(i), and see CRPD Committee, 'General comment No 5 on Article 5: Equality and non-discrimination', 31 August 2017.

[48] Art. 27(1)(g).

The concept of reasonable accommodation is defined in the CRPD as the 'necessary and appropriate modification and adjustments not imposing a disproportionate or undue burden, where needed in a particular case, to ensure to persons with disabilities the enjoyment or exercise on an equal basis with others of all human rights and fundamental freedoms'.[49] The CRPD creates State obligations to ensure that persons with disabilities can access all rights on an equal basis with others in all fields, including those other than employment. For example, the right to vote will be meaningful for some people with mental health issues only if the State allows the voter to take a support person into the voting booth, or allows kerb-side voting so that a person with social anxiety need not leave their car. Dismantling of legal barriers is also required, such as amending systems that deprive a person of legal capacity and render them unable in law to vote.[50]

The chapter now turns to examine in some detail three clusters of rights of particular relevance to community mental health practitioners: the right to health, the right to live in the community, and the right to legal capacity.

Right to health

The right to health is located in Article 12 of the International Covenant on Economic, Social and Cultural Rights and finds its place in Article 25 of the CRPD. This provision provides that States 'recognize that persons with disabilities have the right to the enjoyment of the highest attainable standard of health without discrimination on the basis of disability', which by definition includes on the basis of a mental health problem. Specifically, States should '[p]rovide persons with disabilities with the same range, quality and standard of free or affordable health care and programmes as provided to other persons'.[51] This includes sexual and reproductive health and population-based public health programmes. The CRPD also mandates the provision—although not the forcible provision—of 'health services needed by persons with disabilities specifically because of their disabilities, including early identification and intervention as appropriate, and services designed to minimize and prevent further disabilities, including among children and older persons'.[52] Taken together with Article 19 of the CRPD which sets out the right to live in the community, it is clear that Article 25 requires States to provide mental health services in the community.

Article 25 of the CRPD lays out entitlements to ensure the highest attainable standard of physical and mental health. As Professor Paul Hunt (then UN Special Rapporteur on the Right to Health) stated a year before the CRPD was adopted, such entitlements for persons with mental health issues include obligations on each State to:

> ensure a full package of community-based mental health care and support services conducive to health, dignity, and inclusion, including medication, psychotherapy, ambulatory services, hospital care for acute admissions, residential facilities, rehabilitation for persons with psychiatric disabilities, programmes to maximize the independence and skills of persons with intellectual disabilities, supported housing and employment, income support, inclusive and appropriate education for children with intellectual disabilities, and respite care for families looking after a person with a mental disability 24 hours a day. In this way, unnecessary institutionalization can be avoided.[53]

This language anticipates that of Article 19 of the CRPD (which is examined in the next section of this chapter) in setting out a range of community alternatives which need to be provided so as to avoid institutionalization.

Professor Hunt picks up on a crucial point for community mental health practitioners, namely that:

> the right to health includes an entitlement to the underlying determinants of health, including adequate sanitation, safe water and adequate food and shelter. Persons with mental health issues are disproportionately affected by poverty, which is usually characterized by deprivations of these entitlements'.[54]

In some countries institutions provide water, food, and shelter where such necessities may not be available to a person with mental health issues in the community. That such basic elements to sustain life are provided in institutions but not in the community is no justification for the existence of, and reliance on, institutions. In localities where mental health services are institutional in nature, the language of human rights provides a tool for users of mental health services and those who care for them to advocate for access to the full range of human rights on an equal basis with others in the community. In this sense the right to health goes well beyond access to treatments for mental health issues.

This was confirmed in 2017 by Dainius Puras, the then UN Special Rapporteur on the Right to Health, who described the right to health as 'a powerful guide for States towards a paradigm shift that is recovery and community-based, promotes social inclusion and offers a range of rights based treatments and psychosocial support at primary and specialized care levels'.[55] Puras went on to observe that:

> [i]n many parts of the world, community care is not available, accessible, acceptable and/or of sufficient quality (often limited to psychotropic medications). The largest concentration of mental hospitals and beds separated from regular health care is in higher-income countries, a cautionary note for lower and middle-income countries to forge a different path and shift to rights-based mental health care.

Health services are classically considered to lie within the 'economic, social or cultural rights' grouping, and as such, the right is subject to 'progressive realization'. This means that States must have a plan to implement the right and take demonstrable steps year-on-year to progressively realize the full implementation of the right to health, so that progress can be measured. The right to health includes entitlements, ensuring that people with mental health issues have access to health care services, including services which assist in recovery from

---

[49] CRPD, Art. 2. For a more comprehensive discussion of reasonable accommodation, see General Comment 6, Equality and Non-Discrimination, section V.D (2018), available at https://www.ohchr.org/en/hrbodies/crpd/pages/gc.aspx

[50] See the European Court of Human Rights judgment in the case of *Alajos Kiss v. Hungary*, Application No. 38832/06, judgment 20 May 2010.

[51] CRPD, Art. 25(a).

[52] CRPD, Art. 25(b).

[53] Report of the Special Rapporteur on the right of everyone to the enjoyment of the highest attainable standard of physical and mental health, Paul Hunt to the UN Commission on Human Rights (2005), ref: E/CN.4/2005/51, para. 43.

[54] Hunt, para. 45.

[55] Dainius Puras, 'Report of the Special Rapporteur on the right of everyone to the enjoyment of the highest attainable standard of physical and mental health: mental health', A/HRC/35/21, 28 March 2017, para. 76.

mental ill health. As well as entitlements, the right to health also contains freedoms. For people with mental health issues, freedom often means that others should respect a decision to consent to or refuse mental health treatment. Professor Hunt considers forced psychiatric treatment to be 'one of the most important human rights issues relating to mental disability',[56] which is 'intimately connected with a vital element of the right to health: the freedom to control one's health and body'.[57]

The CRPD makes specific reference to the concept of 'consent to treatment' in two places, first by providing that 'no one shall be subjected without his or her free consent to medical or scientific experimentation'.[58] This prohibition sits in the provision setting out the absolute ban on torture and other forms of ill-treatment. Second, consent to treatment is set out in the provision on the right to health, an element of which is that States should '[r]equire health professionals to provide care of the same quality to persons with disabilities as to others, including on the basis of free and informed consent'.[59] This right should be achieved by a variety of activities including human rights awareness-raising,[60] training, and standard-setting. In the context of community mental health, it may be helpful to read this provision jointly with the provision prohibiting discrimination on the basis of disability.[61]

Puras has called for 'rights-based treatment responses' in mental health, noting that:

> Coercion, medicalization and exclusion, which are vestiges of traditional psychiatric care relationships, must be replaced with a modern understanding of recovery and evidence-based services that restore dignity and return rights holders to their families and communities. People can and do recover from even the most severe mental health conditions and go on to live full and rich lives.[62]

Given this combination, it is difficult to see that any infringement on the right of any patient to consent would be justified for people with mental health issues, when it would not be so justified for people without such a condition. On this basis, community treatment orders—legal requirements to accept psychiatric treatment in the community—must become suspect, at least when they concern people with capacity to consent to treatment: there is no comparable mechanism for somatic treatments. Puras' recommendation that 'effective psychosocial interventions in the community should be scaled up and the culture of coercion, isolation and excessive medicalization abandoned', adds weight to the argument. Where it has encountered community treatment orders (such as in the UK), the CRPD Committee has expressed concern about 'involuntary, compulsory treatment and detention both inside and outside hospitals on the basis of actual or perceived impairment'.[63] Any reliance on incapacity as a ground for restricting the right to consent is further likely to be difficult if not impossible, as will be discussed later in this chapter.

Of direct relevance to community mental health practitioners, the CRPD obliges States to ensure that health services are provided 'as close as possible to people's own communities, including in rural areas'.[64] From a right to health perspective, this means bringing mental health 'closer to primary care and general medicine, integrating mental health with physical health, professionally, politically and geographically'.[65] It is this vision of community living to which the chapter now turns.

Right to live in the community

An innovative feature of the CRPD is that unlike other human rights treaties, it is both specific and absolute about inclusion. Article 19 of the CRPD obliges States to 'recognize the equal right of all persons with disabilities to live in the community, with choices equal to others'. The article further specifies that States 'shall take effective and appropriate measures to facilitate full enjoyment by persons with disabilities of this right and their full inclusion and participation in the community, including ensuring the following three particular elements:

1. Persons with disabilities have the opportunity to choose their place of residence and where and with whom they live on an equal basis with others and are not obliged to live in a particular living arrangement.
2. Persons with disabilities have access to a range of in-home, residential, and other community support services, including personal assistance necessary to support living and inclusion in the community, and to prevent isolation or segregation from the community.
3. Community services and facilities for the general population are available on an equal basis to persons with disabilities and are responsive to their needs.

In its General Comment No. 5, the CRPD Committee expands on each of these, and on the overall direction of the Article. Institutional care is anathema to living in the community, where the person must be enabled to 'to exercise choice and control over their lives and make all decisions concerning their lives'.[66] Community support services are to be viewed as a right, and should be flexible enough to accommodate the needs and lifestyle of the individual, rather than organized around the convenience of service providers.

Living in the community does not operate in isolation, and other CRPD provisions should be flagged to ensure that people are included into the community rather than stuck at home, being as isolated and bored at home as in an institution. The right to personal mobility (Article 20), the right to work and employment (Article 27), the right to participation in cultural life (Article 30), and the right to be free from exploitation and abuse (Article 16) are all relevant.

---

[56] Hunt, para. 83.
[57] Hunt, para. 83.
[58] CRPD, Art. 15(1).
[59] CRPD, Art. 25(d).
[60] This wording links with Article 6 of the CRPD which sets out awareness-raising obligations throughout society of the rights of persons with disabilities, including people with mental health problems.
[61] CRPD, Art. 5.
[62] Dainius Puras, 'Report of the Special Rapporteur on the right of everyone to the enjoyment of the highest attainable standard of physical and mental health: mental health', A/HRC/35/21, 28 March 2017, para. 81.
[63] CRPD Committee, Concluding observations on the initial report of the United Kingdom of Great Britain and Northern Ireland, 3 October 2017, CRPD/C/GBR/CO/1, para. 34. See also Newton-Howes (2019).
[64] CRPD, Art. 25(c).
[65] Puras, para. 78.
[66] General Comment 5, para II.A.16. Available at https://www.ohchr.org/en/hrbodies/crpd/pages/gc.aspx. See also Lewis and Richardson (2020).

Right to legal capacity

The CRPD provides a new approach to equality before the law, by significantly restricting the scope of traditional decision-making regimes.[67]

The preamble to the CRPD recognizes the 'importance for persons with disabilities of their individual autonomy and independence, including the freedom to make their own choices,'[68] and the treaty rejects the comprehensive and routine deprivations of rights based on blanket findings of 'incapacity', often, historically and to this day in some parts of the world, based on remarkably flimsy evidence consisting little more than a psychiatric diagnosis.

In many jurisdictions, the law allows the relatives of a person with mental health issues, or a local government official, to apply to a court to have that person's legal capacity restricted partially or deprived totally. The person is placed under (what in many countries is called) guardianship of someone else who is empowered to take decisions for and on behalf of the adult with mental health issues. The case of Britney Spears being under 'conservatorship' is a recent well-known case of the human rights abuses inherent in guardianship systems (Smith, 2021). Courts and other bodies that interpret 'old paradigm' human rights instruments that pre-date the CRPD—such as the European Convention on Human Rights—have introduced increased procedural safeguards for these mechanisms, but they have not done away with them.[69]

The CRPD demands a shift away from this approach. People who need support in exercising legal capacity are to be provided with the supports which they need,[70] rather than having their rights taken away.

Significantly, in the view of the CRPD Committee, this new approach extends not merely to judicial and similar processes that remove decision-making authority from individuals on a large scale. It also extends to situations where capacity is determined on a decision-by-decision basis, such as the Mental Capacity Act 2005 in England and Wales.[71] Essentially, the view is that if mental disability (be it mental health difficulty, learning difficulty, dementia, brain injury, or other cognitive disability) is in whole or in part, directly or indirectly, a factor in determining the right of an individual to make a decision, the system is discriminatory and in violation of Article 12 of the CRPD.

Decisions must instead be made consistent with the will and preferences of the person with disabilities, or consistent with the best approximation of those will and preferences if the individual's views are really not known or knowable. An assessment of objective 'best interests' is not part of the picture. While there may perhaps be some discretion in determining what a person's 'real' will and preferences actually are, *any* restriction of Article 12 rights requires that safeguards be put in place to ensure that any restrictions on decision-making 'respect the rights, will and preferences of the person, are free of conflict of interest and undue influence, are proportional and tailored to the person's circumstances, apply for the shortest time possible and are subject to regular review by a competent, independent and impartial authority or judicial body'.[72] There can be little doubt that this constitutes a significant shift in approaches to decision-making by people with disabilities and requires root and branch law and policy reform, and service delivery arrangements at the community level.

The CRPD Committee makes a compelling case for its position. Legal capacity is crucial for people with mental health issues in the community. Without it, there are significant barriers to making decisions in areas of life which others take for granted. These may include taking decisions about one's own finances and property, about where and with whom to live, about working, signing contracts, forming relationships and entering into sexual relations, bringing up children, voting and standing for election, writing a will, joining associations and political parties, and accessing courts and other legal mechanisms. In this sense, legal capacity is not simply 'inextricably linked'[73] to other rights, but acts as a gatekeeper of other rights. Without providing the right to legal capacity and supports for those who access them, it is likely that full and equal participation in the community will never be achieved.

Community mental health practitioners will perhaps be most cognizant of how legal capacity is connected with the right to consent to or refuse treatment, a topic outlined in the 'Right to health' section, above. Any reliance on incapacity as a ground for restricting the right to informed consent needs to be consistent with the right to legal capacity in Article 12 of the CRPD.

Implementation of Article 12 of the CRPD poses a significant practical challenge in community mental health provision. So much relies on the provision of support in decision-making, but development of appropriate supported decision-making structures—mechanisms which really do work to promote the articulation of the will and preferences of the individual and meet the CRPD's other requirements—are still at best embryonic. The Article 12 rights are vital, and change clearly needs to happen, but it is less clear what the optimal ways forward are. There is a wide space for mental health practitioners, working with other stakeholders and in particular with people with disabilities, to engage in the development of those new processes.

Conclusion

The last section of this chapter speaks directly to community mental health practitioners and sets out ideas about how they can play a part in ensuring that the CRPD is implemented so that their clients benefit from the range of rights set out in the treaty.

At the micro level, practitioners can develop their own understanding by reading about the CRPD in journal articles, on the internet, and joining discussion forums. They can distribute copies

---

[67] CRPD, Art. 12.
[68] CRPD, perambulatory para. (n).
[69] See, for example, the European Court of Human Rights judgments *Shtukaturov v. Russia* (Application no. 44009/05, judgment on the merits 27 March 2008 and judgment concerning just satisfaction 4 March 2010) and *Salontaji-Drobnjak v. Serbia* (Application No. 36500/05, judgment 13 October 2009); *Stanev v. Bulgaria* (Application no. 36760/06, judgment of 17 April 2012), and *A-MV v. Finland* (application no. 53251/13, judgment of 23 June 2017).
[70] CRPD, Art. 12(3).
[71] General Comment 1, para 15. Available at https://www.ohchr.org/en/hrbodies/crpd/pages/gc.aspx. Regarding the CRPD and the Mental Capacity Act 2005, see, e.g. Bartlett (2020).

[72] CRPD, Art. 12(4).
[73] CPRD Committee, General Comment No. 1, para. 31.

to their community mental health teams, and professionals with whom they work: social workers, mental health nurses, paramedics, hospital-based colleagues, lawyers, and judges. Practitioners can play an important role in raising awareness about the CRPD at the local level by giving copies of the Convention to clients, as well as their carers and families.[74] After all, the human rights implementation at the local level in individual human interactions is as important as law reform domestically and discussions at the UN in New York and Geneva.

In 2021, the WHO published 'Guidance on community mental health services: promoting person-centred and rights-based approaches',[75] which provides an array of practical mechanisms for clinicians to implement CRPD values in community psychiatric practice. Free online training on human rights and mental health that incorporates the CRPD values is also available through the WHO's QualityRights initiative.[76] Both these sources are available in multiple languages, and are suitable for clinicians at all stages of their careers, other professional and non-professional carers, and people with lived experience. They are obvious starting points for translating the broader values discussed in this chapter into concrete improvements.

Within organizations that deliver community support services to people with mental health issues, practitioners could discuss the CRPD with colleagues and see how the local service can make changes to bring the services better in line with the CRPD. Practitioners could engage in a conversation with their clients and ask how they would like the practitioners to change in order that the CRPD is being implemented for them. In this way, practitioners breathe life into the CRPD provisions on involvement of persons with disabilities in the implementation of services.[77] Practitioners can encourage their clients to join local advocacy groups in order to be active in improving services and holding their government to account. Practitioners could ensure that people with mental health issues are given the opportunity to serve on decision-making boards that monitor services and provide improvement recommendations. Practitioners could work together with colleagues and people with mental health issues to develop codes of practice for particular rights issues which impact their work.

In their dealings with regional or national government, practitioners can use their platform to call for the advancement of human rights. Mental health practitioners are usually more politically powerful than their clients, and while they should not speak 'for' their clients, they can use their connections and platforms to support the voices of people with mental health issues. Practitioners can help open doors to decision-makers, ombudsman offices, and foreign embassies. They can speak the language of the CRPD in meetings with decision-makers and call directly for legislative and policy reforms, for the development of services to enable people with disabilities to live in the community, and for adequate resources to be allocated.

Practitioners could feed into the changes abroad by asking their government (in countries that are donors) to ensure that all development funding is accessible for people with disabilities, and that there is a specific focus on the rights of people with mental health issues in particular. Practitioners in aid-recipient countries can play a valuable role in supporting their clients and their representative organizations to track development financing and ensuring inclusion of their clients.[78]

This chapter has outlined how the CRPD sets forth a set of guiding principles and lays out specific State obligations for implementation. The Convention is now over a decade old, and governments should be implementing its provisions. In rejecting the caveats of previous mental illness-specific texts and the hesitancy of previous human rights instruments, the CRPD represents the political coming of age of the disability rights movement, of which people with psychosocial disabilities, users, ex-users, and survivors of psychiatry are part. The inclusion of the right to health, the right to live in the community, and the right to legal capacity, each without discrimination on the basis of disability, is a step change in international law. Community mental health practitioners have a crucial role to play in being part of the implementation initiatives, as well as holding the State accountable for progressing its obligations to respect, protect, and fulfil 'the equal right of all persons with disabilities to live in the community, with choices equal to others'.[79] It is a core right for all human beings and it is an invitation for community mental health practitioners to advocate for, and be, the change.

FURTHER READING

Bantekas, I., Stein, M., & Anastasiou, D. (2018). *The UN Convention on the Rights of Persons with Disabilities.* Oxford: Oxford University Press. [A detailed exploration of all elements of the CRPD. Meticulously referenced, but not an introductory text!]

Schulze, M. (2010). *Understanding the UN Convention on the Rights of Persons with Disabilities.* New York: Handicap International. https://www.ebookmakes.com/pdf/understanding-the-un-convention-on-the-rights-of-persons-with-disabilities-a-handbook-on-the-human-rights-of-persons-with-disabilities/ [A piece-by-piece introduction to the CRPD, and how it fits with the rest of international law.]

Szmukler, G. (2017). The UN Convention on the Rights of Persons with Disabilities: 'rights, will and preferences' in relation to mental health disabilities. *International Journal of Law and Psychiatry,* **54**, 90–97. [A thoughtful exploration of the tensions in CRPD implementation.]

World Health Organization (2021). Guidance on community mental health services: promoting person-centred and rights-based approaches. https://www.who.int/publications/i/item/9789240025707

World Health Organization (n.d.). QualityRights e-training on mental health. https://www.who.int/teams/mental-health-and-substance-use/policy-law-rights/qr-e-training

---

[74] See preambulatory paragraph (x) of the CRPD which states that 'the family is the natural and fundamental group unit of society and is entitled to protection by society and the State, and that persons with disabilities and their family members should receive the necessary protection and assistance to enable families to contribute towards the full and equal enjoyment of the rights of persons with disabilities'.

[75] Available online at https://www.who.int/publications/i/item/9789240025707

[76] Available online at https://www.who.int/teams/mental-health-and-substance-use/policy-law-rights/qr-e-training

[77] See CRPD perambulatory para. (o) as well as Art. 4(3).

[78] See CRPD, Art. 32 on international cooperation.

[79] CRPD, Art. 19.

REFERENCES

Bartlett, P. (2020). At the interface between paradigms: English mental capacity law and the CRPD. *Frontiers in Psychiatry*, **11**, 570735.

de Beco, G., Quinlivan, S., & Lord, J. E. (Eds.) (2019). *The Right to Inclusive Education in International Human Rights Law* (Cambridge Disability Law and Policy). Cambridge: Cambridge University Press.

Lewis, O. & Pathare, S. (2020). Chronic illness, disability and mental health. In: Gostin, L. & Meier, B. (Eds.), Foundations of Global Health and Human Rights, Oxford: Oxford University Press.

Oliver O. & Richardson, G. (2020). The right to live independently and be included in the community. International Journal of Law and Psychiatry, **69**, 101499.

Newton-Howes, G. (2019). Do community treatment orders in psychiatry stand up to principalism: considerations reflected through the prism of the Convention on the Rights of Persons with Disabilities. Journal of Law, Medicine & Ethics, **47**, 126–133.

Smith, A. (2021). Britney Spears conservatorship: the human rights perspective. *Human Rights Pulse*, 27 October. https://www.humanrightspulse.com/mastercontentblog/britney-spears-conservatorship-the-human-rights-perspective

UN Press Release (2009). Secretary General hails adoption of landmark convention on rights of people with disabilities. UN Press Release, 13 December, ref: SG/SM/10797, HR/4911, L/T/4400.

Treatment pressures, coercion, and compulsion

George Szmukler and Paul S. Appelbaum

Introduction

In the last half of the twentieth century and beginning of the twenty-first century, psychiatrists and other mental health clinicians became increasingly sensitive to the effects and implications of treatment that was not fully consensual. The number of psychiatric inpatients declined in many countries by more than two-thirds during that period. Many have tightened their procedures and standards for involuntary commitment (Appelbaum, 1997; Dressing & Salize, 2004). Mental health systems have generally worked harder to protect patients' liberty interests, and to avoid circumstances in which non-consensual treatment occurs.

Nonetheless, the nature of mental illness—with patients frequently manifesting denial of the need for care—and the public's concerns about the propensity of mentally ill persons to injure others or themselves, will probably make it impossible for non-consensual treatment ever to be abandoned completely. Indeed, with the movement to community care, new mechanisms for exerting pressures on patients have developed in services such as assertive community treatment (Stein & Santos, 1998). A major focus of assertive community treatment—usually targeted at persons with chronic mental illness who are considered likely to drift away from care—is to prevent defaulting from treatment, since loss of contact is likely to lead to relapse and readmission to hospital. Treatment is brought assertively *to* the patient making disengagement difficult. 'Compliance' or 'adherence' with medication is often a central issue. In the background also remains the possibility of compulsory admission to hospital.

This chapter has three aims:

1. To outline a spectrum of treatment pressures in contemporary practice, drawing ethically relevant distinctions between them
2. To consider when the exercise of such treatment pressures can be justified
3. To suggest approaches aimed at reducing the need for treatment pressures in community mental health services.

A range of treatment pressures

The term 'coercion' is often used almost synonymously with pressures exerted by one person (or organization) on another with the intention of making the latter act in accordance with the wishes of the former. We prefer to use the less moralized term 'treatment pressures'; as we shall see, 'coercion' is best applied to specific types of pressure. Within the concept of 'treatment pressures' we cover the whole range of interventions aimed at inducing patients to accept treatment which they have initially declined or seem likely to decline. We seek to identify morally relevant distinctions within the range of treatment pressures. We are only considering treatment pressures involving mental health professionals, not pressures exerted by family and friends.

Here, we attempt to build on our earlier work (Szmukler & Appelbaum, 2008), to outline a hierarchy of pressures for which commensurate justifications must be provided. Our spectrum of pressures is as follows:

- Persuasion
- Interpersonal leverage
- Inducements
- Threats
- Compulsory treatment (in the community or as an inpatient).

Persuasion

Least problematic is *persuasion*, an appeal to reason. The discussion revolves around an appraisal of the benefits and risks of treatment based on the evidence and the patient's life situation. There is a respect for the patient's arguments. The process does not go beyond a debate.

Interpersonal leverage

Since the clinician (key worker, case manager), especially in assertive community treatment programmes, may have established a relationship with the patient broader in scope and more intimate than a traditional patient–clinician relationship, opportunities for other kinds of pressure arise. Key workers engage with patients in their ordinary community settings to help with many basic skills, for example, budgeting, shopping, cleaning. The key worker may act as an advocate in accessing a range of community services. The patient may develop a significant degree of emotional dependency, enabling the exercise of *interpersonal leverage*. The patient may wish to please someone who has proved helpful or agree to a clinician's proposal in reaction to the clinician's disappointment when a treatment suggestion is rejected.

Inducement and threat

The next level of pressure arises with the introduction of conditional 'if … then' propositions. *If* the patient accepts treatment A, *then* the clinician will do X; or *if* the patient does not accept treatment A, the clinician will do Y. At this point, application of the term *coercion* is likely to be considered. A helpful account by Wertheimer (1987) argues that *threats* coerce but *offers* generally do not:

> The crux of the distinction between threats and offers is that A makes a threat when B will be worse off than in some relevant baseline position if B does not accept A's proposal, but that A makes an offer when B will be no worse off than in some relevant baseline position if B does not accept A's proposal. (p. 204)

Therefore, the key to what counts as a coercive proposal is to properly fix the *baseline*. Wertheimer favours a '*moral baseline*' and gives an example to clarify this concept: A comes upon B who is drowning. A proposes to rescue B on condition that B pays A a large sum of money. There are no other potential rescuers. Has A made a threat or an offer? The answer depends on where we set the baseline. Under a moral test, the key issue is whether A is *morally required* (ought) to rescue B (or whether B has a *right* to be rescued by A). If A is morally required to rescue B, then B's baseline includes a right to be saved by A. A's proposal is therefore a threat. On the other hand, if A is not morally required to rescue B, then A's proposal is an offer.

A threat thus anticipates making the recipient worse off according to the proposed moral baseline, while an offer—even if declined—typically does not. Threatening to remove something to which the subject is *entitled* (e.g. a housing benefit determined by legal decree; assistance with an application for a disability living allowance) makes the subject worse off if they do not accede. An offer of something which is not an entitlement but is in the nature of extra assistance (e.g. the offer of an introduction to a sympathetic second-hand furniture dealer who gives special discounts) made on condition that the patient complies with the treatment would, if rejected, not make the patient worse off compared with the relevant moral baseline—what their position would have been if the offer had never been made. Conditional access to monetary benefits (statutory entitlements), as occurs when some patients in the US have a 'representative payee' under Supplemental Security Income/Social Security Disability Insurance who only gives the patients their benefits when they comply with treatment, is on this account coercive (Elbogen et al., 2003). When it is proposed to a mentally ill person before a Mental Health Court that the usual custodial sentence will be suspended if the person accepts treatment (Goodale et al., 2013), this is an offer. If rejected by the person, they are no worse off than if the offer were never made—a custodial sentence is the standard punishment (Steadman et al., 2001).

Baselines other than 'moral' have been proposed. A 'legal' baseline has been proposed by Bonnie and Monahan (2005). This is more easily defined than a 'moral' baseline, but has the disadvantage of relativity—even in a single country, if it should have different legislatures governing some domains.

A variety of other interventions have been documented in community mental health that may fall along the inducements/threats spectrum. These include access to housing (Robbins et al., 2006), visitation for non-custodial parents or rights to custody (Busch & Redlich, 2007), and release from or avoidance of confinement via probation or parole (Skeem et al., 2006). All may be conditioned on adherence to treatment recommendations, including avoidance of intoxicating substances.

Allied to threats is *deception*. Failing to correct a patient's misconception about the consequences of not accepting treatment may be coercive. Some outpatient commitment orders may depend for their effectiveness on a patient's misapprehension that transgression of the order will result in rehospitalization or enforced treatment, though it may only permit conveying to a treatment facility or an assessment for compulsory inpatient treatment.

In our hierarchy of pressures, we thus place *offers* (or inducements) before *threats*. Only the latter would count as *coercive*, as would presumably the exercise of compulsion in treatment described below.

Acts which resemble 'coercion': 'exploitation' and 'unwelcome predictions'

A distinction can be made between a coercive threat and exploitation (Rhodes, 2000; Wertheimer, 1987, 1996). Exploitation involves an offer that nevertheless takes unfair advantage of a person in a difficult predicament. Rhodes considers the example of a homeless person in a cold climate who is offered a warm apartment but at a very high rent. The threat is a 'background threat', and not of the landlord's doing. The key issue is the moral baseline. On Wertheimer's account, exploitation, while often morally questionable, is not 'coercive'. Is it the person's 'right' in this example to be offered a room at a 'fair' rent? Most would say no. Further, exploitative offers, in some sense, expand possibilities for the recipient; if the offer is not accepted, the person is no worse off than they would have been if the offer had not been made. Both the exploiter and the person exploited can derive advantage from an exploitative offer (a warm room for the former and a larger income for the latter). The harm lies in taking *unfair advantage* of a person who is at a disadvantage.

If a clinician were to say to a patient that stopping medication will result in involuntary admission to hospital, a distinction can be drawn between this being an *unwelcome prediction*—a statement of fact, over which the clinician has no control—or a threat. Much depends on the factual basis of the prediction; the past history may indicate repeated similar instances that have resulted in a compulsory admission. Whether the clinician will be an instigator of the event is also relevant. A prediction of an unwelcome event, based on sound evidence, would not be considered 'coercive'. However, a clear line between a threat and an unwelcome prediction may be difficult to draw in practice.

Problematic inducements

Inducements can be problematic. The lure of an offer may be so powerful an inducement that the patient is no longer able to engage in a rational process of weighing the risks and benefits of a decision. An example of a potentially problematic inducement is a proposal to pay non-compliant patients with a psychosis to accept treatment (Claassen, 2007). It has been argued that it is an offer and therefore not 'coercive'. Yet the results of a survey of clinicians in the UK revealed a widely held intuition that the practice is unethical (Claassen, 2007). There may be a number of explanations for this. First, the transaction involves an exchange of 'goods' involving what might be seen as 'incommensurable values', that is, values that cannot be measured on a single metric, one good being in a higher, and thus separate, domain than the other. Selling a child is a stark example. Such an exchange corrupts or degrades the higher value. In paying patients to take medication, money could be seen as being exchanged for an aspect of respect for the person—that is, there is a failure to respect a patient's agency in deciding what is in their best interests (assuming the patient has capacity). Further, placing the 'goods' of money versus an aspect of human flourishing on the same metric degrades or corrupts the value of the latter. Second, there may be a possibility of exploitation. It is the patient's vulnerability, psychological or material—often both—which would induce an acceptance of the offer. As noted above, in exploitation one party gains unfairly at the expense of the one who is exploited (even though the exploited may still derive some gain) (Mayer, 2007). Who gains here? A significant motive for monetary inducements may be to reduce costs to the health service by preventing relapse and rehospitalization, although there may also be benefit to a patient who is induced to be compliant and thus avoids relapse. Third, there is an issue concerning the fairness of paying non-treatment-adherent patients but not treatment-adherent patients. There is also a range of other problems—for example, ensuring treatment adherence actually occurs, and how possible it would be in practice for payment to be terminated. While inducements may in the wider society be less coercive than threats, in the special setting of mental healthcare, their failure to respect a patient's agency, often already undermined through their marginalization in society, raises the need for special attention when their use is being considered (for a more detailed discussion of the issues see Szmukler, 2009, 2019).

Compulsion

Next in our hierarchy of pressures is *compulsion* (backed up by legally authorized force). As the locus of treatment has shifted to the community and concerns about non-adherence to treatment have grown, a number of jurisdictions have introduced *outpatient commitment* orders. Three major types can be discerned:

1. As a substitute for hospital admission: the outpatient commitment order is considered a less restrictive alternative to compulsory inpatient admission when alternatives to compulsory treatment have been exhausted.
2. To facilitate earlier discharge from hospital (a form of conditional discharge): although the patient may not be well enough for full discharge and requires continued treatment under compulsion, this can be obtained in the community as a less restrictive alternative to the hospital.
3. To prevent relapse: this type of order is applied where there is a proven history of relapse secondary to discontinuation of treatment, usually medication, and relapse is believed to be associated with significant risk to the patient or others.

Outpatient commitment orders carry varying powers (Dawson, 2005). Some allow recall of the patient for compulsory treatment as an inpatient. Others are limited to forced medication 'in the community', usually achieved by conveying the patient to a clinic where an injection is administered. Still others only permit non-compliant patients to be brought involuntarily to a clinic to be subject to persuasion, leverage, inducements, or threats; coercive treatment per se is not authorized. (This is typically the situation in the US, although there is some variation among the states (Appelbaum, 2001).) Outpatient commitment orders also vary in the range of conditions attached to the order (e.g. specification of clinician, clinic, frequency of reviews, treatments, residence) and their duration (Dawson, 2005).

Finally, there is the option of *compulsory admission to hospital*.

Objective and subjective 'coercion'

An important dimension in thinking about treatment pressures, including coercion, involves the distinction between 'objective' and 'subjective' aspects (Hiday, 1992; Hoge et al., 1997; Lidz et al., 1995). The subjective experience of feeling coerced may not follow an 'objective' schema such as the one outlined above. Indeed, the results of studies of patients' perceived coercion can seem counterintuitive. Involuntary as opposed to voluntary hospitalization does not necessarily predict subjective coercion at the individual patient level, nor does being placed on outpatient commitment compared with receiving voluntary outpatient services (Swartz et al., 2009). Patients' perceptions of how fairly they have been treated and the motives of decision-makers may be more influential in their subjective sense of coercion than actual legal status. From the patient's perspective, this may be the most important issue in coercion. Approaches to reducing the need for coercion (discussed below) may also be effective in minimizing subjective coercion.

However, for the clinician seeking to act ethically in pressing a reluctant patient to accept treatment, morally relevant distinctions of an 'objective' kind can be helpful in making justifiable decisions. The hierarchy we have outlined is an attempt to meet this need, but it will require adjustment to take account of a particular patient's preferences and values. Within the domain of *compulsory treatment* there may be variations in restrictions on autonomy or choice, as well as of the subjective experience of constraint.

Justifications for exercising treatment pressures

Two types of justification are usually offered for applying treatment pressures on a patient who declines:

1. Treatment is in the patient's 'best interests' (or 'health or safety'), or
2. Treatment is needed for the protection of others.

If a hierarchy of treatment pressures on reluctant patients is defined as above, then one would ask for a stronger justification the more coercive the pressure to be exerted:

Justification in the best interests of the patient

Before the focus on treatment in the community, the major form of treatment pressure revolved around compulsory treatment in hospital, or its threat. Criteria for involuntary admission embodied in mental health legislation generally rely, at least in part, on evidence of substantial dangers to the patient's health or safety. In the community, however, a wider spectrum of risks or degrees of danger is identified by professionals in closer proximity to the daily lives of their patients. They may suffer from physical disorders that require treatment they are incapable of seeking. A hard-won tenancy may be jeopardized by the patient's failure to take care of an apartment. Significant supportive relationships may be on the verge of breaking down. Criteria of the type set down in mental health legislation governing involuntary hospitalization are simply not sensitive to the broader range of 'risk' encountered in community settings. Nor are they sensitive to 'values' differences in the complex multicultural societies of today, and their role in determining what might be in a person's 'best interests'.

Linking justifications for treatment pressures in the spectrum outlined above to the continuum of risks seen in the community thus requires a broader, more comprehensive ethical framework. It must be able to deal with questions of 'value'.

We outline two 'best interests' frameworks, one deriving from an analysis of decision-making capacity (or mental competence), the other from an analysis of 'paternalistic' actions (Gert et al., 2006). The former framework is more commonly invoked and may appear in mental health law.

A framework based on 'capacity' and 'best interests'

'Mental incapacity' is assuming an increasing emphasis in justifying interventions against a patient's will, in psychiatry as well as in general medicine where it has been long established (Dawson & Szmukler, 2006; Grisso & Appelbaum, 1998). As for physical disorders, it is difficult in psychiatry to argue for treatment against a person's wishes unless that person lacks the capacity (or 'competence', used by us synonymously) to make treatment decisions for themselves. Definitions of decision-making capacity vary, but common elements are the ability to understand and retain information relevant to the decision (including the consequences of deciding one way or the other), and the ability to use that information to make a decision. The latter includes the ability to 'appreciate' that the information applies to the patient's predicament, the ability to reason with that information, and the ability to exercise a choice (Grisso & Appelbaum, 1998; Legislation.gov.uk, 2005).

Only if the patient lacks capacity would treatment against a patient's wishes be considered (so-called soft paternalism); but a further test must also be passed—that treatment is in the patient's 'best interests'. Definitions of 'best interests' are difficult, but the UK Law Commission (1995) proposed practical guidance for deciding on the matter, now incorporated in the Mental Capacity Act 2005 (Legislation.gov.uk, 2005). Included, for example, is that regard should be given to the following:

The assessor must:

- so far as reasonably practicable, permit and encourage the person to participate, or to improve their ability to participate, as fully as possible
- consider as far as is reasonably ascertainable: (1) the person's past and present wishes and feelings (and any relevant written statements made with capacity); (2) the person's beliefs and values that would be likely to influence their decision if they had capacity; and (3) other factors that they would be likely to consider if they were able to do so
- take into account, if practicable and appropriate, the views of: (1) anyone named by the person to be consulted; (2) anyone caring for the person or interested in their welfare; (3) any done of a lasting power of attorney; and (4) any deputy appointed by the court—as to what would be in the person's best interests and, in particular the matters mentioned above
- consider whether the purpose for which any action or decision is required can be as effectively achieved in a manner less restrictive of the person's freedom of action.

A framework based on 'paternalism'

Gert et al. (2006) propose that a person is acting paternalistically towards another if their action benefits the other; their action involves violating a moral rule with regard to the other; and their action does not have the other's past, present, or immediately forthcoming consent. Their approach to 'paternalistic' actions may be helpful. In justifying a paternalistic act, a series of pertinent questions can elicit the 'morally relevant facts':

1. What are the moral rules that would be violated if the clinician were to act against the patient's wishes (e.g. limiting freedom of choice, causing psychological pain)?
2. What are the harms thus perpetrated on the patient and for how long will they last?
3. What is the seriousness of the harms to be avoided through the paternalistic intervention (e.g. death, disability, and worsening of the psychiatric disorder), and what is their likelihood?
4. What are the relevant beliefs and desires of the person toward whom a rule is being violated (e.g. religious beliefs)?
5. Are there any alternative actions that would be preferable?

Based on these facts, further questions come into play:

6. How does the clinician rank the two sets of harms compared to the patient?
7. Is the patient's preference when comparing the harms to be avoided with the harms to be incurred, irrational—that is, does the patient have a rational reason to prefer an outcome with apparently greater harms?
8. Can the clinician advocate publicly for their ranking of the harms to be perpetrated compared to those to be avoided? Would most rational people agree that this kind of moral violation should in such circumstances be universally allowed?

A decision to exercise a specific treatment pressure in a specific circumstance would depend on a balance informed by the answers to these questions, although no algorithm exists to allow these determinations to be made in a rigorous (or possibly even replicable) way.

Whatever framework is adopted, we insist that if community mental health teams are to exercise their powers to intervene in patients' lives in an ethical manner, an appropriate framework is required. Professionals should be as well versed in using such a framework as they are in assessing 'technical' problems, for example, the likely benefits of interventions such as medication or psychological treatments.

The application of a framework such as one described above suggests that the degree of pressure to be used should be the minimum necessary, and that the justification should be stronger the more one moves along the spectrum from persuasion to direct force.

These principles should also be considered in relation to involuntary outpatient commitment. As discussed above, blunt criteria similar to those used in mental health legislation are difficult to apply when a wide spectrum of risk is identified by professionals in close and frequent contact with patients in the community. If outpatient commitment is an alternative to admission to hospital or is used to facilitate earlier discharge, criteria for terminating the order are essential. The criteria could be based on one of the frameworks above, for example, recovery of capacity to make treatment decisions or the compulsory treatment no longer being in the best interests of the patient.

United Nations Convention on the Rights of Persons with Disabilities

At this point we must draw attention to a significant change, regarded by some as a 'paradigm shift', in the legal landscape in respect of coercive interventions in mental healthcare. The United Nations Convention on the Rights of Persons with Disabilities (CRPD), adopted in 2006, is the most recent stipulation, specifically tailored, of the rights of persons with disabilities, based on the principles of human dignity, equality, non-discrimination, autonomy, and social participation and inclusion (United Nations, 2006). It requires that persons with a disability be treated on an 'equal basis with others'. Most authorities accept that persons with a mental disorder treated within the mental health system are considered to have a disability under the CRPD.

Interpretations issued by the United Nations Committee set up to monitor the implementation of the Convention insist that non-consensual treatment of people with mental health (or 'psychosocial') disabilities is a violation of the treaty (United Nations, 2014). It states that support in the exercise of legal capacity must respect the 'rights, will and preferences' of persons with disabilities and should never amount to 'substitute decision-making'—that is, a decision made by another person in the place of the person with a disability (not appointed by the person, done against their will, and not based on their own 'will and preferences'). The Committee claims that with appropriate support (that the Convention obliges States to provide), people with disabilities will be able to express their 'will and preferences'. Where this may prove difficult, the Committee states that one should aim for a 'best interpretation' of the person's 'will and preferences', consulting those who know the person. The Committee proposes, even where there is a risk to the person or to others in association with a disability, coercive measures are nevertheless in breach of the Convention. This 'authoritative' (but not considered in international law 'legally binding') interpretation of the CRPD has been contested vigorously (Appelbaum, 2019; Dawson, 2015; Freeman et al., 2015).

Nevertheless, the CRPD challenges us to think again about justifications for coercive interventions. By examining the meaning of the terms 'will' and 'preference', one of us has argued there may be a place under the CRPD for non-consensual treatment when a person's 'preferences'—as expressed in treatment choices in the moment—seriously contradict the person's 'will'—manifest in the person's deeply held and generally stable beliefs, values, commitments, or conception of the good (Szmukler, 2019). An 'advance directive' provides a clear model of this construction. The person's 'will', expressed when well, leads to an instruction that a 'preference' predicted to be expressed at a future time when the person is ill and which is incongruent with the 'will', should not be respected. This construction may also be helpful in cases where the determination of decision-making capacity and best interests is difficult. In assessing the person's ability to 'appreciate' and 'reason' with the information provided by the clinician, a significant disjunction between the person's 'will' and a currently expressed 'preference'—one which seriously threatens the 'will'—may point, first, to an impairment of decision-making capacity, and second, to what would constitute an intervention in the person's 'best interests'—essentially one aiming to facilitate or give effect to the person's 'will' (their deeply held values and commitments).

Justification based on protection of others

'Protection of others' is a common criterion for involuntary hospitalization, and generally also for outpatient commitment. However, in a community setting, the definition of risk to others is in danger of expansion; just as there is a spectrum of risk to the well-being of the patient, so is there one for risk to others. In a climate of concern that the safety of the public is threatened, pressures from community members to intervene may intensify. Patients may become subject to treatment pressures under a potentially broad interpretation of the 'protection of others'.

The 'protection of others' is often confused with health interests. However, they are conceptually distinct (Culver & Gert, 1982). When others seek authority to determine what is in a patient's best interests, the legitimacy of their request depends on the patient's lack of capacity to make decisions about the patient's welfare or health. In contrast, the protection of others does not turn on capacity, but on factors such as the risk of harm and its seriousness.

Viewed thus, the fact that 'preventive' detention on the grounds of risk of harm to others is generally restricted only to those with a mental disorder is difficult to defend, although the likelihood of personal benefit from the intervention is often invoked. The likelihood of serious violence is higher in many more non-mentally disordered persons, for example, those who regularly become assaultive when intoxicated or who habitually perpetrate domestic violence. Yet we do not force preventive interventions on such persons before they have been convicted of an offence. It has been argued that separate generic 'dangerousness' legislation would be the most appropriate measure for preventing violence if that is deemed a significant societal goal (Campbell & Heginbotham, 1991; Szmukler & Holloway, 1998), though such law would be unacceptable in most liberal societies and a violation of many human rights conventions or charters.

Predicting serious violence is also subject to a major limitation that carries significant ethical implications. Incidents of serious violence by persons with a mental disorder are rare. The prediction of rare events inherently lacks accuracy. The very best predictive instruments available, even when tested in research settings, have a false-positive rate of well over 90% if the base rate of serious violence is 1% in the patient population (Large & Nielssen, 2017; Szmukler, 2003). If the risk of violence were to lead to coercive interventions, the moral cost of unnecessarily infringing the liberty of a large number of patients to prevent harm by a few is very difficult to justify.

We are left with some thorny issues. Society demands a degree of social control from mental health services. As services move into the community and see at close quarters the lives of their patients and those around them, dilemmas around risk may become especially problematic. The potential for community mental health teams to expand activities directed at social control must be recognized. A dialogue between those advocating on behalf of patients with mental illness and a community often fearful of such persons is essential (and urgent) if abuses are to be avoided.

Implications for forensic services

The management of offenders with a mental disorder needs also to be considered. Offenders with a mental disorder are frequently subject to differential treatment when compared with 'non-disordered' offenders who have committed a similar offence. This may involve the duration of their deprivation of liberty when detained in a hospital on a court order and the nature and duration of their subsequent restrictions when discharged. The offender with a mental disorder is often subject to their order for much longer than the length of the usual sentence imposed on the non-disordered offender. This differential treatment is predicated on a presumed link between the mental disorder and the offence, with an assumption that effective control of the disorder and its symptoms will reduce the likelihood of reoffending. However, studies suggest that even among people with serious mental disorders, most acts of violence are not causally linked to the underlying disorder but arise from other sources (Skeem et al., 2016), calling into question this approach. Differential restrictions on offenders with mental disorders can be eliminated if the court order imposed on the offender were for a duration commensurate with the normal sentence for a similar offence with a similar degree of seriousness imposed on a non-disordered offender. If involuntary mental health care should still be warranted on expiration of the order, this would then need to be under a civil order. Such changes would to some extent accord with the CRPD's requirement that persons with a disability must be treated 'on an equal basis with others', though a disagreement about involuntary treatment would remain (Szmukler, 2020).

Reducing the need for treatment pressures

Services can employ a range of measures to reduce the need for exerting pressures on patients to accept treatment. Unfortunately, few of these have been evaluated formally.

Make services as acceptable and attractive to users as possible

Traditionally, mental health service users have had little say in how services ostensibly created to help them are implemented. For services to become more responsive to patients' needs, an active, not token, involvement of service users in their planning is required (Pilgrim & Waldron, 1998). Users can make crucial contributions as members of management committees where they ensure that discussion, service developments, and evaluations of quality and outcomes are seen from users', as well as providers' perspectives (Millar et al., 2016; Rose et al., 2003).

Enhance patients' involvement in planning their own care

Patients are likely to feel less coerced the more they play an active role in determining their treatment. Initiatives employing *advance statements* (Henderson et al., 2008b) have provided evidence that their use may reduce the need for 'coercive' interventions.

In the UK, 'crisis cards' originated as a service user/voluntary sector initiative to facilitate access to an advocate and to state patients' preferences for care during an emergency when they might be too unwell to express their wishes clearly (Sutherby & Szmukler, 1998). 'Crisis cards' have usually been drawn up by the patient alone, without discussion with the mental health team. They have not proved popular.

The idea of the 'crisis card' was developed into the *joint crisis plan* (JCP) (Sutherby et al., 1999). Here the content of the card, though still ultimately determined by the patient, is negotiated with the treatment team when the patient is able to make competent judgements about what is in their best interests. An important aspect of the JCP is the independent 'facilitator' whose role it is to make sure the patient's voice is heard.

Sutherby et al. (1999) reported on the introduction of crisis cards and JCPs in London. Participation was offered to patients with a psychotic illness at high risk of relapse. They chose to include a wide range of information including diagnosis, current treatment, contact information for carers and professionals, first signs of relapse and the preferred treatment, treatment preferences and refusals for established relapses, indications for admission, and practical requests (e.g. who should take care of domestic arrangements in case of admission). A majority of the patients reported feeling empowered in determining details of their care. Subsequently, a randomized controlled trial of JCPs involving 160 patients with a psychosis showed that by 15 months' follow-up, the rate of compulsory admissions was halved in the group completing JCPs (Henderson et al., 2004). Again, the effects of drawing up a JCP on patients' attitudes to treatment were, in the main, positive (Henderson et al., 2008a). Although a larger multicentre randomized controlled study in England involving 569 patients failed to find a significant reduction in compulsory admissions (Thornicroft et al., 2013), this was attributed to a lesser degree of service provider 'buy-in' across 64 mental health teams. However, a meta-analysis of all trials of JCPs found a significant reduction of involuntary admissions by 23% (de Jong et al., 2016).

Another form of 'advance statement' is a *psychiatric advance directive* (PAD). All states in the US permit advance directives to be written for health care in general (including psychiatric care), and 25 states have statutes creating specific provisions for psychiatric advance directives (National Resource Center on Psychiatric Advance Directives, 2021). Advance directives are in principle legally binding, although some PAD statutes stipulate that the patient's wishes may be overridden if they violate 'accepted standards of care'. How this should be interpreted is not clear (Appelbaum, 2004; Swanson et al., 2006). The directives in a PAD may be of three kinds: first, specified treatments that are refused or requested; second, statements about personal values, attitudes, or general preferences that may be used as a guide for those making decisions about treatment; and third, nomination of a person to act a 'substitute' or 'proxy' decision-maker. PAD statutes presume that the patient had decision-making capacity when a PAD was made, in the absence of evidence to the contrary, and their utility is predicated on the assumption that the circumstances in which the PAD is triggered are those that were anticipated.

A variant of the PAD process, termed a *facilitated PAD* (F-PAD), has been introduced following research revealing a low incidence of patients who say they desire a PAD actually completing one. Practical complexities in their execution may act as deterrents to their adoption. In an F-PAD process, a trained facilitator explains what a PAD involves and, if the patient chooses to opt for one, assists with its completion (Swanson et al., 2006b). The service provider may also be asked to become involved.

A randomized controlled study of F-PADs has indeed shown that facilitation results in a highly significant increase in the number of patients who decide to formulate a PAD (61% vs 3% of controls). At 1-month follow-up, those with an F-PAD reported a much better working alliance with their clinicians and were more likely to say that they received the services they needed (Swanson et al., 2006b). The number of 'coercive interventions' over the succeeding 2 years for those who completed a PAD was considerably fewer compared to patients who did not (Swanson et al., 2008), including for those patients who had suffered a loss of capacity during the crisis.

Thus, there is emerging evidence that some forms of 'advance statement' could significantly reduce the number of situations in which clinicians need to act against a patient's competent preferences. Many of the ethical dilemmas discussed above occur precisely at such times of crisis. Independent facilitation, either in a JCP or an F-PAD, may be a critical factor. However, for reasons that may relate to lack of information, absence of support, and hesitance of clinicians, PADs have not been widely adopted in practice (Swartz et al., 2021).

Use approaches to reduce levels of perceived coercion

Applying the principles derived from studies such as the MacArthur Foundation-funded coercion project (Hoge et al., 1997; Lidz et al., 1995), though so far untested, may reduce the need for actual coercion as well as patients' 'perceived' coercion. Where situations with the potential for coercive interactions arise, principles of 'procedural justice' can be borne in mind—treating the patient with respect and fairness, giving them a 'voice' and taking seriously what is said, and avoiding 'negative pressures' such as threats or force.

Use pressure or coercion only when it is necessary

Using pressures or coercive measures on patients only when justified and to a degree commensurate with the risks to the patient's best interests should minimize their use. The multidisciplinary team is an invaluable resource for ethical decision-making of this kind since the impact of proposed interventions on the values at stake can be tested across a range of team members' perspectives. The views of informal and other formal caregivers should also be considered.

Conclusion

The scope for exerting pressures for treatment on reluctant patients is probably as great in the modern era of community care as it ever was. New forms exist, while ways of thinking about compulsory treatment hallowed by time and convention are not adequate to deal with the subtle gradations of risk and distinctions among interventions relevant to community psychiatry. We strongly suggest that being adept at using an ethical framework for deciding when a specific treatment pressure is justified should be a core skill of members of community mental health teams. If community mental health services are to flourish within complex, multicultural, and ever-changing societies, they will need to rest on sound ethical foundations. The history of psychiatry, an enterprise in which questions of value are always to the fore, shows that a swing of the moral pendulum is never far away (Appelbaum, 1994).

REFERENCES

Appelbaum, P. S. (1991). Advance directives for psychiatric treatment. *Hospital and Community Psychiatry*, **42**, 983–984.

Appelbaum, P. S. (1994). *Almost a Revolution: Mental Health Law and the Limits of Change*. New York: Oxford University Press.

Appelbaum, P. S. (1997). Almost a revolution: an international perspective on the law of involuntary commitment. *Journal of American Academy of Psychiatry and the Law*, **25**, 135–148.

Appelbaum, P. S. (2001). Thinking carefully about outpatient commitment. *Psychiatric Services*, **52**, 347–350.

Appelbaum, P. S. (2004). Law and psychiatry: psychiatric advance directives and the treatment of committed patients. *Psychiatric Services*, **55**, 751–752.

Appelbaum, P. S. (2019). Saving the UN Convention on the Rights of Persons with Disabilities—from itself. *World Psychiatry*, **18**, 1–2.

Bonnie, R. J. & Monahan, J. (2005). From coercion to contract: reframing the debate on mandated community treatment for people with mental disorders. *Law and Human Behavior*, **29**, 485–503.

Busch, A. & Redlich, A. (2007). Patients' perception of possible child custody or visitation loss if not adherent to psychiatric treatment. *Psychiatric Services*, **58**, 999–1002.

Campbell, T. & Heginbotham, C. (1991). *Mental illness: Prejudice, Discrimination and the Law*. Aldershot: Dartmouth.

Claassen, D. (2007). Financial incentives for antipsychotic depot medication: ethical issues. *Journal of Medical Ethics*, **33**, 189–193.

Claassen, D., Fakhoury, W., Ford, R., & Priebe, S. (2007). Money for medication—financial incentives to improve medication adherence in Assertive Outreach patients. *Psychiatric Bulletin*, **31**, 4–7.

Culver, C. N. & Gert, B. (1982). *Philosophy in Medicine: Conceptual and Ethical Issues in Medicine and Psychiatry*. Oxford: Oxford University Press.

Dawson, J. (2005). *Community Treatment Orders: International Comparisons*. Dunedin: Otago University Press.

Dawson, J. (2015). A realistic approach to assessing mental health laws' compliance with the UNCRPD. *International Journal of Law and Psychiatry*, **40**, 70–79.

Dawson, J. & Szmukler, G. (2006). Fusion of mental health and incapacity legislation. *British Journal of Psychiatry*, **188**, 504–509.

de Jong, M. H., Kamperman, A. M., Oorschot, M., Priebe, S., Bramer, W., van de Sande, R., et al. (2016). Interventions to reduce compulsory psychiatric admissions: a systematic review and meta-analysis. *JAMA Psychiatry*, **73**, 657–664.

Dressing, H. & Salize, H. J. (2004). Compulsory admission of mentally ill patients in European member states. *Social Psychiatry and Psychiatric Epidemiology*, **39**, 797–803.

Elbogen, E., Swanson, J., Swartz, M., & Wagner, H. (2003). Characteristics of third-party money management for persons with psychiatric disabilities. *Psychiatric Services*, **54**, 1136–1141.

Freeman, M. C., Kolappa, K., de Almeida, J. M., Kleinman, A., Makhashvili, N., Phakathi, S., et al. (2015). Reversing hard won victories in the name of human rights: a critique of the General Comment on Article 12 of the UN Convention on the Rights of Persons with Disabilities. *Lancet Psychiatry*, **2**, 844–850.

Gert, B., Culver, C. M., & Clouser, K. D. (2006). *Bioethics: A Systematic Approach* (2nd ed.). New York: Oxford University Press.

Goodale, G., Callahan, L., & Steadman, H. G. (2013). What can we say about mental health courts today? *Psychiatric Services*, **64**, 298–300.

Grisso, T. & Appelbaum, PS. (1998). *Assessing Competence to Consent to Treatment: A Guide for Physicians and Other Health Professionals*. New York: Oxford University Press.

Henderson, C., Flood, C., Leese, M., Thornicroft, G., Sutherby, K., & Szmuckler, G. (2004). Effect of joint crisis plans on use of compulsory treatment in psychiatry: single blind randomised controlled trial. *BMJ*, **329**, 136.

Henderson, C., Flood, C., Leese, M., Thornicroft, G., Sutherby, K., & Szmukler, G. (2008a). Views of service users and providers on joint crisis plans: single blind randomized controlled trial. *Social Psychiatry and Psychiatric Epidemiology*, **44**, 369–376.

Henderson, C., Swanson, J. W., Szmukler, G., Thornicroft, G., & Zinkler, M. (2008b). A typology of advance statements in mental health care. *Psychiatric Services*, **59**, 63–71.

Hiday, V. A. (1992). Coercion in civil commitment: process, preferences, and outcome. *International Journal of Law & Psychiatry*, **15**, 359–377.

Hoge, S. K., Lidz, C. W., Eisenberg, M., Gardner, W., Monahan, J., Mulvey, E. P., et al. (1997). Perceptions of coercion in the admission of voluntary and involuntary psychiatric patients. *International Journal of Law & Psychiatry*, **20**, 167–181.

Large, M. & Nielssen, O. (2017). The limitations and future of violence risk assessment. *World Psychiatry*, **16**, 25–26.

Law Commission (1995). *Mental Incapacity* (Report No. 231). London: HMSO.

Legislation.gov.uk (2005). Mental Capacity Act 2005. https://www.legislation.gov.uk/ukpga/2005/9/section/3

Lidz, C., Hoge, S., Gardner, W., Bennett, N., Monahan, J., Mulvey, E., et al. (1995). Perceived coercion in mental hospital admission: pressures and process. *Archives of General Psychiatry*, **52**, 1034–1039.

Mayer, R. (2007). What's wrong with exploitation. *Journal of Applied Philosophy*, **24**, 137–150.

Millar, S., Chambers, M., & Giles, M. (2016). Service user involvement in mental health care: an evolutionary concept analysis. *Health Expectations*, **19**, 209–221.

National Resource Centre on Psychiatric Advance Directives (2021). State by state info. https://www.nrc-pad.org/states/

Pilgrim, D. & Waldron, L. (1998). User involvement in mental health service development: how far can it go? *Journal of Mental Health*, **7**, 95–104.

Robbins, P., Petrila, J., LeMelle, S., & Monahan, J. (2006). The use of housing as leverage to increase adherence to psychiatric treatment in the community. *Administration and Policy in Mental Health and Mental Health Services Research*, **33**, 226–236.

Rhodes, M. (2000). The nature of coercion. *Journal of Value Inquiry*, **34**, 369–381.

Rose, D., Fleischman, P., Tonkiss, F., Campbell, P., & Wykes, T. (2003). *User and Carer Involvement in Change Management in a Mental Health Context: Review of the Literature*. London: NHS Service Delivery and Organisation R&D Programme.

Skeem, J., Emke-Francis, P., & Eno Louden, J. (2006). Probation, mental health, and mandated treatment: a national survey. *Criminal Justice & Behavior*, **33**, 158–184.

Skeem, J., Kennealy, P., Monahan, J., Peterson, J., & Appelbaum, P.S. (2016). Psychosis uncommonly and inconsistently precedes violence among high-risk individuals. *Clinical Psychological Science*, **4**, 40–49.

Steadman, H., Davidson, S., & Brown, C. (2001). Mental health courts: their promise and unanswered questions. *Psychiatric Services*, **52**, 457–458.

Stein, L. I. & Santos, A. B. (1998). *Assertive Community Treatment of Persons with Severe Mental Illness*. New York: Norton.

Sutherby, K. & Szmukler, G. (1998). Crisis cards and self-help crisis initiatives. *Psychiatric Bulletin*, **22**, 4–7.

Sutherby, K., Szmukler, G. I., Halpern, A., Alexander, M., Thornicroft, G., Johnson, C., et al. (1999). A study of 'crisis cards' in a community psychiatric service. *Acta Psychiatrica Scandinavica*, **100**, 56–61.

Swanson, J. W., McCrary, S. V., Swartz, M. S., Elbogen, E. B., & Van Dorn, R. A. (2006a). Superseding psychiatric advance directives: ethical and legal considerations. *Journal of the American Academy of Psychiatry and the Law*, **34**, 385–394.

Swanson, J. W., Swartz, M. S., Elbogen, E. B., Van Dorn, R. A., Wagner, H. R., Moser, L. A., et al. (2006b). Facilitated psychiatric advance directives: a randomized trial of an intervention to foster advance treatment planning among persons with severe mental illness. *American Journal of Psychiatry*, **163**, 1943–1951.

Swanson, J. W., Swartz, M. S., Elbogen, E. B., Van Dorn, R. A., Wagner, H. R., Moser, L. A., et al. (2008). Psychiatric advance directives and reduction of coercive crisis interventions. *Journal of Mental Health*, **17**, 255–267.

Swartz, M. S., Swanson, J. W., Easter, M. M., & Robertson, A. G. (2021). Implementing psychiatric advance directives: the transmitter and receiver problem and the neglected right to be deemed incapable. *Psychiatric Services*, **72**, 219–221.

Swartz, M. S., Swanson, J. W., Steadman, H. J., Robbins, P. C., & Monahan, J. (2009). *New York State Assisted Outpatient Treatment Program Evaluation*. Durham, NC: Duke University School of Medicine. http://www.omh.state.ny.us/omhweb/resources/publications/aot_program_evaluation/index.html

Szmukler, G. (2003). Risk assessment: 'numbers' and 'values'. *Psychiatric Bulletin*, **27**, 205–207.

Szmukler, G. (2009). Financial incentives for patients in the treatment of psychosis. *Journal of Medical Ethics*, **35**, 224–228.

Szmukler, G. (2019). 'Capacity', 'best interests', 'will and preferences' and the UN Convention on the Rights of Persons with Disabilities. *World Psychiatry*, **18**, 34–41.

Szmukler, G. (2020). Offenders with a mental impairment under a 'fusion law': non-discrimination, treatment, public protection. *International Journal of Mental Health and Capacity Law*, **26**, 35–51.

Szmukler, G. & Appelbaum, P. S. (2008). Treatment pressures, leverage, coercion, and compulsion in mental health care. *Journal of Mental Health*, **17**, 233–244.

Szmukler, G. & Holloway, F. (1998). Mental health legislation is now a harmful anachronism. *Psychiatric Bulletin*, **22**, 662–665.

Thornicroft, G., Farrelly, S., Szmukler, G., Birchwood, M., Waheed, W., Flach, C., et al. (2013). Clinical outcomes of joint crisis plans to reduce compulsory treatment for people with psychosis: a randomised controlled trial. *Lancet*, **381**, 1634–1641.

United Nations (2006). Convention on the Rights of Persons with Disabilities. https://www.un.org/development/desa/disabilities/convention-on-the-rights-of-persons-with-disabilities/convention-on-the-rights-of-persons-with-disabilities-2.html

United Nations (2014). Committee on Convention on the Rights of Persons with Disabilities: general comment on article 12: equal recognition before the law. https://www.ohchr.org/en/documents/general-comments-and-recommendations/general-comment-no-1-article-12-equal-recognition-1

Wertheimer, A. (1987). *Coercion*. Princeton, NJ: Princeton University Press.

Wertheimer, A. (1996). *Exploitation*. Princeton, NJ: Princeton University Press.

SECTION 6
Stigma and discrimination

30. **Public knowledge and awareness about mental illnesses** *313*
    Anthony F. Jorm

31. **Reducing stigma and discriminatory behaviour** *321*
    Petra C. Gronholm, Dristy Gurung, Sarah J. Parry, Nisha Mehta, and Graham Thornicroft

Public knowledge and awareness about mental illnesses

Anthony F. Jorm

Introduction

For major physical health problems, like cancer and cardiovascular disease, members of the public typically have considerable knowledge about what they can do for prevention or early intervention, or have knowledge of treatments and services available. For example, in the area of cardiovascular disease, there is widespread knowledge about modifiable risk factors like smoking and exercise, people know the value of screening and treatment for hypertension and high cholesterol, many people have the first aid skills to apply cardiopulmonary resuscitation in an emergency, and some would know the warning signs of a stroke and the need to call an ambulance immediately.

Knowledge about mental disorders in the community has generally lagged behind that for major physical diseases. This is surprising given the high prevalence of mental disorders. Community surveys in many countries show high rates, with 1-year prevalence rates of 10–19% and lifetime prevalence rates of 18–36% being typical (Kessler et al., 2009). This high prevalence means that the whole population will either be personally affected by a mental disorder or have close contact with other people who are. Given the high exposure to mental disorders in the population, it can be argued that everyone needs some knowledge and skill to take action to improve community mental health.

The concept of mental health literacy

The term *mental health literacy* has been coined to draw attention to this neglected area. This is defined as 'knowledge and beliefs about mental disorders which aid their recognition, management or prevention' (Jorm et al., 1997, p. 182). Note that mental health literacy is more than just knowledge about mental disorders; rather, it is knowledge that a person can use to guide action to benefit their own mental health or that of others. As shown in **Figure 30.1**, there is a hypothesized link from mental health literacy to behaviours that benefit the mental health of oneself or others, and this behaviour change in turn leads to improved mental health.

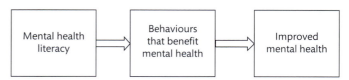

Figure 30.1 Hypothesized link from mental health literacy to behaviours that benefit mental health.

All of the following are examples of mental health literacy:

- Recognition of developing disorders which can guide early help-seeking
- Knowledge of the range of professional help and effective treatments available
- Knowledge of effective self-help strategies
- Knowledge and skills to access quality mental health information
- Knowledge and skills to give mental health first aid
- Knowledge of risk factors and causes that can be used to guide preventive action.

For people who have a mental disorder, mental health literacy would also involve knowledge and skills for self-management, while for family members it would also involve knowledge and skills of how to be a supportive caregiver. However, this chapter focuses on aspects of mental health literacy that apply to the community as a whole, rather than on those more appropriate to people who have a mental disorder or who provide family support to someone with a mental disorder.

Recognition of developing disorders which can guide early help-seeking

Community surveys of mental disorders show that many people do not get professional help. In developed countries, 36–50% of people with a mental disorder have not received treatment in the previous 12 months, while in less-developed countries the rate of non-treatment is 76–85% (WHO World Mental Health Consortium, 2004). Even when professional help is sought, there may be long delays. The length of delay typically varies with the type and severity of the disorder. For example, for anxiety disorders delays of many years are common (Christiana et al., 2000), whereas for psychotic disorders delays of months will be more typical (Howes et al., 2021).

Delays in recognition are important because early intervention with mental disorders may be associated with a better outcome. With psychotic disorders, many studies have shown that a longer duration of untreated psychosis is associated with worse outcome (Howes et al., 2021). There is also some evidence that duration of untreated depression is associated with worse outcomes (Ghio et al., 2014).

Delays in help-seeking are affected by the knowledge a person with a mental disorder has about recognition. For example, a study of people being treated for anxiety or mood disorders found an average delay of 8.2 years (Thompson et al., 2008). Most of this delay was due to a failure to recognize that the symptoms were due to a mental disorder. The average time to recognize the problem as a mental disorder was 6.9 years and it then took an average of 1.3 years between recognition and help-seeking.

Community surveys in many countries have shown that there are deficiencies in recognition of mental disorders. A typical methodology used in these surveys is to present a case vignette of a person with a mental disorder and ask the respondent what they think is wrong with the person. The results differ from country to country and may depend on local community awareness activities. For example, in Australia, 77% of adults applied the label 'depression' to a vignette of a person who was depressed and suicidal, compared to only 35% of the Japanese public (Jorm et al., 2005a). By contrast, the term 'stress' was applied more in Japan than in Australia. The conceptualization of the problem as a mental disorder versus a life problem can affect help-seeking preferences. For example, people who conceptualize the problem as 'depression' are less likely to think it is helpful to deal with the problem on one's own (Jorm et al., 2006b).

An additional factor contributing to under-recognition is that mental disorders often first develop during adolescence and early adulthood (Kessler et al., 2009). This is a period of life where the knowledge and experience of mental disorders may be less developed and assistance may be needed from family or other supporters to recognize the problem. When a young person recognizes a pattern of symptoms as a mental disorder, they are more likely to choose appropriate help and treatment (Wright et al., 2012). Furthermore, if a young person with a mental disorder attends an appointment with a general practitioner (GP), the GP is more likely to detect it if the young person conceptualizes their problem as a mental disorder (Haller et al., 2009).

While early recognition of mental disorders may have benefits, caution is needed about unnecessary labelling that may lead to stigma. Sometimes labelling a person as having a 'mental illness' can lead others to avoid or otherwise stigmatize them. Labelling needs to be a positive act that gives a person with a mental disorder earlier treatment and better support, rather than a negative one that leads to avoidance and discrimination.

Knowledge of the range of professional help and effective treatments available

Once a person with a mental disorder recognizes the problem and decides they need help, they need to know about the range of professional help available and what treatments are likely to be helpful.

Surveys have been carried out in many developed countries looking at public beliefs about sources of help and types of treatment (Angermeyer et al., 2005; Dahlberg et al., 2008; Jorm et al., 2000a, 2005b; Kermode et al., 2009; Lauber et al., 2001; Magliano et al., 2004; Wang et al., 2007). While many findings are country specific, there are some that apply across many countries. These include:

- family and friends are viewed very positively as a source of help, often ahead of health professionals
- psychiatric medications are seen negatively by many people because of concerns that they do not treat the underlying causes and can cause dependence
- psychological treatments such as counselling are viewed very positively for a wide range of disorders
- beliefs about GPs as a source of help for mental disorders are very positive in most countries, but appear to be influenced by the type of health care system operating and the perceived appropriateness of GPs for mental health treatment
- a significant minority of the population believes that it is helpful to deal with mental disorders on one's own.

A particular concern is where beliefs about treatments diverge from those of professionals and from what the evidence shows is effective. This is seen most clearly with psychiatric medications. For example, in Germany, only 11% of the public give medication as their first choice of treatment for depression and only 15% as their first choice for schizophrenia (Riedel-Heller et al., 2005). In Australia, around a quarter of the public see antidepressants as likely to be harmful for a person with depression, while in Canada antidepressants are rated at a similar level to non-evidence-based treatments such as vitamins (Wang et al., 2007). Having negative views about medications can have major effects on the benefit received from these treatments. For example, depressed patients who have negative views about antidepressants are less likely to be prescribed these medications, less likely to fill prescriptions, and less likely to benefit overall (Pyne et al., 2005). If patients are to get the full benefit of evidence-based health care, community beliefs need to be concordant with the evidence.

Fortunately, community beliefs can be changed. In both Germany and Australia, repeat community surveys show that attitudes towards treatments for mental disorders, including medication, have become more favourable over time (Angermeyer et al., 2018; Reavley & Jorm, 2012). Even so, there is considerable room for further improvement.

Knowledge of effective self-help strategies

Self-help strategies are those that a person can use to deal with mental health problems on their own. Sometimes self-help strategies will be used under the guidance of a health professional (e.g.

using a website that teaches how to apply cognitive behavioural therapy). However, most self-help is informal and carried out without any professional guidance. Self-help strategies are very commonly used by members of the public to deal with disabling symptoms. For example, in an Australian community sample, the following strategies were commonly used to deal with depression and anxiety symptoms: alcohol to relax, pain relievers, physical activity, help from friends and family, holidays, and time off work (Jorm et al., 2000b). Some of these strategies are supported by evidence as likely to be helpful (e.g. physical activity), but others may be counterproductive (e.g. heavy use of alcohol can exacerbate anxiety and depression).

Community surveys show that the public believe in the effectiveness of self-help strategies, often more so than in professional interventions. This preference for self-help extends to more severe mental disorders like schizophrenia, as well as for common ones like depression. Self-help interventions that are endorsed as helpful across a number of countries include exercise, getting out and about more, taking vitamins, reading self-help books, getting support from family and friends, and consulting a website (Reavley & Jorm, 2012; Wang et al., 2007).

Self-help strategies are not an effective substitute for professional treatments of mental disorders. However, they can play a very useful role in dealing with anxiety and depressive symptoms that do not reach a diagnostic threshold. Such subthreshold symptoms are very common in the community and cause much disability, but do not justify the use of scarce mental health professional care. It has been proposed that informal self-help strategies that have evidence of effectiveness (such as exercise) should be widely promoted in the community in order to prevent the development of subthreshold symptoms into clinical disorders (Jorm & Griffiths, 2006). Morgan and Jorm (2009) have produced a list of self-help strategies that could be usefully promoted, based on a review of the available evidence of effectiveness and the consensus of clinicians and consumers. These include physical activity, better sleep practices, scheduling regular activities, seeking support from others, and learning relaxation methods. A randomized controlled trial of email messages to promote these self-help strategies found that they were effective in changing behaviour and reducing depressive symptoms in people with subthreshold depression (Morgan et al., 2012).

Knowledge and skills to give mental health first aid

When a person develops a mental disorder, this will often be recognized by other people in their social network. Whether these others provide appropriate support and encourage appropriate help-seeking may be important to the person's recovery. There is evidence that people with mental disorders are more likely to seek help if someone else suggests it (Cusack et al., 2004; Vogel et al., 2007). There is also evidence that receiving good social support is associated with a better outcome for the person with a mental disorder (Keitner et al., 1995) and is protective against the development of post-traumatic stress disorder following a traumatic event (Charuvastra & Cloitre, 2008). Such findings illustrate the importance of improving the community's knowledge and skills in mental health first aid. *Mental health first aid* is the initial help provided by a person's social network when they are developing a mental health problem, experiencing the worsening of an existing mental health problem or are in a mental health crisis (e.g. are suicidal).

There is only limited evidence from community surveys on mental health first aid knowledge. Australian national surveys have shown that many people see the value of listening to the person, providing support and information, and of encouraging professional help-seeking, although there are significant minorities who do not (Rossetto et al., 2014). However, they are less likely to know what to do in a crisis, such as when the person has suicidal thoughts. Furthermore, many members of the public do not see it as helpful to ask a person with a mental disorder about suicidal feelings, despite the overwhelming consensus of mental health professionals that this is appropriate (Jorm et al., 2008; Nicholas et al., 2020). A particular concern is evidence from the US that many young people say that they would not tell a responsible adult if a friend disclosed suicidal intentions (Dunham, 2004).

Knowledge of risk factors and causes that can be used to guide preventive action

Public knowledge of how to prevent mental disorders has received scant research attention. Nevertheless, a German survey on public attitudes to the prevention of depression showed that 75% agreed that prevention of depression is possible and around half of these said that they would take part in prevention programmes (Schomerus et al., 2008). Strategies that were approved of by over 90% of the population included stable friendships, enjoyable leisure activities, family support, thinking positively, disclosing oneself to a confidant, activities that increases self-confidence, and meaningful activities.

Given these data showing public interest in taking preventive action, it is interesting that there has been so little health promotion activity in this area, in great contrast to the situation with major physical diseases. To some extent, this may be because there is less consensus about modifiable risk factors for mental disorders. However, there is evidence from longitudinal studies showing a number of risk and protection factors for depression that adolescents can modify in their own lives, including reducing substance use, dieting, and negative coping strategies, and adopting a healthy weight, diet, and sleep pattern (Cairns et al., 2014).

Parents can also be key prevention agents. There is evidence from longitudinal studies on what parents can do to reduce their adolescent children's risk of depression and anxiety disorders, and their risk of problem drinking. Parental factors associated with increased risk of both depression and anxiety include less warmth, more conflict between the parents, overinvolvement, and aversiveness (Yap et al., 2014). Parental factors associated with adolescent alcohol misuse include parental provision of alcohol, favourable parental attitudes towards alcohol, and parental drinking. Protective factors for alcohol misuse are parenting monitoring of their child, having a good-quality parent–child relationship, parental support for the child, and involvement in the child's life (Yap et al., 2017).

Finding quality mental health information

In order to take effective action, the community needs to know how to find quality mental health information. Community surveys show that books, the internet, and professional experts are all seen as suitable sources by many people (Jorm et al., 2005b; Reavley & Jorm, 2012). Print media have been a traditional source, but increasingly the internet has become the primary source for health information. A US national survey found that 70% of adults who were internet users used the internet as their first source of health information (Prestin et al., 2015), while a survey of European Union countries found that an average of three-quarters of internet users searched for health-related information over the previous 12 months (Bachl, 2016). A survey of German psychiatric patients found that 71% used the internet for mental health-related reasons. The content accessed was most commonly information on mental disorders (58%), medication (44%), and mental health services (39%); less commonly used were platforms with other patients (20%) and platforms with mental health professionals (17%) (Kalckreuth et al., 2014).

While there is considerable information available to the public, there has been concern about its variable quality. One study found that the quality of information was lower for psychiatry websites than for other areas of medicine (Daraz et al., 2019). When information on different types of mental disorders was examined, the quality was found to be higher for schizophrenia, bipolar disorder, and dysthymia, and lower for phobia, anxiety, and panic disorder (Grohol et al., 2014). A study of depression websites found that the quality varied greatly, but information on pharmacological treatments was generally better than on other treatment options (Walsh et al., 2018). The best depression websites were BC Health Guide, Blue Pages, Mayo Clinic, Royal College of Psychiatry, and WebMD. A general problem with information websites is that they tend to have a high reading grade level, making them less accessible to people with a lower level of education (Grohol et al., 2014; Walsh et al., 2018). Fortunately, the most popular search engines, Google and Bing, tend to rank better quality sites higher, which means that their search results can largely be trusted (Grohol et al., 2014).

Public support for improving services

In many countries, mental health services are not supported by public funds at a level that satisfies the needs of service users, their families, or the clinicians who work in these services. Public knowledge and awareness may be an important factor in persuading policymakers to devote more resources to mental health services. This is well illustrated by a community survey in Germany where members of the public were asked about what diseases should get a reduction in services if the health care budget had to be cut (Schomerus et al., 2006). In general, mental disorders were more often favoured for cuts than physical diseases, with alcoholism heading the list, followed by depression and schizophrenia. Cancer and myocardial infarction were seldom selected for cuts. The most important determinant of whether an area should be cut was the perceived severity of the disorder. This finding shows the importance of promoting to the public the large contribution that mental disorders make to a country's burden of disease.

Interventions to improve public knowledge and awareness

There have been programmes in many countries to improve public knowledge and awareness. However, many of these have no or limited evaluation. Described here are some programmes that have been evaluated against a control condition of some kind.

Population interventions

Beyond Blue

Beyond Blue is an Australian national organization which aims to increase community awareness and reduce stigma around depression and related disorders. It started in 2000 and is primarily funded by the federal and state governments. Beyond Blue has used a variety of means to achieve its community awareness aims, including frequent contacts with the media, advertising campaigns, high-profile supporters, sponsored community activities, and a popular website. A national survey of adults in 2004–2005 showed that awareness of Beyond Blue was very high (62%) and that there was a high level of exposure to depression through the media (Highet et al., 2006). However, because some Australian states did not initially provide funding for Beyond Blue, exposure to its work was higher in some parts of the country than in others. A comparison of changes in depression literacy showed that the high-exposure states had greater change than the low-exposure states (Jorm et al., 2005a, 2006a). In particular, there was greater ability to recognize depression, more positive beliefs about the benefits of some treatments, increased belief in the benefits of help-seeking in general, greater awareness of depression in self or others, and greater awareness of discrimination against depressed people.

European Alliance Against Depression

In Germany, the Nuremberg Alliance Against Depression involved four components: interventions with GPs, a public campaign (poster, leaflets, events), interventions with community facilitators (e.g. clergy, teachers, police), and interventions with consumers and their relatives (Dietrich et al., 2010). The intervention was run in 2001–2002 in Nuremberg, with the city of Wurzburg serving as a comparison. To evaluate the intervention, surveys were carried out before during and after the campaign in both cities. These showed increased awareness of depression, with the effects being stronger in people directly or indirectly affected by depression. For example, there was an improvement in attitudes to antidepressants and a decline in the belief that depression is due to a lack of self-discipline. The evaluation also showed a reduction in suicidal acts in Nuremberg compared to Wurzburg. This intervention has now been extended to 17 European countries and is called the European Alliance Against Depression.

An evaluation of this approach in four other European countries (Germany, Portugal, Ireland, and Hungary) compared intervention regions with control regions in each country (Kohls et al., 2017). The public awareness campaigns were found to reduce personal depression stigma, and people who were aware of the campaign reported more openness towards seeking professional help than those who were unaware of it. However, a reduction in suicidal acts was only found in Portugal (Hegerl et al., 2019).

Treatment and Intervention in Psychosis (TIPS)

TIPS was a programme based in one region of Norway designed to reduce the duration of untreated psychosis in first-episode schizophrenia (Joa et al., 2008). The programme had two components: availability of easy access detection teams and a large-scale information campaign to raise awareness of early recognition of psychosis to the public, schools, and GPs. Before the campaign began, the duration of untreated psychosis was 16 weeks and this reduced to 5 weeks during intervention. However, after the campaign stopped, the duration of untreated psychosis increased back to 15 weeks, despite the continuing availability of the easy access detection teams. These findings show that community awareness is critical to improving early intervention for people with schizophrenia.

More recently, the TIPS approach has been extended to detect young people with mental health problems who are at high risk of transitioning to psychosis (rather than those currently experiencing psychosis) (Joa et al., 2021). In this Prevention of Psychosis study, members of the general public in an area of Norway received targeted information on mental health in adolescence. In addition, there were targeted education programmes for teachers, GPs, and others working in community health care with adolescents. Although this programme increased the detection of young people at risk, it fell far short of its target, indicating that a more intensive programme is needed to have a substantial impact on detection of young people with earlier and milder mental health problems.

Compass Strategy

The Compass Strategy was a community awareness campaign targeting young people aged 12–25 in one region of Australia from 2001 to 2003 (Wright et al., 2006). The aim was to encourage earlier detection and treatment of mental disorders during the stage of life when these disorders often have first onset. A variety of methods were used to convey messages, including cinema, radio, newspapers, youth magazines, posters, brochures, postcards, a website, an information line, and training for professionals who might facilitate earlier help-seeking. To evaluate the programme, community surveys of young people were carried out in the intervention region and in an adjacent comparison region. Although the campaign was of relatively short duration and of moderate intensity, a number of aspects of mental health literacy increased more in the intervention region.

Interventions based in educational institutions

High schools have been a popular setting for mental health education, both because mental health problems often have first onset during adolescence and the convenient setting that schools provide for universal intervention. A review of evaluations of mental health literacy interventions in high schools found that these generally involve an educational approach delivered by teachers and that they were effective in improving mental health literacy (Seedaket et al., 2020). An example of a successful school-based intervention is the 'Mental Health is For Everyone' programme in Norway (Skre et al., 2013). This is a 3-day educational programme for students in grades 8–10 that is taught by teachers. The course includes individual tasks, group tasks and plenary sessions, and illustrative video material. A particular effort was made to make the tasks varied and engaging for adolescents. An evaluation study found improvements compared to a control group in symptom profile identification, prejudiced beliefs, and knowledge about where to seek help.

There has also been work to improve the mental health literacy of university students, who are in a high-risk age group. A review of evaluation research on these interventions found that a variety of approaches have been tried, including face-to-face training, online resources, videos, and printed materials (Reis et al., 2021). These interventions have covered mental illness in general, as well as a range of specific disorders. However, apart from mental health first aid training (see following section), the effects of these interventions were weak and inconsistent.

Mental health first aid training

A mental health first aid course has been developed in Australia to train members of the public to give early help to people developing a mental disorder and to give assistance in mental health crisis situations, such as when a person is suicidal, self-injuring, having a panic attack, being severely out of contact with reality, or having had a traumatic experience (Jorm et al., 2019). This programme has been tailored for various age and cultural groups and has been widely disseminated globally. A review of 18 randomized controlled trials evaluating this type of training found benefits in mental health first aid knowledge, recognition of mental disorders, and beliefs about effective treatments. Improvements were also observed in confidence in helping a person with a mental health problem, intentions to provide first aid, and in the amount of help provided to a person with a mental health problem (Morgan et al., 2018).

One variant on mental health first aid training focuses on training high school students in how to support their peers with mental health problems, including if their peer is suicidal. A randomized controlled trial of this type of training found that it produced improvements in ability to recognize suicidality in a peer and in intentions to assist a suicidal peer, and that these changes were still present 12 months after the training finished (Hart et al., 2020).

Web-based interventions

Websites are now an important source of mental health information and have been the subject of a number of randomized controlled trials. A review of these studies found variable results (Brijnath et al., 2016). Most were found to improve mental health literacy, and some improved help-seeking intentions and improved mental health. The more successful interventions were those that involved a structured programme with users guided through a series of sequential steps and used the potential of the internet for participant interaction. Two web interventions that stood out for their effectiveness were BluePages (https://bluepages.anu.edu.au/), which provides information about depression, and moodgym (https://moodgym.com.au/), which provides cognitive behavioural therapy in an educational format.

Conclusion

Across many countries, deficiencies have been found in mental health literacy which limit the ability of the public to take action for prevention, early intervention, uptake of evidence-based treatment, self-help, first aid, and support for better mental health services. While there is some evidence that improvements are possible, this is an area that has not seen the large investment in health education and promotion that has occurred with cancer and heart disease.

REFERENCES

Angermeyer, M. C., Breier, P., Dietrich, S., Kenzine, D., & Matschinger, H. (2005). Public attitudes toward psychiatric treatment: an international comparison. *Social Psychiatry and Psychiatric Epidemiology*, **40**, 855–864.

Angermeyer, M. C., Matschinger, H., & Schomerus, G. (2018). Attitudes towards psychiatric treatment and people with mental illness: changes over two decades. *British Journal of Psychiatry*, **203**, 146–151.

Bachl, M. (2016). Online health information seeking in Europe: do digital divides persist? *Studies in Communication and Media*, **5**, 427–453.

Brijnath, B., Protheroe, J., Mahtani, K. R., & Antoniades, J. (2016). Do web-based mental health literacy interventions improve the mental health literacy of adult consumers? Results from a systematic review. *Journal of Medical Internet Research*, **18**, e165.

Cairns, K. E., Yap, M. B. H., Pilkington, P. D. & Jorm, A. F. (2014). Risk and protective factors for depression that adolescents can modify: a systematic review and meta-analysis of longitudinal studies. *Journal of Affective Disorders*, **169**, 61–75.

Charuvastra, A. & Cloitre, M. (2008). Social bonds and posttraumatic stress disorder. *Annual Review of Psychology*, **59**, 301–328.

Christiana, J. M., Gilman, S. E., Guarding, M., Mickelson, K., Morselli, P. L., Olfson, M., & Kessler, R. C. (2000). Duration between onset and time of obtaining initial treatment among people with anxiety and mood disorders: an international survey of members of mental health patient advocate groups. *Psychological Medicine*, **30**, 693–703.

Cusack, J., Deane, F. P., Wilson, C. J., & Ciarrochi, J. (2004). Who influence men to go to therapy? Reports from men attending psychological services. *International Journal of Advances in Counselling*, **26**, 271–283.

Dahlberg, K. M., Waern, M., & Runeson, B. (2008). Mental health literacy and attitudes in a Swedish community sample—investigating the role of personal experience of mental health care. *BMC Public Health*, **8**, 8.

Daraz, L., Morrow, A. S., Ponce, O. J., Beuschel, B., Farah, M. H., Katabi, A., et al. (2019). Can patients trust online health information? A meta-narrative systematic review addressing the quality of health information on the internet. *Journal of General Internal Medicine*, **34**, 1884–1891.

Dietrich, S., Mergl, R., Freudenberg, P., Althaus, D., & Hegerl, U. (2010). Impact of a campaign on the public's attitudes towards depression. *Health Education Research*, **25**, 135–150.

Dunham, K. (2004). Young adults' support strategies when peers disclose suicidal intent. *Suicide and Life-Threatening Behavior*, **34**, 56–65.

Ghio, L., Gotelli, S., Marcenaro, M., Amore, M., & Natta, W. (2014). Duration of untreated illness and outcomes in unipolar depression: a systematic review and meta-analysis. *Journal of Affective Disorders*, **152-154**, 45–51.

Grohol, J. M., Slimowicz, J., & Granda, R. (2014). The quality of mental health information commonly searched for on the internet. *Cyberpsychology, Behavior, and Social Networking*, **17**, 216–221.

Haller, D. M., Sanci, L. A., Sawyer, S. M., & Patton, G. C. (2009). The identification of young people's emotional distress: a study in primary care. *British Journal of General Practice*, **59**, e61–e70.

Hart, L. M., Cropper, P., Morgan, A. J., Kelly, C. M., & Jorm, A. F. (2020). Teen Mental Health First Aid as a school-based intervention for improving peer support of adolescents at risk of suicide: outcomes from a cluster randomised crossover trial. *Australian & New Zealand Journal of Psychiatry*, **54**, 382–392.

Hegerl, U., Maxwell, M., Harris, F., Koburger, N., Mergl, R., Székely, A., et al. (2019). Prevention of suicidal behaviour: results of a controlled community-based intervention study in four European countries. *PLoS One*, **14**, e0224602.

Highet, N. J., Luscombe, G. M., Davenport, T. A., Burns, J. M., & Hickie, I. B. (2006). Positive relationships between public awareness activity and recognition of the impacts of depression in Australia. *Australian and New Zealand Journal of Psychiatry*, **40**, 55–58.

Howes, O. D., Whitehurst, T., Shatalina, E., Townsend, L., Onwordi, E. C., Mak, T. L. A., et al. (2021). The clinical significance of duration of untreated psychosis: an umbrella review and random-effects meta-analysis. *World Psychiatry*, **20**, 75–95.

Joa, I., Bjornestad, J., Johannessen, J. O., Langeveld, J., Stain, H. J., Weibell, M., & Hegelstad, W. T. V. (2021). Early detection of ultra high risk for psychosis in a Norwegian catchment area: the two year follow-up of the prevention of psychosis study. *Frontiers in Psychiatry*, **12**, 573905.

Joa, I., Johannessen, J. O., Auestad, B., Friis, S., McGlashan, T., Melle, I., et al. (2008). The key to reducing duration of untreated first psychosis: information campaigns. *Schizophrenia Bulletin*, **34**, 466–472.

Jorm, A. F., Angermeyer, M. C., & Katschnig, H. (2000a). Public knowledge of and attitudes to mental disorders: a limiting factor in the optimal use of treatment services. In: Andrews, G. & Henderson, S. (Eds.), *Unmet Need in Psychiatry: Problems, Resources, Responses* (pp. 399–413). Cambridge: Cambridge University Press.

Jorm, A. F., Christensen, H., & Griffiths, K. M. (2005a). The impact of beyondblue: the national depression initiative on the Australian public's recognition of depression and beliefs about treatments. *Australian and New Zealand Journal of Psychiatry*, **39**, 248–254.

Jorm, A. F., Christensen, H., & Griffiths, K. M. (2006a). Changes in depression awareness and attitudes in Australia: the impact of beyondblue: the national depression initiative. *Australian and New Zealand Journal of Psychiatry*, **40**, 42–46.

Jorm, A. F. & Griffiths, K. M. (2006). Population promotion of informal self-help strategies for early intervention against depression and anxiety. *Psychological Medicine*, **36**, 3–6.

Jorm, A. F., Kelly, C. M., Wright, A., Parslow, R. A., Harris, M. G., & McGorry, P. D. (2006b). Belief in dealing with depression alone: results from community surveys of adolescents and adults. *Journal of Affective Disorders*, **96**, 59–65.

Jorm, A. F., Kitchener, B. A. & Reavley, N. J. (2019). Mental Health First Aid training: lessons learned from the global spread of a community education program. *World Psychiatry*, **18**, 142–143.

Jorm, A. F., Korten, A. E., Jacomb, P. A., Christensen, H., Rodgers, B., & Pollitt, P. (1997). 'Mental health literacy': a survey of the public's ability to recognise mental disorders and their beliefs about the effectiveness of treatment. *Medical Journal of Australia*, **166**, 182–186.

Jorm, A. F., Medway, J., Christensen, H., Korten, A. E., Jacomb, P. A., & Rodgers, B. (2000b). Public beliefs about the helpfulness of interventions for depression: effects on actions taken when experiencing anxiety and depression symptoms. *Australian and New Zealand Journal of Psychiatry*, **34**, 619–626.

Jorm, A. F., Morgan, A. J., & Wright, A. (2008). First aid strategies that are helpful to young people developing a mental disorder: beliefs of health professionals compared to young people and parents. *BMC Psychiatry*, **8**, 42.

Jorm, A. F., Nakane, Y., Christensen, H., Yoshioka, K., Griffiths, K. M., & Wata, Y. (2005b). Public beliefs about treatment and outcome of mental disorders: a comparison of Australia and Japan. *BMC Medicine*, **3**, 12.

Kalckreuth, S., Trefflich, F., & Rummel-Kluge, C. (2014). Mental health related internet use among psychiatric patients: a cross-sectional analysis. *BMC Psychiatry*, **14**, 368.

Keitner, G. I., Ryan, C. E., Miller, I. W., Kohn, R., Bishop, D. S., & Epstein, N. B. (1995). Role of the family in recovery and major depression. *American Journal of Psychiatry*, **152**, 1002–1008.

Kermode, M., Bowen, K., Arole, S., Joag, K., & Jorm, A. F. (2009). Community beliefs about treatments and outcomes of mental disorders: a mental health literacy survey in a rural area of Maharashtra, India. *Public Health*, **123**, 476–483.

Kessler, R. C., Aguilar-Gaxiola, S., Alonso, J., Chatterji, S., Lee, S., Ormel, J., et al. (2009). The global burden of mental disorders: an update from the WHO World Mental Health (WMH) surveys. *Epidemiologia e Psichiatria Sociale*, **18**, 23–33.

Kohls, E., Coppens, E., Hug, J., Wittevrongel, E., Van Audenhave, C., Koburger, N., et al. (2017). Public attitudes toward depression and help-seeking: impact of the OSPI-Europe depression awareness campaign in four European regions. *Journal of Affective Disorders*, **217**, 252–259.

Lauber, C., Nordt, C., Falcato, L., & Rössler, W. (2001). Lay recommendations on how to treat mental disorders. *Social Psychiatry and Psychiatric Epidemiology*, **36**, 553–556.

Magliano, L., Fiorillo, A., De Rosa, C., Malangone, C., & Maj, M. (2004). Beliefs about schizophrenia in Italy: a comparative nationwide survey of the general public, mental health professionals, and patients' relatives. *Canadian Journal of Psychiatry*, **49**, 322–330.

Morgan, A. J. & Jorm, A. F. (2009). Self-help strategies that are helpful for sub-threshold depression: a Delphi consensus study. *Journal of Affective Disorders*, **115**, 196–200.

Morgan, A. J., Jorm, A. F., & Mackinnon, A. J. (2012). Email-based promotion of self-help for subthreshold depression: Mood Memos randomised controlled trial. *British Journal of Psychiatry*, **200**, 412–418.

Morgan, A. J., Ross, A., & Reavley, N. J. (2018). Systematic review and meta-analysis of Mental Health First Aid training: effects on knowledge, stigma, and helping behaviour. *PLoS One*, **13**, e0197102.

Nicholas, A., Niederkronthaler, T., Reavley, N., Pirkis, J., Jorm, A., & Spittal, M. J. (2020). Belief in suicide prevention myths and its effect on helping: a nationally representative survey of Australian adults. *BMC Psychiatry*, **20**, 303.

Prestin, A., Vieux, S. N., & Chou, W. S. (2015). Is online health activity alive and well or flatlining? Findings from 10 years of the Health Information National Trends Survey. *Journal of Health Communication*, **20**, 790–798.

Pyne, J. M., Rost, K. M., Farahati, F., Tripathi, S. P., Smith, J., Willams, D. K., et al. (2005). One size fits some: the impact of patient treatment attitudes on the cost-effectiveness of a depression primary-care intervention. *Psychological Medicine*, **35**, 839–854.

Reavley, N. J. & Jorm, A. F. (2012). Public recognition of mental disorders and beliefs about treatment: changes in Australia over 16 years. *British Journal of Psychiatry*, **200**, 419–425.

Reis, A. C., Saheb, R., Moyo, T., et al. (2021). The impact of mental health literacy training programs on the mental health literacy of university students: a systematic review. *Prevention Science*, No-Specified. doi:https://dx.doi.org/10.1007/s11121-021-01283-y

Riedel-Heller, S. G., Matschinger, H., & Angermeyer, M. C. (2005). Mental disorders—who and what might help? Help-seeking and treatment preferences of the lay public. *Social Psychiatry and Psychiatric Epidemiology*, **40**, 167–174.

Rossetto, A., Jorm, A. F., & Reavley, N. J. (2014). Quality of helping behaviours of members of the public towards a person with a mental illness: a descriptive analysis of data from an Australian national survey. *Annals of General Psychiatry*, **13**, 2.

Schomerus, G., Angermeyer, M. C., Matschinger, H., & Riedel-Heller, S. G. (2008). Public attitudes towards prevention of depression. *Journal of Affective Disorders*, **106**, 257–263.

Schomerus, G., Matschinger, H., & Angermeyer, M. C. (2006). Preferences of the public regarding cutbacks in expenditure for patient care: are there indications of discrimination against those with mental disorders? *Social Psychiatry and Psychiatric Epidemiology*, **41**, 369–377.

Seedaket, S., Turnbull, N., Phajan, T., & Wanchai, A. (2020). Improving mental health literacy in adolescents: systematic review of supporting intervention studies. *Tropical Medicine and International Health*, **25**, 1055–1064.

Skre, I., Friborg, O., Breivik, C., Johnsen, L. I., Arnesen, Y. & Wang, C. E. A. (2013). A school intervention for mental health literacy in adolescents: effects of a non-randomized cluster controlled trial. *BMC Public Health*, **13**, 873.

Thompson, A., Issakidis, C., & Hunt, C. (2008). Delay to seek treatment for anxiety and mood disorders in an Australian clinical sample. *Behaviour Change*, **25**, 71–84.

Vogel, D. L., Wade, N. G., Wester, S. R., Larson, L., & Hackler, A. H. (2007). Seeking help from a mental health professional: the influence of one's social network. *Journal of Clinical Psychology*, **63**, 233–245.

Walsh, K., Pryor, T. A. M., Reynolds, K. A., Walker, J. R., & The Mobilizing Minds Research Group (2018). Searching for answers: how well do depression websites answer the public's questions about treatment choices? *Patient Education and Counseling*, **102**, 99–105.

Wang, J. L., Adair, C., Fick, G., Lai, D., Evans, B., Perry, B. W., et al. (2007). Depression literacy in Alberta: findings from a general population sample. *Canadian Journal of Psychiatry*, **52**, 442–449.

WHO World Mental Health Survey Consortium (2004). Prevalence, severity, and unmet need for treatment of mental disorders in the World Health Organization World Mental Health Surveys. *Journal of the American Medical Association*, **291**, 1581–1590.

Wright, A., Jorm, A. F., & Mackinnon, A. J. (2012). Labels used by young people to describe mental disorders: which ones predict effective help-seeking choices? *Social Psychiatry and Psychiatric Epidemiology*, **47**, 917–926.

Wright, A., McGorry, P. D., Harris, M. G., Jorm, A. F., & Pennell, K. (2006). Development and evaluation of a youth mental health community awareness campaign: the Compass Strategy. *BMC Public Health*, **6**, 215.

Yap, M. B. H., Cheong, T. W. K., Zaravinos-Tsakos, F., Lubman, D. I., & Jorm, A. F. (2017). Modifiable parenting factors associated with adolescent alcohol misuse: a systematic review and meta-analysis of longitudinal studies. *Addiction*, **112**, 1142–1162.

Yap, M. B. H., Pilkington, P. D., Ryan, S. M., & Jorm, A. F. (2014). Parental factors associated with depression and anxiety in young people: a systematic review and meta-analysis. *Journal of Affective Disorders*, **156**, 8–23.

# Reducing stigma and discriminatory behaviour

Petra C. Gronholm, Dristy Gurung, Sarah J. Parry, Nisha Mehta, and Graham Thornicroft

Defining stigma

The term stigma (plural stigmata) was originally used to refer to an indelible dot left on the skin after stinging with a sharp instrument, sometimes used to identify vagabonds or slaves. The resulting mark led to the metaphorical use of 'stigma' to refer to stained or soiled individuals were who in some way morally diminished. In modern times stigma has come to mean 'any attribute, trait or disorder that marks an individual as being unacceptably different from the 'normal' people with whom he or she routinely interacts, and that elicits some form of community sanction' (Goffman, 1963).

Understanding stigma

There is a voluminous literature on stigma with hundreds of scientific papers covering the topic of stigma of mental illness. The most complete model of the component processes of stigmatization has five key components (Link et al., 2004):

1. Labelling, in which personal characteristics are signalled or noticed as conveying an important difference
2. Stereotyping, which is the linkage of these differences to undesirable characteristics
3. Separating, the categorical distinction between the mainstream/normal group and the labelled group as in some respects fundamentally different
4. Emotional reactions, towards (e.g. anger, irritation, anxiety, pity, and fear) and within (e.g. embarrassment, shame, fear, alienation, anger) the labelled group
5. Status loss and discrimination: devaluing, rejecting, and excluding the labelled group.

The three core issues

We shall consider later what needs to be done to allow people with mental illnesses a full opportunity for social participation. First of all, we need to have a clear map to know where we are and where we want to go.

Stigma theories have not been enough to understand the feelings and experiences of people with mental illness, nor to know what practical steps are needed to reverse social exclusion. Rather, stigma can be seen as an overarching term that contains three important elements (Thornicroft, 2006; Thornicroft et al., 2007):

- Problems of knowledge (ignorance)
- Problems of attitudes (prejudice)
- Problems of behaviour (discrimination).

These domains will now be discussed in turn.

Ignorance: the problem of knowledge

Ignorance reflects a lack of accurate information about mental illness, which can lead to misconceptions about what mental illnesses are and how persons with mental illness should be helped. Ignorance can also contribute towards perpetuated unhelpful common beliefs, or myths, about, for example, what people with mental illness are like or what they are capable of doing.

Some of these myths reflect negative stereotyped views, such as the belief that persons with mental illness pose a threat to others. It is a common misunderstanding that there would be an association between mental illness and violence (Ahonen et al., 2019). Impressions and narratives in the media and the general public often imply mental health conditions as a potential precursor for violence and dangerous behaviours (Ahonen et al., 2019). In fact, persons with mental illness are more likely to be the victim of violence than the perpetrator (Simpson et al., 2022). This misconception is common particularly in relation to people with schizophrenia, who are often assumed to be violent, unpredictable, or dangerous (Gwarjanski & Parrott, 2018).

Other inaccurate beliefs include the assumption that mental illnesses are contagious (Kohrt et al., 2020) or a result of supernatural causes like curses (Potts & Henderson, 2021). Some issues with knowledge reflect a lack of understanding of treatment, for example, that mental illness cannot be treated or that it can only be treated with strong medication, and that psychological counselling is only as helpful as generic advice (Kohrt et al., 2020).

The public level of knowledge about mental illnesses and their treatments has been conceptualized as 'mental health literacy' (Jorm et al., 1997). Despite how an unprecedented volume of information about mental health problems is available in the public domain, the level of general knowledge about mental illnesses remains relatively poor (Furnham & Swami, 2020). Commonly, older people are less knowledgeable than younger people (Ahonen et al., 2019; Piper et al., 2018). A person's level of mental health literacy is likely to influence their perceived need for help, which is a key barrier for seeking treatment for mental health conditions globally (Andrade et al., 2014). Indeed, low mental health literacy is associated with reduced help-seeking for mental health problems (Schnyder et al., 2017). Studies also report an association between mental health literacy and stigma (Svensson & Hansson, 2016; Yin et al., 2020).

Given the links between knowledge, mental health literacy, and stigma, a number of anti-stigma efforts have focused on reducing stigma through education-based strategies aiming to correct misconceptions and improve mental health literacy (Kohrt et al., 2020; Walsh & Foster, 2021). However, approaches focused on 'mental health literacy' or the improvement of knowledge alone does not seem to be sufficient to reduce stigma. In fact, anti-stigma strategies focused on debunking myths and providing facts can be inefficient or even increase stigma (Dobson & Wolf, 2022). The need to consider the concept of stigma beyond the role of knowledge alone is also evident in how groups such as health care providers—who generally have a high level of factual knowledge regarding mental illness—are not free from stigma (Kohrt et al., 2020).

Prejudice: the problem of negative attitudes and emotions

If ignorance is the first great hurdle faced by people with mental illness, prejudice is the second. This is reflective of a problem of negative attitudes and emotional reactions towards mental illnesses and people affected by them.

Although the term prejudice has been used extensively in some groups which undergo particular disadvantage, for example, minority ethnic groups, it has not always been employed in relation to people with mental illness (Corrigan et al., 2001). For almost a century, social psychologists were focused on thoughts (cognition) rather than feelings (affect) (Bogardus, 1925). In particular, they have long been interested in stereotypes (widely held and fixed images about a particular type of person), and degrees of social distance to such stereotypes (Fiske, 1998). These stereotypes are related to the problem of ignorance and reflect a lack of awareness and common misconceptions, and myths regarding mental illness, its treatment, and people affected by mental health conditions.

Reactions of rejection do not usually involve only negative thoughts, but also negative feelings such as anxiety, anger, resentment, hostility, distaste, or disgust (Link et al., 2004). In fact, prejudice may more strongly predict discrimination (negative behaviours to a specific category of people) than do stereotypes (Dovidio et al., 1996).

First, so-called gut level prejudices (Fiske, 1998) may stem from anticipated group threats, or in other words, how far a member of an 'out-group' is seen to threaten the goals or the interests of the person concerned. Perceiving possible harm may provoke anger (if the person is seen to threaten harm), fear (if the harm is in the certain future), anxiety (if the harm is in the uncertain future), or sadness (if the harm is in the past) (Fiske, 1998; Thornicroft, 2006). Some writers have made a distinction between 'hot' prejudices, in which strong emotions are more prominent than negative thoughts, and 'cold' forms of rejection, for example, in failing to promote a member of staff, when stereotypes are activated in the absence of negative feelings (Fiske, 2003).

Second, emotional reactions may be a consequence of direct contact with the 'target' group. This may be experienced as discomfort, anxiety, ambivalence, or as a rejection of intimacy (Crocker et al., 1998). Such feelings have been shown to be stronger in individuals who have a relatively authoritarian personality, and among people who tend to believe that the world is basically just (and so that people get what they deserve) (Crandall & Eshleman, 2003). Emotional aspects of rejection have been studied extensively in the fields of HIV/AIDS (Herek et al., 2002) and in those conditions which produce visible marks which contravene aesthetic conventions (Hahn, 1988), such as the use of catheters or colostomies (Wilde, 2003). Investigations into emotional reactions in relation to people with mental illness started comparatively later (Angermeyer et al., 2010), with fear of violence the most frequently explored reaction.

Attitudes towards mental illnesses, people affected by them, and also attitudes towards help-seeking, have been examined in various world regions (Cremonini et al., 2018; Hartini et al., 2018; Mathias et al., 2018; Nohr et al., 2021; Yuan et al., 2017) at a general population level, and also among specific groups such as young people (DuPont-Reyes et al., 2019; Radez et al., 2021), health care providers, and others (Forbes et al., 2013).

For example, more positive community attitudes towards people with mental illness predicted more positive help-seeking attitudes in Cuban and German samples (Nohr et al., 2021). In North India, community attitudes reflecting a belief that a person will recover from their mental illness and return to normal life were associated with reduced preference for social distance (Mathias et al., 2018). A study among health care professionals in Italy found that although attitudes towards mental illness were overall positive, differences could be observed between different professional groups, districts, and care unit types (Cremonini et al., 2018). For example, nursing professionals in general held less positive attitudes than social workers, professional educators, and health care assistants, and staff at day care mental health centres held more positive attitudes than health care professionals within mental health wards. Negative attitudes towards mental health and help-seeking are a key barrier to seeking and accessing care for mental health problems among children and adolescents (Radez et al., 2021) and also parents (Reardon et al., 2017). UK military personnel were found to have overall slightly less positive attitudes towards mental illness than the general community (e.g. more agreement with statement 'People with mental illness have the same rights to a job as everyone else') but more positive attitudes regarding causes of mental illness (e.g. more disagreement with statement 'One of the main causes of mental illness is a lack of self-discipline and willpower') (Forbes et al., 2013).

Discrimination: the problem of rejecting behaviour

Discrimination reflects the behaviours towards, and the actual experiences of, people with mental illness: for example, social rejection or withdrawal, and loss of opportunities and limited access to social roles.

For a long time this aspect of stigma remained underexamined (Gronholm et al., 2017; Thornicroft et al., 2016), with most research attention focused primarily on discussing and assessing stigma in terms of knowledge and attitudes towards mental illness. However, it could be argued that behaviours are the most meaningful outcome to consider from the perspective of people affected by stigma (Evans-Lacko et al., 2011; Rose et al., 2007; Rüsch et al., 2009). It has been reported that the experience of discrimination can be as disabling or even worse than the impact of the mental illness itself (Thornicroft et al., 2016, 2022), and global studies have demonstrated that discrimination across a number of life domains is a common experience for most people experiencing mental ill health (Lasalvia et al., 2013; Thornicroft et al., 2009).

One reason for the paucity of research examining discrimination is the challenge of assessing this domain of stigma. There have, however, been instruments and approaches developed specifically to capture behavioural aspects of stigma. These range from brief self-report questionnaires to longer interview-based assessment tools, and even some role-play-based instruments to capture behaviours reflective of discrimination (Bakolis et al., 2019; Brohan et al., 2013; Evans-Lacko et al., 2011; Kohrt et al., 2015).

More recently, attention regarding discrimination has shifted to also consider so-called microaggressions, that is, intentional and unintentional brief and commonplace subtle dismissals that communicate hostile, derogatory, and negative slights and insults towards a person (Barber et al., 2020). Initially, microaggressions were explored primarily in relation to racial discrimination (Sue et al., 2007), but have since been considered also in relation to other marginalized groups, such as women, sexual minorities, and people with disabilities (Sue, 2013). The emerging study of microaggressions also in relation to people affected by mental illness reflects the increased attention and nuance with which discrimination in relation to mental illness is considered.

Global patterns of stigma and discrimination

It has been well documented that mental health-related stigma is one of the biggest barriers to treatment not just in high-income countries, but also in low- and middle income countries (LMICs) (Mascayano et al., 2015). Over the years, stigma has been identified as a universal phenomenon that is apparent in all cultures and societies. Various studies from different regions of Asia and Africa have shown high prevalence of mental health-related stigma. In a cross-sectional survey conducted in 39 countries, 79% of the participants reported experiencing discrimination in at least one domain of life as measured by the Discrimination and Stigma Scale (DISC) (Lasalvia et al., 2013). Similarly, another study using population-wide data from 16 countries (three in the Americas, five in Asia, seven in Europe, and one each in Oceania and Africa) showed prevalence of perceived stigma to be 13.5% overall (Alonso et al., 2008). The prevalence was higher in developing countries (22.1%) than in the developed countries (11.7%). In China, the prevalence of stigma among health professionals, public, patients, and their relatives ranged from 40% to 70% which is higher than those reported in high-income countries (Xu et al., 2018). In an Indian study, however, negative discrimination was reported as lower than in high-income countries but the reporting of anticipated discrimination was in line with those from high-income countries (Koschorke et al., 2014).

Contradictory to past claims that non-Western societies experience lower discrimination and stigma experiences, a wide body of evidence in recent years from LMICs has shown that mental illness-related stigma, discrimination, and human rights abuses is common, making it a global phenomenon (Gurung et al., 2022; Lasalvia et al., 2013; Sorsdahl et al., 2012). This shows that not all studies capture the cross-cultural drivers and context-specific manifestations of stigma and discrimination. Although stigma is a global phenomenon, its drivers and manifestations may vary according to the cultural and sociopolitical context (Yang et al., 2014). The understanding of mental health and illness and presentation of symptoms varies according to different cultures, making stigma and its measurement more complex. It is important to understand the processes of stigma and discrimination, and context-specific factors affecting them in LMICs as existing evidence comes from mostly high-income settings in the Western and Northern parts of the world, which may not be applicable in other areas (Ikwuka et al., 2016).

Different cultures conceptualize mental health differently and so the factors that drive or facilitate mental health stigma may vary. For example, in Ethiopia, mental illness is considered to be caused by evil spirits due to violation of holy rules (Girma et al., 2022). The supernatural attribution of stigma is also present in most of the South Asian communities. In Nepal, for example, mental illness is considered to be an outcome of bad karma or sins committed in past life (Gurung et al., 2022). In the majority of countries in Europe and the US, however, the cause of mental illness is considered to be illness of genetics or brain disease (Schomerus et al., 2012). Japanese populations, on the other hand, identify schizophrenia as a consequence of weak character and not an organic brain condition (Tateyama et al., 1998). Cultural norms and beliefs also characterize the concept of 'normal' and 'abnormal'. In some South Asian cultures, for example, hearing voices and talking to 'spirits' during a state of 'possession' may be a common occurrence during cultural ritual (Sapkota et al., 2014), while this might be considered as 'abnormal' in other communities.

This difference in cultural values towards mental illness is also highlighted in a review (Yang et al., 2014). In some African communities, mental illness is considered to be a form of punishment for having practised 'satanism'. Personhood or adulthood of such communities is attached to moral values of being able to take care of parents and family. Loss of ability to do so due to mental illness prevents the community treating the person as a proper functioning adult. In Latin communities, the concept of 'machismo' or men as primary protector and provider in a family, means that not fulfilling those roles drive stigma towards men with mental illness. In most LMIC communities, people with mental illness are often associated with 'dangerous' and 'unpredictable' behaviour and therefore stigma is driven by fear of harm (Mascayano et al., 2016). In some communities, such as in Lebanon, people with mental illness are often viewed as a burden on society and so not deserving of sympathy (Aramouny et al., 2020).

These drivers and facilitators of mental illness-related stigma based on a community's cultural beliefs determine the different ways stigma is manifested. In countries such as Mongolia and Siberia, mental illness is perceived to be a personal weakness, and so the public is less willing to provide benefits for their sick role (Dietrich et al., 2004). Several studies from India highlighted the stigma manifestation in prospects of marriage. In a comparative study conducted in Bangalore and London, concerns around mental illness affecting marital prospects were prominent in Bangalore while the concern was not brought up by participants in London (Weiss et al., 2010). In communities where productivity and economic contribution mattered most, people with mental illness were perceived to be burdensome by family members, leading to divorces or abandonment in the street (Yang et al., 2014).

Such manifestations of stigma and discrimination towards people with mental illness are shown to have impacts on personal, health, socioeconomic, and structural levels. In communities where mental illness is perceived to be hereditary, this causes shame and discrimination not just to the person but to their entire family. This is also true for communities where mental illness is associated with sins committed in past life or by forefathers. Such stigma and discrimination have been associated with feelings of low self-esteem, suicidality, and self-harm (Eliasson et al., 2021; Xu et al., 2018). Studies conducted in Nigeria and India report a high level of perceived stigma and discrimination, which often leads to the concealment of illness by individuals and family members (Oshodi et al., 2014; Shrivastava et al., 2011). This concealment or lack of disclosure in turn may affect help-seeking, access, and adherence to treatment (Upadhaya et al., 2020).

Besides cultural factors, a country's historical and socioeconomic factors such as poverty and access to care may also drive how people with mental illness are perceived and how they are treated (Thornicroft et al., 2009). In a study conducted in 27 European counties, people with mental illness experienced more social exclusion during times of economic hardships (Evans-Lacko et al., 2013). This intersectionality is also seen in consequences of stigma as the impact of discrimination on job opportunities among people with mental illness would be far more severe and devastating for those living in low-resource settings and where social welfare systems are dysfunctional. Similarly, historical injustice and ill-treatment of people with mental illness by the government or the health system can influence the public's stigmatizing attitude.

These cultural and socioeconomic differences in the manifestations and consequences of stigma highlight the need for further research which takes into account context-specific meanings and explanations of mental illness and stigma (Yang et al., 2014). Culture and context need to be considered not only in understanding the process of stigma but also in the efforts to reduce stigma. Understanding and measuring these factors that shape stigma in different cultural contexts may help inform the development of effective and context-specific interventions.

Interventions to reduce stigma at the public level

Three main strategies have been used to reduce public stigma: protest, education, and contact (Corrigan et al., 2001). Protest, by stigmatized individuals or members of the public who support them, is often applied against stigmatizing public statements, such as media reports and advertisements. Many protest interventions, for example, against stigmatizing advertisements or soap operas, have successfully suppressed negative public statements and for this purpose they are clearly very useful (Wahl, 1995). However, it has been argued (Corrigan & Penn, 1999) that protest is not effective for improving attitudes towards people with mental illness. Education interventions aim to diminish stigma by replacing myths and negative stereotypes with facts, and have reduced stigmatizing attitudes among members of the public. However, research on educational campaigns suggests that behaviour changes are often not evaluated, and the degree of change achieved is both limited and may fade quickly. The third strategy is personal contact with persons with mental illness. In a number of interventions in secondary schools, education and personal contact have been combined (Pinfold et al., 2003). Contact appears to be the more efficacious part of the intervention. Factors that create an advantageous environment for interpersonal contact and stigma reduction include equal status among participants, a cooperative interaction, and institutional support for the contact initiative.

For both education and contact, the content of anti-stigma programmes matters. Biogenetic models of mental illness are often highlighted because viewing mental illness as a biological, mainly inherited problem, may reduce shame and blame associated with it. Evidence supports this optimistic expectation (i.e. that a biogenetic causal model of mental illness will reduce stigma) in terms of reduced blame. However, focusing on biogenetic factors may increase the perception that people with mental illness are fundamentally different, and thus biogenetic interpretations have been associated with increased social distance, perceptions of mental illness as more persistent, serious, and dangerous, and with more pessimistic views about treatment outcomes (Phelan et al., 2006). Therefore, a message of mental illness as being 'genetic' or 'neurological' may be overly simplistic and unhelpful for reducing stigma.

Anti-stigma initiatives can take place nationally as well as locally. National campaigns often adopt a social marketing approach, whereas local initiatives usually focus on target groups.

National-level campaigns

An example of a large multifaceted national campaign is *Time To Change* in England (Henderson & Thornicroft, 2009). It combines mass media advertising and local initiatives. The latter try to facilitate social contact between members of the general public and mental health service users as well as targeting specific groups such as medical students and teachers. The programme is evaluated by public surveys assessing knowledge, attitudes, and behaviour, and by measuring the amount of experienced discrimination reported by people with mental illness. Similar initiatives in other countries, such as *See Me* in Scotland (Dunion & Gordon, 2005), *Like Minds, Like Mine* in New Zealand (Vaughan & Hansen, 2004), or the World Psychiatric Association anti-stigma initiative (Sartorius & Schulze, 2005) in, among many other countries, Japan, Brazil, and Egypt, have reported positive outcomes.

Local-level strategies

In local communities or health and social care economies, the initiatives in Table 31.1 are suggested to promote the social inclusion of people with mental illness.

Interventions to reduce stigma at the person level—target groups

In terms of national policy, a series of changes are necessary which span governmental ministries, the non-governmental and independent sector, along with service user and professional groups. This is a vision of a long-term approach addressing individual and systemic/structural discrimination (Corrigan et al., 2004) through a coordinated, multisectoral programme of action to promote the social inclusion of people with mental illness. Further social marketing approaches, the adaptation of advertising methods for a social good rather than for the consumptions of a commodity, are increasingly often being used (Dunion & Gordon, 2005; Sullivan et al., 2005). In the anti-stigma network of the World Psychiatric Association (called 'Open the Doors'), for example, interventions have been applied to specific target groups such as medical staff, journalists, schoolchildren, police, employers, and church leaders (Sartorius & Schulze, 2005).

Working professionals

For some people with mental illness, allowance needs to be made at work for their personal requirements. In parallel with the modifications made for people with physical disabilities, people with mental illness-related disabilities may need what are called 'reasonable adjustments' in relation to the anti-discrimination laws. In practice, this can include the following measures:

- Having a quieter work place with fewer distractions for people with concentration problems, rather than a noisy open plan office, and a rest area for breaks
- Giving longer or more frequent supervision than usual to give feedback and guidance on job performance
- Allowing a person to use headphones to block out distracting noise
- Creating flexibility in work hours so that they can attend their health care appointments, or work when not impaired by medication
- Funding an external job coach for counselling and support, and to mediate between employee and employer
- Providing a buddy/mentor scheme to provide on-site orientation and assistance
- Writing clear person specifications, job descriptions, and task assignments to assist people who find ambiguity or uncertainty hard to cope with
- Making contract modifications to specifically allow whatever sickness leave is required by people likely to become unwell for prolonged periods
- Providing a more gradual induction phase, for example, with more time to complete tasks, for those who return to work after a prolonged absence, or who may have some cognitive impairment
- Improving disability awareness in the workplace to reduce stigma and to underpin all other accommodations
- Reallocating marginal job functions which are disturbing to an individual
- Allowing use of accrued paid and unpaid leave for periods of illness.

Further, community bodies need to act to promote the social inclusion of people with mental illnesses. The following initiatives address discrimination in the workplace, and misinformation about mental health issues (Wheat et al., 2010).

- Employers' federations should inform employers of their legal obligations under existing disability laws towards people with mental illnesses.
- Employers in the health and social care sector, when recruiting, should make explicit that a history of mental illness is a valuable attribute for many roles.
- Mental health services should work with employers and business confederations to ensure that reasonable accommodations and adjustments in the workplace are made for people with mental illness.
- The education, health, and police authorities and commissioners should provide well-evaluated interventions to increase integration with, and understanding of, people with mental illness

Table 31.1 Initiatives to promote social inclusion of people with mental illness at local community level

Action	By
Introduction of supported work schemes	Mental health services with specialist independent sector providers
Psychological treatments to improve cognition, self-esteem, and confidence	Mental health and general health services
Health and social care explicitly give credit to applicants with a history of mental illness when hiring staff	Health and social care agencies
Provision of reasonable adjustments/accommodations at work	Mental health providers engaging with employers and business confederations
Inform employers of their legal obligations under disability laws	Employers' confederations
Deliver and evaluate the widespread implementation of targeted interventions with targeted groups including schoolchildren, police, and health care staff	Education, police, and health commissioning and providing authorities
Provide accurate data on mental illness recovery rates to mental health practitioners	Professional training and accreditation organizations
Implementation of measures to support care plans negotiated between staff and consumers	Mental health provider organizations and consumer groups

to targeted groups such as schoolchildren, police, and health care staff.
- Professional training and accreditation organizations should ensure that mental health practitioners are fully aware of the actual recovery rates in mental illness.

The development of psychological services designed to support people in or seeking work are important. Many people with mental illness experience demoralization, reduced self-esteem, loss of confidence, and sometimes depression (Hayward et al., 2002). It is therefore likely that support programmes assisting people with mental illness to gain employment will need to assess whether structured psychological treatment is also needed (Brown et al., 2004). Furthermore, mental health staff may increasingly see the need to widen their remit from direct treatment provision, to also intervening for local populations (Thornicroft et al., 2010), for example, through mental health awareness campaigns with local programmes which are targeted to specific groups.

Health care professionals

A key target group is health care professionals. People with lived experience surprisingly often describe that their experiences of general health care and mental health care staff reveal levels of ignorance, prejudice, and discrimination that they find deeply distressing. This has been confirmed in several international studies, including a review of interventions aimed at reducing stigmatizing knowledge, attitudes, and behaviours in health care professionals (Henderson et al., 2014). Based on the principle 'catch them young', several programmes have given anti-stigma interventions to medical students (Deb et al., 2019; Lethem, 2004). As is usual in the field of stigma and discrimination, there is more research describing stigma than assessing which interventions are effective. In Japan, one study found that the traditional medical curriculum led to mixed results: students became more accepting of mentally ill people and mental health services, and more optimistic about the outlook with treatment, but there was no impact on their views about how far people with mental illness should have their human rights fully observed (Mino et al., 2000). Positive changes in all of these domains were achieved with a 1-hour supplementary educational programme (Mino et al., 2001). Studies have also reviewed evidence on interventions to reduce mental illness stigma among medical and nursing students in LMICs (Heim et al., 2019).

It appears that psychiatrists may not be in the best position to lead such educational programmes. Studies in Switzerland found no overall differences between the general public and psychiatrists in terms of social distance to mentally ill people. Psychiatry itself tries to walk the narrow tightrope between the physical/pharmacological and psychological/social poles (Luhrmann, 2000). Clinicians who keep contact with people who are unwell, and who selectively stop seeing people who have recovered, may therefore develop a pessimistic view of the outlook for people with mental illnesses (Burti & Mosher, 2003). On balance, there is mixed evidence about whether psychiatrists can be seen as stigmatizers or destigmatizers (Schlosberg, 1993). In 2020, a pilot study evaluating the impact of an anti-stigma intervention for psychiatrists in Mexico showed promising results (Lagunes-Cordoba et al., 2022). Mental health nurses also been found to have more and less favourable views about people with mental illness than the general public (Caldwell & Jorm, 2001).

Nurses, like the general population, tend to be more favourable if they have a friend who is mentally ill, in other words if there is a perceived similarity and equality with the person affected (Sadow et al., 2009).

In this case, what should mental health staff do? Direct involvement in the media is a vital route that professionals can use more often, with proper preparation and training. They also need to set their own house in order by promoting information within their training curricula, continuing professional development (continuing medical education), and relicensing/revalidation procedures which ensures that they have accurate information, for example, on recovery (Crisp, 2004).

Further, in future, practitioners need to pay greater attention to what consumers and family members say about their experiences of discrimination, for example, in relation to work or housing. It is clear that consumer groups increasingly seek to change the terms of engagement between mental health professionals and consumers, and to move from paternalism to negotiation (Chamberlin, 2005). Strategies to support shared decision-making include crisis plans (Sutherby et al., 1999), which seem able to reduce the frequency of compulsory treatment (Henderson et al., 2004); advance directives (Swanson et al., 2006); shared care agreements (Byng et al., 2004); and consumer-held records (Lester et al., 2003). The key issue is that many consumers want direct participation in their own care plans.

Going into the public advocacy domain, staff in mental health systems may well develop in future a direct campaigning role. A practical approach is for local and national agencies to set aside their differences and to find common causes. In some areas such coordinating groups are called forums, peak bodies, alliances, or consortia. What they have in common is a recognition that what they can achieve together, in political terms, is greater that their individual impact. Core issues able to unite such coalitions are likely to be parity in funding, the use of disability discrimination laws for people with mental illness-related disabilities, and the recognition of international human rights conventions in practice (Thornicroft & Rose, 2005).

Interventions to reduce stigma at the policy level

Setting international standards for national polices can be a useful intervention. For example, the World Health Organization (WHO) has published standards to guide countries in producing or revising mental health laws (WHO, 2005). This covers advice on:

- access to care
- confidentiality
- assessments of competence and capacity
- involuntary treatment
- consent
- physical treatments
- seclusion
- restraint
- privacy of communications
- appeals against detention
- review procedures for compulsory detention.

In 2020, 75% of countries in the WHO member states had a mental health policy (WHO, 2021). Generally, lower-income countries are more likely to have older legislation and in 2007, 20–30% of LMICs did not have mental health legislation or policies (Thornicroft & Rose, 2005).

In the European Union, for example, anti-discrimination laws are now mandatory under the Article 13 Directive (Bartlett et al., 2006). Such laws must make illegal all discrimination in the workplace on grounds that include disability, and also set up institutions to enforce these laws. The time is therefore right to share experience between different countries on how successful such laws have been to reduce discrimination against people with mental illness, and to understand more clearly what is required both for new legislation elsewhere, and for amendments to existing laws that fall short of their original intentions.

International collaborations, for example, the Indigo Network (Thornicroft et al., 2019), have been set up to promote collaboration of research experts committed to reducing stigma and discrimination relating to mental illness. Furthermore, initiatives like the Lancet Commission on Stigma and Discrimination in Mental Health (Thornicroft et al., 2022) provide a platform for sharing up-to-date evidence on the effectiveness of interventions. International organizations, such as the WHO, can also contribute towards better care and less discrimination by indicating the need for national mental health policies, and by giving guidance on their content. In Europe, Health Ministers have signed a Mental Health Declaration and Action Plan which set the following priorities:

- Foster awareness of mental illness
- Tackle stigma, discrimination, and inequality
- Provide comprehensive, integrated care systems
- Support a competent, effective workforce
- Recognize the experience and knowledge of services users and carers.

In 2015, mental health was included specifically for the first time in the sustainable development goals, recognizing mental health as a priority for global development (Votruba & Thornicroft, 2016; Votruba et al., 2014). The Covid-19 global pandemic has further contributed to an increasing recognition of the importance of prioritizing mental health policy and legislation.

Conclusion

The strongest evidence at present for active ingredients to reduce stigma refers to direct social contact with people with mental illness (Mehta et al., 2015; Thornicroft et al., 2016, 2022). At the national level, there is evidence that a carefully coordinated approach based on using social marketing techniques, namely advertising and promotional methods designed to achieve a social good rather than sales of a commodity, have shown benefit in countries around the world (Global Anti-Stigma Alliance, n.d.; Potts & Henderson, 2021). The challenge in the coming years is to generate further evidence, in particular from LMICs, and to identify which interventions are most cost-effective in reducing the social exclusion of people with mental illness (Gronholm et al., 2017).

If we deliberately shift focus from stigma to discrimination in this way, there are a number of advantages. First, attention moves from intentions to actual behaviour, not if an employer *would* hire a person with mental illness, but if he or she *does*. Second, interventions can be tried and tested to change behaviour towards people with mental illness, without *necessarily* changing knowledge or feelings towards such people. Third, people who have a diagnosis of mental illness can expect to benefit from all the relevant anti-discrimination provisions and laws in their country or jurisdiction, or a basis of parity with people with physical disabilities. Fourth a discrimination perspective requires us to change viewpoint from that of the person within the 'in-group' to that of the person in the 'out-group', namely people with mental illness. In sum, this means sharpening our sights upon injustice and human rights as experienced by people with mental illness.

REFERENCES

Ahonen, L., Loeber, R., & Brent, D. A. (2019). The association between serious mental health problems and violence: some common assumptions and misconceptions. *Trauma Violence & Abuse*, **20**, 613–625.

Alonso, J., Buron, A., Bruffaerts, R., He, Y., Posada-Villa, J., Lepine, J. P., et al. (2008). Association of perceived stigma and mood and anxiety disorders: results from the World Mental Health Surveys. *Acta Psychiatrica Scandinavica*, **118**, 305–314.

Andrade, L. H., Alonso, J., Mneimneh, Z., Wells, J. E., Al-Hamzawi, A., Borges, G., et al. (2014). Barriers to mental health treatment: results from the WHO World Mental Health (WMH) Surveys. *Psychological Medicine*, **44**, 1303–1317.

Angermeyer, M. C., Anita, H., & Herbert, M. (2010). Emotional reactions to people with mental illness. *Epidemiologia e Psichiatria Sociale*, **19**, 26–32.

Aramouny, C., Kerbage, H., Richa, N., Rouhana, P., & Richa, S. (2020). Knowledge, attitudes, and beliefs of catholic clerics' regarding mental health in Lebanon. *Journal of Religion and Health*, **59**, 257–276.

Bakolis, I., Thornicroft, G., Vitoratou, S., Rüsch, N., Bonetto, C., Lasalvia, A., et al. (2019). Development and validation of the DISCUS scale: a reliable short measure for assessing experienced discrimination in people with mental health problems on a global level. *Schizophrenia Research*, **212**, 213–220.

Barber, S., Gronholm, P. C., Ahuja, S., Rüsch, N., & Thornicroft, G. (2020). Microaggressions towards people affected by mental health problems: a scoping review. *Epidemiology and Psychiatric Sciences*, **29**, 1–11.

Bartlett, P., Lewis, O., & Thorold, O. (2006). *Mental Disability and the European Convention on Human Rights*. Leiden: Martinus Nijhoff.

Bogardus, E. S. (1925). Social distance and its origins. *Journal of Applied Sociology*, **9**, 216–226.

Brohan E, Clement S, Rose D, Sartorius N, Slade M, Thornicroft G. (2013). Development and psychometric evaluation of the Discrimination and Stigma Scale (DISC). *Psychiatry Research*, **208**, 33–40.

Brown, J. S. L., Elliott, S. A., Boardman, J., Ferns, J., & Morrison, J. (2004). Meeting the unmet need for depression services with psycho-educational self-confidence workshops: preliminary report. *British Journal of Psychiatry*, **185**, 511–515.

Burti, L. & Mosher, L. R. (2003). Attitudes, values and beliefs of mental health workers. *Epidemiologia e Psichiatria Sociale*, **12**, 227–231.

Byng, R., Jones, R., Leese, M., Hamilton, B., McCrone, P., & Craig, T. (2004). Exploratory cluster randomised controlled trial of shared care development for long-term mental illness. *British Journal of General Practice*, **54**, 259–266.

Caldwell, T. M. & Jorm, A. F. (2001). Mental health nurses' beliefs about likely outcomes for people with schizophrenia or depression: a comparison with the public and other healthcare professionals. *Australian and New Zealand Journal of Mental Health Nursing*, **10**, 42–54.

Chamberlin, J. (2005). User/consumer involvement in mental health service delivery. *Epidemiologia e Psichiatria Sociale*, **14**, 10–14.

Corrigan, P. W., Edwards, A. B., Green, A., Diwan, S. L., & Penn, D. L. (2001). Prejudice, social distance, and familiarity with mental illness. *Schizophrenia Bulletin*, **27**, 219–225.

Corrigan, P. W., Markowitz, F. E., & Watson, A. C. (2004). Structural levels of mental illness stigma and discrimination. *Schizophrenia Bulletin*, **30**, 481–491.

Corrigan, P. W. & Penn, D. L. (1999). Lessons from social psychology on discrediting psychiatric stigma. *The American Psychologist*, **54**, 765–776.

Corrigan, P. W., River, L. P., Lundin, R. K., Penn, D. L., Uphoff-Wasowski, K., Campion, J., et al. (2001). Three strategies for changing attributions about severe mental illness. *Schizophrenia Bulletin*, **27**, 187–195.

Crandall, C. S. & Eshleman, A. (2003). A justification-suppression model of the expression and experience of prejudice. *Psychological Bulletin*, **129**, 414–446.

Cremonini, V., Pagnucci, N., Giacometti, F., & Rubbi, I. (2018). Health care professionals attitudes towards mental illness: observational study performed at a public health facility in Northern Italy. *Archives of Psychiatric Nursing*, **32**, 24–30.

Crisp, A. H. (Ed.) (2004). *Every Family in the Land: Understanding Prejudice and Discrimination Against People with mental Illness* (rev. ed.). London: The Royal Society of Medicine Press.

Crocker, J., Major, B., & Steele, C. (1998). Social stigma. In: Gilbert, D., Fiske, S. T., Lindzey, G. (Eds.), *The Handbook of Social Psychology* (4th ed, pp. 504–533). Boston, MA: McGraw Hill.

Deb, T., Lempp, H., Bakolis, I., Vince, T., Waugh, W., Henderson, C., et al. (2019). Responding to experienced and anticipated discrimination (READ): anti-stigma training for medical students towards patients with mental illness—study protocol for an international multisite non-randomised controlled study. *BMC Medical Education*, **19**, 1–9.

Dietrich, S., Beck, M., Bujantugs, B., Kenzine, D., Matschinger, H., & Angermeyer, M. C. (2004). The relationship between public causal beliefs and social distance toward mentally ill people. *Australian and New Zealand Journal of Psychiatry*, **38**, 348–354.

Dobson, K. S. & Wolf, S. (2022). 'Myths and facts' campaigns are at best ineffective and may increase mental illness stigma. *Stigma and Health*, 25 February.

Dovidio, J. F., Brigham, J., Johnson, B., & Gaertner, S. (1996). Stereotyping, prejudice and discrimination: another look. In: McCrae, N., Stangor, C., & Hewstone, M. (Eds.), *Stereotypes and Stereotyping* (pp. 276–319). New York: Guilford.

Dunion, L. & Gordon, L. (2005). Tackling the attitude problem. The achievements to date of Scotland's 'see me' anti-stigma campaign. *Mental Health Today*, **March**, 22–25.

DuPont-Reyes, M. J., Villatoro, A. P., Phelan, J. C., Painter, K., & Link, B. G. (2020). Adolescent views of mental illness stigma: an intersectional lens. *American Journal of Orthopsychiatry*, **90**, 201–211.

Eliasson, E. T., McNamee, L., Swanson, L., Lawrie, S. M., & Schwannauer, M. (2021). Unpacking stigma: meta-analyses of correlates and moderators of personal stigma in psychosis. *Clinical Psychology Review*, **89**, 102077.

Evans-Lacko, S., Knapp, M., McCrone, P., Thornicroft, G., & Mojtabai, R. (2013). The mental health consequences of the recession: economic hardship and employment of people with mental health problems in 27 European Countries. *PLoS One*, **8**, e69792.

Evans-Lacko, S., Rose, D., Little, K., Flach, C., Rhydderch, D., Henderson, C., et al. (2011). Development and psychometric properties of the Reported and Intended Behaviour Scale (RIBS): a stigma-related behaviour measure. *Epidemiology and Psychiatric Sciences*, **20**, 263–271.

Fiske, S. T. (1998). Stereotyping, prejudice and discrimination. In: Gilbert, D., Fiske, S., Lindzey, G. (Eds.), *The Handbook of Social Psychology* (4th ed., pp. 357–411). Boston, MA: McGraw Hill.

Fiske, S. T. (2003). Social cognition and social perception. *Annual Review of Psychology*, **44**, 155–194.

Forbes, H. J., Boyd, C. F. S., Jones, N., Greenberg, N., Jones, E., Wessely, S., et al. (2013). Attitudes to mental illness in the U.K. military: a comparison with the general population. *Military Medicine*, **178**, 957–965.

Furnham, A. & Swami, V. (2020). Mental health literacy: a review of what it is and why it matters. *International Perspectives in Psychology: Research, Practice, Consultation*, **7**, 240–257.

Girma, E., Ketema, B., Mulatu, T., Kohrt, B. A., Wahid, S. S., Heim, E., et al. (2022). Mental health stigma and discrimination in Ethiopia: evidence synthesis to inform stigma reduction interventions. *International Journal of Mental Health Systems*, **16**, 1–18.

Global Anti-Stigma Alliance (n.d.). Time To Change: what we do. https://www.time-to-change.org.uk/about-us/what-we-do/our-global-work/global-anti-stigma-alliance

Goffman, E. (1963). *Stigma: Notes on the Management of Spoiled Identity*. New York: Simon & Schuster, Inc.

Gronholm, P. C., Henderson, C., Deb, T., & Thornicroft, G. (2017). Interventions to reduce discrimination and stigma: the state of the art. *Social Psychiatry and Psychiatric Epidemiology*, **52**, 249–258.

Gurung, D., Poudyal, A., Wang, Y. L., Neupane, M., Bhattarai, K., Wahid, S. S., et al. (2022). Stigma against mental health disorders in Nepal conceptualised with a 'what matters most' framework: a scoping review. *Epidemiology and Psychiatric Sciences*, **31**, e11.

Gwarjanski, A. R. & Parrott, S. (2018). Schizophrenia in the news: the role of news frames in shaping online reader dialogue about mental illness. *Health Communication*, **33**, 954–961.

Hahn, H. (1988). The politics of physical differences: disability and discrimination. *Journal of Social Issues*, **44**, 39–47.

Hartini, N., Fardana, N. A., Ariana, A. D., & Wardana, N. D. (2018). Stigma toward people with mental health problems in Indonesia. *Psychology Research and Behavior Management*, **11**, 535.

Hayward, P., Wong, G., Bright, J. A., & Lam, D. (2002). Stigma and self-esteem in manic depression: an exploratory study. *Journal of Affective Disorders*, **69**, 61–67.

Heim, E., Henderson, C., Kohrt, B. A., Koschorke, M., Milenova, M., & Thornicroft, G. (2019). Reducing mental health-related stigma among medical and nursing students in low- and middle-income countries: a systematic review. *Epidemiology and Psychiatric Sciences*, **29**, e28.

Henderson, C., Flood, C., Leese, M., Thornicroft, G., Sutherby, K., & Szmukler, G. (2004). Effect of joint crisis plans on use of compulsory treatment in psychiatry: single blind randomised controlled trial. *BMJ*, **329**, 136–138.

Henderson, C., Noblett, J., Parke, H., Clement, S., Caffrey, A., Gale-Grant, O., et al. (2014). Mental health-related stigma in health care and mental health-care settings. *Lancet Psychiatry*, **1**, 467–482.

Henderson, C. & Thornicroft, G. (2009). Stigma and discrimination in mental illness: Time to Change. *Lancet*, **373**, 1928–1930.

Herek, G. M., Capitanio, J. P., & Widaman, K. F. (2002). HIV-related stigma and knowledge in the United States: prevalence and trends, 1991–1999. *American Journal of Public Health*, **92**, 371.

Ikwuka, U., Galbraith, N., Manktelow, K., Chen-Wilson, J., Oyebode, F., & Muomah, R. C. (2016). Attitude towards mental illness in southeastern Nigeria: the contradictions of a communitarian culture. *Journal of Community Psychology*, **44**, 182–98.

Jorm, A. F., Korten, A. E., Jacomb, P. A., Christensen, H., Rodgers, B., & Pollitt, P. (1997). Mental health literacy: a survey of the public's ability to recognise mental disorders and their beliefs about the effectiveness of treatment. *Medical Journal of Australia*, **166**, 182–186.

Kohrt, B. A., Jordans, M. J. D., Rai, S., Shrestha, P., Luitel, N. P., Ramaiya, M. K., et al. (2015). Therapist competence in global mental health: development of the ENhancing Assessment of Common Therapeutic factors (ENACT) rating scale. *Behaviour Research and Therapy*, **69**, 11–21.

Kohrt, B. A., Turner, E. L., Rai, S., Bhardwaj, A., Sikkema, K. J., Adelekun, A., et al. (2020). Reducing mental illness in healthcare settings: proof of concept for a social contact intervention to address what matters most for primary care providers. *Social Science & Medicine*, **250**, 112852.

Koschorke, M., Padmavati, R., Kumar, S., Cohen, A., Weiss, H. A., Chatterjee, S., et al. (2014). Experiences of stigma and discrimination of people with schizophrenia in India. *Social Science & Medicine*, **123**, 149–159.

Lagunes-Cordoba, E., Alcala-Lozano, R., Lagunes-Cordoba, R., Fresan-Orellana, A., Jarrett, M., Gonzalez-Olvera, J., et al. (2022). Evaluation of an anti-stigma intervention for Mexican psychiatric trainees. *Pilot and Feasibility Studies*, **8**, 1–11.

Lasalvia, A., Zoppei, S., van Bortel, T., Bonetto, C., Cristofalo, D., Wahlbeck, K., et al. (2013). Global pattern of experienced and anticipated discrimination reported by people with major depressive disorder: a cross-sectional survey. *Lancet*, **381**, 55–62.

Lester, H., Allan, T., Wilson, S., Jowett, S., & Roberts, L. (2003). A cluster randomised controlled trial of patient-held medical records for people with schizophrenia receiving shared care. *British Journal of General Practice*, **53**, 197–203.

Lethem, R. (2004). Mental illness in medical students and doctors: fitness to practice. In: Crisp, A. H. (Ed.), *Every Family in the Land* (pp. 356–364). London: Royal Society of Medicine.

Link, B. G., Yang, L. H., Phelan, J. C., & Collins, P. Y. (2004). Measuring mental illness stigma. *Schizophrenia Bulletin*, **30**:511–541.

Luhrmann, T. (2000). *Of Two Minds*. New York: Vintage Books.

Mascayano, F., Armijo, J. E., & Yang, L. H. (2015). Addressing stigma relating to mental illness in low- and middle-income countries. *Frontiers in Psychiatry*, **6**, 38.

Mascayano, F., Tapia, T., Schilling, S., Alvarado, R., Tapia, E., Lips, W., et al. (2016). Stigma toward mental illness in Latin America and the Caribbean: a systematic review. *Revista Brasileira de Psiquiatria*, **38**, 73–85.

Mathias, K., Kermode, M., Goicolea, I., Seefeldt, L., Shidhaye, R., & San Sebastian, M. (2018). Social distance and community attitudes towards people with psycho-social disabilities in Uttarakhand, India. *Community Mental Health Journal*, **54**, 343–53.

Mehta, N., Clement, S., Marcus, E., Stona, A. C., Bezborodovs, N., Evans-Lacko, S., et al. (2015). Evidence for effective interventions to reduce mental health-related stigma and discrimination in the medium and long term: systematic review. *British Journal of Psychiatry*, **207**, 377–384.

Mino, Y., Yasuda, N., Kanazawa, S., & Inoue, S. (2000). Effects of medical education on attitudes towards mental illness among medical students: a five-year follow-up study. *Acta Medica Okayama*, **54**, 127–132.

Mino, Y., Yasuda, N., Tsuda, T., & Shimodera, S. (2001). Effects of a one-hour educational program on medical students' attitudes to mental illness. *Psychiatry and Clinical Neurosciences*, **55**, 501–507.

Nohr, L., Ruiz, A. L., Sandoval Ferrer, J. E., & Buhlmann, U. (2021). Mental health stigma and professional help-seeking attitudes a comparison between Cuba and Germany. *PLoS One*, **16**, e0246501.

Oshodi, Y. O., Abdulmalik, J., Ola, B., James, B. O., Bonetto, C., Cristofalo, D., et al. (2014). Pattern of experienced and anticipated discrimination among people with depression in Nigeria: a cross-sectional study. *Social Psychiatry and Psychiatric Epidemiology*, **49**, 259–266.

Phelan, J. C., Yang, L. H., & Cruz-Rojas, R. (2006). Effects of attributing serious mental illnesses to genetic causes on orientations to treatment. *Psychiatric Services*, **57**, 382–387.

Pinfold, V., Toulmin, H., Thornicroft, G., Huxley, P., Farmer, P., & Graham, T. (2003). Reducing psychiatric stigma and discrimination: evaluation of educational interventions in UK secondary schools. *British Journal of Psychiatry*, **182**, 342–346.

Piper, S. E., Bailey, P. E., Lam, L. T., & Kneebone, I. I. (2018). Predictors of mental health literacy in older people. *Archives of Gerontology and Geriatrics*, **79**, 52–56.

Potts, L. C. & Henderson, C. (2021). Evaluation of anti-stigma social marketing campaigns in Ghana and Kenya: Time to Change Global. *BMC Public Health*, **21**, 1–14.

Radez, J., Reardon, T., Creswell, C., Lawrence, P. J., Evdoka-Burton, G., & Polly, W. Why do children and adolescents (not) seek and access professional help for their mental health problems? A systematic review of quantitative and qualitative studies. *European Child & Adolescent Psychiatry*, **30**, 183–211.

Reardon, T., Harvey, K., Baranowska, M., O'Brien, D., Smith, L., & Creswell, C. (2017). What do parents perceive are the barriers and facilitators to accessing psychological treatment for mental health problems in children and adolescents? A systematic review of qualitative and quantitative studies. *European Child & Adolescent Psychiatry*, **26**, 623–647.

Rose, D., Thornicroft, G., Pinfold, V., & Kassam, A. (2007). 250 labels used to stigmatise people with mental illness. *BMC Health Services Research*, **7**, 97.

Rüsch, N., Corrigan, P. W., Wassel, A., Michaels, P., Olschewski, M., Wilkniss, S., et al. (2009). Ingroup perception and responses to stigma among persons with mental illness. *Acta Psychiatrica Scandinavica*, **120**, 320–328.

Sadow, D., Ryder, M., & Webster, D. (2009). Is education of health professionals encouraging stigma towards the mentally ill? *SSM—Population Health*, **11**, 657–665.

Sapkota, R. P., Gurung, D., Neupane, D., Shah, S. K., Kienzler, H., & Kirmayer, L. J. (2014). A village possessed by 'witches': a mixed-methods case–control study of possession and common mental disorders in Rural Nepal. *Culture, Medicine and Psychiatry*, **38**, 642–668.

Sartorius, N. & Schulze, H. (2005). *Reducing the Stigma of Mental Illness: A Report from a Global Association*. Cambridge: Cambridge University Press.

Schlosberg, A. (1993). Psychiatric stigma and mental health professionals (stigmatizers and destigmatizers). *Medicine and Law*, **12**, 409–416.

Schnyder, N., Panczak, R., Groth, N., & Schultze-Lutter, F. (2017). Association between mental health-related stigma and active help-seeking: systematic review and meta-analysis. *British Journal of Psychiatry*, **210**, 261–268.

Schomerus, G., Schwahn, C., Holzinger, A., Corrigan, P. W., Grabe, H. J., Carta, M. G., et al. (2012). Evolution of public attitudes about mental illness: a systematic review and meta-analysis. *Acta Psychiatrica Scandinavica*, **125**, 440–452.

Shrivastava, A., Johnston, M. E., Thakar, M., Shrivastava, S., Sarkhel, G., Sunita, I., et al. (2011). Impact and origin of stigma and discrimination in schizophrenia: patient perceptions. *Stigma Research and Action*, **1**, 11.

Simpson, A. I. F., Penney, S. R., & Jones, R. M. (2022). Homicide associated with psychotic illness: what global temporal trends tell us about the association between mental illness and violence. *Australian and New Zealand Journal of Psychiatry*, **56**, 1384–1388.

Sorsdahl, K., Stein, D. J., & Myers, B. (2012). Negative attributions towards people with substance use disorders in South Africa: variation across substances and by gender. *BMC Psychiatry*, **12**, 1–8.

Sue, D. (2013). *Microaggressions and Marginality: Manifestation, Dynamics, and Impact*. Hoboken, NJ: John Wiley & Sons.

Sue, D. W., Capodilupo, C. M., Torino, G. C., Bucceri, J. M., Holder, A. M. B., Nadal, K. L., et al. (2007). Racial microaggressions in everyday life: implications for clinical practice. *The American Psychologist*, **62**, 271–286.

Sullivan, M., Hamilton, T., & Allen, H. (2005). Changing stigma through the media. In: Corrigan, P. W. (Ed.), *On the Stigma of Mental Illness: Practical Strategies for Research and Social Change* (pp. 297–312). Washington, DC: American Psychological Association.

Sutherby, K., Szmukler, G. I., Halpern, A., Alexander, M., Thornicroft, G., Johnson, C., et al. (1999). A study of 'crisis cards' in a community psychiatric service. *Acta Psychiatrica Scandinavica*, **100**, 56–61.

Svensson, B. & Hansson, L. (2016). How mental health literacy and experience of mental illness relate to stigmatizing attitudes and social distance towards people with depression or psychosis: a cross-sectional study. *Nordic Journal of Psychiatry*, **70**, 309–313.

Swanson, J., Swartz, M., Ferron, J., Elbogen, E., & van Dorn, R. (2006). Psychiatric advance directives among public mental health consumers in five U.S. cities: prevalence, demand, and correlates. *Journal of the American Academy of Psychiatry and the Law*, **34**, 43–57.

Tateyama, M., Asai, M., Hashimoto, M., Bartels, M., & Kasper, S. (1998). Transcultural study of schizophrenic delusions. Tokyo versus Vienna and Tübingen (Germany). *Psychopathology*, **31**, 59–68.

Thornicroft, G. (2006). *Shunned: Discrimination Against People with Mental Illness*. Oxford: Oxford University Press.

Thornicroft, G., Bakolis, I., Evans-Lacko, S., Gronholm, P. C., Henderson, C., Kohrt, B. A., et al. (2019). Key lessons learned from the INDIGO global network on mental health related stigma and discrimination. *World Psychiatry*, **18**, 229–230.

Thornicroft, G., Brohan, E., Rose, D., Sartorius, N., & Leese, M. (2009). Global pattern of experienced and anticipated discrimination against people with schizophrenia: a cross-sectional survey. *Lancet*, **373**, 408–415.

Thornicroft, G., Mehta, N., Clement, S., Evans-Lacko, S., Doherty, M., Rose, D., et al. (2016). Evidence for effective interventions to reduce mental-health-related stigma and discrimination. *Lancet*, **387**, 1123–1132.

Thornicroft, G., Rose, D., Kassam, A., & Sartorius, N. (2007). Stigma: ignorance, prejudice or discrimination? *British Journal of Psychiatry*, **190**, 192–193.

Thornicroft, G., Rose, D., & Mehta, N. (2010). Discrimination against people with mental illness: what can psychiatrists do? *Advances in Psychiatric Treatment*, **16**, 53–59.

Thornicroft, G. & Rose, D. (2005). Mental health in Europe. *BMJ*, **330**, 613–614.

Thornicroft, G., Sunkel, C., Aliev, A. A., Baker, S., Brohan, E., Davies, K., et al. (2022). The Lancet Commission on ending stigma and discrimination in mental health. *Lancet*, **400**, 1438–1480.

Upadhaya, N., Regmi, U., Gurung, D., Luitel, N. P., Petersen, I., Jordans, M. J. D., et al. (2020). Mental health and psychosocial support services in primary health care in Nepal: perceived facilitating factors, barriers and strategies for improvement. *BMC Psychiatry*, **20**, 1–13.

Vaughan, G. & Hansen, C. (2004). 'Like Minds, Like Mine': a New Zealand project to counter the stigma and discrimination associated with mental illness. *Australasian Psychiatry*, **12**, 113–117.

Votruba, N., Eaton, J., Prince, M., & Thornicroft, G. (2014). The importance of global mental health for the Sustainable Development Goals. *Journal of Mental Health*, **23**, 283–286.

Votruba, N. & Thornicroft, G. (2016). Sustainable development goals and mental health: learnings from the contribution of the FundaMentalSDG global initiative. *Global Mental Health*, **3**, e26.

Wahl, O. F. (1995). *Media Madness: Public Images of Mental Illness*. New Brunswick, NJ: Rutgers University Press.

Walsh, D. A. B. & Foster, J. L. H. (2021). A call to action. A critical review of mental health related anti-stigma campaigns. *Frontiers in Public Health*, **8**, 1–15.

Weiss, M. G., Jadhav, S., Raguram, R., Vounatsou, P., & Littlewood, R. (2010). Psychiatric stigma across cultures: local validation in Bangalore and London. *Anthropology & Medicine*, **8**, 71–87.

Wheat, K., Brohan, E., Henderson, C., & Thornicroft, G. (2010). Mental illness and the workplace: conceal or reveal? *Journal of the Royal Society of Medicine*, **103**, 83.

Wilde, M. H. (2003). Life with an indwelling urinary catheter: the dialectic of stigma and acceptance. *Qualitative Health Research*, **13**, 1189–1204.

World Health Organization (2021). *WHO Mental Health Atlas 2020*. Geneva: World Health Organization.

World Health Organization (2005). *WHO Resource Book on Mental Health, Human Rights and Legislation*. Geneva: World Health Organization.

Xu, X., Li, X. M., Zhang, J., & Wang, W. (2018). Mental health-related stigma in China. *Issues in Mental Health Nursing*, **39**, 126–134.

Xu, Z., Müller, M., Lay, B., Oexle, N., Drack, T., Bleiker, M., et al. (2018). Involuntary hospitalization, stigma stress and suicidality: a longitudinal study. *Social Psychiatry and Psychiatric Epidemiology*, **53**, 309–312.

Yang, L. H., Chen, F. P., Sia, K. J., Lam, J., Lam, K., Ngo, H., et al. (2014). 'What matters most': a cultural mechanism moderating structural vulnerability and moral experience of mental illness stigma. *Social Science & Medicine*, **103**, 84–93.

Yang, L. H., Thornicroft, G., Alvarado, R., Vega, E., & Link, B. G. (2014). Recent advances in cross-cultural measurement in psychiatric epidemiology: utilizing 'what matters most' to identify culture-specific aspects of stigma. *International Journal of Epidemiology*, **43**, 494–510.

Yin, H., Wardenaar, K. J., Xu, G., Tian, H., & Schoevers, R. A. (2020). Mental health stigma and mental health knowledge in Chinese population: a cross-sectional study. *BMC Psychiatry*, **20**, 1–10.

Yuan, Q., Picco, L., Chang, S., Abdin, E., Chua, B. Y., Ong, S., et al. (2017). Attitudes to mental illness among mental health professionals in Singapore and comparisons with the general population. *PLoS One*, **12**, e0187593.

SECTION 7
Policies and the funding

32. **Shaping national mental health policy** 333
    Harvey Whiteford and Sandra Diminic

33. **Funding of mental health services** 341
    Dan Chisholm, Martin Knapp, and Shari Jadoolal

Shaping national mental health policy

Harvey Whiteford and Sandra Diminic

Introduction

From the perspective of those at the service delivery coalface, national mental health policy often seems a remote activity unrelated to their daily responsibilities. The concept of national policy can be vague and how it is formed opaque. The time taken from the beginnings of policy formulation to adoption and implementation can seem extraordinarily long. When national policy does become relevant it is often because it is driving change that the clinician or service manager finds confronting and difficult. It is therefore easy to be cynical about government policy, but most of us still want and expect explicit national mental health policy, the implementation of which drives improved services for people with mental illness and their families. For the creation of good policy, those working outside of government bureaucracies need to better understand, and be able to exert influence on, the policymaking process.

The aim of this chapter is to describe the policy development cycle and the factors that shape national mental health policy. A good understanding of these should enhance the capacity of service providers and others to influence the content and effectiveness of mental health policy. At the outset it is important to provide a caveat. This chapter is most relevant to countries that operate a democratic system of government. While many of the concepts discussed in the chapter will apply to policy development in any country with an organized system of government, the assumptions that underpin the policy cycle described in the chapter are most applicable in a democratically governed society.

Also at the outset, it is important to clarify the term *policy* which is often used to describe different things, such as government decisions, government programmes, and/or the political process. The following definition applies to the way the term policy is used in this chapter: 'policy is deciding at any time and place what objectives and substantive measures should be chosen in order to deal with a particular problem, issue or innovation' (Dimock et al., 1983, p. 40). In this chapter, the discussion is limited to government policy. The private for-profit and not-for-profit sectors also make policy for their own purposes and while many of the principles described here might be relevant, there are also many differences beyond the scope of this chapter.

The public policy cycle has been well documented and health policy analysis is an important area for academic research (Walt et al., 2008). Roberts and colleagues (2003) developed a five-part policy cycle (**Figure 32.1**) that has been applied to health. Understanding the components of the cycle—problem identification, development of a policy option, policy adoption, policy implementation, and policy evaluation—and the factors that influence and shape them should improve our ability to exert influence on the policy content and outcomes. The description of these five components as a cycle should not be taken to imply that the policy process is uniform and sequential. Policy development and implementation is anything but linear, and flexibility is essential in the policy process. In addition to the impact of the policy environment on the process of policy development, it is essential to consider other aspects of the policy process in each phase. For example, it is important for policy development to be influenced by an understanding of implementation and for evaluation to be considered very early in the cycle. This chapter is primarily concerned with *shaping* national policy and will therefore concentrate on the first two components of the policy cycle: problem identification and development of a policy option. It is nevertheless important to understand how these two steps relate to the adoption, implementation, and revision of mental health policy.

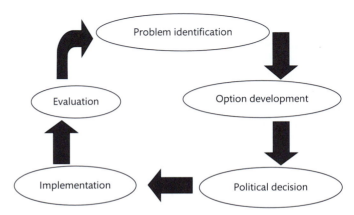

Figure 32.1 Generic policy cycle as identified by Roberts et al. (2003).
Source: Roberts, M., Hsiao, W., Berman, P., & Reich, M. (2003). *Getting Health Reform Right: A Guide to Improving Performance and Equity*. Oxford: Oxford University Press.

For economically more developed countries, many improvements in the quality of life for people with mental illness have come from improvements in welfare and health care more generally (Frank & Glied, 2006). Conversely, for those countries in economic decline and/or in conflict, the mental health of the population and services for those with mental illness usually suffer (Charlson et al., 2019; Jacob et al., 2007). The national economic and security situations notwithstanding, it is important to identify what action can be taken within the mental health sector, including in low- and middle-income countries, to improve mental health (Saraceno et al., 2007). Having a national policy on mental health is widely seen as fundamental to promoting mental health in the population and delivering effective mental health services (World Health Organization (WHO), 2005a). A review of the health and mental health policy literature identifies the context within which policy development takes place, the factors that influence the process and shape the content of the policy, the factors that impede or facilitate implementation of the policy, and the extent to which an evidence base informs policy (Baker, 1996; Lee et al., 2002; Walt 1994; WHO, 2005b)

Problem identification

For an understanding of what shapes mental health policy, it is most important to appreciate what problem or problems the policy is intended to address. Government policy, including mental health policy, is developed in response to real or perceived issues or problems. The identification of any particular problem as needing policy attention occurs within the wider social, economic, historical, and political environment. A problem that those working in mental health services think is deserving of government attention may not necessarily appear the most prominent from a government perspective. For example, the fact that the majority of people with depression in a population do not access treatment might not be a priority for a busy mental health service. However, governments may take a different view about people who do not, or cannot, get treatment and may see improving access to care as a priority needing policy attention.

Among the many demands being made on government, how does one particular issue, in our case mental health, become identified as needing policy attention? These demands, and therefore the factors shaping policy, can arise from inside, or from forces external to, the country. With respect to the latter, international agencies can be influential, particularly in developing countries where international expectations are articulated and development or aid funding is linked to policy attention to a particular area. For example, by highlighting the importance of mental health in *The World Health Report 2001* and subsequent *Comprehensive Mental Health Action Plan 2013–2030* (WHO, 2021c), the WHO made it harder for national governments to ignore this area of health. The potential ranking of country resources allocated to mental health in the WHO's *Mental Health Atlas* (WHO, 2021a) can attract internal and external criticism to those countries with low resource allocation, thereby applying pressure to the government to increase resources.

International aid agencies and development banks, with their focus on social and economic development and poverty reduction, can greatly influence the content of health policy by the conditions attached to their aid and loans. To the extent that their focus includes mental health and related disability and psychosocial development, national governments will consider mental health more seriously. The relationship between poverty and mental health (Ridley et al., 2020) has allowed poverty reduction funding to be linked to improving mental health, through both promotion of psychosocial development at a population level and the improvement of treatment services (Flisher et al., 2007). Impaired mental health adversely impacts many other health conditions and opportunities can be found to improve outcomes in a range of physical health areas by employing strategies to improve mental health (Prince et al., 2007). At a more macro level, when it is possible to link action on mental health to achievement of high level goals, such as the United Nations Sustainable Development Goals (Votruba & Thornicroft, 2016), further expectations and opportunities are created for government action.

Some international agencies focus on post-conflict redevelopment and human rights issues and here there have also been opportunities to incorporate a focus on mental health policy and services (Piachaud, 2008). The history of stigma, human rights violations, and social exclusion of people with mental illness (Patel et al., 2006) has led to international efforts to reform mental health legislation and services. For example, major efforts have been made in eastern Europe to reform mental health legislation encouraged by the European Union and United Nations (Knapp et al., 2007). The WHO QualityRights initiative provides training and guidance materials to support countries to prioritize human rights within their mental health systems and services (Funk & Bold, 2020; WHO, 2019). The WHO has also published guidance to support person-centred and human rights-based approaches within community mental health services (WHO, 2021b).

New and influential research findings can also provide a base from which policy-relevant arguments for attention to mental health can be made. The publication of the Global Burden of Disease Studies since 1996 showing mental disorders to be one of the leading causes of health-related disability in most countries (GBD 2019 Mental Disorders Collaborators, 2022; Murray et al., 1996) and a seminal *Lancet* series of articles (Horton, 2007) outlining the need for increased action in mental health both raised the expectation that governments would do more in the area of mental health. International professional organizations such as the World Psychiatric Association (http://www.wpanet.org), non-government organizations such as the World Federation for Mental Health (https://wfmh.global/) and United for Global Mental Health (https://unitedgmh.org/), and advocacy movements such as the Movement for Global Mental Health (http://www.globalmentalhealth.org) can and do apply external pressure on governments to address mental health issues. These movements may have contributed to the significantly higher profile of mental health internationally in recent years (Collins & Saxena, 2016); however, there are continued calls to advocate for improvements to mental health care on national and international political agendas (United for Global Mental Health, 2022).

Complementing these external influences, demand on national governments to address a particular issue arises from inside the country. Most governments feel the need to respond to the demands of their citizens. Information about the needs of individuals within a country can be effective in advocating for mental health resources. For example, the World Mental Health Survey Initiative (https://www.hcp.med.harvard.edu/wmh/) has undertaken surveys in over

25 countries using the WHO Composite International Diagnostic Interview, identifying the prevalence of mental disorders, the disability caused by these disorders, and services utilized (or not utilized) by those with the disorders. Dissemination of findings such as these within the country highlights the extent of the health need, and the gap between need and services.

In response to such evidence, WHO member states have adopted the WHO's *Comprehensive Mental Health Action Plan 2013–2020* (WHO, 2021c) which sets clear actions and indicators for national and international agencies to promote mental health and wellbeing and improve mental health services. The WHO also provides a range of guidance to support such action, including the Mental Health Gap Action Programme aimed at scaling up care for mental, neurological, and substance use disorders (https://www.who.int/teams/mental-health-and-substance-use/treatment-care/mental-health-gap-action-programme). The increasing recognition of the economic burden of mental illness, especially in terms of lost productivity, has also been a factor spurring action in some countries (Saxena et al., 2007) especially when there is seen to be a positive economic return on investing in treatment of mental disorders (WHO, 2013).

The first author's experience as mental health specialist at the World Bank was that there were four major mental health areas of focus that influenced governments to seek World Bank loans that included a mental health component. The first two of these were high-profile public health issues—suicide and substance abuse. Both had received adverse media attention and were emotive topics that the government came to believe were necessary areas for policy attention. The third area was to address the mental health consequences of conflict or natural disasters. Again, populations having experienced conflict or a natural disaster were in media focus and were attractive targets for donor countries and organizations with considerable non-governmental organization engagements. The fourth area was to facilitate the reorganization of services to move resources from institutional to community care. Here governments were persuaded that reform of services, including a more cost-effective use of existing resources, could lead to better outcomes for more patients with mental illness.

Roberts and colleagues (2003) highlight two mechanisms that determine how these issues can receive selective attention within a country. First, cultural norms and social attitudes in a country provide a set of filters that selectively focus on or divert public and government attention. Attitudes that devalue and minimize the importance of any issue will result in attention being diverted away. A mental health example is the poor living conditions, inadequate quality of care, and human rights abuses in psychiatric hospitals during much of the last century. For decades, these circumstances were not seen as warranting intervention. A change in societal attitudes saw the extension of the human rights movement to encompass individuals with mental illness, legitimize, and later require government action in the form of a major policy shift to either improve conditions in these hospitals or to close wards or even hospitals.

Social norms and attitudes continue to change. The deinstitutionalization that resulted in part from the new policy position is now facing its own backlash. Societal focus has shifted from patient abuse and neglect in institutions to community safety and the 'right' to treatment for mental illness. The right to treatment often means increased access to inpatient care. A parallel changing of norms and attitudes underpins the fluctuations in the threshold for involuntary detention in our Mental Health Acts. When societal focus is on individual liberty, the threshold for involuntary detention and treatment is higher. When the focus is on 'right to treatment' and public safety, the threshold for involuntary detention and treatment is lower.

The second mechanism identified by Roberts et al. (2003) relates to the role of 'issue entrepreneurs'. These individuals or groups are advocates who promote attention to their issue. They highlight and promote the issue as needing attention until it emerges from the societal filters as a problem needing policy attention. These advocates may be political or special interest lobby groups within the community. Their motives vary. Some groups form on the basis of a conviction about the need to improve a particular area and these individuals or groups often have a stake in that area. In mental health, there are professional groupings (e.g. national associations of psychiatrists or psychologists) and consumer and carer groupings. Sometimes these groupings form a coalition and increase their ability to influence government policy (Whiteford et al., 2016).

Advocates target those who they believe can deliver the decisions they want and these are usually elected or appointed politicians. The motives of these politicians and their staff are usually a mixture of genuine interest and party and/or electoral politics. The balance between these motives is often not clear to the advocacy groups and the willingness of politicians to become involved in particular issues can be influenced by the electoral cycle, with a need to placate activists and minimize adverse publicity in an election year. Advocates need to understand the different roles of politicians, their staff, and government officials and public servants in their country. It is generally expected that the departmental officials (a bureaucracy whose members are called public servants in many countries) implement the policies of the government of the day. However, most governments do not come to power with a detailed action plan for how they will deal with mental health. Even when mental health is part of a political party's health policy statement, there is usually little detail about mental health and much room for interpretation. The officials in the ministry of health and related ministries (such as social services, justice, housing, and education) do most of this interpretation. these officials hold the corporate history about government programmes and prepare submissions with options (and often costings of those options) for ministers and governments to consider. They can therefore facilitate or impede problem identification (and policy adoption and implementation). Given departmental officials generally hold the keys to making the machinery of government work, it is important for issue entrepreneurs to understand the role these officials play in having matters considered by the government.

The interaction between the social filters and the efforts of advocates produces fluctuating patterns in the process of problem definition and in this the incentives and behaviour of the media can play an important role (Miller, 2007). The reporting of issues by the media can highlight important problems needing attention or create the perception of a problem where none really exists (Meurk et al., 2015). This is especially true in countries where there is less government control of the media. While a 'free press' is an important element of democratic societies, the media is not unbiased or without its own distorting of facts. The media focus can be captured by scandal and/or personalities, which at its worst is called tabloid journalism. Information is often presented in a way that will sell media products. However, the media can also be an important avenue for disseminating information and improving community knowledge. Nevertheless, there is a herd pattern found among the media. Competitive media outlets can feel compelled to cover a story simply because other outlets are doing so, but the interest in the issue can quickly fade. Mental health advocates have to be patient as their issue cycles in and out of public attention and different perspectives on the issue are presented as problems at different times.

Development of a policy option

Once it has been agreed that a problem exists and needs to be addressed, policymakers have to find a way of doing this. Sometimes the option for fixing the problem is predetermined. This occurs when the government has been elected with a mandate to take certain action. However, this is uncommon in mental health and it is usually after a government has formed that solutions to various problems need to be found. How a solution is chosen from among a range of options is policy development.

Governments may try to craft a policy solution in a very generic way. Decision research suggests that decisions about resource allocation by governments are influenced by knowledge of the need and effectiveness of service options, perceptions of resource scarcity, the political ideology of individual decision-makers, and perceptions of responsibility for the recipient's problems that require service (Corrigan & Watson, 2003).

Solutions to improving service delivery can be sought by considering health as an industry with inputs, processes, outputs, and outcomes and applying industry solutions to problems of quality, equity, and efficiency. Historically, mental health services have been measured by counting inputs (numbers of staff or beds) or processes and activities (number of occupied bed days or number of outpatient services provided). In industry, routine outcome measures are considered essential in order to measure efficiency and allow customer feedback and benchmarking. Mental health has historically been disadvantaged by the lack of outcome measures that can be easily collected, that are clinically relevant to the clinician and consumer, and able to be used in cost-effectiveness analyses. However, recent decades have seen major advances in these areas with the introduction of routine outcome measures and the development of methodologies for cost-effectiveness of mental health interventions (Chisholm, 2005; McDaid et al., 2019).

Governments often start by looking at what other jurisdictions or countries have chosen to do in response to similar problems. In mental health policy and service development there is an established and growing evidence base for what services work and when (De Silva & Ryan, 2016; WHO, 2005a). Whether a policy option is being imported from another jurisdiction or from another industry or is developed generically, it is necessary to arrive at a consensus on the option to be chosen. Achieving this consensus requires the government to consider the possible options and choose from among them. In many countries this choice will be informed by stakeholder consultation. Choosing the stakeholders to consult is important, because excluding any major group from the process will create ill will and potential opposition. It is nearly always better to have all stakeholders involved in the process, even if it is considered that this will result in time-consuming debate and even enmity. Subsequent political support may depend, in large part, on the extent of stakeholder consultation and support for any particular option.

Stakeholder analysis is a recognized methodology used to determine the position of relevant groups and individuals both inside and outside government who are likely to influence the policy choice and the success of its implementation (Sturm, 1999). Stakeholder analysis includes interest group analysis and bureaucratic analysis and has been refined to the extent that software exists to do the analysis (Reich, 1996).

Mental health reform also requires complementary action in areas outside health. A challenge for national mental health policy is clarifying what policy should be endorsed and action taken in portfolios such as social services, housing, education, police, and justice. The correct policy settings in these areas can greatly improve outcomes for people with mental illness and overcome fragmentation between components of the health, housing, and social services systems (Hogan, 2008); the government officials and stakeholders from these sectors cannot be excluded from consideration when mental health policy options are being developed.

The opinions of identified stakeholders and views of the general population (often considered to be expressed through the media) sometimes agree. While major policy shifts are often adopted because they fit well with the interests of these major stakeholders, overriding the findings of any stakeholder analysis is the question of whether an option presented as a policy position is politically feasible. The position of experts in the stakeholder community and politics can clash when the two come to irreconcilable conclusions. The debate about needle exchange programmes is an example (Collins & Coates, 1989). The scientific data supported the use of such programmes but in many countries the political view was that they would be unpopular with the electorate. This leads us to consider how the decision is made to adopt a policy, and this decision is political.

Political decision

The environment of political decision-making is complex. Factors such as the relative power of each player (politicians, advisors, government officials, and major stakeholders) in the political landscape, the positions taken by them, and the intensity of commitment for or against the policy all come into play. Within the political sphere, these players include not only the health minister, but also their staff, other key ministers (especially the minister responsible for finance) and their staff, and the head of the government (e.g. the premier or prime minister) and their social policy or health policy adviser. Senior bureaucrats and advisory bodies in each of these departments are often exceptionally influential through the advice they give to the minister's office. Successfully negotiating a coalition of support from among these players usually involves bargaining and trade-offs. Throughout the process of negotiation, the content of a policy will be modified, because compromise is usually necessary to achieve consensus.

In trying to arrive at a decision about adopting a policy, the politicians and their advisors will often scan the stakeholder and community landscape to assess the degree of support the policy will have. Determining this is made difficult in health and mental health by levels of complexity. It is necessary to consider the impact of a policy change on other parts of the system because it may be necessary to make multiple changes at the same time in order to achieve the right policy outcome. Failure to do this can undermine the success of good policy decisions in another area. For example, the policy of closing long-stay hospital beds was often accompanied by a policy to expand community-based mental health services. However, the lack of community-based accommodation for patients discharged from the hospitals, often the responsibility of the housing department, seriously undermined the mental health policies (Whiteford, 1994).

Another component of this complexity is the concentrated costs, and power, of select groups such as the medical and nursing professions. The potential beneficiaries of a policy, for example consumers, are generally less powerful and less well organized. The closure of a ward in a psychiatric hospital with the savings going to community-based services is likely to bring a more vigorous response from the staff who are to be affected in the hospital than the potential beneficiaries of the community services.

To create the necessary support for a policy to be adopted, it can be useful to align it with symbols that are seen as ideologically unchallengeable and which would have widespread community support. Community mental health care was aligned with 'least restrictive care'. Concepts such as the 'right' to treatment and 'equity' in access to care were introduced to generate support for the relevant policies.

Sometimes it is also a matter of reframing the explanation around the policy to ensure political adoption. During the revision of mental health legislation in Australia, a policy debate arose about legislation permitting patients to be involuntarily treated in private hospitals. This position was initially seen in Australia as unsupportable because of the perception that the private sector would profit from patients being treated in hospital against their will. With over a third of the population at the time having private health insurance and wanting treatment with the psychiatrist of their choice, the policy position was reframed to argue that a person with mental illness, who had chosen and paid for their private health insurance, should be allowed to remain with the psychiatrist (and hospital) of their choice even when (or especially when) their illness was at its worst. With this reframing of the context, the policy became politically acceptable and was adopted. Perceptions of policy reform are matters of values as well as facts. Political decision-making is about emotion as well as data.

Policy implementation

Many policies are developed and adopted but not implemented. Government options are actually quite limited and in reality they have only five main levers available (Lee et al., 2002; Musgrove, 1996). These are information collection and dissemination; the financing system that determines how resources are collected and who has access to them; the payment system that determines on what terms these resources are made available to individuals and organizations; the organization of the health system in both the distribution of services and how they respond to consumer demands; and the regulatory system, which imposes a set of constraints on services (e.g. how providers are trained and accredited, how any health or pharmaceutical insurance schemes operate, and regulations that cover the private sector). The specific levers available to different levels of government will vary depending on the governance arrangements for the health system (Meurk et al., 2017).

Successful implementation requires an implementation plan and there are many excellent texts on strategic planning (Bryson, 2004; Swayne et al., 2006). A discussion on strategic planning is outside the scope of this chapter but it is important to emphasize that policy implementation is much more likely to be successful if it has the support of those professional and community organizations that came together to ensure that the policy was adopted in the first place (Shen et al., 2017). In addition, forging new alliances consolidates support and enhances implementation.

The central government, if it has sufficient financial resources, can tie funding allocations to the implementation of the policy (and the provision of agreed data to allow monitoring of the policy implementation), as can regional or state governments with funding going to districts or local health care organizations. The information lever is important as there needs to be agreement to collect data on national progress in implementing the policy. National indicators need to be drawn from data collected around the country at service delivery sites and considerable effort is needed to develop nationally consistent data definitions and collection so comparable data from different parts of the country can be aggregated. National reports on progress should be public documents and benchmarks that can be used as a form of accountability.

Policy implementation requires sustained effort over time. During the implementation stage, which is often over a 5- or 10-year time span, the political party in power when the policy was adopted may well change. However, if the coalition of stakeholders remains largely intact and there is public expectation for change then progress should continue. There is, however, always a risk that new governments, with their need to have policies which distinguish them from the party they replaced, will attempt to prematurely change the direction of the implementation. This is just one reason why the implementation of policy virtually never goes as planned. It is also an argument for attempting to gain bipartisan support for the policy when it is developed. Flexibility is essential for responding and adapting to emerging issues, which can create barriers and opportunities.

There are many examples of the key elements of mental health service programmes (Pirkis et al., 2007; Thornicroft & Tansella, 2004), including the WHO's Mental Health Gap Action Programme (https://www.who.int/teams/mental-health-and-substance-use/treatment-care/mental-health-gap-action-programme) which provides advice on scaling up services for mental, neurological, and substance use disorders, especially within low- and middle-income countries. Each country can adapt the available evidence for their own circumstances. At a local level, implementation of national policy will also tend to be piecemeal in response to specific problems and resources idiosyncratic to the local environment (Garfield, 2009).

Evaluation

The shaping of national mental health policy should be shaped by an evaluation of the successes and failures of implementing existing policy. However, as noted earlier, many polices remain largely unimplemented and even fewer are evaluated in a way that would inform a revised national policy. By the time an evaluation is due to be conducted (at the end of 5 or 10 years), many of the politicians and government officials originally involved in its development will have moved to different areas. During the implementation, organizations that supported the policy may have wilted (or grown), and those who opposed it may be stronger. The environment will be different. For an evaluation to have credibility, it must be as transparent and independent as possible. This means finding people to undertake the evaluation who can demonstrate objectivity. With the availability of higher-quality independent data, it is possible to have the evaluation done by representatives of the key stakeholders.

The results of the evaluation should be used to revise the policy. In revising policy or developing successive implementation plans, it is important to resist the temptation to neglect those areas that have been successful and focus primarily on areas that have been less well addressed. There will always be criticism that areas were neglected and the temptation to expand the policy implementation agenda once the policy is revised is enormous. While the policy can and should be broad, it is important to ensure that in policy implementation scarce resources remain focused on key areas where the best outcomes can be achieved. If the effort is diffuse and resources spread too widely, effectiveness will be diluted, with a loss of credibility for the policy.

Conclusion

Policy development, adoption, implementation, and evaluation are often seen as political and bureaucratic exercises out of the reach of clinicians, consumers, and others in the mental health sector. Some of the factors influencing the five stages are summarized in Table 32.1. It is important that the perspectives of clinicians and those who

Table 32.1 Examples of factors influencing the policy cycle

Stage of the cycle	Influencing factors	
Problem identification	Primarily internal influences	*Citizens:* - Changes in cultural norms/social attitudes; public opinion *Media:* - Focus on high-profile areas such as substance use, suicide, and conflict *Advocates and stakeholders:* - Agendas depending on priorities specific to each group *New information:* - New research and data inform problem identification *Other factors:* - Mental health receives focus because of its relationship to physical health priorities (e.g. HIV) - Mental health issues recognized following conflict or natural disaster
	Primarily external influences	*International agencies:* - Government responds to leadership of an agency (e.g. WHO) - Aid/loans linked to health policy and/or outcomes - Government responds to criticism, e.g. of inadequate spending or human rights issues
Option development	*Policy mandate and ideology:* - Public government commitments including in election platform - Governments accept responsibility for a solution *Political feasibility and sustainability:* - Governments seek re-election *Cost:* - Governments seek cost-effective solutions to problems - Resources are available *Experience of other jurisdictions* *Available knowledge and evidence* *Stakeholder opinion* *Implementation design:* - project scope, process, performance measurement, impact on rest of health system and other sectors	
Decision-making	Assessment of electoral acceptance Intensity of political commitment Relative power of advocates in government, bureaucracy, and community Harnessing stakeholders for long-term sustainability	
Implementation	*Information collection and dissemination:* - Funding tied to data collection and reporting requirements *Financing system* (how resources are collected) *Payment system* (how resources are distributed) *Organization of the broader health system* *Impact of the broader health regulatory system* *Development of implementation plan:* - Stakeholders involved in implementation design - Include performance monitoring and reporting for transparency	
Evaluation	Designed at the time of policy development and/or implementation Conducted independent of those implementing policy utilizing a transparent process Use to inform future and revised policy	

use services and their families and carers be brought to the policy process so decisions are made more on the basis of relevance and less on the basis of political expediency and ideology. In doing this, it is necessary for information from those intimately engaged in research and service delivery to be communicated in a way that can be assimilated by individuals in government who are unfamiliar with the technical detail. It is often necessary to reframe the information or reduce it to what may seem overly simplistic or inexact summaries.

Mental health professionals should have an advantage in the policy arena because they are trained in systems thinking. Many government policies outside of health can impact the mental health of populations or the delivery of mental health services. Mental health professionals should understand the context within which policy is framed, as well as the resources needed, the interrelated components of provision and the outcomes that need to be achieved. However, they must be prepared to enter an arena where their opinions are not automatically accepted and which is not only unfamiliar but operates at times in a way that they may find disturbingly irrational.

REFERENCES

Baker, C. (1996). *The Health Care Policy Process*. London: Sage Publications.

Bryson, J. M. (2004). *Strategic Planning for Public and Nonprofit Organizations: A Guide to Strengthening and Sustaining Organizational Achievement* (3rd ed.). San Francisco, CA: Jossey-Bass Publishers.

Charlson, F., van Ommeren, M., Flaxman, A., Cornett, J., Whiteford, H., & Saxena, S. (2019). New WHO prevalence estimates of mental disorders in conflict settings: a systematic review and meta-analysis. *Lancet*, **394**, 240–248.

Chisholm, D. (2005). Choosing cost-effective interventions in psychiatry: results from the CHOICE programme of the World Health Organization. *World Psychiatry*, **4**, 37–44.

Collins, C. & Coates, T. (1989). Science and health policy: can they cohabit or should they divorce? *American Journal of Public Health*, **90**, 1389–1390.

Collins, P. Y. & Saxena, S. (2016). Action on mental health needs global cooperation. *Nature*, **532**, 25–27.

Corrigan, P. W. & Watson, A. C. (2003). Factors that explain how policy makers distribute resources to mental health services. *Psychiatric Services*, **54**, 501–507.

De Silva, M. J. & Ryan, G. (2016). Global mental health in 2015: 95% implementation. *Lancet Psychiatry*, **3**, 15–17.

Dimock, M. E., Dimock, M. O., & Fox, G. M. (1983). *Public Administration*. New York: Holt, Rinehart and Winston.

Flisher, A. J., Lund, C., Funk, M., Banda, M., Bhana, A., Doku, V., et al. (2007). Mental health policy development and implementation in four African countries. *Journal of Health Psychology*, **12**, 505–516.

Frank, R. G. & Glied, S. A. (2006). *Better but Not Well: Mental Health Policy in the United States since 1950*. Baltimore, MD: Johns Hopkins University Press.

GBD 2019 Mental Disorders Collaborators (2022). Global, regional, and national burden of 12 mental disorders in 204 countries and territories, 1990–2019: a systematic analysis for the Global Burden of Disease Study 2019. *Lancet Psychiatry*, **9**, 137–150.

Funk, M. & Bold, N. D. (2020). WHO's QualityRights initiative: transforming services and promoting rights in mental health. *Health and Human Rights*, **22**, 69–75.

Garfield, R. (2009). Mental health policy development in the states: the piecemeal nature of transformational change. *Psychiatric Services*, **60**, 1329–1335.

Hogan, M. F. (2008). Transforming mental health care: realities, priorities and prospects. *Psychiatric Clinics of North America*, **31**, 1–9.

Horton, R. (2007). Launching a new movement for mental health. *Lancet*, **370**, 806.

Jacob, K. S., Sharan, P., Mirza, I., Garrido-Cumbrera, M., Seedat, S., Mari, J. J., et al. (2007). Mental health systems in countries: where are we now? *Lancet*, **370**, 1061–1077.

Knapp, M., McDaid, D., Mossialos, E., & Thornicroft, G. (2007). *Mental Health Policy and Practice across Europe*. Maidenhead: Open University Press.

Lee, K., Buse, K., & Fustukian, S. (2002). *Health Policy in a Globalising World*. Cambridge: Cambridge University Press.

McDaid, D., Park, A.-L., & Wahlbeck, K. (2019). The economic case for the prevention of mental illness. *Annual Review of Public Health*, **40**, 373–389.

Meurk, C., Harris, M., Wright, E., Reavley, N., Scheurer, R., Bassilios, B., et al. (2017). Systems levers for commissioning primary mental health care: a rapid review. *Australian Journal of Primary Health*, **24**, 29–53.

Meurk, C., Whiteford, H., Head, B., Hall, W., & Carah, N. (2015). Media and evidence-informed policy development: the case of mental health in Australia. *Contemporary Social Science*, **10**, 160–170.

Miller, G. (2007). Mental health and the mass media: room for improvement. *Lancet*, **370**, 1015–1016.

Murray, C. J. L. & Lopez, A. D. (Eds.) (1996). *The Global Burden of Disease and Injury Series, Volume 1: A Comprehensive Assessment of Mortality and Disability from Diseases, Injuries, and Risk Factors in 1990 and Projected to 2020*. Cambridge, MA: Harvard University Press.

Musgrove, P. (1996). *Public and Private Roles in Health: Theory and Financing Patterns*. Washington, DC: World Bank.

Patel, V., Saraceno, B., & Kleinman, A. (2006). Beyond evidence: the moral case of international mental health. *American Journal of Psychiatry*, **163**, 1312–1315.

Piachaud, J. (2008). Globalization, conflict and mental health. *Global Social Policy*, **8**, 315–334.

Pirkis, J., Harris, M., Buckingham, B., Whiteford, H. A., & Townsend-White, C. (2007). International planning directions for provision of mental health services. *Administration and Policy in Mental Health and Mental Health Services Research*, **34**, 377–387.

Prince, M., Patel, V., Saxena, S., Maj, M., Maselko, J., Phillips, M., & Rahman, A. (2007). No health without mental health—a slogan with substance. *Lancet*, **370**, 859–877.

Reich, M. R. (1996). Applied political analysis for health policy reform. *Current Issues in Public Health*, **2**, 186–191.

Ridley, M., Rao, G., Schilbach, F., & Patel, V. (2020). Poverty, depression, and anxiety: causal evidence and mechanisms. *Science*, **370**, eaay0214.

Roberts, M., Hsiao, W., Berman, P., & Reich, M. (2003). *Getting Health Reform Right: A Guide to Improving Performance and Equity*. Oxford: Oxford University Press.

Saraceno, B., van Ommeren, M., Batniji, R., Cohen, A., Gureje, O., Mahoney, J., et al. (2007). Barriers to improvement of mental health services in low-income and middle-income countries. *Lancet*, **370**, 1164–1174.

Saxena, S., Thornicroft, G., Knapp, M., & Whiteford, H. A. (2007). Resources for mental health: scarcity, inequity, and inefficiency. *Lancet*, **370**, 878–889.

Shen, G. C., Eaton, J., & Snowden, L. R. (2017). Mainstreaming mental health care in 42 countries. *Health Systems & Reform*, **3**, 313–324.

Sturm, R. (1999). What type of information is needed to inform mental health policy? *Journal of Mental Health Policy and Economics*, **2**, 141–144.

Swayne, L. E., Duncan, W. J., & Ginter, P. M. (2006). *Strategic Management of Health Care Organizations* (5th ed.). Oxford: Blackwell publishers.

Thornicroft, G. & Tansella, M. (2004). Components of a modern mental health service: a pragmatic balance of community and hospital care: overview of systematic evidence. *British Journal of Psychiatry*, **185**, 283–290.

United for Global Mental Health (2022). Global mental health advocacy roadmap for 2022–2023. https://unitedgmh.org/mental-health-2022-global-local

Votruba, N. & Thornicroft, G. (2016). Sustainable development goals and mental health: learnings from the contribution of the FundaMentalSDG global initiative. *Global Mental Health*, **3**, E26.

Walt, G. (1994). *Health Policy: An Introduction to Process and Power*. Johannesburg: Witwatersrand University Press.

Walt, G., Shiffman, J., Schneider, H., Murray, S. F., Brugha, R., & Gilson, L. (2008). 'Doing' health policy analysis: methodological and conceptual reflections and challenges. *Health Policy and Planning*, **23**, 308–317.

Whiteford, H. A. (1994). Intersectoral policy reform is critical to the national mental health strategy. *Australian Journal of Public Health*, **18**, 342–344.

Whiteford, H. A., Meurk, C., Carstensen, G., Hall, W., Hill, P., & Head, B. W. (2016). How did youth mental health make it onto australia's 2011 federal policy agenda? *SAGE Open*, **6**, 4.

World Health Organization (2005a). *Mental Health Declaration for Europe: Facing the Challenges, Building Solutions*. Copenhagen: World Health Organization.

World Health Organization (2005b). *Mental Health Policy, Plans and Programmes (Updated Version 2)* (Mental Health Policy and Service Guidance Package). Geneva: World Health Organization.

World Health Organization (2013). Investing in mental health: evidence for action. https://www.who.int/publications/i/item/9789241564618

World Health Organization (2019). QualityRights materials for training, guidance and transformation. https://www.who.int/publications/i/item/who-qualityrights-guidance-and-training-tools

World Health Organization (2021a). Mental health Atlas. https://www.who.int/publications/i/item/9789240036703

World Health Organization (2021b). Guidance on community mental health services: promoting person-centred and rights-based approaches. https://www.who.int/publications/i/item/9789240025707

World Health Organization (2021c). Comprehensive mental health action plan 2013–2030. https://www.who.int/publications/i/item/9789240031029

33

Funding of mental health services

Dan Chisholm, Martin Knapp, and Shari Jadoolal

Introduction

Whether it is a case of setting out to develop, reorientate, or just maintain existing levels of community-based mental health services, policymakers and planners will run up against the inconvenient but inescapable question of resource constraints. How much money will it take, for example, to build up service coverage and capacity, to introduce effective new intervention strategies, to overhaul prevailing modes of service delivery, or to cater for the changing needs of the population? Decisions made at this strategic level of mental health policy and planning exert a powerful influence over the extent to which those people in need of services will actually be able to access and use them, and will shape the way in which provision is organized and paid for.

Mental health financing is a far-reaching topic that not only addresses the specific question of what services to purchase and how, but also more normative questions around how much *should* be allocated to (say) community mental health care (e.g. what can be afforded, given the extent of mental health and broader other health needs in the population?), as well as equity issues (e.g. are funding arrangements fair, in the sense that people in need are not prevented from accessing services on financial grounds?). Indeed, alongside meeting the reasonable expectations of service users and actualizing mental health improvements in the population, fair financing does or should represent a key goal of a mental health system (World Health Organization (WHO), 2010). In this chapter, we endeavour to cover these diverse questions under several central financing themes—resource generation and revenue collection, risk pooling and financial protection, plus resource allocation and purchasing—to highlight key funding issues that need to be considered when planning, implementing, or evaluating community mental health services.

Mental health care and market failure

Prior to discussion of these key mental health financing themes, however, we should ask whether individuals should be left to purchase the health services and goods that they need or desire—just like many other commodities such as groceries or transport—or whether there are particular reasons for some kind of collective action or state intervention when it comes to mental health services. In short, is there justification for state intervention in the financing (or provision) of mental health care? There are in fact a number of well-established 'market failures' that commonly arise in the context of health care; that is, reasons why 'regular' market forces cannot be relied upon to achieve socially acceptable outcomes. These include undesired spillover effects (such as the spread of infectious disease within and across populations), and the information imbalance that often exists between the consumer (service user) and supplier of care (health professional). Such distortions to the 'equilibrium' of the mental health care market can lead to the undersupply of essential services, excessive prices, or reduced quality of care for consumers, and—of most concern—unmet individual needs and poor quality of life. Overarching these problems, there is the inherent uncertainty around a person's future health status, which makes it hard for individuals to predict when they will need to use and pay for health care.

Mental health and other chronic conditions present a range of market failures that are accentuated in comparison to other disorders (Watts & Segal, 2009). For example, while antisocial behaviours induced by use of illicit drugs would constitute a negative spillover effect that justifies some form of public intervention, for many mental health problems such negative spillover effects are not a major concern (i.e. most of the costs or consequences of illness are 'internalized'—they mainly affect the person experiencing poor mental health). On other grounds, however, mental disorders are especially prone to market failure, perhaps most obviously in terms of information deficits—many people with mental health needs may temporarily lack insight into their condition—leading to lower demand than is both personally and socially optimal: individuals may be unaware of their condition and therefore not seek appropriate treatment. The result will be an undersupply of services that only collective action can redress. For those with an identified condition, the pervasive stigma attached to mental illness produces a further check on the demand for services. In addition, there is ample international evidence to indicate that mental ill health is associated with impoverishment, either as a result of a drift by those with mental health problems towards more socially disadvantaged circumstances (due to impaired levels of psychological or social functioning), or a greater exposure to adverse life events (Funk et al., 2012; Patel & Kleinman, 2003).

There are also problems when it comes to paying for or insuring against mental illness, particularly chronic or lifelong conditions such as schizophrenia or bipolar affective disorder (Watts & Segal, 2009). Uninsured individuals or households face potentially ruinous costs associated with health care expenditures and forgone work opportunities, while those with or seeking voluntary health insurance (sometimes called 'private' insurance) plans may find themselves excluded or restricted from receiving the services they need. The latter problem of 'adverse selection' occurs because private insurance companies strive to keep premiums competitive by removing or limiting entitlements for high-cost conditions. Conversely, where mental health care *is* covered, policy holders may use more services than they really need because they feel entitled to do so (the problem of 'moral hazard').

In summary, there are sufficiently strong arguments to argue for a collective or public response to mental health problems in the population. As we discuss below, the exact nature of that response or action—for example, the extent to which governments actually pay for or deliver services—can and does vary considerably, depending on prevailing notions of social choice in a country, as well as existing health system structures and constraints.

Resource generation, revenue collection, and risk pooling

Resource needs for mental health

Providing community-based mental health services involves putting together human, physical capital, and other resource inputs to deliver interventions and services capable of improving mental health and related outcomes (WHO, 2009). Accordingly, a basic initial requirement of any mental health system is the assessment of what resources are needed to deliver services to the target population and meet programme goals. The first logical step in such an exercise is to ascertain what resources are currently available (numbers of mental health professionals, inpatient beds, day care places, etc.), followed by an epidemiologically driven appraisal of expected service needs and costs at target levels of service coverage (see **Figure 33.1** for an example).

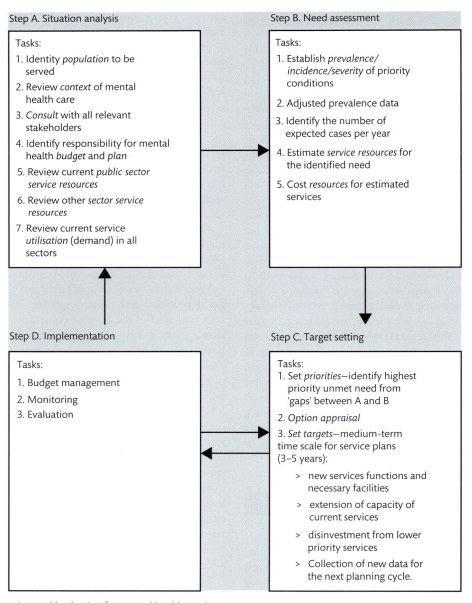

Figure 33.1 Steps in planning and budgeting for mental health services.
Source: World Health Organization (2003). *Planning and Budgeting to Deliver Service for Mental Health* (Mental health Policy and Service Guidance Package—Module 3). Geneva: World Health Organization.

Funding sources for mental health

Alongside the articulation of programme goals and a viable financial plan for meeting them, consideration needs to be given to how revenues will be sourced to pay for salaries, medications, consumables, information systems, and capital infrastructure. Revenue collection is the process by which the health system obtains financial contributions from households, firms, and organizations (plus donors, where applicable). Revenues can be collected in various ways: general taxation, (mandated) social health insurance, voluntary (private) health insurance, out-of-pocket payments, and donations (Chisholm et al., 2019).

All insurance mechanisms share the goal of spreading the risk of having to pay for services across all members of the pool of contributors. Social health insurance is more specifically organized around mandatory contributions by employees and their employers, and is found in many countries of Europe, Asia, and Latin America. In contrast, general taxation applies to all taxpayers, not just those in employment: the UK's NHS, for example, is funded out of general taxation. Voluntary insurance represents the predominant financing mechanism for most citizens in the US, but there are special (publicly financed) schemes for the indigent and the older people. In many other (mainly lower-income) countries of the world, but also for uninsured subpopulations of higher-income countries, out-of-pocket payments represent the most common means by which health service use is paid for. Table 33.1 provides a summary of some of the distinctive features of these different funding mechanisms, although, as will be made apparent, most countries tend to have in place a combined financing model.

Broadly speaking, the sources of funding for mental health services reflect the pattern for health care in general (Dixon et al., 2006; WHO, 2021). Accordingly, people with mental health service needs living in countries with predominantly tax- or insurance-based systems pay only a small amount or nothing at all at the point of accessing services, while those in countries without such provisions must rely on current household income as their primary funding source. Even in mental health systems adequately financed through prepayment contributions, it is common practice for patients or service users to be charged a small fee (a so-called co-payment) at the point of use. This charge—which may be waived for certain services or individuals (such as people with low incomes or debilitating health conditions)—is levied in order to counter the aforementioned problem of 'moral hazard', whereby fully paid-up members of a 'risk pool' have an incentive to use more services than they strictly need.

> **Box 33.1** Financial resources needed to deliver mental health care in low- and middle-income countries
>
> A new module of the United Nations strategic planning OneHealth Tool was applied to three priority mental and neurological disorders in six low- and middle-income countries. Analysis showed that in four of the countries (Ethiopia, India, Nepal, and Uganda), the cost of delivering key interventions for psychosis, depression, and epilepsy at existing treatment coverage is estimated at US $0.06–0.33 per head of total population per year (in Nigeria and South Africa it is US $1.36–1.92). By comparison, the projected cost per capita at target levels of coverage approaches US $5 per capita in Nigeria and South Africa, and ranges from US $0.14 to $1.27 in the other four countries.
>
> From Chisholm et al. (2017).

The lack of complete or reliable local epidemiological and resource data has thwarted such efforts in many countries, but that is now changing with the generation of national-level mental health profiles and epidemiological estimates (see, e.g. WHO's Mental Health Atlas project (WHO, 2021) and the Global Burden of Disease Results tool (available at http://ghdx.healthdata.org)). While such profiles may not provide all the detailed information needed by mental health planners to develop community-based services at the national level, they do clearly reveal both the extent of need in the population and the paucity of human and financial resources available to meet these needs. Many lower-income countries in fact devote less than 2% of their total health budgets to mental health, and the poorer the country (measured in terms of average annual income per capita), the more likely they are to allocate a smaller proportion to the mental health sector (WHO, 2021).

How much a country *should* be spending on mental health is a question often posed (Lim et al., 2008) but rarely answered, owing to the complex landscape that needs to be mapped out, the multidimensional goals of a mental health system, and data limitations. All too often, budget allocations for mental health are based on little more than historical precedent (i.e. last year's allocation, plus or minus an incremental amount). Ultimately, however, such budgetary estimates should be based on an assessment of population mental health needs and associated resource implications. Analytical tools and methods for resource need estimation and financial planning have been developed in many countries and also internationally (e.g. the United Nations inter-agency OneHealth Tool) and have been used, for example, to estimate the cost of scaling up the delivery of a specified package of mental health care in the context of low- and middle-income countries (Chisholm et al., 2017) (Box 33.1).

Table 33.1 Characteristics of different health insurance mechanisms

	National insurance	Social insurance	Voluntary insurance	No insurance
Collection method	General taxation	Employee premiums	Household premiums	Cash (out-of-pocket)
Legal status	Mandatory	Mandatory for workers	Voluntary	None
Pre-paid population	Everyone	Workers only	Those able to pay	None
Fairness/equity	Progressive	Neutral	Regressive	Regressive
Adverse selection	No	No (if working)	Yes	N/A
Moral hazard (users)	Yes	Yes	Yes	N/A
Co-payments	Few	Some	Many	N/A

Knapp, M. R. J. & McDaid, D. (2007). The Mental Health Economics European Network. *Journal of Mental Health*, 16, 157–165.

In low-income populations, such fees also have this general intent (as well as shifting some of the financial burden to consumers) but can also have the more negative consequence of putting off potential users in real need of care. Accordingly, there are quite strong equity arguments for abandoning user fees for socioeconomically disadvantaged or other vulnerable groups in the population, including those facing challenging mental health problems.

Fairness in financing mental health

Funding mental health services via mandatory tax-based contributions provides the opportunity to gear payments according to ability to pay; that is, by stipulating contributions as a fixed proportion of income, higher-income groups end up 'putting more into the pot' than those with lower incomes. Such a system is described as *progressive*. By contrast, it is widely acknowledged that out-of-pocket payments represent a *regressive* form of health financing—they penalize those least able to afford care—and represent an obvious channel through which impoverishment may occur (Wagstaff et al., 2020; WHO, 2010). Specifically, they lead in many cases to health spending levels that have been labelled 'catastrophic' because they cause households to reallocate their budgets away from other essential needs such as education, food, and housing. For example, a survey of household economic costs associated with behavioural health conditions was conducted in six low- and middle-income countries: households with mentally ill members reported catastrophic health expenses accounting for 10% or more of their income or 40% of their ability to pay (Lund et al., 2019). In high-income nations such as Canada, by comparison, out-of-pocket spending does not represent a substantial source of financial burden for most service users, as health care expenditures are often supplemented by private insurance (Baird, 2016).

Among prepayment mechanisms, and as noted already, non-state insurance markets throw up some challenges in the context of mental health services, in particular the issue of adverse selection. For example, in Malaysia, health services are provided via a hybrid system where public care coexists alongside voluntary health insurance schemes. However, many insurance companies do not offer to insure individuals with mental illness or cover psychiatric service costs, which might dissuade people from getting help or force them to pay out of pocket (Hanafiah & Van Bortel, 2015). Even with its parity laws, major disparities remain in the US with respect to equitable coverage for mental illness. Regardless of the parity rules for out-of-network treatment, cost-sharing for privately insured enrolees with mental illnesses may cause excessive financial hardship and represent access to care hurdles (Xu et al., 2019). That is why the mandatory nature of national insurance schemes is so important, since relaxing this rule provides higher earners with an incentive to opt out and secure for themselves an insurance plan that potentially offers more personalized or responsive care arrangements. An obvious knock-on effect of such opting out is that there is then less money to go round for those left in the insured pool, with predictable adverse consequences for service quality and coverage.

Overall, it is safe to say that prepayment mechanisms such as national or social insurance represent a more equitable approach for safeguarding at-risk populations from the adverse financial consequences of mental health conditions compared to out-of-pocket expenditures. Furthermore, it can be noted that by mandating universal health insurance, key problems of voluntary or social insurance such as adverse selection can be avoided, and contributions can be geared according to ability to pay.

Despite the desirability of universal health coverage, many countries are being hampered from moving towards this goal by a variety of constraining factors, including weak taxation systems and governance structures, inefficient use of existing resources, plus the high transaction costs associated with any fundamental reform. Indeed, in countries with weak (income) tax collection and/or a large informal economy, tax-based financing may not generate sufficient resources for mental health service provision at the population level, which is why many countries have considered social health insurance as a more viable means by which at least one large segment of the population can be covered (often public employees based in urban areas). By so doing, however, such schemes explicitly exclude those working (unpaid) in the household or in the informal sector (which in many countries is very substantial) as well as those unable to work due to long-term or recurrent illness or disability; these gaps in coverage represent a significant shortcoming given the well-known association between low socioeconomic status or poverty and the incidence of mental disorder (Lund et al., 2011) and, indeed, that income inequality itself negatively may affect mental health (Silva Ribeiro et al., 2017).

Mental health care: a mixed economy of financing and provision

Although in certain cases the principal funder may also be the predominant provider, it is more common in the mental health sector to find a 'mixed economy' of financing and provision, in which funding from the various possible sources is expended across an assortment of public, private, and also voluntary or non-governmental agencies. Many service delivery models explicitly involve non-governmental actors or sectors, since the specific arguments in favour of state funding of mental health services (negative spillover effects, information failures) do not apply equally to the state *provision* of mental health services. The precise roles performed by these different providers depends on the prevailing legal, economic, and institutional frameworks of a country, and may also have historical or sociocultural determinants. To illustrate, the role of the non-governmental sector might be quite substantial in a low-income country with a weak state health system—as non-governmental organizations (NGOs) or private providers attempt to fill the void left by state provision—but quite limited in the context of strong state control and provision. International donors (state and non-state) can be especially major contributors to mental health system resources in some countries (Iemmi, 2019).

Cross-classification of funding and provider types generates a simple matrix representation of the interconnections characterizing pluralist care systems and their constituent transactions (Table 33.2). What would go into such a matrix? The simplest task would be to list services (such as inpatient facilities, community nurses, primary care doctors, and sheltered work schemes) in the appropriate provider-funding cells of the matrix. More demanding but also more informative would be to record the volumes of provision and/or the total funding or expenditure amounts. Given the multiplicity of service types potentially active in supporting people with mental health problems, it would be preferable if the completed matrix spanned

Table 33.2 Mixed economy of mental health care

Revenue collection (funding)	Mode or sector of provision			
	Public/state sector	Voluntary/NGO	Private (for profit)	Informal sector
General taxation	1. Psychiatric wards in general or specialized hospitals 2. Psychiatric outpatient clinics 3. Mental health care at primary health care level 4. Community-based residential care 5. Contribution to mental health promotion activities	State-level contribution to NGO partners providing outreach services	State-contracted residential care in the community	Grants or pensions to people with longer-term psychosocial disabilities
Social insurance	–	–	–	–
Voluntary insurance	–	–	Contributions/premia for voluntary (private) insurance	–
Charitable donations	1. NGO providing sheltered employment in state-run facilities 2. International donors supporting services in low- and middle-income countries (e.g. philanthropies)	1. Mental health promotion and advocacy 2. Mental health and psychosocial support services	–	Grants to support households facing adversity
External donors	Governmental development assistance (to low-income countries) for mental health services	Support to NGOs working in crises and emergencies	–	–
Out-of-pocket spending	Contribution to medication or consultation costs (co-payments for those able to pay, e.g. fixed fee per prescription medication)	–	Fee-for-service payments to private practitioners	Fee-for-service payments to informal care practitioners
No exchange	–	–	–	Family- and community-level support

Knapp, M., McDaid, D., Mossialos, E., & Thornicroft, G. (2007). *Mental Health Policy and Practice across Europe.* Buckingham: Open University Press.

a range of sectors, not being confined to the (narrow) health care system.

Table 33.2 provides some illustrations of the types of links that might be found in a mental health system. In this hypothetical example (for a lower-income country), financing of the mental health system comes mainly from general taxation but is complemented by contributions from international donors and charitable foundations, as well as via fees or copayments paid by users of the system to service providers. On the provision side, the state sector is primarily responsible for running government-run hospitals and outpatient services, while non-governmental agencies (whether for-profit or not) carry out activities in their own right, both on the open market and under contract with state sponsors. Mapping the mental health system in this way—even if only descriptively—generates an informative overview of who is doing what now and can be a useful template against which to consider (for example) the development of or movement towards community-based mental health services.

Paying for mental health care

Following on from questions around how to generate sufficient resources for mental health and to protect the sick against the spectre of financial catastrophe or impoverishment, there remains the central issue of how, where, and to whom should available funds be most appropriately channelled for the purpose of delivering services to the population in need. Several mechanisms are possible, each with their own underlying incentives, processes, and implications.

Perhaps the most straightforward scenario to consider is one in which both funding and provision of services are controlled by the same agency (most typically a ministry of health). In this case, funds that have been collected (via taxation) can be allocated directly to government-run services at the subnational level, most simply on a per capita basis (i.e. budgets are set in proportion to population size alone). Since the budget is fixed, there is strong pressure to keep overall expenditures under this set amount (i.e. there is very little flexibility for providers to increase their income beyond what has been allocated). However, such a mechanism overlooks the potentially large variations in mental health need at the subnational level: for example, regions with large cities might be expected to have a larger or more complex case mix than more rural regions. Accordingly, a few countries in Europe and elsewhere have constructed allocation formulae to better capture these expected variations and better anticipate actual mental health service funding requirements. Budgets can then be based on a fixed fee per person enrolled into the mental health service of a defined catchment area.

The extent to which fixed budgets should be devolved to providers is a commonly recurring financing issue. In principle, devolved budgets and purchasing should increase the likelihood that decision-making is sensitive to user needs and preferences. Through their everyday work, health care professionals should be well placed to recognize individual and (local) community needs and wants, and hopefully to respond to them. Consequently, devolution of financial responsibilities could be one way to help a health system be more needs-led, although devolved budget holders would need to have the right information, skills, autonomy, and incentives if they are to budget flexibly, effectively, and efficiently. However, a devolved budget holder may have less information than a central budget holder, fewer technical resources to process what information they have, and less of a financial cushion in the event of a mistaken decision. In India, for example, health spending amounting to 4.6% of gross domestic product is delegated by the central government to individual states, but less than 1% of that overall health spending is for mental health (Rathod et al., 2017). Holding the budget centrally may leave an organization better placed to pool and spread risks, to wield its purchasing power to achieve better price/contract deals, and to use non-price interventions such as subsidies and contracts linked to investment to improve quality. Centralized budgeting might also make it easier to respond strategically to area-wide needs, whether in terms of purchasing, investment, or shaping of the broader system.

A further concern around allocating public funds *directly* to state providers is that it provides limited incentives for maintaining or improving the quality of services being delivered. This is because providers are essentially free of competition for those funds and can consequently operate without any real fear of 'losing business' (to use a market-based analogy). There is also the risk that professionals or managers pursue their own rather than nationally mandated objectives. There is therefore increasing interest in—and implementation of—performance-based financing of health services, which links the prospective allocation of resources to the quantity and quality of service provision (via legally binding contracts). (A better approach still would be to link resource allocation to the actual meeting of needs—i.e. the achievement of better health and quality of life—but this is inherently complex to set up.)

In countries where both financing and provision rest mainly with the state, such as in the UK, incentive-based funding has been introduced artificially via the imposition of a virtual market in health care, consisting of purchasers or commissioning agencies on the one hand—who are charged with assessing and meeting the needs of a defined population—and (hospital, community, or primary care) providers on the other hand, who compete with each other for the available resources. In countries where social or private insurance systems are in place, the contract is between the insurance agency and a range of public as well as private providers.

The main contract types are described in **Box 33.2**. One central choice in contract specification is the degree of flexibility, particularly with respect to prices. While a predetermined price has the advantage of predictability to the purchaser, the provider may experience cost changes that leave their net revenue (their profits if they are in the commercial sector) uncertain. Moreover, predetermined prices are not responsive to the individual needs of users. Providers may thus not have the incentive to tailor the services they supply to specific individual circumstances; in particular, they may not offer more intensive treatment and support to those with greater needs. Flexible prices shift some of the risk back to the purchasers and offer greater incentives to providers to respond to the changing care circumstances.

An alternative mechanism for paying providers is based on 'fee for service', whereby a fixed price is agreed beforehand (e.g. with social insurance or sickness funds) and reimbursed retrospectively following the provision of a service, such as an outpatient consultation or an overnight inpatient stay. In this case, there is a clear incentive for providers to deliver as much care as they can handle,

> **Box 33.2** Types of contract between purchasers and providers
>
> - *Block contracts* link service specifications and reimbursement to provider facilities—for instance, buying a defined number of inpatient places—and payment is made regardless of whether the service is used. Because block contracts guarantee a level of revenue, small or risk-averse providers may be prepared to accept lower payments in return for predictability. However, purchasers run the risk of having either too few or too many places in the facilities that turn out to be needed. The larger the purchaser (or the purchasing budget), the lower the risk of a mismatch between demand and capacity.
> - *Spot and call-off contracts* are price-by-case arrangements in that the individual service user is the basis for reimbursement: the provider is only paid if the client uses the service. Purchasers sometimes prefer the flexibility that comes from spot purchasing, but risk paying a premium for this, particularly in markets for highly specialized services. Spot contracts are usually more expensive to operate than block contracts because the latter offer economies of scale in drafting and negotiation. These contracts have a price band set prior to purchase, negotiated by a centralized purchaser, and occasionally with some variation to allow for the needs of individual users. Local decision-makers or care managers or other decentralized agents then call off services from the contract. Spot and call-off contracts shift more of the financial risk onto providers.
> - *Cost-and-volume contracts* are combinations of block and price-by-case arrangements. A guaranteed level of service is purchased; beyond that level, additional reimbursement is made according to the number of users. There is also the possibility of more easily building in other contingencies.

since the more they do, the more they receive. Although that does not represent a problem for many essential services, it *can* lead to the overprovision of other, less essential services or even the unnecessary prescription of drugs. Examples in the context of mental health services might include an unduly long duration of stay in hospital, or the medicalization of—and subsequent drug prescription for—emotional or behavioural problems in childhood and adolescence. Such an inbuilt incentive to produce or even induce services for which there is strongest demand or highest return—irrespective of the outcomes that they generate—has the potential to undermine other services that are more clinically important or economically efficient. In countries where such a payment model is in place—typically those with social health insurance and mostly private providers, like many countries in central and eastern Europe—there is a consequent need to specify national priorities and develop clinical treatment guidelines that specify normal limits of reimbursable service provision. Accordingly, the main role of government in this context is to formulate national mental health policy and service development strategies, put in place regulatory structures, and monitor the overall performance of the mental health system.

Financing the move towards community-based mental health care

Community-based mental health services form one critical component of a comprehensive mental health system (Thornicroft & Tansella, 2013), bringing as they do more accessible and responsive care to those in need than does hospital-based care (such as outreach and rehabilitation services, for example). In a great many countries, however, the transition to a community-based service model is moving slowly. This is due in no small part to negative social perceptions of mental illness and a lack of political will, but there are also constraints of a financial nature. Over and above the more general health financing objective of moving people with mental health problems away from reliance on out-of-pocket payments towards prepayment funding schemes, therefore, there is the more specific challenge of how to move funds for mental health away from institutionally focused services and channel them into the development of community-based care.

At the heart of the funding conundrum for community mental health care is the pre-existing and continuing financial commitment to large-scale hospital institutions for persons with long-term mental health problems. Dating back many generations, governments throughout the world invested in the construction and maintenance of asylums for mentally ill people. With the advent of antipsychotic drugs and the growing emphasis on human rights, together with realization (through research) of the dire standards in many institutions, such a model of care has been increasingly discredited, and many countries began a process of deinstitutionalization that is continuing to this day. Nevertheless, in most regions of the world, mental hospitals continue to consume a large proportion of the (government) mental health budget and account for at least three-quarters of total bed capacity (WHO, 2021).

The reasons for this prevailing situation include a lack of strong leadership or political will and the protection of vested interests (in the status quo). Over and above these barriers, efforts to change the balance of mental health care have been hindered by a lack of appropriate transitional funding. Transitional or dual funding is clearly required over a period in order to build up appropriate community-based services *before* residents of long-term institutions can be relocated. Since such relocation of former inpatients is a gradual movement, it is usually some years before the old institution can be closed (and any proceeds from the sale of land and buildings recouped, as well as staff redeployed to new service configurations). However, governments are typically hesitant about putting such dual funding in place because of concerns that they will not be able to recoup much of the additional investment they put into the development and maintenance of community-based services (Knapp & Wong, 2020).

Accordingly, where deinstitutionalization has occurred, new funding has generally been patchy and inadequate, resulting in inappropriate care arrangements for a proportion of former inpatients, with the attendant risk that a poorly funded community-based system will fail the people it is intended to support. For mental health policymakers seeking to move towards community-based mental health care, it is therefore crucial to present an evidence-based case not only on the grounds of equity, human rights, and user outcomes, but also on the grounds of financial feasibility over a defined transitional period. In addition, it may also be possible to bring arguments of economic efficiency to bear—or at least cost neutrality—although that will depend on the specific needs of the individuals to be relocated and the time span over which this happens (Knapp et al., 2021).

A further funding issue relating to the move from hospital towards community-based mental health care concerns the greater multiplicity of providers and their respective roles, in particular the shifting of responsibilities and associated funding from health to social care and housing systems. Where previously the financial responsibility for long-term institutional care of people with chronic mental health problems clearly rested with the health system, care arrangements in the community typically extend to social or other welfare services (including supported housing and vocational rehabilitation). In the many countries where access or entitlement to these social services is subject to some form of means testing, individuals whose care would have been paid for by the state under the terms of national or social health insurance may now find themselves having to pay substantially towards that care. It is therefore important that sufficient safeguards are in place—via payment exemption schemes for people meeting a certain threshold level of physical or mental disability, for instance—to protect against such instances of unfair financing for health.

Another plausible mechanism in this regard would be to provide self-directed care financing to users, whereby shared decision-making is made through equal contributions between service users and clinicians (Thomas et al., 2019). Self-directed care uses personal budgets or public funds to purchase goods or services that aid users to remain outside traditional institutions. It goes beyond person-centred care and gives users the ultimate decision-making authority that will best facilitate their mental health and wellness goals (Snethen et al., 2016).

To go one step further, there is an increasing need for—and pressure on—governments to re-fashion their planning and financing towards an economy of well-being, including the promotion and protection of mental well-being as a policy goal in its own right. In 2019, New Zealand introduced its first well-being budget, which focuses resource allocation away from standard metrics of economic output such as gross domestic product to a wider range of valued outcomes, including human health, safety, and flourishing (https://budget.govt.nz/budget/2021/wellbeing). Such a policy directive incentivizes interdepartmental or intersectoral working and enlivens efforts to tackle the social and other underlying determinants of mental health, including childhood adversity, poverty, and social inequality.

Conclusion

While the pursuit of improved health and well-being in the population should unquestionably be the overarching goal of a mental health system, a further objective is to ensure that the financial risks faced by each household in society with respect to mental health are distributed fairly, for example, according to their ability to pay (Dixon et al., 2006; WHO, 2003b, 2010). In order to fully meet these objectives, it is necessary to raise and pool enough funds upfront so that a comprehensive set of services can be provided to those in need (without regard to income status, ethnicity, age, and so on). In addition, it is incumbent on governments to ensure that available resources for mental health service provision—wherever those contributions may come from—are used to best effect across the range of intervention strategies, service levels, and provider sectors that make up the mixed economy of mental health care.

Earlier in this chapter we reviewed the case for collective action or state intervention concerning the funding of mental health services and argued that there is solid justification (especially on the grounds of information failure and stigmatized attitudes to mental illness). We might go further and point out that since mental health is an integral part of health, and since health is an integral component of social well-being and happiness, governments would do well to realign their priorities away from those whose primary intent revolves around the creation or retention of wealth towards those that clearly promote societal well-being (and in so doing tackle prominent causes of unhappiness, such as depression and anxiety). Viewed from this broader perspective of what a society should be trying to achieve, it is quite evident that most countries are letting themselves down—often quite badly—when it comes to providing decent and equitable care for their mentally ill populations. It is a sad fact that annual mental health spending in many countries continues to fall far below $1 per capita or just a fraction of 1% of total health expenditure (Mackenzie & Kesner, 2016). That is equivalent to putting a very low price on human happiness or psychological well-being.

Generating new resources for mental health is therefore of paramount significance in countries with weak or underfunded mental health systems, and a critical step towards building a functional, community-based mental health system. As illustrated in **Figure 33.1**, estimation of the additional human, physical, and financial capital needed to develop, or scale up prioritized services or interventions is one task that can usefully be undertaken to demonstrate the existing funding gap and to provide a starting point for discussions of how it could be bridged over time. Persuading national governments or international donors to make the large-scale investments needed nevertheless remains a massive challenge. In other, mainly higher-income settings, the shortfall in resources is less stark, and the focus is more likely to be around the reconfiguration of services and associated reallocations of existing resources.

In terms of revenue collection and risk pooling, national insurance was identified as the most likely route to universal coverage, while 'pay-as-you-go' payment mechanisms are clearly the most inequitable. All countries therefore need to try to minimize the contribution of out-of-pocket payments and shift as much as the population to prepayment mechanisms such as social or national insurance. How collected resources are used to purchase services is a much more flexible and nuanced question, however. The main mechanisms that we reviewed—each subject to its own set of incentives and limitations—included retrospective fee-for-service payments, direct allocation to decentralized providers, and performance-based contracting. Direct (devolved) payments to service users offer a new option in some contexts. Given the ever-increasing concern with cost inflation in the health sector, it seems likely that interest in and implementation of performance-based contracting between providers and insurers of all kinds will only increase over time. Where insurance-based systems are found wanting, not-for-profit NGOs can go some way to filling the void left by state-sponsored provision. Finally, we sounded some specific words of warning around the economics of deinstitutionalization, where again there may be financial incentives at work which can act *against* the desired goal of comprehensive community-based care that is accessible to all in need.

REFERENCES

Baird, K. E. (2016). The financial burden of out-of-pocket expenses in the United States and Canada: how different is the United States? *SAGE Open Medicine*, **4**, 2050312115623792.

Chisholm, D., Docrat, S., Abdulmalik, J., Alem, A., Gureje, O., Gurung, D., et al. (2019). Mental health financing challenges, opportunities and strategies in low- and middle-income countries: findings from the Emerald project. *British Journal of Psychiatry Open*, **5**, e68.

Chisholm, D., Heslin, M., Docrat, S., Nanda, S., Shidhaye, R., Upadhaya, N., et al. (2017). Scaling-up services for psychosis, depression and epilepsy in sub-Saharan Africa and South Asia: development and application of a mental health systems planning tool (OneHealth). *Epidemiology and Psychiatric Sciences*, **26**, 234–244.

Dixon, A., McDaid, D., Knapp, M., & Curran, C. (2006). Financing mental health services in low- and middle-income countries. *Health Policy and Planning*, **21**, 171–182.

Funk, M., Drew, N., & Knapp, M. (2012). Mental health, poverty and development. *Journal of Public Mental Health*, **11**, 166–185.

Hanafiah, A. N. & Van Bortel, T. (2015) A qualitative exploration of the perspectives of mental health professionals on stigma and discrimination of mental illness in Malaysia. *International Journal of Mental Health Systems*, **9**, 10.

Iemmi, V. (2019). Sustainable development for global mental health: a typology and systematic evidence mapping of external actors in low-income and middle-income countries. *BMJ Global Health*, **4**, e001826.

Knapp, M. R. J., Cyhlarova, E., Comas-Herrera, A., & Lorenz-Dant, K. (2021). *Crystallising the Case for Deinstitutionalisation: COVID-19 and the Experiences of Persons with Disabilities*. London: Care Policy and Evaluation Centre, London School of Economics and Political Science.

Knapp, M. & Wong, G. (2020). Economics and mental health: the current scenario. *World Psychiatry*, **19**, 3–14.

Lim, K. L., Jacobs, P., & Dewa, C. (2008). *How Much Should We Spend on Mental Health?* (IHE Report). Alberta: Institute of Health Economics. http://www.ihe.ca/documents/Spending%20on%20Mental%20Health%20Final.pdf

Lund, C., De Silva, M., Plagerson, S., Cooper, S., Chisholm, D., Das, J., et al. (2011). Poverty and mental disorders: breaking the cycle in low-income and middle-income countries. *Lancet*, **378**, 1502–1514.

Lund, C., Docrat, S., Abdulmalik, J., Alem, A., Fekadu, A., Gureje, O., et al. (2019). Household economic costs associated with mental, neurological and substance use disorders: a cross-sectional survey in six low-and middle-income countries. *BJPsych Open*, **5**, 3.

Mackenzie, J. & Kesner, C. (2016). *Mental Health Funding and the SDGs: What Now and Who Pays?* London: Overseas Development Institute. https://odi.org/en/publications/mental-health-funding-and-the-sdgs-what-now-and-who-pays/

Patel, V. & Kleinman, A. (2003). Poverty and common mental disorders in developing countries. *Bulletin of the World Health Organization*, **81**, 609–615.

Rathod, S., Pinninti, N., Irfan, M., Gorczynski, P., Rathod, P., Gega, L., & Naeem, F. (2017). Mental health service provision in low- and middle-income countries. *Health Services Insights*, **10**, 1178632917694350.

Silva Ribeiro, W., Bauer, A., Rezende Andrade, M., York-Smith, M., Pan, P. M., Pingani, L., et al. (2017). Income inequality and mental illness-related morbidity and resilience: a systematic review and meta-analysis. *Lancet Psychiatry*, **4**, 554–562.

Snethen, G., Bilger, A., Maula, E. C., & Salzer, M. S. (2016). Exploring personal medicine as part of self-directed care: expanding perspectives on medical necessity. *Psychiatric Services*, **67**, 883–889.

Thomas, E. C., Zisman-Ilani, Y., & Salzer, M. S. (2019). Self-determination and choice in mental health: qualitative insights from a study of self-directed care. *Psychiatric Services*, **70**, 801–807.

Thornicroft, G. & Tansella, M. (2013). The balanced care model: the case for both hospital-and community-based mental healthcare. *British Journal of Psychiatry*, **202**, 246–248.

Wagstaff, A., Eozenou, P., & Smitz, M. (2020). Out-of-pocket expenditures on health: a global stocktake. *The World Bank Research Observer*, **35**, 123–157.

Watts, J. J. & Segal, L. (2009). Market failure, policy failure and other distortions in chronic disease markets. *BMC Health Services Research*, **9**, 1–6.

World Health Organization (2003). *Planning and Budgeting to Deliver Services for Mental Health* (Mental Health Policy and Service Guidance Package—Module 3). Geneva: World Health Organization.

World Health Organization (2009). *Improving Health Systems and Services for Mental Health*. Geneva: World Health Organization.

World Health Organization (2010). *Health System Financing: The Path to Universal Coverage*. Geneva: World Health Organization.

World Health Organization (2021). *Mental Health Atlas 2020*. Geneva: World Health Organization. https://www.who.int/publications/i/item/9789240036703

Xu, W. Y., Song, C., Li, Y., & Retchin, S. M. (2019). Cost-sharing disparities for out-of-network care for adults with behavioral health conditions. *JAMA Network Open*, **2**, 11.

SECTION 8
Assessing the evidence for effectiveness

34. **Research designs and evaluating treatment interventions** 353
    Peter Tyrer

35. **Qualitative research methods in mental health** 361
    Rob Whitley

36. **Developing evidence-based mental health practices** 369
    Kim T. Mueser and Robert E. Drake

37. **Implementing guidelines** 375
    Amy Cheung, Simon Gilbody, and Jeremy Grimshaw

Research designs and evaluating treatment interventions

Peter Tyrer

Introduction

New treatments are constantly being introduced to all forms of psychiatry and for most of these the setting in which the treatment is administered is not of special importance. Thus, the introduction of a new and effective drug for a mental disorder will require similar testing in hospital, community, or other settings and does not require special description here. However, all treatments given in the community have a common problem associated with them, compliance, or what is now more appropriately termed 'concordance' or 'adherence' (Mullen, 1997). Because treatment in the community can rarely be supervised satisfactorily, a great deal depends on the motivation of individual patients to continue whatever intervention is being given without the need to be closely monitored. Increasingly, therefore, the evaluation of community treatment is going to involve (1) some check on whether the treatment is being given appropriately and (2) if not, whether additional treatments are able to be introduced to improve concordance and adherence. Treatments to improve compliance have now been introduced for the major psychoses and shown to be effective (Kemp et al., 1996, 1998; Perry et al., 1999) and these approaches are likely to impinge increasingly on those working in the community and be among the areas of competence being evaluated for such workers.

The word 'evaluation' is now being used increasingly to describe any type of description of an intervention, and more and more it is being used inappropriately with regard to community treatments. The word 'evaluate' is a mathematical expression originally used to give a numerical value to something which previously had no such value. It is still used in this sense in related expressions such as 'evaluable', but increasingly it has been broadened in use to describe any form of assessment, whether or not it is quantified accurately.

Three key questions

Before discussing different forms of evaluation of community treatment it is necessary to establish what type of evaluation is proposed in any one instance, and this is common to evaluations of all treatments in medicine. Up to three main questions are normally being asked in such evaluations and it is important not to blur these because doing so creates confusion. The three questions are as follows:

- Is the treatment (or service) effective (i.e. does it serve the purpose of the treatment or service)?
- Does the treatment work in conditions of ordinary practice (i.e. is it efficacious)?
- Is the treatment cost-effective (i.e. it is worth spending the money required for its implementation)?

Is the treatment effective?

There is no point in any treatment being introduced to clinical practice in medicine unless it is an improvement on no treatment. The first prerequisite of any putative treatment is therefore to develop its efficacy. The way by which such efficacy can be demonstrated has been the subject of considerable dispute over past years. Since the pioneering paper by Schwartz and Lellouch in 1967 (see 'Phase 3: randomized controlled trials'), a distinction has been made between explanatory and pragmatic trials of treatment effectiveness. Most, if not all, treatments in community psychiatry are determined by pragmatic trials as the circumstances in which treatments are given in ordinary practice may be very different from those which demonstrate the efficacy of a treatment. Such comparisons can be carried out in any setting but may not be necessarily appropriate to ordinary practice. For example, some years ago Soloff and colleagues demonstrated that haloperidol in relatively low dosage (around 7 mg a day) was superior to both antidepressants and placebo tablets in patients with borderline personality disorder treated in a penitentiary. There were no drop-outs from care because all the patients were in a locked environment and, not surprisingly, all patients took their medication as prescribed (Soloff et al., 1986). The prerequisite of efficacy had been established but this is no guarantee that in ordinary clinical usage the treatment would be appropriate for the general population of people with borderline personality disorder. Examination of all the data, as for example in the National Institute for Health and Care Excellence guidelines (National Collaborating Centre for Mental Health, 2009), has shown no good evidence of benefit and the guideline suggests that antipsychotic drugs should be avoided in the treatment of this condition.

Nevertheless, this explanatory phase of investigation is needed to show that the treatment confers benefit; without it there can be no confidence that the treatment is effective. However, in community psychiatry this may have to be carried out by designs that are very different from those in pragmatic trials.

Is the treatment efficacious in practice?

In a pragmatic trial, the circumstances in which the treatment would be used in ordinary clinical practice are being tested and these may be very different from those appertaining in an explanatory trial. Pragmatic trials are more relevant to community mental health services and are also favoured by evidence-based medicine, now accepted as the best way of choosing treatments. A distinction is sometimes made between the words 'effective' and 'efficacious' in this context. If the treatment is superior to a control treatment it can be said to show 'efficacy', but it is only when it has been tested in ordinary circumstances of clinical practice and shown to be superior to other treatments that it can be regarded as 'efficacious'. This might stretch interpretation of the English language too far. 'Effective' refers to the ability of a treatment to bring about a desired effect, and this is virtually the same as 'efficacious', something 'that produces, or is certain to produce, the intended effect (i.e. effective)' (*Shorter Oxford English Dictionary*; Little et al., 1973). The definition of a good service need not therefore be strictly determined by the results of a randomized controlled trial, and although such trials should never be regarded as redundant or unnecessary, evaluation can be greatly reinforced by a range of other sources of information (for review, see Thornicroft & Tansella, 1999, pp. 101–105).

Cost-effectiveness

It is no longer satisfactory to merely demonstrate the effectiveness of a treatment. If the cost of this is so much greater than that of existing treatments, and the gain only a small advance, it is difficult to justify its introduction except on a very limited scale. It is fortunate that most treatments in community psychiatry are relatively cheap compared with the high cost of inpatient services. A substantial part of cost-effectiveness of community treatments is the demonstration that inpatient care is reduced as a consequence of introducing the treatment. Even if the reduction in inpatient care is only modest, in most cases it would be more than sufficient to make the cost of treatment less than the alternative (Byford et al., 2010; Knapp & Beecham, 1990).

Stages of evaluation

All evaluations in community psychiatry are complex interventions (ones in which two or more interventions are involved, even if they are not always specified). So it might be thought, for instance, that the assessment of a drug treatment in the community using a placebo comparison was a simple intervention, as the drug/placebo comparison in a randomized trial is now a standard allegedly 'gold standard' comparison. But it is not simple. Whereas in an inpatient sample the administration of the drug can largely be assured in the community, there is no certainty that patients will take the medication as prescribed. Many other interventions have up to ten different components that could all be tested in their own right but in practice are very difficult to tease out from others. In most evaluations in the community the key interventions can be regarded as a set of variables which commonly include (1) the setting, (2) the personnel involved in the interventions, (3) the specific tested intervention (which may itself have several components), (4) the nature of any relevant comparison treatment, and (5) the relationships between the treaters and the treated. This is a little more complicated than is commonly discussed in the evaluation of complex health interventions, but the principles are the same, and follow a graded process occurring in a set of phases (Campbell et al., 2000), somewhat similar to the phases that have now become common parlance in the evaluation of new drugs. I will take the example of one relatively recent community treatment that has now completed all these phases, assertive community treatment (ACT), to illustrate each of these.

Phase 0: preclinical or theoretical phase

In the first stage of evaluation, it is legitimate to think broadly about an issue and decide whether it is an important subject to examine and research, and then to think about the methods that might be employed. Thus, to take our exemplar, ACT, there was great concern in the 1960s about the pathological effects of hospital treatment in those with any form of illness that persisted. The nasty eight-syllable word, 'institutionalization', appeared in the literature as a complicating pathology in those who stayed for any time in hospital (Barton, 1966), and so it was natural to look for alternatives in the community. ACT grew from this wish; if people could be engaged in treatment outside hospital, preferably in their own homes, the perils of the institution might be avoided. Stein and Test put this notion forward in 1964 and tested it out some years later (Marx et al., 1973). It had a clear theoretical base and was feasible—it was treatment without the institution, probably the core of community psychiatry.

Phase 1: modelling

In this phase the effects of a new intervention or treatment are described and, to some extent, measured before and after its introduction and an idea of its likely effect size obtained. This goes beyond simple description and gives some idea of the impact of the new intervention. However, most open studies exaggerate the degree of change created by the new intervention and invariably further studies show that its impact is considerably less. Nevertheless, these studies serve a valuable purpose in demonstrating (1) the intervention is feasible in clinical practice, (2) is more likely to have a positive impact than a negative one, and (3) gives some idea of its relative advantages and disadvantages. Other improvements that can be made in such studies include (1) reduction in numbers of other treatments that are given so confounding is less, (2) formal assessment using rating scales at the beginning and end of the treatment period so that change is measured more precisely, (3) better selection of patients for treatment, and (4) formal pre-post designs that give some notion of the benefits of the treatment.

In the case of ACT these initial modelling studies were carried out in the 1970s (Marx et al., 1973; Stein & Santos, 1998) and showed that the risks of treating people with severe mental illness outside hospital were much less than the benefits.

Phase 2 or exploratory trial

In this phase the information gathered in phase 1 is used to develop what appears to be the most optimal form of intervention and to test this in an appropriate study design with a comparison treatment or intervention. This can involve merely testing aspects of the treatment such as acceptability and practicality as these are part of the mix of complex interventions described above. It may also be tested with user groups at this stage in order to develop a strong case for the trial within the community of patients likely to be treated.

Researchers are usually advised to carry out a pilot randomized controlled trial at this stage as this offers many advantages: it informs the development of a definitive trial by helping to decide if a large trial is feasible, the data collected help in deciding the sample size of a larger trial, and problems in recruitment and retention of subjects can be identified and corrected. The pilot trial also has greater scope. Austin Bradford Hill, the inventor of the randomized trial, always pointed out that a good trial answered a 'precisely framed question' but at the stage of the exploratory trial it is often far from certain what that question is. There is sometimes a tendency in the definitive evaluation of complex interventions to either rush to the main research question too early in enquiry or to test out many questions simultaneously; the pilot trial offers the opportunity to be more flexible and choose a different primary research question when the main trial plan is formulated.

There is also a range of interventions that fall short of the requirements of the true randomized controlled trial. These include quasi-randomization in that randomization of the population does not take place but other measures are introduced to make the groups as similar as possible at baseline. The problems of randomization are prominent when community services are being compared (an der Heiden, 1996; Thornicroft et al., 1998).

Phase 3: randomized controlled trials

In the last stage of comparison the new treatment is compared with a standard treatment under the rigorous conditions of a randomized controlled trial. While this has always been the 'gold standard' whereby any new treatment is to be judged, it is important not to be carried away by the scientific arguments for using such trials (which are incontrovertible) without considering alternatives which may be more appropriate *at that particular time in the development of the treatment*. Randomized controlled trials are still relatively new to medicine and particularly to psychiatry and the first major studies, of the treatment of schizophrenia in the US (Casey et al., 1960) and of depression in the UK (Clinical Psychiatry Committee, Medical Research Council, 1965), are still within my experience in psychiatry.

Attitudes towards the randomized controlled trial have changed markedly in the last 25 years because of the distinction made between pragmatic and explanatory trials of interventions (Schwartz & Lellouch, 1967). Before this time, all was invested in the explanatory trial, a tightly organized and controlled trial of highly selected individuals who were homogeneous for the condition being treated and who were likely to complete the course of treatment. The findings of these studies were then generalized to routine clinical practice. Schwartz and Lellouch pointed out that this approach was not valid. The explanatory trial was 'aimed at understanding whether a difference existed between two treatments' whereas the pragmatic trial 'aimed at decision by answering the question "which of the two treatments should we prefer?"' (Schwartz & Lellouch, 1967). It is this question that is at the heart of any service evaluation and it is asked at a later stage than the explanatory trial.

Johnson (1998) has pointed out that, despite long use of the randomized controlled trial in psychiatry, it continues to be used inefficiently and often wrongly. There are greater problems with psychiatric disorders (and with psychiatric patients) than in other medical conditions and these include (1) problems of achieving reliable diagnoses, (2) the difficulties of maintaining blind assessments, (3) the common practice of simultaneously giving many treatments, and (4) the difficulties in selecting control groups, particularly for psychosocial treatments. However, these do not excuse the generally laxity of design and poor presentation and interpretation of findings. Johnson recommends that those involved in carrying out clinical trials of treatment interventions in psychiatry should follow seven principles when choosing a suitable design: (1) choose no more than two outcome variables, (2) concentrate on obtaining follow-up information on all randomized patients on a few occasions rather than many, (3) use a multicentre design wherever possible, (4) ensure that the entry criteria are as broad as possible so that the results are likely to be generalizable, (5) forget power calculations and aim to recruit at least 100 patients for analysis in each treatment group, (6) develop the strategy for analysis *before* the trial database is 'unblinded' to reveal treatments, and (7) use recently introduced statistical modelling techniques to enable analysis of all available data rather than restrict this to those with full follow-up information (Everitt, 1995).

Individual randomization may not always be appropriate in mental health service evaluation. For example, if an intervention is directed towards a team intervention, cluster randomization is frequently used and this will affect the numbers needed to show benefit (these are usually larger than when individual randomization is made) (Kerry & Bland, 1998) and may pose important ethical issues (Edward et al., 1999). Randomized incomplete block designs have also been used when full randomized studies are not deemed to be possible.

Because it is rarely possible to blind both patients and investigators in trials of community mental health services there is great potential for bias. Attempts to minimize bias need to be made explicit and one way of ensuring this is to make the investigating (research) team independent of the service providers. The characteristics of those who refuse to participate or who drop out at an early stage of evaluation are likely to differ from those who participate throughout and should be recorded.

The sample size necessary for a trial is dependent on the power calculation which relies on estimating the difference between the effects of two or more interventions and the likely variance of the data. This may be possible if an exploratory trial has been carried out using the same design but in most instances there is a great deal of guesswork in making such estimations. In practice, many investigators work backwards. They estimate how many patients they are likely to have available for treatment and then work out the power calculations to fit these figures. This was not the purpose for which power calculations were introduced and the recommendation of Johnson (1998) that investigators should aim for a minimum of 100 patients in each arm of the trial is a better solution.

In the case of ACT the influential trial that demonstrated its efficacy was published in 1980 and was carried out in the state of Wisconsin in the US (Stein & Test, 1980; Weisbrod et al., 1980).

This indicated both marked clinical efficacy and cost-savings and ACT was adopted with varying degrees of enthusiasm across the US (Stein & Santos, 1998).

Phase 4: dissemination and implementation

This final phase is sometimes neglected by researchers who feel their work has been done when they complete their main trials. The growth of research and development in health service research has achieved greater prominence because of the failure to implement advances quickly enough; this was the main impetus behind the development of the Cochrane Collaboration (now known as Cochrane). Part of this phase is equivalent to post-marketing surveillance after the introduction of a new drug and it is fair to add that health service interventions have been slow to introduce this adequately. However, it has a role in the establishment of audit.

Audit is often undervalued by experienced research workers who are used to working with good resources and no time pressures. However, audit is the best way of ensuring that the benefits of research advance are not only disseminated to clinical practice but are also maintained. In clinical practice, good audit ensures quality control so that sound practice is maintained.

Patient preference

Although randomized trials provide the best evidence of efficacy for treatments, such as a comparison of new drugs in which patient preference is a very minor factor, the situation is different for many psychosocial treatments or those in which drugs and other treatments are being compared. In a consumer society, the issue of patient preference in respect of treatment is coming more to the fore. This is particularly true in community settings. One common example is the prescription of antipsychotic drugs in schizophrenia. Although the evidence for the efficacy of these drugs in schizophrenia is overwhelming there is still a large minority of patients who prefer to take other forms of treatment, particularly 'alternative therapies' of unproven and doubtful value. In my personal experience, the strong personal belief of such patients that these treatments are the only valid ones does have an influence on response to treatment which goes far beyond the simple placebo effect for the preferred treatment and the nocebo effect (Tyrer, 1991) of the rejected one. The nocebo effect (i.e. the expectation that a treatment will harm) is now as prevalent as the placebo effect in clinical practice. Sixty-five years ago, new treatments were mainly 'wonder drugs' that led to marvel, amazement, and the expectation of improvement. Now we have a more sophisticated and informed population that is likely to look up all the adverse effects on the internet before agreeing to start treatment.

There is also the possibility that there are important interactions between an individual's preferences and the effects of treatment, yet in the standard randomized controlled trial these are not detected. If these are important, the results of the randomized controlled trial may be wrongly attributed to the specific content of the intervention alone (McPherson et al., 1997). As a consequence of this there is increasing interest in non-experimental methods in the assessment of efficacy of treatments (Wennberg, 1988) and in different research designs that take account of patient preferences (or indeed, other people's preferences such as clinicians). Brewin and Bradley (1989) proposed a partially randomized patient-centred design for psychosocial treatments in which patients who had strong preferences for a particular treatment were allocated to it whereas those who had no particular preference were randomly allocated in the usual way. The problem with this approach is that it breaks one of the fundamental principles of the randomized controlled trial, ensuring equivalent populations for all factors apart from the treatments under consideration. If, as has been shown to be the case, patients who have strong preferences differ from others in their level of education and other potentially important factors (Feine et al., 1998) then their results cannot be compared satisfactorily with others.

This does not mean that patient preference trials are inappropriate but it is probably preferable to avoid contaminating the randomized controlled trial by attempting to combine randomization and patient preference in one design. If a patient preference trial is carried out independently of a randomized controlled trial then the results can be compared and policy decisions made after taking account of both sets of findings (Wennberg et al., 1993).

Choice of evaluation for different treatments

Although circumstances vary greatly, it is possible to list the most appropriate forms of evaluation for different treatments (Table 34.1). For most drug treatments it is preferable to concentrate on randomized controlled trials as the main method of evaluation as, despite their difficulties in community settings, the ability to make treatments more or less double-blind is a major advantage. However, when multiple drug treatments are being evaluated it is almost impossible to get adequate numbers of patients to test hypotheses adequately and in these circumstances it is better to carry out audit studies and introduce standards to reduce the extent of polypharmacy (Wressell et al., 1990).

For psychosocial interventions the choice is not so straightforward; the difficulties in ensuring blind assessment (or even masked

Table 34.1 Common psychiatric treatments and their evaluation in community psychiatry

Treatment	Problems of community evaluation	Most common form of evaluation
Single drug therapy	Adherence	Randomized controlled trial
Multiple drug therapy	Adherence	Audit
Psychodynamic therapy	Choice of outcomes	Preference and randomized controlled single-blind trials
Behaviour therapy	Choice of outcomes	Single-blind trials
Cognitive therapy	Treatment fidelity	Single-blind trials
Mixed drug and psychological therapies	Choice of control populations	Trials of complex design with insufficient numbers but with opportunities for combining data in meta-analyses
Policy change	Most changes are statutory so little opportunity for adequate controls	(Unsatisfactory) before-after comparisons

assessment when a small amount of information sometimes is leaked) are often very great. For treatments such as psychotherapy, patient preference should be taken into account more and be linked to single-blind trials, whereas for more clearly defined therapies such as cognitive and behaviour therapy it is appropriate to concentrate on good single-blind trials with tightly defined outcomes.

In the settings of ordinary community practice many treatments are given simultaneously, both pharmacological and non-pharmacological. It has to be admitted that the process of evaluation here is not satisfactory and no sleight of hand in the form of complex assessment procedures and designs can conceal this. At the same time, it is quite clear that the solutions to therapeutic questions in these settings are much more important than for most single treatments. It is reasonable to attempt such evaluations only if the investigators are prepared to combine data from several interventions in analysing data. Thus drug and psychological treatments could be combined separately prior to analysis and interactions examined. Ideally studies should be multicentre ones in which sufficient numbers can be generated to test several hypotheses but for many involved in such research the special circumstances of their own community settings seem to make them reluctant to pool resources in this way. As a consequence, we have a large number of small-scale studies carried out in different settings with silly differences in methodology which prevent data from being combined or meta-analysis from being carried out successfully. Organizations such as the European Network for Mental Health Service Evaluation (ENMESH) could play an important part in fostering a common basis for evaluation that could aid such multicentre studies.

In all countries of the world we now have to accept that medical services are rationed to some extent and any treatment in the community that is more expensive than other treatments, even if it is more effective, has a hard task in getting preference. In practice, most treatments in community psychiatry do not demonstrate such clear-cut advantages over the best of existing treatments, and the most frequent scenario is that a number of treatments produce equivalent clinical findings but the one that does it most cheaply is the one that is recommended for adoption. In many cases the treatment might appear to be more expensive than the comparison ones but if it saves money by reducing admissions to hospital it would turn out to be cheaper overall. Thus, for example, the atypical neuroleptic drugs are much more expensive than the standard antipsychotic drugs but the case has been made for their adoption in clinical practice because, overall, they save money (Aitcheson & Kerwin, 1997; Guest et al., 1996).

Although cost is an obvious target for outcome measurement it is fraught with difficulties in analysis. Almost invariably costs show a grossly skewed distribution with few outliers costing a very large amount of money and many others costing very little if intervention had been minimal. In terms of analysis, non-parametric statistics are appropriate and yet these data do not deal with real figures. Mean costs constitute real resources whereas median costs are hypothetical even though they are more appropriate for statistical analyses. One of the consequences of this is that most analyses of costs tend to be poorly carried out (Barber & Thompson, 1998) and much more rigour is needed in the analysis of data. In our personal work we found the statistical technique called the 'bootstrap method' (Efron & Tibshirani, 1993) to be an appropriate way of dealing with cost

Outcome measures

Although it would be wrong to think that community mental health practice leads to a different set of outcomes than other forms of treatment, there is a recurring set of themes involved in community care which has to be borne in mind to process an evaluation. These themes will be discussed in order of importance. This is also relevant in view of the tendency of evaluations of community treatment to attempt to measure large numbers of outcomes on the grounds that all can contribute to the overall effect of a treatment policy.

Cost

Although at various times during the move towards community care emphasis has been placed on improving the quality of life for patients, destigmatizing the mentally ill, and promoting the dignity of self-sufficiency, the major reason why community care has been promoted in psychiatry is that it is considerably cheaper than hospital care. This is illustrated in **Figure 34.1** in which the relative costs of providing care for a population of psychotic patients was recorded over 1 year. The figures shown that, even when community care is specifically focused upon in the practice, its costs are completed dwarfed by the costs of inpatient care. Thus the best-resourced team in the study (Early Intervention Service (EIS)) shown in **Figure 34.1** still accounted for a much smaller proportion of the total budget than inpatient care despite accounting for a large fraction of the cost of community care in the study. The slogan 'a week in hospital is worth a year in the community' is essentially true even when considerable input is given to the community services.

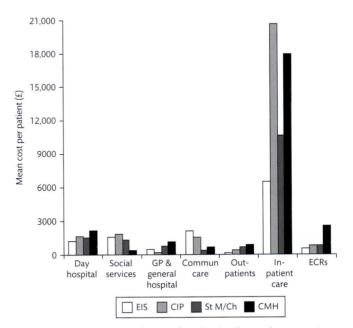

Figure 34.1 Comparison of costs of randomly allocated community-oriented and hospital-orientated care over 1 year for 144 patients with recurrent psychotic disorder, illustrating the much greater expense of hospital inpatient care compared with community services (derived from Tyrer et al., 1998). CIP, community intervention project (community team); CMH, Central Middlesex Hospital (hospital team); ECR, extra-contractual referral (inpatient care away from parent hospital); EIS, early intervention service (community team); St M/Ch, St Mary's/St Charles Hospital (hospital team).

data and this allows arithmetic means to be used in analysis despite skewing of the data (Evans et al., 1999).

Generalizability

Good evaluations of treatment lead to findings that can be used widely across a range of settings. In standard research trial methodology this is achieved by broad entry criteria to studies so that the population treated is representative of all those at risk and dropout rates are kept as low as possible so that the intervention can be analysed within this representative population. Unfortunately, it is in this area that many interventions in community psychiatry lead to problems. Community interventions are very dependent on setting. A drug treatment should have its effects shown in all people who take the agent as prescribed, and comparison with a dummy pill under controlled conditions makes it fairly easy to take out the effects of non-specific factors that are independent. Community interventions, including drugs, are different. In the case of drug treatment there is the problem of adherence, particularly with conditions such as schizophrenia, and with different forms of non-drug management, including psychological treatment, there are often great differences between the effectiveness of the personnel concerned and the nature of the 'control' condition in a randomized trial.

The control arm of most community psychiatric interventions is not a placebo—it is another complex intervention. The trouble is that the control group, often called 'treatment as usual', given greater respectability by the initials, TAU, implying it is an independent (Greek) symbol, is anything but a genuine control. The trouble is, it is often assumed to be, and so leads to confusion. Burns (2009) eloquently sounds what he hopes will be the death knell of TAU when he restates this position to make sure it cannot be forgotten. Fundamentally, he argues, 'when we conduct [these] community psychiatry studies of complex interventions, we are comparing two interventions and should treat them equally'. An obvious point, but do we listen? No we don't, or at least, not until now. So we have had to go through interminable arguments about why ACT is so much worse in the UK, with claims that it shows less treatment fidelity that its US gold standard, even though the real reason has been clear for all to see. I am not the greatest at predicting the future but I wrote 25 years ago that:

> Unlike drug/placebo comparisons, in which the effects of placebo are roughly similar whatever the year, complex psychosocial interventions such as those in a mental health service are changing constantly. I can predict with some confidence that the Cochrane review showing such excellent findings with regard to superiority of ACT in randomized controlled trials will show steadily decreasing benefits of ACT in future revisions. (Tyrer, 2000)

Yes, indeed it has, and simple straightforward community mental health team management does just as well (Malone et al., 2007).

This does not mean that treatment fidelity is unimportant. It can be, particularly in less complex interventions. It is tested most often in studies of psychological treatments that can be formally defined, such as cognitive therapy, but it could equally well be addressed in all forms of treatment, including drug therapy. In respect of drug therapy, treatment fidelity is primarily concerned with compliance, adherence, or concordance. Although this is true of all forms of treatment it is the essential element in drug treatment since the consumption of the medication constitutes the essential part of treatment fidelity. Pharmacokinetic differences may lead to the drug being less effective in some people compared with others, but these are in no way under the voluntary control of the patient or therapist. In community comparisons of drug treatment, it is very difficult to be certain of adherence to treatment, since simple measures such as counting of tablets after each course of treatment does not guarantee that those which have been taken have been consumed by the patient, and the detection of drugs which can be tested in the urine or in other body fluids does not guarantee that the drug concerned has been taken in regular dosage over the total course of treatment.

What seems to be most important in ensuring compliance is education and knowledge. The more a patient knows about the reasons for a treatment and the consequences of not taking it, the more likely they are to comply with a treatment regime. One of the reasons why cognitive and behavioural approaches have been so valuable in recent years is that they essentially involve a collaborative approach with the patient which involves an explanation as to why treatment is necessary and which the patient has to adopt if treatment is to proceed successfully (Kemp et al., 1996, 1998; Perry et al., 1999). The best way to achieve adherence is still far from clear and unfortunately compliance or adherence therapy has not proved to be successful in a larger trial (Gray et al., 2006).

For psychological treatments the variance in treatment fidelity may be much greater. If we regard the basic unit of community treatment as the community mental health team, it is clear there is a wide range of experience and knowledge across the range of treatments available and most team members will not be capable of giving psychological treatment competently without training and periodic refresher courses. The standard way of determining treatment fidelity in psychosocial interventions is to record interviews and, ideally, have them rated blind by an independent assessor. Although this is a perfectly reasonable procedure to adopt, it is important to realize that it may interfere with the therapeutic session, may not always be representative of all parts of treatment since the therapist and patient know they are being monitored, and it is not usually representative of ordinary practice. It merely tests whether patient and therapist are *capable* of carrying out treatment in a proper manner; it does not confirm that this treatment is being given consistently in this way. Such measures also beg the question, 'What do we do with the results when treatment fidelity is not satisfactory?' In ordinary practice there is, as yet, no standard way of ensuring that patients are treated by competent therapists (e.g. Kingdon et al., 1996).

Summary

The methodology of evaluation of community treatments is still a young area of science. However, we have moved far from following in the paths of John Conolly at Hanwell and Edward Charlesworth at Lincoln 175 years ago when they removed constraint and encouraged rehabilitation as the first stage of community treatment. These initiatives had face validity in that they illustrated that patients with mental illness could have a much better quality of life when the right intervention was given. We have become much better informed in the last few years and have moved a long way from the stage of what Thornicroft and Tansella term 'naïve community mental health' in which the chant of the animals in Orwell's *Animal Farm* 'four legs good, two legs bad' could be paraphrased as 'community treatment good, hospital treatment bad'. Thornicroft and Tansella (2004) suggest a more balanced approach:

> In recent years there has been a debate between those who are in favour of the provision of mental health treatment and care in hospitals, and those who prefer to use primarily or even exclusively community settings, in which the two forms of care are often seen as incompatible. This false dichotomy can now be replaced by an approach that balances both community services and modern hospital care. (p. 288)

There is also an urgent need to develop new approaches that are not as time-consuming, expensive, and limited in scope as the randomized controlled trial. It is likely that progress will be made more effectively integrating qualitative and quantitative approaches in this regard. Above all, we need to be aware of the 'saboteur of setting'—the undermining of excellent evidence of a valuable new treatment or form of management by what may first appear as a minor difference in place but which on close examination proves to be a major cruncher.

REFERENCES

Aitcheson, K. J. & Kerwin, R. W. (1997). Cost-effectiveness of clozapine. *British Journal of Psychiatry*, **171**, 125–130.

An der Heiden, W. (1996). Experimental and quasi-experimental design in evaluative research. In: Knudsen, H. C. & Thornicroft, G. (Eds.), *Mental Health Service Evaluation* (pp. 143–155). Cambridge: Cambridge University Press.

Barber, J. & Thompson, S. G. (1998). Analysis and interpretation of cost data in randomised controlled trials: review of published studies *BMJ*, **317**, 1195–1200.

Barton, R. (1966). *Institutional Neurosis*. London: Butterworth/Heinemann.

Brewin, C. R. & Bradley, C. (1989). Patient preferences and randomised clinical trials. *BMJ*, **299**, 313–315.

Burns, T. (2009). The end of the road for treatment-as-usual studies? *British Journal of Psychiatry*, **195**, 5–6.

Byford, S., Sharac, J., Lloyd-Evans, B., Gilburt, H., Osborn, D. P. J., Leese, M., et al. (2010). Alternatives to standard acute in-patient care in England: readmissions, service use and cost after discharge. *British Journal of Psychiatry*, **197**, s20–s25.

Campbell, M., Fitzpatrick, R., Haines, A., Sandercock, P., Spiegelhalter, D., & Tyrer, P. (2000). A framework for the design and evaluation of complex interventions to improve health. *BMJ*, **321**, 694–696.

Casey, J. F., Lasky, J. J., Klett, C. J., & Hollister, L. E. (1960). Treatment of schizophrenic reactions with phenothiazine derivatives. *American Journal of Psychiatry*, **117**, 97–105.

Clinical Psychiatry Committee, Medical Research Council (1965). Clinical trial of the treatment of depressive illness. *BMJ*, **1**, 881–886.

Edwards, S., Braunholtz, D., Stevens, A., & Lilford, R. (1999). Ethical issues in the design and conduct of cluster RCTs. *BMJ*, **318**, 1407–1409.

Efron, B. & Tibshirani, R. J. (1993). *An Introduction to the Bootstrap*. London: Chapman and Hall.

Evans, K., Tyrer, P., Catalan, J., Schmidt, U., Davidson, K., Dent, J., et al. (1999). Manual-assisted cognitive–behaviour therapy (MACT): a randomised controlled trial of a brief intervention with bibliotherapy in the treatment of recurrent deliberate self-harm. *Psychological Medicine*, **29**, 19–25.

Everitt, B. S. (1995). The analysis of repeated measures: a practical review with examples. *The Statistician*, **44**, 113–135.

Feine, J. S., Awad, M. A., & Lund, J. P. (1998). The impact of patient preference on the design and interpretation of clinical trials. *Community Dental and Oral Epidemiology*, **26**, 70–74.

Gray, R., Leese, M., Bindman, J., Becker, T., Burti, L., David, A., et al. (2006). Adherence therapy for people with schizophrenia: European multicentre randomised controlled trial. *British Journal of Psychiatry*, **189**, 508–514.

Guest, J. S., Hart, W. N., Cookson, R. S., & Lindstrom, E. (1996). Pharmaco-economic evaluation of long-term treatment with risperidone for patients with chronic schizophrenia. *British Journal of Medical Economics*, **10**, 59–67.

Johnson, T. (1998). Clinical trials in psychiatry: background and statistical perspective. *Statistical Methods in Medical Research*, **7**, 209–234.

Kemp, R., Hayward, P., Applewhaite, G., Everitt, B., & David, A. (1996). Compliance therapy in psychotic patients: randomised controlled trial. *BMJ*, **312**, 345–349.

Kemp, R., Kirov, G., Applewhaite, G., Everitt, B., Hayward, P., & David, A. (1998). Randomised controlled trial of compliance therapy. 18-month follow-up. *British Journal of Psychiatry*, **172**, 413–419.

Kerry, S. M. & Bland, J. M. (1998). Analysis of a trial randomised in clusters. *BMJ*, **316**, 54.

Kingdon, D., Tyrer, P., Seivewright, N., Ferguson, B., & Murphy, S. (1996). The Nottingham Study of Neurotic Disorder: influence of cognitive therapists on outcome. *British Journal of Psychiatry*, **169**, 93–97.

Knapp, M. & Beecham, J. (1990). Costing mental health services. *Psychological Medicine*, **20**, 893–908.

Little, W., Fowler, H. W., & Coulson, J. (Revised and edited by Onions, C. T.) (1973). *Shorter Oxford English Dictionary*. Oxford: Clarendon Press.

Malone, D., Newton-Howes, G., Simmonds, S., Marriott, S., & Tyrer, P. (2007). Community mental health teams (CMHTs) for people with severe mental illnesses and disordered personality. *Cochrane Database of Systematic Reviews*, **3**, CD000270.

Marx, A. J., Test, M. A., & Stein, L. I. (1973). Extrohospital management of severe mental illness. Feasibility and effects of social functioning. *Archives of General Psychiatry*, **29**, 505–511.

McPherson, K., Britton, A. R., & Wennberg, J. E. (1997). Are randomised controlled trials controlled? Patient preferences and unblind trials. *Journal of the Royal Society of Medicine*, **90**, 652–656.

Mullen, P. D. (1997). Compliance becomes concordance. *BMJ*, **314**, 691–692.

National Collaborating Centre for Mental Health (2009). *Borderline Personality Disorder: The NICE Guideline on Treatment and Management*. National Clinical Practice Guideline No. 78. London: British Psychological Society & Royal College of Psychiatrists.

Perry, A., Tarrier, N., Morriss, R., McCarthy, E., & Limb, K. (1999). Randomised controlled trial of efficacy of teaching patients with bipolar disorder to identify early symptoms of relapse and obtain treatment. *BMJ*, **318**, 149–153.

Schwartz, D. & Lellouch, J. (1967). Explanatory and pragmatic attitudes in therapeutic trials. *Journal of Chronic Diseases*, **20**, 637–648.

Soloff, P. H., George, A., Nathan, R. S., Schulz, P. M., Ulrich, R. F., & Perel, J. M. (1986). Progress in pharmacotherapy of personality disorders: a double blind study of amitriptyline, haloperidol and placebo. *Archives of General Psychiatry*, **43**, 691–697.

Stein, L. I. & Santos, A. B. (1998). *Assertive Community Treatment of Persons with Severe Mental Illness*. London: Norton Books.

Stein, L. I. & Test, M. A. (1980). Alternative to mental hospital treatment. I. Conceptual model, treatment program, and clinical evaluation. *Archives of General Psychiatry*, **37**, 392–397.

Thornicroft, G., Strathdee, G., Phelan, M., Holloway, F., Wykes, T., Dunn, G., et al. (1998). Rationale and design: the PRiSM Psychosis Study. *British Journal of Psychiatry*, **173**, 363–370.

Thornicroft, G. & Tansella, M. (1999). *The Mental Health Matrix: A Manual to Improve Services*. Cambridge: Cambridge University Press.

Thornicroft, G. & Tansella, M. (2004). Components of a modern mental health service: a pragmatic balance of community and hospital care. Overview of systematic evidence. *British Journal of Psychiatry*, **185**, 283–290.

Tyrer, P. (1991). The nocebo effect—poorly known but getting stronger. In: Dukes, M. N. G. & Aronson, J. K. (Eds.), *Side Effects of Drugs Annual 15* (pp. 19–25). Amsterdam: Elsevier.

Tyrer, P. (2000). Effectiveness of intensive treatment in severe mental illness. *British Journal of Psychiatry*, **176**, 492–493.

Weisbrod, B. A., Test, M. A., & Stein, L. I. (1980). Alternative to mental hospital treatment. II. Economic benefit–cost analysis. *Archives of General Psychiatry*, **37**, 400–405.

Wennberg, J. E. (1988). Non-experimental methods in the assessment of efficacy. *Medical Decision Making*, **8**, 175–176.

Wennberg, J. E., Barry, M. J., Fowler, F. J., & Mulley, A. (1993). Outcomes research, PORTs, and health care reform. *Annals of the New York Academy of Sciences*, **703**, 52–62.

Wressell, S. E., Tyrer, S. P., & Berney, T. P. (1990). Reduction in antipsychotic drug dosage in mentally handicapped patients: a hospital study. *British Journal of Psychiatry*, **157**, 101–106.

35
Qualitative research methods in mental health

Rob Whitley

Introduction

Qualitative research is a broad umbrella term describing a constellation of research methods and paradigms that rely on the collection, analysis, and interpretation of non-numeric data. Qualitative research attempts to access the whole gamut of human experience by documenting and analysing knowledge, beliefs, behaviours, attitudes, and emotions of specific groups and subpopulations. Qualitative research in mental health usually relies on (1) a series of *in-depth interviews* with individuals from a group of interest, for example, people with a mental illness participating in an innovative psychosocial rehabilitation programme to better understand their experience therein (Whitley et al., 2021); (2) a series of *focus groups* held with different stakeholders on a topic of psychiatric interest, for example, with clinicians, patients, and family members to understand the nature and impact of stigma associated with mental illness (Schulze & Angermayer, 2003); or (3) *ethnographic observation* in a naturalistic setting such as an inpatient ward to better understand the overall patient experience as well as underlying staff–patient dynamics (Goffman, 1961; Rosenhan, 1973). These three methods can be used in combination. This is known as *triangulation* and is considered a very strong approach as it gives greater perspective and insight into a problem, discussed in detail below.

The aims of qualitative research

At root, qualitative approaches share an attempt to understand individuals and groups in context, and are often used in three specific manners. First, qualitative research is used to understand individuals' or groups' generic or specific interaction with core societal institutions such as the education system, health system, or criminal justice system. Why do boys drop out of high school at a higher rate than girls? Why are certain ethno-racial minorities more distrustful of the police than the majority population? Why do immigrants use conventional mental health services at a lower rate than non-immigrants? These are the kind of research questions that can be answered by an intelligently designed qualitative research project that assesses relations between individuals and societal institutions.

Second, qualitative research can be deployed to understand the lived day-to-day experience of a specific subpopulation living in a particular social context—exploring just how they behave and experience the world around them at the micro-level, meso-level, and macro-level. What is it like to be a full-time carer for someone with Alzheimer's disease? How do people with schizophrenia experience the social world post hospitalization? What is psychiatric training like for female residents? These are the kind of questions that can be answered through this type of qualitative research.

Third, qualitative research is often used in a very focused manner, in order to evaluate a programme or intervention, or as a needs assessment for a group of people. What are the health needs of elderly immigrants with dementia living in inner-city London? How does a physical exercise intervention influence the social and emotional well-being of people with severe mental illness? What are the barriers and facilitators to implementing a new psychosocial intervention at a routine mental health clinic?

Qualitative research is often concerned with questions of 'Why?', 'What?', and 'How?' Qualitative researchers are particularly interested in reasons given by different stakeholders for actions; these are critically assessed by the researcher who will make appropriate inferences based on their knowledge of the data, the context, and the existing literature.

Malinowski (1990) argued that qualitative research aims to understand a phenomenon from a 'native' point of view that, above all, attempts to document and understand subjective meaning and experience. This involves eliciting as much information as possible about an individual, a group of individuals, their worldview, and their sociocultural context. In the famous words of Clifford Geertz (1973), the researcher aims to construct a 'thick description' of the group and phenomena under study. As such, the researcher should immerse themselves in the context in which research participants live their lives, which allows for the generation of the desired 'thick description'.

The 'thick description' per se serves a very important function. It brings to life the experience of a group, often a group that is marginalized, stigmatized, and misunderstood. It documents challenges and concerns faced by the group in daily life, which can include challenges interacting with the health care system. This information can be used by health service planners to create more accessible, appropriate, and culturally competent services. The 'thick description' also serves a second function. It is often used to generate a hypothesis or theory that can be tested in new rounds of data collection (Glaser & Strauss, 1967). For example, a seminal study explored the experience and meaning of stigma by comparing data from focus groups of patients with schizophrenia, their relatives, and health professionals. The 'thick description' of stigma allowed the authors to theorize that stigma is dimensional and that appropriate interventions should be targeted to these various dimensions (Schulze & Angermayer, 2003). In this manner, stand-alone qualitative studies can build up a local 'substantive' theory, which is provisional and open to further testing. As more and more studies are conducted, their results can be compared and integrated to generate more general and more conclusive 'formal' theory (Glaser & Strauss, 1967).

Table 35.1 Broad differences between typical forms of qualitative and quantitative research

	Qualitative	Quantitative
Epistemology	Inductive	Deductive
Study design	Data driven	Theory driven
Departure point	Research question	Hypothesis
Sample size	Smaller	Larger
Analytical units	Words (and behaviours)	Numbers
Analytical process	Repeated iterations during data collection	End-point analysis once all data is gathered
Workload	More back-end work analysis is lengthy	More front-end, especially in recruitment and execution

Note: these are somewhat simplified for the purposes of summary. For example, multisite qualitative studies have large samples, and many epidemiological surveys are not hypothesis driven. This table should be considered a 'rough guide' rather than definitive.

Reprinted with permission from the *American Journal of Psychiatry*, (copyright 2009), American Psychiatric Association, first appeared in Whitley, R. (2009). Introducing psychiatrists to qualitative research: a guide for instructors. *Academic Psychiatry*, 33(3), 252–255.

The design and execution of qualitative research

The design and execution of qualitative research, if done rigorously, is largely similar to that of quantitative research. The same a priori thought and discussion that goes into the development and design of a quantitative study should also occur in a qualitative study. Like quantitative research, qualitative research is a detailed endeavour, requiring adherence to certain methodological canons. Namely, an innovative research question should be formulated in the light of literature review. A study should be designed that is capable of answering the research question. This should take account of the financial, temporal, and human resources available to the investigator. The study should be executed in a timely manner. Incoming data should be interpreted and written up for publication. Stringent training and quality assurance procedures should be in place throughout. All studies should have professional qualitative experts in leadership, supervisory, and/or consultancy roles, just as quantitative studies often require input from professional statisticians or advanced methodological expertise (Whitley, 2009).

Though there is much overlap between qualitative and quantitative research, there are also a number of differences, which are summarized in **Table 35.1**. Those trained mainly in quantitative research will likely be wedded to a positivist model of research that emphasizes the importance of large sample sizes, predictive statistics, reliability, and external validity. Those trained mainly in qualitative research will likely be wedded to more interpretive-constructivist models of research that emphasize small sample sizes, thick description, context particularities, and internal validity (Whitley & Crawford, 2005).

It is important to understand some of these broad differences in orientation. Three major differences relate to hypothesis testing, sample size, and design modification. First, qualitative research is rarely hypothesis driven, but is generally inductive in orientation. Data is explored in light of a research question, rather than tested against a predefined hypothesis or a predefined theory. This is because qualitative research generally aims to broadly understand a phenomenon of interest (e.g. the impact of psychiatric institutionalization) or a subpopulation of interest (e.g. low-income single mothers), rather than precisely test an extant theory (Whitley, 2007). The second difference relates to sample size. Though a few studies have large numbers of participants (mostly cross-site), generally qualitative studies have a small sample, commonly between 20 and 40 participants (e.g. Boucher et al., 2019; Whitley & Zhou, 2020). Some studies have fewer than 20 participants—though these are frequently longitudinal in design, meaning that the desired thick description is achieved by following a cohort over time (e.g. Brom et al., 2017; Corepal et al., 2018). The careful and judicious study of lived experience in a sample that is smaller than quantitative studies on the same topic is considered optimal in qualitative research as it reaches an intimate depth of knowledge unattainable through survey methods or other quantitative techniques (Pope & Mays, 1995). Third, it should be noted that interim analysis and subsequent modification of design is encouraged in qualitative research, which is rarely seen in epidemiological or survey research. This allows the researcher to hone in an area of interest that may not have been obvious from the outset, allowing the researcher to follow new leads in the data collection process.

Another major difference between qualitative and quantitative research is the difference between 'front-end' and 'back-end' work (Miles & Huberman, 1994). Quantitative research can involve an enormous amount of 'front-end' work, for example, in the setting up and implementation of a randomized control trial. However, once all the data is gathered in, 'back-end' work may be relatively light, in that statistical packages can be used to help test the hypothesis under observation. In qualitative research, 'front-end' work may be relatively less intense, as researchers recruit a relatively small sample of people and conduct a relatively small number of interviews or focus groups to understand a phenomenon, often with the assistance of helpful clinics, community groups, or peer support organizations. The most challenging part of qualitative research may come at the analysis and interpretation stage, that is, during the 'back-end' of research, which can be extremely lengthy. Audio recordings of interviews and focus groups need to be transcribed and should be read (and listened to) many times. Transcripts will need to be coded, meaning that sentences and paragraphs are extracted and categorized into cross-cutting themes. Emerging codes might need to be pruned, merged, and finessed into super-ordinate categories, and once this process is completed, a detailed empirically grounded theory can be produced (Glaser & Strauss, 1967). Computer-assisted qualitative data analysis software may help expedite some of these processes; however, this is an organizational aid and does not conduct the analysis in itself. The researcher still needs to categorize, code, and link data, without losing sight of the overall dataset. Moreover, all results should be ensconced into the wider background literature, which should also be considered in the interpretation of results and generation of new theory. This can be a lengthy process.

Qualitative research in community mental health

Qualitative research has its roots in sociology and anthropology. However there is also a strong tradition of qualitative research within psychiatry and community mental health in particular (Davidson et al., 2008). Qualitative research has been judiciously employed throughout the history of psychiatry, and can trace its lineage back to seminal figures such as Karl Jaspers and Melanie Klein. It continues to be a methodology of choice for those investigating important domains of contemporary community psychiatry such as psychosocial recovery, stigma, cultural competence, gender issues, and service utilization.

Psychiatric deinstitutionalization is one of the developments that was heavily influenced by qualitative research. One of the most influential and well-known studies in psychiatric history was Rosenhan's (1973) 'being sane in insane places'. This is one of the few qualitative papers ever to be published in the prestigious journal *Science*. It was written in 1973 when there were around 200,000 inpatients in US psychiatric institutions. This led to concerns about overdiagnosis and iatrogenesis. Rosenhan explored this matter by employing 'sane' research assistants as 'pseudopatients' to present at psychiatric hospitals, pretending that they heard a voice. This was the only 'psychiatric' complaint given by participants. All were admitted into the hospital. Once admitted, length of hospitalization averaged 19 days. While in the hospitals, pseudopatients engaged in classic participant observation. They experienced and witnessed many 'depersonalizing' events, for example, being sworn at or ignored by staff. This paper has had a huge impact, being cited over 4000 times. It raised questions of the validity of psychiatric diagnostic techniques, as well as the efficacy and humanity of psychiatric hospitalization.

The results of Rosenhan's research were consistent with those of Goffman's, whose best-selling book *Asylums* (1961) described and analysed some of the depersonalizing and stultifying effects of psychiatric institutionalization. In this book, Goffman provided a 'thick description' of life in an asylum, and then formulated a grounded super-ordinate concept from his work known as 'the total institution'. This described places where individuals therein were deprived of control and agency, living their lives under strict rules and routines, and included places such as mental hospitals, boarding schools, and military barracks. Goffman's work was based on 2 years' participant observation at a psychiatric institution where he was ostensibly 'Assistant Athletic Director', but was actually engaged in ethnographic research. Again, Goffman's work strongly influenced the movement for deinstitutionalization, and the transformation towards community care.

When deinstitutionalization finally arrived, it demanded a new research question: 'What is it like for people with severe mental illness to live in the community?' This question has been the focus of intense qualitative study since then. Estroff's (1981) monograph, *Making It Crazy*, gives a thick description of life in the community for recently discharged people with severe mental illness, based on two years' ethnographic observation with clients receiving outpatient services. Her book richly chronicles the trials and tribulations of living in the community in the context of fragmented services, and patient strategies for surviving and 'making it' in the community. The book cast light on the desperation of many people receiving 'community care' in the context of fragmented and patchy service provision in the post-institutionalization era.

Antonovsky's (1979) classic qualitative study of stress, coping, and thriving among holocaust survivors in the new Israeli society raised awareness of medicine's 'pathological emphasis', which tends to ignore the multifarious ways people live meaningful lives after experiencing severe trauma and adversity. This work somewhat presaged the strengths-based focus of the emerging recovery paradigm, now common in community mental health (Slade et al., 2014; Tse et al., 2016). This paradigm is frequently investigated through qualitative methods, which are ideally placed to elicit and analyse the lived experience of people in recovery from severe mental illness. For example, Deegan (2005) found through qualitative study the importance of everyday activities that give life meaning and purpose in facilitating recovery (e.g. reading, studying, working, and parenting) and that these activities often outweighed clinical services in subjective importance as catalysts of recovery. Similarly, Boucher et al. (2019) found that people with severe mental illness create their own healing landscapes which can include parks, churches, and other local community spaces, which are visited and utilized regularly in order to better foster recovery.

Certain variables have become the frequent focus of attention in qualitative research focused on mental health. These include gender (Affleck et al., 2018), housing (Voisard et al., 2021), employment (Poremski et al., 2016), religion/spirituality (Whitley, 2012), stigma (Arthur & Whitley, 2015), social support (Davidson, 2003), and community integration (Ware et al., 2007). Some qualitative studies in psychiatry are published as books, especially those that are anthropologically informed (e.g. Jenkins & Csordas, 2020; Lester, 2019; Myers, 2015). However, most are published as refereed articles in scientific journals. Respected journals which regularly publish qualitative research relevant to community mental health include the *British Journal of Psychiatry*, the *Community Mental Health Journal*, *Culture, Medicine & Psychiatry*, the *International Journal of Social Psychiatry*, *Psychiatric Services*, and the *Psychosocial Rehabilitation Journal*. Any reader interested in perusing a qualitative study in some aspect of community psychiatry can consult the current issue of one of the above journals, and they will likely find at least one qualitative study within. This raises an important question. If the novice reader was to conduct such an exercise and find a relevant qualitative study, just how could they differentiate a rigorous qualitative study from a study lacking in rigour? This question is explored in the next section.

Criteria of rigour in qualitative research

When conducting or evaluating a quantitative study, certain criteria of rigour can be deployed to assess the strength and contribution of the study. Two concepts which are central to quantitative research are validity and reliability, both arising out of the positivist framework in which most quantitative research is conducted. Reliability refers to the repeatability of findings—will the same findings be produced in separate repeated studies? An important distinction in reliability is that drawn between inter-rater reliability and test–retest reliability. Inter-rater reliability refers to the extent which two individual raters agree on measurement scores within a study. Test–retest reliability refers to the stability of findings over time—will the same study with the same instruments find similar results with the same participants at different points in time?

Validity refers to the strength of the conclusions and presented findings of a study in relation to the study processes, for example, that it is accurately measuring what it is purporting to measure. An important distinction is that drawn between internal and external validity. External validity refers to the strength of any generalizations that can be made to contexts beyond that of the study. Internal validity refers to the strength of any inferences and conclusions within the study itself, for example, how well what is measured fits with existing knowledge or theory.

Many qualitative researchers have convincingly argued against the application of quantitative criteria of rigour to qualitative research (Barbour & Barbour, 2003; Lincoln & Guba, 1985; Pope & Mays, 1995; Whitley & Crawford, 2005). This is because the social world is constantly in flux, and that it is illogical to expect test–retest reliability in such circumstances. Giddens' (1987) well-known 'double hermeneutic' indeed posits that lay people are constantly interpreting the results of social science studies, and adjusting their behaviour accordingly. Likewise, an axiom of much social science is that dynamics and processes are locally grounded and it is fallacious to expect to see similar processes elsewhere. Thus an inability to replicate a qualitative study over time and place does not invalidate it in the least; it may simply reflect changing contexts. As such, many qualitative researchers have argued that criteria of rigour used to assess quantitative research must not be used when assessing qualitative research (Strauss & Corbin, 1990). Instead, other frameworks have developed criteria of rigour that are specific to qualitative research.

Lincoln and Guba (1985) posit a four-dimensional framework that can be used to assess what they call the *trustworthiness* (i.e. rigour) of qualitative research. *Credibility* refers to the 'degree of confidence in the "truth" that the findings of a particular inquiry have for the subject with which—and context within which—the inquiry is carried out' (Erlandson et al., 1993, p. 29). Credibility is thus somewhat similar to internal validity. *Transferability* refers to the extent to which a study's findings can be applied in other contexts or to other people in a similar context. This concept is thus similar to external validity. *Dependability* refers to the extent to which study replication with similar participants and similar contexts would produce similar findings. This concept is somewhat similar to reliability. *Confirmability* refers to the degree to which study findings are the product of a systematic methodology and analysis, and not of the biases of the researcher. This concept is somewhat similar to objectivity.

Hammersley (1992) posits two criteria of rigour for qualitative research: *validity* and *relevance*. He states that validity can be assessed by identifying the main claims of a study, and assessing the supporting evidence in favour of these claims. This assessment will also include examination of underlying design, methodology, and analytical approach. Relevance refers to an examination of whether the research is addressing issues of societal and/or local concern. If the study is producing knowledge which has no public or local relevance, it is deemed not to be rigorous. Giacomini and Cook (2000) concur with Hammersley, though they also emphasize the importance of clinical relevance in health services qualitative research. In agreement with this position is Malterud (2001), who also emphasizes the importance of validity and relevance. However, she also posits the importance of *reflexivity* as a criterion of rigour. This addresses a critique of qualitative research that it is reliant on the subjective interpretation of data by one or a few researchers, meaning that the analytical processes can be coloured by the personal biases, narratives, and agendas of lead researchers. Malterud argues that researchers should thus make a conscious effort to declare their own background and position in disseminated research, ensuring that the effect of the researcher is attended to systematically at every step of the research process. This is known as 'positionality', and allows the researcher and the reader to systematically reflect on the investigator's role in underlying knowledge production.

It should be stated that some scholars, often known as 'anti-realists' or 'post-modernists' have criticized the creation of the above criteria of rigour for qualitative research. Smith and Heshusius (1986) critique the underlying assumption that there are social and cultural realities that exist independent of the researcher. They argue that such criteria betray the critical and interpretative nature of qualitative research. Additionally, the presented criteria of rigour are considered to have only a superficial difference from the traditional positivistic criteria of validity and reliability. As such, these criteria are sometimes rejected as being pseudo-positivistic. This arguments states that researchers can attempt to offer an interpretation of participants' perspectives which do not reflect a single underlying reality, precisely because (according to this argument) there is no single underlying reality to represent.

This epistemological position is somewhat extreme and not adhered to by the vast majority of qualitative researchers in psychiatry who may be labelled as 'critical realists'. This describes an approach where scholars assume the existence of reality, with the awareness that such realities are often socially constructed and are by no means inevitable or immutable. Such a foundation allows for the critical conduct of qualitative research in psychiatry. Researchers can attempt to explore, document, and analyse realities through use of ethnographic observation, focus groups, and individual interviews. They can evaluate the rigour of such attempts using concepts of validity, relevance, credibility, transferability, dependability, and confirmability. This position of critical realism is one espoused herein. As such, rigorous qualitative research should be conducted with strong efforts to enhance validity, relevance, credibility, transferability, dependability, and confirmability. Fortunately, there are a battery of processes and techniques that are commonly used by qualitative researchers to facilitate such rigour. In the next section, the most common techniques and strategies are outlined.

Techniques and strategies to enhance rigour

Techniques and strategies to enhance rigour can be applied at various stages of the research project. In appraising the rigour of qualitative research, readers can assess the level to which such techniques and strategies have been followed. These techniques and strategies can be applied in the design stage, the execution stage, and the analysis/dissemination stage. The following list of techniques and strategies is distilled from various seminal texts on rigour in qualitative research including Lincoln and Guba (1985), Erlandson et al. (1993), Hammersley (1992), and Glaser and Strauss (1967).

A strong method of enhancing validity and credibility is through a method known as *triangulation*. This term derives from orienteering and navigation, where people can work out their exact location by taking a compass bearing from a number of visible reference points (e.g. a church steeple, a lighthouse, and another prominent landmark). By the same logic, qualitative researchers strive to use different reference points to explore the phenomena under study, in order to get a truer sense of the said phenomena.

There are three different forms of triangulation commonly used in qualitative research, namely (1) methodological triangulation, (2) participant triangulation, and (3) investigator triangulation. Methodological triangulation means using two or more methods to investigate the research question. For example, a study that uses focus groups, in-depth interviews, and participant observation is stronger than a study that relies on one of those methods, as the use of multiple methods obtains different perspectives on a problem under study.

Participant triangulation means collecting data from different types of participant. For example, a study of mental health stigma could involve collecting data from service users, family members, and clinicians. This would thicken the description of the phenomena under study, giving a wider expanse of data from which inferences can be made. The different perspectives gathered can be compared and contrasted, and any varying findings integrated to deepen the analysis. The degree of confidence in the key findings of the study increases where there is convergence from these various data sources (Erlandson et al., 1993).

Investigator triangulation refers to having individuals from different disciplinary backgrounds working on data collection and data analysis. For example, a study of mental health recovery could be led by a research team comprising a psychiatrist, a sociologist, an anthropologist, a social worker, and a pharmacologist. All could bring unique perspectives to the collection and analysis of data, and would mitigate the potential for bias or myopic thinking on a topic under consideration. In short, triangulation can be built into the design of a study in various ways and is a strong signifier of thoughtful planning and rigorous thinking.

Another factor which plays a strong role in rigour is *sampling*. As previously mentioned, sample sizes in qualitative research vary, but a very small sample should be cause for concern—unless it has been followed up longitudinally using in-depth ethnographic methods. For example, a cross-sectional qualitative study that has fewer than ten interviews, or fewer than four focus groups may lack validity, dependability, and transferability. On the other hand, very large samples may also be cause for concern as this could indicate superficiality in the analysis, as it may be difficult for researchers to become intimately acquainted with the large amounts of raw data found in a large sample (Miles & Huberman, 1994). A sample of between 20 and 40 participants is an acceptable rule of thumb in qualitative research. Another factor important to bear in mind is the nature and scope of the sample. Homogeneity in qualitative samples is often encouraged, as this allows for an in-depth understanding of the subpopulation under study, as well as credibility of results. Samples which are sociodemographically or clinically heterogeneous should be treated with caution as they may lack validity, credibility, and dependability, unless they are based on a single unifying concept (e.g. experience of stigma). Another exception to this rule is when the researcher explicitly attempts to compare and contrast across certain sociodemographic or clinical domains, for example, a gender-based analysis examining differences between men and women undergoing a psychosocial rehabilitation intervention, or a sociologically informed analysis comparing the role of religion/spirituality in fostering recovery among different ethno-racial groups.

Another factor related to design, execution, and analysis is whether the research was conducted by a *multidisciplinary team*: the aforementioned 'investigator triangulation'. A multidisciplinary team brings various forms of expertise and perspective to the research project. Sociologists or anthropologists can provide conceptual and methodological expertise, whereas psychiatrists or social workers can provide clinical and other practical expertise. In mixed-methods studies, epidemiologists and statisticians may also join the team to provide expertise in their respective domains. Such collaboration ensures that elementary errors are not made in the research process and that proper methodological procedures have been followed.

In the execution of research, issues of *training and supervision* of research assistants, graduate students, and junior researchers is paramount. Conducting ethnographic observation in a busy clinic is a different skill than administering a 12-item questionnaire to an individual in a university office. As such, qualitative research papers should show convincing evidence that interviewers, analysts, and project leaders have the sufficient training and experience to conduct the research. This might involve outlining the qualifications and prior experience of data collectors and analysts, as well as what kind of on-the-job training (and by whom) was received.

Another important factor related to training is supervision. How closely were data collectors and analysts supervised? How often did senior researchers shadow research assistants in the field to ensure they were following recommended procedure? Were recordings of interviews and focus groups listened to by senior researchers, and appropriate feedback given to the junior researchers? Affirmative answers to these types of questions suggest rigour, enhancing validity and dependability.

A number of analytical techniques can be used to enhance rigour. A well-known technique is known as *multiple coding*, and involves a number of different individuals coding the same transcripts or pieces of data. Emergent themes can then be compared between different individual coders, and triangulated for consistency, convergence, or discrepancy. The rationale for multiple coding is that various members of the research team (especially those from different disciplinary backgrounds) may differentially perceive underlying themes. For example, discussion of the influence of religion on recovery may be interpreted differently by a cultural anthropologist than by a clinical psychologist. Likewise, a finding that is agreed upon by four analysts from different backgrounds is more credible than a finding derived from a single person.

Another technique commonly employed in the analysis stage is known as *respondent validation* or *member checking*. This refers to a process whereby key themes and findings from a qualitative study are presented to the original research participants, whose opinions on the accuracy of these themes are garnered. For example, researchers might conclude from the raw data of a qualitative study that access to psychiatric care is enhanced when it is integrated with physical health care services. This can be presented to the original participants who can state whether they agree or disagree with this emerging theory. An advantage of this technique is that it can prevent inaccurate portrayals of research participants. It can enhance validity by ensuring conclusions are agreed upon by the people being researched. A disadvantage is that this technique can lead to overly bland or flattering accounts, in that researchers may be tempted to produce a sanitized version of events to avoid offending participants.

Another analytical technique that is often used as a check on rigour is known as *negative (or deviant) case analysis*. This refers to a researcher paying conscious and explicit attention to cases which deviate from the principal findings of the overall study. For example, a needs assessment for carers of people with Alzheimer's disease might find huge gaps in need for most participants, but a minority of participants might not have these gaps. A sensitive research team will interrogate the data to understand why some people have less needs—do they instead rely on family, or friends, or churches, or the like for support? What is it about this subgroup that makes them different? This will then be presented in the results and appropriately discussed.

A final method of evaluating the rigour of a qualitative study is to assess how well the study is ensconced in the existing literature, as well as its use (and contribution to) theory. A good qualitative study should be well ensconced in the existing literature. Other relevant and formative studies should be debated in the introduction and in the discussion. It should be clear how the present study moves this literature forward and advances knowledge on the topic. The findings should also be related to wider social theory. Studies in social and cultural psychiatry often produce findings related to myriad policy or societal factors beyond psychiatry. This may include factors as diverse as gender policy, fair employment legislation, housing provision, the role of religion in the public sphere, and the use (or credibility) of alternative medicine. An astute qualitative researcher will situate their results in the appropriate social theory, in order to assist thinking and policymaking in this regard. Again, teamwork is a factor that can enhance these processes.

Conclusion

Qualitative research has a strong tradition in psychiatry. It continues to make a valuable contribution to the discipline's development. That said, it is worth stating that much qualitative research is of questionable quality. However, this usually reflects lack of judgement, training, experience, or interpretive acuity in the investigators, rather than something inherently defective in the method itself. Where properly applied, qualitative research may be very well suited to answer some of the innovative questions arising out of contemporary community psychiatry. These include questions related to recovery-oriented care, mental health service evaluation, and the enhancement of gender-sensitive and person-centred medicine.

FURTHER READING

Fortunately, there are many pedagogical resources available for people particularly interested in qualitative research. Numerous 'how to do qualitative research' textbooks exist which can be recommended to students dependent upon their level of study (e.g. Corbin & Strauss, 2015). All these resources give helpful advice on the conduct and evaluation of qualitative research. Many of the journals listed in this book chapter publish qualitative research articles. They can be surveyed regularly by the interested reader. Numerous brief summaries of qualitative research in the health sciences have been published in key journals. These are useful resources for those planning, conducting, or evaluating qualitative research. Some of these journal articles are listed below.

Buston, K., Parry-Jones, W., Livingston, M., Bogan, A., & Wood, S. (1998). Qualitative research. *British Journal of Psychiatry*, **172**, 197–199.

Corbin, J. & Strauss, A. (2015). *Basics of Qualitative Research: Techniques and Procedures for Developing Grounded Theory* (4th ed.). Thousand Oaks, CA: Sage.

Davidson, L., Ridgway, P., Kidd, S., Torpor, A., & Borg, M. (2008). Using qualitative research to inform mental health policy. *Canadian Journal of Psychiatry*, **53**, 137–144.

Malterud, K. (2001). Qualitative research: standards, challenges, and guidelines. *Lancet*, **358**, 483–488.

Malterud, K. (2001). The art and science of clinical knowledge: evidence beyond measures and numbers. *Lancet*, **358**, 397–400.

Pope, C. & Mays, N. (1995). Reaching the part other methods cannot reach: an introduction to qualitative methods in health and health services research. *BMJ*, **311**, 42–45.

Whitley, R. & Crawford, M. (2005). Qualitative research in psychiatry. *Canadian Journal of Psychiatry*, **50**, 108–114.

REFERENCES

Affleck, W., Thamotharampillai, U., Jeyakumar, J., & Whitley, R. (2018). 'If one does not fulfil his duties, he must not be a man': masculinity, mental health and resilience amongst Sri Lankan Tamil refugee men in Canada. *Culture, Medicine, and Psychiatry*, **42**, 840–861.

Antonovsky, A. (1979). *Health, Stress and Coping*. San Francisco, CA: Jossey-Bass.

Arthur, C. M. & Whitley, R. (2015). 'Head take you': causal attributions of mental illness in Jamaica. *Transcultural Psychiatry*, **52**, 115–132.

Barbour, R. S. & Barbour, M. (2003). Evaluating and synthesizing qualitative research: the need to develop a distinctive approach. *Journal of Evaluation in Clinical Practice*, **9**, 179–186.

Boucher, M.-E., Groleau, D., & Whitley, R. (2016). Recovery and severe mental illness: the role of romantic relationships, intimacy and sexuality. *Psychiatric Rehabilitation Journal*, **39**, 180–182.

Boucher, M.-E., Groleau, D., & Whitley, R. (2019). Recovery from severe mental illness in Québec: the role of culture and place. *Health & Place*, **56**, 63–69.

Brom, L., De Snoo-Trimp, J.C., Onwuteaka-Philipsen, B. D., Widdershoven, G. A., Stiggelbout, A. M., & Pasman, H. R. W. (2017). Challenges in shared decision making in advanced cancer care: a qualitative longitudinal observational and interview study. *Health Expectations*, **20**, 69–84.

Corepal, R., Best, P., O'Neill, R., Tully, M. A., Edwards, M., Jago, R., et al. (2018). Exploring the use of a gamified intervention for encouraging physical activity in adolescents: a qualitative longitudinal study in Northern Ireland. *BMJ Open*, **8**, e019663.

Davidson, L. (2003). *Living Outside Mental Illness: Qualitative Studies of Recovery in Schizophrenia*. New York: NYU Press.

Davidson, L., Ridgway, P., Kidd, S., Torpor, A., & Borg, M. (2008). Using qualitative research to inform mental health policy. *Canadian Journal of Psychiatry*, **53**, 137–144.

Deegan, P. E. (2005). The importance of personal medicine: a qualitative study of resilience in people with psychiatric disabilities. *Scandinavian Journal of Public Health*, **33**, 29–35.

Erlandson, D. A., Harris, E. L., Skipper, B., & Allen, S. D. (1993). *Doing Naturalistic Inquiry: A Guide to Methods*. Newbury Park, CA: Sage Publications.

Estroff, S. E. (1981). *Making it Crazy: An Ethnography of Psychiatric Clients in an American Community*. Berkeley, CA: University of California Press.

Geertz, C. (1973). *The Interpretation of Cultures*. New York: Basic Books.

Giacomini, M. K. & Cook, D. J. (2000). Users' guides to the medical literature: XXIII. Qualitative research in health care A. Are the result of the study valid? *JAMA*, **284**, 357–362.

Giddens, A. (1987). *Social Theory and Modern Sociology*. Cambridge: Polity Press.

Glaser, B. & Strauss, A. (1967). *The Discovery of Grounded Theory*. Chicago, IL: Aldine.

Goffman, E. (1961). *Asylums*. New York: Doubleday.

Hammersley, M. (1992). *What's Wrong with Ethnography?* London: Routledge.

Jenkins, J. H. & Csordas, T. J. (2020). *Troubled in the Land of Enchantment: Adolescent Experience of Psychiatric Treatment*. Oakland, CA: University of California Press.

Lester, R. J. (2019). *Famished: Eating Disorders and Failed Care in America*. Oakland, CA: University of California Press.

Lincoln, Y. & Guba, E. (1985). *Naturalistic Inquiry*. Thousand Oaks, CA: Sage.

Malinowski, B. (1990). *A Scientific Theory of Culture and Other Areas*. Raleigh, NC: University of North Carolina Press.

Malterud, K. (2001). Qualitative research: standards, challenges, and guidelines. *Lancet*, **358**, 483–488.

Mays, N. & Pope, C. (1995). Rigour and qualitative research. *BMJ*, **311**, 109–112.

Miles, M. & Huberman, A. (1994). *Qualitative Data Analysis*. Thousand Oaks, CA: Sage.

Myers, N. L. (2015). *Recovery's Edge: An Ethnography of Mental Health Care and Moral Agency*. Nashville, TN: Vanderbilt University Press.

Pope, C. & Mays, N. (1995). Reaching the parts other methods cannot reach: an introduction to qualitative methods in health and health services research. *BMJ*, **311**, 42–45.

Poremski, D., Whitley, R., & Latimer, E. (2016). Building trust with people receiving supported employment and housing first services. *Psychiatric Rehabilitation Journal*, **39**, 20.

Rosenhan, D. L. (1973). Being sane in insane places. *Science*, **179**, 250–258.

Schulze, B. & Angermeyer, M. C. (2003). Subjective experience of stigma. A focus group study of schizophrenic patients, their relatives and mental health professionals. *Social Science & Medicine*, **56**, 299–312.

Slade, M., Amering, M., Farkas, M., Hamilton, B., O'Hagan, M., Panther, G., et al. (2014). Uses and abuses of recovery: implementing recovery-oriented practices in mental health systems. *World Psychiatry*, **13**, 12–20.

Smith, J. K. & Heshusius, L. (1986). Closing down the conversation: the end of the quantitative-qualitative debate among educational inquirers. *Educational Researcher*, **15**, 4–12.

Strauss, A. L. & Corbin, J. (1990). *Basics of Qualitative Research*. Thousand Oaks, CA: Sage.

Tse, S., Tsoi, E. W., Hamilton, B., O'Hagan, M., Shepherd, G., Slade, M., et al. (2016). Uses of strength-based interventions for people with serious mental illness: a critical review. *International Journal of Social Psychiatry*, **62**, 281–291.

Voisard, B., Whitley, R., Latimer, E., Looper, K., & Laliberté, V. (2021). Insights from homeless men about PRISM, an innovative shelter-based mental health service. *PLoS One*, **16**, e0250341.

Ware, N. C., Hopper, K., Tugenberg, T., Dickey, B., & Fisher, D. (2007). Connectedness and citizenship: redefining social integration. *Psychiatric Services*, **58**, 469–474.

Whitley, R. (2007). Mixed-methods studies. *Journal of Mental Health*, **16**, 697–701.

Whitley, R. (2009). Introducing psychiatrists to qualitative research: a guide for instructors. *Academic Psychiatry*, **33**, 252–255.

Whitley, R. (2012). 'Thank you God': religion and recovery from dual diagnosis among low-income African Americans. *Transcultural Psychiatry*, **49**, 87–104.

Whitley, R. & Crawford, M. (2005). Qualitative research in psychiatry. *Canadian Journal of Psychiatry*, **50**, 108–114.

Whitley, R., Sitter, K. C., Adamson, G., & Carmichael, V. (2021). A meaningful focus: investigating the impact of involvement in a participatory video program on the recovery of participants with severe mental illness. *Psychiatric Rehabilitation Journal*, **44**, 63–69.

Whitley, R. & Zhou, J. (2020). Clueless: an ethnographic study of young men who participate in the seduction community with a focus on their psychosocial well-being and mental health. *PLoS One*, **15**, e0229719.

Developing evidence-based mental health practices

Kim T. Mueser and Robert E. Drake

Introduction

Effective interventions for individuals with severe mental illnesses such as schizophrenia and bipolar disorder have emerged rapidly over the past 60 years. Numerous pharmacological and psychosocial interventions are now available to ameliorate the symptoms of mental illnesses, to enhance people's functional abilities, and to improve their quality of life (Keepers et al., 2021; Nathan & Gorman, 2015). Further, clinical research studies frequently evaluate combinations of multiple therapeutic approaches (Jindal & Thase, 2003; Kopelowicz & Liberman, 2003). To a large extent, progress reflects a profound shift in developing, testing, and implementing therapies. Current interventions are designated as *evidence based* because they have been demonstrated to be effective under scientific conditions (Sackett et al., 1997).

Evidence-based practices

Evidence in health care research denotes reliable, valid information that has been developed using rigorous scientific methods. Scientific evidence involves a hierarchy of conditions, some more rigorous than others, but in general differs from expert opinion or anecdotal information because scientific evidence is systematically and deliberately collected under specific conditions designed to control or minimize the effects of bias and other influences. For example, scientific methods include allocation to treatment condition by random assignment, monitored interventions, and standardized assessment procedures. These scientific procedures reduce the possibility of false conclusions and maximize the reliability and validity of observations and inferences. In other words, evidence collected under scientific conditions tends to be highly reproducible—to predict what will happen to other clients who receive similar treatments in the future or in other settings.

First consider this simple example. An individual who experienced depression for several months gradually recovered to a normal mood. He might attribute the recovery to a change in diet, to a new relationship, to taking vitamins, to sleeping better, to increased sun exposure, or numerous other experiences, including treatment, that temporally coincided with feeling better. This is anecdotal evidence. At the same time, his therapist might attribute the recovery to avoiding alcohol for 2 weeks, to dream interpretation, to a new medicine, or to any number of other possible interventions. This too is anecdotal evidence. These attributions are unlikely to be reproducible in other depressed clients.

Now consider this contrast. The same depressed individual participated in a randomized controlled trial (RCT) in which he was assigned by chance to psychotherapy A rather than to psychotherapy B. He was one of the 80% of clients in psychotherapy A who recovered from depression within 6 weeks, while only 20% in psychotherapy B recovered. His recovery was documented by self-report, by interviews with an assessor who was unaware of which intervention he received and who used a standardized instrument, and by documented sleep pattern. In this situation, many personal characteristics and coinciding events during treatment would be controlled by the experimental conditions. We could therefore be more confident in attributing the client's recovery to psychotherapy A because other clients who received this treatment were much more likely to improve than those receiving psychotherapy B, suggesting that the attribution would likely be reproducible in other people with depression. If the results were in fact replicated in several RCTs, we would consider psychotherapy A to be an *evidence-based treatment*.

The primary problem with relying on personal experience, personal observation, or anecdotal reports is that these types of evidence are highly subject to bias and systematic distortion (Kahneman, 2011; Kahneman et al., 1982). For example, people tend to notice and remember information that supports their pre-existing beliefs rather than to be unbiased scientists. Good science involves the use of rigorous methods to overcome these natural tendencies.

Science does not gainsay the value of personal experiences, individual observations, and anecdotal reports. All provide valuable insights about potentially effective interventions. In fact, all current classes of psychiatric medications were discovered serendipitously by careful observations. Similarly, the growing literature by consumers on the lived experience of recovery (Deegan, 1988; Leete, 1989; Saks, 2007) provides important phenomenological information that may lead to effective interventions. For example, supported employment was largely developed and refined according to reports from clients about their vocational experiences (Becker & Drake, 2003). Science often makes use of accidental discoveries by one person.

Evidence-based practices (EBPs) are interventions for which there is a solid scientific basis demonstrating their effectiveness in helping clients or patients to attain valued outcomes. *Best practices*, on the other hand, usually refer to a consensus of individuals in the field as to which interventions are most effective. Best practice recommendations are often made in treatment areas for which there is limited rigorous research to guide more empirically based judgements as to the optimal intervention. Best practices are sometimes biased by the current beliefs or theories of experts, by the prejudices of guild organizations (e.g. professional groups), or by the marketing of industry. Best practices are often proven incorrect by scientific research. Thus, consistent scientific evidence of effectiveness is required to establish an EBP.

Criteria for evidence-based practices

Numerous groups and organizations have developed standardized criteria for establishing EBPs (e.g. American Psychological Association Presidential Task Force on Evidence Based Practices, 2006; Hunsley et al., 1999; Sackett et al., 1997). A broad consensus has emerged on the importance of the following criteria: transparency of the review process, standardization of the intervention, controlled research (e.g. RCTs), replication across multiple investigator teams, and impact on meaningful outcomes.

The criteria (e.g. how to find evidence, what qualifies as evidence, and how to judge quality of evidence) and the process of review (e.g. who reviews the evidence) should be transparent—open to the field and to the public for observation and discussion. The methods should be described in sufficient detail that independent reviewers can replicate the findings.

An intervention should be standardized so that it can be replicated elsewhere by other clinicians. Standardization typically involves a manual that clearly defines the practice and measures to confirm that the intervention adheres to principles and guidelines (i.e. fidelity). Standardization includes detailed criteria and procedures for assessment, treatment, and outcome measurement. Measures of therapist adherence and treatment fidelity can quantify the accuracy of the implementations to the intended model (Bond et al., 2012; Mueser et al., 2003; Durbin et al., 2019).

The most rigorous methodological design to evaluate an intervention is the RCT, in which clients are randomly assigned (i.e. by chance) to receive one of two or more interventions (which can include 'treatment as usual' or 'waiting list' control groups) and are then followed up and evaluated after treatment by unbiased assessors to measure important outcomes. Due to random assignment to treatment conditions, significant differences between groups in outcomes can be attributed to the treatment rather than to other factors, such as unobserved or unknown pre-treatment differences between the groups. However, recruitment of inappropriate clients, high attrition, low participation in services, and other problems can undermine the basic assumptions of RCTs (Drake et al., 1994; Metcalfe & Drake, 2022). Several RCTs consistently demonstrating the effectiveness of an intervention constitute very strong evidence.

While RCTs represent the strongest research design for evaluating treatment effectiveness, they are often difficult or impossible to conduct in real-world clinical settings. A less rigorous alternative to the RCT is the quasi-experimental design, in which clients receiving different treatments are compared to one another, but treatment allocation is not by random assignment (Shadish et al., 2002). For example, clients in one mental health centre receive one treatment and are compared to clients in another centre who receive a different treatment. The most significant limitation of quasi-experimental studies such as this is that the clients in the different treatment groups may differ in important ways that could affect different outcomes. Nevertheless, quasi-experimental designs often provide valuable information regarding the effectiveness of an intervention. Another less rigorous research design alternative to RCTs is the *multiple baseline research design* (Barlow et al., 2008). This approach is usually studied to evaluate the benefit of specific components of treatment in individual clients by first obtaining a stable baseline over several assessments, and then systematically adding treatment components one at a time to evaluate their unique contributions to the overall treatment goals. By varying the length of the no-treatment period and number of assessments conducted over baseline between subjects, stronger inferences can be drawn that the treatment components are contributing to any improvements observed in the outcome measures.

Replication means that more than one study finds similar positive effects. Replication is fundamental to research because similar results across multiple studies are unlikely to be due to chance. Reviews also insist that different investigators replicate the findings to minimize the possibility of investigator bias.

Effective interventions should improve important goals or outcomes that are meaningful to clients, such as symptoms, associated functional impairments, or quality of life. Many outcomes are unequivocally important. People with mental illnesses do not want to be overwhelmed by symptoms or side effects, and nearly all want to live independently, have meaningful work, and have close friends. Other outcomes are more difficult to define. For example, demonstrating that social skills training improves social skills within a treatment group rather than relationships in the community is probably insufficient (Heinssen et al., 2000).

Developing an evidence-based practice

The process of developing an EBP has received limited attention. For example, Onken, Rounsaville, and colleagues described a three-stage approach: (1) feasibility and pilot testing, (2) RCTs of the intervention, and (3) studies to demonstrate generalizability and implementation (Onken et al., 1997; Rounsaville et al., 2001). Interventions that have passed the first two stages are considered EBPs. Mueser and Drake (2005) previously proposed a four-step process, which we elaborate here: (1) articulating the problem, (2) identifying possible treatments, (3) pilot testing the intervention, and (4) evaluating the intervention in RCTs.

1. Articulating the problem

All interventions begin with a problem for which an effective treatment is needed. The problem area should be regarded as meaningful (e.g. a distressing symptom that does not respond to standard treatment or a significant functional impairment). The problem should be defined and measured in a reliable and valid way (Nunnally, 1978). Reliable measurement involves reproducibility: inter-rater reliability (i.e. different observers see the same thing), internal reliability (e.g. different items on a scale are related to one another), and test–retest reliability (i.e. showing stability of the measure over relatively brief periods of time in the absence of intervention). For example, valid measurement corresponds to related measures or behavioural indices and is sensitive to change. Developing an effective intervention requires reliable and valid measures of important outcomes.

Some interventions have broad goals (e.g. reducing hospitalization, incarceration, and homelessness), while others have narrow goals (e.g. independent living skills or competitive employment). General outcomes are often difficult to assess (e.g. quality of life), whereas a narrow behavioural target is often assessed more easily and reliably (e.g. employment).

Defining the target population broadly has the advantage of maximizing the number of individuals who may potentially benefit from an intervention, but most interventions are effective only for subgroups. Intervention development includes identifying specifically the individuals who might benefit. For example, people who refuse medications are inappropriate for a medication trial, and those without interest in working should not be in a trial of vocational services. Research often starts narrowly and expands to more general populations.

2. Identifying possible treatments

New interventions are developed by several different approaches: (1) using theories regarding the problem area, (2) using theories of behaviour change, (3) adapting successful interventions used with other populations, (4) adapting successful interventions used for other problems, or (5) discovering interventions serendipitously.

Psychotherapy based on relational frame theory exemplifies the first approach (Hayes et al., 2001). According to this theory, humans' capacity for language and thought enables them to interpret and respond to their thoughts as though they were real-world experiences rather than symbolic representations. Based on this theory, acceptance and commitment therapy (Hayes et al., 2012) teaches clients to accept rather than trying to control unpleasant thoughts and feelings, which are largely beyond their control.

Extending social skills training based on social learning theory (Bandura, 1969) to a wide range of social problems (Mueser et al., 2024), and using motivational interviewing based on the stages of change concept (Prochaska & DiClemente, 1984) to addictive disorders (Miller & Rollnick, 2023) illustrate the second approach. The crux of social learning theory is that people learn from observing others' behaviour, as well as from the consequences of their behaviour. Social skills training involves the systematic teaching of social behaviours through a combination of modelling skills, role-playing, receiving positive and corrective feedback, and practising skills in natural situations. Based on the observation that changes towards healthier behaviour tend to occur through a sequence of distinct stages (pre-contemplation, contemplation, preparation, behaviour change, and maintenance), motivational interviewing helps people articulate their personal goals and explore the steps and barriers to achieving those goals, thereby enhancing the client's own motivation to address substance use problems.

The Individual Placement and Support model of supported employment represents the third approach (Becker & Drake, 2003). Individual Placement and Support was adapted from successful supported employment approaches for individuals with developmental disabilities (Wehman & Moon, 1988). Employment specialists work collaboratively with mental health treatment teams to help clients find and succeed in competitive jobs that match their personal preferences.

Adaptations of assertive community treatment (Stein & Santos, 1998) follow the fourth approach. Originally developed to address the problem of frequent hospitalizations and poor psychosocial functioning, assertive community treatment has subsequently been used to address several other problems, such as homelessness (Lehman et al., 1997), substance use disorders (Essock et al., 2006), and involvement in the criminal justice system (Lamberti et al., 2017).

Finally, serendipity has been the dominant model for developing pharmacological interventions for mental illness. Although this seems less likely to occur for complex psychosocial interventions, many rehabilitation interventions stem from observing techniques that clients have discovered themselves. For example, the teaching of coping skills to manage persistent psychotic symptoms (Mueser et al., 2002) was initially based on naturalistic studies that demonstrated that clients with schizophrenia often develop their own strategies for coping with distressing symptoms (Alverson et al., 1995; Falloon & Talbot, 1981).

3. Pilot testing the intervention

Pilot testing an intervention establishes feasibility and potential. Secondary goals include standardizing the intervention and developing a measure of fidelity. Pilot testing typically involves providing the intervention to a small number of clients and observing the targeted outcomes. Prior to formal pilot testing, researchers try the intervention with a few clients to examine suitability, mode of delivery, intensity, and need for modifications. Once these aspects are clear, researchers must establish feasibility.

Feasibility includes acceptability and retention. Acceptability refers to the willingness of individuals to participate in an intervention, while retention involves staying in treatment long enough to achieve benefits. Interventions can only be effective if clients are willing to join and participate. Although experts disagree, a dropout rate (proportion of participants not receiving a sufficient dose of intervention) of less than 20% is the goal, and dropouts above 30% can be problematic. Establishing the feasibility of an intervention is often not a matter of conducting a single pilot study, but rather is frequently an integral part of the ongoing process of treatment development. Treatments are often created through an iterative process that involves modifying and honing the intervention based on the results of multiple small pilot studies until it is clearly feasible. Because the amount of time and the number of trials required to satisfactorily establish the feasibility of an intervention are usually unknown, investigators may save time and money by using open clinical trial study designs at this stage of the research, in which all participants receive the intervention under development, rather than controlled study designs in which valuable resources are diverted to recruiting and assessing control groups.

Pilot studies also examine the intervention's potential to improve the targeted outcomes. Researchers disagree about the need for a control group during this stage of pilot testing. Those who use a pre–post–follow-up design without a control group must interpret improvements in selected outcomes as meaningful compared to expectations. If functioning in targeted problem areas is relatively stable without treatment, improvements following the intervention can be attributed to the intervention. However, most psychiatric problems fluctuate over time, so improvements could be due to natural history. Controlled research designs that include a comparison group, such as RCTs or quasi-experimental studies, provide stronger evidence, but often lack sufficient statistical power to detect significant differences (Bartels et al., 2004). Researchers should therefore state from the outset that the pilot study aims to show that some clients benefit and to estimate the likely magnitude of the change (called the effect size), not to show statistical significance. However, researchers should also be cautioned that effect size calculations based on relatively small pilot studies are often inaccurate and should not be used to estimate the sample size needed to achieve similar effects in a larger and more adequately powered RCT (Kraemer et al., 2006).

Standardizing a manual

The pilot study is usually based on an outline of the intervention programme or a draft of the manual. Because valuable experience delivering the intervention is gained during the pilot study, a formal treatment manual can readily be written based on the pilot. When a draft of a manual exists prior to the pilot study, some modifications are usually made after the study is completed based on the additional clinical experience. The specificity of manuals varies greatly from one project to another and depends partly on the nature of the intervention. Most treatment manuals include information to orient clinicians to the nature of the problem, as well as some conceptual foundations to the intervention. Specific guidelines are provided regarding the logistics of the intervention, identification of individuals for whom the intervention is designed, curriculum, activities, and guidance for handling common problems. Manuals often provide clinical vignettes to illustrate treatment principles and incorporate specific instruments for assessment and monitoring clinical outcomes. The length of treatment manuals varies widely, depending on the complexity of the intervention.

During pilot testing, researchers also need to establish methods to verify that an intervention is delivered in a manner consistent with the treatment model. Such verification is crucial to conducting a rigorous assessment of the intervention. Researchers must first establish that the intervention has been implemented as intended before determining its effects. Expert judgements are often used to establish fidelity. In this method, a recognized expert on the intervention obtains information regarding the implementation (e.g. by observing live treatment sessions or listening to audio recordings of sessions, reviewing case notes, and conducting interviews) and provides feedback regarding the degree of adherence to the model. Alternatively, specific behavioural anchor points for rating adherence can be used to train raters and make fidelity ratings. Objective fidelity ratings avoid the expense and potential bias of expert ratings. Fidelity scales have become the standard in the field (Bond & Drake, 2020). They provide specific information needed to address implementation problems and to explore the relationship between fidelity and outcome.

In addition to the importance of fidelity scales in conducting rigorous research on an intervention and for addressing implementation problems, they can also be used to train clinicians in an intervention, especially when fidelity assessments are based on discrete recordings of treatment sessions. For example, early in the process of training clinicians, frequent fidelity assessments can be conducted on treatment sessions (e.g. weekly), with the quantitative results of the assessment along with qualitative feedback and suggestions for improvement provided back to clinicians in a timely fashion, and integrated as needed into supervision (Lu et al., 2012; Mueser et al., 2019). Incorporating routine and frequent fidelity assessments into the training of clinicians enables them to more rapidly modify and hone their behaviour in accordance with the principles and defining elements of an intervention.

4. Evaluating the intervention in randomized controlled trials

Rigorous evaluation is the sine qua non for evidence-based interventions. In this section, we briefly address several of the most crucial aspects of RCTs, including the experimental design, the selection of a control group, inclusion/exclusion criteria for the target population, the setting for the trial, and the choice of outcome measures.

The RCT is considered superior to other research designs because it controls for group equivalence. Many important variables are unknown or unobserved, and quasi-experimental designs almost inevitably compare non-equivalent groups. The most common type of RCT is when individuals are randomized to an experimental or control intervention (or more than two interventions), and routine assessments are conducted to evaluate and compare the outcomes of the different groups.

A variant to the individual RCT is the cluster RCT, in which clinicians, treatment teams, or mental health centres are randomly assigned to provide the experimental intervention or the control intervention, and all the clients (who consent to research) treated by each clinician/team/centre receive the intervention that the clinician (or team or centre) was randomized to provide (Meurer & Lewis, 2015). In several circumstances, the cluster RCT may be a preferable or more practical alternative to the individual RCT research design. First, training clinicians in some interventions might be expected to alter their behaviour when working with clients, even when they are not deliberately trying to implement the intervention. For example, training clinicians in a brief motivational interviewing intervention (one or two sessions) to reduce problematic alcohol or drug use could alter how they work with clients with substance use problems, regardless of whether they are participating in a study or following a specific treatment protocol. In these circumstances, the experimental intervention should be delivered by trained clinicians, and the control treatment (or treatment as usual) should be delivered by clinicians who have not been trained in the intervention. This can be accomplished using an individual RCT design in treatment settings in which clients can be randomized to different treatment groups initially, and then assigned to either a trained or untrained clinicians depending on the randomization. However, in some settings assigning clients to different clinicians following individual randomization to a treatment group may not be feasible. For example, in an outpatient substance use disorder treatment programme in which most individuals receive one to three counselling sessions, new clients may be assigned to clinicians based on caseload and availability so that assignment by individual randomization is not possible. In these circumstances, a cluster RCT design, in which half of the clinicians are randomized to be trained and provide the experimental intervention and the other half are not, is a viable alternative.

A second circumstance in which the cluster RCT design may be preferable is when evaluating complex interventions involving more than one treatment provider. For example, early intervention services for first-episode psychosis are typically team-based, multicomponent programmes involving treatment elements such as pharmacological management, cognitive behaviour therapy, family psychoeducation, and supported employment and education (Correll et al., 2018). The involvement of several different people working together to implement an intervention in a treatment setting may make it difficult or impossible to maintain a 'treatment as usual' condition at the same agency, especially if those individuals providing the new programme continue to have clinical responsibility for treating other clients at the agency. In such circumstances, a cluster RCT design can be used to randomize agencies to provide an early intervention programme or usual services to individuals with early psychosis (Kane et al., 2016).

In selecting the comparison group for an RCT, the common options are an equally intensive intervention, a less intensive intervention, treatment as usual, placebo treatment, or no treatment (e.g. a waiting list). Each option has advantages and disadvantages. In practice, the selection reflects pragmatic considerations as well as the specific research question.

Pilot work should guide selection of the inclusion and exclusion criteria for the RCT. These criteria inevitably involve a trade-off between efficacy and effectiveness. Efficacy studies use narrowly defined clients to maximize the chance of finding significant differences, whereas effectiveness studies use broad criteria to maximize real-world applicability, or generalizability. Regardless, informed consent must ensure that the clients understand the study and are willing to participate.

Similar considerations influence site selection because location will affect transferability to other settings. Clinical trials conducted in routine mental health centres rather than in university clinics (i.e. the effectiveness design) maximize potential for applicability to the kinds of settings in which most people receive treatment. By contrast, efficacy studies are often conducted in highly controlled settings, with specially trained clinicians and other constrained conditions for the sake of isolating and controlling the treatment intervention. Traditionally, interventions have been tested first in efficacy trials and then in effectiveness trials. Recently, however, interventions are increasingly developed and tested under effectiveness conditions to ensure generalizability from the outset. Of course, recruitment, training, high-fidelity implementation, retention, and assessment challenge researchers in multifarious ways.

Measurement should address outcomes, implementation/process, and theory. Outcome measures assess the goals of the intervention (e.g. work, quality of social relationships, symptom severity, relapses, and hospitalization), as identified and measured since the earliest steps of developing an EBP. Primary outcomes reflect the most important targets, while secondary outcomes include areas that may be improved by changes in the primary outcomes. For example, the primary outcome of supported employment is working, measured by percentage of clients who are employed, number of hours they are working, and wages they are earning. Employment may also affect secondary outcomes such as self-esteem, symptoms, and life satisfaction.

Implementation and process measures assess whether the interventions were provided as intended and whether clients received the interventions. These measures can be broadly divided into those that evaluate fidelity to the treatment model and those that record clients' exposure to treatment. Treatment exposure measures include information such as the number, duration, and time of treatment contacts.

RCTs can also provide valuable information regarding how an intervention works, how theoretical constructs interact with functional outcomes, and how different outcomes are related. Theory testing and development can guide the refinement of an intervention to enhance effectiveness.

Summary

EBPs are scientifically validated interventions that help people with mental illnesses to achieve improvements in meaningful areas of their lives. Developing and establishing an EBP requires attention to scientific detail, considerable time, and multiple steps. We have described the major steps as (1) articulation of the problem area, (2) identification of possible treatments, (3) pilot testing the intervention, and (4) controlled evaluation of the intervention.

REFERENCES

Alverson, M., Becker, D. R., & Drake, R. E. (1995). An ethnographic study of coping strategies used by people with severe mental illness participating in supported employment. *Psychosocial Rehabilitation Journal*, **18**, 115–128.

American Psychological Association Presidential Task Force on Evidence-Based Practice (2006). Evidence-based practice in psychology. *American Psychologist*, **61**, 271–285.

Bandura, A. (1969). *Principles of Behavior Modification*. New York: Holt, Rinehart and Winston, Inc.

Barlow, D. H., Nock, M., & Hersen, M. (2008). *Single Case Experimental Designs: Strategies for Studying Behavior Change* (3rd ed.). Boston, MA: Addison-Wesley.

Bartels, S. J., Forester, B., Mueser, K. T., Miles, K. M., Dums, A. R., Pratt, S. I., et al. (2004). Supported rehabilitation and health care management of older persons with severe mental illness. *Community Mental Health Journal*, **40**, 75–90.

Becker, D. R. & Drake, R. E. (2003). *A Working Life for People with Severe Mental Illness*. New York: Oxford University Press.

Bond, G. R. & Drake, R. E. (2020). Assessing the fidelity of evidence-based practices: history and current status of a standardized measurement methodology. *Administration and Policy in Mental Health and Mental Health Services Research*, **47**, 874–884.

Bond, G. R., Peterson, A. E., Becker, D. R., & Drake, R. E. (2012). Validating the revised Individual Placement and Support Fidelity Scale. *Psychiatric Services*, **63**, 758–763.

Correll, C. U., Galling, B., Pawar, A., Krivko, A., Bonetto, C., Ruggeri, M., et al. (2018). Comparison of early intervention services vs treatment as usual for early-phase psychosis: a systematic review, meta-analysis, and meta-regression. *JAMA Psychiatry*, **75**, 555–565.

Deegan, P. E. (1988). Recovery: the lived experience of rehabilitation. *Psychosocial Rehabilitation Journal*, **11**, 11–19.

Drake, R. E., Becker, D. R., & Anthony, W. A. (1994). The use of a research induction group in mental health services research. *Hospital and Community Psychiatry*, **45**, 487–489.

Durbin, J., Selick, A., Langill, G., Cheng, C., Archie, S., Butt, S., & Addington, D. (2019). Using fidelity measurement to assess quality of early psychosis intervention services in Ontario. *Psychiatric Services*, **70**, 840–844.

Essock, S. M., Mueser, K. T., Drake, R. E., Covell, N. H., McHugo, G. J., Frisman, L. K., et al. (2006). Comparison of ACT and standard case management for delivering integrated treatment for co-occurring disorders. *Psychiatric Services*, **57**, 185–196.

Falloon, I. R. H. & Talbot, R. E. (1981). Persistent auditory hallucinations: coping mechanisms and implications for management. *Psychological Medicine*, **11**, 329–339.

Hayes, S. C., Barnes-Holmes, D., & Roche, B. (Eds.). (2001). *Relational Frame Theory: A Post-Skinnerian Account of Human Language and Cognition*. New York: Kluwer Academic/Plenum Publishers.

Hayes, S. C., Strosahl, K. D., & Wilson, K. G. (2012). *Acceptance and Commitment Therapy: An Experiential Approach to Behavior Change* (2nd ed.). New York: Guilford Publications.

Heinssen, R. K., Liberman, R. P., & Kopelowicz, A. (2000). Psychosocial skills training for schizophrenia: lessons from the laboratory. *Schizophrenia Bulletin*, **26**, 21–46.

Hunsley, J., Dobson, K. S., Johnson, C., & Mikail, S. F. (1999). Empirically supported treatments in psychology: implications for Canadian professional psychology. *Canadian Psychologist*, **40**, 289–302.

Jindal, R. K. & Thase, M. E. (2003). Integrating psychotherapy and pharmacotherapy to improve outcomes among patients with mood disorders. *Psychiatric Services*, **54**, 1484–1490.

Kahneman, D. (2011). *Thinking, Fast and Slow*. New York: Farrar, Straus and Giroux.

Kahneman, D., Slovic, P., & Tversky, A. (1982). *Judgment Under Uncertainty: Heuristics and Biases*. New York: Cambridge University Press.

Kane, J. M., Robinson, D. G., Schooler, N. R., Mueser, K. T., Penn, D. L., Rosenheck, R. A., et al. (2016). Comprehensive versus usual care for first episode psychosis: two-year outcomes from the NIMH RAISE Early Treatment Program. *American Journal of Psychiatry*, **173**, 362–372.

Keepers, G. A., Fochtmann, L. J., Anzia, J. M., Benjamin, S., Lyness, J. M., Mojtabai, R., et al. (2021). *The American Psychiatric Association Practice Guideline for the Treatment of Patients with Schizophrenia* (3rd ed.). Washington, DC: American Psychiatric Association.

Kopelowicz, A. & Liberman, R. P. (2003). Integrating treatment with rehabilitation for persons with major mental illnesses. *Psychiatric Services*, **54**, 1491–1498.

Kraemer, H. C., Mintz, J., Noda, A., Tinklenberg, J., & Yesavage, J. A. (2006). Caution regarding the use of pilot studies to guide power calculations for study proposals. *Archives of General Psychiatry*, **63**, 484–489.

Lamberti, J. S., Weisman, R. L., Cerulli, C., Williams, G. C., Jacobowitz, D., Mueser, K. T., et al. (2017). A randomized controlled trial of the Rochester Forensic Assertive Community Treatment model. *Psychiatric Services*, **68**, 1016–1024.

Leete, E. (1989). How I perceive and manage my illness. *Schizophrenia Bulletin*, **15**, 197–200.

Lehman, A. F., Dixon, L. B., Kernan, E., & DeForge, B. (1997). A randomized trial of assertive community treatment for homeless persons with severe mental illness. *Archives of General Psychiatry*, **54**, 1038–1043.

Lu, W., Yanos, P. T., Gottlieb, J. D., Duva, S. M., Silverstein, S. M., Xie, H., et al. (2012). Using fidelity assessments to train clinicians in the CBT for PTSD program for clients with serious mental illness. *Psychiatric Services*, **63**, 785–792.

Metcalfe, J. & Drake, R. E. (2022). Measuring participation in individual placement and support in the Supported Employment Demonstration project. *Administration and Policy in Mental Health*, **49**, 521–529.

Meurer, W. J. & Lewis, R. J. (2015). Cluster randomized trials: evaluating treatments applied to groups. *JAMA*, **313**, 2068–2069.

Miller, W. R. & Rollnick, S. (Eds.) (2023). *Motivational Interviewing: Preparing People for Change* (4th ed.). New York: Guilford Publications.

Mueser, K. T., Bellack, A. S., Gingerich, S., Agresta, J., & Fulford, D. (2024). *Social Skills Training for Schizophrenia: A Step-by-Step Guide* (Third ed.). Guilford Press.

Mueser, K. T., Corrigan, P. W., Hilton, D., Tanzman, B., Schaub, A., Gingerich, S., et al. (2002). Illness management and recovery for severe mental illness: a review of the research. *Psychiatric Services*, **53**, 1272–1284.

Mueser, K. T. & Drake, R. E. (2005). How does a practice become evidence-based? In: Drake, R. E., Merrens, M., & Lynde, D. L. (Eds.), *Evidence-Based Mental Health Practice: A Textbook* (pp. 217–242). New York: John Wiley.

Mueser, K. T., Meyer-Kalos, P., Glynn, S. M., Lynde, D. W., Robinson, D. E., Gingerich, S., et al. (2019). Implementation and fidelity assessment of the NAVIGATE treatment program for first episode psychosis in a multi-site study. *Schizophrenia Research*, **204**, 271–281.

Mueser, K. T., Noordsy, D. L., Drake, R. E., & Fox, L. (2003). *Integrated Treatment for Dual Disorders: A Guide to Effective Practice*. New York: Guilford Press.

Nathan, P. & Gorman, J. M. (Eds.). (2015). *A Guide to Treatments That Work* (4th ed.). New York: Oxford University Press.

Nunnally, J. (1978). *Psychometric Theory* (2nd ed.). New York: McGraw Hill.

Onken, L. S., Blaine, J. D., & Battjes, R. (1997). Behavioral therapy research: a conceptualization of a process. In: Henngler, S. W. & Amentos, R. (Eds.), *Innovative Approaches for Difficult to Treat Populations* (pp. 477–485). Washington, DC: American Psychiatric Press.

Prochaska, J. O. & DiClemente, C. C. (1984). *The Transtheoretical Approach: Crossing the Traditional Boundaries of Therapy*. Homewood, IL: Dow-Jones/Irwin.

Rounsaville, B. J., Carroll, K. M., & Onken, L. S. (2001). A stage model of behavioral therapies research: getting started and moving on from stage I. *Clinical Psychology: Science and Practice*, **8**, 133–142.

Sackett, D. L., Richardson, W. S., Rosenberg, W., & Haynes, R. B. (1997). *Evidence-Based Medicine*. New York: Churchill Livingstone.

Saks, E. R. (2007). *The Center Cannot Hold*. New York: Hyperion.

Shadish, W. R., Cook, T. D., & Campbell, D. T. (2002). *Experimental and Quasi-Experimental Designs for Generalized Causal Inference*. Boston, MA: Houghton Mifflin.

Stein, L. I. & Santos, A. B. (1998). *Assertive Community Treatment of Persons with Severe Mental Illness*. New York: Norton.

Wehman, P. & Moon, M. S. (1988). *Vocational Rehabilitation and Supported Employment*. Baltimore, MD: Paul Brookes.

37

Implementing guidelines

Amy Cheung, Simon Gilbody, and Jeremy Grimshaw

Introduction

According to the Institute of Medicine (2011), clinical practice guidelines are 'statements that include recommendations, intended to optimize patient care, that are informed by a systematic review of evidence and an assessment of the benefits and harms of alternative care options'. Guidelines translate complex scientific research about what is known about a specific disorder or set of disorders, whether it is regarding screening, diagnosis, or management, into practical guidance for healthcare professionals and service users. Compared to systematic reviews, they provide a broad overview of the management of a disorder or of an intervention to enhance individual patient encounters (Eccles et al., 2012; Shekelle et al., 2012; Woolf et al., 2012).

Guidelines may be used as the evidence base for quality improvement activities in health care organizations. Guidelines can also provide the evidence base for other interventions to improve practice (such as part of a computerized decision support tool) (Eccles et al., 2012; Shekelle et al., 2012; Woolf et al., 2012). For example, many North American primary care clinics have adapted the 'Guidelines for adolescent depression in primary care' as the basis for improving depression care for their adolescent patients which has also been incorporated into a web-based decision support tool for paediatricians (CHADIS; www.chadis.com) (Cheung et al., 2007; Zuckerbrot et al., 2007). Guidelines are also a good source of information for medical education initiatives. There are many examples of educational activities based on mental health guidelines. One example is the McMaster Mental Health Modules, which is the basis of new curricula for training family physicians. Finally, guidelines can be used to solve clinical problems that come up as part of patient encounters, for example, when embedded in online clinical decision support tools such as the Child Health Improvement through Computer Automation (CHICA) system for maternal depression which has been shown to be effective in improving screening for maternal depression compared to physician assessment alone (Carroll et al., 2013).

The use of guidelines should lead to improved outcomes for service users and their families. However, the quality of guidelines can be variable and mental health professionals and organizations need to identify those that are valid prior to implementation. Developing guidelines can be challenging with many methodological issues such as how to interpret conflicting research data. The Institute of Medicine (2011) established standards for clinical practice guidelines development. These standards include managing conflict of interest as well as establishing guidelines for rating strength of evidence/recommendations.

However, guidelines are not self-implementing; mental health organizations need to actively disseminate and implement guidelines to ensure their effective uptake. Several frameworks have been developed to address the activities required to implement guidelines effectively, from identifying the need for guidelines in the first place through to monitoring and feedback into future quality improvement activities. One leading framework by Graham and colleagues (2006), which aims to engineer improvements in health care settings, is readily applicable to the whole process of implementing guidelines (**Figure 37.1**). Its components are as follow:

- Identification of a problem that needs addressing
- Identification, review, and selection of the knowledge or research relevant to the problem (e.g. practice guidelines or research findings)
- Adaptation of the identified knowledge or research to the local context
- Assessment of barriers to using the knowledge
- Selection, tailoring, and implementation of interventions to promote the use of knowledge (i.e. implement the change)
- Monitoring knowledge use
- Evaluation of the outcomes of using the knowledge
- Sustaining ongoing knowledge use.

This chapter will describe how mental health professionals and organizations can follow these steps to implement guidelines to improve clinical care. Resources to assist in this process are also listed at the end of the chapter.

Identification of a problem that needs addressing

Among mental health professionals, patient encounters in the clinical setting or participation in routine continuing medical education may identify areas of suboptimal care. Among mental health organizations, problems could be identified following a critical

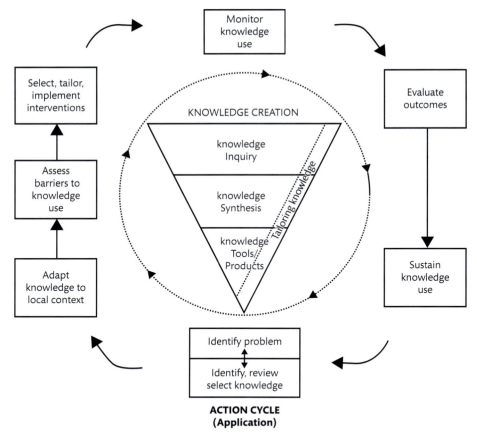

Figure 37.1 The knowledge to action process framework.

incident or routine audit. Health care professionals and organizations may also be prompted to change their practice following the publication of a new guideline or as part of continuous quality improvement strategy.

Identification, review, and selection of the knowledge or research relevant to the problem

Identification of guidelines

Many guidelines are not published in peer-reviewed publications and even among those that are, they can be difficult to identify in bibliographic databases. Fortunately, there are many resources available to help mental health professionals and organizations. Some common resources for guidelines are listed at the end of this chapter. Generally, these resources can be divided into two categories:

1. Organizations that produce guidelines such as the UK National Institute for Health and Care Excellence (NICE; www.nice.org.uk), and the US American Academy of Child and Adolescent Psychiatry (AACAP; www.aacap.org). NICE is one of the largest guideline programmes in the world and produces guidelines that are implemented throughout England and Wales's NHS. This includes a programme of developing guidelines for mental health care, led by mental health clinicians (Kendall & Pilling, 2004). The two most prominent psychiatric associations in North America, the American Psychiatric Association and the American Academy of Child and Adolescent Psychiatry (AACAP), both produce their own guidelines based on research evidence and expert opinion. The AACAP guidelines, also known as practice parameters, are developed through several stages including a literature review, an expert review, and a review by AACAP's membership for input and feedback.

2. Organizations that catalogue external guidelines. For example, the ECRI Guidelines Trust (https://guidelines.ecri.org) catalogues existing guidelines but does not endorse or recommend the use of any specific guidelines. Guidelines are summarized and appraised against the US National Academy of Medicine 'Standards of Trustworthy Guidelines'. The trustworthiness of each guideline is shown through the 'Transparency and Rigor Using Standards of Trustworthiness' (TRUST) score card.

Review and selection of guidelines

Guidelines may be specific to a psychiatric disorder across the lifespan (e.g. bipolar disorder) or generalized for mental health care (NICE, 2014). Generally, guidelines are more likely to be valid if they are produced by a national or regional guideline multidisciplinary group based upon systematic reviews of relevant evidence. Multidisciplinary groups tend to provide a more balanced perspective than unidisciplinary groups because the diversity of perspectives within the guideline development group allows for (1) resolution of legitimate conflicts over values (e.g. importance of outcomes such as mortality versus quality of life), (2) interpretation of the available data, and (3) credibility to support implementation of the guidelines after development (Lomas, 1991). These multidisciplinary groups should include service user and carer involvement (or have a mechanism of ensuring their input) (NICE, 2014, section 3). In fact, involvement of users and carers is much more advanced in mental health than in other areas of health care.

Guidelines are also more likely to be valid if the rationale and strength of evidence underlying recommendations is made explicit. Guidelines should be developed based on a recognized grading system to determine not only the strength of the underlying evidence but also the trade-offs between the benefits and the risks, burden, and costs of implementing a specific recommendation in clinical practice. A systematic approach to grading evidence minimizes bias and highlights the uncertainty around the trade-off between risks and benefits by the strength of a recommendation. An example of commonly used system is Grading of Recommendations Assessment, Development and Evaluation (GRADE) (Balshem et al., 2011; Guyatt et al., 2011).

In general, guidelines for psychiatric disorders are developed based on a combination of expert opinion and scientific evidence since these disorders and their management are not generally well studied. As a result, the explicit link between the strength of the evidence and recommendations is even more important in the field of mental health.

Frequently, there may be several competing guidelines and mental health professionals and organizations must determine which one is the most appropriate to follow based on considerations of the quality and relevance of the available guidelines. Fortunately, there are tools available to help with this process. The AGREE II instrument (www.agreecollaboration.org) is a validated instrument used internationally to appraise the quality of guidelines that comprises 23 criteria that map onto six domains and has been translated into several languages (Box 37.1) (Brouwers et al., 2010a, 2010b). While the AGREE II instrument is probably the gold standard for appraising guidelines, it may be too unwieldy and time-consuming for individual mental health professionals to quickly assess the likely quality of guidelines in day-to-day practice. In this case, there are several simple strategies that professionals and organizations can use to determine whether a set of guidelines is valid. First, we would suggest that professionals and organizations avoid guidelines that do not explicitly discuss their development. Without information on the development methods, it is not possible to determine whether the guidelines are valid. Second, the 'Users' Guides to the Medical Literature' series contains a guide to interpret and use clinical guidelines (Alonso-Coello et al., 2017; Hayward et al., 1995; Wilson et al., 1995). This guide describes a series of questions to help professionals and organizations to appraise guidelines. In general, the professionals and/or organization should assess the trustworthiness of a guideline and its applicability to patients in their clinical setting. In mental health, these options and outcomes will look different compared to those for other areas of medicine. In mental health, practice options should include psychological, social, and biological treatments. Outcomes in mental health should focus on improved functioning and quality of life rather than hard outcomes such as mortality. The professionals and/or organizations should also be convinced that a comprehensive literature review has been conducted. Relevant databases for mental health include Medline, the Cumulative Index to Nursing and Allied Health Literature (CINAHL), and PsychINFO.

Finally, developers must consider implementability during the development of guidelines. Recent research has focused on developing frameworks for the implementation of existing guidelines. Gagliardi et al. (2011) examined how existing guidelines could be modified to facilitate implementation. A summary of their findings is included in Table 37.1. The table provides a framework on how to develop guidelines that are more accessible and user-friendly. The authors also suggest alternate versions of the same guidelines for different purposes. However, further research is needed to evaluate the effectiveness of how these strategies might influence guidelines use.

Adaptation of the identified knowledge or research to the local context

There are specific issues that need to be considered when adapting and implementing guidelines in mental health including (1) diagnosis and diagnostic heterogeneity, (2) individual tailoring of psychological treatments and individual expertise of practitioners, (3) course of mental health problems, and (4) mental health practitioners' responsibilities to protect the wider public as well as their patients (Kendall & Pilling, 2004). First, although the diagnoses of mental illness have been operationalized, concerns regarding validity of the diagnostic criteria has impacted the evidence base available to guide clinical care. In particular, some diagnostic groups are too broad and overinclusive while others are too restrictive and/or do not give consideration to co-occurring illnesses. For example, broader diagnostic groups such as depression and anxiety limit our understanding of the effectiveness of specific treatments due to the heterogeneity of those included in this large group. Conversely, research on very restrictive diagnostic categories such as anorexia nervosa and bulimia have also limited our understanding of a larger service user group who may have disordered eating as well as common comorbid conditions.

Second, the application of psychological treatments is dependent on the psychological make-up of an individual, the expertise of an individual practitioner, and the interaction between the two. However, evaluations of such interventions have not accounted for these factors and have instead utilized only quantitative methodology for evaluating pharmacological treatments. Hence, we have limited understanding of the true impact of such interventions. Only recently have more appropriate methodologies such as mixed qualitative–quantitative methods been developed and utilized.

Third, the episodic and often unpredictable natural course of mental illnesses is unlike other physical illnesses. This has impacted our ability to better understand the effectiveness of interventions in altering the trajectory of mental illnesses.

Box 37.1 Domains of the AGREE instrument

1. Scope and purpose
2. Stakeholder involvement
3. Rigour of development
4. Clarity and presentation
5. Applicability
6. Editorial independence.

Table 37.1 Final framework for guideline implementability

Domain	Element	Examples
Usability	Navigation	Table of contents
	Evidence format	Narrative, tabulated, or both
	Recommendation format	Narrative, graphic (algorithms) or both; recommendation summary (single list in full or summary version)
Adaptability	Alternate versions	Summary (print, electronic for PDA); patient (tailored for patients/caregivers); published (journal)
Validity	Number of references	Total number of distinct references to evidence upon which recommendations are based
	Evidence graded	A system is used to categorize quality of evidence supporting each recommendation
	Number of references	Total number of distinct recommendations (sub-recommendations considered same)
Applicability	Individualization	Clinical information (indications, criteria, risk factors, drug dosing) that facilitates application of the recommendations explicitly highlighted as tips or practical issues using subtitles or text boxes, or summarized in tables and referred to in recommendations or narrative contextualizing recommendations
Communicability	Patient education or involvement	Informational or educational resources for patients/caregivers, questions for clinicians to facilitate discussion, or contact information (phone, fax, email, or URL) to acquire informational or educational resources
Accommodation	Objective	Explicitly stated purpose of guideline (clinical decision-making, education, policy, quality improvement)
	Users	Who would deliver/enable delivery of recommendations (individuals, teams, departments, institutions, managers, policymakers, internal/external agents), who would receive the services (patients/caregivers)
	Users' needs/values	Identification of stakeholder needs, perspectives, interests, or values
	Technical	Equipment or technology needed, or the way services should be organized to deliver recommendations
	Regulatory	Industrial standards for equipment or technology, or policy regarding their use
	Human resources	Type and number of health professionals needed to deliver recommended services
	Professional	Education, training, or competencies needed by clinicians/staff to deliver recommendations
	Impact	Anticipated changes in workflow or processes during/after adoption of recommendations
	Costs	Direct or productivity costs incurred as a result of acquiring resources or training needed to accommodate recommendations, or as a result of service reductions during transition from old to new processes
Implementation	Barriers/facilitators	Individual, organizational, or system barriers that are associated with adoption
	Tools	Instructions, tools, or templates to tailor guideline/recommendations for local context; Point-of-care templates/forms (clinical assessment, standard orders)
	Strategies	Possible mechanisms by which to implement guideline/recommendations
Evaluation	Monitoring	Suggestions for evaluating compliance with organization, delivery, and outcomes of recommendations, including programme evaluation, audit tools, and performance measures/quality indicators

Source: Gagliardi, A. R., Brouwers, M. C., Palda, V. A., et al. (2011). How can we improve guideline use? A conceptual framework of implementability. *Implementation Science*, 6, 26. https://doi.org/10.1186/1748-5908-6-26

Finally, mental health professionals and organizations have the dual responsibility of caring for individuals with mental illness as well as protecting the public such as through involuntary detention. Having a good evidence base for those who are under involuntary detention is particularly important. Each of these specific issues poses further difficulties in the successful implementation of mental health guidelines by professionals and organizations.

Other issues facing mental health professionals and organizations in the adaptation and implementation of guidelines include whether they should use existing guidelines (and if so, how to determine when/how to adapt existing ones to fit a clinical need) or develop new ones. Adapting existing guidelines is often the most efficient method when no existing guidelines directly address the needs of a particular clinical setting (Graham et al., 2002). An international collaboration, ADAPTE, was developed to promote the development and use of clinical practice guidelines through the adaptation of existing guidelines (www.adapte.org): 'The group's main endeavour is to develop and validate a generic adaptation process that will foster valid and high-quality adapted guidelines as well as the users' sense of ownership of the adapted guideline.' The ADAPTE collaboration outlines a framework for the adaptation of existing guidelines. In general, recommendations should not be modified if they are supported by very strong evidence (e.g. the use of mood stabilizers in managing symptoms of mania) while recommendations with less evidence may be more appropriate to modify to the local circumstances (e.g. providing education around substance use). The adaptation of guidelines should also be done by a multidisciplinary group of health professionals as this composition ensures the delivery of better health care.

Finally, although professionals and organizations may be tempted to only adapt individual recommendations that have the strongest evidence base, this process may lead to problems with implementation. For example, organizations could decide to screen for individuals with prodromal symptoms of psychosis due to evidence that early identification will improve prognosis (Phillips et al., 2005). However, if there are no additional resources provided to these families and individuals, the likelihood of them continuing in follow-up will be low given the lack of overt symptoms of psychosis or significant impairment in functioning. Therefore, mental health professionals and organizations must look at the logic chain of implementing a set of guidelines to ensure that the overall change in a clinical setting is successful, leading to improved practices or outcomes.

Barriers to using the knowledge

French and colleagues (2012) proposed a four-step systematic approach for developing change interventions that can be widely applied to diverse settings/clinical issues. It recognizes that clinical practice guideline implementation strategies need to address the specific barriers and lever facilitators that mental health organizations and healthcare professionals face in order to change clinician behaviour and improve patient outcomes (Grimshaw et al., 2006; Weinmann et al., 2007). Barriers can occur at the healthcare system, healthcare organization, peer group, individual professional, and professional–patient interaction levels. Many existing theoretical models and frameworks can facilitate the identification of barriers and enablers. The Consolidated Framework for Implementation Research (Figure 37.2) identifies constructs in five domains (intervention characteristics, outer setting, inner setting, characteristics of individuals, and process) that have been associated with effective implementation and that can be used to assess potential barriers (Damschroder et al., 2009). Successful implementation often requires key actors (clients, patients, healthcare, and other professionals, managers, policymakers) to change their behaviours. The Theoretical Domains Framework (TDF) synthesizes psychological theories and identifies 14 domains (Atkins et al., 2017; Michie et al., 2005; Patey et al., 2017) that influence behaviours and has been widely used to determine barriers and facilitators to implementation (Table 37.2) (Patey et al., 2017). Finally, there is increasing recognition of the importance of *non-reflective processes* (habits, routines) as a driver of healthcare professional behaviours (Sladek et al., 2006) and the need for different approaches to addressing these when they represent barriers (Pottoff et al., 2009).

There are several current examples of barriers in mental health. With the development of new drugs that have significant side effects, monitoring of them has become a critical issue. A common example is the inability of mental health professionals to remember a specific protocol for the initiation and follow-up of a prescription medication, such as the use of atypical antipsychotics which is associated with weight gain, diabetes, and hyperlipidaemia. Despite these potential adverse outcomes, mental health professionals often forget to monitor for them (domain of 'Memory, attention, and decision processes'; Mackin et al., 2007). An example related to non-reflective processes is the use of 'as-required' medications for psychiatric inpatients overnight when staffing is limited. There is often an overuse of these medications from routines developed in the clinical units to sedate 'agitated' inpatients despite evidence of frequent overuse (Castel, n.d.).

Selection, tailoring, and implementation of interventions to promote the use of knowledge

There is substantial evidence that passive dissemination of guidelines alone is unlikely to optimize clinical care. This has led to the development of a broad range of interventions to promote the use of knowledge in clinical settings. These include professional interventions (e.g. distribution of educational materials, academic detailing, reminders, and audit feedback), organizational interventions (e.g. changing staff roles), financial interventions, regulatory interventions, or a combination of these interventions (e.g. multifaceted) (Grimshaw et al., 2012). The choice of dissemination and implementation strategies should be informed by the perceived barriers, identification of potential strategies based upon consideration of their ability to overcome likely barriers, and evidence of their effectiveness and practical considerations (such as available resources and logistical issues). However, often little consideration is given to these factors; instead, most interventions are selected based on 'common

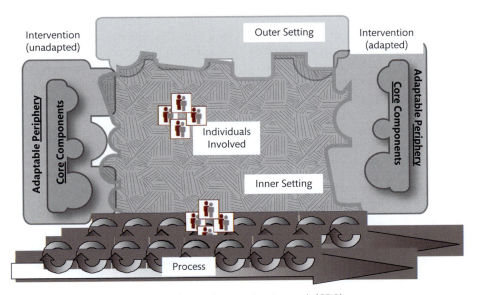

Figure 37.2 Major domains of the Consolidated Framework for Implementation Research (CFIR).
Source: Damschroder, L. J., Aron, D. C., Keith, R. E., et al. (2009). Fostering implementation of health services research findings into practice: a consolidated framework for advancing implementation science. *Implementation Science*, 4, 50. https://doi.org/10.1186/1748-5908-4-50

Table 37.2 The Theoretical Domains Framework

Knowledge	Existing procedural knowledge, knowledge about guidelines, knowledge about evidence and how that influences what the participants do
Skills	Competence and ability about the procedural techniques required to perform the behaviour
Social/professional role and identity	Is the behaviour something the participant is supposed to do or someone else's? (When discussing 'we'/the collective)
	Boundaries between professional groups
Beliefs about capabilities	Perceptions about competence and confidence in doing the behaviour
Beliefs about consequences	Perceptions about outcomes and advantages and disadvantages of performing the behaviour or previous experiences that have influenced whether the behaviour is performed or not
Motivation and goals	Priorities, importance, commitment to a certain course of actions or behaviours
	Intentions
Memory, attention, and decision processes	Attention control, decision-making, memory, i.e. is the target behaviour problematic because people simply forget?
Environmental context/resources	How factors related to the setting in which the behaviour is performed (e.g. people, organizational, cultural, political, physical, and financial factors) influence the behaviour
Social influences	External influence from other people, views of other professions, patients, and families, doing what you are told and how that influences what you do
Emotion	How feelings, affect (positive or negative) may influence behaviour
Behavioural regulation	Ways of doing things that relate to pursuing and achieving desired goals, standards, or targets
	Strategies the participants have in place to help them perform the behaviour
	Strategies the participants would like to have in place to help them
Nature of the behaviours	What is the participant's history of the behaviour, have they any experience (done it often or not at all in the past), is the behaviour routine or automatic?

Source: Patey, A. M., Curran, J. A., Sprague, A. E. et al. (2017). Intermittent auscultation versus continuous fetal monitoring: exploring factors that influence birthing unit nurses' fetal surveillance practice using theoretical domains framework. *BMC Pregnancy Childbirth*, 17, 320. https://doi.org/10.1186/s12884-017-1517-z

sense'. This 'common-sense' approach for developing interventions has only shown modest changes in clinician behaviours and, more importantly, in patient outcomes (Gagliardi et al., 2011; Graham et al., 2002).

Emerging research suggests that the use of theory-based behavioural change interventions may be most effective in changing provider behaviour. The four-step systematic approach for developing change interventions using the TDF, can be widely applied to diverse clinical settings (Phillips et al., 2005). After identifying the relevant barriers to uptake, interventions targeting these barriers can be developed (Table 37.2). The TDF framework identified what specific beliefs and domains need to be addressed to inform the selection of behavioural change techniques and design of interventions. A targeted intervention for behavioural change must be 'locally relevant and likely to be feasible' (Phillips et al., 2005).

For example, in the study to improve disclosure of the diagnosis of dementia, intervention mapping was used to link the identified factors (social influence, beliefs about capability) influencing the behaviours with appropriate behaviour change techniques (Foy et al., 2007). The resulting intervention included behaviour change techniques that targeted the specific factors (persuasive communication targeting social influence and graded tasks (i.e. starting with easy tasks first) targeting beliefs about capabilities) (Eccles et al., 2009).

Similar to interventions developed using the TDF that have specific mechanisms of action and assumptions underpinning their use, there are interventions that can target habits and routines. Figure 37.3 outlines common strategies that can create new habits or routines, or disrupt old ones (Potthoff et al., 2022).

There is a substantial evidence base about the effects of different behaviour change interventions across all areas of clinical practice. The Cochrane Effective Practice and Organisation of Care group supported over 160 systematic reviews of interventions to improve health care delivery and health care systems. Table 37.3 summarizes key findings from these systematic overviews and reviews across all clinical behaviours—most interventions are effective under some circumstances usually resulting in moderate improvements in clinical care. This reinforces the need to carefully select interventions based upon the factors identified above (Grimshaw et al., 2001). There is less specific evidence about the effects of interventions to improve mental health practice. Although there has been more focus recently on the trustworthiness of mental health guidelines, there have been very few guidelines examined for implementation effectiveness (Bennett et al., 2018). Girlanda and colleagues (2013) reviewed guideline implementation strategies in specialist mental health care settings and found that few have shown any effective uptake. Similarly, Gilbody and colleagues (2003) conducted a systematic review to examine the impact of educational and organizational interventions to improve depression management in primary care and found that education and passive dissemination strategies were not very effective. However, organizational changes were more effective. Gilbody and colleagues later examined the higher costs associated with these interventions (2006).

Monitoring knowledge use and evaluation of outcomes

Once a set of guidelines has been implemented, there should be a detailed monitoring process to determine uptake and outcomes

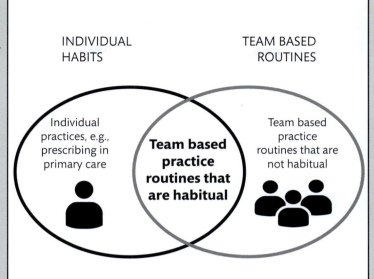

Figure 37.3 Common strategies that can create new habits or routines, or disrupt old ones.
Source: Potthoff, S., Kwasnicka, D., Avery, L., et al. (2022). Changing healthcare professionals' non-reflective processes to improve the quality of care. *Social Science & Medicine*, 298, 114840. https://doi.org/10.1016/j.socscimed.2022.114840

including changes in behaviour, patient outcomes, and provider outcomes. For example, this may include a chart audit several months after the implementation of new guidelines to determine whether practice has changed and patient outcomes have improved. Unfortunately, detailed monitoring such as chart audits cannot be sustained over time given the required additional resources. Therefore, over time, less resource-intensive methods for monitoring and evaluation of outcomes will have to be used such as the analyses of data drawn from databases such as electronic medical records or computerized physician order entry systems, once these become more widespread.

Outcome selection should be informed by all the stakeholders including patients. The recent move towards patient-oriented research has seen significant involvement of people with lived experience in mental health research. This includes not only embedding people with lived experience on research and clinical teams/units but has also influenced what outcomes are considered most important when evaluating the effectiveness of interventions. This should be taken into consideration when examining the impact of guidelines implementation.

Sustaining ongoing knowledge use

After the implementation of guidelines into clinical practice, how does one sustain ongoing knowledge use? First, organizations need to develop processes and policies that promote the sustained use of new knowledge. For example, the responsibility of keeping up to date regarding changes in best practice need to be delegated to someone within the organization, and resources need to be dedicated to the dissemination of these changes. Other resources are also needed to maintain existing incorporation of best practices such as ongoing reminders to professionals. Therefore, professionals and organizations must be prepared and well-resourced to handle these potential barriers to sustained uptake of knowledge.

Once guidelines have been translated into clinical practice, professionals and organizations also need to monitor the emergence of new knowledge that might make guideline recommendations out of date. While this is often undertaken by guideline development agencies, mental health organizations likely need to share some responsibility for this. Furthermore, although there is often concern about guidelines becoming out of date, there is good evidence that guidelines do not generally become out of date quickly. In fact, new evidence that may emerge and shift recommendations are generally related to major clinical trials, therefore allowing for a much less labour-intensive process (limited search strategies for new literature) to update older guidelines. Several resources are available to professionals and organizations interested in learning more about this process (Shekelle et al., 2001).

Table 37.3 Summary of key findings from overviews of reviews

Intervention (key reference) (Definition of intervention based upon Bero, 2007)	Barriers addressed	Effectiveness	Resource considerations	Practical considerations
Printed educational materials (Giguère et al., 2020) (Distribution of published or printed recommendations for clinical care, including clinical practice guidelines, audiovisual materials, and electronic publications)	Individual professional knowledge, (attitudes)	84 studies with 32 RCTs Moderate effect across health conditions Median ARD (PEM compared to no intervention) was 0.04 (or 4% absolute improvement) (range 0.1–0.9)	Relatively inexpensive	Commonly used in healthcare settings
Educational meetings—didactic (Forsetlund et al., 2021) (Health care providers who have participated in *didactic* conferences, lectures, workshops, or traineeships)	Individual professional knowledge	215 RCTs included 65 comparisons Generally effective Slight improvement in desired practice compared to no intervention Median adjusted RD was 6.9% (interquartile range 0.30–13%)	Relatively inexpensive	Commonly used in healthcare settings
Educational meetings—interactive (Forsetlund et al., 2021) (Health care providers who have participated in *interactive* conferences, lectures, workshops, or traineeships)	Individual professional and peer group knowledge, attitudes, and skills	3 RCTs of interactive educational meetings vs didactic Uncertain effect	Modest expense (usually higher facilitator-to-participant ratio than didactic activities)	Commonly used in healthcare settings
Educational outreach (O'Brien et al., 2007) (Use of a trained person who met with providers in their practice settings to give information with the intent of changing the provider's practice)	Individual professional knowledge, attitudes using a social marketing approach (Soumerai & Avorn, 1990)	69 RCTs Generally effective Prescribing behaviours: median effect size across 17 comparisons 4.8% absolute improvement, (interquartile range 3.0–6.5%) Other behaviours: median effect across 17 comparisons 6.0% absolute improvement, (interquartile range 3.6–16.0%)	Relatively expensive due to employment of academic detailers (although can still be efficient) (Mason et al., 2001)	Used in some health care systems. Typically aim to get maximum of 3 messages across in 10–15 minutes (using approach tailored to individual health care provider) and use additional strategies to reinforce approach (Soumerai & Avorn, 1990) Typically focus on relatively simple behaviours in control of individual physician, e.g. choice of drugs to prescribe
Local opinion leaders (Flodgren et al., 2019)	Individual professional and peer group knowledge, attitudes (skills)	18 RCTs Generally effective Median adjusted RD was 10.8% absolute improvement (interquartile range 3.5–14.6%)	Moderately expensive due to need to survey target population for each condition	May be effective alone or in combination with other interventions
Audit and feedback (Ivers et al., 2012) (Any summary of clinical performance of health care over a specified period of time)	Individual professional (and peer group) awareness of current performance	140 RCTs Generally effective Median adjusted RD was 4.3% across 82 high-quality comparisons (interquartile range 0.5–16%) Larger effects seen if baseline performance is low	Resources required largely relate to costs of data abstraction. May be relatively cheap if data can be abstracted by routine administrative systems	Effectiveness may be dependent on a number of factors including baseline performance
Computerized decision support (Kwan et al., 2020)	Individual professional—memory, attention, decision-making	108 RCTs Generally effective Increased patients receiving desired care by 5.8% (95% confidence interval 4.0–7.6%) In trials reporting clinical endpoints, proportion of patients achieving guideline-based targets increased by a median of 0.3% (inter quartile range −0.7% to 1.9%)	For some processes of care such as vaccinations and screening, a small increase could translate into significant benefit at the population level	For some, processes of care connected to a small change in adherence might not justify implementation and contribution to clinicians' frustration with electronic health records

Table 37.3 Continued

Intervention (key reference) (Definition of intervention based upon Bero, 2007)	Barriers addressed	Effectiveness	Resource considerations	Practical considerations
Multifaceted interventions overview (Squires et al., 2014) (An intervention including two or more components)	Target multiple barriers of the included intervention components	25 reviews of RCTs Generally not more effective compared to single-component interventions Krushal–Wallis test p = 0.18 for studies with no intervention control groups and p = 0.69 for studies with multiple intervention control group	More costly than single interventions and may be less effective	Need to carefully consider how to combine interventions to ensure additive or synergistic effects (e.g. interventions that include components that target same barriers may not be additive/synergistic)

Borrowed and updated with permission from Jeremy M. Grimshaw, Holger J. Schünemann, Jako Burgers, Alvaro A. Cruz, John Heffner, Mark Metersky, and Deborah Cook on behalf of the ATS/ERS Ad Hoc Committee on Integrating and Coordinating Efforts in COPD Guideline Development. Integrating and Coordinating Efforts in Chronic Obstructive Pulmonary Disease (COPD) Guideline Development. An Official ATS/ERS Workshop Report. *Proc Am Thorac Soc.* 2012: 9(5);298–303.

References cited:

Bero, L., Eccls, M., Grilli, R., Grimshaw, J., Gruen, R.I., Mayhew, A., et al (2007). Cochrane Effective Practice and Organisation of Care Group. About The Cochrane Colaboration (Cochrane Review Groups (CRGs)), [Issue 4. Art. No.: EPOC]

Flodgren, G., O'Brien, M., Parmelli, E., & Grimshaw, J. (2019). Local opinion leaders: effects on professional practice and health care outcomes. *Cochrane Database of Systematic Reviews*, 6, CD000125.

Forsetlund, L., O'Brien, M., Forsen, L., et al. (2021). Continuing education meetings and workshops: effects on professional practice and healthcare outcomes. *Cochrane Database of Systematic Reviews*, 9, CD003030.

Giguère, A., Zomahoun, H. T., Carmichael, P.-H., et al. (2020). Printed educational materials: effects on professional practice and healthcare outcomes. *Cochrane Database of Systematic Reviews*, 8, CD004398.

Ivers, N., Jamtvedt, F., Flottorp, S., et al. (2012). Audit and feedback: effects on professional practice and health care outcomes. *Cochrane Database of Systematic Reviews*, 6, CD000259.

Kwan, J., Lo, L., Ferguson, J., et al. (2020). Computerised clinical decision support systems and absolute improvements in care: meta-analysis of controlled clinical trials. *BMJ*, 370, m3216.

Mason, J., Freemantle, N., Nazareth, I., et al. (2001). When is it cost-effective to change the behavior of health professionals? *JAMA*, 286, 2988–2992.

O'Brien MA, Rogers S, Jamtvedt G, et al. (2007). Educational outreach visits: effects on professional practice and health care outcomes. *Cochrane Database of Systematic Reviews*, 4, CD000409.

Soumerai, S. B. & Avorn, J. (1990). Principles of educational outreach ('academic detailing') to improve clinical decision making. *JAMA*, 263, 549–556.

Squires, J., Sullivan, K., Eccles, M., et al. (2014). Are multifaceted interventions more effective than single-component interventions in changing health-care professionals' behaviours? An overview of systematic reviews. *Implementation Science*, 9, 152.

Summary

Although guidelines can be used to improve patient care, successful uptake and sustained change in practice based on new knowledge requires active interventions. There are several steps that mental health professionals and organizations can follow to improve the implementation of guidelines in clinical settings. After identifying an area of clinical practice requiring improvement, professionals and organizations need to find and adapt or in rare instances, develop guidelines that are appropriate for their setting. The identification of barriers to effective uptake is also a critical step in this process so that professionals and organizations can tailor their implementation strategies to overcome specific barriers. Finally, the ongoing use of knowledge requires changes in processes and policies as well as resources to maintain improvements and perhaps to keep up to date with new emerging knowledge.

Although this area of research in mental health is still in its infancy and the evidence for the implementation of mental health guidelines is limited, there is a broader literature that can inform the work of professionals and organizations interested in improving clinical care.

Acknowledgements

We would like to acknowledge the contributions of Paula Whitty and Martin Eccles who co-authored the original version of this chapter.

ELECTRONIC GUIDELINE RESOURCES

Mental health specific

American Academy of Child and Adolescent Psychiatry practice parameters: https://www.aacap.org/aacap/Resources_for_Primary_Care/Practice_Parameters_and_Resource_Centers/Home.aspx

American Psychiatric Association: https://psychiatry.org/psychiatrists/practice/clinical-practice-guidelines

Canadian Network for Mood and Anxiety Treatments: http://www.canmat.org/

GENERAL (INCLUDES ALL MEDICAL DISORDERS)

Australia National Health and Medical Research Council: http://www.nhmrc.gov.au/guidelines/index.htm

Canadian Medical Association Clinical Practice Guidelines Infobase: www.cma.ca/cpgs/index/html

National Institute for Health and Care Excellence: http://www.nice.org.uk

Scottish Intercollegiate Guidelines Network: http://www.sign.ac.uk/

REFERENCES

Alonso-Coello, P., Oxman, A. D., Moberg, J., Brignardello-Petersen, R., Akl, E. A., Davoli, M., et al. (2017). GRADE evidence to decision (EtD) frameworks: a systematic and transparent approach to making well informed healthcare choices 2. Clinical practice guidelines. *Gaceta Sanitaria*, **32**, e1–e167.

Atkins, L., Francis, J., Islam, R., O'Connor, D., Patey, A., Ivers, N., et al. (2017). A guide to using the theoretical domains framework of behaviour change to investigate implementation problems. *Implementation Science*, **12**, 77.

Balshem, H., Helfand, M., Schünemann, H. J., Oxman, A. D., Kunz, R., Brozek, J., et al. (2011). GRADE guidelines: 3. Rating the quality of Evidence. *Journal of Clinical Epidemiology*, **64**, 401–406.

Bennett, K., Courtney, D., Duda, S., Henderson, J., & Szatmari, P. (2018). An appraisal of the trustworthiness of practice guidelines for depression and anxiety in children and youth. *Depression and Anxiety*, **35**, 530–540.

Brouwers, M., Kho, M., Browman, G., Burgers, J. S., Cluzeau, F., Feder, G., et al. (2010a). Development of the AGREE II, part 1: performance, usefulness and areas for improvement. *Canadian Medical Association Journal*, **182**, 1045–1052.

Brouwers, M., Kho, M., Browman, G., Burgers, J. S., Cluzeau, F., Feder, G., et al. (2010b). Development of the AGREE II, part 2: assessment of validity of items and tools to support application. *Canadian Medical Association Journal*, **182**, E472–E478.

Carroll, A., Biondich, P., Anand, V., Dugan, T. M., & Downs, S. M. (2013). A randomized controlled trial of screening for maternal depression with a clinical decision support system. *Journal of the American Medical Informatics Association*, **20**, 311–316.

Castel, S. (n.d.). *Implementing Treatment Monitoring Guidelines for Atypical Antipsychotics and Mood Stabilizers*. Sunnybrook Medical Services Alternative Funding Plan Association Grant.

Cheung, A., Zuckerbrot, R. A., Jensen, P. S., Ghalib, K., Stein, R. K., Laraque, D., et al. (2007). Guidelines for adolescent depression in primary care—GLAD PC—part II. *Pediatrics*, **120**, e1313–e1326.

Damschroder, L., Aron, D., Keith, R., Kirsh, S. R., Alexander, J. A., & Lowery, J. C. (2009). Fostering implementation of health services research findings into practice: a consolidated framework for advancing implementation science. *Implementation Science*, **4**, 50.

Eccles, M., Foy, R., Johnston, M., Johnston, M., Bamford, C., Grimshaw, J. M., et al. (2009). Improving professional practice in the disclosure of a diagnosis of dementia: a modeling experiment to evaluate a theory-based intervention. *International Journal of Behavioral Medicine*, **16**, 377–387.

Eccles, M. P., Grimshaw, J. M., Shekelle, P., Schünemann, H. J., & Woolf, S. (2012). Developing clinical practice guidelines: target audiences, identifying topics for guidelines, guideline group composition and functioning and conflicts of interest. *Implementation Science*, **7**, 60.

Foy, R., Francis, J. J., Johnston, M., Eccles, M., Lecouturier, J., Bamford, C., & Grimshaw, J. (2007). The development of a theory-based intervention to promote the appropriate disclosure of a diagnosis of dementia. *BMC Health Services Research*, **7**, 207.

French, S. D., Green, S. E., O'Connor, D. A., Lemieux-Charles, L., & Grimshaw, J. M. (2012). Developing theory-informed behaviour change interventions to implement evidence into practice: a systematic approach using the Theoretical Domains Framework. *Implement Sci*, **7**, 38.

Gagliardi, A. R., Brouwers, M. C., Palda, V. A., Lemieux-Charles, L., & Grimshaw, J. M. (2011). How can we improve guideline use? A conceptual framework of implementability. *Implementation Science*, **6**, 26.

Gilbody, S., Bower, P., & Whitty, P. M. (2006). The costs and consequences of enhanced primary care for depression: a systematic review of randomized economic evaluations. *British Journal of Psychiatry*, **189**, 297–308.

Gilbody, S., Whitty, P., Grimshaw, J., & Thomas, R. (2003). Educational and organizational interventions to improve the management of depression in primary care: a systematic review. *JAMA*, **289**, 3145–3151.

Girlanda, F., Fiedler, I., Ay, E., Barbui, C., & Koesters, M. (2013). Guideline implementation strategies for specialist mental healthcare. *Current Opinion in Psychiatry*, **26**, 369–375.

Graham, I. D., Harrison, M. B., Brouwers, M., Davies, B. L., & Dunn, S. (2002). Facilitating the use of evidence in practice: evaluating and adapting clinical practice guidelines for local use by health care organizations. *Journal of Obstetric, Gynecologic, and Neonatal Nursing*, **31**, 599–611.

Graham, I. D., Logan, J., Harrison, B., Straus, S. E., Tetroe, J., Caswell, W., & Robinson, N. (2006). Lost in knowledge translation: time for a map? *Journal of Continuing Education in the Health Professions*, **26**, 13–24.

Grimshaw, J., Eccles, M., MacLenna, G., MacLennan, G., Ramsay, C., Fraser, C., & Vale, L. (2006). Toward evidence-based quality improvement. *Journal of General Internal Medicine*, **21**(Suppl. 2), 514–520.

Grimshaw, J. M., Shirran, L., Thomas, R., Mowatt, G., Fraser, C., Bero, L., et al. (2001). Changing provider behavior: an overview of systematic reviews of interventions. *Medical Care*, **39**(8 Suppl. 2), II2–II45.

Grimshaw, J. M., Schünemann, H. J., Burgers, J., Cruz, A. A., Heffner, J., Metersky, M., Cook, D., & ATS/ERS Ad Hoc Committee on Integrating and Coordinating Efforts in COPD Guideline Development (2012). Disseminating and implementing guidelines: article 13 in Integrating and coordinating efforts in COPD guideline development. An official ATS/ERS workshop report. *Proceedings of the American Thoracic Society*, **9**, 298–303.

Guyatt, G., Oxman, A. D., Aki, E. A., Kunz, R., Vist, G., Brozek, J., et al. (2011). GRADE guidelines: 1. Introduction—GRADE evidence profiles and summary of table findings. *Journal of Clinical Epidemiology*, **64**, 383–394.

Hayward, R. S. A., Wilson, M. C., Tunis, S. R., Bass, E. B., & Guyatt, G. (1995). Users' guides to the medical literature. VII. How to use clinical practice guidelines. A. Are the recommendations valid? *JAMA*, **274**, 570–574.

Institute of Medicine (2011). Clinical practice guidelines we can trust. March 23. http://www.iom.edu/Reports/2011/Clinical-Practice-Guidelines-We-Can-Trust.aspx

Kendall, T. & Pilling, S. (2004). The National Collaborating Centre for Mental Health. In: Whitty, P. & Eccles, M. (Eds.), *Clinical Practice Guidelines in Mental Health* (pp. 81–92). Oxford: Radcliffe Publishing.

Lomas, J. (1991). Making clinical policy explicit: legislative policy making and lessons for developing practice guidelines. *International Journal of Technology Assessment in Health Care*, **13**, 35–39.

Mackin, P., Bishop, D. R., & Helen, M. O. (2007). A prospective study of monitoring practices for metabolic disease in antipsychotic-treated community psychiatric patients. *BMC Psychiatry*, **7**, 28.

Michie, S., Johnston, M., Abraham, C., Lawton, R., Parker, D., Walker, A. & 'Psychological Theory' Group. (2005). Making psychological theory useful for implementing evidence based practice: a consensus approach. *Quality and Safety in Health Care*, **14**, 6–33.

National Institute for Health and Care Excellence (2014). Developing NICE guidelines: the manual NICE process and methods [PMG20]. https://www.nice.org.uk/process/pmg20/chapter/introduction (updated 2024)

Patey, A., Curran, J., Sprague, A., Francis, J. J., Driedger, S. M., Légaré, F., et al. (2017). Intermittent auscultation versus continuous fetal monitoring: exploring factors that influence birthing unit nurses' fetal surveillance practice using theoretical domains framework. *BMC Pregnancy Childbirth*, **17**, 320.

Phillips, L. J., McGorry, P. D., Yung, A. R., McGlashan, T. H., Cornblatt, B., & Klosterkötter, J. (2005). Prepsychotic phase of schizophrenia and related disorders: recent progress and future opportunities. *British Journal of Psychiatry*, **187**, s33–s44.

Potthoff, S., Kwasnicka, D., Avery, L., Finch, T., Gardner, B., Hankonen, N., et al. (2022). Changing healthcare professionals' non-reflective processes to improve the quality of care. *Social Science & Medicine*, **298**, 114840.

Potthoff, S., Rasul, O., Sniehotta, F., Marques, M., Beyer, F., Thomson, R., et al. (2009). The relationship between habit and health care professional behaviour in clinical practice: a systematic review and meta-analysis. *Health Psychology Review*, **13**, 73–90.

Shekelle, P., Eccles, M., Grimshaw, J., & Woolf, S. H. (2001). When should clinical guidelines be updated? *BMJ*, **323**, 255–257.

Shekelle, P., Woolf, S., Grimshaw, J. M., Schünemann, H. J., & Eccles, M. P. (2012). Developing clinical practice guidelines: reviewing, reporting, and publishing guidelines; updating guidelines; and the emerging issues of enhancing guideline implementability and accounting for comorbid conditions in guideline development. *Implementation Science*, **7**, 62.

Sladek, R., Phillips, P., & Bond, M. (2006). Implementation science: a role for parallel dual processing models of reasoning? *Implementation Science*, **1**, 12.

Weinmann, S., Koesters, M., & Becker, T. (2007). Effects of implementation of psychiatric guidelines on provider performance and patient outcome: systematic review. *Acta Psychiatrica Scandinavica*, **115**, 420–433.

Wilson, M. C., Hayward, R. S. A., Tunis, S. R., Bass, E. B., & Guyatt, G. (1995). Users' guides to the medical literature. VII. How to use clinical practice guidelines. B. What are the recommendations and will they help you in caring for your patients? *JAMA*, **274**, 1630–1632.

Woolf, S., Schunemann, H. J., Eccles, M., Grimshaw, J. M. & Shekelle, P. (2012). Developing clinical practice guidelines: types of evidence and outcomes; values and economics, synthesis, grading, and presentation and deriving recommendations. *Implementation Science*, **7**, 61.

Zuckerbrot, R. A., Cheung, A., Jensen, P. S., Stein, R. K., Laraque, D., & GLAD PC Steering Group (2007). Guidelines for adolescent depression in primary care—GLAD PC—part I. *Pediatrics*, **120**, e1299–e1312.

SECTION 9
Global mental health

38. **The global burden of disease and the mental health of communities** *389*
    Daniel V. Vigo, Laura Jones, Rifat Atun, and Graham Thornicroft

39. **Planning mental health care at the national level** *401*
    Nicole Votruba, Melvyn Freeman, Eleni Misganaw, Keshav Desiraju, and Charlotte Hanlon

40. **Contributions of religious, alternative, and complementary practitioners** *417*
    Olatunde Ayinde and Oye Gureje

41. **Planning and implementing community services for a district: the case of PRIME** *425*
    Crick Lund, Erica Breuer, Arvin Bhana, Carrie Brooke-Sumner, Mark Jordans, Nagendra Luitel, Girmay Medhin, Vaibhav Murhar, Juliet Nakku, Olivia Nalwadda, Inge Petersen, Medhin Selamu, Rahul Shidhaye, Joshua Ssebunnya, Mark Tomlinson, Charlotte Hanlon, and Vikram Patel

42. **Mental health aspects of epidemics and pandemics** *439*
    Akin Ojagbemi and Oye Gureje

43. **'Mental health' in low- and middle-income countries** *449*
    R. Srinivasa Murthy

44. **Overcoming impediments to community mental health in low- and middle-income countries** *461*
    Benedetto Saraceno, Mark van Ommeren, and Rajaie Batniji

38

The global burden of disease and the mental health of communities

Daniel V. Vigo, Laura Jones, Rifat Atun, and Graham Thornicroft

Introduction: the global burden of disease

Despite constituting the most disabling of all disorder groups (Institute for Health Metrics and Evaluation, 2018; Murray et al., 2012), and producing the largest economic impact of all non-communicable diseases (Atun, 2015; GBD 2015 DALYs and HALE Collaborators, 2016), mental illnesses have been historically neglected by decision-makers and funders. As indicated in Chapter 5 of this book, just 10% of people with major depressive disorder are estimated to receive effective treatment coverage, as indicated by a study of a broad sample of countries at various income levels, even though major depressive disorder, and mental disorders in general, are widely acknowledged as leading causes of disability worldwide (GBD 2017 Disease and Injury Incidence and Prevalence Collaborators, 2018). In addition to disability, depressed individuals are at greater risk for death from suicide, heart disease, stroke, and cancer (Alonso et al., 2013; Prince et al., 2007), and the economic costs of mental disorders are enormous as reflected in healthcare utilization, use of social services, loss of productivity in the workplace, and loss of income and benefits for families (Bloom et al., 2011; Trautmann et al., 2016; Vigo, 2019; Vigo et al., 2016). Yet, policymakers and health systems are failing to address the needs of individuals with mental illness.

The reasons for this imbalance between burden and spending are many and varied, including, among others, stigma and discrimination towards people with mental disorders, insufficient knowledge about effective and cost-effective interventions, and undercounting of the multiple burdens associated with mental illness (Henderson et al., 2014; Lasalvia et al., 2013; Saxena et al., 2007; Thornicroft et al., 2009; Vigo, 2019). This last aspect, the systematic underestimation of the burden, is due to the pervasive methodological limitations of the epidemiological frameworks widely used to quantify burden of mental illness.

A well-established metric widely used to measure burden of disease is the disability-adjusted life year (DALY) used, among others, by the Global Burden of Disease (GBD) Study. The DALY is a composite metric of disease burden, calculated by the addition of years lived with disability (YLDs) and years of life lost (YLLs) (Murray et al., 2012). Longitudinal analysis of disease burden shows that an epidemiological transition has largely shifted the global burden of disease from communicable, maternal, childhood, and nutritional diseases to non-communicable diseases, particularly in high- (HICs) and middle-income countries (MICs) (Atun, 2015; GBD 2015 DALYs and HALE Collaborators, 2016; GBD 2017 Disease and Injury Incidence and Prevalence Collaborators, 2018).

A large component of this growing non-communicable disease burden is attributable to a relatively small number of disorders affecting mental health (Alonso et al., 2013; Prince et al., 2007) that have substantial adverse health, social, and economic consequences (Bloom et al., 2011; Prince et al., 2007; Trautmann et al., 2016; Vigo et al., 2016). Despite these well-established facts, many GBD estimates using DALYs still undercount the burden attributable to disorders affecting mental health due to methodological limitations that disproportionately affect mental disorders and produce an underestimation of the disease burden caused by these disorders (Vigo et al., 2016, 2022).

We have developed an alternative methodology that partially corrects the methodological shortcomings of the approach used by GBD Study. Using this alternative methodology, our estimate yields a total burden attributable to mental disorders that more than doubles the GBD estimates for 2019: from 4.9% to 13.0% of the total burden of disease worldwide as measured by DALYs (Vigo et al., 2022).

Methods

Our methodology involves the re-analysis of GBD Study outputs to re-estimate the burden of mental, neurological, substance use disorders, and suicide (MNSS). In order to do this, 2019 disaggregated sex- and age-specific burden of disease data (DALYs and YLDs) were downloaded from the Global Health Data Exchange (ghdx.healthdata.org) for four locations: global, low-income countries (LICs), MICs, and HICs. Following the extraction of data, mental health-related burden was re-estimated with adjustments to specifically include the following conditions, which are excluded from GBD estimates (GBD 2019 Mental Disorders Collaborators,

2022): self-harm and suicide, specific neurological disorders (Alzheimer's disease and other dementias, idiopathic epilepsy, and headache disorders), drug use disorders, alcohol use disorder and resulting physical harms (liver cancer due to alcohol use, alcoholic cardiomyopathy, and cirrhosis due to alcohol use), and an estimation for somatic symptom disorder with prominent pain based on the assumption that a fraction of musculoskeletal disorders without anatomical correlates are in fact part of the highly prevalent syndrome classified by different nosologies as pain disorder (*Diagnostic and Statistical Manual of Mental Disorders*, fourth edition (DSM-IV) and International Classification of Diseases, tenth revision) or somatoform disorder with prominent pain (DSM-5) (estimated using the following equation: 1/3[low back pain + neck pain + other musculoskeletal disorders/2]). This burden is collectively referred to as MNSS. In every instance in which YLDs or DALYs were added to the MNSS aggregation, they were subtracted from their initial group in the GBD aggregation, so the overall classification remained exhaustive and mutually exclusive (Vigo et al., 2016, 2020).

Following re-estimation, the burden of disease was analysed at several levels of disorder classification. Firstly, overall DALY and YLD burden was examined for the GBD Level 1 groupings of disorders (GBD 2017 DALYs and HALE Collaborators, 2018): (a) injuries, (b) communicable, maternal, neonatal, and nutritional diseases, and (c) non-communicable diseases, with an emphasis on MNSS as a portion of non-communicable diseases. These results are visually displayed in this chapter as treemaps, which use the colour, size, and position of nested rectangles to convey relative importance.

An age-based analysis was subsequently performed, where DALYs were examined across the lifespan. This was done firstly for all GBD Level 2 groupings of non-communicable diseases (e.g. MNSS, cardiovascular diseases, etc.) in the context of the other two GBD Level 1 groupings that form the total burden of disease (injuries and communicable, maternal, etc.). Second, a lifespan analysis focusing on the disorders that comprise the MNSS grouping was also performed. These results are shown as stacked area charts with 5-year age groups on the x-axis and percentage of total burden on the y-axis.

Finally, MNSS disorders were ranked separately for men and women based on age-standardized rates of DALYs. These analyses were all undertaken with global estimates, as well as the estimates for LICs, lower-middle-income countries (LMICs), upper-middle-income countries (UMICs), and HICs.

Results

The global burden of disease

We start by considering the disease burden of MNSS in the context of all human disorders, with the understanding that only a holistic consideration of needs can lead to a rational allocation of resources.

Globally, non-communicable disorders account for the vast majority of the disease burden measured in DALYs: 65.2% of the total disease burden is due to these conditions, while communicable, maternal, neonatal, and nutritional disorders cause 26.4%, and injuries cause 8.5%. As can be expected, this burden is not homogeneously distributed across countries of different income levels. In HICs, non-communicable disorders are at the top, injuries in the middle, and communicable, maternal, neonatal, and nutritional at the bottom of the disease burden rankings. Whereas, in LICs, the latter are at the top, non-communicable disorders are in the middle, and injuries are ranked at the bottom. Disorder groupings in LMICs and UMICs follow roughly the same rank order as the global sample, with communicable, maternal, neonatal, and nutritional disorders tied with injuries at the bottom in UMICs (see **Figure 38.1** for details).

The disease burden of MNSS also shows large variations in terms of proportions across income levels: globally, it accounts for 13% of the burden. In HICs, the relative burden of MNSS is more than three times the burden in LICs (20.8% vs 6.7%). As we will indicate in the section covering the burden of MNSS in men and women, these differences in proportions are not caused by low absolute burden in LICs, but by the staggering burden of communicable, maternal, and neonatal disorders in LICs, which crowd out other disorder groupings: **Figure 38.1** shows that the relative burden of communicable, maternal, and neonatal disorders in LICs is 12.6 times the proportion in HICs.

As described in the 'Methods' section, our framework partially corrects for the usual absence of YLLs in DALY estimates for mental disorders by capturing deaths due to dementia, substance use, and suicide. However, many deaths caused directly or indirectly by other MNSS are still unaccounted, such as deaths due to severe mental disorders (schizophrenia and bipolar disorders) and increased all-cause mortality due to MNSS. With the goal of presenting a more nuanced picture of the disease burden of MNSS, we also analysed how the burden of disability (excluding mortality) is distributed globally and across countries of different income levels.

The picture of disability globally is less heterogeneous when analysed by country income level: 80.6% of global YLDs are caused by non-communicable disorders, ranging from 67.0% in LICs to 87.7% in HICs. The ranking of the main disorder groupings is the same globally, in MICs (both LMICs and UMICs), and in LICs: non-communicable diseases at the top, communicable, maternal, neonatal, and nutritional disorders second, and injuries third. In HICs, communicable, maternal, neonatal, and nutritional disorders are at the bottom of the ranking, accounting for 3.8% of the total burden, further highlighting the different stages of the epidemiological transition across country income levels.

Figure 38.2 shows that MNSS cause 28.6% of global disability, with a range of between 26.7% in LICs and 31.0% in HICs. Of note, this constitutes a much larger fraction than communicable, maternal, neonatal, and nutritional disorders plus injuries globally, in MICs (both LMICs and UMICs) and in HICs. Even more striking is that the disability caused by MNSS is almost the same as that caused by communicable, maternal, neonatal, and nutritional disorders in LICs (25.9% vs 26.4%).

The global burden of disease across the life course

An analysis of the burden of MNSS across the life course of individuals indicates that, globally, MNSS rapidly surpass a fifth of the total disease burden (at around 10 years of age) and remain above that threshold until after 40 years old, peaking at 28% of total burden between 20 and 30 years of age. The picture is very dissimilar in LICs vs HICs, again, as a result of these groups of countries being, in general,

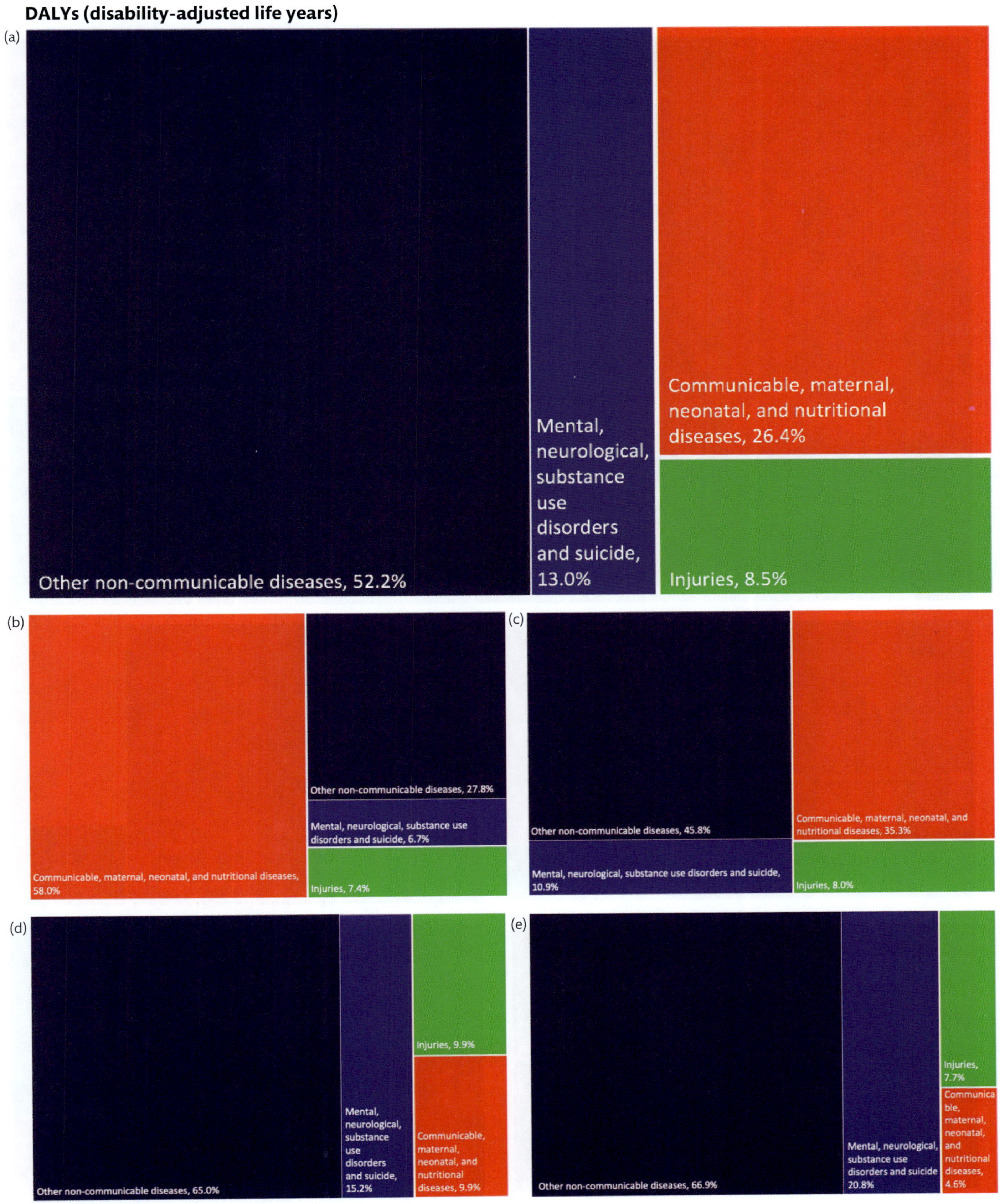

CHAPTER 38 The global burden of disease and the mental health of communities

DALYs (disability-adjusted life years)

(a)
- Other non-communicable diseases, 52.2%
- Mental, neurological, substance use disorders and suicide, 13.0%
- Communicable, maternal, neonatal, and nutritional diseases, 26.4%
- Injuries, 8.5%

(b)
- Communicable, maternal, neonatal, and nutritional diseases, 58.0%
- Other non-communicable diseases, 27.8%
- Mental, neurological, substance use disorders and suicide, 6.7%
- Injuries, 7.4%

(c)
- Other non-communicable diseases, 45.8%
- Communicable, maternal, neonatal, and nutritional diseases, 35.3%
- Mental, neurological, substance use disorders and suicide, 10.9%
- Injuries, 8.0%

(d)
- Other non-communicable diseases, 65.0%
- Mental, neurological, substance use disorders and suicide, 15.2%
- Injuries, 9.9%
- Communicable, maternal, neonatal, and nutritional diseases, 9.9%

(e)
- Other non-communicable diseases, 66.9%
- Mental, neurological, substance use disorders and suicide, 20.8%
- Injuries, 7.7%
- Communicable, maternal, neonatal, and nutritional diseases, 4.6%

Figure 38.1 Overall DALY disease burden distribution globally (A), and in low-income (B), lower-middle-income (C), upper-middle-income (D), and high-income (E) countries.

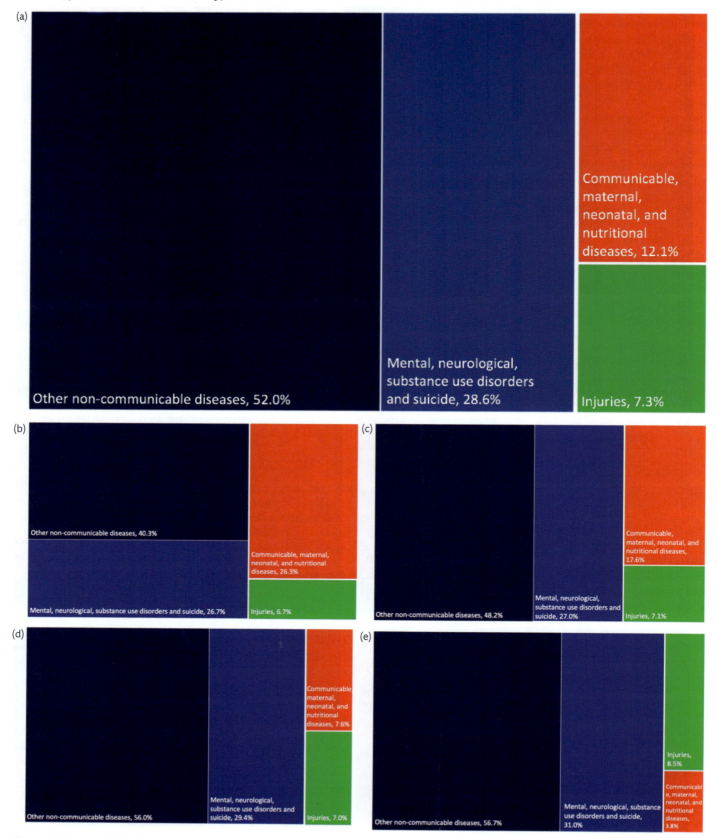

Figure 38.2 Overall YLD disease burden distribution globally (A), and in low-income (B), lower-middle-income (C), upper-middle-income (D), and high-income (E) countries.

in different phases of an epidemiological transition. In LICs, communicable, maternal, neonatal, and nutritional disorders still cause the vast majority of the disease burden during childhood, crowding out the relative impact of MNSS during youth and adulthood. MNSS, however, still reach nearly a fifth of total disease burden between 15 and around 30 years of age.

By contrast, in HICs, the rapid relative increase of the burden caused by MNSS crowds out every other disorder grouping: it surpasses a fifth of all burden around 10 years of age and remains above that threshold until nearly 60 years of age. In fact, it goes well above a third of total burden before 15, reaching nearly half the total burden between 20 and 30 years old (see Figure 38.3 for details). Interestingly, the other non-communicable disease groups show a similar pattern globally, in LICs, and in MICs (both LMICs and UMICs), with cardiovascular disorders replacing MNSS as the largest cause of burden during older adulthood. In HICs, however, neoplasms cause the largest share of the burden between approximately 55 and 75 years of age. The changes in the distribution of disease burden across the lifetime in LMICs and UMICs occur in a continuum between the extremes seen in LICs and HICs, as could be expected.

Focusing now on how the burden of MNSS varies across the life course, the following considerations emerge from a population health perspective. Of note, the pattern is quite similar globally, in LICs, LMICs, and UMICs, while the pattern in HICs appears distinct.

Until 4 years of age, the burden is caused by epilepsy, autism spectrum disorders, and developmental disabilities. In LICs, LMICs, and UMICs, more than 50% of the MNSS burden is caused by epilepsy, whereas in HICs more than 50% is caused by autism. Between 5 and 15 years old, conduct, anxiety, and headache disorders cause the majority of the MNSS burden. Around 15 years of age, a pattern emerges globally and remains stable until, approximately, 75 years of age (with the exception of HICs, as we will note below): common mental disorders (including anxiety, depression, somatoform disorders, and self-harm/suicide) dominate the picture, with around 50% of the MNSS burden; substance use disorders capture an increasing share of the burden (between 10% and 20% during the same period), with drug use initially more prevalent and gradually replaced by alcohol use; headache disorders emerge as a large and pervasive source of burden (also approximately 10–20% during these years); and severe mental disorders (schizophrenia and bipolar disorders) cause around 10% of the burden throughout this period.

In HICs, however, the extra burden caused by drug use disorders (which reaches 30% of the MNSS burden around 30 years of age) crowds out all others, starting around 15 years of age and lasting well into the fifties, when the typical global pattern mentioned above emerges. Finally, neurocognitive disorders start gaining prominence around 50 years of age, and rapidly increase to become the largest cause of MNSS burden around 75 years of age and causing almost the totality in the older age groups (see Figure 38.4 for details).

Differential distribution of the MNSS burden in men and women

An analysis of the age-standardized DALY burden of MNSS shows distinct patterns—with noteworthy similarities and differences—between the sexes and country income levels (GBD data do not include self-identified gender-specific data, so gender-specific analysis is not possible). Overall, for both men and women the age-standardized burden of MNSS appears lowest in UMICs. In men, the following four disorders are present in the top five globally and across income levels: alcohol use disorders, self-harm and suicide, depressive disorders, and somatic symptom disorder with prominent pain. Globally, in UMICs, LMICs, and in LICs, headache disorders are also in the top five, whereas in HICs, drug use disorders are the top cause of disease burden in men. In women, the top five disorders globally and across income levels include the following four: headache, depressive, anxiety disorders, and somatic symptom disorder with prominent pain. In HICs, drug use disorders are also a top-five cause of burden in women, whereas globally, in UMICs and LICs, Alzheimer's disease is within the top five causes of burden. In LMICs, self-harm and suicide is the fifth cause of burden in women. The full rankings of MNSS for men and women globally and per income level are shown in Table 38.1.

Discussion

These previously unpublished analyses show that MNSS are the largest cause of YLDs of any disorder grouping globally and across country income levels (even surpassing communicable, maternal, neonatal, and nutritional disorders—a much broader and higher-level grouping—in LICs). Despite the challenges to estimating mortality resulting from mental disorders, MNSS are also among the largest causes of DALYs, most notably in HICs, where they cause nearly three times the level of burden from injuries and nearly five times the burden of communicable, maternal, neonatal, and nutritional disorders.

Several limitations have to be considered when interpreting these data. YLDs only capture impairment of 'within the skin' functions (i.e. sensory, motor, cognitive, and emotional dysfunction) but they do not capture broader impacts such as loss of quality of life, impaired social functioning, economic losses, etc. Furthermore, YLLs only capture causes of death recorded in death certificates. Hence, deaths resulting from mental disorders are very likely to be underestimated despite our corrections. Finally, our own approach has limitations: we include all forms of suicide and self-harm within MNSS, although some suicides (arguably a very small minority) may not be considered pathological (e.g. euthanasia in the context of terminal illness); and our estimation of somatoform disorders or somatic symptom disorders with prominent pain are only captured indirectly, as a fraction of musculoskeletal disorders without anatomical correlates.

Despite these limitations, our findings have important implications for community mental health services, and community health services in general. They add to the mounting evidence that MNSS should be a societal priority addressed largely at the primary care and community level, due to their prominent place as major causes of disease burden to society.

If governments were to follow evidence-based priority setting for health systems, which recommends that funding allocation for health services should be 'proportionate to burden', then MNSS should receive 13% of the funds globally allocated to health, with a range of 7% of the total health funding in LICs to 21% in HICs (World Health Organization, 2003, 2013). Needless to say, expenditures on mental

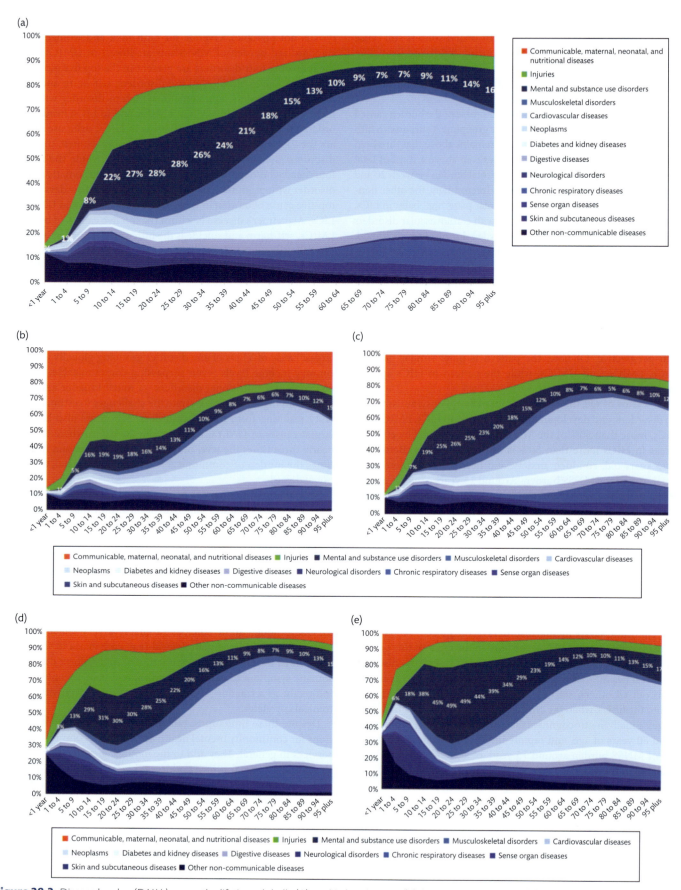

Figure 38.3 Disease burden (DALYs) across the lifetime globally (A), and in low-income (B), lower-middle-income (C), upper-middle-income (D), and high-income (E) countries. x-axis, age-group; y-axis, percentage of total DALYs in the country for both sexes.

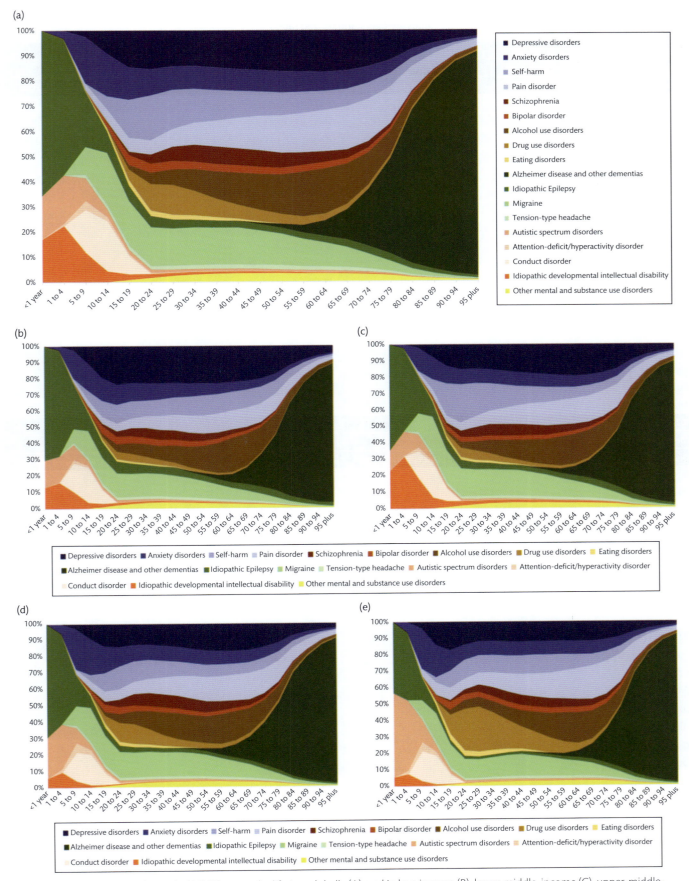

Figure 38.4 Disease burden (DALYs) of MNSS across the lifetime globally (A), and in low-income (B), lower-middle-income (C), upper-middle-income (D), and high-income (E) countries. x-axis, age-group; y-axis, percentage of total DALYs in the country for both sexes.

Table 38.1 Ranking of sex-specific burden (DALYs) of MNSS disorders (A) globally, in low-income (B), lower-middle income (C), upper middle income (D), and high-income countries (E). Values are age-standardized rates

A. Globally

Men		Women	
Disorder	DALYs per 100,000	Disorder	DALYs per 100,000
MNSS (all disorders)	4208	MNSS (all disorders)	4051
Alcohol use disorders	636	Headache disorders	725
Self-harm and suicide	577	Depressive disorders	702
Depressive disorders	452	Somatic symptom disorder with prominent pain	494
Headache disorders	440	Anxiety disorders	445
Somatic symptom disorder with prominent pain	365	Alzheimer's disease and other dementias	361
Alzheimer's disease and other dementias	304	Self-harm and suicide	274
Anxiety disorders	275	Drug use disorders	178
Drug use disorders	272	Schizophrenia	172
Schizophrenia	196	Alcohol use disorders	162
Idiopathic epilepsy	187	Idiopathic epilepsy	15
Other mental disorders	126	Bipolar disorder	109
Bipolar disorder	101	Other mental disorders	86
Conduct disorder	87	Idiopathic developmental intellectual disability	57
Autism spectrum disorder	85	Eating disorders	49
Idiopathic developmental intellectual disability	59	Conduct disorder	48
Eating disorders	25	Autism spectrum disorder	27
Attention-deficit/hyperactivity disorder	20	Attention-deficit/hyperactivity disorder	8

B. LICs

Men		Women	
Disorder	DALYs per 100,000	Disorder	DALYs per 100,000
MNSS (all disorders)	4271	MNSS (all disorders)	3814
Depressive disorders	676	Depressive disorders	940
Alcohol use disorders	642	Headache disorders	584
Self-harm and suicide	610	Anxiety disorders	409
Headache disorders	379	Alzheimer's disease and other dementias	375
Somatic symptom disorder with prominent pain	324	Somatic symptom disorder with prominent pain	349
Alzheimer's disease and other dementias	310	Idiopathic epilepsy	207
Idiopathic epilepsy	296	Self-harm and suicide	205
Anxiety disorders	288	Alcohol use disorders	182
Schizophrenia	146	Schizophrenia	130
Other mental disorders	126	Bipolar disorder	119
Bipolar disorder	119	Other mental disorders	87
Drug use disorders	102	Drug use disorders	70
Conduct disorder	89	Conduct disorder	51
Autism spectrum disorder	81	Idiopathic developmental intellectual disability	47
Idiopathic developmental intellectual disability	56	Autism spectrum disorder	29
Eating disorders	14	Eating disorders	24
Attention deficit hyperactivity disorder	12	Attention deficit hyperactivity disorder	4

Table 38.1 Continued

C. LMICs			
Men		**Women**	
Disorder	DALYs per 100,000	Disorder	DALYs per 100,000
MNSS (all disorders)	4053	MNSS (all disorders)	3963
Alcohol use disorders	610	Headache disorders	727
Self-harm and suicide	599	Depressive disorders	715
Depressive disorders	496	Somatic symptom disorder with prominent pain	478
Headache disorders	472	Anxiety disorders	382
Somatic symptom disorder with prominent pain	335	Self-harm and suicide	374
Alzheimer's disease and other dementias	278	Alzheimer's disease and other dementias	314
Anxiety disorders	250	Idiopathic epilepsy	182
Idiopathic epilepsy	210	Schizophrenia	157
Schizophrenia	194	Alcohol use disorders	148
Other mental disorders	120	Drug use disorders	102
Drug use disorders	111	Idiopathic developmental intellectual disability	98
Idiopathic developmental intellectual disability	98	Bipolar disorder	88
Bipolar disorder	91	Other mental disorders	84
Conduct disorder	86	Conduct disorder	49
Autism spectrum disorder	68	Eating disorders	34
Eating disorders	20	Autism spectrum disorder	26
Attention deficit hyperactivity disorder	13	Attention deficit hyperactivity disorder	5
D. UMICs			
Men		**Women**	
Disorder	DALYs per 100,000	Disorder	DALYs per 100,000
MNSS (all disorders)	3952	MNSS (all disorders)	3782
Alcohol use disorders	656	Headache disorders	700
Self-harm and suicide	486	Depressive disorders	641
Headache disorders	415	Anxiety disorders	472
Depressive disorders	383	Somatic symptom disorder with prominent pain	461
Somatic symptom disorder with prominent pain	340	Alzheimer's disease and other dementias	383
Alzheimer's disease and other dementias	326	Schizophrenia	182
Anxiety disorders	285	Self-harm and suicide	173
Drug use disorders	249	Alcohol use disorders	157
Schizophrenia	198	Drug use disorders	150
Idiopathic epilepsy	152	Idiopathic epilepsy	123
Other mental disorders	122	Bipolar disorder	106
Bipolar disorder	92	Other mental disorders	85
Autism spectrum disorder	86	Eating disorders	46
Conduct disorder	85	Conduct disorder	44
Attention deficit hyperactivity disorder	30	Autism spectrum disorder	25
Eating disorders	25	Idiopathic developmental intellectual disability	20
Idiopathic developmental intellectual disability	22	Attention deficit hyperactivity disorder	12

(*continued*)

Table 38.1 Continued

E. HICs			
Men		**Women**	
Disorder	DALYs per 100,000	Disorder	DALYs per 100,000
MNSS (all disorders)	5306	MNSS (all disorders)	5122
Drug use disorders	880	Headache disorders	867
Self-harm and suicide	724	Depressive disorders	807
Alcohol use disorders	673	Somatic symptom disorder with prominent pain	676
Somatic symptom disorder with prominent pain	503	Anxiety disorders	598
Depressive disorders	478	Drug use disorders	535
Headache disorders	448	Alzheimer's disease and other dementias	353
Anxiety disorders	335	Self-harm and suicide	243
Alzheimer's disease and other dementias	295	Alcohol use disorders	227
Schizophrenia	216	Schizophrenia	199
Other mental disorders	147	Bipolar disorder	171
Bipolar disorder	147	Eating disorders	131
Autism spectrum disorder	138	Idiopathic epilepsy	110
Idiopathic epilepsy	132	Other mental disorders	91
Conduct disorder	92	Conduct disorder	50
Eating disorders	49	Autism spectrum disorder	33
Attention deficit hyperactivity disorder	29	Idiopathic developmental intellectual disability	19
Idiopathic developmental intellectual disability	19	Attention deficit hyperactivity disorder	10

health and substance use services are much lower than the burden of disease would justify, and, in terms of official development assistance, miniscule (Vigo et al., 2016).

From a life-course perspective, we found that MNSS are particularly burdensome during the working years, causing between a fifth and half the total disease burden depending on country income level (in LICs and HICs, respectively). Focusing on which specific MNSS are more burdensome for each age group, we detected relevant patterns that should inform decision-making in terms of resource allocation and training of both general and mental health providers. Primary care providers and paediatricians treating newborns, infants and toddlers should focus on detecting, treating, or referring epilepsy, autism spectrum disorders, and developmental disabilities. In the case of older children, they should focus on anxiety, headache, and conduct disorders.

General providers should be capable of detecting, treating, or referring adolescents and adults with depressive, anxiety, somatoform disorders, and self-harmful behaviours, as well as drug and alcohol use. Also, to detect and refer people with new onset of severe mental disorders such as schizophrenia and bipolar disorders. And after 60–65 years old, new onset of neurocognitive disorders such as Alzheimer's disease should be the focus of all general and mental health providers. Important differences can also be observed between women and men, but also similarities. In fact, globally and across countries of different income levels, a large fraction of the MNSS disease burden in both sexes is caused by depressive and somatoform disorders, in addition to more specific sex- and country income level-related patterns that include substance use disorders (especially in men and in HICs), self-harm and suicide (especially in men), headache disorders, anxiety disorders, and Alzheimer's disease (especially in women).

A final note on the most devastating MNSS epidemic of our time: in HICs, opioid use disorders are already the leading cause of death and disability in young people (due to widespread use of high potency synthetic opioids), so health systems need to urgently diversify treatment options and develop an intersectoral approach to an epidemic that has proven intractable for more than a decade. And in LICs and MICs, health systems should urgently prepare for the likely increase in the penetration of synthetic opioids. In some countries there is already a baseline opioid consumption (e.g. Iran) that will eventually be tragically amplified by synthetic opioids that are becoming ever more powerful, cheaper, and easier to produce locally. In most other LICs and MICs, where baseline consumption of opioids is low, there is a major risk that synthetic opioids could emerge as purposeful contaminants of non-opioids (stimulants, party drugs) with the goal of expanding demand and maximizing profits by leveraging the unparalleled addictive nature of opioids. At the time of writing, the first such case suddenly emerged in Argentina, where 20 people died overnight due to one batch of fentanyl-contaminated cocaine (Krausz et al., 2021). This is the third time in history that opioids are primed to create a global level crisis, which we hope will not catch global health systems off guard, as they did in many HIC health systems with devastating outcomes.

In summary, MNSS represent the largest global cause of disability and one of the largest causes of disability and mortality combined, regardless of country income level. Our analysis corrects for some of the usual limitations of other disease burden estimations, and provide decision-makers with a less biased picture of the extent and the distribution of burden across the life course, as well as stratified by country income level and sex. These estimates can help governments with resource allocation and health system prioritization decisions, as well as to develop concrete training programmes for primary and community health providers.

Acknowledgements

DV is supported by Health Canada (HC), by the Canadian Institutes of Health Research (CIHR), and by Vancouver Coastal Health (VCH).

GT is supported by the National Institute for Health Research (NIHR) Applied Research Collaboration South London at King's College London NHS Foundation Trust, by the NIHR Asset Global Health Unit award, and the NIHR Hope Global Health Group award. GT is also supported by the Guy's and St Thomas' Charity for the On Trac project (EFT151101), and by the UK Medical Research Council (UKRI) in relation to the Emilia (MR/S001255/1) and Indigo Partnership (MR/R023697/1) awards.

The views expressed are those of the author(s) and not necessarily those of HC, CIHR, VCH, the NHS, the NIHR or the Department of Health and Social Care.

REFERENCES

Alonso, J., Chatterji, S., & He, Y. (Eds.). (2013). *The Burdens of Mental Disorders: Global Perspectives from the WHO World Mental Health Surveys*. Cambridge: Cambridge University Press.

Atun, R. (2015). Transitioning health systems for multimorbidity. *Lancet*, **386**, 721–722.

Bloom, D. E., Cafiero, E. T., Jan-Llopis, E., Abrahams-Gessel, S., Bloom, L. R., Fathima, S., et al. (2011). The global economic burden of noncommunicable diseases. PGDA Working Papers 8712, Program on the Global Demography of Aging. https://ideas.repec.org/p/gdm/wpaper/8712.html

GBD 2015 DALYs and HALE Collaborators (2016). Global, regional, and national disability-adjusted life-years (DALYs) for 315 diseases and injuries and healthy life expectancy (HALE), 1990–2015: a systematic analysis for the Global Burden of Disease Study 2015. *Lancet*, **388**, 1603–1658.

GBD 2017 DALYs and HALE Collaborators (2018). Global, regional, and national disability-adjusted life-years (DALYs) for 359 diseases and injuries and healthy life expectancy (HALE) for 195 countries and territories, 1990–2017: a systematic analysis for the Global Burden of Disease Study 2017. *Lancet*, **392**, 1859–1922.

GBD 2017 Disease and Injury Incidence and Prevalence Collaborators (2018). Global, regional, and national incidence, prevalence, and years lived with disability for 354 diseases and injuries for 195 countries and territories, 1990–2017: a systematic analysis for the Global Burden of Disease Study 2017. *Lancet*, **392**, 1789–1858.

GBD 2019 Mental Disorders Collaborators (2022). Global, regional, and national burden of 12 mental disorders in 204 countries and territories, 1990–2019: a systematic analysis for the Global Burden of Disease Study 2019. *Lancet Psychiatry*, **9**, 137–150.

Henderson, C., Noblett, J., Parke, H., Clement, S., Caffrey, A., Gale-Grant, O., et al. (2014). Mental health-related stigma in health care and mental health-care settings. *Lancet Psychiatry*, **1**, 467–482.

Institute for Health Metrics and Evaluation (2018). Protocol for the Global Burden of Diseases, Injuries, and Risk Factors Study (GBD). https://www.healthdata.org/sites/default/files/files/Projects/GBD/GBD_Protocol.pdf

Krausz, R. M., Westenberg, J. N., Mathew, N., Budd, G., Wong, J. S. H., Tsang, V. W. L., et al. (2021). Shifting North American drug markets and challenges for the system of care. *International Journal of Mental Health Systems*, **15**, 86.

Lasalvia, A., Zoppei, S., Van Bortel, T., Bonetto, C., Cristofalo, D., Wahlbeck, K., et al. (2013). Global pattern of experienced and anticipated discrimination reported by people with major depressive disorder: a cross-sectional survey. *Lancet*, **381**, 55–62.

Murray, C. J., Ezzati, M., Flaxman, A. D., Lim, S., Lozano, R., Michaud, C., et al. (2012). GBD 2010: design, definitions, and metrics. *Lancet*, **380**, 2063–2066.

Prince, M., Patel, V., Saxena, S., Maj, M., Maselko, J., Phillips, M. R., & Rahman, A. (2007). No health without mental health. *Lancet*, **370**, 855–877.

Saxena, S., Thornicroft, G., Knapp, M., & Whiteford, H. (2007). Resources for mental health: scarcity, inequity, and inefficiency. *Lancet*, **370**, 878–889.

Thornicroft, G., Brohan, E., Rose, D., Sartorius, N., & Leese, M. (2009). Global pattern of experienced and anticipated discrimination against people with schizophrenia: a cross-sectional survey. *Lancet*, **373**, 408–415.

Trautmann, S., Rehm, J., & Wittchen, H. (2016). The economic costs of mental disorders. *EMBO Reports*, **17**, 1245–1249.

Vigo, D. V. (2019). Disease burden and government spending on mental, neurological, and substance use disorders, and self-harm: cross-sectional, ecological study of health system response in the Americas. *Lancet Public Health*, **4**, e89–e96.

Vigo, D., Jones, L., Atun, R., & Thornicroft, G. (2022). The true global disease burden of mental illness: still elusive. *Lancet Psychiatry*, **9**, 98–100.

Vigo, D., Jones, L., Thornicroft, G., & Atun, R. (2020). Burden of mental, neurological, substance use disorders and self-harm in North America: a comparative epidemiology of Canada, Mexico, and the United States. *Canadian Journal of Psychiatry*, **65**, 87–98.

Vigo, D., Thornicroft, G., & Atun, R. (2016). Estimating the true global burden of mental illness. *Lancet Psychiatry*, **3**, 171–178.

World Health Organization (2003). *The WHO Mental Health Policy and Service Guidance Package*. Geneva: World Health Organization.

World Health Organization (2013). *Mental Health Action Plan 2013–2020*. Geneva: World Health Organization.

39

Planning mental health care at the national level

Nicole Votruba, Melvyn Freeman, Eleni Misganaw, Keshav Desiraju, and Charlotte Hanlon

Dedication

While writing this Chapter our co-author and colleague, Keshav Desiraju, very sadly passed away. Keshav was the Health Secretary to the Union government of India in 2013-14 and brought to this Chapter not only a deep passion for mental health, but an understanding of planning for better mental health from the position of a person at the pinnacle of a country's health administration. He fully appreciated the competing needs of many priority health areas, but had insight into the neglect of mental health and why careful national planning and resourcing is so important to mental health attaining its "rightful" place in health. His wisdom and broad knowledge and experience are, we hope, reflected in this Chapter. MHSRIP.

Introduction

National mental health care planning is a substantial step towards achieving equitable, fair, good-quality, human rights oriented, and affordable mental health care, as well as the prevention of mental health conditions and the promotion of mental well-being. While planning for mental health can suggest and include all processes required to deliver a range of interventions and services, and thus include the development of mental health policy and legislation (as these are part of the 'planning process'), in this chapter we focus primarily on the plans that are required for effective implementation. These are often based on already developed policy or laws. However, mental health planning can also take place in the absence of a formal policy or legislation.

This chapter aims to support countries to develop a comprehensive mental health care plan that can reduce the large burden of mental health conditions and improve the lives of people living with mental health conditions, their families, and their carers. The term 'mental health condition' is used in this chapter to refer to mental health issues for which a person may require some form of care. This includes both people with a diagnosed mental health problem and those with manifestations of mental distress who do not necessarily have a formal diagnosis. The nature of 'care' includes interventions that can be delivered in a range of settings, including outside the health system. Based on their population burden and/or association with human rights violations, the World Health Organization (WHO) has prioritized particular mental health conditions for action, including depression, anxiety, psychosis, bipolar disorder, alcohol and substance use problems, dementia, child mental health problems, suicidal thoughts and behaviours, and others (WHO, 2016).

This chapter will first describe why mental health is relevant to national planners, how national mental health planning is nested within the global policy context, and why better national mental health planning is needed. It will then explain what national mental health planning is, highlight relevant essential approaches and elements to inform national mental health planning, and outline the necessary steps for developing a national mental health plan. Strategies to overcome frequent challenges will be given and recommendations for successful national planning for mental health care will be presented. Case studies of what works and what does not in integration of mental health care planning will be presented. The chapter concludes with a brief summary.

How is mental health relevant to national planners?

There is accumulating recognition of the high prevalence and burden of mental health conditions globally, contributing to at least 13% of all disability-adjusted life years (GBD 2019 Mental Disorders Collaborators, 2022; Vigo et al., 2022). Pervasive global treatment and care gaps persist, leaving up to 90% of people with mental health conditions without the care they need (Pathare et al., 2018). The lack of access to appropriate and timely care contributes to poorer quality of life, human rights violations, worse physical health, and a high excess mortality in people with mental health conditions, including from suicide (Drew et al., 2011; Liu et al., 2017). Planners in every country of the world need to work out the best way to respond to this high level of unmet need.

Effective mental health planning is also vital for other national health priorities. Mental health conditions are frequently comorbid with physical health conditions. When depression occurs in a person who has any chronic infectious (e.g. HIV, tuberculosis (TB)), non-communicable disease (e.g. hypertension, diabetes), or neglected tropical disease, the prognosis of both conditions is worse (Kuper, 2020; Stein et al., 2019). The SARS-CoV-2 (Covid-19) pandemic that started in 2020 has also underlined the critical and bidirectional links that exist between mental health and physical health. The WHO estimates a 15% increase in depression and anxiety worldwide due to the pandemic (COVID-19 Mental Disorders Collaborators, 2021), while people with mental health conditions are at higher risk of more severe Covid-19 infection and poorer outcomes (Vai et al., 2021) and less likely to access vaccines (Kumar et al., 2021). This highlights how health planners need to plan for better mental health in order to achieve better population health in general.

Mental health conditions are also heavily interrelated with poverty, leading to reduced economic productivity and worse socioeconomic status and food security for affected households (Lund et al., 2018). Country development efforts will be undermined by a high burden of untreated mental health conditions. Investments in treatment of depression and anxiety have been shown to be cost saving through their impacts on economic productivity: estimates indicate that for every $1 investment there is a $2–$3 return in economic benefit (Chisholm et al., 2016). Framing national mental health plans as 'pro-poor' and underlining the economic ramifications of inaction can be persuasive arguments to motivate national action.

The substantial contributions of social determinants to the development, course, and outcomes of mental health conditions also mean that planners can achieve national mental health benefits through action in non-health sectors. Poverty, violence, climate change, and displacement of people are potent risk factors for poor mental health (Lund et al., 2018). A multisectoral approach to national mental health care planning can ensure that mental health considerations are integrated into plans for other sectors, for example, poverty reduction or climate change mitigation plans, and leverage additional resources and impacts for mental health (WHO, 2022).

A further key motivation for national planning is to uphold the human rights of people with mental health conditions. Stigma and discrimination are pervasive, often directly linked to violations of the human rights of people with mental health conditions and inhibiting progress in improving their lives. For people with intersecting identities associated with disadvantage, such as ethnic minority status, disability, marginalized sexual orientation, or gender identity, the stigma linked to mental health conditions can reinforce and exacerbate discrimination. Abuse of people with mental health conditions is widespread, both in health and social services facilities as well as in communities and homes. Planning for mental health, therefore, needs to include structural responses to address exclusion and abuse. Lack of access to health care, including economic and geographic access, are further human rights violations that require careful attention from mental health planners.

Several publications have highlighted the evidence for, and the urgency of, global action for mental health planning (Chisholm et al., 2007; Fisher et al., 2012; Kessler et al., 2011; Kohn et al., 2004; Patel et al., 2007; Vigo et al., 2016; WHO, 2022). The Lancet Commission on global mental health and sustainable development has emphasized that planning should not just address access to care, but also respond to the vast gaps in quality of care and the pressing need for prevention to reduce the global burden of mental conditions (Patel et al., 2018).

The need for effective national mental health planning is, therefore, evident. On the face of it, the global situation is promising, with most, but not all, countries reporting the existence of national plans. Three-quarters of WHO member states have a stand-alone national mental health plan or strategy, 57% have a stand-alone mental health law (increase from 51% in 2014), and 46% have updated their mental health policy or plan since 2017 (WHO, 2021a). However, existing national plans are often not being translated into effective and transformative interventions and services. In this chapter we focus on national planning that maximizes the chance of achieving beneficial action on the ground.

National mental health planning within the global policy context

The large and growing burden of mental health conditions and the inter-relationships between mental health and other sectors require country-level strategic, planned, systemwide decision-making and action. These country-level planning processes take place within a wider global policy context that national planning teams will need to recognize and respond to. A major contributor to current global policies is 'global mental health'. Global mental health is an evolving field of policy, practice, and research, driven by a diverse group of stakeholders, including people with LE of mental health conditions and their carers, academics, policymakers, planners, non-governmental organizations (NGOs), and the WHO, based on the fundamental principles of evidence on effective interventions and safeguarding the human rights of people with mental conditions (Collins, 2020).

WHO member states have endorsed a Comprehensive Mental Health Action Plan (WHO, 2021b) that provides a framework for national planning. Taking a life-course approach, the Action Plan aims to achieve mental health equity for people with mental health conditions, through universal health coverage and stresses the importance of prevention. It has four major objectives: (1) more effective leadership and governance for mental health; (2) the provision of comprehensive, integrated mental health and social care services in community-based settings; (3) implementation of strategies for promotion and prevention; and (4) strengthened information systems, evidence, and research. Since 2013, countries are now incorporating these objectives and associated targets and indicators into national policies and planning and will need to deliver and report back on them by 2030 (Table 39.1).

In addition to the WHO's Comprehensive Mental Health Action Plan, a number of global treaties have been adopted to guide countries' actions and plans for improving mental health in their populations. As early as 1990, the Caracas Declaration of Mental Health and Human Rights stressed a clear need for community-based services that are linked with primary care and called on countries to establish laws and policies to guide restructuring of the services and ensure human and civil rights of people living with mental health conditions, paving the way for global conventions. The United Nations (UN) adopted the Convention on the Rights of Persons with Disabilities (CRPD) in 2007 as a substantial global treaty to protect the rights and dignity of persons with disabilities and ensure their legal, social, and political equality. The CRPD specifically emphasizes parity between psychosocial disability (including that resulting from mental health conditions) and physical disability, offering a paradigm shift from the biomedical model to a social and human rights-based model. The CRPD is a crucial global policy and should be at the heart of national health planning. Increasingly, global mental health has become service user led, particularly since the

Table 39.1 Mental health objectives, targets, and indicators in key global policies

Objectives	Targets	Indicators
Comprehensive Mental Health Action Plan (WHO, 2021b)		
Objective 1. To strengthen effective leadership and governance for mental health	Global Target 1.1 80% of countries will have developed or updated their policy or plan for mental health in line with international and regional human rights instruments, by 2030	Indicator 1.1.1. Existence of a national policy or plan for mental health that is being implemented and in line with international human rights instruments
	Global Target 1.2 80% of countries will have developed or updated their law for mental health in line with international and regional human rights instruments, by 2030	Indicator 1.1.2. Existence of a national law covering mental health that is being implemented and in line with international and regional human rights instruments
Objective 2. To provide comprehensive, integrated, and responsive mental health and social care services in community-based settings	Global Target 2.1 Service coverage for mental health conditions will have increased at least by half, by 2030	Indicator 2.1.1. Proportion of persons with psychosis who are using services over the past 12 months (%) Indicator 2.1.2 Proportion of people with depression who are using services over the past 12 months (%)
	Global Target 2.2 80% of countries will have doubled number of community-based mental health facilities, by 2030	Indicator 2.2.1. Number of community-based mental health facilities
	Global Target 2.3 80% of countries will have integrated mental health into primary health care, by 2030	Indicator 2.3.1. Existence of a system in place for integration of mental health into primary health care
Objective 3. To implement strategies for promotion and prevention in mental health	Global Target 3.1 80% of countries will have at least two functioning national, multisectoral mental health promotion and prevention programmes, by 2030	Indicator 3.1.1. Functioning programmes of multisectoral mental health promotion and prevention in existence
	Global Target 3.2 The rate of suicide will be reduced by one-third, by 2030	Indicator 3.2.1. Suicide mortality rate (per 100,000 population)
	Global Target 3.3. 80% of countries will have a system in place for mental health and psychosocial preparedness for emergencies and/or disasters, by 2030	Indicator. Existence of a system in place for mental health and psychosocial preparedness for emergencies/disasters
Objective 4. To strengthen information systems, evidence, and research for mental health	Global Target 4.1. 80% of countries will be routinely collecting and reporting at least a core set of mental health indicators every 2 years through their national health and social information systems, by 2030	Indicator 4.1.1. Core set of identified and agreed mental health indicators routinely collected and reported every 2 years
	Global Target 4.2. The output of global research on mental health doubles, by 2030	Indicator 4.2.1. Number of published articles on mental health research (defined as research articles published in the databases)
UN Sustainable Development Goals (UN, 2017)		
SDG3. Health	Target 3.4. Prevention, treatment, and promotion of mental health	Indicator 3.4.2. Suicide mortality rate
	Target 3.5. Substance abuse	Indicator 3.5.1. Coverage of treatment interventions Indicator 3.5.2. Harmful use of alcohol
	Target 3.8. Universal health coverage	Indicator 3.8.1. Coverage of essential health services Indicator 3.8.2. Proportion of population with large household expenditures on health as a share of total household expenditure or income

Movement for Global Mental Health was born in 2007, an alliance of people with mental conditions and practitioners that is championing mental health, service scale-up, and integration into community care (www.globalmentalhealth.org). Increasingly, networks of people with LE arise and are growing, such as the Global Mental Health Peer Network (www.gmhpn.org). The 2015 UN Sustainable Development Goals (SDGs) include the promotion of mental health and the prevention of mental and substance use disorders and universal health coverage as global development targets (Table 39.1).

Since 2008, the WHO's Mental Health Gap Action Programme (mhGAP) supports countries with evidence-based guidance for scaling up care for people with mental health conditions. mhGAP guidance includes an operational guide on district-level planning, delivery, and monitoring of mental health care (WHO, 2018b); an intervention guide (mhGAP-IG) of evidence-based, clinical guidance for non-specialist health settings, which is designed for use by doctors, nurses, other health workers (WHO, 2016); and an mhGAP community toolkit which provides guidance on multisectoral community provision needed to optimize mental health (WHO, 2019). A joint WHO–OHCHR guideline, *Mental Health, Human Rights and Legislation: Guidance and Practice*, provides direction for adopting, amending, and implementing legislation related to mental health (WHO, 2023). These WHO initiatives and resources provide a strong foundation for national planning, but an effective national plan needs to be locally owned, feasible, acceptable, and tailored to local needs.

Since the first *World Health Report* in 2001 dedicated to mental health (WHO, 2001b), countries report every 3 years on their progress on key indicators. The WHO Mental Health Atlas collates this information which serves as a benchmark for countries to assess their performance against key concerns relevant to planning (WHO, 2001a, 2021a). This includes a requirement to provide regularly updated country data on mental health policies, legislation, financing, human resources, services, and information systems. The recent *World Mental Health Report: Transforming Mental Health for All* summarizes global evidence, highlights gaps, and gives guidance and examples for transformation for mental health (WHO, 2022).

While influenced by the global policy context, local conditions and culture must be taken into account when developing national plans. Global mental health and international policies and guidelines are not necessarily always welcomed uncritically within countries. A controversy has emerged around perceptions that global mental health may push a neocolonial agenda, for instance, focusing on its roots in colonial tropical medicine, uncritical imposition of Western concepts of mental health and illness and their treatments, and on human rights violations linked to the political abuse of psychiatry (Whitley, 2015). There are calls for more culturally rooted approaches to mental health planning, greater engagement with the key local stakeholders, ranging from people with LE of mental health conditions to traditional healers, to capture the maximum breadth of views and needs, and to broaden the focus from biomedical interventions to 'whole-of-society' approaches (Kola et al., 2021).

Across the world and various cultural settings, researchers, policymakers, practitioners, and service users in global mental health are providing ever-increasing experience and evidence on effective, evidence-based interventions and service models that are found to be affordable, cost-effective, and appropriate to narrow the care, treatment, quality, and prevention gaps in mental health. In an ever more connected and interrelated world, unavoidably, the global mental health and policy context is shaping national policy. There is a substantial opportunity for more South–South and South–North learning and experience sharing, and learning from grass roots movements, for example, the BasicNeeds programme (https://basicneedsghana.org/).

In summary, global conventions, policies, and movements provide an essential backdrop for national mental health planning, but effective county plans will need to translate these global imperatives into something that is contextually relevant, feasible, and locally owned.

Gaps in existing national mental health planning

The global context for scaling up and improving mental health services with well-formulated policies and plans means that countries are well set to take action. Indeed, substantial progress for mental health has been achieved in recent years. However, in almost all countries across the world, serious gaps prevail and mental health care planning remains inadequate.

In part this reflects the limited power of global mental health policy to influence national plans. For instance, the recommendations by WHO, which are ultimately endorsed by its own member states, are guidance only. Thus, the implementation, if taken forward on a national level, is often slow and inadequate. Similarly, the UN SDGs are non-binding goals, and their completion is voluntary by nations; however, they are regarded as an honorary achievement. So, while many countries strive to achieve the targets and indicators, it is their decision which they pick, and many will choose those targets that are most achievable, which may not necessarily be those relating to mental health.

The latest WHO Atlas report of progress in implementing the WHO Action Plan notes that, overall, the measured progress and expected rates were not achieved satisfactorily (WHO, 2021a). In spite of steady progress in adoption of policy, plans, and laws, mental health services across the world remain unequally available and accessible, and resources insufficiently allocated. Significant gaps are noted between existing policies, plans, and legislation, and the actual reality of implementation, resources allocation, and monitoring of progress.

Crucial questions that remain for global mental health and national level planners are why are we not where we should be according to global agreements and guidance from WHO, and often with national policy commitments and even plans in place? What does it take to get to where we want to be? What does it take (in addition) to establish an adequate mental health focus in countries? To address these questions, we first start by considering what effective national mental health plans need to include.

Principles underpinning national mental health planning

The process of developing a plan is as important as the plan itself, to set the direction, establish relationships and ensure that relevant voices are heard, and to achieve buy-in from key stakeholders. Mental health service planners and policymakers need to have (1) a clear vision of what they wish to achieve in mental health, and (2) a plan mapping this out and how it will be achieved. The principles that underlie their vision must be stated unambiguously and reflected in the plan.

In this section we will focus on the principles that should inform national mental health planning, and in the following section (see 'Key elements of mental health planning') we will discuss the recommended elements and best practice guidance that will help to achieve an effective plan.

Nothing about us without us—involvement of people with lived experience

At the centre of all mental health care planning are people with LE would be preferable, I think of mental health conditions, their families, and their carers. The voices of people with LE are crucial in shaping and taking decisions on health policy, care planning, and services. Their involvement needs to be continuous and meaningful, and not tokenistic. However, due to structural barriers to involvement, pervasive stigma, and long-standing marginalization of many people with LE, involvement can be difficult to achieve in practice. Planners need to consider how people with LE can be supported to be involved. This could mean, for example, convening a series of smaller consultation workshops with people with LE to supplement a larger stakeholder workshop where some people with LE may be less comfortable to speak. Providing resources to support the running of representative associations for people with LE and advocates may also be necessary. To address potential financial barriers, people with LE should be remunerated for their time and any expenses incurred. Crucially, people with LE should be involved early in the process, when decisions are still being made, and not just to give their approval to finalized plans.

See **Box 39.1** for a case study example of some of the opportunities and barriers to meaningful involvement of mental health service users in national planning in Ethiopia.

Rights-based approach to mental health

A key principle of mental health care planning is the respect of human rights, which means that all strategies, actions, and interventions for care, prevention, and promotion must uphold the

> **Box 39.1** Case study 1: service user involvement in national planning in Ethiopia
>
> The importance of involving mental health service users and caregivers in the improvement of the healthcare system is being acknowledged by stakeholders around the world, both in theory and in practice with varying pace across countries (Tambuyzer et al., 2014).
>
> Service user involvement is in general a new practice especially in low- and middle-income countries such as Ethiopia. Let alone in planning exercises at national level, service users are not even involved in their personal treatment plans. These are normally discussed with caregivers or simply administered by the medical staff with no discussion at all with the people experiencing the mental health problem who are directly affected.
>
> In Ethiopia, mental health services are organized by primary, secondary, and tertiary level. The health posts and health centres constitute the primary level. General hospitals are at secondary level and specialized hospitals are the highest tier of mental health services. There is no mental health policy but a National Mental Health Strategic Plan (NMHSP), which sets out a road map for the coming five years. In the revision of this Plan, service users were involved through their association, the Ethiopian Mental Health Service Users Association (MHSUA).
>
> The NMHSP intends to engage mental health care users at different levels. It recognizes the advocacy role service users and other civil organizations can play in creating more effective and accountable policies, laws, and services for mental health in a manner consistent with international and regional human rights instruments. It also recognizes the importance of involving them in identifying community needs and appropriate interventions. The role of lived experience is also highlighted in the fight against stigma and discrimination.
>
> The establishment of the MHSUA is acknowledged as an opportunity to build on in the NMHSP's SWOT analysis. This is a milestone for the historically voiceless service users in the country. The NMHSP also recognizes service users, their organizations, and the community as one of the stakeholders on which depends the effective implementation of the NMHSP. In addition, peer support delivered by service users is considered as one of the treatment options in the 'Optimal Mix of Mental Health Service' in the NMHSP.
>
> Ethiopia does not have a specific mental health legislation, but a Health Act is at draft stage, where mental health issues are addressed in few sections. The MHSUA was not invited to any of the consultation sessions even though they specifically asked the legal directorate to be involved in the discussion. It required a lot of personal effort by members of the MHSUA to access the draft and forward comments in a written letter copying the minister's office for greater visibility.
>
> Although the NMHSP sets out a requirement to involve service users at the planning and implementation stages, this usually does not happen or occurs in a tokenistic way which is not useful to highlight their perspectives. There is a lot to be done to ensure that service users are meaningfully engaged so that the desired change can occur at all levels.

principles enshrined in CRPD and existing international and regional human rights laws and instruments (WHO, 2021b). A rights-based approach to mental health care also means enabling and supporting people living with mental conditions in their decision-making and in taking control of their own lives and health, including the empowerment of champions and peer-support groups. Planning mental health care also needs to take an equity lens, ensuring that people have access to mental health care, delivery, prevention, promotion, and recovery according to their needs and without discrimination against vulnerable groups (Kola et al., 2021). The WHO's QualityRights initiative provides a toolkit of resources to train and guide inclusion of rights-based approaches to mental health care, to combat stigma and discrimination, to reform national policies and legislation in line with the CRPD and other global human rights standards, and to assess and monitor outcomes (WHO, 2012). Planners may also wish to initiate a process to develop or reform legislation to protect the rights of people with mental health conditions alongside the development of a national plan if such legislation is not already in place. Even without the framework of legislation, planners can also include targets and indicators into their plans that will allow them to track, review, and respond to rights violations. Comprehensive guidance and examples for adopting, amending, and implementing legislation related to mental health is available in the WHO (2023) publication *Mental Health, Human Rights and Legislation: Guidance and Practice*.

Parity between physical and mental health

People should have access to quality health care based on need, and with consideration of parity of mental and physical health services. This means that mental health and physical health should be valued and considered in equal terms (Millard & Wessely, 2014). Although the preamble to the WHO Constitution of 1946 defines mental health as equal to physical health (WHO, 2006), mental health globally does not have equal status in priority, quality, access to services, funding, and resources as physical health does. National funding for mental health across the globe is significantly lower than that for the proportionally equivalent burden of physical health. A massive gap persists for people with mental health conditions, with mortality being 20 years higher for men, and 15 years for women, compared to men and women who do not have a mental health conditions (Thornicroft, 2011).

Mental health conditions have wider effects on people, society, and the economy, in particular for severe and chronic conditions, where it is often difficult to separate mental conditions from physical conditions. Therefore, parity of esteem (of mental and physical health) is difficult to measure and challenging to be translated into plans and legislation (Millard & Wessely, 2014). While equal funding according to the relative prevalence and burden of metal health conditions will be an important step, parity of physical health requires more than just resources. Critically, it will mean that an equal status and respect should be achieved for people living with mental health conditions, their families, carers, and health care providers, as well as for research, compared to physical health conditions. This includes addressing excess mortality, quality of care, access to services, stigma and discrimination, development of treatments and therapies, and monitoring and evaluation of interventions. The WHO Mental Health Action Plan provides a comprehensive guideline for planners, how to take steps towards achieving parity of esteem (WHO, 2021b).

People-centred and recovery-oriented care

People-centred care means taking the perspectives of people with LE, their carers, and their communities into account, focusing on their comprehensive needs, and including them as beneficiaries and participants of the health systems and care delivery (WHO, 2018a). The process of national mental health planning should include these stakeholders and consider their needs for information and how they can be involved in ongoing governance of local mental health plan implementation. A people-centred plan will necessarily be multisectoral (see 'Multisectoral collaboration and action') as the needs of people with mental health conditions go beyond what the health system can supply. People-centred care also requires planners to institute structures to facilitate greater involvement of individual people with LE in decisions about their care, including advanced directives and supported decision-making. Effective people-centred care also needs to consider the cultural context of mental health care, supporting people with LE to integrate different sources of healing that are meaningful to supporting their recovery.

The concept of 'personal recovery' captures the journey that a people with LE takes to overcome or live with the challenges that mental health conditions bring, seeking to achieve outcomes that are of value to them. The national mental health plan needs to be orientated around supporting people with LE to achieve what matters most to them, and not be narrowly focused on clinical symptom control and protection. Personal recovery does not necessarily mean that an individual is in remission from symptoms. For example, personal recovery goals might include being able to work, feeling part of a community, or be related to an individual's spiritual life. Achieving this through national mental health planning may require changes to mental health training of health workers, grassroots efforts to empower people with LE to advocate for their valued goals, and coordination of input from non-biomedical healers to care.

Integrated and community-based care

Provision of comprehensive, integrated, and responsive mental health and social care services in community-based settings is more accessible and affordable for people with mental health conditions and their families. Care that is 'close to home' helps to maximize social support and promote recovery. Care in non-institutional settings is also less likely to involve coercion or other violations of human rights. Integration of care upholds the principle of parity between mental health and physical health care.

Integration of mental health into primary and general health care services can be done in a number of different ways, but the principle is that mental health care is an integral part of health care and is, therefore, everybody's business. This means that planners need to consider what role each health (and social care) worker will play in mental health care and ensure that their training, supervision, competencies, and job specifications are aligned with these expectations.

Mental health must be integrated into all health programmes and must be included as part of the plans for these programmes. In addition to the WHO's mhGAP programme that integrates mental health with physical health within primary care (see 'National mental health planning within the global policy context'), given high comorbidities with HIV, TB, non-communicable diseases, and maternal health, for example, mental health needs to be included in the care plans of these diseases. Integration of mental health into primary health care is recommended as an important contribution to achieving universal health coverage. This approach requires at least the following to be in place (WHO, 2021a): (1) guidelines for mental health integration into primary health care are available and adopted at the national level; (2) pharmacological and psychosocial interventions for mental health conditions are available and provided at the primary care level; (3) health workers at primary care level receive training on the management of mental health conditions; and (4) mental health specialists are involved in the training and supervision of primary care professionals.

It is important for countries to plan care for people with a range of different conditions. Integrated health services should provide people with a continuum of care, from health promotion, disease prevention, and management to rehabilitation services, which are coordinated and delivered beyond the health sector and according to their changing needs throughout the life course (WHO, 2018a).

A 'whole-of-society' approach

Mental health plans should be embedded within a wider population perspective or 'whole-of-society' approach to allow a country to meet the mental health needs of their population (Purtle et al., 2020). Population-based approaches to mental health will need to include three areas for national planning: (1) social, economic, and environmental policy interventions (to be implemented by legislators and public agency directors); (2) public health practice interventions (to be implemented by public health department officials); and (3) health care system interventions (to be implemented by hospital and health care system leaders).

As previously described in the section 'National Mental health planning within the global policy context', mental health conditions are heavily interrelated with social determinants. Social determinants describe the influence of contextual factors that influence mental health, and they include a broad range of social, economic, structural, and environmental factors (Lund et al., 2018). Social adversities and inequalities commonly cluster in particular populations, interacting with both physical and mental health as 'syndemics' (Mendenhall et al., 2017). Planners need to recognize where syndemics may be operating in their own populations and plan for an adequate response. Syndemic-informed planning will integrate understanding of how to address complex interrelationships between pathophysiology, socioeconomic conditions, health system structures, and cultural context, to achieve better design and implementation of prevention and intervention programmes. For example, historically disadvantaged ethnic groups may face structural barriers to accessing care, while exposed to persistent poverty, unsafe neighbourhoods, and poor nutrition. National mental health planners may need to develop innovative care models, for example, involving community outreach and coordination of economic and nutrition interventions alongside broader efforts to address political marginalization.

Key elements of mental health planning

Clear, feasible mental health care plans are the link between commitment and action. A national mental health plan may be based on a well-designed mental health policy/ies, or countries may start off with a mental health strategy which is nested within an overarching health policy and/or even other policies, such as social care, or development/poverty reduction. Developing a mental health plan means setting priorities for the major strategies to achieve and implement the mental health policy, and to establish the estimated time frame and required resources. The mental health plan should clearly outline in detail how the policy/ies and their objectives will be implemented (WHO, 2009).

Planners must know how to design, implement, and scale up services and other interventions for mental health and to work with a range of stakeholders and sectors to achieve better mental health for all.

A vision for national mental health planning

The essence of national health planning is to translate the vision of what is desired for mental health in a country into reality. While the key areas that countries need to address are highlighted in the WHO Global Action Plan, national plans are needed to contextualize these objectives and translate them into implementable programmes through which the targets can be met. Critically, the latter three objectives of the Plan (to achieve improved care, prevention and promotion, and information and research) will require those appointed or elected into leadership and governance positions (the first objective) to develop, in collaboration with key stakeholders, focused and realizable mental health plans, as these are the key to concrete change. If there is no effective leadership in a country then appointing and training such leadership may also become part of the plan.

Logically, a national mental health policy and legislation should be in place prior to the development of an implementation plan, as this will greatly facilitate the concrete requirement for planning. However, many countries still have no, or very basic, mental health policies or legislation in place, and changes or improvements may be needed before effective mental health plans can be developed and implemented. On the other hand, in some contexts, policies and legislation can be developed in parallel with a plan. Legislation in particular may take a long time to get enacted and should not be an impediment to action in national mental health planning. In any event, before concrete planning begins, it is essential that the country knows what it wants to achieve and the broad principles of how this will be done. For example, before concrete planning can begin, the country must have decided on fundamental directions for mental health. A country may have a vision to utilize a primarily community mental health care approach rather than an emphasis on hospital care (see 'Gaps in existing national mental health planning'). Other fundamental decisions may be to integrate mental health into general health care or to have prioritized specific conditions to focus on initially. A vision needs to capture the multisectoral nature of any mental health response, and to indicate how non-health policy and planning areas, such as economics and finance, work and pensions, education, justice, family, security, and development, can be harnessed to achieve mental health goals.

What is in a plan?

Whereas a mental health policy is supposed to define the aims, a mental health care plan translates these policy aims into action. A national mental health plan is a clear guide on taking national health policies into strategies and breaking these down into activities to ensure their implementation. The plan defines specific action, targets, and indicators to measure the progress and outcomes and sets a clear time frame (Funk & Drew, 2015). The plan will outline how the country will realize and promote the priority areas. Policy and planning areas may vary in different countries and regions and at different time periods, but the WHO has identified several areas of action that have been involved in most of the policies and plans developed over the past 20 years (Saraceno et al., 2005). To be effective, mental health planning needs to simultaneously plan to realize the following areas:

- Coordination
- Financing
- Legislation and human rights
- Organization of services (**Figure 39.1**)
- Human resources and training
- Promotion, prevention, treatment, and rehabilitation
- Essential drug procurement and distribution
- Advocacy
- Quality improvement
- Information systems
- Research and evaluation of policies and services
- Intersectoral collaboration.

Recommended structures for mental health systems and services

A national plan should envision how a mental health system will be structured, as well as the organization and mix of services that are required to achieve the goal of population mental health. The mental health system is part of the overall health system. Recommendations for high-quality health systems thus apply to the mental health system (Kruk et al., 2018). The WHO's 'building blocks' for health system strengthening provide a framework for critical areas which are relevant also for mental health (WHO, 2007). At its core, the mental health system needs to be for people (see 'Multisectoral collaboration and action'), equitable, efficient, and resilient. The mental health system should be able to inspire confidence and deliver improved mental health and economic benefits (at individual, household, and country level). The foundation for this is to:

- respond to population mental health needs and expectations (identified through situation analyses, epidemiological studies, and consultative processes)
- ensure governance structures and processes are in place where needed (e.g. policies, legislation, and health insurance that includes mental health conditions; administrators and leaders orientated to mental health)
- link mental health care to relevant platforms (e.g. within health care, education, prisons, and traditional and religious healing)
- expand, equip, and support the mental health workforce (e.g. specialist mental health workers from different disciplines (psychiatrists, psychologists, social workers, psychiatric nurses, counsellors), general health workers trained for task-shared care, and lay workers for community-based rehabilitation)
- establish structures to avail necessary interventions, including psychological and social interventions alongside medication and core laboratory investigations
- ensure relevant information and data are collected and used to allow assessment of the performance of the mental health system, as well as providing input for improvement.

Building on these foundations and integral to achieving the desired outcomes of a mental health system, there needs to be careful attention to supporting the delivery of competent care, standardizing and improving care processes, and ensuring a positive user experience of care.

The WHO has proposed a pyramid of the optimal mix of services to deliver population mental health (WHO, 2009) (**Figure 39.1**). This

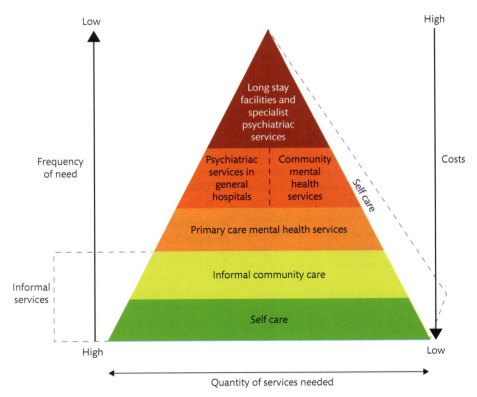

Figure 39.1 WHO service organization pyramid for an optimal mix of services for mental health.
Source: World Health Organization (2009). *Improving Health Systems and Services for Mental Health*. Geneva: World Health Organization.

pyramid emphasizes that the largest component of mental health care occurs outside of formal mental health services; for example, through the things that individuals and communities do to promote and support mental health (self-care, social support, and social inclusion) and non-biomedical approaches to healing. Even within the health system, most mental health care should be delivered through primary and general health care settings (e.g. through task-shared models of care). The WHO mhGAP resources are designed for these tiers of the pyramid. Thus, most people with a mental health condition do not need to directly see a mental health specialist. For those who do need more specialist input, outpatient care will be the most common, and only a minority will need more assertive community mental health team input or inpatient care or long-term residential care. This model of the mix of services has profound implications for the distribution of funding for mental health care and may require planning for the scaling down of psychiatric institutions.

Prevention and promotion

Recognizing that social and economic factors are critical to improved mental health outcomes is fundamental. Promoting mental health and preventing the development of mental health conditions are prerequisites for achieving mental health for all. Planning for mental health should hence embrace prevention and promotion, including acting on the social determinants of mental health (distal mental health promotion) as well as more proximal interventions such as parenting and anti-bullying programmes. Improved care and services that promote human rights and are available, affordable, appropriate, acceptable, and accessible and that take the full needs of people into account are similarly essential to achieving mental health for all. Mental health plans are embedded within a wider population health approach. They also need to keep the appropriate balance between efforts for mental health care of those with mental health conditions and prevention/promotion activities. Mental health planning is not an issue that concerns the department of health alone but affects almost all government departments and therefore requires intersectoral collaboration.

Multisectoral collaboration and action

In order to address the social determinants of mental health, mental health planning needs to develop integrated, cross-sectoral approaches and strategies. This means, in the case of poverty, for instance, that mental health planning needs to both plan for integrated approaches that reach people living in poverty, and that close links and collaborative approaches and planning need to be developed that specifically focus on poverty, together with the respective ministries and government departments, such as the ministry of finance, ministry of work and pensions, and ministry of education. In a socioeconomic environment where poverty is not addressed, the impact of singular mental health poverty interventions is unlikely to achieve sustainable population changes. Therefore, in order to improve mental health, poverty reduction will need to be addressed in an integrated way, in intersectoral collaboration, with individual leads by both ministries and departments in their policies and plans. It will need to be specified in mental health plans who will be responsible for initiating and establishing regular, intersectoral meetings with all relevant departments and sectors. Without this level of detail, plans easily become ideas rather than concrete realities.

Due to the interconnected nature of mental health with many socioeconomic factors, there is a critical need for truly integrated, multisectoral approaches for mental health planning and cross-governmental working (Patel et al., 2018). The sectors most relevant for intersectoral collaboration are those that provide services by welfare, religious, education, housing, employment, workplace, criminal justice, police, and other social services (Saraceno et al., 2005). The rights and responsibilities for mental health should be distributed across these sectors, including their financing. This does not imply that resources should be taken away from direct mental health interventions as these also benefit other sectors.

Mental health conditions put an excessive economic burden on society and across all sectors, beyond mental health services and care. Costs in other sectors occur as a consequence of people's mental conditions, and vice versa, the impact of other sectors does affect mental health outcomes. For instance, it has been found that in the criminal justice sector, for every £1 incurred in the health care sector as a consequence of drug dependency, an additional £13 was incurred in the criminal justice sector (Healey et al., 1998). Mental health interventions can, for instance, increase the impact of poverty reduction programmes, whereas providing mental health care can reduce food insecurity (Tirfessa et al., 2020).

At the same time, though, interventions in other sectors help to reduce mental health conditions and hence the need for services. For example, reducing poverty would lead to less care needs, while school-based mental health programmes would similarly result in better mental health and hence less people requiring care. The health sector, though, cannot take over the roles and responsibilities of other sectors from either a resource or a skills perspective, and therefore it is incumbent on these sectors to implement programmes that impact positively on mental health. The costs for and benefits that occur in non-health sectors have been defined as intersectoral costs and benefits. They are essential for health economics analyses and have been reported from a wide range of sectors, such as the labour, family, and criminal justice sector (Chisholm et al., 2016; Janssen et al., 2020) and different steps along the care pathway, such as recovery and prevention (Drost et al., 2013; Jørgensen et al., 2020).

Developing a mental health plan at the national level

An outline of mental health planning at the national level

Every country and context is different and all guidance will need to be adapted to the country-specific social, economic, cultural, and other contexts. However, some general principles and suggested steps for developing a national level mental health care plan are as follows (adapted from WHO (2009)):

Preparatory steps
Step 1: Determine the strategies and time frames
Step 2: Set indicators and targets
Step 3: Determine major activities
Step 4: Determine the costs and the resources available and budget accordingly
Step 5: Monitoring and evaluation.

Preparatory steps

Some preparatory steps may need to be considered, according to the country context. To start with, it will be necessary to gain an understanding of the national and district-level policy landscape and to clarify how the new plan can speak to existing plans and priorities. Conducting a situational analysis can be helpful, by assessing the population, context, stakeholders and their roles in the mental health planning process, resources (existing and needed) both from the mental health and other sectors, and service utilization (WHO, 2009).

Particularly, planners need to identify the key stakeholders and organizations/institutions who are and/or need to be engaged in the planning process, which include people with LE, health care providers, doctors, nurses, professional associations and special interest groups, and representatives from other government sectors. People who can be engaged in delivering mental health care at different levels of the health system need to be identified and brought into the network.

A SWOT analysis (strengths, weaknesses, opportunities, and threats) can be helpful to understand how existing policies (social care, poverty reduction, school-based health, etc.) provide opportunities or constrain options, and to develop a basis for strategic planning (Rajan, 2016).

A mapping exercise can help planners to identify existing resources and locations where further resources might be leveraged, for instance, in the sectors of HIV, non-communicable diseases, or maternal care. It may also be necessary to map out key social determinants for mental ill health in the specific context/country and to identify potential syndemics that need a coordinated response, and in particular in relation to vulnerable populations, and to identify local data which will need to inform the definition and achievement of the strategies.

A number of key drivers of population mental health can be mapped to inform national planning:

1. Relevant health issues include:
    - patterns of substance use
    - burden of chronic illness—HIV, TB (especially multidrug-resistant TB), and non-communicable diseases, all of which are strongly associated with mental health conditions
    - known suicide rates.
2. Social determinants include:
    - conflict and internally displaced persons
    - occupational drivers of poor mental health
    - poverty
    - sex/gender-based violence
    - child maltreatment
    - trauma exposures (e.g. linked to societal violence, high accident levels).

These drivers of population health should be considered by countries and addressed by their mental health plans. Policies and plans that address mental health indirectly and reduce psychosocial stress factors (e.g. through reducing poverty or traumatic events such as sex/gender-based violence), may have the greatest impact on population mental health (Purtle et al., 2020).

Step 1: Determine the strategies and time frames

Starting with the *elements of national mental health planning* (see above) which will have been defined and specified in the mental health policy, the first step is to formulate the core strategies and time frames for each area of action (Saraceno et al., 2005, p. 46). The strategies need to be checked and adapted to be coherent and coordinated so that they meet the key policy objectives. Consultations and negotiations with stakeholders and experts, including people living with mental health conditions, will be carried out to formulate and prioritize the strategies, often using SWOT analysis, looking to identify the strengths/weaknesses of the existing mental health system and the opportunities for/threats to the mental health policy and plans.

For each of the strategies, a time frame will be defined, clarifying start and end year/month. Some strategies will be permanently in place and others will only be required for a specific period. Budget constraints will need to be taken into consideration to ensure that resources and capacities allow for the strategies that have been identified to be fully implemented.

Step 2: Set indicators and targets

The next step is to break the strategies down and define targets and indicators for each strategy. The targets and indicators need to be clear and explicit, and state precisely what will be achieved within given time frames. All targets need to be measurable, specify indicators of how the achievement and completion of the target will be measured and assessed, and align with international reporting requirements where possible.

Step 3: Determine major activities

Next, for each strategy, detailed activities need to be defined that will ensure that and how the strategy will be realized. The mental health plan will list all activities that are planned, who is the named person responsible for the completion of the activity, the start, end, and duration of each activity, and a timeline of activities that clarifies which are carried out simultaneously and which follow on from each other. The expected outputs of each activity will be specified along with what the potential obstacles and delays are that could inhibit the realization of the activity.

Step 4: Determine the costs and the resources available and budget accordingly

The next and critical step in the mental health plan is to ensure that the implementation of all strategies is based on solid and available resources. Therefore, the costs of each activity need to be calculated and a summary of total cost of the plan for each year need to be established. The WHO OneHealth Tool was developed to support mental health planning, using an integrated approach, which means not assuming all costs were new costs (e.g. some people already employed, facilities already built), and also showing the expected return on investment in terms of health lives (Chisholm et al., 2017). The costs will include capital investments, recurring costs, human resources, consumables, and others. A key requirement will be to understand the capacity of the existing mental health workforce, both specialist and non-specialist health care workers.

Next, who will fund the resources required for the plan and each of the strategies needs to be defined. It is common in most countries to use mixed structures for health financing, which include varying proportions of state funding (general taxation), social insurance, donors, private insurance, and out-of-pocket payments. The funding should not be derived from the health sector alone, but is a multisectoral investment, and mental health expenditures will be required from a number of different government sectors (education, labour, justice, housing, etc.) as explained above (see 'Multisectoral collaboration and action'), while additional contributions will come from NGOs, service user/family organizations, and private donors/institutions (Chisholm et al., 2019). The time frames may need to be adjusted according to the available resources for different years.

Step 5: Monitoring and evaluation

Continuous monitoring and evaluation of the implementation of the mental health plan and strategies is essential and annual cycles of replanning and adjusting of resources and time frames will be required.

Strategies to overcome frequent challenges

Many countries have developed good mental health policies and plans, yet the implementation of the strategies often presents challenges which can lead to failure of the programmes or plans. Frequent challenges are highlighted here and strategies that can support countries in their design and implementation of a national mental health care plan, in particular ensuring that it fits the country context, continuous co-creation, and collaboration with stakeholders.

Contextualize the national mental health care plan

Many countries develop a perfect, idealistic policy, which is translated into the ideal national plan; yet, when it comes to implementation, the realities of district policies, plans, and funding present major challenges. Frequently, the plan does not sufficiently consider the specific context and conditions for enabling the implementation of the plan and strategies.

In order to ensure from the development phase that the national-level mental health care plan fits as best as possible the specific needs and context of the country, and to facilitate its implementation in practice, it is essential to contextualize it to the specific country settings, and regional and local differences. Mental health plans will differ across countries, depending on their resources, socioeconomic context, existing mental health services, and level of integration into primary health care to date. For instance, details, strategies, and indicators for mental health plans will differ for low- and middle-income countries compared to high-income countries and may also differ between planning for mental health in an urban area relative to a rural area. A careful assessment of the country-specific context, mental health needs, and social, economic, and cultural conditions is required from the start of developing the plan (and already at policy stage), and throughout the plan design and implementation phase. In particular, an assessment of mental health-related stigma and discrimination is needed, and the situation and level of involvement of people with LE of mental conditions. Another important contextual factor to consider is the existing and future funding for mental health care, and which structures, programmes, and stakeholders will be involved, under which premises. Many countries face differences in regional and local contexts for mental health care, for instance, because of religious minorities, regions of conflict, and poverty. A good mental health plan

Collaborate with stakeholders throughout

A further challenge that many countries face when developing and implementing their mental health plan is the involvement of all the key stakeholders. Many plans are at risk, or fail, because the people who are supposed to carry out the plan and who are affected by the strategies have not been sufficiently part of the development of the plan, may even not be aware of the plan, not be in line with its strategies, or are unable to carry it out for a number of reasons, such as lack of resources, lack of training, or others.

In order to properly contextualize plans, and more generally to ensure that plans are not just plans for the sake of developing mental health care plans, it is critical to collaborate and co-create the national mental health care plan together with all relevant stakeholders and to maintain their involvement throughout the implementation of the plan and strategies. Co-creation with stakeholders prevents the plan from failing to match reality of systems, services, and people in place to carry out the work. Involving stakeholders from the beginning is also critical to gain their buy-in, by developing the strategies jointly and continuous collaboration will help to mobilize and sustain their involvement throughout. The engagement and relationships with stakeholders need to be actively initiated and will include people from across the system, covering all areas of the optimal mix of services for mental health from specialist services, long-stay facilities, community mental health services, psychiatric/psychological services in general hospitals, mental health services through primary health care, informal community care, and self-care (WHO, 2003).

See **Box 39.2** for an example of how collaboration at both the national and provincial level was essential for developing a workable plan to decentralize mental health care in South Africa.

This means involving policymakers, planners, with the mental health workforce, both formal and informal, traditional/faith healers, academics, and others. Particularly important is the inclusion and collaboration with people with LE of mental conditions, their families, and caregivers. Co-creation and collaboration also require enabling all stakeholders to participate and contribute, which will include remuneration for time and transport costs, training and empowerment of service users to enable their active involvement, and careful consideration of power differences and stigmatizing attitudes towards people with LE and how to overcome/address these throughout.

Create a supportive network for a system change

Oftentimes, it can be very challenging to engage other stakeholders for action for mental health, and in particular for other sectors to take responsibility for mental health activities within their remit. With budget and resource constraints across all sectors, many mental health plans struggle to gain support and initiative from other sectors to commit funding and workforce to cross-linked mental health-related actions.

Box 39.2 Case study 2: multilevel planning for decentralized implementation—a case study from South Africa

Responsibility for health in South Africa, like many countries around the world, occurs at different levels. The national department of health has responsibility for mental health legislation and policy and must monitor and evaluate national outputs and outcomes, while provinces (of which there are nine) are required to implement this policy and to provide the budgets and other resources for this, such as human resources, physical facilities, and medication. In turn, primary health care, including district hospital care, is decentralized to district health authorities (52 in total) to be implemented through district health systems. Given this structure, it is critical that national planning neither runs ahead of, nor falls behind, provincial and district realities. This includes human and financial resource availability and affordability as well as the willingness and readiness of provinces and districts to implement national plans.

Prior to South Africa adopting its National Policy Framework and Strategic Plan 2013–2020, it underwent extensive consultation with key stakeholders such as people with LE, professional bodies, NGOs, and with mental health providers at primary, secondary, and tertiary levels. It was then adopted by the National Health Council. Critically, this body comprises of the national minister *and* their provincial counterparts and therefore had the support of both national and provincial governments. Among the key decisions taken in this policy framework were that general hospitals would be expanded to include mental health/psychiatry and that district mental health teams would be set up in each district. The latter was seen as a critical element to achieve the goal of decentralizing mental health services into communities and the scaling down of psychiatric hospitals. Clear roles and responsibilities were set out for these teams and included conducting a situation analysis of mental health needs and service resources in the district population, and developing an action plan for promotion, prevention, treatment, and recovery for that district; establishing routine ongoing training and supervision and care pathways; integrating mental health into services such as HIV, maternal health, and chronic diseases; and building capacity for users (service users, their families) to provide appropriate self-help and peer-led services, such as support groups, facilitated by NGOs. A consensus was reached by all stakeholders that unless there was a team of people in each district that was responsible for planning and ensuring implementation of mental health services in the district, including the integration into primary health care, that mental health would remain neglected and that a number of the objectives outlined in the policy would remain theoretical only.

By the end of the policy period 40 regional and district general hospitals in South Africa had a psychiatric unit, with a total of 1665 beds. These units are largely run by medical officers with support provided by psychiatrists from specialized psychiatric hospitals. One hundred and eighty-eight general hospitals (of a total of 315 public hospitals in the country) were designated to conduct 72-hour assessment of involuntary mental health care users. This reflects relatively good progress on implementation of the national policy. On the other hand, only 11 districts out of 52 had established a district mental health team. Most districts said that lack of resources was the main reason why no team had been established.

This case study illustrates that if a policy and plan is to translate from paper into changed lives, getting full commitment from all levels of governance and implementation partners into the adoption of a policy is critical. However, it also illustrates that buy-in, even genuine buy-in from the level of implementation, does not necessarily translate into change, especially where demands for resources are also being made from other health areas, as happened in South Africa over this time period. Ongoing advocacy and lobbying for implementation of a mental health plan is needed from well before the plan is drafted but must continue throughout its duration, otherwise other priorities are likely to take precedence. Those responsible for mental health at a national level also need to use their monitoring and evaluation functions to keep pressure on lower levels where implementation is slow or not happening at all.

It is critically important to engage all sectors in a system-wide change, including commitments to change policies and legislation and integration of mental health across their own plans. The ministry of health, the health districts, and the leads of the mental health plan will need to actively drive the information, dissemination, and advocacy for the new strategies. They will need to raise awareness that mental conditions not only cause very significant suffering to people with mental health conditions, their families, and communities but also contribute a significant proportion of the global burden of disease (disability-adjusted life years). Mental health planners also will need to raise awareness and action for addressing the cross-links of mental health conditions with other health priorities and sectors, and the financial and resource needs and demands that are existing. Lastly, they will need to generate political support and funding across all sectors and stakeholders.

The WHO Comprehensive Mental Health Action Plan 2013–2030 proposes that all countries set up a functional mental health unit or coordination mechanism(s) in the health ministry, with an allocated budget and responsibility for strategic planning, coordination, needs assessment, inter-ministerial, and multisectoral collaboration and service evaluation for mental health across the life course. This would appear to be a minimum requirement for national mental health planning. Ideally, though, national planning requires a competent group of public health and mental health experts to lead, manage, and drive planning efforts. Moreover, these individuals need to be drawn from, or established in, all levels of the health system and beyond, and include service users, to create a supportive network that can drive the system change from within (Saraceno et al., 2005). At the level of the ministry of health, a multidisciplinary team will be ideal, and should include psychiatrists, public health physicians, psychologists, psychiatric nurses, social workers, and occupational therapists. At the health district level, a similar setup to the ministry of health would be ideal, but importantly including a mental health professional. At community level, the teams should have a coordinator that will be assigned for several hours per week to public health and management. At primary care level, each facility/team should also have a dedicated mental health coordinator.

The aim of the collaboration is also to be able to engage key stakeholders and committed individuals to create a 'coalition of the willing', which will be established within a supportive organization. Relationships are the central, most critical mechanism in the process of getting mental health evidence into policy and practice, and the active and sustained engagement of key stakeholders is critical to reinforce intersectoral collaboration (Votruba et al., 2021). The aim is to establish a system that is sustainable beyond individuals leaving and changing institutions. Interactions and collaborations between and across all levels need to be actively driven and include a clear and strong involvement of people with LE, and ideally beyond the health system, to include policy, media, and external stakeholders. This will also be helpful to recognize and benefit from catalysts or other opportunities that might present for mental health cross-links within the wider context. The EVITA (Evidence to Policy Advocacy framework) can be a helpful tool to support the process of engagement and networking throughout the mental health planning process and for increasing visibility of mental health across the network (Votruba et al., 2021). A series of workshops (theory of change) can help to provide strategic direction for policy and programmes, by defining the aims and strategies, clarifying the challenges, and identifying what else is needed to implement the changes (Breuer et al., 2016).

See **Box 39.3** for an example of how NGOs in Nepal helped to form a collaboration of stakeholders to galvanize national mental health planning.

Guidelines and materials

A number of guidelines and advice exist for developing a mental health care plan at national level. The WHO has produced a comprehensive guidance package of manuals to assist policymakers and planners in developing and improving national policy, plans and programmes, the *Mental Health Policy and Service Guidance*, of which in particular the 2005 updated module on 'Mental Health Policy, Plans and Programmes' provides very clear and straightforward guidance (Saraceno et al., 2005). Though this document is relatively old, the guidance for developing and implementing a mental health plan remains current. This module is complemented in a report entitled *Improving Health Systems and Services for Mental Health* (WHO, 2009). It presents guidance on organization of mental health services, based on the WHO model of optimal mental health care and other principles for organizing mental health services, gives support in planning and budgeting for mental health, quality improvement, human resources/workforce and training, information systems, financing, psychotropic medication, psychological and psychosocial interventions, and helpful checklists for evaluating mental health plans (and policy and legislation). The package on 'Organization of services for mental health' gives useful guidance on the overall integration of mental health services into the general health system and into primary care (WHO, 2003). Another helpful resource for national-level integration is the report on 'Integrating mental health into primary care' which provides guidance and case studies on how to successfully integrate mental health into primary care and highlights ten common principles which are central for achieving integrated mental health care (Funk, 2008).

Helpful guidance is also provided by the WHO 'Assessment Instrument for Mental Health Systems' (WHO-AIMS), a tool that helps collect essential information on the mental health system of a country/region, which aims to improve mental health systems and to provide a baseline for monitoring the change (WHO, 2005). The WHO 'Guidance on community mental health services' provides information and support to planners for developing or transforming the mental health system and developing community mental health services that are aligned with international human rights standards and focus on recovery (WHO, 2021c).

In addition, much learning can be drawn from country reports and case studies and the specific challenges they faced (Minoletti & Zaccaria, 2005). Throughout this chapter, we also present a number of case reports (see **Box 39.1**: a case study from Ethiopia; **Box 39.2**, a case study from South Africa; and **Box 39.3**, a case study from Nepal).

Recommendations for successful planning at national level

See **Box 39.4**.

Box 39.3 Case study 3: non-governmental organizations driving the planning agenda in Nepal

NGOs in Nepal have played an essential role in mental health systems strengthening (Upadhaya et al., 2014). NGOs have contributed to the capacity building of paraprofessionals, service delivery, research, and advocacy work in the mental health sector. NGOs have increasingly contributed to national planning and policymaking, evidenced by their continuous collaboration and involvement in governmental activities and decision-making processes.

This rise in involvement of NGOs has, however, been a slow and uphill process with national conflict, natural disasters (such as the 2015 earthquake), and increased international interest in mental health acting as a catalyst. In Nepal, the WHO's mhGAP was first implemented through the Program for Improving Mental Health Care (PRIME), led by an NGO (the Transcultural Psychosocial Organization (TPO) Nepal) working in close collaboration with government stakeholders. A baseline situation analysis identified key gaps in existing systems of care (Luitel et al., 2015). Prioritization exercises and theory of change workshops conducted with the government stakeholders then helped to respond to this situation to develop a district mental health care plan. This provided the foundations for development of a community mental health care package endorsed by the government.

Alongside this work, the 'Emerging mental health systems in low- and middle-income countries' (Emerald) project was implemented to study and improve mental health systems alongside the PRIME project (Thornicroft et al., 2019). Again NGO led (by TPO Nepal), this project conducted a series of studies and activities to help identify barriers and provide recommendations to strengthen the mental health systems in Nepal. This included development of mental health indicators for routine data collection in the health facilities, costing of mental health care and sustainable financing mechanisms for sustainable mental health services, and highlighting the importance of involvement of stakeholders including people with LE in national mental healthcare policy and planning processes.

In the aftermath of the 2015 earthquake, which caused the loss of about 9000 lives in Nepal, there was an increased international response in the psychosocial and mental health sector as part of 'building back better' initiatives (Chase et al., 2018). This shifted the government's focus on psychosocial and mental health care to centre stage. The government and NGOs collaborated with local stakeholders including policymakers, security personnel, community-based organizations, local saving and credit cooperatives, and other community groups to effectively plan and deliver psychosocial and mental health care services, drawing directly on lessons learned through PRIME. During this period, the international NGOs working in mental health, advocacy groups formed by people with LE, and the WHO advocated for revision of mental health policy, inclusion of psychotropic drugs in the free drug list, and appointment of a focal point for mental health in the ministry of health. Through such efforts, 11 psychotropic drugs were added to the government's free drug list, mental health training curricula were developed for different cadres of government health workers, a national focal person for mental health was appointed, and a national budget was secured for implementation of community mental health programmes. More recently, the ministry of health has endorsed mental health strategy and action plans (2020) that were developed together with stakeholders from NGOs, advocacy groups, and mental health departments of national academic institutions.

This case study highlights the contribution made by NGOs in Nepal over the years to mainstream mental health. When NGOs actively involve government stakeholders and local community groups in the planning and implementation of their mental health programmes, this not only creates buy-in but also helps to achieve sustainable scale-up of such programmes at national level.

Case study courtesy of Dristy Durung, TPO Nepal, Kathmandu, Nepal; Health Service and Population Research (HSPR) Department, Institute of Psychiatry, Psychology, and Neuroscience (IOPPN), King's College London, London, UK.

Box 39.4 Ten recommendations for successful national mental health plans

1. Involve all the key players from the beginning of the planning process, national and regional, to ensure buy-in throughout.
2. Actively facilitate the early and active inclusion and contribution of People with LE of mental health conditions so that the plan upholds their rights and meets their needs.
3. Include civil society groups, faith-based organizations, and NGOs in mental health, and draw on their resources.
4. Establish a robust mechanism to ensure multisectoral collaboration early on—if possible chaired by a senior government minister.
5. Identify champions to raise and maintain motivation across all stakeholders for implementation of a plan and increase awareness through sustained and coordinated advocacy.
6. Plan for national needs, priorities, and contexts rather than for a global audience, while also making sure to design the plan to achieve the global policy targets that a national plan is expected to achieve.
7. Draw on best practice from around the world—link with mental health planners from other countries and review published evidence to find out what is working well in neighbouring countries with similar challenges and opportunities.
8. Ensure that the plan has time frames, a budget, and a designated lead per section who must be held accountable for implementation.
9. Monitor and evaluate how well a plan is working so that it can be improved.
10. Ensure that a national programme to reduce stigma and discrimination is rolled out alongside the implementation of the plan.

Conclusion

This chapter presents a brief overview of the what and how of planning mental health care on a national level. Even though most countries have some level of mental health plan, the effective implementation could often be improved. Principles and approaches are presented that help planners ensure that mental health care plans are following a multisectoral, needs-based strategy, are rights based, community based, and integrated. Partnering with people with LE and facilitating their engagement throughout the planning and implementation and evaluation process will be critical to realize people-centred care and to reduce stigma. An outline of essential steps for a mental health plan and strategies to overcome challenges, together with guidance materials, should support planners in taking the plan into action.

The aim of this chapter was to give policymakers and planners guidance on why and how to develop a mental health care plan, and information and resources to take their work further. Many countries are working hard to develop suitable plans for mental health care, and yet there are many challenges in the complex system that may affect or hinder successful implementation. In particular, stigma is a complex and pervasive factor influencing the implementation of national mental health care plans and will require additional efforts from planners and others. Finally, some of the limitations of national planning are that even good plans may not necessarily change things on the ground, immediately or at all. Hopefully some of the main challenges can be avoided, and new learnings in the future will contribute to greater effectiveness in mental health plans and their implementation.

REFERENCES

Breuer, E., De Silva, M. J., Shidaye, R., Petersen, I., Nakku, J., Jordans, M. J., et al. (2016). Planning and evaluating mental health services in low- and middle-income countries using theory of change. *British Journal of Psychiatry*, **208**(Suppl 56), s55–s62.

Chase, L. E., Marahatta, K., Sidgel, K., Shrestha, S., Gautam, K., Luitel, N. P., et al. (2018). Building back better? Taking stock of the post-earthquake mental health and psychosocial response in Nepal. *International Journal of Mental Health Systems*, **12**, 1–2.

Chisholm, D., Docrat, S., Abdulmalik, J., Alem, A., Gureje, O., Gurung, D., et al. (2019). Mental health financing challenges, opportunities and strategies in low- and middle-income countries: findings from the Emerald project. *BJPsych Open*, **5**, e68.

Chisholm, D., Flisher, A., Lund, C., Patel, V., Saxena, S., Thornicroft, G., & Tomlinson, M. (2007). Scale up services for mental disorders: a call for action. *Lancet*, **370**, 1241–1252.

Chisholm, D., Heslin, M., Docrat, S., Nanda, S., Shidhaye, R., Upadhaya, N., et al. (2017). Scaling-up services for psychosis, depression and epilepsy in sub-Saharan Africa and South Asia: development and application of a mental health systems planning tool (OneHealth). *Epidemiology and Psychiatric Sciences*, **26**, 234–244.

Chisholm, D., Sweeny, K., Sheehan, P., Rasmussen, B., Smit, F., Cuijpers, P., & Saxena, S. (2016). Scaling-up treatment of depression and anxiety: a global return on investment analysis. *Lancet Psychiatry*, **3**, 415–424.

Collins, P. Y. (2020). What is global mental health? *World Psychiatry*, **19**, 265–266.

COVID-19 Mental Disorders Collaborators (2021). Global prevalence and burden of depressive and anxiety disorders in 204 countries and territories in 2020 due to the COVID-19 pandemic. *Lancet*, **398**, 1700–1712.

Drew, N., Funk, M., Tang, S., Lamichhane, J., Chávez, E., Katontoka, S., et al. (2011). Human rights violations of people with mental and psychosocial disabilities: an unresolved global crisis. *Lancet*, **378**, 1664–1675.

Drost, R., Paulus, A., Ruwaard, D., & Evers, S. (2013). Inter-sectoral costs and benefits of mental health prevention: towards a new classification scheme. *Journal of Mental Health Policy and Economics*, **16**, 179–186.

Fisher, J., Cabral de Mello, M., Patel, V., Rahman, A., Tran, T., Holton, S., & Holmes, W. (2012). Prevalence and determinants of common perinatal mental disorders in women in low- and lower-middle-income countries: a systematic review. *Bulletin of the World Health Organization*, **90**, 139G–149G.

Funk, M. (2008). *Integrating Mental Health into Primary Care: A Global Perspective*. Geneva: World Health Organization.

Funk, M. K., & Drew, N. J. (2015). Mental health policy and strategic plan. *EMHJ-Eastern Mediterranean Health Journal*, **21**, 522–526.

GBD 2019 Mental Disorders Collaborators (2022). Global, regional, and national burden of 12 mental disorders in 204 countries and territories, 1990–2019: a systematic analysis for the Global Burden of Disease Study 2019. *Lancet Psychiatry*, **9**, 137–150.

Healey, A., Knapp, M., Astin, J., Gossop, M., Marsden, J., Stewart, D., et al. (1998). Economic burden of drug dependency: social costs incurred by drug users at intake to the National Treatment Outcome Research Study. *British Journal of Psychiatry*, **173**, 160–165.

Janssen, L. M. M., Pokhilenko, I., Evers, S., Paulus, A. T. G., Simon, J., Konig, H. H., et al. (2020). Exploring the identification, validation, and categorization of the cost and benefits of criminal justice in mental health: the PECUNIA project. *International Journal of Technology Assessment in Health Care*, **36**, 418–425.

Jørgensen, K., Rasmussen, T., Hansen, M., Andreasson, K., & Karlsson, B. (2020). Recovery-oriented intersectoral care in mental health: as perceived by healthcare professionals and users. *International Journal of Environmental Research and Public Health*, **17**, 8777.

Kessler, R. C., Aguilar-Gaxiola, S., Alonso, J., Chatterji, S., Lee, S., Ormel, J., et al. (2011). The global burden of mental disorders: an update from the WHO World Mental Health (WMH) surveys. *Epidemiologia e Psichiatria Sociale*, **18**, 23–33.

Kohn, R., Saxena, S., Levav, I., & Saraceno, B. (2004). The treatment gap in mental health care. *Bulletin of the World Health Organization*, **82**, 858–866.

Kola, L., Kohrt, B. A., Acharya, B., Mutamba, B. B., Kieling, C., Kumar, M., et al. (2021). The path to global equity in mental health care in the context of COVID-19. *Lancet*, **398**, 1670–1672.

Kruk, M. E., Gage, A. D., Arsenault, C., Jordan, K., Leslie, H. H., Roder-DeWan, S., et al. (2018). High-quality health systems in the Sustainable Development Goals era: time for a revolution. *Lancet Global Health*, **6**, e1196–e1252.

Kumar, S., Pathare, S., & Esponda, G. M. (2021). COVID-19 vaccine prioritisation for individuals with psychoses. *Lancet Psychiatry*, **8**, 751.

Kuper, H. (2020). Disability, mental health, stigma and discrimination and neglected tropical diseases. *Transactions of the Royal Society of Tropical Medicine and Hygiene*, **115**, 145–146.

Liu, N. H., Daumit, G. L., Dua, T., Aquila, R., Charlson, F., Cuijpers, P., et al. (2017). Excess mortality in persons with severe mental disorders: a multilevel intervention framework and priorities for clinical practice, policy and research agendas. *World Psychiatry*, **16**, 30–40.

Luitel, N. P., Jordans, M. J., Adhikari, A., Upadhaya, N., Hanlon, C., Lund, C., & Komproe, I. H. (2015). Mental health care in Nepal: current situation and challenges for development of a district mental health care plan. *Conflict and Health*, **9**, 1.

Lund, C., Brooke-Sumner, C., Baingana, F., Baron, E. C., Breuer, E., Chandra, P., et al. (2018). Social determinants of mental disorders and the Sustainable Development Goals: a systematic review of reviews. *Lancet Psychiatry*, **5**, 357–369.

Mendenhall, E., Kohrt, B. A., Norris, S. A., Ndetei, D., & Prabhakaran, D. (2017). Non-communicable disease syndemics: poverty, depression, and diabetes among low-income populations. *Lancet*, **389**, 951–963.

Millard, C. & Wessely, S. (2014). Parity of esteem between mental and physical health. *BMJ*, **349**, g6821.

Minoletti, A. & Zaccaria, A. (2005). The National Mental Health Plan in Chile: 10 years of experience. *Revista panamericana de salud publica/Pan American Journal of Public Health*, **18**, 346–358.

Patel, V., Araya, R., Chatterjee, S., Chisholm, D., Cohen, A., De Silva, M., et al. (2007). Treatment and prevention of mental disorders in low-income and middle-income countries. *Lancet*, **370**, 991–1005.

Patel, V., Saxena, S., Lund, C., Thornicroft, G., Baingana, F., Bolton, P., et al. (2018). The Lancet Commission on global mental health and sustainable development. *Lancet*, **392**, 1553–1598.

Pathare, S., Brazinova, A., & Levav, I. (2018). Care gap: a comprehensive measure to quantify unmet needs in mental health. *Epidemiology and Psychiatric Sciences*, **27**, 463–467.

Purtle, J., Nelson, K. L., Counts, N. Z., & Yudell, M. (2020). Population-based approaches to mental health: history, strategies, and evidence. *Annual Review of Public Health*, **41**, 201–221.

Rajan, D. (2016). Situation analysis of the health sector. In: Schmets, G., Rajan, D., & Kadandale, S. (Ed.), *Strategizing National Health in the 21st Century: A Handbook* (pp. 103–157). Geneva: World Health Organization.

Saraceno, B., Funk, M., & Minoletti, A. (2005). *Mental Health Policy, Plans and Programmes (Updated Version 2)*. Geneva: World Health Organization.

Stein, D. J., Benjet, C., Gureje, O., Lund, C., Scott, K. M., Poznyak, V., & van Ommeren, M. (2019). Integrating mental health with other non-communicable diseases. *BMJ*, **364**, l295.

Tambuyzer, E., Pieters, G., & Van Audenhove, C. (2014). Patient involvement in mental health care: one size does not fit all. *Health Expectations*, **17**, 138–150.

Thornicroft, G. (2011). Physical health disparities and mental illness: the scandal of premature mortality. *British Journal of Psychiatry*, **199**, 441–442.

Tirfessa, K., Lund, C., Medhin, G., Selamu, M., Birhane, R., Hailemichael, Y., et al. (2020). Impact of integrated mental health care on food insecurity of households of people with severe mental illness in a rural African district: a community-based, controlled before–after study. *Tropical Medicine & International Health*, **25**, 414–423.

Thornicroft, G. & Semrau, M. (2019). Health system strengthening for mental health in low-and middle-income countries: introduction to the Emerald programme. *BJPsych Open*, **5**, 5.

United Nations (2017). Global indicator framework for the Sustainable Development Goals and targets of the 2030 Agenda for Sustainable Development. https://unstats.un.org/sdgs/indicators/indicators-list/

Upadhaya, N., Luitel, N. P., Koirala, S., Adhikari, R. P., Gurung, D., Shrestha, P., et al. (2014). The role of mental health and psychosocial support nongovernmental organisations: reflections from post conflict Nepal. *Intervention*, **12**(Suppl. 1), 113–128.

Vai, B., Mazza, M. G., Delli Colli, C., Foiselle, M., Allen, B., Benedetti, F., et al. (2021). Mental disorders and risk of COVID-19-related mortality, hospitalisation, and intensive care unit admission: a systematic review and meta-analysis. *Lancet Psychiatry*, **8**, 797–812.

Vigo, D., Jones, L., Atun, R., & Thornicroft, G. (2022). The true global disease burden of mental illness: still elusive. *Lancet Psychiatry*, **9**, 98–100.

Vigo, D., Thornicroft, G., & Atun, R. (2016). Estimating the true global burden of mental illness. *Lancet Psychiatry*, **3**, 171–178.

Votruba, N., Grant, J., & Thornicroft, G. (2021). EVITA 2.0, an updated framework for understanding evidence-based mental health policy agenda-setting: tested and informed by key informant interviews in a multilevel comparative case study. *Health Research Policy and Systems*, **19**, 35.

Whitley, R. (2015). Global mental health: concepts, conflicts and controversies. *Epidemiology and Psychiatric Sciences*, **24**, 285–291.

World Health Organization (2001a). Atlas of mental health resources in the world 2001. https://apps.who.int/iris/handle/10665/66910

World Health Organization (2001b). *The World Health Report 2001: Mental Health: New Understanding, New Hope*. Geneva: World Health Organization.

World Health Organization (2003). Organization of services for mental health (Mental health policy and service guidance package). https://iris.who.int/handle/10665/333104

World Health Organization (2005). *Assessment Instrument for Mental Health Systems—WHO-AIMS Version 2.2*. Geneva: World Health Organization.

World Health Organization (2006). Constitution of the World Health Organization. https://www.who.int/publications/m/item/constitution-of-the-world-health-organization

Word Health Organization (2007). Everybody's business: strengthening health systems to improve health outcomes: WHO's framework for action. https://extranet.who.int/mindbank/item/2068

World Health Organization (2009). *Improving Health Systems and Services for Mental Health*. Geneva: World Health Organization. https://www.who.int/publications/i/item/9789241598774

World Health Organization (2012). WHO QualityRights Toolkit: assessing and improving quality and human rights in health and social care facilities. https://apps.who.int/iris/handle/10665/66910

World Health Organization (2016). mhGAP intervention guide for mental, neurological and substance use disorders in non-specialized health settings: mental health Gap Action Programme (mhGAP). Version 2.0. https://www.who.int/publications/i/item/9789241549790

World Health Organization (2018a). Continuity and coordination of care: a practice brief to support implementation of the WHO Framework on integrated people-centred health services. https://www.who.int/publications/i/item/9789241514033

World Health Organization (2018b). *mhGAP Operations Manual: Mental Health Gap Action Programme (mhGAP)*. Geneva: World Health Organization. https://www.who.int/publications/i/item/mhgap-operations-manual

World Health Organization (2019). *Community mhGAP Toolkit Field Test Version: Mental Health Gap Action Programme (mhGAP)*. Geneva: World Health Organization. https://www.who.int/publications/i/item/the-mhgap-community-toolkit-field-test-version

World Health Organization (2021a). *Mental Health Atlas 2020*. Geneva: World Health Organization. https://www.who.int/publications/i/item/9789240036703

World Health Organization (2021b). *Comprehensive Mental Health Action Plan 2013–2030*. Geneva: World Health Organization.

World Health Organization (2021c). *Guidance on Community Mental Health Services: Promoting Person-Centred and Rights-Based Approaches*. Geneva: World Health Organization.

World Health Organization (2022). *World Mental Health Report: Transforming Mental Health for All*. Geneva: World Health Organization.

World Health Organization (2023). *Mental Health, Human Rights and Legislation: Guidance and Practice*. Geneva: World Health Organization.

40

Contributions of religious, alternative, and complementary practitioners

Olatunde Ayinde and Oye Gureje

Introduction

Globally, there is a large array of health and healing practices that are complementary or alternative to allopathic health approaches. Many of these practices are informed by religious practices and beliefs and are best described as faith healing. Some other forms of complementary and alternative health practices do not have clear identification with religion but are nevertheless often strongly influenced by spiritualism. The focus of this chapter is to describe different approaches of mental health care that are based on religious precepts or on spiritualism, the philosophies underpinning such practices, and the contexts in which the services are used. The chapter also discusses the contributions of the practitioners to global mental health, including their potential role in attempts to scale up mental health services. While it is recognized that religious, alternative, and complementary practitioners are common in both high-income countries (HIC) as well as in low- and middle-income countries (LMICs), this chapter will pay particular attention to their importance in the provision of mental health care in LMICs.

Religion or spirituality plays a major role in the lives of large sections of many communities across the world. Other than being a vehicle through which people commonly express their belief in the salience of spirituality to human existence, religious practices also often provide important and powerful sources of comfort, opportunities for building social networks, as well as providing and receiving social support. Even though spirituality is a distinct construct from religiosity (Upenieks & Ford-Robertson, 2022), the concepts are often used interchangeably since there is a broad and important overlap between the two, with religious practices and activities relating to expression of faith traditions being commonly regarded as demonstrating spirituality. There is a long history of connection between religion, spirituality, and mental health (Hirshbein 2020, 2021). Important examples of the link include the importance of religion in the historical use of moral therapy in mental institutions as well as more recent collaboration of psychiatrists with pastoral care practitioners. In general, research provides important evidence of the link between religiosity or spirituality with mental as well as physical health. It is therefore not surprising that mental health care has commonly been sought from faith healers in many parts of the world (Camp, 2011; Weber & Pargament, 2014).

The importance of faith and other complementary health providers in the provision of mental health care is likely to grow in the years to come, especially in settings with low resources for mental health services. The burden of disease attributable to mental, neurological and substance use disorders is large globally (GBD 2019 Mental Disorders Collaborators, 2022; Whiteford et al., 2015), and recent evidence suggests that this burden will continue to rise in the coming years as a result of rapid population growth in many parts of the world (GBD 2019 Mental Disorders Collaborators, 2022). Large treatment gaps also exist for these disorders globally, but especially in LMICs, where as high as 90% of persons suffering from mental disorders do not receive any treatment in a given year in some parts of the world (Demyttenaere et al., 2004; Wang et al., 2007). In nearly all countries, and especially in LMICs, there is significant scarcity of mental health professionals who are required to provide quality services for mental disorders, and this scarcity in human resources is projected to persist for many more years (Liu et al., 2017; World Health Organization (WHO), 2018). In addition to the shortage of trained mental health professionals, there is also between-region as well as urban–rural disparity in the distribution of the available workers. For example, the WHO African region has the second lowest number of psychiatrists per capita in the world, with the ratio of psychiatrists to the population being less than one per 1,000,000 in most of the countries in the region (WHO, 2018). Reflecting what Saxena et al. (2007) called 'widespread systemic and long term neglect of resources for mental health in LMIC', many rural areas and urban slums in these countries are without any mental health services at all. As noted by Orr and Bindi (2017), some of this gap is filled by a variety of treatment approaches that fall outside of mainstream orthodox services. Even though these approaches often do not meet the standards of what is recognized as evidence-based care as provided by orthodox medicine, they nevertheless serve some of the needs of the population in the cultures in which they exist. Religious, alternative, and complementary practitioners, including those commonly referred to as traditional healers, generally belong to this unorthodox group. As a group, they play a major role in the delivery of health care (including mental health care) in all countries, but especially in LMICs, and are often the main mental health care providers in many African countries (Burns & Tomita, 2015; Esan et al., 2018; Gureje et al., 2015). Indeed, these non-allopathic healthcare providers have been providing mental health services for hundreds of years in many cultures and are recognized as important partners in current efforts to close the mental health treatment gap in community settings (Gureje et al., 2015). These practitioners are widely available, are close to the community they service, and commonly provide services that are culturally acceptable to their clients.

Definitions of terms and categories of healers

Religious, traditional, complementary, and alternative healing approaches are diverse, and vary by cultural and geographical boundaries. In a narrative review, Gureje et al. (2015) identified two broad categories of alternative healing systems, according to published literature: traditional medicine as practised in LMICs, and complementary and alternative medicine (CAM) as practised in HICs. Traditional medicine is commonly as old as the culture in which a particular variant is found, and has been defined as 'the sum total of the knowledge, skill, and practices based on the theories, beliefs, and experiences indigenous to different cultures, whether explicable or not, used in the maintenance of health as well as in the prevention, diagnosis, improvement or treatment of physical and mental illness' (World Health Organization, 2013). Traditional medicine relies on indigenous beliefs about the causation and treatment of diseases, is often associated with a particular ethnolinguistic group, culture, and religion, and is practised widely in many countries (Incayawar et al., 2009). In a recent survey by the WHO (2019), indigenous traditional medicine is used in more than 80% of the 133 member countries surveyed. Traditional medicine is commonly based on indigenous religions.

On the other hand, there are also healing approaches that are based on religions that are not indigenous to but are widely practised in specific geographical regions. For example, on the African continent, there are healing approaches that are based on Islam and Christianity, the two dominant non-indigenous religions in the region (Kaba, 2005). Even though both groups are grounded in faith, it is common to refer to the practitioners of the former as traditional healers and the latter as faith healers (Esan et al., 2018; Gureje et al., 2015; Ojagbemi & Gureje, 2020). In general and within the faith healing category, healers exist on a continuum; there are healers whose practices are based strictly on their interpretations of their holy books, as is the case for the charismatic Pentecostal pastors and prophets found in the prayer camps in Ghana, for example (Read, 2017), where the predominant mode of healing is prayer, use of holy water, and exorcism. Also, there are Islamic healers in many Muslim communities in North Africa, Europe, and the Middle East, whose causal attributions of mental illness revolve around evil spirits (jinn) and satanic entities (shaytaan), and who rely on the recitation of Qur'anic verses to exorcise malevolent spirits (Dein & Illaiee, 2013; Gaw, 1993). However, because beliefs and values are dynamic and people mingle within populations and travel across ethnic and geographical boundaries, healing approaches that are based on syncretic beliefs and values evolve. This is the case for some religious groups, such as the Aladura Church Movement in Nigeria (Dada, 2014), the Gnawa cults in Morocco, and Candomblé in Afro-Caribbean countries (Ward, 2004) in which the tenets of non-indigenous religions, such as Christianity or Islam, are combined with local traditional religious beliefs and practices.

Notwithstanding these apparent differences, there are significant similarities and overlaps in the explanatory models of illness among the various groups of healers. For example, the belief in demonic possession as a cause of mental illness is a feature of almost all traditional religions in Africa, as well as it is in Islam and Christianity. In a survey across regions in Nigeria, Kenya, and Ghana, Esan et al. (2018) found a variety of traditional and faith healers (TFHs) such as herbalists, diviners, Christian faith healers, and Islamic faith healers who shared broadly similar beliefs about the causation of mental illness.

The WHO defines CAM as 'a broad set of health care practices that are not part of that country's own tradition or conventional medicine and are not fully integrated into the dominant health-care system' (WHO, 2013). CAM 'includes a range of resources that encompasses health systems, modalities, and practices and their accompanying theories and beliefs, apart from those intrinsic to the predominant health-care system of a society or culture in a given historical period', as well as 'resources perceived by their users as associated with positive health outcomes' (Institute of Medicine, 2005).

The term CAM has been used in a number of different ways. In the broad sense, CAM is the umbrella term encompassing all healing practices outside of conventional medicine, including traditional and faith healing. Complementary and alternative practitioners (CAPs) may include the American Indian shaman in Guatemala, the Mullah in Morocco, the acupuncturist in China, the sangoma in South Africa, the traditional healer in Ghana, and the Pentecostal healer in Nigeria (Ojagbemi & Gureje, 2020). In the narrow sense, CAM often refers to traditional medicine when adopted outside of its traditional culture (Gureje et al., 2015). In this sense, CAM is described as being alternatives to or as complementary healing modalities used alongside conventional medicine (Barrett, 2003).

In many HICs, acupuncture, chiropractic, herbal medicine, and homeopathy are among the more prominent examples of CAM (Barrett, 2003). In whichever sense it is used, CAM is often regarded as being distinct from biomedicine (allopathy, orthodox, regular, modern, conventional, mainstream or Western medicine), and is thought to satisfy demands that are not met by conventional medicine. In some countries, the boundaries between CAM and conventional medicine are beginning to blur, as medical schools, general practitioners, and hospitals begin to offer some of the CAM modalities along with conventional medicine, and national regulatory bodies acknowledge and license some of them (Incayawar et al., 2009).

As noted earlier, as a broad generalization, TFHs provide services in LMICs as well as among minority groups in many HICs, while CAM providers in the narrow sense tend to be less culture specific in their distribution (Gureje et al., 2015). Irrespective of the specificities of their practice, CAPs commonly share an emphasis on holistic approach to health and illness than do conventional medical practitioners (Incayawar et al., 2009). Their approaches make less distinction between mind and body, such that in addition to attending to physical health complaints, they also seek to attend to psychological, social, and spiritual aspects of illness. Given that persons with mental disorders commonly also have psychosocial problems, such as relational and family dysfunction, they therefore tend to value this holistic approach to care (Mbwayo et al., 2013).

Cosmologies, philosophies, and explanatory models underlying complementary and alternative medicine practices

Western medicine evolved from the Greek Hippocratic system and onwards to modern biomedicine, and is generally secular. Within that tradition, the mental health specialty attempts to expand its emphasis from a purely disturbed physiology to a broader psychosocial understanding of the causes, manifestations, and consequences of mental illness (Kuriyama, 1999; Leslie & Young, 1992). On the other hand, CAM, including traditional and faith healing, has evolved from different cultural, historical, and philosophical traditions, too numerous to mention. Nevertheless, it is a worthwhile venture to explicate on the cosmology and philosophy of traditional and faith healing as practised in sub-Saharan Africa, as a prototype and then draw some parallels with the philosophies underlying other healing approaches.

Faith and traditional healing approaches are commonly based on ethnic/national identity, as well as religion, spirituality, the concept of the self, and beliefs related to bodily functions (Incayawar et al., 2009). For example, in the African context, ethnicity, religion, and the self are the three dimensions of the collective identity of a person (Kpanake, 2018), such that a complete state of well-being can only exist if the self (physical person, body parts, body fluids, etc.), social agency (their kin and community), and spirit agency (deities, divinities, spirits, etc.) are in harmony. Deities, divinities, spirits, and ancestors, as well as members of one's family and community—and even animals and inanimate objects—form one unbroken web of connectedness, the balance of which is required to maintain physical, mental, social, spiritual, and communal well-being (Ayinde et al., 2021a). A disconnect in any of this complex web of spiritual and physical relationships—personal transgression against a spiritual entity, breaking of communal taboos, disagreement with a neighbour with access to spiritual powers such as witchcraft—are believed to lead to personal, family, and communal misfortune or ill health, including mental illness. Because the medicine man understands this inter-connectedness, he is therefore not just a healer, he is the one to consult to find out who to marry for a successful and fruitful union, which ancestor is behind a failing career, or who has afflicted a family member with mental illness (Peltzer, 2009).

The traditional healer is also a psychotherapist and a community mobilizer. Their prayers and invocations, rituals, and symbolism not only repair fractured relationships across the physical–spiritual planes, but also become useful in repairing broken relationships and communities. They are the one trusted by deities and ancestors to broker peace between unseen forces and humans.

It is interesting to note that despite the dominance of the two Abrahamic religions on the African continent, with traditional religion often being relegated to the background, especially in formal and official circles and interactions, traditional healers continue to play a prominent role in the lives of modern-day Africans. Scholars of religion have argued that religious conversions are often never complete (Nadel, 1954), and while converting to Islam and Christianity, Africans either hold on to their old religions at the subconscious level, while professing the adopted religion publicly, or they simply create syncretic forms of these adopted religions, thus giving room for the rich songs, dance, ritual, and active emotional display characteristic of traditional African religions (Dada, 2014). This process is facilitated by the fact that there is a great deal of overlap in the explanatory model of illness and healing elements among adherents of traditional religions and the Abrahamic religions: all agree that mental illness can be caused through witchcraft and evil spirits, which are amenable to prayers, invocation, and exorcism. It is therefore not surprising that there are healers who combine elements of one or more religious traditions in their routine (Esan et al., 2018).

Explanatory models are culturally determined processes of making sense of illness and symptoms, formulating causal attributions, help-seeking, and expectations of outcome of treatment (Dinos et al., 2017). These frameworks define how individuals and their families respond to episodes of illness. It is sometimes the case that patients and their family members hold multiple and conflicting explanatory models simultaneously (Bhikha et al., 2012; Read, 2017). Explanatory models are an important determinant of a pathway to care, treatment preferences, compliance with treatment, as well as satisfaction with treatment received (Callan & Littlewood, 1998).

It has been said that explanatory models of mental illness, among other factors, play a major part in the practice and patronage of traditional and faith healing in LMICs. While Western medicine recognizes biological and psychosocial aetiology of mental illness, in many societies, especially those in LMICs, belief in the supernatural causation of mental illness is common (Ayinde et al., 2021b; Bhikha et al., 2012; Burns & Tomita, 2015; Gureje et al., 2015; Ojagbemi & Gureje, 2020; Patel, 1995). In addition, both healers and help seekers across LMICs also believe in biological causation of mental illness such as abuse of psychoactive substance, head trauma, and heredity, as well as psychosocial ones such as poverty, family conflict, and bereavement (Ayinde et al., 2021b). In a study among patrons of TFHs in Nigeria, Ghana, and Kenya, there was a surprising overlap across the three countries on the supernatural aetiology of mental illness, with the suggested causal attributions including spiritual attack, demonic possession, retribution for crimes or bad behaviour, breaking communal taboos, witchcraft, curses, failure to obey communal norms such as paying bride price, and so on (Ayinde et al., 2021b). Also in that study and contrary to the usual division of models into supernatural and biopsychosocial ones, participants endorsed a complex array of causal attributions, spanning multiple categories, sometimes complementary and sometimes contradictory.

Even when beliefs in biological and psychosocial models were expressed, many help aseekers claimed that the sufferer was susceptible to the biological agent through supernatural means in the first instance or that the illness started as a 'spiritual attack' (Ayinde et al., 2021b; Kpobi et al., 2018). Sometimes, it is believed, witches can take advantage of an illness with primary biomedical cause and either make it worse or run a chronic unremitting course. Among other causal attributions that have been reported in Africa is the belief that mental illness can be contagious and be transmissible through body fluids (Ojagbemi & Gureje, 2020). Studies have shown that these various causal models of mental illness are commonly held in the community. In one nationally representative survey of 5315 Nigerians, 54% believed that mental illness can be due to possession by evil spirits (Africa Polling Institute & EpiAfric, 2020). It is not surprising therefore that users of traditional and faith healing services share these beliefs and commonly approach the healer for the explanations of the causes of their mental illness, an understanding of which biomedical practitioners may lack (Patel et al., 1997). As reported by Abo (2011), some patients consult traditional healers specifically to find out why their illness occurred in the first instance. Therefore, in seeking help from TFHs, expectation is not limited to the treatment for the illness; equally important is the need to gain understanding of why the mental illness occurred, which communal taboo may have been broken, which spirit has been offended, or which social and spiritual relationship has broken down, and to thereby get to the root cause of the illness.

Prevalence of use, reasons for, and pattern of patronage of complementary and alternative practitioners

CAPs play a major role in the care itinerary of persons with mental illness and their families, globally, and especially in LMICs. In 2013, it was estimated that 100 million Europeans and many more in other continents used traditional CAM for various health reasons, including mental health (Barnes et al., 2008; EICCAM, 2008). In many LMICs, and especially sub-Saharan Africa, TFHs are the main providers of mental health services, especially for persons with severe mental illness. In one study from Nigeria, up to 60% of those who consult TFHs for a variety of health reasons do so because of mental illness (Odinka et al., 2014). Studies of pathways to mental health care in LMICs have shown that up to 90% of patients presenting with psychosis in outpatient departments of teaching hospitals and community mental health centres had consulted TFHs at some point in their illness itinerary (Gureje et al., 2015).

There are multiple reasons persons with mental disorders and their relatives decide when and where help is sought, and when to switch healers or combine services of different types of healers (Ayinde et al., 2021b; Burns & Tomita, 2015). Some of these are supply-side factors, such as availability and cost, while some are demand-side factors, such as access, attitude, shared beliefs, and preferences. In many LMICs, both healers and their patrons share a common explanatory model of mental illness, and this shared currency is an important reason for the choice of TFHs in the management of mental illness, adherence to their prescriptions, as well as satisfaction with their services (Ayinde et al., 2021b; Callan & Littlewood, 1998; Patel et al., 1997).

Second, TFHs are widely available and accessible, and are close to the community. The number of TFHs in sub-Saharan Africa, for example, may be about 100 times that of biomedical practitioners (WHO, 2002). In a survey of TFH facilities in Nigeria, Ghana, and Kenya, these facilities were found to have two- to tenfold the admission capacity of conventional mental health facilities (Esan et al., 2018).

Third, there are rural–urban disparities in the distribution of biomedical mental health services and trained mental health practitioners, such that fewer of them are available in rural areas where most of the population in LMICs reside. Where mental health services are available in rural areas and urban slums, such services are either too costly for most help seekers, with services being paid for out of pocket, or facilities are too far and transportation is a barrier to access (Burns & Tomita, 2015).

Considerable research has gone into the pattern of service use by persons seeking help from TFHs. Plurality appears to be the predominant pattern of use. Tomita and Burns (2015) point out that in many LMICs, especially in sub-Saharan Africa, pathways to mental healthcare are not simple, but are 'complex and recursive' (Burns & Tomita 2015), with persons with mental disorders and their families seeking help concurrently or consecutively from different categories of providers within biomedical and non-orthodox services (Ayinde et al., 2021b; Campbell-Hall et al., 2010; Read, 2017). In one study, patrons of TFHs claim the reasons for plurality in help-seeking include perceived non-improvement of symptoms with biomedical care, poor or inadequate communication from biomedical practitioners, and perceptions that illness is of supernatural origin or of dual origin (physical and supernatural) (Ayinde et al., 2021b). Patrons also believed that the healing obtained from biomedical facilities is incomplete as they do not address a lot of their existential anxieties as well as relationship breakdown and restoration of loss occasioned by illness. Participants in the study also cited several reasons why they abandoned biomedical care for TFHs, including perceived supernatural aetiology of illness, non-satisfaction with biomedical care, referral to a TFH by a biomedical practitioner who shared a supernatural causal attribution with the client, lack of improvement in symptoms, side effects of orthodox medications, cost of orthodox medications, and use of derogatory language by hospital staff.

It would therefore be too simplistic to think that persons with mental illness and their families use non-orthodox mental health services because of non-availability of biomedical care alone. In certain contexts, they are used not just as alternatives or in addition to biomedical care but in other contexts, as the only source of available help.

Practice characteristics of traditional and faith healers

TFHs typically have undergone some form of training, often spanning several years, before commencing their practice. This includes informal apprenticeship with relatives or non-relatives, as well as formal training at pastoral institutes or herbal institutes. In some instances, they have undergone no training at all, and claim to have been initiated into the profession by ancestral spirits, or following cure of their illness by another healer or a combination these. Categories of healers include herbalists, diviners, and faith healers of both Christian and Muslim persuasion as well as witchcraft practitioners. In some cases, categories are not exclusive and may overlap. Esan et al. (2018) reported the presence of Christian and Muslim herbalists in Nigeria, Kenya, and Ghana. Many healers are generalists, treating both physical and mental illness, while some specialize in the treatment of mental disorders. The range of persons with mental illness commonly in the care of traditional healers includes those with psychosis, severe mood disorders, puerperal mental disorders, and epilepsy, as well as those with alcohol and substance use disorders.

Assessment, diagnosis, and treatment of mental disorders

The management of mental disorders by TFHs begins with assessment and diagnosis. Assessment approaches include a combination of history taking and observation of the patient. Healers may also use divination to obtain supernatural revelation of the cause of illness and this approach may include clairvoyance, tossing of artefacts, use of mirrors, animal sacrifice, trance, and prayers. Some of the diagnostic constructs may map onto those used in conventional psychiatry (Makanjuola, 1987). In traditional medicine, the emphasis is not so much on the symptoms and signs of illness, as the perceived supernatural cause of the illness, and the psychosocial circumstance of the sufferer at the time of diagnosis (Gessler et al., 1995; Incayawar, 2008; Jones, 2000). For this reason, many of the labels used reflect the presumed aetiology of the condition (Cohen et al., 2016; Makanjuola, 1987).

As earlier noted, traditional and faith healing, especially in sub-Saharan Africa, is much broader than the resolution of symptoms and restoration of function. Of particular importance are subjective qualitative changes in the meaning, relationships, and self-image of the help seeker (Nortje et al., 2016; van der Watt et al., 2018). Treatment approaches are often based on the indigenous faiths, beliefs, knowledge, and practices of the culture of the population being served, making the treatments more culturally sensitive and acceptable to the clients and their families (Abbo, 2011; Ayinde et al., 2021b; Kpobi and Swartz, 2018; Mbwayo et al., 2013). Similarly, faith healing may also be informed by the scriptural specifications of the Abrahamic religion on which the healers base their practice. Given that religion is a central feature in the lives of most persons in LMICs, with up to 99% of the population in some countries admitting that religion plays an important part in their lives (Gallup Inc., 2010), it is not surprising that faith and spirituality feature prominently in the healing process of most persons with mental illness in these countries (Ayinde et al., 2021a, 2021b; Read, 2017).

TFH treatment modalities are often eclectic in nature, with wide overlap between and among categories of healers (Makanjuola & Jaiyeola, 1987). The use of rituals is common across healers, while the use of holy water, anointing oil, spiritual bath, vigils, fasting, music, and dance is popular among Christian faith healers (Ayinde et al., 2021b; Esan et al., 2018; Gureje et al., 2015). Herbal concoctions, herbal snuff, use of ritual oil, animal sacrifice, ingestion of animal parts and blood, animal sacrifice, scarification marks, special food to eat and others to avoid as taboos, as well as abstaining from sexual intercourse are treatment approaches among traditional healers and Islamic healers. Prayers, invocations, and reading from holy books and exorcism are also common approaches in faith healing facilities.

Harmful practices and human right abuses

Harmful treatment practices have been the most consistent concern of researchers and policymakers in the discourse on integrating TFH services into the formal health system of countries where healers play prominent role in mental health delivery (van der Watt et al., 2017). Studies of treatment practices in TFH facilities have documented practices such as beating, shackling, confinement to a room, starvation, denial of water, exposure to the elements, overcrowding, cohabitation of sexes, and sleeping on bare floor (Esan et al., 2018). Despite these inhumane practices, studies among users of TFH services have often found that the respondents expressed satisfaction with the overall care they receive and are tolerant of the practices (Ayinde et al., 2021b; Mbwayo et al., 2013; Patel et al., 1997), possibly because such practices are considered as a necessary part of care or because of a lack of understanding of what constitutes standard of care leading to a general reduction in expectation.

Nevertheless, there is good evidence that TFHs can be trained to minimize such harmful practices in the delivery of care (Gureje et al., 2020). Therefore, part of the formal oversight of TFHs and licensing of their practices ought to include the importance of eliminating such treatment approaches. Similarly, it will be important to educate and empower users of the services of TFHs to demand quality and safety standards in their care (Ayinde et al., 2021b).

Effectiveness and quality of care

Several studies have examined the effectiveness of CAP services. In a systematic review of evidence of the impact of the services of CAPs, Nortje et al. (2016) found 32 published papers, most from HICs, and of which only two are randomized controlled trials. The authors found little evidence for efficacy of CAP treatment of severe mental disorders. However, they found some papers that reported efficacy of TFH intervention that was similar to studies of primary psychiatry care for common mental health conditions such as depression, anxiety, and somatization, as well as interpersonal and social difficulties. It would appear that the effect of some of the interventions for common mental health conditions might be mediated by ritual and ceremony acting through catharsis, cognitive restructuring, change in family structures, restoration of community identity, and social cohesion (Kirmayer, 2004). In view of the evidence that users of TFH services often perceive them as effective even when objective evidence is less clear, it has been suggested that perhaps subjecting traditional and faith healing services to biomedical-style evaluation may be inappropriate (Mills & White, 2017). The view has been canvassed that outcomes as defined by the users of these services may be different from those of biomedical practitioners and that the former should be given greater attention (White et al., 2016). While Western medicine focuses on symptom remission, functioning, and quality of life, CAPs and their patrons are more interested in subjective qualitative changes in bodily functions, as well as family cohesion and community healing and integration (Nortje et al., 2016). It is possible that this is in keeping with lay or cultural concept of healing and recovery.

Implications for legislation, policy, research, training, and practice

In view of the importance of TFH in the provision of mental health services in LMICs, with the majority of them practising outside of the formal health system, there have been calls for some form of oversight of their practice. Services that are widely utilized such as those of the healers need to have certain standards of safety, if not efficacy. TFHs themselves have often expressed the fear that some of the secrets of their trade might be 'stolen' by Western practitioners in the process of collaboration, and have sought to have formal regulation of their practice as a way of protecting their methods and approaches (Campbell-Hall et al., 2010; van der Watt et al., 2017).

As at 2018, 64% of the member states of WHO had laws or regulations on herbal medicines. More than 85% of the member states in the African and South East Asia regions had a national policy on traditional and CAM, with the corresponding figures in the Western pacific and Eastern Mediterranean being 63% and 43%, respectively (WHO, 2019). For the Americas and European regions, the figures stood at 31% and 21% respectively, indicating the relative level of importance of these healing approaches in these regions.

In calling for more research on the effectiveness of TFH services, some researchers have advocated outcomes that incorporate multidimensional measures such as those that assess subjective experiences of satisfaction with service by users, measures that are not always sufficiently emphasized in conventional biomedical designs of randomized controlled trials (Orr & Bindi, 2017). Similarly, continued training as well as regulation, possibly embedded in the registration of TFH groups and licencing of the practitioners, may be useful in improving the quality of their practices.

Collaboration between biomedical practitioners and traditional and faith healers

The continued patronage and popularity of TFHs in LMICs has often been discussed from the premise of the role this may play in the delay of users accessing orthodox and presumably more effective mental health service where such services are available (Burns & Tomita, 2015). As a panacea, some authors have suggested trying to improve referral practices from TFHs to conventional mental health practitioners. However, it has also been argued that if all persons who patronize TFHs were efficiently referred to conventional mental health services, the existing capacities of the formal health system would fall far too short to meet the need, especially in LMICs (Burns, 2014). The more feasible approach would be to scale up mental health services through collaboration with TFHs, using resources that already exist in the community and are easily accessible and widely available. Moreover, studies have reported high level of satisfaction among patrons of TFHs, indicating that there are elements that users of these services find useful (Ayinde et al., 2021b; van der Watt et al., 2018). Indeed, the WHO, policymakers, and researchers working in regions with scarce human resources for mental health have advocated for the integration of TFHs into the formal health systems of their countries (Gureje, 2009; Gureje et al., 2015, 2019). However, there continue to be barriers for the successful implementation of this proposal. Among biomedical practitioners, objections have included the difference in the worldviews between TFHs and biomedical practitioners, non-standardization of TFH interventions, poor evidence base, and harmful practices (Campbell-Hall et al., 2010; Chipolombwe & Muula, 2005).

TFHs have also expressed some mistrust towards their biomedical colleagues and governments (van der Watt et al., 2017). Specifically, TFHs have often expressed their displeasure with the lack of recognition from government and disrespect from biomedical practitioners (Campbell-Hall et al., 2010; Sorsdahl et al., 2010; van der Watt et al., 2017). Healers also expressed the fear that Western medical practitioners might steal their trade secrets (Campbell-Hall et al., 2010; Sorsdahl et al., 2010; van der Watt et al., 2017). Other barriers to collaboration might also be connected with a power imbalance between the two groups and an understandable cultural struggle between old traditional values and modern aspirations (Del Casino, 2004).

In developing collaboration between healers and biomedical practitioners, it has been suggested that among the steps that need to be taken will include engendering mutual respect between the two categories of practitioners, educating each group about each other's healing approach, and training both groups to collaborate (van der Watt et al., 2017), including providing specific training to TFHs on how to avoid the use of harmful treatment practices (Ayinde et al., 2021b).

This approach was tested in a groundbreaking randomized controlled trial by Gureje et al. (2020). In this cluster randomized trial, conducted in Nigeria and Ghana, clusters of primary care clinics and neighbouring TFH facilities were randomized to intervention group (collaborative shared care) and enhanced care as usual. Intervention consisted of clinical support by primary care providers to respond to the medical needs of patients who were admitted in TFH facilities and were primarily being cared for by TFHs through the administration of medications for psychotic symptoms as well as treatment of any co-occurring physical conditions. Also included in the collaborative shared care was clinical support to improve services on a continuous basis through interactions and engagements of the primary care providers with TFHs, patients, and their relatives. The enhanced care as usual did not have any formal collaboration components, but both groups of providers were trained separately on ways to avoid inhumane and potentially harmful treatment practices. Over 6 months, patients in the intervention arm had significantly better improvement in symptoms compared to the control arm. The collaborative shared care was also cost-effective. Harmful practices were reduced significantly in both arms of the study. This study provides strong evidence that not only is it feasible for TFHs to collaborate with biomedical practitioners in LMIC settings, but that such collaborations can lead to improved patient outcomes and can be cost-effective. More studies are needed to replicate these findings as well as to extend them by investigating implementation science parameters of adoption, maintenance, and sustainability. The findings of such studies will be important as governments in sub-Saharan Africa strive to find a way to give effect to the often-stated policy aspiration of integrating healers into mainstream mental health system.

Religion and spirituality are central to the ways of life of many people around the world. It is therefore not surprising that healing practices informed by religion and spirituality are prominent in several communities. In LMICs, these practices take on greater importance because of the gap in formal mental health service that healers fill. Even though their practices are often outside of the realm of scientific understanding and may not always be objectively demonstrably effective, they are valued by members of the community and certainly seem to provide aspects of healing and recovery that people see as important.

REFERENCES

Abbo, C. (2011). Profiles and outcome of traditional healing practices for severe mental illnesses in two districts of Eastern Uganda. *Global Health Action*, **4**, 7117.

Africa Polling Institute & EpiAfric (2020). Mental health in Nigeria survey. https://africapolling.org/wp-content/uploads/2020/01/Mental-Health-in-Nigeria-Survey-Report.pdf

Ayinde, O. O., Fadahunsi, O., Kola, L., Malla, L.O., Nyame, S., Okoth, R.A., et al. (2021b). Explanatory models, illness, and treatment experiences of patients with psychosis using the services of traditional and faith healers in three African countries: similarities and discontinuities. *Transcultural Psychiatry*, **60**, 521–536.

Ayinde, O., Ojagbemi, A., Makanjuola, V., & Gureje, O. (2021a). African religions, spirituality, and mental health healing practices. In: Moreira-Almeida, A., Mosqueiro, B. P., & Bhugra, D. (Eds.), *Spirituality and Mental Health across Cultures* (pp. 277–92). Oxford: Oxford University Press.

Barnes, P. M., Bloom, B., & Nahin, R. L. (2008). Complementary and alternative medicine use among adults and children: United States, 2007. *National Health Statistics Report*, **12**, 1–23.

Barrett, B. (2003). Alternative, complementary, and conventional medicine: is integration upon us? *Journal of Alternative and Complementary Medicine*, **9**, 417–427.

Bhikha, A. G., Farooq, S., Chaudhry, N., & Husain, N. (2012). A systematic review of explanatory models of illness for psychosis in developing countries. *International Review of Psychiatry*, **24**, 450–462.

Burns, J. K. (2014). The burden of untreated mental disorders in KwaZulu-Natal Province—mapping the treatment gap. *South African Journal of Psychiatry*, **20**, 5.

Burns, J. K. & Tomita, A. (2015). Traditional and religious healers in the pathway to care for people with mental disorders in Africa: a systematic review and meta-analysis. *Social Psychiatry and Psychiatric Epidemiology*, **50**, 867–877.

Callan, A. & Littlewood, R. (1998). Patient satisfaction: ethnic origin or explanatory model? *International Journal of Social Psychiatry*, **44**, 1–11.

Camp, M. E. (2011). Religion and spirituality in psychiatric practice. *Current Opinion in Psychiatry*, **24**, 507–513.

Campbell-Hall, V., Petersen, I., Bhana, A., Mjadu, S., Hosegood, V., Flisher, A. J., & MHaPP Research Programme Consortium (2010). Collaboration between traditional practitioners and primary health care staff in South Africa: developing a workable partnership for community mental health services. *Transcultural Psychiatry*, **47**, 610–628.

Chipolombwe, J. & Muula, A. S. (2005). Allopathic health professionals' perceptions towards traditional health practice in Lilongwe, Malawi. *Malawi Medical Journal*, **17**, 131.

Cohen, A., Padmavati, R., Hibben, M., Oyewusi, S., John, S., Esan, O., et al. (2016). Concepts of madness in diverse settings: a qualitative study from the INTREPID project. *BMC Psychiatry*, **16**, 388.

Dada, A. O. (2014). Old wine in new bottle. *Black Theology*, **12**, 19–32.

Dein, S. & Illaiee, A. S. (2013). Jinn and mental health: looking at jinn possession in modern psychiatric practice. *The Psychiatrist*, **37**, 290–293.

Del Casino, V. J. (2004). (Re)placing health and health care: mapping the competing discourses and practices of 'traditional' and 'modern' Thai medicine. *Health and Place*, **10**, 59–73.

Demyttenaere, K., Bruffaerts, R., Posada-Villa, J., Gasquet, I., Kovess, V., Lepine, J. P., et al. (2004). Prevalence, severity, and unmet need for treatment of mental disorders in the World Health Organization World Mental Health Surveys. *JAMA*, **291**, 2581–2590.

Dinos, S., Ascoli, M., Owiti, J. A., & Bhui, K. (2017). Assessing explanatory models and health beliefs: an essential but overlooked competency for clinicians. *BJPsych Advances*, **23**, 106–114.

EICCAM (2008). European Information Centre for Complementary & Alternative Medicine. https://www.antroposofischegeneeskunde.be/wp-content/uploads/eiccam-brochure-nov-2008.pdf

Esan, O., Appiah-Poku, J., Othieno, C., Kola, L., Harris, B., Nortje, G., et al. (2018). A survey of traditional and faith healers providing mental health care in three sub-Saharan African countries. *Social Psychiatry and Psychiatric Epidemiology*, **54**, 395–403.

Gallup Inc. (2010). Religiosity highest in world's poorest nations. *Gallup.com*, 31 August. https://news.gallup.com/poll/142727/religiosity-highest-world-poorest-nations.aspx

Gaw, A. (1993). *Culture, Ethnicity, and Mental Illness*. Arlington, VA: American Psychiatric Publishing.

GBD 2019 Mental Disorders Collaborators (2022). Global, regional, and national burden of 12 mental disorders in 204 countries and territories, 1990–2019: a systematic analysis for the Global Burden of Disease Study 2019. *Lancet Psychiatry*, **9**, 137–150.

Gessler, M. C., Msuya, D. E., Nkunya, M. H., Schär, A., Heinrich, M., & Tanner, M. (1995). Traditional healers in Tanzania: sociocultural profile and three short portraits. *Journal of Ethnopharmacology*, **48**, 145–160.

Gureje, O. (2009). WPA-WHO policy roundtable. *WPA News*, December. Geneva: World Psychiatric Association.

Gureje, O., Appiah-Poku, J., Bello, T., Kola, L., Araya, R., Chisholm, D., et al. (2020). Effect of collaborative care between traditional and faith healers and primary health-care workers on psychosis outcomes in Nigeria and Ghana (COSIMPO): a cluster randomised controlled trial. *Lancet*, **396**, 612–622.

Gureje, O., Nortje, G., Makanjuola, V., Oladeji, B. D., Seedat, S., & Jenkins, R. (2015). The role of global traditional and complementary systems of medicine in the treatment of mental health disorders. *Lancet Psychiatry*, **2**, 168–177.

Gureje, O., Seedat, S., Kola, L., Appiah-Poku, J., Othieno, C., Harris, B., et al. (2019). Partnership for mental health development in Sub-Saharan Africa (PaM-D): a collaborative initiative for research and capacity building. *Epidemiology and Psychiatric Sciences*, **28**, 389–396.

Hirshbein, L. (2020). Religion and spirituality, meaning, and faith in American psychiatry from the 19th to the 21st century. *Journal of Nervous and Mental Disease*, **208**, 582–586.

Hirshbein, L. (2021). Why psychiatry might cooperate with religion: the Michigan Society of Pastoral Care, 1945–1968. *Journal of the History of the Behavioral Sciences*, **57**, 113–129.

Incayawar, M. (2008). Efficacy of Quichua healers as psychiatric diagnosticians. *British Journal of Psychiatry*, **192**, 390–391.

Incayawar, M., Wintrob, R., Bouchard, L., & Bartocci, G. (Eds.) (2009). *Psychiatrists and Traditional Healers: Unwitting Partners in Global Mental Health*. West Sussex: John Wiley & Sons.

Institute of Medicine (2005). *Complementary and Alternative Medicine in the United States*. Washington, DC: National Academies Press.

Jones, R. (2000). Diagnosis in traditional Maori healing: a contemporary urban clinic. *Pacific Health Dialog*, **7**, 17–24.

Kaba, A. J. (2005). The spread of Christianity and Islam in Africa: a survey and analysis of the numbers and percentages of Christians, Muslims and those who practice indigenous religions. *Western Journal of Black Studies*, **29**, 553.

Kirmayer, L. J. (2004). The cultural diversity of healing: meaning, metaphor and mechanism. *British Medical Bulletin*, **69**, 33–48.

Kpanake, L. (2018). Cultural concepts of the person and mental health in Africa. *Transcultural Psychiatry*, **55**, 198–218.

Kpobi, L. & Swartz, L. (2018). 'That is how the real mad people behave': beliefs about and treatment of mental disorders by traditional medicine-men in Accra, Ghana. *International Journal of Social Psychiatry*, **64**, 309–316.

Kpobi, L., Swartz, L., & Keikelame, M. J. (2018). Ghanaian traditional and faith healers' explanatory models for epilepsy. *Epilepsy and Behavior: E&B*, **84**, 88–92.

Kuriyama, S. (1999). *The Expressiveness of the Body and the Divergence of Greek and Chinese Medicine*. New York: Zone Press.

Leslie, C. & Young, A. (1992). Introduction. In: Leslie, C. &Young, A (Eds.), *Paths to Asian Medical Knowledge* (pp. 1–18). Berkeley, CA: University of California Press.

Liu, J. X., Goryakin, Y., Maeda, A. Bruckner, T., & Scheffler, R. (2017). Global health workforce labor market projections for 2030. *Human Resources for Health*, **15**, 11.

Makanjuola, R. O. (1987). Yoruba traditional healers in psychiatry. I. Healers' concepts of the nature and aetiology of mental disorders. *African Journal of Medicine and Medical Sciences*, **16**, 53–59.

Makanjuola, R. O. & Jaiyeola, A. A. (1987). Yoruba traditional healers in psychiatry. II. Management of psychiatric disorders. *African Journal of Medicine and Medical Sciences*, **16**, 61–73.

Mbwayo, A., Ndetei, D., Mutiso, V., & Khasakhala, L. I. (2013). Traditional healers and provision of mental health services in cosmopolitan informal settlements in Nairobi, Kenya. *African Journal of Psychiatry*, **16**, 134–140.

Mills, C. & White, R. (2017). 'Global mental health spreads like bush fire in the Global South': efforts to scale up mental health services in low- and middle-income countries. In: White, R. G., Jain, S., & Orr, D. M. R., et al. (Eds.), *The Palgrave Handbook of Sociocultural Perspectives on Global Mental Health* (pp. 187–209). New York: Palgrave Macmillan.

Nadel, S. F. (1954). *Nupe Religion* (pp. 232-258). New York: Routledge.

Nortje, G., Oladeji, B., Gureje, O., & Seedat, S. (2016). Effectiveness of traditional healers in treating mental disorders: a systematic review. *Lancet Psychiatry*, **3**, 154–170.

Odinka, P. C., Oche, M., Ndukuba, A. C., Muomah, R. C., Osika, M. U., Bakare, M. O., et al. (2014). The socio-demographic characteristics and patterns of help-seeking among patients with schizophrenia in south-east Nigeria. *Journal of Health Care for the Poor and Underserved*, **25**, 180–191.

Ojagbemi, A. & Gureje, O. (2020). The importance of faith-based mental healthcare in African urbanized sites. *Current Opinion in Psychiatry*, **33**, 271–277.

Orr, D. M. & Bindi, S. (2017). Medical pluralism and global mental health. In: White, R., Jain, S., Orr, D., Read, U. (Eds.), *The Palgrave Handbook of Sociocultural Perspectives on Global Mental Health* (pp. 307–328). London: Palgrave Macmillan.

Patel, V. (1995). Explanatory models of mental illness in sub-Saharan Africa. *Social Science & Medicine*, **40**, 1291–1298.

Patel, V., Simunyu, E., & Gwanzura, F. (1997). The pathways to primary mental health care in high-density suburbs in Harare, Zimbabwe. *Social Psychiatry and Psychiatric Epidemiology*, **32**, 97–103.

Peltzer, K. (2009). Utilization and practice of traditional/complementary/alternative medicine (TM/CAM) in South Africa. *African Journal of Traditional, Complementary, and Alternative Medicines*, **6**, 175–185.

Read, (2017). 'Doctor sickness' or 'pastor sickness'? Contested domains of healing power in the treatment of mental illness in Kintampo, Ghana. In: Basu, H., Littlewood, R., Steinforth, A. S. (Eds.), *Spirit & Mind* (pp. 167–188). Münster: LIT Verlag.

Saxena, S., Thornicroft, G., Knapp, M., & Whiteford, H. (2007). Resources for mental health: scarcity, inequity, and inefficiency. *Lancet*, **370**, 878–889.

Sorsdahl, K., Stein, D. J., Flisher, A. J. (2010). Traditional healer attitudes and beliefs regarding referral of the mentally ill to Western doctors in South Africa. *Transcultural Psychiatry*, **47**, 591–609.

Upenieks, L. & Ford-Robertson, J. (2022). Changes in spiritual but not religious identity and well-being in emerging adulthood in the United States: pathways to health sameness? *Journal of Religion and Health*, **61**, 4635–4673.

Wang, P. S., Aguilar-Gaxiola, S., Alonso, J., Angermeyer, M. C., Borges, G., Bromet, E. J., et al. (2007). Use of mental health services for anxiety, mood, and substance disorders in 17 countries in the WHO world mental health surveys. *Lancet*, **370**, 841–850.

Ward, K. (2004). African traditional religion. In: Palmer, M. (Ed.), *World Religions: A Comprehensive Guide to the Religions of the World* (pp. 86–92). London: Times Books.

van der Watt, A., Nortje, G., Kola, L., Appiah-Poku, J., Othieno, C., Harris, B., et al. (2017). Collaboration between biomedical and complementary and alternative care providers: barriers and pathways. *Qualitative Health Research*, **27**, 2177–2188.

van der Watt, A., van de Water, T., Nortje, G., Oladeji, B. D., Seedat, S., Gureje, O., & Partnership for Mental Health Development in Sub-Saharan Africa (PaM-D) Research Team (2018). The perceived effectiveness of traditional and faith healing in the treatment of mental illness: a systematic review of qualitative studies. *Social Psychiatry and Psychiatric Epidemiology*, **53**, 555–566.

Weber, S. R. & Pargament, K. I. (2014). The role of religion and spirituality in mental health. *Current Opinion in Psychiatry*, **27**, 358–363.

White, R. G., Imperiale, M. G., & Perera, E. (2016). The capabilities approach: fostering contexts for enhancing mental health and well-being across the globe. *Globalization and Health*, **12**, 16.

Whiteford, H. A., Ferrari, A. J., Degenhardt, L., Feigin, V., & Vos, T. (2015). The global burden of mental, neurological and substance use disorders: an analysis from the Global Burden of Disease Study 2010. *PLoS One*, **10**, e0116820.

World Health Organization (2002). *WHO Traditional Medicine Strategy 2000-2005*. Geneva: World Health Organization.

World Health Organization (2013). *WHO Traditional Medicine Strategy, 2014–2023*. Geneva: World Health Organization.

World Health Organization (2018). *Mental Health Atlas 2017*. Geneva: World Health Organization.

World Health Organization (2019). *Who Global Report on Traditional and Complementary Medicine 2019*. Geneva: World Health Organization.

41
Planning and implementing community services for a district
The case of PRIME

Crick Lund, Erica Breuer, Arvin Bhana, Carrie Brooke-Sumner, Mark Jordans, Nagendra Luitel, Girmay Medhin, Vaibhav Murhar, Juliet Nakku, Olivia Nalwadda, Inge Petersen, Medhin Selamu, Rahul Shidhaye, Joshua Ssebunnya, Mark Tomlinson, Charlotte Hanlon, and Vikram Patel

Introduction

Districts are a key administrative health unit for implementing and scaling up community-based mental health services, when faced with the enormous care gap for mental disorders in low-resource settings. By developing district-level mental health care plans (MHCPs), planners and local stakeholders can test the feasibility and acceptability of mental health care in local settings, while simultaneously developing models that can be scaled up to larger populations.

The Programme for Improving Mental health carE (PRIME) was a UK Department for International Development-funded research programme consortium, which was led from the University of Cape Town, and worked in five low- and middle-income countries: Ethiopia, India, Nepal, South Africa, and Uganda from 2011 to 2019. Consortium partners included the London School of Hygiene and Tropical Medicine, King's College London, UK, and the World Health Organization (WHO).

The aim of PRIME was to implement and evaluate district-level MHCPs in low-resource settings, with a view to generating lessons for the further scale-up of much needed mental health care (Lund et al., 2012). In each country, the PRIME teams were led by a research team at a local university or non-governmental organization (NGO), which worked in partnership with the Ministry of Health. Each country selected a 'district demonstration site', from which lessons could be generated to inform future scaling up of mental health services in each country, and potentially beyond. Through an extensive local consultation process, the PRIME teams developed district-level MHCPs, which were implemented over a 3-year period. The focus of the plans was on providing care for priority mental, neurological, and substance use (MNS) disorders: psychosis, epilepsy, depression, and alcohol use disorders (AUD), although not all countries address all of these disorders.

The PRIME district plans included the implementation of the WHO mental health Gap Action Programme Intervention Guide (mhGAP-IG) (WHO, 2016b), adapted to the local settings, with additional components of evidence-based psychosocial interventions in primary care and community settings (Hanlon et al., 2016). The teams employed rigorous evaluation methods, incorporating five main study designs (De Silva et al., 2016): (1) formative research, including a situational analysis of each district, qualitative studies, and consultation with local stakeholders; (2) repeat community surveys to assess changes in population-level treatment coverage; (3) repeat facility surveys to assess changes in detection and treatment of priority disorders; and (4) treatment cohorts, with nested qualitative studies, to assess improvements in clinical symptoms, disability, and economic outcomes for people who received care in the PRIME sites. Some countries also nested randomized controlled trials in their evaluations, to address specific research questions. In all countries, theory of change was employed extensively as a planning, consultation and evaluation tool (Breuer et al., 2016).

In this chapter, we describe the development, implementation, and evaluation of district MHCPs in the five PRIME countries, and reflect on key lessons that can inform the scale-up of community-based mental health services in low-resource settings. Although we emphasize the community-based mental health service level in the districts, these cannot be separated from services in primary care clinics, which were designed to be strongly linked to the community setting in each site.

Ethiopia

Context

In Ethiopia, the development of a scalable district MHCP took place just after the publication of the first National Mental Health Strategy in 2012 (Federal Democratic Republic of Ethiopia Ministry of Health, 2012). At the national level there was momentum during this period to expand access to mental health care across the country. The Federal Ministry of Health partnered with Amanuel Specialised Mental Hospital (the only dedicated psychiatric hospital in the country) and the WHO to plan scale-up of the WHO's mental health Gap Action Programme (mhGAP). A national-level stakeholder committee decided priority mental health conditions for expanding treatment coverage (psychosis, bipolar disorder, epilepsy, depression, and AUD), projected the human resource requirements, adapted the mhGAP-IG, and conducted a proof-of-concept study evaluating the impact of training of health workers in mhGAP-IG (Federal Democratic Republic of Ethiopia Ministry of Health & World Health Organization, 2013).

These Ministry of Health activities to promote mental health at the national level were the foundation for PRIME in Ethiopia. The Strategy gave PRIME a mandate to approach district health officials and engage them in mental health care planning. Through close working with the Ministry of Health, the PRIME Ethiopia team learned lessons from the early pilot with mhGAP. Importantly, the early mhGAP pilot showed that non-specialist health workers could be successfully trained, but that the number of cases treated was much lower than expected, especially for psychosis (Federal Democratic Republic of Ethiopia Ministry of Health and World Health Organization, 2013). This pointed to important demand-side challenges and an urgent need for rigorous implementation research.

Sodo district, in the Gurage Zone of the Southern Nations Nationalities and Peoples' Region of Ethiopia, was selected as the PRIME implementation district. Sodo is located approximately 100 km south of Addis Ababa, the capital city of Ethiopia, and is a very rural district: over 90% of the inhabitants live outside of towns. At the time of starting PRIME, there was no mental health care available in the district, for a population of over 160,000 people, and no mental health research had ever been conducted in that district. The neighbouring districts had hosted the well-known Butajira epidemiological studies which investigated the course and outcome of people with severe mental disorder (Alem et al., 2009; Fekadu et al., 2015; Kebede et al., 2003; Shibre et al., 2014a, 2014b). This meant that there was some legacy of mental health awareness and care. Nonetheless, mental health services in Butajira were limited to an outpatient clinic staffed by psychiatric nurses that was 35 km away from the population of Sodo. This situation is typical of the rest of Ethiopia, where most mental health care outside of the major cities is delivered by psychiatric nurses in outpatient clinics linked to general hospitals.

Developing the district mental health care plan

Participatory planning of the district MHCP for Sodo began with establishment of a Community Advisory Board (CAB). Members of the CAB included officials from the district health, social affairs, and women's affairs sections, as well as religious leaders, police, and education representatives, NGOs engaged in community-based work, and caregivers of people with mental health conditions. As the mental health activities in the district became established, the CAB also included representation of people with lived experience of mental illness. Due to the low background awareness about mental health, in the first meeting of the CAB, the PRIME Ethiopia team explained what was known about mental illness and its impacts in Ethiopia, drawing on data from the neighbouring districts. The CAB members were receptive and expressed a motivation to work with PRIME to expand access to care. Even at that early stage the CAB expressed its particular concern about excessive alcohol use within the district, as well as the plight of those with severe mental illness who were destitute.

Alongside regular meetings with the CAB, the PRIME team then embarked on a period of intensive formative research to understand the opportunities and barriers to expanding access to mental health care. The focus was on achieving contextual fit, acceptability, feasibility, and potential to be scalable and sustainable. Taking a strengths-based approach, the PRIME team mapped the rich social and cultural resources that existed in Sodo district and identified over 150 traditional healers, 164 churches and mosques, 401 religious groups, 51 micro-finance institutions, and multiple social associations, including an average of five *eddir* groups (traditional funeral associations) per subdistrict (Selamu et al., 2015). In keeping with the concerns raised by the CAB, this exercise also identified two traditional bars per subdistrict of 2000–3000 adults. The burden of AUD in the population was confirmed in a population-level survey (n = 1485), which revealed overall prevalence of AUD of 13.9% (25.8% in men, 2.4% in women) (Zewdu et al., 2019). This was coupled with a high treatment gap of 87% for AUD. The same survey also showed high levels of population distress and low levels of social support: 14.1% had moderate/severe depression or anxiety symptoms and 13.8% expressed suicidal ideation, attempts, or plans (Fekadu et al., 2014).

A situation analysis of health system readiness identified important potential barriers, including absence of structures to supervise, monitor, and evaluate mental health care, and very limited availability of essential psychotropic medication (Hanlon et al., 2014). However, the extensive primary health care (PHC) network (including community health extension workers and health volunteers) and public health orientation of the health system were identified as opportunities for mental health integration. Furthermore, service models for people with chronic care needs, in particular for tuberculosis and HIV, were present in theory, even if not fully implemented, and could provide a blueprint for mental health care. Qualitative exploration with key stakeholders, including those with lived experience and their caregivers, underlined that impoverishment and social exclusion of people with mental illness were overriding concerns (Hailemariam et al., 2016). An integrative model of continuing care for people with severe mental illness was developed, emphasizing the important roles of community members and linkage with traditional and religious healers to achieve valued aspects of recovery (Mall et al., 2017).

The formative phase study findings fed into a participatory process with the CAB and other stakeholders to develop a theory of change for how clinical and social outcomes of people with mental health conditions could be improved (Hailemariam et al., 2015). This theory of change was then translated into a multilevel, multisectoral district MHCP (Fekadu et al., 2016). The main components of the Ethiopia plan are summarized in **Table 41.1**.

Table 41.1 Key components of the Ethiopia district mental health care plan

	Expected role	Intervention
Community level		
Community advisory board (CAB)	• Ensure multisectoral planning • Generate support for the plan in the community • Provide a collaborative link to religious healers • Ensure local ownership of the plan • Lead implementation and troubleshooting to overcome implementation barriers	• Established CAB and facilitated meetings every 6 months
Community health extension workers	• Detect and refer people with probable psychosis or epilepsy • Outreach to those who drop out of care • Detection and referral for patients with medication side effects • Raise community awareness about mental health problems and availability of care • Mobilize the community to address social needs	• 114 health extension workers trained for 2 days in case recognition and supporting people to access care
Primary care facility level		
Clinicians	• Follow evidence-based guidelines for the assessment and treatment of people with mental health conditions according to mhGAP-IG	• 150 primary care facility clinicians trained for 5 days in mhGAP followed by 5 days of on-the-job training
Other general facility staff members	• Provide non-stigmatizing support for people with mental health conditions to enter the facility and navigate care	• 0.5-day awareness-raising training
Pharmacists and pharmacy assistants	• Safe dispensing of psychotropic medication and capacity to provide support to health workers when prescribing	• 2-day training in safe dispensing and prescribing of psychotropic medications
Specialist mental health care		
Psychiatric nurses in general hospital	• Supervise and train primary health care workers in mhGAP-IG • Provide consultation on complex cases	• 5-day training in supervision of primary health care workers and orientation to new care model
Health system strengthening		
District mental health focal person and facility managers	• Coordinate and monitor implementation of plan • Procure essential psychotropic medications and monitor stock-outs • Track availability of trained staff and coordinate additional training • Coordinate supervision of trained staff	• Mentored by PRIME intervention coordinator
Psychiatrists and psychiatric nurses	• Provide mhGAP training and supervision	• Utilization of project psychiatrists and psychiatric nurses in the absence of mental health specialists in the district
Senior primary health care workers	• Provide facility-based supervision of mental health care integrated within existing supervisory framework	• Train and support senior health workers to be supervisors
Involvement of people with lived experience	• Involvement of people with lived experience in planning and monitoring quality	• Nested projects to empower and facilitate involvement (Abayneh et al., 2020)
Registration books	• Track service utilization (new cases and follow-up) for different types of mental health condition to (1) promote ongoing engagement in care (and linkage with community health extension workers), and (2) provide data for monitoring and quality improvement	• Project format introduced as routine indicators inadequate for planning and monitoring care

Implementing the plan

The plan was implemented in a sequential way. First, all facility-based PHC workers in eight health centres who were involved in patient care were trained in first-line mental health care (using mhGAP-IG) and a reliable supply of essential psychotropic medications was established. Only after this was achieved were community health extension workers and other community members trained in community-based case detection. This was to avoid the situation when help-seeking was increased before the facility was ready to provide care. PRIME staff, especially the intervention coordinator, worked closely with the district mental health focal person and PHC facility heads to support the implementation process. This included initial procurement of medication by PRIME and working alongside managerial staff to enable them to take over this process and establish revolving drug funds to ensure sustainable supplies. The PRIME intervention coordinator also oversaw the facility-based registration system for recording contacts with people with mental health conditions. As the national health management information system indicators did not differentiate between mental health conditions, a project-led mechanism for capturing these data was necessary. The data were then fed into quality improvement activities with facility staff to tackle the emerging problem of low detection of depression and high drop-out from care for people with psychosis. PRIME also tracked the number of mhGAP-trained staff available in facilities and worked with managers to coordinate further rounds of mhGAP training and refresher training. PRIME worked closely with the district to develop sustainable approaches to ongoing supervision of primary care staff who were trained in mhGAP. In the absence of mental health staff in the district, PRIME employed a psychiatric nurse to provide supervision to each facility on a regular basis (initially more frequent and reducing to monthly). Seeing the need to have specialist mental health workers to support the programme on an ongoing basis, the district sponsored a general nurse to be trained as a psychiatric nurse. The district also identified high-performing general health workers to be trained as mental health supervisors.

Impacts of the plan

The MHCP achieved high treatment coverage for people with psychosis, with over 80% of the estimated number of people with psychosis in the community engaging with the new primary care-based service (300 people) (Hailemariam et al., 2020). Over a 12-month follow-up period, there were significant improvements in clinical and functional outcomes, reduction in experience of discrimination, and reduced experience of restraint (from 25% to 12%) (Hanlon et al., 2019). These findings from PRIME have been supported by a randomized controlled trial of a similar model of task-shared care which was shown to be non-inferior to mental health care delivered by psychiatric nurses (Hanlon et al., 2022). Economic benefits of the PRIME MHCP were also seen, in terms of improved household income (Hailemichael et al., 2022) and improved food security (Tirfessa et al., 2020). Out-of-pocket health care costs for people with psychosis reduced significantly over time, especially driven by reduced costs accessing traditional and religious healing (Chisholm et al., 2020). These impacts were evident to the community and helped to increase commitment to the programme by families with a person with psychosis, the CAB, community members, and health care professionals. Inspired by the changes that were seen in some people with severe mental illness, community members made extraordinary efforts to help homeless people with psychosis to access care and support, including for their basic needs for food and shelter.

Important benefits of the MHCP were also seen for people with epilepsy (Catalao et al., 2018). For both people with psychosis and people with epilepsy, respondents especially valued the proximity of care. However, they reported unmet psychosocial needs. Ongoing engagement in care was also a challenge due to the costs of repeated clinic visits and medication, and an expectation of cure rather than chronic care (Hailemariam et al., 2017). Many people with psychosis and epilepsy continued to access traditional or religious healing, although this was not reported as an important driver of non-engagement or drop-out from care. Mortality was also high in both groups over the follow-up period, indicating an urgent need to improve physical health care. Nested within PRIME in Ethiopia was a randomized controlled trial of community-based rehabilitation (the 'RISE' trial) for people with psychosis whose functioning remained impaired after 6 months of engagement with primary care-based mental health care. In RISE, adding community-based rehabilitation significantly improved functioning after 12 months, indicating that add-on interventions can have value for those who have more enduring disability (Asher et al., 2022).

The PRIME MHCP in Ethiopia was less successful in meeting the needs of people with depression or AUD. mhGAP training failed to lead to any improvement of the extremely low levels of detection of depression in PHC facilities (Fekadu et al., 2017). Qualitative exploration indicated that normalization of depressive symptoms as understandable in the context of social adversities was an important reason for low detection, alongside preferred alternative religious and cultural explanations for depressive symptoms (Tekola et al., 2021). Differing manifestations of depressive symptoms in this context were also identified as important.

Very few people with AUD were detected after implementation of the MHCP. However, among those who received a brief intervention for AUD, there was evidence of reduced use of alcohol and reduced alcohol-related harms, translating into important impacts on the person's life (Zewdu et al., 2022). Acceptability of care for AUD was relatively lower than for other conditions, however, due to perceptions that problems with alcohol were a social problem rather than within the purview of the health care system.

Important lessons learned

The impacts of PRIME in Ethiopia were beyond our expectations, even if much more still needs to be done. The successes were due largely to the commitment of the community leaders and the CAB members. Without their early and ongoing engagement, the programme would have had little community support. The CAB took ownership of the programme and played an essential role in troubleshooting the frequent implementation barriers. Visible benefits to those with overt mental illness fuelled the momentum. Seeing people who the community had all but given up on resuming their place in society was a powerful testament to the benefits of care. This in turn was assisted by high-level national policy support throughout.

Nonetheless, there were clear failures in expanding care to people with depression or AUD. In the case of depression, our team has been prompted to go 'back to basics' and develop deeper understanding of the concept of depression in this setting and appropriate ways to detect and provide acceptable care. For AUD, health officials still have high levels of concern about the detrimental effects of alcohol in Sodo. Stakeholder consultation indicates that community-based approaches to detection and treatment may be a more acceptable approach, alongside increased awareness about AUD in the community in general.

We went into PRIME knowing that demand-side barriers were important and only partially managed to address this gap. Subsequent work to empower people with lived experience of mental health conditions to advocate for better and more accessible services indicates that mobilization of service users could be a vital aspect of increasing the demand for care (Abayneh et al., 2020). The community-level activities of the MHCP could also have been strengthened in the areas of awareness raising activities, livelihoods initiatives, and efforts to facilitate ongoing engagement in care.

Health system bottlenecks to sustaining the district MHCP were substantial, and yet are potentially surmountable with sufficient political commitment. Any new health programme needs health system supports, in terms of appropriate indicators for monitoring, holding health workers and districts accountable through regular programme review, integration of mental health into existing supervisory systems, and making mental health part of the role expectation for every health worker. There is only so much a project can do to overcome system barriers, but PRIME Ethiopia has shown ways in which system barriers can be addressed to achieve a functioning district mental health service.

Conclusions

A community-based model of integrated mental health care in Ethiopia helped to make care more accessible and delivered clear benefits for people with severe mental illness and epilepsy. More needs to be done to understand how to better meet the needs of people with depression and AUD. Close working with communities and those with lived experience of mental illness in planning and implementing new care models is essential for success.

India

Context

In India, the PRIME MHCP was implemented and evaluated in Sehore district in Madhya Pradesh. The state of Madhya Pradesh is situated in the central part of India, has a population of 72.5 million, and it was one of the priority states for UK aid due to its poor general health indicators. Sehore is a neighbouring district of the city of Bhopal which is the state capital. It has a population of 1.3 million which is predominantly rural (81% of the population lives in the villages). Sehore was selected because it was one of the districts where the District Mental Health Programme (a flagship component of the National Mental Health Programme) was implemented and therefore the infrastructure to develop, implement, and scale up the MHCP was already in place.

During the formative phase (August 2011–March 2014), a comprehensive situational analysis was undertaken to understand the context (Shidhaye et al., 2015), followed by a series of theory of change workshops, a qualitative study with key stakeholders, and pilot implementation in one community health centre (CHC). In Madhya Pradesh, a district has several administrative blocks. A CHC is located at the block level and the district hospital is located at the district headquarters. A CHC caters to a population of around 150,000.

The situational analysis primarily helped the PRIME team to identify a range of major health system challenges in developing and implementing the MHCP. The first and foremost challenge was the lack of political will resulting in an extremely low priority accorded to mental health by the local decision-makers and state-level planners, and major challenges related to overall governance and financing of mental health services. Poor intersectoral coordination between various departments responsible for implementation of mental health programmes had resulted in underutilization of allocated funds from the federal government. Very little funds were allocated within the state budget and activities essential for mental health service delivery were not included in the Project Implementation Plans submitted to the National Rural Health Mission. The second major challenge was around human resources which were not just scarce but highly inequitably distributed. The almost complete lack of psychiatric nurses, psychiatric social workers, and occupational therapists precluded development of any collaborative care models for service delivery. The third challenge was poor community participation and ownership of the mental health programme. This was particularly important as the reduction in the treatment gap depends both on the supply of accessible mental health services as well as on demand for and utilization of mental health services by the community. Absence of a robust monitoring framework and non-integration of mental health indicators with general health management information systems was identified as the fourth major challenge.

Developing the district mental health care plan

The PRIME India MHCP was developed in partnership with the Department of Health Services, Government of Madhya Pradesh, and other key stakeholders. The MHCP had seven packages and they were broadly divided into enabling and service delivery packages (Shidhaye et al., 2016). Each package was further broken down into components and for each, a number of steps for their implementation were identified.

The enabling packages comprised of cross-cutting interventions that would ensure the smooth implementation of core mental health service delivery packages. There were three enabling packages: programme management, capacity building, and community mobilization. The four service delivery packages were awareness for mental disorders, identification, treatment, and recovery. The core service delivery packages were related to the delivery of mental health services for the three priority disorders: depression, psychosis, and AUD.

There was a dynamic interplay between the enabling and service delivery packages. A few illustrative examples are described below. Two important service delivery packages were identification and treatment of people with priority mental disorders. This could begin only when medical officers, paramedical staff, and frontline workers were trained in evidence-based interventions, using the WHO mhGAP-IG. The capacity-building package ensured this by not only providing the initial training but also continuous supportive supervision which helped in maintaining and enhancing the skills and competencies acquired during the initial training. The interlinked activities related to capacity-building and identification and treatment were supported by simultaneously functioning programme management package. This package included human and financial resource management, supply chain management of essential psychotropic drugs, and a well-functioning information system. Engagement with the general community members and mobilizing users, carers, and other community members to advocate for rights-based delivery of mental health services was the objective of a community mobilization package (one of the enabling packages). This, along with awareness (a service delivery package) simultaneously increased the demand for mental health services. Thus, the enabling packages served as a foundation for service delivery packages of the MHCP.

The MHCP was implemented in three CHCs in the Sehore district. These three CHCs were situated in towns, but mostly served the rural population and on average there are 1600 outpatients (including adults and children) per month.

Programme management activities related to governance, human resource management, and drug procurement and supply chain management started in March 2014. Training of medical officers, community health workers (Accredited Social Health Activists), and case managers was conducted from March 2014 to July 2014. The health management information system was established in the last week of July 2014. The MHCP service delivery packages became operational in August 2014 and regular process data was collected from 1 August 2014 until the end of the implementation phase (31 August 2016).

Mental health services were delivered on both health care and community platforms at the CHC and village level, respectively. The mental health case managers employed by PRIME played a very important role in implementation of the MHCP. At the health care-platform level, they coordinated provision of mental health services in 'Mann-Kaksha', a room in each CHC that was allocated for the mental health programme. At the community-platform level, the case managers visited villages that were in the catchment areas of their respective CHCs to provide services.

Impacts of the plan

We found that the PRIME MHCP did not have a significant impact on contact coverage (treatment seeking) for depression (14.8% at the baseline and 10.5% at the follow-up) and AUD (7.7% at the baseline and 7.3% at the follow-up) (Shidhaye et al., 2019a). In the health facilities (CHCs), the MHCP had a small impact on detection and initiation of treatment for depression and AUD (9.7% for depression and 17.8% for AUD compared with 0% for both at the baseline). People with depression who received care as part of the MHCP had higher rates of response (i.e. reduction in PHQ-9 score by 50% compared to the baseline; 52.2% in the treatment group vs 26.9% in the comparison/usual care group), early remission (i.e. PHQ-9 <10 at 3 months; 70.2% in the treatment group vs 44.8% in the comparison/usual care group) and recovery (i.e. PHQ-9 <10 at 12 months but not at 3 months; 56.1% in the treatment group vs 28.5% in the comparison/usual care group), but there was no impact of treatment on their functioning.

Important lessons learned

Nevertheless, implementation of the MHCP in Sehore district demonstrated that it is feasible to establish structures (e.g. Mann-Kaksha) and operationalize various processes to integrate mental health services in primary care (Shidhaye et al., 2019b). The key lessons from the multilevel case study were as follows: (1) clear 'process maps' of clinical interventions as well as implementation steps were very helpful in monitoring/tracking the progress; (2) in addition to the training of service providers, implementation support from an external team to provide clinical supervision and address the implementation barriers is important; (3) enabling packages of the MHCP played a crucial role in strengthening the health systems and improving the context/settings for implementation; and (4) lack of incentives for community health workers (Accredited Social Health Activists in the case of India) led to poor delivery of services at the community-platform level.

Conclusions

Design, implementation, and evaluation of the PRIME MHCP during the period 2011–2019, contributed to several important policy shifts in state of Madhya Pradesh.

1. *Scaling up of mental health services*: in late 2015 and early 2016, after a number of consultations with the PRIME India team, the Government of Madhya Pradesh decided to scale up the mental health programme in all 51 districts in the state covering a population of 75 million (Kokane et al., 2017). The PRIME implementation model, especially the 'Mann-Kaksha', was at the core of this effort. This programme was led by the Department of Health Services with significant inputs from the PRIME India team. Two nurses in each of the 51 district hospitals were trained in screening of priority mental disorders and provision of psychosocial interventions and one medical officer from each of these district hospitals received a month-long training in diagnosis and treatment of mental disorders. Operationalization of 'Mann-Kaksha' to strengthen mental health services was awarded as a best practice by the National Health Mission (Ministry of Health and Family Welfare, 2017).

2. *Health systems integration*: until 2014, mental health programmes were led by the Department of Medical Education whereas all other health programmes were under the Department of Health Services. This led to fragmentation of services. The scaled-up mental health programme is now included under the National Health Mission, which oversees implementation of all public health programmes in the state. A senior level official of the rank of the Deputy Director of Health Services was appointed to oversee implementation of mental health services across the state.

3. *Sustainable financing of the mental health programme*: the situational analysis found that there was no allocation of funds by the state government for mental health programmes until 2011 and even the funds allocated by the central government were underutilized. With the scale-up of mental health programmes across the state, the situation has changed substantially. The state government now allocates a dedicated budget every year to support state-wide scale-up of mental health services. This is unprecedented in the Indian context as most of the other states rely solely on the central government funds released as part of the District Mental Health Programme which are, in turn, often inadequate and delayed in disbursement, posing a major barrier in programme implementation.

Nepal

Context

In Nepal, like most low- and middle- income countries, there is a scarcity of mental health services outside the urban centres (Luitel et al., 2015). The National Mental Health Policy of 1996 emphasized community mental health programmes, but systematic implementation of the policy into practice had not yet occurred when the PRIME programme initiated its activities in 2011.

The district MHCP developed and implemented in Chitwan, Nepal, comprised interventions at community, health facility, and health service organization levels, following the blueprint that was developed for the PRIME consortium (Jordans et al., 2016). The core of the MHCP was to integrate mental health services into PHC, following WHO's mhGAP-IG (WHO, 2016a), and we demonstrated largely positive results in doing so in Nepal (Jordans et al., 2019b).

However, we recognized early on the importance of the community-level interventions for the Nepal context. This is because health workers have very limited time to provide the more time-consuming psychological interventions, there is a lack of confidential space at PHC facilities, and demand-side barriers prevent people with mental health problems seeking help from PHC providers (Brenman et al., 2014). As a result, we emphasized two approaches to strengthening community-based services that were part of the district MHCP in Nepal. First, community gatekeepers were identified to play a role in proactive case detection to increase help-seeking. Second, we included a cadre of community psychosocial counsellors to provide psychological treatments in both PHC facilities, where confidential space is available, and in community settings.

Proactive case detection

Under-detection of mental health problems is one of the key demand-side barriers for the scaling up of mental health care (Jordans et al., 2015). Low literacy and high levels of stigma prevent the use of universal screening methods to aid detection, as do the lack of valid self-report instruments for serious mental illness. Community case-finding has been advocated as a strategy to increase access to mental health care. In response, we developed the Community Informant Detection Tool (CIDT) in Nepal, which is a method of proactive case detection that enables lay people in the community (i.e. gatekeepers) to assist in the identification of people with potential depression, psychosis, AUD, and epilepsy. The tool consists of context-sensitive vignettes, combined with illustrations, describing prototypes of the mentioned mental health conditions, that are easy to understand by low-literacy populations. Those using the tool are asked to gauge the extent to which any member of the community matches a prototype, followed by two simple questions about perceived impaired daily functioning and perceived need for support for the identified individual. Following positive responses to the questions, the community gatekeeper encourages the person to seek support from the nearby PHC centre (where health workers have been trained in mhGAP). Female community health volunteers (FCHV), the least specialized level of health care providers in the health system in Nepal, are well respected in the community and have access to vulnerable populations (especially women) who are less likely to visit formal health services. In the PRIME MHCP, female community health volunteers are trained in case detection and referral using the CIDT. In studies we have demonstrated that female community health volunteers are accurate in approximately two-thirds of the cases they detect, when compared to structured clinical interviews by a psychiatrist (Jordans et al., 2015), and that approximately two-thirds of those detected using the CIDT actually go on to seek mental health care (Jordans et al., 2017). When implementing this in our district-wide implementation of the PRIME MHCP, we were able to demonstrate the effectiveness of this approach, resulting in a 50% increase in help-seeking in the areas where the CIDT was being used compared to those where it was not being used (Jordans et al., 2020). The tool has since been endorsed and adopted by the government of Nepal Ministry of Health and Population, as part of the newly developed comprehensive community mental health care package. With increasing attention and initiatives globally for making mental health care available, we argue that this should go hand in hand with efforts to increase access to, and engagement with, those services. The CIDT has been demonstrated to be a tool that can contribute to efforts to overcoming the treatment gap.

Psychological interventions by community psychosocial counsellors

In the absence of mental health specialists, health workers were trained as part of the PRIME MHCP to provide mental health care (consisting of brief emotional support, psychoeducation, and provision of psychotropic medicines when indicated), but often lacked the time for full-blown multisession psychological interventions. In Nepal, we therefore included community counsellors as an integral part of Nepal's MHCP to ensure that psychological interventions are provided. Paraprofessional counsellors were trained to provide support in health facilities and the community, specifically the Healthy Activity Programme (HAP) for depression (Chowdhary et al., 2016) and Counselling for Alcohol Problems (CAP) for alcohol use problems (Nadkarni et al., 2017). From our evaluation of these services, we learned that the community-based counsellor-delivered HAP was an effective intervention for depression, above and beyond health worker delivered mhGAP-based care—an effect that was sustained and increased at 12 months (Jordans et al., 2019a). For people with alcohol use problems, the counsellor-delivered CAP did not result in significantly better outcomes when compared to health worker-provided psychosocial and pharmacological treatment (Jordans et al., 2019a).

Important lessons learned

The study and our experience lend support for the inclusion of psychological treatments as part of the roll-out of mhGAP guidelines for depression, provided by dedicated community-based counsellors (or comparable cadre of service providers). The absence of a position for counsellors in the Nepal health care system at present, however, is a challenge for sustaining psychological interventions. Advocacy is therefore needed for a long-term mental health strategy and programme that includes a cadre of service providers dedicated to providing psychological interventions. We believe this is an important safeguard against over-medicalization of mental health care using the mhGAP, given the above-mentioned limited time per patient for most primary health workers.

South Africa

Context

With mental illness being regarded as a chronic condition, albeit with acute episodes, the national Department of Health directed the PRIME programme in South Africa to work in a district which was piloting a model for integrated chronic disease management. The rationale was that this approach would help us to understand how best identification and management of mental health could be included in this model. The model included introduction of different streams for patients attending PHC facilities that included a chronic care stream, the use of an integrated set of chronic care guidelines—Primary Care 101, later called Adult Primary Care, as well as the introduction of ward-based community health worker outreach teams linked to PHC facilities (Mahomed et al., 2014). The site was the Dr Kenneth Kaunda District in the North West Province.

Development of the district mental health care plan

The formative phase of the PRIME-South Africa programme resulted in the development of a district MHCP focused on integration of common mental disorders into the chronic care stream within PHC facilities, as this was identified as a notable gap during the situational analysis (Petersen et al., 2016). Another notable gap identified was the paucity of psychosocial rehabilitation programmes for stabilized mental health service users with severe mental illness who had been down-referred to PHC facilities for follow-up care following discharge from hospital as part of the national policy imperative for deinstitutionalization (Department of Health, 2013). The PRIME-South Africa MHCP thus also addressed the need for community-based psychosocial rehabilitation for these service users, with a focus on schizophrenia (Petersen et al., 2016). In addition, at the community level, community health worker outreach teams already in the system were identified as existing human resources who could assist with the promotion of mental health, detection and referral of family members within communities with mental health problems, adherence support, and tracing non-adherent mental health service users to link them back into care in line with their roles for other conditions (Petersen et al., 2016).

Implementing the plan

Adopting a task-sharing collaborative care approach, PHC nurses' capacity to assess and diagnose common mental disorders in chronic care patients was strengthened through training in a supplementary mental health Adult Primary Care module. This incorporated mhGAP guidelines as well as a module in clinical communication skills to assist nurses with a person-centred approach to care. Referral pathways for treatment were strengthened through the introduction of a co-located counselling service for mild to moderate depressive symptoms provided by lay counsellors, trained in an eight-session manualized counselling intervention drawing on cognitive behavioural techniques (Petersen et al., 2016). This was in addition to the existing referral pathways to PHC doctors and mental health specialists, who were a scarce resource within PHC settings. With regard to addressing the gap in psychosocial rehabilitation services for service users with severe mental illness, auxiliary social workers, working for a state-subsidized mental health NGO in the district, were identified through the situational analysis as potential facilitators of the planned community-based psychosocial rehabilitation programme. In-depth qualitative interviews with service users and their caregivers informed the development of a group-based psychosocial rehabilitation programme comprising 12 sessions that included psychoeducation, adherence support, coping skills for conflict, coping skills for stigma and discrimination, income generation activities, substance abuse, contributing to the running of the household, and money management (Brooke-Sumner et al., 2014). Sessions accommodated non-medical explanatory models of illness and built on the significance of religion in recovery. A training manual for auxiliary social workers to facilitate the sessions as well as a facilitators guide were developed to support the programme.

Impacts of the plan

The collaborative care model for patients with comorbid common mental disorders was evaluated under real-world conditions across four large facilities in one subdistrict through a quasi-experimental design and shown to improve detection of common mental disorders and reduce depressive symptoms among patients with chronic conditions (Petersen et al., 2019). Exposure to a greater number of counselling sessions was found to optimize clinical depression outcomes, with patients having better clinical outcomes on their depressive scores (Selohilwe et al., 2019). This was followed by a pragmatic cluster randomized controlled trial targeting hypertensive patients with comorbid depression, where the intervention group with the strengthened Adult Primary Care mental health module and clinical communication skills as well as co-located lay counselling service was found to be neither superior nor inferior to care as usual. Low exposure of the trial participants in the intervention group to depression treatment was a limitation of the trial (Petersen et al., 2021a). Qualitative comparative analysis of process indicators collected alongside the trial indicates the importance of ensuring programme fidelity for achieving implementation outcomes (Janse van Rensburg et al., 2021). The collaborative care package has since been repackaged for broader scale-up through the Southern African Mental health INTegration (SMhINT) project in the province of KwaZulu-Natal. Implementation science is being used to understand how the innovation and the health system need to be strengthened to be enabling of implementation and scale-up within routine PHC services (Petersen et al., 2020, 2021b).

In relation to the psychosocial rehabilitation programme for service users with severe mental disorders, the intervention was pre-piloted with a small group of service users with stable conditions attending one PHC facility, with qualitative interviews informing revisions to the programme prior to a pilot evaluation across four large facilities servicing one subdistrict. Forty-four service users were enrolled in the pilot evaluation using a single cohort group design. Results were promising in respect of improved functionality and reduced internalized stigma (Brooke-Sumner et al., 2018). Follow-up qualitative data revealed improved self-esteem and increased illness knowledge, reduced risk taking, reduced social isolation and improved pro-social behaviour, improved financial management and engagement in income generation activities, as well as improved acceptance by the community (Brooke-Sumner et al., 2018). However, the need for the groups to be ongoing and provide longer-term support was identified by participants (Brooke-Sumner et al., 2018). Building on these findings, the programme has been further adapted to include a peer support component to promote ongoing support. This adapted programme is currently being evaluated through a randomized control trial in the Eastern Cape, supported by multiplier funding.

One of the main challenges encountered by the PRIME project in the development, implementation, and scaling up of mental health services at the community level was the weak intersectoral collaboration within the community subsystem. The community subsystem includes community health workers, who interface with PHC facilities, households, community structures such as faith-based organizations, NGOs, civic groups, local political structures, and other sectors, particularly social work services at a community level (Schneider & Lehmann, 2016). Reintegration of discharged mental health service users into the community is particularly hamstrung by the division of responsibilities for community mental health care between sectors and lack of coordination between sectors. The Department of Health is responsible for ongoing medical care, whereas the Department of Social Development is responsible for psychosocial rehabilitation, housing, and disability grants. Qualitative investigation with stakeholders from these sectors as part of PRIME led to recommendations for improving this intersectoral work (e.g. role clarification, provision of a focal person to coordinate collaboration, and improving communication and referrals between sectors) (Brooke-Sumner et al., 2016).

These strategies, however, remain challenging to implement. As a consequence, many mental health service users are lost to care upon discharge. This contributes to South Africa's 'revolving door' problem, with close to 25% of mental health service users being readmitted to hospital within 3 months of a previous discharge (Docrat et al., 2019). A further notable challenge at a community level is low mental health literacy. This reduces demand for mental health services and fuels mental health stigma, adding an additional challenge for reintegration of mental health service users into the community, while also leading to low levels of help-seeking by people with mental health problems (Egbe et al., 2014). The need for population-level anti-stigma interventions is indicated as is the need for psychoeducation on the causes, signs, and symptoms as well as care and treatment options for mental health problems.

Important lessons learned

1. Integration of care for common mental disorders into chronic care platforms at PHC level using a collaborative task-sharing approach is possible within resource-constrained settings. However, effectiveness within routine PHC is compromised by poor uptake and fidelity to the integration package.
2. Implementation science research is required to understand how the health system needs strengthening to be more enabling of uptake of integrated mental health care within routine chronic care in PHC settings.
3. In this regard, systems-strengthening interventions that strive towards people-centred care and include mental health within this approach from the outset may help to stop mental health being viewed as an add-on.
4. Strengthening the community subsystem to optimize intersectoral collaboration; strengthening the linkages between PHC facilities and the community subsystem; and strengthening mental health literacy to improve demand for services as well as to enable reintegration of services users with severe mental illness within communities following discharge are indicated.

Uganda

Context

The district MHCP for Uganda was developed to operationalize the National Health Policy Framework (2011–2030) and the then National Health Policy (2010–2015) which prioritized strengthening the health system in line with decentralization; reconceptualizing, organizing supervision and monitoring of health systems at all levels; establishing a functional integration within the public and private sector; and addressing the human resource crisis.

In Uganda, Kamuli was the district pilot site for the MHCP and the implementation area for PRIME. Kamuli was chosen out of 135 districts in Uganda because it is typical of the many rural districts in Uganda with inadequate staffing and limited mental health care service provision in PHC. Kamuli is located in Eastern Uganda, approximately 155 km from the national referral mental hospital (Butabika). The district has a total population of 490,255 of whom 96% reside in rural areas and 58% live in poverty.

Developing the district mental health care plan

As part of the work of PRIME, we developed a district MHCP for the district demonstration site in Kamuli district, in a bid to operationalize the national mental health policy framework at service delivery level. The plan was structured within the broad objectives of the national Ugandan mental health programme, namely providing equitable access to quality mental health care, strengthening the engagement of communities, promoting the integration of mental health into PHC, protecting the human rights of people with MNS disorders, changing the negative attitudes and misperceptions of the population as regards MNS disorders through community sensitization, and strengthening the workforce for MNS disorders in the district.

Prior to its development, a situational analysis and formative research were conducted to gather views and perceptions of various stakeholders. This was followed by theory of change workshops involving several stakeholders within the district (including service users, health service providers, health managers, planners, and political administrators), during which a theory of change map for the MHCP was developed. The plan had five packages of care, delivered at three levels of health service delivery, including community level, health facility level, and health organization/management level (Table 41.2).

The five packages included Awareness and Knowledge enhancement, Detection of disorders, Treatment, Recovery, and Programme Management (Kigozi et al., 2016). At each level of service delivery, the stakeholders identified the various components under each package, the objective, the primary providers (their roles and responsibilities), the activities to undertake, tools to use, and the methods of delivery. The plan further provided details on the different input, process, output, and outcome indicators, and how the evaluation would be done.

Packages of care at community level

At the community level, three packages of care were provided, including awareness and knowledge enhancement, detection, and recovery. The first component under awareness and knowledge enhancement was community sensitization and anti-stigma mobilization. Here the aim was to raise the community's awareness about mental health and psychosocial problems, reduce stigma towards people with mental health problems in the community, and increase support and demand for mental health services including perinatal mental health services. The primary providers were members of the Village Health Teams, whose role was to sensitize the communities on mental health issues through community sensitization meetings, distribution of information, education, and communication materials and radio talk-shows; as well as the mental health coordinator, who supervised the Village Health Teams. The other providers included the PHC workers, such as nurses, midwives, and health inspectors. The second component was training of the members of the Village Health Teams to be able to identify and offer basic psychosocial support to people with MNS disorders in the community. The primary providers were the mental health specialists in the district, supported by the specialists/national trainers from the Ministry of Health. These would organize and conduct training workshops for the Village Health Team members as well as supervision.

Table 41.2 Packages of care in the Uganda district mental health care plan

	Packages				
	Awareness and Knowledge Enhancement	Detection	Treatment	Recovery	Programme management
1. Health organization	1.1 Engagement/advocacy/ mental health literacy				2.1. Drug supply chain management 2.2. Health management information systems 2.3. Human resource support, motivation, and supervision 2.4. Capacity building 2.5. Routine monitoring and evaluation
2. PHC health facility	1.1. Standardized in-service training	2.2. Screening and assessment	3.1. Psychotropic medication 3.2. Basic psychosocial support	4.1. Continuing care	
3. Community	1.1. Community sensitization/ anti-stigma/mobilization 1.2. Training of Village Health Team workers	2.1. Community detection		4.1. Outreach/ adherence support 4.2. Community-based rehabilitation	

The second package at this level was community detection, for which the objective was to increase detection and referral of persons with mental health problems within the community. The primary providers were members of the Village Health Teams, whose role was to identify and support people with mental health problems in the community. Other providers included community leaders as well family members of persons with mental health problems, who would identify and make referrals to the health facilities.

The third package at this level was recovery, with two components. The first was outreach and adherence support provided by PHC nurses, midwives, Village Health Team members, as well as the mental health coordinator. The objective was to ensure adherence to mental health treatments and provide continuing psychosocial support to persons with mental illness. This was provided through outreach activities in the community, supportive counselling, psychoeducation, and documenting and reporting non-adherence to treatment. The second component was community-based rehabilitation, for which the providers were Village Health Team members and community development officers. The objective was to provide community-based rehabilitation to persons with MNS disorders by providing peer and livelihood support as well as linking them to available community-based livelihood programmes. Under this component, the service users were trained in advocacy, self-management, and entrepreneurship skills, mobilized and supported to form user support groups, attached to the main health facilities.

Impacts of the plan

Implementation of the plan resulted in increased clinical detection of depression for adults attending the clinics in the short term (Nakku et al., 2019). There was also a significant reduction in symptom severity and functional impairment among those who received care in primary care clinics over 12 months during the implementation of the plan. There was a negligible change in population-level treatment coverage for people with depression and AUD in the district. This consequently resulted in reduced stigma and discrimination, and increased support for people with mental health problems (Nakku et al., 2019).

The training of members of the Village Health Teams increased their capacity and competence to identify and offer basic psychosocial support to people with MNS disorders in the community. This resulted in increased case detection of persons with mental health problems within the community and referral to the health facilities.

The engagement, advocacy, and increased demand for services that resulted made a case for addressing the human resource gap, and consequently more mental health specialists were recruited and deployed at various health facilities. The engagement at community level facilitated the formation of user support and peer groups. With the support of the health workers, these groups provided a platform for continuing psychosocial support and community-based rehabilitation of persons with MNS disorders. With the mobilization through these groups, users were able to access and benefit from the services by the existing structures, including the livelihood support services in the district (Nakku et al., 2019).

Important lessons learned

From our experience in implementing the district MHCP, there are a couple of lessons which might be helpful for those wishing to implement and scale up community mental health services at district level. First is the importance of devoting the necessary resources and support for the programme. Creating demand for services alone does not guarantee change and sustainability of the health system improvements. Rather, it requires more inputs including resources, monitoring, and supervision. Second, community-level mental health programmes should also explore and consider the factors that influence the decision to contact a health care provider by people with mental disorders. There is a need to understand the nature and quantity of interventions required to improve help-seeking in the community if interventions are to make the desired impact.

Conclusion

The experience from PRIME has shown that there are a number of advantages to a district-level approach for planning and delivering community mental health care in low-resource settings. First, there are opportunities to adopt a population health approach, measuring not only the impacts of community-based services on individual service users, but also impacts on processes of delivering care and on population coverage. Second, district approaches allow for integrated planning that links community with primary care and health management levels, and supports the integration of mental health into other general health services. Third, this approach provides an opportunity for collaborative planning and engagement of stakeholders, such as through the use of theory of change methods. Finally, district-level planning provides an opportunity to address both demand-side and supply-side constraints on community mental health service delivery.

PRIME has also generated a number of planning, implementation, and evaluation tools which can be disseminated and adapted for scale-up of mental health care in low-resource settings. Further work is needed to ensure that these tools are disseminated to other countries wishing to scale up community-based mental health care in low-resource settings. From a methodological perspective, further research is needed on optimal implementation science methods to evaluate the implementation and scaling up of community mental health care in low-resource settings. With growing public and policy awareness of the importance of mental health in the Covid-19 era, there is now strong interest in providing affordable, accessible, acceptable, and effective mental health services in communities. The materials from PRIME provide resources that can hopefully assist in meeting this urgent need.

REFERENCES

Abayneh, S., Lempp, H., Alem, A., Kohrt, B., Fekadu, A., & Hanlon, C. (2020). Developing a theory of change model of service user and caregiver involvement in mental health system strengthening in primary health care in rural Ethiopia. *International Journal of Mental Health Systems*, **14**, 51.

Alem, A., Kebede, D., Fekadu, A., Shibre, T., Fekadu, D., Beyero, T., et al. (2009). Clinical course and outcome of schizophrenia in a predominantly treatment-naive cohort in rural Ethiopia. *Schizophrenia Bulletin*, **35**, 646–654.

Asher, L., Birhane, R., Weiss, H. A., Medhin, G., Selamu, M., Patel, V., et al. (2022). Community-based rehabilitation intervention for people with schizophrenia in Ethiopia (RISE): results of a 12-month cluster-randomised controlled trial. *Lancet Global Health*, **10**, e530–e542.

Brenman, N. F., Luitel, N. P., Mall, S., & Jordans, M. J. D. (2014). Demand and access to mental health services: a qualitative formative study in Nepal. *BMC International Health and Human Rights*, **14**, 1–10.

Breuer, E., De Silva, M. J., Shidaye, R., Petersen, I., Nakku, J., Jordans, M. J., et al. (2016). Planning and evaluating mental health services in low- and middle-income countries using theory of change. *British Journal of Psychiatry*, **208**(Suppl. 56), s55–s62.

Brooke-Sumner, C., Lund, C., & Petersen, I. (2014). Perceptions of psychosocial disability amongst psychiatric service users and caregivers in South Africa. *African Journal of Disability*, **3**, 146.

Brooke-Sumner, C., Lund, C., & Petersen, I. (2016). Bridging the gap: investigating challenges and way forward for intersectoral provision of psychosocial rehabilitation in South Africa. *International Journal of Mental Health Systems*, **10**, 21.

Brooke-Sumner, C., Selohilwe, O., Mazibuko, M. S., & Petersen, I. (2018). Process evaluation of a pilot intervention for psychosocial rehabilitation for service users with schizophrenia in North West Province, South Africa. *Community Mental Health Journal*, **54**, 1089–1096.

Catalao, R., Eshetu, T., Tsigebrhan, R., Medhin, G., Fekadu, A., & Hanlon, C. (2018). Implementing integrated services for people with epilepsy in primary care in Ethiopia: a qualitative study. *BMC Health Services Research*, **18**, 372.

Chisholm, D., Garman, E., Breuer, E., Fekadu, A., Hanlon, C., Jordans, M., et al. (2020). Health service costs and their association with functional impairment among adults receiving integrated mental health care in five low- and middle-income countries: the PRIME cohort study. *Health Policy and Planning*, **35**, 567–576.

Chowdhary, N., Anand, A., Dimidjian, S., Shinde, S., Weobong, B., Balaji, M., et al. (2016). The Healthy Activity Program lay counsellor delivered treatment for severe depression in India: systematic development and randomised evaluation. *British Journal of Psychiatry*, **208**, 381–388.

De Silva, M. J., Rathod, S. D., Hanlon, C., Breuer, E., Chisholm, D., Fekadu, A., et al. (2016). Evaluation of district mental healthcare plans: the PRIME consortium methodology. *British Journal of Psychiatry*, **208**(Suppl. 56), s63–s70.

Department of Health (2013). *Mental Health Policy Framework and Strategic Plan*. Pretoria: Department of Health.

Docrat, S., Besada, D., Cleary, S., Daviaud, E., & Lund, C. (2019). Mental health system costs, resources and constraints in South Africa: a national survey. *Health Policy Plan*, **34**, 706–719.

Egbe, C. O., Brooke-Sumner, C., Kathree, T., Selohilwe, O., Thornicroft, G., & Petersen, I. (2014). Psychiatric stigma and discrimination in South Africa: perspectives from key stakeholders. *BMC Psychiatry*, **14**, 191.

Federal Democratic Republic of Ethiopia Ministry of Health (2012). *National Mental Health Strategy, 2012/13–2015/16*. Addis Ababa: Federal Ministry of Health.

Federal Democratic Republic of Ethiopia Ministry of Health & World Health Organization (2013). *mhGAP in Ethiopia. Proof of concept*. Addis Ababa: Federal Ministry of Health.

Fekadu, A., Hanlon, C., Medhin, G., Alem, A., Selamu, M., Giorgis, T., et al. (2016). Development of a scalable mental healthcare plan for a rural district in Ethiopia. *British Journal of Psychiatry*, **208**(Suppl. 56), s4–s12.

Fekadu, A., Medhin, G., Kebede, D., Alem, A., Cleare, A., Prince, M., et al. (2015). Excess mortality in severe mental disorders: a 10-year population-based cohort study in rural Ethiopia. *British Journal of Psychiatry*, **206**, 289–296.

Fekadu, A., Medhin, G., Selamu, M., Giorgis, T. W., Lund, C., Alem, A., et al. (2017). Recognition of depression by primary care clinicians in rural Ethiopia. *BMC Family Practice*, **18**, 56.

Fekadu, A., Medhin, G., Selamu, M., Hailemariam, M., Alem, A., Giorgis, T. W., et al. (2014). Population level mental distress in rural Ethiopia. *BMC Psychiatry*, **14**, 194.

Hailemariam, M., Fekadu, A., Medhin, G., Prince, M., & Hanlon, C. (2020). Equitable access to mental healthcare integrated in primary care for people with severe mental disorders in rural Ethiopia: a community-based cross-sectional study. *International Mental Health Systems*, **13**, 78.

Hailemariam, M., Fekadu, A., Prince, M., & Hanlon, C. (2017). Engaging and staying engaged: a phenomenological study of barriers to equitable access to mental healthcare for people with severe mental disorders in a rural African setting. *International Journal for Equity in Health*, **16**, 156.

Hailemariam, M., Fekadu, A., Selamu, M., Alem, A., Medhin, G., Giorgis, T. W., et al. (2015). Developing a mental health care plan in a low resource setting: the theory of change approach. *BMC Health Services Research*, **15**, 429.

Hailemariam, M., Fekadu, A., Selamu, M., Medhin, G., Prince, M., & Hanlon, C. (2016). Equitable access to integrated primary mental healthcare for people with severe mental disorders in Ethiopia: a formative study. *International Journal for Equity in Health*, **15**, 121.

Hailemichael, Y., Hailemariam, D., Tirfessa, K., Docrat, S., Alem, A., Medhin, G., et al. (2022). The effect of expanded access to mental health care on economic status of households with a person with a mental disorder in rural Ethiopia: a controlled before-after study. *International Journal of Mental Health Systems*. Advance online publication. https://doi.org/10.21203/rs.3.rs-1006902/v1.

Hanlon, C., Fekadu, A., Jordans, M., Kigozi, F., Petersen, I., Shidhaye, R., et al. (2016). District mental healthcare plans for five low- and middle-income countries: commonalities, variations and evidence gaps. *British Journal of Psychiatry*, **208**(Suppl. 56), s47–s54.

Hanlon, C., Luitel, N. P., Kathree, T., Murhar, V., Shrivasta, S., Medhin, G., et al. (2014). Challenges and opportunities for implementing integrated mental health care: a district level situation analysis from five low- and middle-income countries. *PLoS One*, **9**, e88437.

Hanlon, C., Medhin, G., Dewey, M. E., Prince, M., Assefa, E., Shibre, T., et al. (2022). Efficacy and cost-effectiveness of task-shared care for people with severe mental disorders in Ethiopia (TaSCS): a single-blind, randomised, controlled, phase 3 non-inferiority trial. *Lancet Psychiatry*, **9**, 59–71.

Hanlon, C., Medhin, G., Selamu, M., Birhane, R., Dewey, M., Tirfessa, K., et al. (2019). Impact of integrated district level mental health care on clinical and social outcomes of people with severe mental illness in rural Ethiopia: an intervention cohort study. *Epidemiology and Psychiatric Sciences*, **29**, e45.

Janse Van Rensburg, A., Kathree, T., Breuer, E., Selohilwe, O., Mntambo, N., Petrus, R., et al. (2021). Fuzzy-set qualitative comparative analysis of implementation outcomes in an integrated mental healthcare trial in South Africa. *Global Health Action*, **14**, 1940761.

Jordans, M. J. D., Kohrt, B. A., Luitel, N. P., Komproe, I. H., & Lund, C. (2015). Accuracy of proactive case finding for mental disorders by community informants in Nepal. *British Journal of Psychiatry*, **207**, 501–506.

Jordans, M. J. D., Luitel, N. P., Baron, E., Kohrt, B. A., Rathod, S. D., Shrestha, P., et al. (2019a). Effectiveness of psychological treatments for depression and alcohol use disorder delivered by community-based counsellors: two pragmatic randomized controlled trials within primary health care in Nepal. *British Journal of Psychiatry*, **215**, 485–493.

Jordans, M. J. D., Luitel, N. P., Kohrt, B. A., Lund, C., & Komproe, I. (2017). Proactive community case finding to facilitate treatment seeking for mental disorders, Nepal. *Bulletin of the World Health Organization*, **95**, 531–536.

Jordans, M. J. D., Luitel, N. P., Kohrt, B. A., Rathod, S. D., Garman, E. C., De Silva, M., et al. (2019b). Community-, facility-, and individual-level outcomes of a district mental healthcare plan in a low-resource setting in Nepal: a population-based evaluation. *PLoS Medicine*, **16**, e1002748.

Jordans, M. J. D., Luitel, N. P., Lund, C., & Kohrt, B. A. (2020). Evaluation of proactive community case detection to increase help seeking for mental health care: a pragmatic randomized controlled trial. *Psychiatric Services*, **71**, 810–815.

Jordans, M. J. D., Luitel, N. P., Pokhrel, P., & Patel, V. (2016). Development and pilot testing of a mental healthcare plan in Nepal. *British Journal of Psychiatry*, **208**, s21–s28.

Kebede, D., Alem, A., Shibre, T., Negash, A., Fekadu, A., Fekadu, D., et al. (2003). Onset and clinical course of schizophrenia in Butajira-Ethiopia. A community-based study. *Social Psychiatry and Psychiatric Epidemiology*, **38**, 625–631.

Kigozi, F. N., Kizza, D., Nakku, J., Ssebunnya, J., Ndyanabangi, S., Nakiganda, B., et al. (2016). Development of a district mental healthcare plan in Uganda. *British Journal of Psychiatry*, **208**(Suppl. 56), s40–s46.

Kokane, A., Chatterji, R., Pakhare, A., Ray, S., Mittal, P., & Arvind, B. (2017). National Mental Health Survey, Madhya Pradesh State Report 2015-2016, *Madhya Pradesh*. Bhopal: All India Institute of Medical Sciences.

Luitel, N. P., Jordans, M., Adhikari, A., Upadhaya, N., Hanlon, C., Lund, C., & Komproe, I. H. (2015). Mental health care in Nepal: current situation and challenges for development of a district mental health care plan. *Conflict and Health*, **9**, 3.

Lund, C., Tomlinson, M., De Silva, M., Fekadu, A., Shidhaye, R., Jordans, M., et al. (2012). PRIME: a programme to reduce the treatment gap for mental disorders in five low- and middle-income countries. *PLoS Med*, **9**, e1001359.

Mahomed, O. H., Asmall, S., & Freeman, M. (2014). An integrated chronic disease management model: a diagnoal approach to health systems strengthening in South Africa. *Journal of Health Care for the Poor and Underserved*, **25**, 1723–1729.

Mall, S., Hailemariam, M., Selamu, M., Fekadu, A., Lund, C., Patel, V., et al. (2017). 'Restoring the person's life': a qualitative study to inform development of care for people with severe mental disorders in rural Ethiopia. *Epidemiology and Psychiatric Sciences*, **26**, 43–52.

Ministry of Health and Family Welfare (2017). *Unlocking New Ideas: Good, Replicable and Innovative Practices*. New Delhi: Ministry of Health and Family Welfare. http://nhm.gov.in/images/pdf/in-focus/MP/Day-1/Coffeetable_Book.pdf

Nadkarni, A., Weobong, B., Weiss, H. A., McCambridge, J., Bhat, B., Katti, B., et al. (2017). Counselling for alcohol problems (CAP), a lay counsellor-delivered brief psychological treatment for harmful drinking in men, in primary care in India: a randomised controlled trial. *Lancet*, **389**, 186–195.

Nakku, J. E. M., Rathod, S. D., Garman, E. C., Ssebunnya, J., Kangere, S., De Silva, M., et al. (2019). Evaluation of the impacts of a district-level mental health care plan on contact coverage, detection and individual outcomes in rural Uganda: a mixed methods approach. *International Journal of Mental Health Systems*, **13**, 63.

Petersen, I., Bhana, A., Fairall, L., Selohilwe, O., Kathree, T., Garman, E., et al. (2019). Evaluation of a collaborative care model for integrated primary care of common mental disorders comorbid with chronic conditions in South Africa. *BMC Psychiatry*, **19**, 107.

Petersen, I., Fairall, L., Bhana, A., Kathree, T., Selohilwe, O., Brooke-Sumner, C., et al. (2016). Integrating mental health into chronic care in South Africa: the development of a district mental healthcare plan. *British Journal of Psychiatry*, **208**(Suppl. 56), s29–s39.

Petersen, I., Fairall, L., Zani, B., Bhana, A., Lombard, C., Folb, N., et al. (2021a). Effectiveness of a task-sharing collaborative care model for identification and management of depressive symptoms in patients with hypertension attending public sector primary care clinics in South Africa: pragmatic parallel cluster randomised controlled trial. *Journal of Affective Disorders*, **282**, 112–121.

Petersen, I., Kemp, C. G., Rao, D., Wagenaar, B. H., Sherr, K., Grant, M., et al. (2021b). Implementation and scale-up of integrated depression care in South Africa: an observational implementation research protocol. *Psychiatric Services*, **72**, 1065–1075.

Petersen, I., Van Rensburg, A., Gigaba, S. G., Luvuno, Z. B. P., & Fairall, L. R. (2020). Health systems strengthening to optimise scale-up in global mental health in low- and middle-income countries: lessons from the frontlines. A re-appraisal. *Epidemiology and Psychiatric Sciences*, **29**, e135.

Schneider, H. & Lehmann, U. (2016). From community health workers to community health systems: time to widen the horizon? *Health Systems & Reform*, **2**, 112–118.

Selamu, M., Asher, L., Hanlon, C., Medhin, G., Hailemariam, M., Patel, V., Thornicroft, G., & Fekadu, A. (2015). Beyond the biomedical: community resources for mental health care in rural Ethiopia. *PLoS One*, **10**, e0126666.

Selohilwe, O., Bhana, A., Garman, E. C., & Petersen, I. (2019). Evaluating the role of levels of exposure to a task shared depression counselling intervention led by behavioural health counsellors: outcome and process evaluation. *International Journal of Mental Health Systems*, **13**, 42.

Shibre, T., Hanlon, C., Medhin, G., Alem, A., Kebede, D., Teferra, S., et al. (2014a). Suicide and suicide attempts in people with severe mental disorders in Butajira, Ethiopia: 10 year follow-up of a population-based cohort. *BMC Psychiatry*, **14**, 150.

Shibre, T., Medhin, G., Alem, A., Kebede, D., Teferra, S., Jacobsson, L., et al. (2014b). Long-term clinical course and outcome of schizophrenia in rural Ethiopia: 10-year follow-up of a population-based cohort. *Schizophrenia Research*, **161**, 414–420.

Shidhaye, R., Baron, E., Murhar, V., Rathod, S., Khan, A., Singh, A., et al. (2019a). Community, facility and individual level impact of integrating mental health screening and treatment into the primary healthcare system in Sehore district, Madhya Pradesh, India. *BMJ Global Health*, **4**, e001344.

Shidhaye, R., Murhar, V., Muke, S., Shrivastava, R., Khan, A., Singh, A., & Breuer, E. (2019b). Delivering a complex mental health intervention in low-resource settings: lessons from the implementation of the PRIME mental healthcare plan in primary care in Sehore district, Madhya Pradesh, India. *BJPsych Open*, **5**, e63.

Shidhaye, R., Raja, A., Shrivastava, S., Murhar, V., Ramaswamy, R., & Patel, V. (2015). Challenges for transformation: a situational analysis of mental health care services in Sehore District, Madhya Pradesh. *Community Mental Health Journal*, **51**, 903–912.

Shidhaye, R., Shrivastava, S., Murhar, V., Samudre, S., Ahuja, S., Ramaswamy, R., & Patel, V. (2016). Development and piloting of a plan for integrating mental health in primary care in Sehore district, Madhya Pradesh, India. *British Journal of Psychiatry*, **208**(Suppl. 56), s13–s20.

Tekola, B., Mayston, R., Eshetu, T., Birhane, R., Milkias, B., Hanlon, C., & Fekadu, A. Understandings of depression among community members and primary healthcare attendees in rural Ethiopia: a qualitative study. *Transcultural Psychiatry*, **60**, 412–427.

Tirfessa, K., Lund, C., Medhin, G., Selamu, M., Birhane, R., Hailemichael, Y., et al. (2020). Impact of integrated mental healthcare on food insecurity of households of people with severe mental illness in a rural African district: a community-based, controlled before-after study. *Tropical Medicine & International Health*, **25**, 414–423.

World Health Organization (2016a). *mhGAP Intervention Guide for Mental, Neurological and Substance Use Disorders in Non-Specialized Health Settings (Version 2.0)*. Geneva: World Health Organization.

World Health Organization (2016b). *mhGAP Intervention Guide Version 2.0*. Geneva: World Health Organization.

Zewdu, S., Hanlon, C., Fekadu, A., Medhin, G., & Teferra, S. (2019). Treatment gap, help-seeking, stigma and magnitude of alcohol use disorder in rural Ethiopia. *Substance Abuse Treatment, Prevention, and Policy*, **14**, 4.

Zewdu, S., Hanlon, C., Fekadu, A., Medhin, G., & Teferra, S. (2022). 'We improved our life because I cut my drinking': qualitative analysis of a brief intervention for people with alcohol use disorder in Ethiopian primary health care. *Journal of Substance Abuse Treatment*, **132**, 108636.

42

Mental health aspects of epidemics and pandemics

Akin Ojagbemi and Oye Gureje

Introduction

A disease outbreak is the occurrence of a greater-than-expected number of cases of the disease in a population and over a period of time (World Health Organization (WHO), 2022). The grouping of disease outbreaks is often based on the extent of geographical spread and most occur as a result of exposure of the population to a hazardous substance or transmissible pathogen. In a few instances, the cause of a disease outbreak may be unknown. For example, the aetiology of Nodding disease outbreaks in East Africa (Tanzania, Uganda, and South Sudan) remains unclear (WHO, 2022).

A disease outbreak may be described as an epidemic when there is a rapid increase in the number of cases of the disease beyond what would normally be expected for a particular geographical area or population (Centres for Disease Control and Prevention, 2012; WHO, 2022). A pandemic is an epidemic extending across many countries and continents of the world (Centres for Disease Control and Prevention, 2012; WHO, 2022). Epidemics are thus large outbreaks of diseases occurring within a geographically restricted area per time, while pandemics are associated with a global spread of the outbreak with little geographical restrictions.

Epidemics and especially pandemics are historical events that significantly impact healthcare delivery systems in the areas affected. This provides a justification for a common consideration of the mental health aspects of the epidemiological phenomena. Partly due to the influence of climate change, population growth and the consequent expansions into previously uninhabited spaces, vector distribution as well as spillover of zoonoses, the number of infectious disease outbreaks has steadily increased globally over the past 30 years. Some notable infectious disease outbreaks in recent history include diphtheria, Ebola, Lassa fever, middle east respiratory syndrome coronavirus (MERS-CoV), monkeypox, plague, Zika, and the severe acute respiratory syndrome (SARS).

On 30 January 2020, the WHO declared the outbreak of a new coronavirus of severe acute respiratory syndrome (SARS-CoV-2) 'a public health emergency of international concern', and later as a pandemic on 11 March 2020 (Cucinotta & Vanelli, 2020). The new coronavirus is responsible for the coronavirus disease (Covid-19), which was first reported in Wuhan, China in December 2019 (Guan & Zhong, 2020). It spread rapidly to all countries and continents of the world. By March 2022, the number of confirmed cases of SARS-CoV-2 infection had reached approximately 460 million globally with over 6 million deaths directly attributable to Covid-19 (Johns Hopkins University Center for Systems Science and Engineering, 2022). The true community prevalence of SARS-CoV-2 infection remains unknown due to the occurrence of asymptomatic cases as well as wide variability in testing capabilities within and across countries (Jones, 2020).

In declaring the outbreak of SARS-CoV-2 as a pandemic, the WHO warned about the potential impact of the spread of the virus on mental health and well-being of the global population (Cucinotta & Vanelli, 2020). In this chapter, we focus on the mental health aspects of infectious disease outbreaks of epidemic or pandemic proportions. In doing this, the chapter takes a cue from the United Nations policy brief advising that countries act and invest on mental health during the Covid-19 crisis as a way of providing safeguards for the population in years to come and as the world confronts any future major disease outbreaks (United Nations, 2020).

Overview of mental health in infectious disease outbreaks

Large outbreaks of highly transmissible infectious diseases often occur suddenly and unexpectedly. Depending on the novelty of the pathogen, the immunity of the population, and the preparedness of the local health care delivery system, including its surveillance systems, the evolution and spread of the infectious agent may be unpredictable. This, in turn may provoke a sense of diminished control of disease spread across the population, as well as a health crisis associated with states of uncertainty in the face of an evident threat. The emotion of fear, which is a functionally adaptive behavioural and perceptual response to a threat, especially when associated with a sense of diminished control (Steimer, 2002), often sets in. The immediate sources of distress in the population faced with an outbreak of a highly transmissible pathogen may include a feeling of vulnerability, fear of getting in contact with individuals who are possibly infected, and concerns about one's health and that of family and friends.

The public health strategies that are often implemented to mitigate the spread of highly transmissible pathogens may include 'spatial' or physical distancing (Abel & McQueen, 2020). This involves maintaining a physical distance from other members of the population. Physical distancing measures may involve closure of educational institutions and workplaces, cancellation of large social gatherings, isolation of suspected or confirmed cases, quarantine of persons in contact with confirmed cases, stay-at-home recommendations, and even mandatory quarantine or 'lockdowns' in some residential areas, towns, cities, or an entire country.

The detrimental impacts of lockdowns and quarantines during pandemics are now well documented (Brooks et al., 2020b; Sommerlad et al., 2022). The containment strategy may have an unintended effect of life disruption, social isolation, loneliness, inactivity, increased access to food and alcohol, loss of income and financial insecurity, limited access to health and social services, as well as reduced social support from family and friends (Xiao et al., 2020). Part of the many effects of social isolation, for example, is that some will spend a lot more time watching television and paying attention to social media. This may be when individuals are exposed to misinformation which, in turn, may further increase the level of uncertainty and unpredictability about the health crisis. Implementation of physical distancing and other containment measures may thus have the potential to transform what could be a normative adaptation to the threats posed by a pathogen into adverse psychological reactions (Qiu et al., 2020). Some of the consequences may include feeling stressed or overwhelmed, tiredness, worry, anger, irritation, lack of motivation, and sleep problems (National Center for Chronic Disease Prevention and Health Promotion, 2021). These outcomes are often associated with both immediate and sustained mental disorders in the population (Karasar & Canli, 2020).

Large disease outbreaks thus create an ideal setting for the onset, recurrence, exacerbation, and maintenance of symptoms and syndromes of mental illnesses in the affected communities. As an example, data obtained from the US Census Bureau's Household Pulse Survey suggest that while approximately one in ten adults had depression or anxiety syndromes before the outbreak of SARS-CoV-2 and Covid-19, about four in ten had reported the mental health conditions within 6 months of the outbreak (Panchal et al., 2021). The increase in mental health conditions during large diseases outbreaks often translates to a rise in the number of people needing mental health services. It highlights the need to find effective strategies for mental health promotion during such outbreaks.

Some studies of large disease outbreaks suggest that most survivors recover from the negative psychological impact of the health crisis and may sometimes lead to unique or shared resilience in the aftermath (Alisic et al., 2014; Kelly, 2020b). For example, observational studies conducted during and after the 2002–2004 SARS outbreak in Hong Kong and Canada suggest that most adverse psychological reactions and mental health consequences of physical distancing and other measures implemented to mitigate disease spread resolved without the need for formal treatments (Lee et al., 2007; Maunder, 2009).

A minority of survivors of large disease outbreaks may develop long-lasting mental health consequences (Alisic et al., 2014; Lee et al., 2007). This group may include members of the population who have endured extended containment measures, those who have narrowly escaped death from contracting the infectious agents, as well as those who have suffered tremendous losses, especially of close family members and friends. Due to official disease containment measures, normal emotional reactions to bereavement and working through grief, including what may be customary rites of mourning or honouring departed loved ones, may sometimes be impossible. In such circumstances, bereavement becomes an even more traumatic experience (Wallace et al., 2020).

Epidemics resulting from infections that affect the central nervous system, especially the brain, may also lead to long-lasting mental health problems. For example, there is evidence that the coronavirus that causes SARS-CoV-2 infection may spread to the brain and that even mild infection may lead to clear evidence of structural changes in the brain (Abbasi, 2022; Douaud et al., 2022). Such changes may manifest as cognitive impairments and other neuropsychiatric conditions (Liu et al., 2022).

Vulnerabilities to the mental health consequences of epidemics and pandemics

Some groups in the population are at elevated risk of the negative mental health impact of large disease outbreaks. Examples may include people who work as frontline health responders, those in lower socioeconomic positions who may be unable to abide by mitigation specifications, and groups that traditionally receive less health service coverage. As well as being at greater risk to exposure to the infection, the mental health and well-being of these sections of the population may also be more frequently overlooked in times of large disease outbreaks when the public health system is overstretched as it grapples with efforts to contain the spread of the pathogen and preserving the lives of affected members of the population.

Low socioeconomic status and economic hardship

Low socioeconomic status and economic hardship have profound influence on mental health across the lifespan (Ojagbemi et al., 2017). Sources of economic hardship in times of large disease outbreaks may include closure of businesses as a physical distancing measure to mitigate spread of the infectious agent. The economic effect may include unemployment, loss of income, inability to meet immediate financial responsibilities, and worries about longer-term financial stability. In many low-resource settings, a large section of the labour force are in the informal sector. Persons in this sector often depend on daily income from petty trading and unskilled labour occupations. Such persons are particularly vulnerable to mitigation strategies, such as lockdowns and physical distancing, that prevent the daily engagement in their occupations. The risk of mental health conditions directly related to worsening of their economic plight is therefore high (Kola et al., 2021; Vigo et al., 2020).

People facing economic hardship or having a low socioeconomic status have a greater likelihood of appraising unpredictable circumstances, such as those imposed by large disease outbreaks, as threatening (E. Chen & Matthews, 2001). The cognitive appraisal of such events in persons facing economic hardship has been linked with heightened emotional states and psychological reactions, including irritation and anger (E. Chen & Matthews, 2001). In addition, many people facing economic hardship in times of large disease outbreaks may need to find work which, in these circumstances, may only be available in dangerous settings such as places with high risk of exposure to the pathogen. The feeling of helplessness in the face of an evident threat as well as pre-existing cognitive bias to such a threat may serve to precipitate new onset or recurrence of mental health conditions. Furthermore, people facing economic hardship are less likely to have access to both physical and mental health services in times of large disease outbreaks (E. Chen & Matthews, 2001; Ojagbemi et al., 2017; Roca et al., 2013).

Ethnic and minority subpopulations

Compared with the general population of most countries, persons in ethnic and minority subpopulations may experience a disproportionate level of burden of both communicable (Williams et al., 2021) and non-communicable diseases (Karim et al., 2021). This high morbidity and mortality burden may be partly explained by socioeconomic disadvantage (Geronimus et al., 2006). Persons in ethnic and minority subpopulations may also have poor access and delivery of health care due to residence in areas of high demand but less supply of needed services as well as actual gaps in treatment seeking (Milam et al., 2020). Some of the barriers to treatment seeking from mainstream mental health systems by such persons may relate to representativeness and multicultural competence of providers, stigmatization, mistrust, and preference for faith-based systems (Ward et al., 2013).

The disparity in morbidity and mortality burden between the general populations and ethnic and minority subpopulations may become more pronounced in times of disaster and large outbreaks of disease (Gu et al., 2020). Many members of ethnic and minority subpopulations live in large households and locations characterized by high population density (Fusaro et al., 2018). These factors make it difficult for people to comply with mitigation strategies for the containment of spread of disease such as physical distancing. Also, access to treatment may be limited for members of such communities who contract the infection. Other vulnerable minority subgroups that are likely to be differentially impacted in times of large outbreaks of disease include migrants as well as persons incarcerated in prisons or who are in juvenile justice systems (Bhopal, 2020; Kinner et al., 2020). In many countries, these institutions are characterized by overcrowded living spaces and lack of safe water supply to ensure regular hygiene. In these circumstances, a higher infectious disease burden, or the fear of contracting the infection in the context of lower access to treatment, are potential causes of increased stress which in turn could increase the risk of mental disorders or lead to a worsening of any pre-existing mental health conditions.

Women

Women commonly have elevated vulnerability to the mental health impact of disasters including those caused by large outbreaks of disease. For example, women are more likely to be exposed to some risk factors for mental health conditions such as domestic violence and household impoverishment which may intensify during lockdowns and stay-at-home strategies (Campbell et al., 2020). It may also be difficult for women to find the needed professional support in these circumstances.

Many health care teams and services may be reconfigured during large outbreaks of infectious disease with some health care workers redeployed to frontlines such as intensive care and isolation units. Women who become pregnant may struggle with decisions about whether to attend regular perinatal hospital visits or not (Almeida et al., 2020). Important sources of psychological distress for such women may include worries about vulnerability to infection and disease because of being pregnant (Brooks et al., 2020c). There may also be worries about transmission of the pathogen to the unborn fetus either during pregnancy or at delivery. In addition, women may be concerned about the risk of pregnancy complications if infected, as well as being separated from their newborn children after birth if neonates were to be admitted in intensive care units. Due to distant social support resulting from some disease mitigation measures, many new mothers who themselves may be dealing with adjustment syndromes related to new family dynamics may find themselves juggling multiple roles with limited help from extended family, grandparents, and friends (Brooks et al., 2020c).

In addition to the stress occasioned by the indirect effects of pandemics, including those related to the mitigation strategies to contain the spread of the infection and some to the fear of contracting the infection, *in utero* spread of infection to the fetus may also be a risk for the later development of mental health conditions for the unborn child. For example, among the long-term consequences of exposure to the 1918 flu pandemic while *in utero* is an elevated risk of developing schizophrenia (Caparros-Gonzalez & Alderdice, 2020; Caparros-Gonzalez et al., 2020).

The economic impact of business failures that often accompany disease mitigation measures may disproportionately affect some economic sectors with high female participation (Dang et al., 2020). These include retail, hospitality, and other services sectors. Women in these sectors are thus more likely to lose their jobs or expect their income to decrease (Dang et al., 2020). In Chile, for example, there was a 12% drop in female participation in the labour force of that country within 5 months of the Covid-19 pandemic (Instituto Nacional de Estadisticas de Chile, 2021). Women who lose their jobs or have a reduced income because of business closure face the prospect of economic hardship and its effect on mental health, including access to needed care and support (Ojagbemi et al., 2017).

Children

Large outbreaks of infectious diseases have implications for children's development in general as well as their mental health and well-being. Sources of psychological distress for children may include closure of schools, parks, and playgrounds as parts of measures to mitigate the spread of the pathogen. Schools create a safe and calm environment for children as well as ensuring routines and the learning of social norms. These factors have a profound influence in promoting good mental health and well-being in children (Department of Education, 2018). A calm and safe school environment has a particular effect of strengthening resilience, a factor that is important for children to effectively navigate the normal stress and hassles of daily life (Brooks et al., 2020a; Department of Education, 2018).

Children from poor backgrounds and who are not in school face the risk of being used by their parents and other adults for purposes of offsetting the effect of economic hardship that families may be experiencing as a result of large infection outbreaks. For instance, children in some poor communities may be deployed as child labour or made to sell merchandise or beg for food and money on the street (Cluver et al., 2020b). Children who find themselves in these circumstances are at increased risk of neglect, of physical and sexual abuse, as well as of the immediate and longer-term mental health consequences (Cluver et al., 2020b). In addition, child abuse and neglect may be less likely to be detected in times of disasters and large outbreaks of disease due to school closures and lack of oversight from teachers and educational systems, as well as a reduction in the activities of child welfare organization and monitoring agencies (Cluver et al., 2020a, 2020b).

Most out-of-school activities for children typically occur outside the home and in group settings, such as in parks or playgrounds. Physical distancing measures that ensure closure of these facilities may thus lead to disruption of the usual lifestyle of children. Those from more resourced backgrounds may resort to online and social media activities which have an attendant effect of increasing screen times and reduced interaction with other members of the family (Ellis et al., 2020). This is compounded by the risk of receiving inaccurate information about the outbreak from online and social media. A study conducted to understand the psychological effect of the 2009 H1N1 swine flu outbreak in Europe observed that children's fear and distress was linked to information received about the outbreaks (Remmerswaal & Muris, 2011). In the same study, a correlation was found between parental fears about the outbreaks and children's psychological distress (Remmerswaal & Muris, 2011).

Older adults

The elderly may be prone to heightened fear of being directly affected by an outbreak of a highly transmissible pathogen (Mehra et al., 2020). This is because older people are more likely to have underlying chronic health conditions such cardiovascular diseases, diabetes, and cancers which are associated with a lowering of immunity. The fear and worry about contracting a rapidly spreading infectious disease could be especially profound among those in institutional care (Armitage & Nellums, 2020). Older people with background health conditions and lowered immunity who then become infected by the pathogen may have worse outcomes of both the infectious disease and the chronic conditions.

Other sources of distress for the elder in times of large outbreaks of infectious diseases may include closure of religious, cultural, and volunteer community organizations, as well as preclusion of face-to-face meetings with families and friends as a part of efforts to mitigate the spread of the pathogen. Social participation in community and family activities are important to the elderly as they serve to stimulate cognitive, motor, and sensory functions as well as self-esteem (Gureje et al., 2014). These activities also promote the well-being of the elderly by ensuring needed social, emotional, and psychological support (Gureje et al., 2014; Ojagbemi et al., 2018). Physical distancing measures to mitigate the spread of infectious disease are likely to bring unexpected change to the routine of older persons and lead to social isolation as well as feelings of loneliness, all of which may negatively affect their mental health (Ojagbemi et al., 2021).

Specific occupational groups

Of all the sectors of the population, people working on the frontline of an infectious disease outbreak are at greater risk of a negative impact on their mental health (Prati & Pietrantoni, 2010). Frontline workers such as health care practitioners, police officers, and people in the armed forces have as their core mission to protect and preserve lives. During an infectious disease outbreak, these workers continuously encounter the threat of acquiring the pathogen, which in may be rapidly transmissible and potentially lethal. As such, many frontline workers may be doing their work under a heightened appraisal of threat and danger to their own lives (Wu et al., 2009). Frontline workers may thus experience the health crisis as especially traumatic (LaFauci Schutt & Marotta, 2011).

People working on the frontline of a large infectious disease outbreak are also more likely to be direct witnesses to the negative effects of such outbreaks including observing people's struggles between life and death and actual traumatic deaths. This is particularly the case for health care professionals such as doctors, nurses, and support staff who are on the frontline of the disease outbreak. These workers may be tasked with offering emotional support to families and friends of affected persons. The constant interaction of frontline workers with people who are directly affected by the pathogen as well as their families may result in 'vicarious traumatization' (Mathieu, 2014). In this situation, the workers may experience adverse psychological reactions similar to those suffered by survivors of disasters and other such traumatic events.

Other common work-related factors affecting the mental health and well-being of frontline workers during a disease outbreak may include adapting to a different work environment, learning new technical skills, managing an increasing workload and experiencing huge performance pressures, sudden surge in workload, limited supply of personal protection equipment especially in less resourced work places, and inadequate protection from contamination (LaFauci Schutt & Marotta, 2011; Lai et al., 2020). Some frontline workers may also lack the tools and equipment required to provide needed services in times of a large disease outbreak. This may lead to frustration from failure to give the required support (Lai et al., 2020). Key stressors for frontline workers in times of large disease outbreaks may thus include burnout (Fessell & Cherniss, 2020) and 'moral injury' (Williamson et al., 2020).

Moral injury, which is more commonly associated with members of the armed forces facing conflicts or war situations (Currier et al., 2018), may occur when people are faced with unexpected traumatic events and are forced to take certain actions which violate their moral code. It may also result from being unable to take applicable actions in these circumstances (Currier et al., 2018). Faced with shortages of supply of needed resources during a large disease outbreak, frontline health care workers may be forced to make difficult decisions about how to prioritize available resources. This situation may result in deaths that would have been preventable in normal circumstances. Additional risk factors for moral injury and burnout among health care workers on the frontline of a large infectious disease outbreak may include inadequate training in disaster management, and dealing with concerns of affected patients and their families who may be distraught, frightened, angry, and uncooperative in these circumstances (Kang et al., 2020; Williamson et al., 2020). Health care workers who may find themselves caring for their own colleagues infected by the pathogen may be especially vulnerable to negative psychological reactions including doubts about their own competence (Maunder et al., 2003). Due to the pressure engendered by the health crisis, frontline health care workers may also endure inadequate support and poor communication from their supervisors or employers (Lai et al., 2020; Williamson et al., 2020).

The workplace pressure that may result from the upsurge in cases of affected persons during epidemics or pandemics and having to work for long hours during such circumstances may be compounded by reduced access of health care workers to their own social support systems (Q. Chen et al., 2020). Many may need to quarantine and isolate from family and friends because of being exposed to the pathogen. Frontline health care workers not needing quarantine may nevertheless be anxious about exposing their family and friends to the pathogen. These circumstances may challenge the coping resources of frontline health care workers and lay the foundation for mental health conditions either during or after the health crisis (Lai et al., 2020; Wu et al., 2009; Zhao et al., 2021).

Persons with pre-existing mental health conditions

Given their higher levels of vulnerability, persons with pre-existing mental health conditions can be expected to be at elevated risk of either a new episode of mental disorder or a worsening of an ongoing episode during an epidemic or a pandemic. Such vulnerability may also be related to the severity of the pre-existing condition with persons with more severe conditions being at particularly higher risk. Even though there were nuanced differences between various groups of patients, a systematic review of 36 studies found that, overall, persons with serious mental illness, consisting of those with affective disorders and schizophrenia, experienced more pronounced symptoms of anxiety, depression, and stress than healthy controls (Fleischmann et al., 2021). While a general impairment of mental health was detectable among persons with serious mental illness, those with affective disorders were more likely to show such evidence than persons with schizophrenia. Heightened risks of further mental health morbidity among persons with pre-existing serious mental illness tend to be associated with young age, poor socioeconomic status, as well as social alienation or isolation.

In general, poor pre-pandemic mental health in the community is strongly associated with not just elevated risks of mental illness, but with a greater effect on the lives of affected persons. Aa analysis of data obtained from 59,482 participants drawn from 12 UK longitudinal studies which collected data before and during the Covid-19 pandemic, found that one standard deviation increase in the level of pre-pandemic psychological distress was associated with major disruptions in health care (access to medication and procedures), as well as in economic activity and housing (Di Gessa et al., 2022).

A bidirectional relationship may exist between mental illness and some large-scale infections in which those who are infected have an elevated risk for mental illness while those with mental illness may also be at elevated risk of contracting the infection. An example of the latter scenario was demonstrated with the Covid-19 pandemic. In an analysis of a nationwide database of electronic records of 61 million adult patients across the 50 states of the US, Wang et al. (2021) found that patients with a diagnosis of a mental disorder had a significantly elevated risk of contracting Covid-19, with the risk being highest among those with depression followed by those with schizophrenia.

Public health response to epidemics and pandemics

Large outbreaks of infectious diseases are major events that impact public health services in unprecedented ways. As discussed in the preceding sections, these events may result in dramatic changes in needs and demands for mental health services and require major reconfiguration of the public mental health systems. The changes necessitated by the health crisis engendered by an infectious disease outbreak may sometimes lead to disruption in mental health service provision especially in settings where resources are lacking to respond to major and unexpected challenges to service provision (WHO, 2020a). Services to rural, ageing, and other vulnerable populations may be especially impacted (Sivakumar et al., 2020).

Public mental health systems need to adapt to new ways of working during large outbreaks of infectious diseases. Among the major required changes may be those relating to the work environments, procedures, tools, technology, and skills required to mitigate the spread of the infection as well as ensuring continuity of mental health care in the context of increased stress for the health care providers (WHO, 2020a). In the wake of the Covid-19 pandemic and some other recent large outbreaks of infectious diseases, several measures became necessary to ensure continuity of mental health care in some affected populations (Alavi et al., 2021). These measures have resulted in the emergence of new interventions, protocols, recommendations, and policies, including those designed to facilitate the need for mental health providers to work remotely (Schiavo, 2020; Sivakumar et al., 2020; WHO, 2020b). Some of these measures provide the template that can be adapted to meet the challenges of future infectious disease outbreaks, taking cognizance of contextual ethical, legal, and cultural considerations.

Reorganization of community mental health services

The exigencies of large outbreaks of infectious diseases may necessitate a reorganization and adaptation of institutions, facilities, and human and material resources within the mental health care system of affected locations. This is important to speedily achieve because people with mental health conditions are more likely to have risk factors such as malnutrition and obesity or overweight, as well as other underlying health conditions including other infectious diseases, diabetes, and cardiovascular and pulmonary morbidities (Jakobsen et al., 2018). These factors place people living with mental health conditions at elevated risks of the worst outcomes of the infectious diseases (Rovers et al., 2020).

The reorganization of the mental health system should be in such a way that facilities providing mental health services are also able to implement preventive measures against the spread of the pathogen as well as to manage patients with symptoms of the infectious disease (Rovers et al., 2020). Therefore, mental health services may have to contend with a modified protocol of operation. This may involve mandating physical distancing measures, wearing of appropriate personal protective equipment, as well as cleaning and disinfection protocols for equipment and premises (Bocher et al., 2020). Depending on the nature of the mental health facility, spaces may have to be restructured in such a way that some areas are dedicated to rapid screening procedures, as well as for suspected cases of the infectious disease (Bocher et al., 2020; Chevance et al., 2020).

Some countries have published specific guidelines for the reorganization of community mental health services especially in regard to infection containment and service delivery. Some of such efforts have been conducted by multidisciplinary groups through a process that include needs assessment, discussions and iterative feedback, and consensus building (Alavi et al., 2021; Guan et al., 2021). Also, national guidelines on remote psychiatric care have been published in some countries as a response to the Covid-19 pandemic (Kelly, 2020a; Scharf and Oinonen, 2020).

Remote access to mental health services

Provision of remote access, through mobile technology, videoconferencing, and electronic databases, is a promising approach to reducing the barrier to mental health services during large outbreaks of infectious diseases. These platforms are suitable for patient consultations as well as to deliver manualized low-intensity interventions and e-prescriptions (Bauerle et al., 2020; Kumar, 2020). Remote access may be especially suitable for patients with mild to moderate symptoms of common mental disorders such as anxiety and depression and those requiring routine follow-ups for such conditions. Patients with this profile form the bulk of people in need of continuity of mental health care in times of large outbreaks of infectious diseases (Kumar, 2020). Some studies have demonstrated comparable outcomes between remote and face-to face therapies for several anxiety, depressive, and somatic symptoms disorders (Andersson et al., 2014). It is thus important for mental health systems to be set up in a way to rapidly transition to remote services during large outbreaks of infectious diseases.

There is very little evidence for the deployment of remote mental health interventions during large outbreaks of infectious diseases that preceded Covid-19. However, in the wake of Covid-19, some existing brief and low-intensity mental health interventions have been remodelled for remote delivery. An example is the modification of an existing brief psychological intervention to suit the unique demands of the Covid-19 pandemic in Malaysia (Ping et al., 2020). The Covid-19-related modifications include a web-based platform incorporating web chat to provide psychological first aid to members of the public experiencing psychological distress. The modified package incorporates cognitive behavioural therapy, acceptance and commitment therapy, dialectical-behavioural therapy, motivational interviewing, early intervention programme, team-based problem-solving, shared decision-making, and validation skills. Each of these forms of therapeutic intervention was designed to be delivered in 15 minutes.

In a study designed to test the effectiveness of a low-intensity electronic mental health intervention during the Covid-19 pandemic conducted in Germany (Bauerle et al., 2020), the authors found a reduction of psychological distress, anxiety, and depressive symptoms, and enhancement of self-efficacy and mindfulness (Bauerle et al., 2021). The intervention package incorporates mindfulness-based stress reduction and cognitive behavioural therapy techniques. Key disadvantages of remotely delivered interventions may include difficulty with maintaining privacy and legal issues (Kumar, 2020).

Specific factors in low- and middle-income countries

Due to factors such as political instability and armed conflicts, inadequate or remotely located health infrastructure, as well as fragile health care systems, there may be a lag in disease surveillance in many low- and middle-income countries (LMICs) (Mboera et al., 2014; Tariq et al., 2019). In these circumstances, some cases of infectious diseases may not come to official or health system attention. A highly transmissible pathogen may thus continue to spread in the community. This could result in a large, unexpected outbreak of the infectious disease. Socioeconomic conditions and vulnerability factors in the populations of many LMICs may exacerbate consequences of infectious disease outbreaks in these locations (Kola et al., 2021; Vigo et al., 2020). The mental health needs in LMICs facing large outbreaks of infectious diseases may be different and potentially more complex than those of higher-income countries (Vigo et al., 2020).

Even though availability and provision of mental health services may vary from one LMIC to another, a common factor across countries is the gap between need for services and availability of resources to meet such needs (Thornicroft et al., 2017). Many LMICs allocate less than 0.5% of their health budgets to mental health (Rathod et al., 2017; WHO, 2018). In addition, specialist mental health staff are few (WHO, 2018). The few available mental health specialists are more often based in a limited number of tertiary hospitals, many of which have little or no capacity for community mental health services (WHO, 2018). Basic medical supplies including personal protective equipment and antidepressants may also not be readily available. As such, mental health systems in many LMICs may be unable to provide the required response in times of large outbreaks of infectious diseases. Of note in this regard is that there may be limited penetration of digital mental health options. Nevertheless, there is evidence to suggest a gradual expansion of digital technology in some LMICs (Taylor Salisbury et al., 2021).

In the wake of Covid-19, governments in some LMICs provided toll-free helplines that could be used by persons in need of mental health assistance. In India, for example, helplines linked callers to a list of videos, advisories, and other resources on coping with stress (Roy et al., 2021). A web portal that incorporates yoga and meditation advice to promote mental health of vulnerable subgroups was also provided.

Some groups working in Sierra Leone during the Ebola outbreak identified barriers and facilitators to effective implementation of mental health programmes during large outbreaks of infectious diseases in LMICs (Sijbrandij et al., 2020). Among the relevant barriers were low literacy, cultural understanding of mental health problems, and lack of resources. A key facilitator of mental health programmes implementation during the Ebola outbreak in Sierra Leone was the availability of trainable frontline primary health care workers. However, brief training towards rapid deployment and implementation of programmes may be better suited for more experienced staff (Sijbrandij et al., 2020; Waterman et al., 2019). Lower cadre or less experienced staff required a longer duration of training (Sijbrandij et al., 2020). Finally, adaptations of training materials to enhance cultural appropriateness was found to be an important factor for successful implementation of mental health programmes during the Ebola outbreaks in Sierra Leone (Waterman et al., 2019).

Conclusion and future directions

The impact of large outbreaks of highly transmissible and potentially lethal infectious diseases on the mental health of affected populations is considerable. This may be partly due to the unexpected nature of such outbreaks and the uncertainty they generate among members of the population. Public health strategies to mitigate disease spread may have several negative but unintended effects, including social isolation, loneliness, alcohol and substance abuse, loss of income and financial insecurity, as well as limited access to health and social services (Xiao et al., 2020). Some of these factors may negatively affect the natural adaptation to the threats posed by the pathogen. The resulting adverse psychological reactions may manifest in the form of new onset, recurrence, or worsening of mental health conditions in affected populations. The increase in mental health conditions during large outbreaks of infectious diseases will commonly translate to a rise in the number of people needing mental health services. The challenge to the public mental health systems is often about how to meet the huge demand in the context of complying with disease containment measures.

The observation in some studies of previous large outbreaks of infectious diseases (Meherali et al., 2021; Remmerswaal & Muris, 2011) is that there is a link between the psychological distress experienced by members of the population and information they received about the crisis. Primary prevention strategies for mental health in times of large outbreaks of infectious diseases ought therefore to include the provision of accurate information about the outbreak. For children, access to context-appropriate educational materials to improve their knowledge about the outbreak is important. These strategies have been directly linked to reduction of uncertainties, fear, and worries engendered by the health crisis among members of the public (Meherali et al., 2021). Furthermore, mental health promotion strategies should include multisectoral mobilization of social support networks. For example, elderly persons and their families should be encouraged to keep regular contacts to minimize social isolation.

Community mental health services should be organized in such a way that they are nimble and adaptable, able to provide immediate and proportionate responses in times of large outbreaks of infectious diseases. The responses should place emphasis on containing the spread of infections as well as providing continuity of mental health care to persons in need, including those with pre-existing mental disorders and those developing new-onset disorders. Community mental health services that are already in place should be appropriately adapted and scaled up, and barriers to accessing such services reduced. This is especially important for vulnerable populations.

While some mental health programmes have been developed or context-adapted in the wake of Covid-19 and other recent large outbreaks of infectious diseases, published evaluations of such programmes are currently limited (Holmes et al., 2020). Preparedness to address public mental health and well-being in the aftermath of Covid-19 and in the event of future large outbreaks of infectious diseases should involve multidisciplinary and multisectoral work to develop new, cost-effective, and context-appropriate interventions, as well as to test and implement programmes that have already been developed in the course of the Covid-19 and previous large outbreaks. Interventions that promote resilience, minimize risks, and support vulnerable populations are especially important in this regard. Given the salience of mitigation strategies in precipitating mental health problems during pandemics, special attention is required to ameliorate the effects of such strategies. For example, in reducing the effects of quarantines, suggestions have been made to limit their duration for no longer than required, provide clear information and rationale for the quarantine, and strive to meet individuals' basic needs (Brooks et al., 2020b).

REFERENCES

Abbasi, J. (2022). Even mild COVID-19 may change the brain. *JAMA*, **327**, 1321–1322.

Abel, T. & McQueen, D. (2020). The COVID-19 pandemic calls for spatial distancing and social closeness: not for social distancing! *International Journal of Public Health*, **65**, 231.

Alavi, Z., Haque, R., Felzer-Kim, I. T., Lewicki, T., Haque, A., & Mormann, M. (2021). Implementing COVID-19 mitigation in the community mental health setting: March 2020 and lessons learned. *Community Mental Health Journal*, **57**, 57–63.

Alisic, E., Zalta, A. K., Van Wesel, F., Larsen, S. E., Hafstad, G. S., Hassanpour, K., & Smid, G. E. (2014). Rates of post-traumatic stress disorder in trauma-exposed children and adolescents: meta-analysis. *British Journal of Psychiatry*, **204**, 335–340.

Almeida, M., Shrestha, A. D., Stojanac, D., & Miller, L. J. (2020). The impact of the COVID-19 pandemic on women's mental health. *Archives of Women's Mental Health*, **23**, 741–748.

Andersson, G., Cuijpers, P., Carlbring, P., Riper, H., & Hedman, E. (2014). Guided internet-based vs. face-to-face cognitive behavior therapy for psychiatric and somatic disorders: a systematic review and meta-analysis. *World Psychiatry*, **13**, 288–295.

Armitage, R. & Nellums, L. B. (2020). COVID-19 and the consequences of isolating the elderly. *Lancet Public Health*, **5**, e256.

Bauerle, A., Graf, J., Jansen, C., Musche, V., Schweda, A., Hetkamp, M., et al. (2020). E-mental health mindfulness-based and skills-based 'CoPE It' intervention to reduce psychological distress in times of COVID-19: study protocol for a bicentre longitudinal study. *BMJ Open*, **10**, e039646.

Bauerle, A., Jahre, L., Teufel, M., Jansen, C., Musche, V., Schweda, A., et al. (2021). Evaluation of the e-mental health mindfulness-based and skills-based 'CoPE It' intervention to reduce psychological distress in times of COVID-19: results of a bicentre longitudinal study. *Frontiers in Psychiatry*, **12**, 768132.

Bhopal, R. (2020). Covid-19: undocumented migrants are probably at greatest risk. *BMJ*, **369**, m1673.

Bocher, R., Jansen, C., Gayet, P., Gorwood, P., & Laprevote, V. (2020). [Responsiveness and sustainability of psychiatric care in France during COVID-19 epidemic]. *Encéphale*, **46**, S81–S84.

Brooks, S. K., Smith, L. E., Webster, R. K., Weston, D., Woodland, L., Hall, I., & Rubin, G. J. (2020a). The impact of unplanned school closure on children's social contact: rapid evidence review. *Euro Surveillance*, **25**, 2000188.

Brooks, S. K., Webster, R. K., Smith, L. E., Woodland, L., Wessely, S., Greenberg, N., & Rubin, G. J. (2020b). The psychological impact of quarantine and how to reduce it: rapid review of the evidence. *Lancet*, **395**, 912–920.

Brooks, S. K., Weston, D., & Greenberg, N. (2020c). Psychological impact of infectious disease outbreaks on pregnant women: rapid evidence review. *Public Health*, **189**, 26–36.

Campbell, A. M., Hicks, R. A., Thompson, S. L., & Wiehe, S. E. (2020). Characteristics of intimate partner violence incidents and the environments in which they occur: victim reports to responding law enforcement officers. *Journal of Interpersonal Violence*, **35**, 2583–2606.

Caparros-Gonzalez, R. A. & Alderdice, F. (2020). The COVID-19 pandemic and perinatal mental health. *Journal of Reproductive and Infant Psychology*, **38**, 223–225.

Caparros-Gonzalez, R. A., Ganho-Avila, A., & Torre-Luque, A. (2020). The COVID-19 pandemic can impact perinatal mental health and the health of the offspring. *Behavioral Sciences*, **10**, 162.

Centres for Disease Control and Prevention (2012). *Section 11: Epidemic disease occurrence*. In: *Principles of Epidemiology in*

Public Health Practice (3rd ed., pp. 1-72–1-79). Atlanta, GA: CDC Division of Scientific Education and Professional Development.

Chen, E. & Matthews, K. A. (2001). Cognitive appraisal biases: an approach to understanding the relation between socioeconomic status and cardiovascular reactivity in children. *Annals of Behavioral Medicine*, 23, 101–111.

Chen, Q., Liang, M., Li, Y., Guo, J., Fei, D., Wang, L., et al. (2020). Mental health care for medical staff in China during the COVID-19 outbreak. *Lancet Psychiatry*, 7, e15–e16.

Chevance, A., Gourion, D., Hoertel, N., Llorca, P. M., Thomas, P., Bocher, R., et al. (2020). Ensuring mental health care during the SARS-CoV-2 epidemic in France: a narrative review. *Encéphale*, 46, 193–201.

Cluver, L., Lachman, J. M., Sherr, L., Wessels, I., Krug, E., Rakotomalala, S., et al. (2020a). Parenting in a time of COVID-19. *Lancet*, 395, e64.

Cluver, L., Shenderovich, Y., Meinck, F., Berezin, M. N., Doubt, J., Ward, C. L., et al. (2020b). Parenting, mental health and economic pathways to prevention of violence against children in South Africa. *Social Science & Medicine*, 262, 113194.

Cucinotta, D. & Vanelli, M. (2020). WHO declares COVID-19 a pandemic. *Acta Bio-Medica*, 91, 157–160.

Currier, J. M., Farnsworth, J. K., Drescher, K. D., McDermott, R. C., Sims, B. M., & Albright, D. L. (2018). Development and evaluation of the expressions of moral injury scale-military version. *Clinical Psychology and Psychotherapy*, 25, 474–488.

Dang, H. A., Huynh, T. L. D., & Nguyen, M. H. (2020). *Does the Covid-19 Pandemic Disproportionately Affect the Poor? Evidence from a Six-Country Survey*. IZA Discussion Paper 13352. Bonn, Germany.

Department of Education (2018). *Mental Health and Behaviours in Schools*. London: Department of Education.

Di Gessa, G., Maddock, J., Green, M. J., Thompson, E. J., Mcelroy, E., Davies, H. L., et al. (2022). Pre-pandemic mental health and disruptions to healthcare, economic and housing outcomes during the COVID-19 pandemic: evidence from 12 UK longitudinal studies. *British Journal of Psychiatry*, 220, 21–30.

Douaud, G., Lee, S., Alfaro-Almagro, F., Arthofer, C., Wang, C., McCarthy, P., et al. (2022). SARS-CoV-2 is associated with changes in brain structure in UK Biobank. *Nature*, 604, 697–707.

Ellis, W. E., Dumas, T. M., & Forbes, L. M. (2020). Physically isolated but socially connected: psychological adjustment and stress among adolescents during the initial COVID-19 crisis. *Canadian Journal of Behavioural Science*, 52, 177–187.

Fessell, D. & Cherniss, C. (2020). Coronavirus disease 2019 (COVID-19) and beyond: micropractices for burnout prevention and emotional wellness. *Journal of the American College of Radiology*, 17, 746–748.

Fleischmann, E., Dalkner, N., Fellendorf, F. T., & Reininghaus, E. Z. (2021). Psychological impact of the COVID-19 pandemic on individuals with serious mental disorders: a systematic review of the literature. *World Journal of Psychiatry*, 11, 1387–1406.

Fusaro, V. A., Levy, H. G., & Shaefer, H. L. (2018). Racial and ethnic disparities in the lifetime prevalence of homelessness in the United States. *Demography*, 55, 2119–2128.

Geronimus, A. T., Hicken, M., Keene, D., & Bound, J. (2006). 'Weathering' and age patterns of allostatic load scores among blacks and whites in the United States. *American Journal of Public Health*, 96, 826–833.

Gu, T., Mack, J. A., Salvatore, M., Prabhu Sankar, S., Valley, T. S., Singh, K., et al. (2020). Characteristics associated with racial/ethnic disparities in COVID-19 outcomes in an academic health care system. *JAMA Network Open*, 3, e2025197.

Guan, I., Kirwan, N., Beder, M., Levy, M., & Law, S. (2021). Adaptations and innovations to minimize service disruption for patients with severe mental illness during COVID-19: perspectives and reflections from an assertive community psychiatry program. *Community Mental Health Journal*, 57, 10–17.

Guan, W. J. & Zhong, N. S. (2020). Clinical characteristics of Covid-19 in China. Reply. *New England Journal of Medicine*, 382, 1861–1862.

Gureje, O., Oladeji, B. D., Abiona, T., & Chatterji, S. (2014). Profile and determinants of successful aging in the Ibadan Study of Ageing. *Journal of the American Geriatrics Society*, 62, 836–842.

Holmes, E. A., O'Connor, R. C., Perry, V. H., Tracey, I., Wessely, S., Arseneault, L., et al. (2020). Multidisciplinary research priorities for the COVID-19 pandemic: a call for action for mental health science. *Lancet Psychiatry*, 7, 547–560.

Instituto Nacional de Estadisticas de Chile (2021). Género y empleo: impacto de la crisis económica por Covid-19. *Boletín Estadístico Instituto Nacional de Estadísticas de Chile*, 8 March, 1–11.

Jakobsen, A. S., Speyer, H., Norgaard, H. C. B., Karlsen, M., Hjorthoj, C., Krogh, J., et al. (2018). Dietary patterns and physical activity in people with schizophrenia and increased waist circumference. *Schizophrenia Research*, 199, 109–115.

Johns Hopkins University Center for Systems Science and Engineering (2022). COVID-19 dashboard. https://coronavirus.jhu.edu/map.html

Jones, D. S. (2020). History in a crisis—lessons for Covid-19. *New England Journal of Medicine*, 382, 1681–1683.

Kang, L., Li, Y., Hu, S., Chen, M., Yang, C., Yang, B. X., et al. (2020). The mental health of medical workers in Wuhan, China dealing with the 2019 novel coronavirus. *Lancet Psychiatry*, 7, e14.

Karasar, B. & Canli, D. (2020). Psychological resilience and depression during the Covid-19 pandemic in Turkey. *Psychiatrica Danubina*, 32, 273–279.

Karim, S., Tamirisa, K., & Chaudhry, H. (2021). Fundamental discussions on race and ethnicity for the cardiology workforce for the United States of America. *Journal of the American Heart Association*, 10, e018884.

Kelly, B. D. (2020a) Emergency mental health legislation in response to the Covid-19 (Coronavirus) pandemic in Ireland: urgency, necessity and proportionality. *International Journal of Law and Psychiatry*, 70, 101564.

Kelly, B. D. (2020b). Plagues, pandemics and epidemics in Irish history prior to COVID-19 (coronavirus): what can we learn? *Irish Journal of Psychological Medicine*, 37, 269–274.

Kinner, S. A., Young, J. T., Snow, K., Southalan, L., Lopez-Acuna, D., Ferreira-Borges, C., & O'Moore, E. (2020). Prisons and custodial settings are part of a comprehensive response to COVID-19. *Lancet Public Health*, 5, e188–e189.

Kola, L., Kohrt, B. A., Hanlon, C., Naslund, J. A., Sikander, S., Balaji, M., et al. (2021). COVID-19 mental health impact and responses in low-income and middle-income countries: reimagining global mental health. *Lancet Psychiatry*, 8, 535–550.

Kumar, T. M. (2020). Community mental health services in India: the pandemic and beyond. *Indian Journal of Social Psychiatry*, 36(Suppl. 1), 168–173.

Lafauci Schutt, J. M. & Marotta, S. A. (2011). Personal and environmental predictors of posttraumatic stress in emergency management professionals. *Psychological Trauma: Theory, Research, Practice, and Policy*, 3, 8–15.

Lai, J., Ma, S., Wang, Y., Cai, Z., Hu, J., Wei, N., et al. (2020). Factors associated with mental health outcomes among health care workers exposed to coronavirus disease 2019. *JAMA Network Open*, **3**, e203976.

Lee, A. M., Wong, J. G., Mcalonan, G. M., Cheung, V., Cheung, C., Sham, P. C., et al. (2007). Stress and psychological distress among SARS survivors 1 year after the outbreak. *Canadian Journal of Psychiatry*, **52**, 233–240.

Liu, Y. H., Chen, Y., Wang, Q. H., Wang, L. R., Jiang, L., Yang, Y., et al. (2022). One-year trajectory of cognitive changes in older survivors of COVID-19 in Wuhan, China: a longitudinal cohort study. *JAMA Neurology*, **79**, 509–517.

Mathieu, F. (2014). Occupational hazards: compassion fatigue, vicarious trauma and burnout. *Canadian Nurse*, **110**, 12–13.

Maunder, R. G. (2009). Was SARS a mental health catastrophe? *General Hospital Psychiatry*, **31**, 316–317.

Maunder, R., Hunter, J., Vincent, L., Bennett, J., Peladeau, N., Leszcz, M., et al. (2003). The immediate psychological and occupational impact of the 2003 SARS outbreak in a teaching hospital. *CMAJ*, **168**, 1245–1251.

Mboera, L. E., Mfinanga, S. G., Karimuribo, E. D., Rumisha, S. F., & Sindato, C. (2014). The changing landscape of public health in sub-Saharan Africa: control and prevention of communicable diseases needs rethinking. *Onderstepoort Journal of Veterinary Research*, **81**, E1–E6.

Meherali, S., Punjani, N., Louie-Poon, S., Abdul Rahim, K., Das, J. K., Salam, R. A., & Lassi, Z. S. (2021). Mental health of children and adolescents amidst COVID-19 and past pandemics: a rapid systematic review. *International Journal of Environmental Research and Public Health*, **18**, 3432.

Mehra, A., Rani, S., Sahoo, S., Parveen, S., Singh, A. P., Chakrabarti, S., & Grover, S. (2020). A crisis for elderly with mental disorders: relapse of symptoms due to heightened anxiety due to COVID-19. *Asian Journal of Psychiatry*, **51**, 102114.

Milam, A. J., Furr-Holden, D., Edwards-Johnson, J., Webb, B., Patton, J. W., Ezekwemba, N. C., et al. (2020). Are clinicians contributing to excess African American COVID-19 deaths? Unbeknownst to them, they may be. *Health Equity*, **4**, 139–141.

National Center for Chronic Disease Prevention and Health Promotion (2021). *Support for Employees*. Atlanta, GA: Centers for Diseases Control and Prevention.

Ojagbemi, A., Abiona, T., Luo, Z., & Gureje, O. (2018). Symptomatic and functional recovery from major depressive disorder in the Ibadan Study of Ageing. *American Journal of Geriatric Psychiatry*, **26**, 657–666.

Ojagbemi, A., Bello, T., & Gureje, O. (2021). The roles of depression and social relationships in the onset and course of loneliness amongst Nigerian elders. *International Journal of Geriatric Psychiatry*, **36**, 547–557.

Ojagbemi, A., Bello, T., Luo, Z., & Gureje, O. (2017). Living conditions, low socioeconomic position, and mortality in the Ibadan Study of Aging. *Journals of Gerontology. Series B, Psychological Sciences and Social Sciences*, **72**, 646–655.

Panchal, N., Kamal, R., Cox, C., & Garfield, R. (2021). The implications of COVID-19 for mental health and substance use. Kaiser Family Foundation. https://www.kff.org/mental-health/issue-brief/the-implications-of-covid-19-for-mental-health-and-substance-use/

Ping, N. P. T., Shoesmith, W. D., James, S., Nor Hadi, N. M., Yau, E. K. B., & Lin, L. J. (2020). Ultra brief psychological interventions for COVID-19 pandemic: introduction of a locally-adapted brief intervention for mental health and psychosocial support service. *Malaysian Journal of Medical Sciences*, **27**, 51–56.

Prati, G. & Pietrantoni, L. (2010). The relation of perceived and received social support to mental health among first responders: a meta-analytic review. *Journal of Community Psychology*, **38**, 403–417.

Qiu, J., Shen, B., Zhao, M., Wang, Z., Xie, B., & Xu, Y. (2020). A nationwide survey of psychological distress among Chinese people in the COVID-19 epidemic: implications and policy recommendations. *General Psychiatry*, **33**, e100213.

Rathod, S., Pinninti, N., Irfan, M., Gorczynski, P., Rathod, P., Gega, L., & Naeem, F. (2017). Mental health service provision in low- and middle-income countries. *Health Services Insights*, **10**, 1178632917694350.

Remmerswaal, D. & Muris, P. (2011). Children's fear reactions to the 2009 swine flu pandemic: the role of threat information as provided by parents. *Journal of Anxiety Disorders*, **25**, 444–449.

Roca, M., Gili, M., Garcia-Campayo, J., & Garcia-Toro, M. (2013). Economic crisis and mental health in Spain. *Lancet*, **382**, 1977–1978.

Rovers, J. J. E., Van De Linde, L. S., Kenters, N., Bisseling, E. M., Nieuwenhuijse, D. F., Oude Munnink, B. B., et al. (2020). Why psychiatry is different—challenges and difficulties in managing a nosocomial outbreak of coronavirus disease (COVID-19) in hospital care. *Antimicrobial Resistance and Infection Control*, **9**, 190.

Roy, A., Singh, A. K., Mishra, S., Chinnadurai, A., Mitra, A., & Bakshi, O. (2021). Mental health implications of COVID-19 pandemic and its response in India. *International Journal of Social Psychiatry*, **67**, 587–600.

Scharf, D. & Oinonen, K. (2020). Ontario's response to COVID-19 shows that mental health providers must be integrated into provincial public health insurance systems. *Canadian Journal of Public Health*, **111**, 473–476.

Schiavo, A. (2020). Happify health designs benefit for remote access to mental health services. Arizent. https://www.benefitnews.com/news/happify-health-designs-benefit-for-remote-access-to-mental-health-services

Sijbrandij, M., Horn, R., Esliker, R., O'May, F., Reiffers, R., Ruttenberg, L., et al. (2020). The effect of psychological first aid training on knowledge and understanding about psychosocial support principles: a cluster-randomized controlled trial. *International Journal of Environmental Research and Public Health*, **17**, 484.

Sivakumar, P. T., Mukku, S. S. R., Kar, N., Manjunatha, N., Phutane, V. H., Sinha, P., et al. (2020). Geriatric telepsychiatry: promoting access to geriatric mental health care beyond the physical barriers. *Indian Journal of Psychological Medicine*, **42**(Suppl.) 41S–46S.

Sommerlad, A., Marston, L., Huntley, J., Livingston, G., Lewis, G., Steptoe, A., & Fancourt, D. (2022). Social relationships and depression during the COVID-19 lockdown: longitudinal analysis of the COVID-19 Social Study. *Psychological Medicine*, **52**, 3381–3390.

Steimer, T. (2002). The biology of fear- and anxiety-related behaviors. *Dialogues in Clinical Neuroscience*, **4**, 231–249.

Tariq, A., Roosa, K., Mizumoto, K., & Chowell, G. (2019). Assessing reporting delays and the effective reproduction number: the Ebola epidemic in DRC, May 2018–January 2019. *Epidemics*, **26**, 128–133.

Taylor Salisbury, T., Kohrt, B. A., Bakolis, I., Jordans, M. J., Hull, L., Luitel, N. P., et al. (2021). Adaptation of the World Health Organization Electronic Mental Health Gap Action Programme Intervention Guide app for mobile devices in Nepal and Nigeria: protocol for a feasibility cluster randomized controlled trial. *JMIR Research Protocols*, **10**, e24115.

Thornicroft, G., Chatterji, S., Evans-Lacko, S., Gruber, M., Sampson, N., et al. (2017). Undertreatment of people with major depressive disorder in 21 countries. *British Journal of Psychiatry*, **210**, 119–124.

United Nations (2020). *United Nations Policy Brief: COVID-19 and the Need for Action on Mental Health*. New York: United Nations.

Vigo, D., Thornicroft, G., & Gureje, O. (2020). The differential outcomes of coronavirus disease 2019 in low- and middle-income countries vs high-income countries. *JAMA Psychiatry*, **77**, 1207–1208.

Wallace, C. L., Wladkowski, S. P., Gibson, A., & White, P. (2020). Grief during the COVID-19 pandemic: considerations for palliative care providers. *Journal of Pain and Symptom Management*, **60**, e70–e76.

Wang, Q., Xu, R., & Volkow, N. D. (2021). Increased risk of COVID-19 infection and mortality in people with mental disorders: analysis from electronic health records in the United States. *World Psychiatry*, **20**, 124–130.

Ward, E. C., Wiltshire, J. C., Detry, M. A., & Brown, R. L. (2013). African American men and women's attitude toward mental illness, perceptions of stigma, and preferred coping behaviors. *Nursing Research*, **62**, 185–94.

Waterman, S., Cole, C. L., Greenberg, N., Rubin, G. J., & Beck, A. (2019). A qualitative study assessing the feasibility of implementing a group cognitive-behavioural therapy-based intervention in Sierra Leone. *BJPsych International*, **16**, 31–34.

Williams, L. D., Tempalski, B., Hall, H. I., Johnson, A. S., Wang, G., & Friedman, S. R. (2021). Trajectories of and disparities in HIV prevalence among Black, White, and Hispanic/Latino high risk heterosexuals in 89 U.S. metropolitan statistical areas, 1992–2013. *Annals of Epidemiology*, **64**, 140–148.

Williamson, V., Murphy, D., & Greenberg, N. (2020). COVID-19 and experiences of moral injury in front-line key workers. *Occupational Medicine*, **70**, 317–319.

World Health Organization (2018). *Mental Health Atlas 2017*. Geneva: World Health Organization.

World Health Organization (2020a). *COVID-19 Disrupting Mental Health Services in Most Countries, WHO Survey*. Geneva: World Health Organization.

World Health Organization (2020b). Helping children cope with stress during the 2019-nCoV outbreak. https://www.who.int/docs/default-source/coronaviruse/helping-children-cope-with-stress-print.pdf

World Health Organization (2022). *Disease Outbreaks: Environment, Climate Change and Health*. Geneva: World Health Organization.

Wu, P., Fang, Y., Guan, Z., Fan, B., Kong, J., Yao, Z., et al. (2009). The psychological impact of the SARS epidemic on hospital employees in China: exposure, risk perception, and altruistic acceptance of risk. *Canadian Journal of Psychiatry*, **54**, 302–311.

Xiao, H., Zhang, Y., Kong, D., Li, S., & Yang, N. (2020). Social capital and sleep quality in individuals who self-isolated for 14 days during the coronavirus disease 2019 (COVID-19) outbreak in January 2020 in China. *Medical Science Monitor*, **26**, e923921.

Zhao, Y. J., Jin, Y., Rao, W. W., Li, W., Zhao, N., Cheung, T., et al. (2021). The prevalence of psychiatric comorbidities during the SARS and COVID-19 epidemics: a systematic review and meta-analysis of observational studies. *Journal of Affective Disorders*, **287**, 145–157.

43

'Mental health' in low- and middle-income countries

R. Srinivasa Murthy

Mental health is critically important to everyone, everywhere. All over the world, mental health needs are high but responses are insufficient and inadequate. The *World mental health report: transforming mental health for all* is designed to inspire and inform better mental health for all. Drawing on the latest evidence available, showcasing examples of good practice from around the world, and voicing people's lived experience, it highlights why and where change is most needed and how it can best be achieved. It calls on all stakeholders to work together to deepen the value and commitment given to mental health, reshape the environments that influence mental health, and strengthen the systems that care for mental health.

World Health Organization, *World Mental Health Report* (2022)

Introduction

During the last decade, from the time of the publication of the first edition of this textbook, there have been major developments in the field of mental health. The most important are the publication of the *World Mental Health Report* (World Health Organization (WHO), 2022); the global launch of the Lancet–World Psychiatric Association Commission 'Time for united action on depression' (Herrman et al., 2022); the indicators to monitor mental health developments in countries globally (Countdown); the Lancet Commission on stigma and discrimination in mental health (Thornicroft et al., 2022); the wide recognition of the increased need for mental health care due to the Covid-19 pandemic; country-level initiatives to develop community mental health care (e.g. in India, Nigeria, and Pakistan); and better understanding of the psychosocial determinants of mental health, opening avenues for action beyond the health services. For mental health, the decade has been a significant one. These developments form the scope of this chapter.

World Mental Health Report, 2022

The latest *World Mental Health Report*, subtitled *Transforming Mental Health for All*, released on 17 June 2022, is a major milestone in the development of mental health in the world (WHO, 2022).

There are seven important reasons to consider this Report as important. Firstly, this Report is from the WHO, where the ministries of health of all countries of the world contribute to policy development and it is the lead organization for health in the world. Secondly, this Report comes 21 years after the last report of October 2001 (WHO, 2001). Thirdly, unlike the 2001 Report which was a *World Health Report* with special focus on mental health, this report is a stand-alone full report on mental health (this Report is twice the size of the 2001 Report). Fourthly, the last two decades have seen major advances in understanding of mental disorders and mental health, especially about the plasticity of the brain and social determinants of health. Fifthly, the Covid-19 pandemic has sensitized the general population, politicians, planners, and the population to the importance of mental health as part of life. Sixthly, the report presents mental health in an engaging and easy-to-read non-technical language, suitable for reading by professionals and non-professionals alike (the more than 70 case studies—innovations, country reports, personal narratives, and graphics—are a special feature of the report). Lastly, the Report is a treat from the design point of view with excellent graphics and photographs. All in all, a significant contribution to the understanding and action towards mental health of the world. This *World Mental Health Report* is designed to inspire and inform the indisputable and urgent transformation required to ensure better mental health for all. While promoting a multisectoral approach, this report is especially written for decision-makers in the

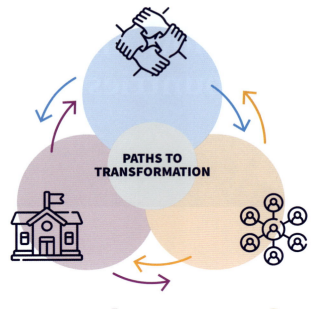

Three transformative paths towards better mental health

 DEEPEN VALUE AND COMMITMENT
- Understand and appreciate intrinsic value
- Promote social inclusion of people with mental health conditions
- Give mental and physical health equal priority
- Intensify engagement across sectors
- Step up investment in mental health

 RESHAPE ENVIRONMENTS
- Reshape physical, social and economic characteristics of different environments for mental health, including
  - homes
  - schools
  - workplaces
  - health care services
  - communities
  - natural environments

 STRENGTHEN MENTAL HEALTH CARE
- Build community-based networks of services
- Move away from custodial care in psychiatric hospitals
- Diversify and scale up care options
- Make mental health affordable and accessible for all
- Promote person-centred, human rights-based care
- Engage and empower people with lived experience

Figure 43.1 Three transformative paths towards better mental health.
Reproduced from *World Mental Health Report: Transforming Mental Health for All*. Geneva: World Health Organization; 2022. Licence: CC BY-NC-SA 3.0 IGO.

health sector. This includes ministries of health and other partners in the health sector who are generally tasked with developing mental health policy and delivering mental health systems and services.

The report is organized around three overarching themes, namely (1) principles and drivers of public mental health, (2) the case for transformation, and (3) mental health reform, in eight chapters: 'Introduction', 'Principles and drivers in public mental health', 'World mental health today', 'Benefits of change', 'Foundations for change', 'Promotion and prevention for change', 'Restructuring and scaling up care for impact', and 'Conclusion'. These are summarized in **Figures 43.1** and **43.2**.

Depression

The global launch of the Lancet–World Psychiatric Association Commission 'Time for united action on depression' on 16 February 2022, reflects the same importance of the COVID-19 pandemic as follows:

> Our task has never felt more urgent. The potentiation by the COVID-19 pandemic of adverse societal factors such as deep-rooted structural inequalities and personal impacts such as social isolation, bereavement, sickness, uncertainty, impoverishment, and poor access to health care has had negative impacts on the mental health of millions of people. It has generated a so-called perfect storm that requires responses at multiple levels. The consequences of the pandemic thus emphasise the need to make the prevention, recognition, and treatment of depression an immediate global priority, which we address through a number of key messages and recommendations. (Herrman et al., 2022, p. 957)

The recommendations call for action at four levels: (1) the community and people living with depression, (2) health care practitioners, (3) researchers and research funders, and (4) decision makers and policymakers.

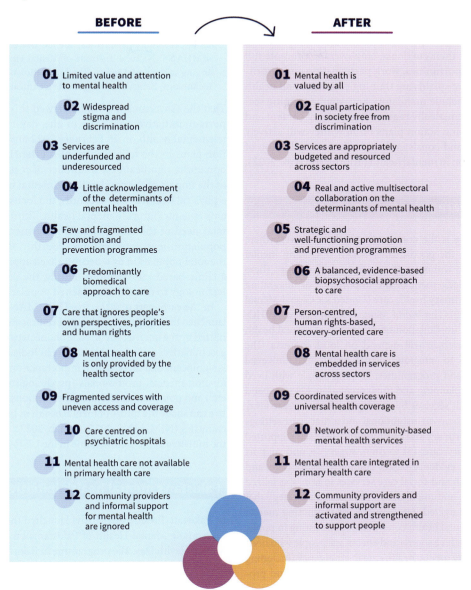

Figure 43.2 Key shifts to transform mental health for all.
Reproduced from *World Mental Health Report: Transforming Mental Health for All*. Geneva: World Health Organization; 2022. Licence: CC BY-NC-SA 3.0 IGO.

Stigma and discrimination

Stigma about persons living with mental illnesses and mental health care has been recognized as a crucial barrier in the area of mental health care (Surgeon General, 1999; WHO, 2001). The Lancet Commission on ending stigma and discrimination in mental health, published in October 2022, is a major contribution (Thornicroft et al., 2022). The Commission recognizes the importance of stigma as a barrier:

> Many people with lived experience of mental health conditions describe stigma as 'worse than the condition itself'. There is clear evidence that we now know how to effectively reduce, and ultimately eliminate, stigma and discrimination. Our Commission makes eight practical, evidence-based and radical recommendations for action to liberate millions of people around the world from social isolation, discrimination and violations of human rights caused by stigma.
> (Kings College London, 2022)

The report provides a comprehensive review of the evidence for effective stigma reduction interventions. The report also finds that social contact between people with and without lived experience of mental health conditions is the most effective way to reduce stigma and discrimination.

Further, the report argues that people with lived experience of mental health conditions must be empowered and supported to play central and active roles in stigma reduction efforts. For this reason, the Commission has made a point to include the voices of people with lived experiences in the form of poems, testimonies, and quotations to fully demonstrate the toll stigma and discrimination take. Experts of the Commission call for immediate, radical action from governments, international organizations, employers, schools, health care providers, and media organizations. The Commission calls on all governments to implement anti-stigma policies, international organizations to issue guidance including decriminalizing suicide, schools to adapt their curricula, employers to promote full access to educational opportunities, work participation and return-to-work programmes, pre-qualifying training courses for all health and social care staff to include mandatory anti-stigma training sessions, and media to systematically remove stigmatizing content and issue policy statements and action plans on how they will actively promote mental health and consistently contribute to reduction of stigma and discrimination in mental health (Thornicroft et al., 2022).

Universal health care policy

Universal health coverage is the concept that everyone, everywhere should be able to access the good-quality health (including mental health) services they need without suffering financial hardship. There is an increasing acknowledgement of the importance of integrating mental health care into primary health care (United for Global Mental Health, 2022; WHO, 2022). The *World Mental Health Report* (WHO, 2022) recognizes that the implantation of integration of mental health with universal health coverage will depend on local contexts. The Report recommends (1) to integrate mental health into universal health coverage policies and programmes, keeping people with lived experience at the core of planning and implementation; (2) to expand coverage for mental health services by shifting the focus of care away from an almost exclusive focus on institutional and tertiary care settings towards evidence-based primary and community care that is supported by institutional and tertiary care; (3) to train, supervise, and support health workers to deliver evidence-based, culturally appropriate, and rights-based mental health and social care services in non-specialized settings; (4) to coordinate and implement a multisectoral strategy that combines universal and targeted interventions for promoting mental health and preventing mental health conditions; (5) investing in public education campaigns to reduce stigma and encourage people who need help to seek it; (6) including mental health care in emergency (including pandemics) preparedness, response and recovery planning, and programmes; and (7) to integrate mental health into health data collection and identify, collate, routinely report, and use core mental health data disaggregated by sex and age in order to improve mental health service delivery, and promotion and prevention strategies

India's mental health initiative

The 1 February 2022 was an important day in the history of mental health care in India. On that day, the Finance Minister of the Government of India, Mrs Nirmala Sitharaman, as part of the annual budget speech, for the first time in the history of budget presentation in Independent India, referred to mental health and allotted funds for the same as follows:

> the pandemic has accentuated mental health problems in people of all ages. Several factors have contributed to a steep rise in depression and anxiety, including restrictions on social contact, lockdowns, economic insecurity, and school and business closures.

Further, she outlined the intervention:

> To better the access to quality mental health counselling and care services, a National Tele-Mental Health programme will be launched—23 nodal centres for telemedical mental health will be operated, with NIMHANS [National Institute of Mental Health and Neurosciences] serving as the nodal centre. The International Institute of Information Technology, Bengaluru will provide technical support.

That the Government of India viewed this commitment as an important initiative was seen in the day-long meeting to launch telemental health on 26 February 2022 and the development of action plans in the following months (The Hindu, 2022). This development is significant for a number of reasons. Firstly, recognition of the impact of the pandemic as a mental health event and not only a physical health event. Secondly, the focus on the social determinants as contributors to mental health. Thirdly, the recognition of the total need of the total population for mental health and focus on population-level interventions. Fourthly, the focus on coverage of the total population by a decentralized approach to care rather than a clinic-based interventions. Fifthly, the utilization of information technology to reach the unreached population.

In the early part of 2023, the TELE-MANAS programme has been launched through five coordinating centres and 51 services centres connected by the internet and mobile phone network. This is one of the biggest initiatives for mental health care in India during the last 50 years. It is significant that there is high importance provided in the programme for non-medical professionals (psychologists, social workers, nurses, etc.) and non-pharmacological interventions. The results of this initiative can shape the future of mental health in India and other developing countries (NIMHANS, 2022a, 2022b, 2022c, 2022d). This is similar to the initiative of the '988' helpline in the US (Miller et al., 2022).

Pakistan's mental health initiatives

In Pakistan, President Arif Alvi launched the President's Programme to Promote Mental Health of Pakistanis on 10 October 2019, World Mental Health Day. The programme in Pakistan emphasizes the role of early-life interventions that promote mental health and prevent mental illness, and calls for a phased implementation of two evidence-based interventions. The first is the WHO Thinking Healthy programme for mothers, a psychosocial intervention delivered by community health workers to high-risk mothers in low-resourced settings. The second intervention is the WHO School Mental Health programme adapted for Pakistan. This programme includes training teachers in skills and strategies to promote mental health in their schools and the early recognition and management of mental health problems. These interventions, to be implemented in one district in the first year, are planned to be rolled out across all four provinces of Pakistan within 5 years. Another aspect of the president's plan is an emphasis on technology to improve access to mental health (Mirza & Rahman, 2019).

New mental health law in Nigeria

Nigeria's National Mental Health Act 2021 was signed into law on 5 January 2023, after two decades of struggle to repeal the outdated, colonial mental health legislation. With this achievement, Nigeria joins the few African countries that have revised or enacted new mental health legislation in accordance with the WHO's call for member countries to use legal reforms to end human rights violations against people with mental health conditions.

The approved law is human rights oriented and clearly outlines the rights of people with mental health conditions. It addresses the limitations of previously proposed mental health bills from 2003, 2013, and 2019 by prohibiting discrimination against people with mental health conditions exercising their fundamental human rights, and by regulating the use of coercive measures. The approved act has provisions, such as the engagement of people with lived experience as peer workers, the development of community mental health services, the development of self-help with digital technologies, and the integration of mental health into disease-specific programmes (e.g. HIV programmes). It also supports collaboration between the Ministry of Health and community mental health services run by non-governmental organizations and faith-based organizations (Aluh et al., 2023).

Covid-19 pandemic and mental health

Similarly, at the level of populations, there is both a threat and an opportunity to rethink mental health. A recent book, described the impact of the Covid-19 pandemic as follows:

> The pandemic has, in this sense, given us an opportunity to make a decisive break from the ethos that has governed our work and caused out burnout over the past fifty years. It's a chance to remake work and reimagine its place in our lives. If we don't take this opportunity, we will slip back into patterns that created the burnout culture in the first place. (Malesic, 2022).

Similarly, Taylor states (2020, 2022):

> The pandemic changed everything about our lives: how we worked, socialised, travelled. Dealing with so many changes at once was a mental challenge for us all ... The pandemic has also taught us the importance of developing resilience—the ability to manage the stressors, large and small, in our lives. Resilience may be one positive legacy of a very tough couple of years.

Major developments in mental health during the last decade

The important aspects of emotional health that are relevant for planning are the following:

- Evidence of the value of daily exercise, adequate restful sleep, nutrition, connectedness, yoga, meditation, and wisdom towards promoting mental health of the population is growing (Gupta, 2021; Jeste, 2020; Lam & Riba, 2016; Murthy, 2020; Srinivasa Murthy, 2021; Varamballly & Gangadhar, 2016).
- For non-syndromal 'distress' associated with stresses of various life situations and associated with chronic medical conditions, benefits can be provided by sharing of feeling, journaling (Pennebaker & Evans, 2014) music/art, thinking differently (WHO, 2020), and spirituality (Koenig, 2012).
- Social networks are vital for mental health: in a longitudinal study, researchers from Harvard and Peking universities analysed 12 years' worth of data from men and women aged 65 years or older and found that loneliness and depressive symptoms appeared to be related risk factors of worsening cognition (Dickens et al., 2013). At the beginning stages of readjustment of relationships, there is likely to be greater confrontation and reduced cohesion.
- A number of environmental interventions like individual exposure to nature or greening of the residential areas and increasing cohesion in the community are beneficial for the mental health of the population (Murthy, 2020).
- Loneliness of old age can be addressed by the use of cultural and spiritual resources (Srinivasa Murthy & Banerjee, 2021).
- Measures that promote resilience and post-traumatic growth can mitigate the negative effects of adverse situations like exposure to disasters/conflicts, severe life-threatening situations like cancer, and result in positive growth of individuals (Southwick & Charney, 2018).
- Changes and stresses of all types are associated with mental health implications (Srinivasa Murthy, 2017).
- Childhood trauma of any type is associated with negative mental health consequences throughout life (Srinivasa Murthy, 2014).
- Domestic violence is associated with higher levels of mental disorders (Begum et al., 2015).
- Inequalities of all types are associated with increased mental disorders. Wilkinson and Pickett (2010, 2017, 2018) present international research studies showing associations with drug abuse, teenage pregnancies, violence, imprisonment, and quality of life. As the movement makes progress, we can expect less inequalities between the sexes and this raises the possibility of reduction of inequality as a contributor to well-being of the total population.
- Urbanization, slums: mobility of populations and urbanization affects mental health through the influence of increased stressors and factors such as an overcrowded and polluted environment, high levels of violence, access to illicit drugs, and reduced social support. In most developing countries, over 10% of the population living in urban areas live in slums. For example, low-paid urban workers often live in crowded spaces with poor basic sanitation, food supplies, and shelter, as well as few—if any—basic governmental and social support services (Srinivasa Murthy, 2018).
- Loneliness: a number of longitudinal studies indicate that loneliness proceeds depression, sleep difficulties, high blood pressure, physical inactivity, functional decline, cognitive impairment, and increased mortality. Physical and mental health components of quality of life were significantly reduced by loneliness. Severe loneliness was associated with reduced patient satisfaction (Musich et al., 2015).

Social determinants of mental health

During last two decades, there has been a revival of the understanding of social factors and mental health. The most recent review of mental health, the World Psychiatric Association–Lancet Psychiatry Commission on the future of psychiatry, summarizes the challenges as follows:

> A large body of evidence shows the importance of social determinants for mental disorders. Societal factors such as social inequality, crime, poverty, poor housing, adverse upbringing conditions, poor education, unemployment, and social isolation are related to

increased rates of mental disorders. The relevance of some social determinants varies across the world. Examples are substantial urbanisation in LMICs [low- and middle-income countries]; increasing social isolation in high-income countries; the changing flow of refugees in some regions; and different levels of economic instability, civil unrest, and inequality between rich and poor people. Most of these social determinants influence physical health problems too, but they can be seen as particularly relevant to psychiatry. (Bhugra et al., 2017, p. 789).

Further, the group, recognized psychiatry in the first quarter of the twenty-first century to be at the cusp of major changes, as follows:

Increased emphasis on social interventions and engagement with societal expectations might be an important area for psychiatry's development. This could encompass advocacy for the rights of individuals living with mental illnesses, political involvement concerning the social risk factors for mental illness, and, on a smaller scale, work with families and local social networks and communities. Psychiatrists should therefore possess communication skills and knowledge of the social sciences as well as the basic biological sciences. (Bhugra et al., 2017, p. 775)

Covid-19 and social determinants

The importance of social determinants of mental health has received support from the country-level experiences of the impact of the pandemic during the last 2 years (2020–2022). The most recent study aimed to quantify the impact of the Covid-19 pandemic on the prevalence and burden of major depressive disorder and anxiety disorders globally in 2020 (COVID-19 Mental Disorders Collaborators, 2021). The study reported a nearly 30% increase in both the disorders. Further, increases in the prevalence of major depressive disorder and anxiety disorders during 2020 were both associated with increasing SARS-CoV-2 infection rates and decreasing human mobility.

In another study, from the US, a longitudinal study of a nationally representative group of US adults ages 18 years and older surveyed in March 2020 and April 2021, called the 'COVID-19 and Life Stressors Impact on Mental Health and Well-being' (CLIMB) study, the prevalence of elevated depressive symptoms persisted from 27.8% in 2020 to 32.8% in 2021. Importantly the central drivers of depressive symptoms were low household income, not being married, and experiencing multiple stressors during the Covid-19 pandemic. The authors conclude, 'Mental health gaps grew between populations with different assets and stressor experiences during the Covid-19 pandemic' (Ettman et al., 2021). American Indian or Alaska Native, Latino, Black, and Asian or Pacific Islander persons were more likely than White persons to have a Covid-19-associated hospitalization, intensive care unit admission, or in-hospital death during the first year of the US Covid-19 pandemic (Acosta et al., 2021).

In a multi-country study, health care workers from nine Eastern Mediterranean Regional countries, working during the Covid-19 pandemic, were assessed: 57.5% had depression, 42.0% had stress, and 59.1% had anxiety. Considering the severity, 19.2%, 16.1%, and 26.6% of participants had severe to extremely severe depression, stress, and anxiety, respectively. Depression, stress, anxiety, and distress scores were significantly associated with participants' residency, having children, pre-existing psychiatric illness, and being isolated for Covid-19. In addition, females, those working in a teaching hospital, and specialists had significantly higher depression and stress scores. Married status, current smoking, diabetes mellitus, having a friend who died with Covid-19, and high Covid-19 worry scores were significantly associated with higher distress scores. The authors urge for immediate implementation of 'special interventions to promote mental well-being among health care workers responding to Covid-19' (Ghaleb et al., 2021).

A recent review entitled 'Screening and interventions for social risk factors' by the US Preventive Services Task Force (Eder et al., 2021) noted that of the interventions studied, 73 addressed multiple social risk domains. The most frequently addressed domains were food insecurity, financial strain, and housing instability. The authors concluded that there is a need for more randomized clinical trials that report health outcomes from social risk screening and interventions.

In a recent paper (Berkessel et al., 2021), the complex interaction of factors like religiosity, lower socioeconomic status, and psychological burden was observed. Using three databases, the relationship between nationalities and religiosity and the psychological burden of poverty was studied. The authors report an interesting finding of psychological burden of lower socioeconomic status, greater in developed nations than in developing ones. This finding suggests that, as national religiosity continues to decline, lower socioeconomic status will become increasingly harmful for psychological well-being. There is an interesting observation in the paper: 'the challenge will be to find alternatives to national religiosity to curb these harmful effects. Such alternatives will not be easily found because national religiosity exerts particularly powerful effects' (Berkessel et al., 2021, p. 4).

The other area of growing concern is the mental health needs of newer groups of personnel like health personnel reporting high levels of burnout (Arnold-Foster, 2022; Hurt, 2021), and caregivers who are becoming the alternate mental health workforce (Srinivasa Murthy, 2016a). On the positive side there have been revisions of the legislation relating to mental health care in a number of countries (e.g. India, Nigeria), higher use of information technology, telemental health and growth of private psychiatry, adding to the increased availability of services.

Policy level developments

The *Mental Health Atlas 2020* (WHO, 2021), published by the WHO every 3 years, is a compilation of data provided by countries around the world on mental health policies, legislation, financing, human resources, availability and utilization of services, and data collection systems. Progress values for 2020 indicate that the targets committed to by WHO member states have not been achieved. There are massive inequalities in the availability of mental health resources and their allocation between high- and low-income countries and across regions. While guidelines for the integration of mental health into primary health care exist and have been adopted in most countries, with activities ongoing for training and supervision, the integration of interventions for service delivery, such as pharmacological and psychosocial interventions for mental health conditions, remains limited. The *Mental Health Atlas 2020* also shows significant limitations in the capacity of countries' mental health information systems to report on specific indicators such as service utilization. The WHO notes that the global targets can be reached in 2030 only if there is a collective global commitment over the next 10 years across member states to make massive investments and expanded efforts at the country level relating to mental health policies, laws, programmes, and services.

In another report of the mental health policies in the Commonwealth countries, Bhugra et al.'s (2019) survey of 52 member countries found that less than half of the countries had a mental health policy. Deinstitutionalization was not seen as a priority in many countries and there was no equity between physical and mental health funding. A major contribution from the WHO is the development of evidence-based mental health intervention material and its adoption by a large number of countries (WHO, 2006, 2016).

The WHO Mental Health Action Plan for 2013–2030 (WHO, 2013) had the following six priorities: universal health coverage, human rights, evidence-based practice, life course approach, multisectoral approach, and empowerment of persons with mental disorders and psychosocial disabilities. Giving global focus to depression in the last few years by making it the theme of the World Health Day, universal coverage for mental health (WHO, 2013), developing caregiver materials for persons with developmental disorders, and initiating suicide prevention are some of the other important initiatives.

Countdown

A significant development in measuring and monitoring mental health of the countries of the world is the United Global Mental Health initiative, 'Countdown' (United for Global Mental Health, n.d.). Countdown Global Mental Health 2030 is the first independent monitoring and accountability mechanism that uses a broad and integrated set of indicators to monitor progress for mental health. This is developed by United for Global Mental Health in partnership with the WHO, UNICEF, GlobalMentalHealth@Harvard, Global Mental Health Peer Network, and *The Lancet*. This is a free and interactive dashboard which lets users search mental health data by country using a range of indicators, combined with an annual monitoring report on what the latest data show. It helps to monitor action to campaign, to advocate, to communicate, and to change policy and practice so that everyone, everywhere is able to exercise their right to the highest attainable level of mental health. The data collection is clustered around three themes: (1) determinants of mental health, (2) factors supporting the demand for mental health care, and (3) factors shaping the strength of the mental health system. These indicators go beyond traditionally defined health indicators and span the entire spectrum of the United Nations Sustainable Development Goals.

Historical developments

The year 2024 is an important time in the history of mental health services in LMICs. It was 50 years ago, in 1974, that the WHO held its first meeting on 'Organization of mental health services in developing countries' at Addis Ababa, Ethiopia (Giel & Harding, 1976; WHO, 1975). The 1975 initiative to outline the need for national-level thinking in developing policies, to integrate mental health with general health care, and involve non-specialists in mental health care as measures to develop mental health care in developing countries was path breaking. What is interesting is that the WHO put these ideas to practice as part of a 6-year, international, seven-country project, 'Strategies for Extending Mental Health Care' (1975–1981) (Harding et al., 1983; Sartorius & Harding, 1983; Srinivasa Murthy & Wig, 1983; Wig et al., 1984). This project is important as a demonstration of the feasibility of integrating mental health care in primary health care in LMICs. The multicentric, 11-country project 'Mental Illness in General Health Care' (Üstün & Sartorius, 1995) was another attempt at demonstrating both the need and feasibility of addressing the common mental disorders at primary health care level. This period was followed by the focus on developing national mental health plans in a number of countries in Asia, the Middle East, Africa, and South America during the next two decades. India was one of the first to develop the National Mental Health Programme (NMHP) in August 1982 (Wig and Murthy, 2018). WHO initiated a number of pilot innovative programmes under 'Nations for Mental Health'. The publication of the *World Health Report 2001* with the subject of 'Mental Health: New Understanding, New Hope' was the next milestone (WHO, 2001). This document boldly presented ten recommendations: provide treatment in primary care; make psychotropic drugs available; give care in the community; educate the public; involve communities, families and consumers; establish national policies, programmes, and legislation; develop human resources; link with other sectors; monitor community mental health; and support more research. This has been covered extensively in the earlier edition of this *Oxford Textbook of Community Mental Health* (Srinivasa Murthy, 2011; Thornicroft et al., 2011)

2017 Lancet Initiative

A challenge faced by many countries is to provide adequate human resources for delivery of essential mental health interventions. The overwhelming worldwide shortage of human resources for mental health, particularly in LMICs, is well established. Kukuma et al, 2017 review the current state of human resources for mental health, needs, and strategies for action. At present, human resources for mental health in countries of low and middle income show a serious shortfall that is likely to grow unless effective steps are taken. Evidence suggests that mental health care can be delivered effectively in primary health care settings, through community-based programmes and task-shifting approaches. Non-specialist health professionals, lay workers, affected individuals, and caregivers with brief training and appropriate supervision by mental health specialists are able to detect, diagnose, treat, and monitor individuals with mental disorders and reduce caregiver burden. We also discuss scale-up costs, human resources management, and leadership for mental health, particularly within the context of low-income and middle-income countries (Bhugra et al., 2011).

World Mental Health Day 2021

In October 2021, as part of the World Mental Health Day 2021 (World Federation for Mental Health: 'Mental Health in an Unequal World' campaign) there were many important country-level initiatives. Some of these include the launch of the 'Countdown Global Mental Health 2030' by Global Mental Health Group, the release of the world *Mental Health Atlas 2020* by the WHO (and the WHO's 'Mental Health for All: Let us Make it a Reality' campaign), and the *State of the World's Children 2021* (UNICEF, 2021) which focused on mental health ('We must change the way we view mental health'). The 270-page report states that children and young people could feel the impact of Covid-19 on their mental health and well-being for many years to come. It focuses on risks and protective factors at critical moments in life and attempts to shed light on the social factors that shape mental health and well-being. The report recognizes that the pandemic is the 'tip of the iceberg' after years of neglecting child mental health.

International collaborative programmes

One of the important developments of the last decade is the launch of action programmes for mental health care in LMICs. Three of them are important, namely, PRIME, EMERALD, and INDIGO.

The aim of the PRogramme for Improving Mental health carE (PRIME) is to generate research evidence on the implementation of district-level mental health care plans for five target mental, neurological, and substance use disorders comprising depression, maternal depression, alcohol use disorders, psychosis, and epilepsy in Ethiopia, India, Nepal, South Africa, and Uganda.

The 'Emerging mental health systems in LMICs' (EMERALD) research programme was a 5-year programme (2012–2017) aimed to improve mental health outcomes in six LMICs in Africa and Asia (Ethiopia, India, Nepal, Nigeria, South Africa, and Uganda) by building capacity and generating evidence to enhance health system strengthening (Semrau et al., 2019). The six recommendations from this project are governance, mental health financing, human resources, service provision, mental health information systems. and knowledge transfer. The project concludes that strengthening of mental health in LMIC countries, requires (1) moving towards universal health coverage for people with mental, neurological, and substance use disorders requires consideration of the resources needed to scale up services and also consideration of the fair and sustainable mechanisms for providing enhanced financial protection to affected households; (2) ensuring that there is a strong focus on capacity building of patients, policymakers, planners, and researchers to support mental health system strengthening; (3) any country that is envisioning the integration of mental health into primary health care should review the requirements and processes across the health system building blocks; and (4) ensuring that routine health information systems include mental health indicators so that mental health care needs and services can be routinely monitored.

Low- and middle-income country experiences

There have been many country-level initiatives utilizing a range of approaches. One of the most popular in this group is the 'Friendship Bench' initiative started in Zimbabwe (Chibanda et al., 2015, 2016; Fernando et al., 2021). It has been extended to other countries like Kenya (Doukani et al., 2021). Other significant country initiatives are in China (Philips et al., 2009), Ethiopia (Johanson et al., 2017), Ghana (Gureje et al., 2021), India (Raykar et al., 2016), Nigeria (Gureje et al., 2021), Uganda (Mugisha et al., 2016; Ssebunnya et al., 2018), and Nepal (Raja et al., 2012). All of these are indications of greater awareness of mental health as a priority, and the recognition for the need for finding country-level solutions. There is a comprehensive and critical review of the LMIC reports in the *World Mental Health Report* (WHO, 2022).

Lessons from mental health care in developed countries

The pandemic has presented challenges of meeting the mental health needs of the population in spite of the much better resources for mental health care. The need for innovation to reach all those who need the care is seen even in developed countries. For example, the launch of the 'Mentally Healthy Nation' by the American Psychiatric Association. The goal of this initiative is significant for the scope of the activity to reach the general public through podcasts to engage the public in conversations about the current mental health crisis. Each episode of 'Mentally Healthy Nation' will be centred around an aspect of mental health that impacts the community, where people live, learn, work, and worship. The goal is to help ease the stigma of mental illness and to reach a more mentally healthy nation. On a similar topic, the new mental health helpline '988' launched in the US in June 2022 (Miller et al., 2022). It can be expected that there will be many innovations in mental health care in the coming decade.

Common themes

The WHO *World Mental Health Report*, in 2022, and the editorial observations of the Lancet–World Psychiatric Association Commission on depression (The Lancet, 2022) reflect the current situation, need, and way forward for mental health for LMICs. The depression report noted that although depression is a common part of the human experience across the life course, there are several reasons why it does not receive sufficient resources and global attention (The Lancet, 2022):

> First, depression, as with mental health conditions in general, has historically been stigmatised. … Second, managing depression is not always straightforward. … Third, depression depends on a combination of biological, social, and psychological factors, and requires domestic policy and investment across sectors, such as health, education, employment, and social services. The Commission calls on the scientific community to adopt a 'multidimensional approach' to develop the cross-disciplinary and collaborative research needed to inform prevention and care. To improve resources and narrow gaps in inequity of care, the Commission calls for a public health perspective on depression. … In sum, the Commission lays out a stark choice: to improve equitable and stigma-free access to interventions for people with depression or to continue to condone indifference to the well-being of the 1 billion people with mental health needs. Governments, donors, and communities must reduce the global burden of depression

through concerted action against stigma and health inequities, and increase their financial and social commitments. Together, the global community must decide to prioritize the emotional wellness of our species. (p. 885)

The progress in the LMICs can be summarized as follows:

Firstly, during the last five decades and more importantly in the last two decades, there has been a sea change in the importance given to mental health in LMICs. There is a shift to recognize the larger mental health needs of the population and include mental health as part of public health programmes.

Secondly, mental health professionals have responded to the challenges of providing mental health care by innovative approaches, relevant to the country situations (community psychiatry in LMICs is not a 'single model' programme but a wide variety of initiatives involving community resources).

Thirdly, the initiatives have been in limited pockets, limited in reach, and have not been adequately supported with funds, by the national governments and international organizations.

Fourthly, extension of the pilot programmes to cover wider population requiring further efforts to develop technical materials (e.g. for families, general public) and at managerial strategies.

Fifthly, there are areas of mental health programme that have not been given adequate attention. The past efforts have laid greater emphasis on care of persons with mental disorders, though there have been smaller-scale attempts at promotion of mental and prevention of mental disorders. The growing recognition of the impact of social changes on the mental health of the population (e.g. childhood trauma, growing suicide rates, domestic violence, inequalities, elderly mental health, migrant populations, displaced populations, etc.) requires that the future mental health programmes should include promotion of mental health, prevention of mental disorders along with mental health care, and rehabilitation of persons with mental disorders.

Sixthly, the undergraduate training of basic doctors is extremely limited. The human resource development to meet the total mental health needs have not been fully addressed.

Seventhly, the issues of rapid social change, along with the many changes in the social institutions like the family, community and the ways to help populations experiencing the ill effects of these changes has still not received adequate attention.

Looking to the future

The WHO *World Mental Health Report* (2022), recognizes 'mental health is critically important for everyone, everywhere' and the challenges to reach the goal of mental health for all, in all countries, more so in LMICs as follows:

> Twenty years after WHO published its landmark *The World Health Report 2001: mental health—new understanding, new hope*, the recommendations made then remain valid today. Yet many advances have been made. Interest in and understanding of mental health has increased. Many countries have established, updated and strengthened mental health policies or plans. Advocacy movements have amplified the voices of people with lived experience of mental health conditions. Informed by research, the field has advanced technically. Numerous practical, evidence-based mental health guidelines, manuals and other tools are now available for implementation. (p. xiii)

There are barriers of availability, accessibility, affordability, and acceptability (the 4As) of mental health care. Throughout human history, relating to mental health, it is the illnesses that have received societal attention. The innovations in LMICs have largely addressed availability of services. Stigma and non-acceptance of mental health care is a major barrier. There is need for 'Making Psychiatry a People's Movement' rather than 'Taking Psychiatry to People'. Self-care for mental health is in the WHO mix of services but has not received the attention that is required (Srinivasa Murthy, 2011, 2016b). However, the recent new understanding about both the positive actions that can promote mental health (exercise, sleep, yoga/meditation, nutrition, and connectedness) and psychological measures by individuals that can address 'distress' (such as skills of sharing of feelings, journaling, listening to music/practice of art, thinking differently and spirituality) offer opportunities to make mental health an integral part of the lives of all people (Gupta, 2021; Jeste, 2020; Koenig, 2012; Lam & Riba, 2016; Murthy, 2020; Srinivasa Murthy, 2016b, 2021; Varambally & Gangadhar, 2016). Such a shift will move mental health from 'deviancy' model to 'normalcy' model. The advances in information technology provide opportunities for information and skills of mental health to reach directly all individuals.

As noted by the WHO *World Mental Health Report* (2022), 'business as usual for mental health simply will not do'. There is a need for a paradigm shift in focus from mental illness to wellness. There is an urgent need for making mental health relevant and the responsibility of each and every member of the society and not limited to persons with illnesses. For such a shift to occur, three levels of changes are needed. Firstly, shifting focus from purely clinical care to public mental health (patients to population). All of the innovations have been mainly focusing on the identification and provision of care for ill persons. A massive movement is needed to address each and every member of the population to give importance to their mental health by their day-to-day actions. When individuals give importance to mental health as part of daily life, there will be less resistance to seek help and lesser tendency to stigmatize mentally ill persons. Secondly, there is an urgent need for research on the utility of the different self-care measures and especially to identify those local, cultural, and religious/spiritual resources relevant and effective for mental health. The current evidence base is limited. Thirdly, as mental health is dependent on multiple factors, there is a need for networking with all stakeholders to address social determinants for better mental health of the population.

The above paradigm shift has many benefits: (1) it increases resources for mental health by many-fold; (2) easy acceptability of care by ill persons when needed; (3) stigma will be minimized; (4) utilization of all community strengths; (5) there is no resource limitation, as all people are the resource; and (6) it will utilize all the wisdom of ages in all communities. The goal should be to address the total population to accept their emotional vulnerability and ways to develop resilience by personal, family, and community actions. The above approaches are especially relevant to LMICs but also applicable to resource-rich countries. Here lies the challenges and opportunities.

REFERENCES

Acosta, A. M., Garg, S., Pham, H., Whitaker, M., Anglin, O., O'Halloran, A., et al. (2021). Racial and ethnic disparities in rates of COVID-19-associated hospitalization, intensive care unit admission, and in-hospital death in the United States from March 2020 to February 2021, *JAMA Network Open*, **4**, e2130479.

Aluh, D. O., Onu, J. U., & deAlmeida, J. N. C. (2023). A new era for mental health care in Nigeria. *Lancet Psychiatry*, **5**, 310–311.

American Psychiatric Association (2021). *Mentally Healthy Nation*. Washington, DC: American Psychiatric Association.

Arnold-Foster, A., Moses, J. D., & Schotland, S. V. (2022). Obstacles to physicians' emotional health—lessons from history. *New England Journal of Medicine*, **386**, 4–5.

Begum, S., Donta, B., Nair, S., & Prakasamm, C. P. (2015). Sociodemographic factors associated with domestic violence in urban slums, Mumbai, Maharastra. *Indian Journal of Medical Research*, **141**, 783–788.

Berkessel, J. B., Gebaue, J. E., Joshanloo, M., Bleidorn, W., Rentfrow, P. J., Potter, J., & Gosling, S. D. (2021). National religiosity eases the psychological burden of poverty. *Proceedings of the National Academy of Sciences of the United States of America*, **118**, e2103913118.

Bhugra, D., Pathare, S., Joshi, R., Kalra, G., Torales, J., & Ventriglio, A. (2019). A review of mental health policies from Commonwealth countries. *International Journal of Social Psychiatry*, **64**, 3–8.

Bhugra, D., Tasman, A., Pathare, S., Priebe, S., Smith, S., Torous, J., et al. (2017). The WPA–Lancet Psychiatry Commission on the Future of Psychiatry. *Lancet Psychiatry*, **4**, 775–818.

Chibanda, D., Bowers, T., Verhey, R., Rusakaniko, S., Abas, M., Weiss, H. A., & Araya, R. (2015). The Friendship Bench programme: a cluster randomised controlled trial of a brief psychological intervention for common mental disorders delivered by lay health workers in Zimbabwe. *International Journal of Mental Health Systems*, **9**, 21.

Chibanda, D., Weiss, H. A., Verhey, R., Simms, V., Munjoma, R., Rusakaniko, S., et al. (2016). Effect of a primary care-based psychological intervention on symptoms of common mental disorders in Zimbabwe. *JAMA*, **316**, 2618–2626.

COVID-19 Mental Disorders Collaborators (2021). Global prevalence and burden of depressive and anxiety disorders in 204 countries and territories in 2020 due to the COVID-19 pandemic. *Lancet*, **398**, 1700–1712.

De Silva, M. J., Rathod, S. D., Hanlon, C., Breuer, E., Chisholm, D., Fekadu, A., et al. (2016). Evaluation of district mental healthcare plans: the PRIME consortium methodology, *British Journal of Psychiatry*, **208**(Suppl. 56), s63–s70.

Dickens, A. P., Richards, S. H., Greaves, C. J., & Campbell, J. L. (2013). Interventions targeting social isolation in older people: a systematic review. *BMC Public Health*, **11**, 647.

Doukani, A., van Dalen, R., Valev, H., Njenga, A., Sera, F., & Chibanda, D. (2021). A community health volunteer delivered problem-solving therapy mobile application based on the Friendship Bench 'Inuka Coaching' in Kenya: a pilot cohort study. *Global Mental Health*, **8**, e9.

Eder, M., Henninger, M., Durbin, S., Iacocca, M. O., Martin, A., Gottlieb, L. M., & Lin, J. S. (2021). Screening and interventions for social risk factors. Technical brief to support the US Preventive Services Task Force. *JAMA*, **326**, 1416–1428.

Ettman, C. K., Cohen, G. H., Abdalla, S. M., Sampson, L., Trinquart, L. L., Castrucci, B. C., et al. (2022). Persistent depressive symptoms during COVID-19: a national, population-representative, longitudinal study of U.S. adults. *Lancet Regional Health Americas*, **5**, 100091.

Fernando, S., Brown, T., Datta, K., Chidhanguro, D., Tavengwa, N. V., Chandna, J., et al (2021). The Friendship Bench as a brief psychological intervention with peer support in rural Zimbabwean women: a mixed methods pilot evaluation. *Global Mental Health*, **8**, e31.

Firth, J., Solmi, M., Wootton, R. E., Vancampfort, D., Schuch, F. B., Hoare, E., et al. (2020). A meta-review of 'lifestyle psychiatry': the role of exercise, smoking, diet and sleep in the prevention and treatment of mental disorders. *World Psychiatry*, **19**, 360–380.

Ghaleb, Y., Lami, F., Al Nsour, M., Rashak, H. A., Samy, S., Khader, Y. S., et al. (2021). Mental health impacts of COVID-19 on healthcare workers in the Eastern Mediterranean Region: a multi-country study. *Journal of Public Health*, **43**(Suppl. 3), iii34–iii42.

Giel, R. & Harding, T. W. (1976). Psychiatric priorities in developing countries. *British Journal of Psychiatry*, **128**, 513–522.

Gupta, S. (2021). *Keep Sharp: Build a Better Brain at Any Age*. London: Hachette.

Gureje, O., Appiah-Poku, J., Bello, T., Kola, L., Araya, R., Chisholm, D., et al. (2021). The effect of collaborative care between traditional/faith healers and primary health care workers to improve psychosis outcome in Nigeria and Ghana (COSIMPO)—a cluster randomized controlled trial. *Lancet*, **396**, 612–622.

Harding, T. W., Climent, C. E., Diop, M., Giel, R., Ibrahim, H. H. A., Ignacio, L. L., et al. (1983). The WHO collaborative study on the strategies for extending mental health care, II: the development of new research methods. *American Journal of Psychiatry*, **140**, 1474–1480.

Herrman, H., Patel, V., Kieling, C., Berk, M., Buchweitz, C., Cuijpers, P., et al. (2022). Time for united action on depression: a Lancet–World Psychiatric Association Commission. *Lancet*, **399**, 957–1022.

Hurt, A. (2022). Physician burnout, depression compounded by COVID: survey. *Medscape*, 21 January. https://www.medscape.com/viewarticle/966996

Jeste, D. (2020). *Wiser: The Scientific Roots of Wisdom, Compassion and What Makes Us Good*. Boulder, CO: Sounds True.

Johanson, K. A., Strand, K. B., Fekadu, A., & Chisholm, D. (2017). Health gains and financial protection provided by the Ethiopian mental health strategy: an extended cost-effectiveness analysis. *Health Policy and Planning*, **32**, 376–383.

Kings College London (2022, 10 October). The Lancet Commission on ending stigma and discrimination in mental health. https://www.kcl.ac.uk/news/the-lancet-commission-on-ending-stigma-and-discrimination-in-mental-health

Koenig, H. G. (2012). Religion, spirituality, and health: the research and clinical implications. *ISRN Psychiatry*, **2012**, 278730.

Kakuma R, Minas H, van Ginneken N, Poz M R D, Desiraju D, Morris J E et al (2011) Human resources for mental health care: current situation and strategies for action, Lancet. 5;378(9803):1654-63. doi: 10.1016/S0140-6736(11)61093-3. Epub 2011 Oct 16.

Lam, L. C. W. & Riba, M. (2016). *Physical Exercise Interventions for Mental Health*. Cambridge: Cambridge University Press.

Malesic, J. (2022). *The End of Burnout: Why Work Drains Us and How to Build Better Lives*. Oakland, CA: University of California Press.

Miller, A. B., Oppenheimer, C. W., Glenn, C. R., & Yaros, A. C. (2022). Preliminary research priorities for factors influencing individual outcomes for users of the US national suicide prevention lifeline. *JAMA Psychiatry*, **79**, 1225–1231.

Mirza, Z. & Rahman, A. (2019). Mental health care in Pakistan boosted by the highest office. *Lancet*, **394**, 2239–2240.

Mugisha, J., Ssebunnya, J., & Kigozi, F. N. (2016). Towards understanding governance issues in integration of mental health into primary health care in Uganda. *International Journal of Mental Health Systems*, **10**, 25.

Murthy, V. H. (2020). *Together: Healing Power of Human Connection in a Sometimes Lonely World*. Noida: Harper Collins.

Musich, S., Wang, S. S., Hawkins, K., & Yeh, C. S. (2015). The impact of loneliness on quality of life and patient satisfaction among older, sicker adults. *Gerontology and Geriatric Medicine*, **1**, 2333721415582119.

NIMHANS (2022a). *Course Content for Tele MANAS Counsellors* (Publication No. 239). Bangalore: NIMHANS.

NIMHANS (2022b). *Facilitator's Manual for Trainers of Tele MANAS Counsellors* (Publication No. 241). Bangalore: NIMHANS.

NIMHANS (2022c). *Operational Guidelines: The Digital Arm of the National Mental Health Programme*. Bangalore: NIMHANS.

NIMHANS (2022d). *Point of Care Guide for Tele MANAS Counsellors* (Publication No. 240). Bangalore: NIMHANS.

Pennebaker, J. W. & Evans, J. F. (2014). *Expressive Writing: Words that Heal*. Enumclaw, WA: Idyll Arbor.

Philips, M., Zhang, J., Shi, Q., Song, Z., Ding, Z., Pang, S., et al. (2009). Prevalence, treatment, and associated disability of mental disorders in four provinces in China during 2001–05: an epidemiological survey. *Lancet*, **373**, 2041–2053.

Raja, S., Underhill, C., Shrestha, P., Sunder, U., Mannarath, S., et al. (2012). Integrating mental health and development: a case study of the basic needs model in Nepal. *PLoS Medicine*, **9**, e1001261.

Raykar, N., Nigam, A., & Chisholm, D. (2016). An extended cost-effectiveness analysis of schizophrenia treatment in India under universal public finance. *Cost Effectiveness and Resource Allocation*, **14**, 9.

Sartorius, N. & Harding, T. T. (1983). The WHO collaborative study on strategies for extending mental health care, I: the genesis of the study. *American Journal of Psychiatry* **140**, 1470–1473.

Semrau, M., Alem, A., Ayuso-Mateos, J. L., Chisholm, D., Gureje, O., Hanlon, C., et al (2019). Strengthening mental health systems in low- and middle-income countries: recommendations from the Emerald programme. *BJPsych Open*, **5**, e73.

Southwick, S. M. & Charney, D. S. (2012). The science of resilience: implications for the prevention and treatment of depression. *Science*, **338**, 79–82.

Southwick, S. M. & Charney, D. S. (2018). *Resilience* (2nd ed.). Cambridge: Cambridge University Press.

Srinivasa Murthy, R. (2011). Mental health services in low and middle income countries. In: Thornicroft, G. & Szmukler, G. (Eds.), *Oxford Textbook of Community Psychiatry* (1st ed., pp. 325–336). Oxford: Oxford University Press.

Srinivasa Murthy, R. (2014). Impact of child neglect and abuse on adult mental health. *Institutionalised Children Explorations and Beyond*, **1**, 150–162.

Srinivasa Murthy, R. (2016a). Caregiving and caregivers: challenges and opportunities in India. *Indian Journal of Social Psychiatry*, **32**, 10–18.

Srinivasa Murthy, R. (2016b). Self care for mental health—the new frontier. In: Saha, G. (Ed.), *Different Strokes* (2nd ed., pp. 87–97). Bhopal: Publication of Indian Psychiatric Society.

Srinivasa Murthy, R. (2018). Globalization, market economy, and mental health. In: Chadda, R. K., Kumar, V., & Sarkar, S. (Eds.), *Social Psychiatry: Principles and Clinical Perspectives* (pp. 508–520). New Delhi: Jaypee Brothers Medical Publishers.

Srinivasa Murthy, R. (2020). COVID-19 pandemic and emotional health: social psychiatry perspective. *Indian Journal of Social Psychiatry*, **36**, S24–S42.

Srinivasa Murthy, R. (2021). Pandemic blues. *The Hindu*, 25 April.

Srinivasa Murthy, R. & Banerjee, D. (2021). Loneliness in older people: from analysis to action. *World Social Psychiatry*, **3**, 120–122.

Srinivasa Murthy, R. & Wig, N. N. (1983). The WHO collaborative study on strategies for extending mental health care, IV: a training approach to enhancing the availability of mental health manpower in a developing country. *American Journal of Psychiatry*, **140**, 1486–1490.

Ssebunnya, J., Kangere, S., Mugisha, J., Docrat, S., Chisholm, D., Lund, C., & Kigozi, F. (2018). Potential strategies for sustainably financing mental health care in Uganda. *International Journal of Mental Health Systems*, **12**, 74.

Surgeon General (1999) US Department of HEALTH And Human Services: Mental health: a report of the Surgeon General. Rockville, MD, US Department of Health and Human Services.

Taylor, S. (2020). *The Psychology of Pandemic: Preparing for the Next Global Outbreak of Infectious Disease*. Newcastle Upon Tyne: Cambridge Scholars Publishing.

Taylor, S. (2022). I wrote the book on the pandemic. Post-Covid will take some getting used to. *The Guardian*, 24 February. https://www.theguardian.com/commentisfree/2022/feb/24/pandemic-psychology-end-covid-pandemic-normal

The Hindu (2022). Mental health in the annual budget: 2022–2023. *The Hindu*, 3 February.

The Lancet (2022). Ensuring care for people with depression. *Lancet*, **399**, 885.

Thornicroft, G., Sunkel, C., Aliev, A. A., Baker, S., Brohan, E., El Chammay, R., et al. (2022). The Lancet Commission on ending stigma and discrimination in mental health. *Lancet*, **400**, 1438–1480.

Thornicroft, G., Szmukler, G., Muesser, K. T., & Drake, R. E. (2011). *Oxford Textbook of Community Mental Health*. Oxford: Oxford University Press.

UNICEF (2021). *The State of the World's Children 2021: On My Mind—Promoting, Protecting and Caring for Children's Mental Health*. New York: UNICEF. https://www.unicef.org/media/114636/file/SOWC-2021-full-report-English.pdf

United for Global Mental Health (n.d.). Countdown global mental health 2030. https://unitedgmh.org/knowledge-hub/countdown2030/

United for Global Mental Health (2022). *Mental Health for All: What Can We Achieve if We Meaningfully Integrate Mental Health into UHC* (UHC Policy Brief series). London: United for Global Mental Health.

Üstün, T. B. & Sartorius, N. (Eds.) (1995). *Mental Illness in General Health Care: An International Study*. Chichester: John Wiley.

Varambally, S. & Gangadhar, B. N. (2016). Yoga-based interventions for the management of psychiatric disorders. In: Lam, L. C. W. & Riba, M. (Eds.), *Physical Exercise Interventions for Mental Health* (pp. 124–146). Cambridge: Cambridge University Press.

Wig, N. N. & Srinivasa Murthy, R. (2018). The birth of national mental health program for India. *Indian Journal of Psychiatry*, **57**, 315–319.

Wig, N. N., Suleiman, M. A., Routledge, R., Murthy, R. S., Ladrido-Ignacio, L., Ibrahim, H. H., et al. (1980). Community reactions to mental disorders. A key informant study in three developing countries. *Acta Psychiatrica Scandinavica*, **61**, 111–126.

Wilkinson, R. & Pickett, K. (2010). *The Spirit Level: Why Greater Equality Makes Societies Stronger*. New York: Bloomsbury.

Wilkinson, R. & Pickett, K. (2017). Inequality and mental illness. *Lancet Psychiatry*, **4**, 512–513.

Wilkinson, R. & Pickett, K. (2018). *The Inner Level: How More Equal Societies Reduce Stress, Restore Sanity and Improve Everyone's Well-Being*. London: Penguin.

World Health Organization (1975). *Organization of Mental Health in Developing Countries* (TRS 564). Geneva: World Health Organization.

World Health Organization (2001). *World Health Report 2001: Mental Health: New Understanding, New Hope*. Geneva: World Health Organization.

World Health Organization (2016). *mhGAP Intervention Guide: Mental Health Gap Action Programme Version 2.0*. Geneva: World Health Organization.

World Health Organization (2013). *Mental Health Action Plan 2013–2030*. Geneva: World Health Organization. https://apps.who.int/iris/handle/10665/89966

World Health Organization (2019). *The WHO Special Initiative for Mental Health (2019–2023): Universal Health Coverage for Mental Health*. Geneva: World Health Organization. https://apps.who.int/iris/handle/10665/310981

World Health Organization (2020). *Doing What Matters in Times of Stress: An Illustrated Guide*. Geneva: World Health Organization.

World Health Organization (2021). *Mental Health Atlas 2020*. Geneva: World Health Organization.

World Health Organization (2022). *World Mental Health Report: Transforming Mental Health for All*. Geneva: World Health Organization.

Overcoming impediments to community mental health in low- and middle-income countries

Benedetto Saraceno, Mark van Ommeren, and Rajaie Batniji

Introduction

As discussed in Chapter 5 by Vigo and colleagues the prevalence of mental disorders across the world—and across low- and middle-income countries (LMICs)—is high. The median rate across the world of having at least one mental disorder in the last year is 10% (WHO World Mental Health Survey Consortium, 2004). The impact of these disorders on disability, other aspects of health, and development is substantial. Yet, the vast majority of people with a mental disorder are not in contact with services that offer mental health care (see Chapter 5). Importantly, the association between severe mental disorder and human rights violations is strong (World Health Organization (WHO), 2001). Even among people with severe mental disorders, few people receive adequate, humane care (WHO, 2001) and discrimination is pervasive (Thornicroft, 2006). It is clear that there is an urgent need to act.

The WHO (2003) developed a mental health policy and planning package to help countries to develop services that provide access to adequate care for people with mental disorder. This package was preceded and followed by evidence-informed and evidence-based advocacy through major publications—such as the *World Health Report 2001* on mental health (WHO, 2001), the *World Mental Health Report* (Desjarlais et al, 1995), *Neurological, Psychiatric, and Developmental Disorders* (Institute of Medicine, 2001), *Disease Control Priorities related to Mental Neurological, Developmental and Substance Abuse Disorders* (WHO & Disease Control Priorities Project, 2006), and the 2007 *Lancet* series on global mental health, and the 2008 mental health Gap Action Plan (WHO, 2008). Although most research evidence on interventions comes from specialized care settings in high-income countries, fortunately there are good indications that much of this evidence generalizes to LMICs (Patel, 2007).

A naïve observer would perhaps expect that with this amount of burden, human rights violations, high-level advocacy, technical guidance, and evidence for interventions, that mental health service development in LMICs is flourishing. Indeed, it should be. Although it is true that some countries have made major strides, the reality, however, has been that mental health service development in most LMICs has been a challenge. This chapter will address some key impediments in developing mental health services in LMICs and will offer strategies to address these impediments.

Financial resources

As in other areas of health (Laxminarayan et al., 2006), to implement evidence-based policy and practice, financial resources are needed. Resources allocated towards mental health care are insufficient or are ineffectively distributed in LMICs (Saxena et al., 2007). There are many explanations for the low levels of financing for mental health. None of these reasons are independent of one other; rather, they interact and together form a formidable block to the allocation of appropriate funds, whether by foreign donors, ministries of health, or ministries of finance. In this section, we will describe a variety of reasons for the lack of funding.

In most countries there is a lack of strong, coordinated, and consistent lobbying and political pressure to increase resources for mental health services. Without strong advocacy, mental health will not be high on the public health agenda and political will and funds will remain inadequate.

This lack of strong advocacy stems from discrepancies about both the intended purpose of advocacy and the differing targets of advocacy. There appear to be two, implicitly stated disagreements regarding the purpose of global mental health advocacy. First, a disagreement on whom to help—some advocates suggest that the goal is to help the severely mentally ill, while others advocate for support for mild mental health problems. Second, among those who agree on which group to focus their advocacy, there is disagreement on how this should be done—some advocates focus on more a medical model, while others call for a combined medical and social model.

To scale up community mental health services, it is extremely helpful to develop a consensus in advocacy messages among the national mental health community (e.g. service providers, professional associations, senior government leaders in mental health, academics, and national policymakers), as fragmentation at this level has prevented action in many settings.

Lobbying efforts towards policy and legislation is important but focusing on legislation and policy alone is insufficient. In reality, successful advocacy is also needed to ensure that these are funded, implemented, and translated into services. Coordinated advocacy groups need to continue their work through and beyond the legislative/policy process.

Mental health financing in countries—which is usually extremely low (see Chapter 33)—may be more likely increased if there was more advocacy from service users, families, and service providers, including non-governmental organizations (NGOs). People with disorders and their families can be a powerful constituency to press for better mental health care with sufficient funding at local levels. Service-providing NGOs, with close community connections, often serve as advocates and coordinating centres for local advocacy. Such local advocacy will go furthest when in concert with appropriately coordinated national-level advocacy.

Part of the reason for the frequent political (and thus financial) inaction on mental health may unfortunately be attributed to the low level of interest from the public in issues of mental health. Stigma and discrimination pose a challenge to mobilizing the community to be involved in advocacy, perhaps making it especially important that people who receive mental health care are involved in lobbying.

Public advocacy will make investment in mental health more politically palatable, though there is a challenge. In developing coordinated advocacy, the interests of different groups (service users, family members, and mental health specialists) may vary greatly within and between groups. For example, different users have been seen to work towards different objectives, ranging from (1) less or no psychiatric interventions to (2) more humane community and socially oriented mental health services to (3) better access to new psychotropic medications. (Indeed, some user organizations are funded by industry while others insist on independence from industry.) Similarly, psychiatrists are not a monolithic group. Opposing advocacy from different stakeholders may result in inaction on the part of governments. Thus, it is necessary to develop a clear consensus and plan for action among the national mental health community. Disagreements on goals to be achieved among a community of mental health specialists limits funding and abilities for policy change. Any internal division among mental health experts and decision-makers is an obstacle to coordinated and effective advocacy.

A prominent explanation for the lack of mental health funding concerns the role of donors and the international community as agenda setters. For example, mental health does not appear in the Millennium Development Goals (MDGs) (Miranda & Patel, 2005). Unfortunately, in several countries, exclusion of mental health from the MDGs has directly obstructed the financing of mental health services by international donors even in countries where national authorities made mental health a priority (e.g. Afghanistan, Rwanda). When international agencies and donors do not prioritize mental health, there is reduced incentive for national policymakers to address this issue. Furthermore, ministry of health staff and funds are often directed towards implementing donor-supported programmes.

Communicable disease, especially HIV/AIDS, has been the funding priority for donors and national leaders, and this has been a barrier to securing funds for mental health services in sub-Saharan Africa. This challenge should be converted into opportunity by integrating mental health services into HIV/AIDS programmes (Freeman, 2000). Rather than compete with communicable disease, integrating mental health care into communicable disease health care programmes may be extremely helpful to funding care for the large percentage of people with mostly mild and moderate common mental disorders. Yet, it is unlikely to provide a solution to the problem of organizing care for people with chronic, severe mental disorders.

There seem to be common, but incorrect, beliefs that mental health interventions are ineffective, economically inefficient, and too costly. Perceptions of cost-ineffective services need to be addressed with evidence and political pressure. It should be noted that any discussion of cost-effectiveness depends greatly on the mental disorder being considered (WHO, 2006). The treatment of severe mental disorders may be relatively less cost-effective but they still may provide good value for money (Chisholm et al., 2008).

Critics of the discussion on cost-efficacy point to the human rights of the mentally ill. Because of the prevalence of human rights violations against people with mental disorders (even at times by the professionals who are supposed to care for them), there is a strong moral case for providing effective and humane mental health care (Patel et al., 2006).

Epidemiological data have highlighted the tremendous global burden of mental disease. It is unclear to what extent epidemiological data are helpful in putting mental health on the agenda. In fact, in many cases such data are easily misunderstood or not very informative (e.g. depression prevalence rates typically do not distinguish between mild and severe depression, which are very different public health issues). Moreover, in some circumstances, rates of poor-quality studies tend to be higher than rates of stronger studies (Steel et al., 2009) and policymakers may be put off by over-advocacy with rates that are not credible. Nonetheless, epidemiological data can have advocacy value if attention to new local evidence prompts health planners to invest in mental health.

Organization of services

The integration of mental health care into general health services occurs mainly in two forms: mental health care delivered by general health workers in primary care settings or through specific programmes addressing physical disease (HIV/AIDS, tuberculosis). Additionally, although not covered here, integration into general health care services could include, for example, liaison psychiatric services in general hospitals.

The term 'dedicated mental health care' is used for mental health care delivered by workers performing full-time mental health work through specific mental health services (e.g. outpatient psychiatry, inpatient care by mental health specialists at general hospitals, and mental hospitals). One could also speak of a hybrid model of general care when a worker's time is fully dedicated to providing mental health care in a primary care clinical setting.

How different types of services are organized/configured/mixed within a mental health system tends to have an impact on the effective treatment coverage of people with diverse mental disorders. A mixed model of care, in which mental health care is available at multiple levels of care, is—without doubt—the ideal, but reflection is needed on how service decision-makers should invest their available, limited resources for mental health care (WHO, 2003).

As described earlier in this book (see Chapter 11), resources and expertise for mental health care need to be geographically decentralized for people to have access to them, and a system needs to be created that makes treatment for acute and chronic mental illness and the corresponding social and rehabilitation services available at the community level. There is thus a need to move staff and financial resources into the community, and this is an enormous challenge. This requires allocation of funds to different regions and subregions of countries, and the funding should cover general mental health clinics covering a range of disorders, rather than vertical programmes for very specific pathologies.

NGOs often play an irreplaceable role in providing community mental health services. However, in some countries NGOs have difficulties in establishing themselves and, even when established, some NGOs may create their own set of problems. In some locations, existing NGOs may be unhelpful by grossly inflating reports on the level and quality of social services that they (the NGOs) provide to the mentally ill. This gives the message that there is no need for the government to invest in mental health, as the NGO already has done all the work.

Like in high-income countries, developing community mental health care in LMICs requires linking mental health more closely with other non-health sector services. Social services are part of, or complementary to, decentralized specialist mental health care, and this should be reflected in the structure of such services. Depending on the setting, linkages that reach beyond the social services sector to traditional and/or religious healers may be appropriate.

Much of the discussion of community involvement in mental health focuses on the crucial role of families and community organizations—especially in rehabilitation, and the need to spread resources and expertise beyond mental health hospitals. There is a need for the 'grassroots' creation and management of mental health programmes, emphasizing collaboration with community members and NGOs. Decentralization and deinstitutionalization—two conceptually distinct but often overlapping processes—open up many opportunities to involve communities and families in mental health care.

Substantial resistance to the decentralization of health resources arises in many countries that have attempted to spread resources to the periphery and to social programmes. Resistance to social services can be substantial, because it involves an understanding of mental disorders outside the medical model.

To assist with these challenges, technical support for LMICs is needed to develop financing schemes for community-based approaches. It is important to understand the separate sectoral costs (e.g. health care, housing, and employment) in attempting to create an integrated, multisectoral mental health programme (WHO, 2003). Problems in mental health financing also arise when mental health policy created at the national level requires financing at the subnational level, where decision-makers may not feel as responsible for implementing national-level policy. This has occurred in South Africa and Pakistan (WHO, 2007).

An important—although often difficult—step in decentralizing mental health resources is downsizing existing mental hospitals (WHO, 2001). Mental hospitals have poor coverage, tend to put people at elevated risk of human rights violations, and absorb a disproportionate amount of resources (WHO, 2001).

Worryingly, some of the most persistent barriers to the implementation of such community programmes appear to be the vested interests of psychiatrists and other hospital workers. These interests can be an obstacle to funding, deinstitutionalization, and the expansion of a mental health workforce. Concerns about job security have delayed moves to community-based care. The staff and leadership of psychiatric institutions are too often willing and able to exert influence that opposes the political will to reform mental health services. Thus, in pursuit of mental health service reform, psychiatrists should be seen as stakeholders, not just as providers.

Financial incentives and professional self-interest have led too many psychiatrists and mental health staff to resist deinstitutionalization and any restructuring of care to the community level, and to oppose expansion of the workforce and public health models of care. Downsizing hospitals can be an understandable threat to the economic and professional interests of those who work in hospitals. Financial and professional guarantees need to be thus put in place for hospital staff during the period of transformation.

In our experience and in that of a range of experts that we interviewed (Saraceno et al., 2007), opposition to downsizing hospitals in favour of community-based care most often comes from trade unions and hospital staff of various levels. It is thus important that the reform process incorporates these groups, so that they may be offered roles in the community-based secondary mental health system. It should be recognized that psychiatrists may also resist attempts to expand the mental health workforce to have non-psychiatrists or non-doctors provide management of mental disorders. Such resistance to changing mental health services is often taken up by professional associations, which makes it difficult to cultivate the united political will to pursue reforms.

Despite much agreement among international mental health experts regarding deinstitutionalization (Saraceno et al., 2007), there often exist some controversy and debate in society—especially when it is implemented in a problematic manner. For example, more than 45 years ago, de-hospitalization (often confused with the complex process of deinstitutionalization) led to many mentally ill persons living on the streets in North America in places where deinstitutionalization was done without the creation of community-based services. Mental health advocates should be clear that talking about closing a hospital leads to understandable resistance and any talk about closing hospitals should be accompanied with a well-communicated, strong plan about developing care in the community.

Downsizing or closing mental hospitals is likely to result in failure if not accompanied with secondary care and community services. Indeed, the likely reason for Brazil's mental health reform's success is the increase of secondary level care that has co-occurred with the decrease of mental hospital beds. The need to downsize mental hospitals thus coexists with the need to develop community mental health services. Challenges to developing community mental health services may transform into challenges to downsizing mental hospitals. Decision-makers are sometimes unwilling to downsize and/

or close mental hospitals—due to the political risk of facing vested interests. Deinstitutionalization is technically complex and cannot occur without adequate community mental health services in place. Thus, any downsizing of mental hospitals should be concurrent with improving community-based inpatient care for the mentally ill. Additional funding will be needed during the transition to community care. Yet, as we discussed earlier, to raise funds unified advocacy is important and this advocacy will be weaker if public health planners and health staff disagree about the need to decentralize. The need for unified, ethical solutions is urgent given the inhumane living conditions in many mental hospitals.

Integration of mental health care in primary health care (PHC) is essential to obtain good coverage. However, poorly executed integration of mental health into primary care leads to undertrained, unsupervised primary care workers who are not sufficiently competent in the care (identification and treatment and/or referral) they are supposed to provide. Even if technically competent in clinical management, they may not know how to manage their time in such a way to find time for mental health care during their working day. Moreover, without appropriate training and supervision, overburdened primary care staff are at risk of increasing their reliance on pharmaceuticals, leading to narrow biomedical support even for people with subthreshold problems. Integrating mental health in PHC thus requires planning (WHO, 2007). Finally, in many LMICs essential psychotropic medicines are often not continuously available at the PHC level—a barrier that hinders appropriate care for those people whose disorders can be effectively treated through medication.

Investment in community mental health services and supervision of PHC workers by mental health specialists is critical to the success of the primary care model. This observation is in line with the WHO (1978) Alma Ata Declaration, which promoted a primary care model 'sustained by integrated, functional and mutually supportive referral systems' as an integral part of a country's health system.

Strengthening the workforce

A commitment to strengthening the mental health workforce by training staff in the community and by expanding the base of providers will require a new role for mental health professionals, one focused on training and supervision, and one that involves the mobilization of families and communities in care and rehabilitation.

Improving the structure of the mental health system in LMICs depends fundamentally on the availability of an adequate mental health workforce. Mental health training needs to move beyond hospitals and universities and beyond theoretical sessions, to a continual process of supervision and mentorship in the community they serve. This applies to the training of psychiatrists, medical officers, and primary care providers, as well as paraprofessionals in mental health. International collaboration for training can be helpful as countries have much to learn from one other. Training through hands-on supervised clinical work is likely of greatest benefit (WHO, 2007). Training in psychiatric hospitals for undergraduate medical students is particularly unhelpful to teach them how to address mental health in primary care settings. It is suggested that training should take place regularly, in clinical settings in the community and under the dedicated supervision of mental health specialists, rather than through one-off workshops. Therefore, mental health support in the community may depend on a shift in the role of mental health experts from clinical care to one of supervision.

Providers in the general health care system—such as community health workers and PHC staff—should be further trained in mental health. Yet, when they are overburdened with other responsibilities, it can be helpful to find, train, and supervise new groups of workers altogether. Training dedicated community mental health workers can be extremely valuable, especially when their roles are recognized and endorsed by governments.

Furthermore, lay individuals in the community can be trained to appropriately refer persons for further care. As for other groups, such training requires adequate post-training supervision from professionals. In particular, it can be valuable to more formally involve families in providing care, and to empower them as advocates. Service users may be involved in care as well, for example, there can be a role for users as staff in supported housing programmes. To best involve families in care, they need the support of trained personnel, who can provide support and guide the use of medications. Family care may be especially useful in rural areas, providing families are given appropriate support by trained mental health staff.

Involving families makes them stakeholders in mental health. The resulting advocacy can have an impact on policy. In addition to involving families, the involvement of service users in advocacy is likely to lead to increased funding for community mental health services to facilitate responsible deinstitutionalization and greater community integration, as we have discussed above. Thus, involving families and users has value both from a human resource and an advocacy perspective.

The involvement of families is complemented by the involvement of the community, and is consistent with using participatory action approaches, which have been common in rural development and which are now also used by some mental health NGOs (Underhill, 2002). Such approaches are also increasingly common in psychosocial programmes in emergencies (Inter-Agency Standing Committee, 2007).

As touched upon earlier, making mental health care broadly available necessitates a supervisory role for mental health specialists. Psychiatrists need to focus their efforts on training other health workers. Developing a broader base of mental health care providers in general health services and in community-based mental services depends on mentorship and community-based training. To restructure care, the specialist must be motivated to switch to a training and supervisory role. This may require financial incentives.

Public mental health leadership

Mental health leaders in LMICs—such as directors of mental health in ministries of health—have responsibility for the complex tasks of increasing funding, making mental health care more broadly available, developing a system for secondary, primary, and community care, and reforming hospitals, among other challenges. Such tasks require not only a familiarity with the needs and possible supports for diverse people with mental disorders, but also population-based, public health vision and skills. The skills for such leadership need to be developed, or sought from outside *psychiatry*, from the academic discipline *public health*.

The rarity of public health-minded approaches in mental health care may be due in part to the nature of existing evidence-based interventions which are mostly at the individual level, and also to the training of mental health leaders that tends to have focused on clinical care only. The rarity of adequate public mental health leadership may also be due to a lack of incentives for psychiatrists to take a public health view, and also to a lack of authority for non-psychiatrists attempting to engage such a view.

Training courses for public mental health leaders are needed. Training leaders in public mental health may greatly improve mental health strategies in LMICs. Examples of such courses include the International Master in Mental Health Policy and Services in Lisbon, Portugal, the Master in Public Mental Health in Cape Town, South Africa, and the Mental Health Leadership and Advocacy Programme short course in Ibadan, Nigeria.

International assistance—laterally with other LMICs or with international agencies—and incentives can play a crucial role to developing public mental health leadership. With concern that any programme should be adapted to local settings, it can be extremely helpful to have lateral, regional, and global cooperation for mentoring and for sharing models of success. International networks—such as the Global Forum for Community Mental Health (http://www.gfcmh.com/)—can also play an important role.

Conclusion

Making mental health services available in the community in LMICs is a must. Community mental health services, compared to institutionalized care, gives greater coverage. Also, community care has a lower risk of human rights violations introduced by the care system. Yet, there are impediments to developing community services, as reviewed in this chapter. In particular, the interests of mental health care providers (and often family members as well) favour institutions. Also, there is the challenge that developing mental health care in the community involves start-up costs, which require a substantial increase in resources, which are most easily raised when key stakeholders agree on how to move to community services.

The formation of national plans for mental health, developed in a participatory manner with service providers and users among other stakeholders, is an excellent vehicle for coordinating advocacy. Such plans are needed not only because good planning helps service development, but also because good plans are a helpful vehicle for fundraising. By functioning as a coherent proposal for services, a national plan, endorsed by the minister of health, can facilitate sound financing from different levels of government and can be used as a proposal to international donors. Such plans can thus break the vicious cycle between lack of unified advocacy and lack of resources.

This chapter also covers other barriers. With respect to human resources, diversifying the mental health workforce is key. Psychiatrists should increasingly move from direct service provision to training/supervising-non psychiatrists (e.g. PHC staff) in mental health care. This change in roles is essential to increase coverage in the community. Incentives—including financial incentives—for such a change in role need to be made available.

The chapter discussed the challenges related to integrating mental health care in PHC, which includes the need for supervision, but also the limited time that PHC providers have for mental health. Greater efforts need to be extended to work with PHC providers on time management for providing mental health care. For example, PHC providers may task shift some of the work by involving community workers or, alternatively, they may dedicate specific—relatively quiet—times of the week to mental health care, during which they schedule appointments with appropriate amount of time for each patient. Making dedicated time for mental health care is justifiable given the high prevalence of mental health problems in PHC (Üstün & Sartorius, 1995).

Psychiatrists will continue to play key roles in many countries and, as mentioned above, they should lead the clinical supervision of mental health treatment in the health sector. Yet, this chapter provides reasons to doubt whether clinicians are best placed to lead mental health services development in countries unless they have a public health training and perspective to facilitate planning at the population level. There is a need for better access to public mental health leadership training for key decision-makers in LMICs.

We end this chapter with two observations and a conclusion. The first observation is that integration of mental health into PHC in rural districts works best if secondary care is in place first so that secondary care mental health experts can supervise the integration into PHC. The second observation is that decentralization from tertiary care to community care works best if secondary care is in place first in order to provide access to care to people who would otherwise go to tertiary care. Accordingly, we conclude that countries should consider prioritizing developing mental health in secondary care (e.g. accessible outpatient mental health clinics staffed by multidisciplinary teams, small acute psychiatry wards in general hospital) to be followed by the important work of integrating mental health at the primary care level and decentralizing the tertiary care level.

Acknowledgements

This chapter is based on a written key informant survey with international experts conducted in 2006–2007 (WHO, 2007). In this chapter, we represent the entire body of lessons we learned from the study. We thank Jessica Mears for her valuable comments on an earlier draft of this chapter.

REFERENCES

Chisholm, D., Gureje, O., Saldivia, S., Villalón Calderón, M., Wickremasinghe, R., Mendis, N., et al. (2008). Schizophrenia treatment in the developing world: an interregional and multinational cost-effectiveness analysis. *Bulletin of the World Health Organanization*, **86**, 542–551.

Desjarlais, R., Eisenberg, L., Good, B., & Kleinman, A. (1995). *World Mental Health: Problems and Priorities in Low-Income Countries*. New York: Oxford University Press.

Freeman, M. (2000). Using all opportunities for improving mental health—examples from South Africa. *Bulletin of the World Health Organization*, **78**, 508–510.

Institute of Medicine (2001). *Neurological, Psychiatric, and Developmental Disorders: Meeting the Challenge in the Developing World*. Washington, DC: National Academy Press.

Inter-Agency Standing Committee (2007). *IASC Guidelines of Mental Health and Psychosocial Support in Emergency Settings*. Geneva: Inter-Agency Standing Committee.

Laxminarayan, R., Mills, A. J., Breman, J. G., Measham, A. R., Alleyne, G., Claeson, M., et al. (2006). Advancement of global health: key messages from the Disease Control Priorities Project. *Lancet*, **367**, 1193–1208.

Miranda, J. J. & Patel, V. (2005). Achieving the Millennium Development Goals: does mental health play a role? *PLoS Medicine*, **2**, e291.

Patel, V., Araya, R., Chatterjee, S., Chisholm, D., Cohen, A., De Silva, M., et al. (2007). Treatment and prevention of mental disorders in low-income and middle-income countries. *Lancet*, **370**, 991–1005.

Patel, V., Saraceno, B., & Kleinman, A. (2006). Beyond evidence: the moral case for international mental health. *American Journal of Psychiatry*, **163**, 1312–1315.

Saraceno, B., van Ommeren, M., Batniji, R., Cohen, A., Gureje, O., Mahoney, J., et al. (2007). Barriers to improvement of mental health services in low-income and middle-income countries. *Lancet*, **370**, 1164–1174.

Saxena, S., Thornicroft, G., Knapp, M., & Whiteford, H. (2007). Resources for mental health: scarcity, inequity, and inefficiency. *Lancet*, **370**, 878–889.

Steel, Z., Chey, T., Silove, D., Marnane, C., Bryant, R. A., & van Ommeren, M. (2009). Association of torture and other potentially traumatic events with mental health outcomes among populations exposed to mass conflict and displacement: a systematic review and meta-analysis. *JAMA*, **302**, 537–549.

Thornicroft, G. (2006). *Shunned: Discrimination against People with Mental Illness*. Oxford: Oxford University Press.

Underhill, C. (2002). Mental health and development: from the local to the global. The involvement of mentally ill people in the development process. *Asian Pacific Disability & Rehabilitation Journal*, **2**, 1–15.

Üstün, T. B. & Sartorius, N. (Eds.) (1995). *Mental Illness in General Health Care: An International Study*. Chichester: John Wiley.

WHO World Mental Health Survey Consortium (2004). Prevalence, severity, and unmet need for treatment of mental disorders in the World Health Organization World Mental Health Surveys. *JAMA*, **291**, 2581–2590.

World Health Organization (1978). 'Declaration of Alma-Ata.' International Conference on Primary Health Care, Alma-Ata, USSR, 6–12 September.

World Health Organization (2001). *World Health Report 2001: Mental Health*. Geneva: World Health Organization.

World Health Organization (2003). *Mental Health Policy and Service Guidance Package*. Geneva: World Health Organization.

World Health Organization (2006). *Dollars, DALYs and Decisions: Economic Aspects of the Mental Health System*. Geneva: World Health Organization.

World Health Organization (2007). *Expert Opinion on Barriers and Facilitating Factors for the Implementation of Existing Mental Health Knowledge in Mental Health Services*. Geneva: World Health Organization.

World Health Organization (2008). *mhGAP Mental Health Gap Action Plan: Scaling Up Care for Mental, Neurological, and Substance Use Disorders*. Geneva: World Health Organization.

World Health Organization & Disease Control Priorities Project (2006). *Disease Control Priorities related to Mental Neurological, Developmental and Substance Abuse Disorders*. Geneva: World Health Organization.

SECTION 10
Looking to the future

45. **Community mental health in the future** 469
    *Graham Thornicroft, Robert E. Drake, Oye Gureje,
    Kim T. Mueser, and George Szmukler*

45

Community mental health in the future

Graham Thornicroft, Robert E. Drake, Oye Gureje, Kim T. Mueser, and George Szmukler

Introduction

Several fundamental tenets inform our approach to community mental health care. First is an understanding of a community's needs for mental health services. Policymakers must appreciate population-based needs to deliver services from a public health perspective. Second, mental health care must balance several opposing forces: the scale of needs against the available resources, and how to invest in which blend of hospital-based and community-based services. Third, mental health services must align with basic human rights and health care values, while also recognizing the clinical duty of care. Fourth, effective mental health care must incorporate evidence-based approaches, including the use of telehealth and digital health resources, and also be cognizant of what types of services are preferred by people with mental health conditions and their family members. Fifth, putting services in place with high fidelity to the evidence needs to be tested by the methods of implementation science. Sixth, community mental health must address the wider range of community supports (including stigma reduction) that address social determinants as well as the narrower domain of mental health services. Finally, systems of care must be flexible enough to evolve as our knowledge of needs, values, evidence-based practices, and implementation science changes over time. This final chapter addresses these tenets, as well as offering an overview of where in our view there have been clear areas of progress or challenge over the last decade since the first edition of this textbook.

The balanced care model

Countries vary widely in how they define, interpret, and implement community-orientated care (Thornicroft et al., 2010; Winkler et al., 2017; World Health Organization (WHO), 2022). Nevertheless, they all must balance competing priorities. Mental health care must align epidemiological needs with the reality of the available resources. From the point of view of the balanced care model (see Chapter 11), most mental health services should be provided in community settings close to the populations served, with the duration of hospital stays reduced to a minimum consistent with recovery, and with inpatient services usually located in acute wards in general hospitals (Thornicroft et al., 2016a).

At the same time, differing priorities apply to low-, medium-, and high-resource settings:

- In low-resource settings, the focus is on establishing and improving the capacity of practitioners in primary health care facilities to deliver mental health care, with limited specialist back-up. Most mental health assessment and treatment occurs, if at all, in primary health care settings or in relation to traditional/religious healers. For example, in Ethiopia most care is provided within the family or in the close community of neighbours and relatives: only 33% of people with persistent major depressive disorder reach either primary health care or traditional healers (Fekadu et al., 2022; Hailemariam et al., 2019). In several other countries in sub-Saharan Africa, a majority of persons with mental disorders, especially severe mental illness, make their first contact with care at the facilities of traditional/religious healers (Esan et al., 2019; Gureje et al., 2015).
- In medium-resource settings, in addition to primary care mental health services, an extra layer of general adult mental health services can be developed as resources allow, in five categories: (1) outpatient/ambulatory clinics; (2) community mental health teams; (3) acute inpatient services; (4) community-based residential care; and (5) work, occupation, and rehabilitation services.
- In high-resource countries, as well as the services described above, more specialized services dedicated to specific patient groups and goals may be affordable in the same five categories. These may include, for instance, specialized outpatient and ambulatory clinics, assertive community treatment teams, intensive case management, early intervention teams, crisis resolution teams, crisis housing, community residential care, acute day hospitals, day hospitals, non-medical day centres, and recovery/employment/rehabilitation services, and these are described in more detail in the chapters of this book.

Work for the 2018 Lancet Commission on global mental health and sustainable development provided an enhancement to the balanced care model by adding a community layer to the model as shown in **Figure 45.1** (Patel et al., 2018). For example, in low-resource

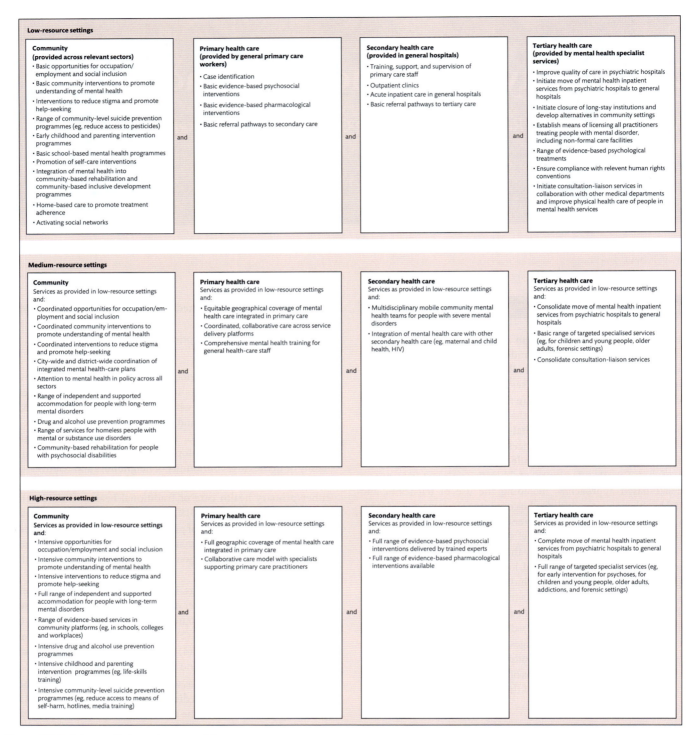

Figure 45.1 Enhanced balanced care model.

Reproduced with permission from Patel, V., Saxena, S., Lund, C., Thornicroft, G., Baingana, F., Bolton, P., Chisholm, D., Collins, P. Y., Cooper, J. L., Eaton, J., Herrman, H., Herzallah, M. M., Huang, Y., Jordans, M. J. D., Kleinman, A., Medina-Mora, M. E., Morgan, E., Niaz, U., Omigbodun, O., Prince, M., Rahman, A., Saraceno, B., Sarkar, B. K., De Silva, M., Singh, I., Stein, D. J., Sunkel, C. & Unutzer, J. (2018). The Lancet Commission on global mental health and sustainable development. *Lancet*, 392, 1553–1598.

settings, the model indicates that before, or in parallel with, access to primary health care for mental health conditions, people may access help and care from the following array of supports in the community: opportunities for occupation/employment and social inclusion; community interventions to promote understanding of mental health; interventions to reduce stigma and promote help-seeking; a range of community-level suicide prevention programmes (e.g. reduce access to pesticides); early childhood and parenting intervention programmes; school-based mental health programmes; promotion of self-care interventions; integration of mental health into community-based rehabilitation; community-based inclusive development programmes; and active social networks.

Human rights and basic health care values

Underpinning the successful implementation of community-orientated mental health care are principles that relate on the one hand to the value of community and on the other to the importance of self-determination and the rights of people with mental illness as persons and citizens (United Nations, 2006) (see Chapter 28). We expect that in the future, community mental health services will increasingly emphasize the importance of supporting and enabling people to recover and to live in, and participate in, the community in a way that maintains their connection with their families, friends, work, and community. This process acknowledges and supports individuals' goals and strengths to further their recovery in their own community (Slade, 2009).

A fundamental principle supporting these values is the notion of people having equitable access to services guided by the United Nations principle of universal health coverage (Hanlon et al., 2019). While recognizing the fact that some people are significantly impaired by their mental health condition, community mental health services seek to foster the service user's rights to self-determination and participation as far as possible in processes involving decisions related to their treatment. These values need to be upheld, often in the face of public pressures to prioritize safety concerns and to re-institutionalize people with mental disorders in hospitals, nursing homes, jails, and prisons.

Various conventions identify and aim to protect the rights of service users as persons and citizens including the United Nations Convention on the Rights of Persons with Disabilities (United Nations, 2006). We strongly endorse these principles and their practical application in the development of community-based services.

Evidence-based approaches

Evidence-based mental health care comprises three fundamental approaches: evidence-based practices, evidence-based decision-making, and quality assurance (Drake et al., 2003). Chapters 34–37 discuss the techniques that are used to develop and validate evidence-based practices. These techniques target specific interventions that are efficacious and effective for specific populations. For example, the evidence indicates that a client with serious mental illness who wants to work should receive supported employment and that a client who experiences serious mental illness and chronic homelessness should receive assertive community treatment and supportive housing (see Chapters 14 and 19).

But evidence-based practices have limits, and many treatment decisions are much more complex than deciding who should receive a basic intervention such as supported employment or assertive community treatment. Mental health clients often have multiple comorbidities, lack basic psychosocial supports, live in communities with limited social capital or mental health resources, or have histories of not benefitting from a series of evidence-based interventions. Often a single, clear best practice does not exist for specific individuals. Instead, several interventions with partial effectiveness, offset by side effects, are available. These decisions require a shared approach to making complex decisions. In such situations the mental health practitioner and the client need to discuss the best scientific information: the practitioner provides expertise on diagnoses, the course of illnesses, and available treatments; and the client offers expertise on personal goals and preferences. Together they negotiate treatment plans that balance these inputs in a process of shared decision-making (Drake et al., 2009, 2010; Ramon et al., 2021; Zisman-Ilani et al., 2017).

At the team, programme, agency, or system level, evidence-based care requires systematic attention to outcomes. Quality is often addressed by training, supervision, and fidelity review (Bond & Drake, 2020). But outcomes must be measured to be certain of quality. Data are systematically gathered on clients, services, and outcomes to assess whether the clients are remaining in services, are receiving services that are appropriate to their needs, and are improving in relation to expected outcomes based on established benchmarks. The process of monitoring data in this fashion to detect problems in the flow of assessment and treatment to improve services is a necessary step for high-quality mental health care.

Implementation science

Implementation differs substantially from intervention. One challenge common to many countries worldwide is the difficulty in putting potentially effective community mental health interventions into large-scale, consistent practice. The science of implementation has expanded considerably over the past decade (Bartels et al., 2022; Thornicroft et al., 2011b).

Policies, plans, and programmes

We have found it helpful in thinking about mental health service developments or reform to consider three levels of change: (1) national *policies* (or provincial or state policies in countries where health policy is set at that level): an overall statement of strategic intent (e.g. over a 5–10-year period) that gives direction to the whole system of mental health care; (2) *implementation plans*: operational documents setting out the specific steps needed to implement the national policy (e.g. what tasks are to be completed, by whom, by when, with which resources, and identifying the reporting lines, and the incentives and sanctions if tasks are completed or not completed); and (3) *mental health programmes*: specific plans either for a local area (e.g. a region or a district) or for a particular sector (e.g. primary care) that specify how one component of the overall care system should be developed.

Scaling up services for whole populations

A further challenge that needs addressing worldwide is the massive gap between population needs for mental health care (true prevalence of mental illness) and what is actually provided in mental health care (treated prevalence) (WHO, 2016), highlighting the importance of scaling up services for whole populations. The substantial burden of mental disorders (see Chapter 38) has not been translated into investments in mental health care. The treatment gap is particularly pronounced in low- and middle-income countries (LMICs), where commonly over 90% of people with mental disorders receive no treatment or care at all, and less than 2% of the health budget is spent on mental health (WHO, 2022).

Similarly, only 10% of global mental health research is directed to the health needs of the 90% of populations living in LMICs, and only a fraction of this research activity is concerned with implementing and evaluating interventions and services (Collins et al., 2011). Methods to estimate resource needs are necessary in scaling up services, as well as a rethinking of professional roles, for instance, in terms of task-shifting (Patel et al., 2018). A valuable approach to the implementation of evidence-based practice is the development and use of treatment guidelines (see Chapter 37). An exemplar of this approach is the WHO Mental Health Gap Action Programme (mhGAP) Intervention Guide, now in use in over 100 countries worldwide (Keynejad et al., 2021; WHO, 2010, 2016).

The community as the context for mental health care: stigma and discrimination

Further common barriers that need to be decisively tackled in the future are mental health-related stigma and discrimination. These pervasive and pernicious problems have many ramifications including exclusion from the workplace, family life, and social life, and also contribute to premature mortality (Mehta et al., 2015; Walker et al., 2015). There is now good evidence from high-income countries to show that social contact between people who do and who do not have experience of mental ill health is the main way to reduce stigma. There is also growing evidence in LMICs that the social contact approach, if carefully and contextually adapted, is also effective in stigma reduction (Li et al., 2019; Maulik et al., 2019; Potts & Henderson, 2021). While further evidence is required specific to LMICs, it is also true that the time is right for large-scale implementation of such stigma reduction programmes (Gronholm et al., 2017; Thornicroft & Sunkel, 2020).

Developing a consensus for change

In most countries, transforming mental health services to focus on community-orientated care has proven a major task. Perhaps the most important factor is the range of people involved in providing services and the recognition that service users and their families should be involved in care planning and service development. In all this has meant that there is a complex mix of people who have an investment in the development and delivery of mental health services, the majority of whom have to be involved when significant change is contemplated. Large- and smaller-scale ventures such as those in the UK, New Zealand, and Australia have proven that the collaborative engagement of a wide variety of supportive stakeholders is critical to successful implementation of community-orientated mental health care.

Change requires the support of politicians, board members and health managers whose primary focus may not be on mental health, clinicians, key members of the community including non-governmental organizations (NGOs), service users and their families, and traditional and religious healers. To involve them in the imperative for change will require different strategies and a change management team that includes people with a variety of expertise and different networks to undertake them. Overall, having clear reasons and objectives for the shift to community-orientated care is essential. Messages should be concise, backed by evidence, and consistent.

Developing consensus for change requires extensive meeting and communicating with people. The main means of communication need to include written material and opportunities to meet with stakeholder groups. Politicians and administrators will require a compelling business case. However, others will need summaries of plans, slide presentations, and the opportunity to meet and work through proposals and concerns. Emails and website information and surveys are now valuable supplements to the process. In all communications the emphasis must be on a willingness to communicate in good faith and to do so openly and honestly to convince people of the benefits of the change process and determination to see it through.

Inevitably, in some cases prejudice and self-interest will have to be confronted. It is helpful, at the beginning of the process, to identify both those who are likely to support change, and those who are likely to oppose it. A willingness to listen to concerns and to find ways of incorporating some concerns into the planning and implementation process is essential because when such an attitude is communicated there is an opportunity for people to feel included in the process. That done, boldness and firmness will communicate to remaining detractors the seriousness of the intent to implement change; it will also encourage supporters to believe that their aspirations for better mental health care will be realized, and thus embolden them in turn.

Engaging stakeholders requires both formal and informal opportunities to meet, receive advice, and work through issues. The establishment of reference groups early in the change process is a key formal mechanism to achieving this. These should include all the key stakeholders in particular service users, families, clinicians, and service providers with the latter being essential to facilitate integrated systems of care further on in the process. While it is important to structure the overall process with formal meetings and communications, it is also important to be willing to convene informal meetings to 'troubleshoot' situations of concern. For practical purposes, the consultation process takes place at a number of levels and should result in an amalgam of 'bottom-up' and 'top-down' contributions to the change process. Reports on progress are an essential way of maintaining trust and generating excitement in the process of successful implementation.

It is important to bear in mind that good mental health services have established processes for ensuring the voices of service users, their families, and community providers are heard on an ongoing basis. It is then not simply a matter of achieving discontinuous change but ongoing quality improvement in which consumers of mental health services know they have a major stake. Without such effective and united consortia, policymakers may find it easy to disregard the demands of a fragmented mental health sector, and instead respond positively to health domains (e.g. HIV/AIDS) which demonstrate the self-discipline of a united approach with a small number of fully agreed priorities.

Mistakes to avoid in implementing community mental health services

Measures must be taken to avoid several key mistakes commonly made in the process of attempting to implement community mental health care. First, a carefully considered sequence of events must link hospital bed closure to community service development. It is important to avoid closing hospital-based services without having successor services already in place to support discharged patients and new referrals, and also to avoid trying to build up community services while leaving hospital care (and budgets) intact. In particular, there needs to be at each stage of a reform process a workable balance between enough (mainly acute beds) and the provision of other parts of the wider system of care that can support people in crisis.

A second common mistake is to attempt system reform without including *all* the relevant stakeholders. Such initiatives especially need to include psychiatrists, who may otherwise feel subject to 'top-down' decision-making and react, either in the perceived interests of patients or in their own interests, by attempting to delay or block any such changes. Other vital stakeholders to be directly included in the process will often include policymakers and politicians, health service planners, service users and carers, service providers including those in state and private practice, national and international NGOs, and those working in alternative, complementary, indigenous, and religious healing traditions, and relevant national and professional associations. Typically, those groups not fully involved in a reform process will make their views known by seeking to undermine the process!

A further frequent error is inappropriately linking the reform of mental health care with narrow ideological or partisan political interests. This tends to lead to instability as a change of government may reverse the policies of their predecessors. Such fault lines of division or fragmentation may also occur, for example, between service reforms proposed by psychologists as opposed to psychiatrists, or between socially and biologically orientated psychiatrists, or between clinicians and service user/consumer groups. Whatever the particular sources of schism, such conflicts weaken the chance that service reforms will be comprehensive, systemic, and sustainable, and they also run the risk that policymakers will refuse to adopt proposals that are not fully endorsed by the whole mental health sector.

Finally, policymakers and mental health administrators often overlook the fact that course of long-term illnesses is more strongly affected by social determinants than treatment. Poverty, poor education, food insecurity, lack of safe housing, unemployment, social isolation, and other social problems are primary drivers of adjustment and cannot be overcome by more and more treatment. Attempting to address social problems with health care is expensive and ineffective. Community mental health and social determinants of adjustment must be addressed simultaneously, usually by integrating mental health care and social services.

Payment systems

A fundamental component in the successful implementation of mental health service provision is that of funding (Chisholm et al., 2019). Funding for mental health services in LMICs tends to be very low. This may be due in part to a stigmatizing attitude towards mental illness, and to an absence of the recognition of the economic benefits that can accrue from improved mental health care. Ideally, the share of its health funding that a country devotes to mental health care will be informed by careful consideration of the comparative health benefits of spending on alternative forms of care. The data needed to carry out such an analysis are, however, typically not available in LMICs.

Furthermore, what funding there is tends to be concentrated on inpatient services—as this entire chapter implicitly presupposes. Correcting this is, initially, a matter of budgetary reallocation: using funds that could have been used for other purposes to increase funding for community-orientated care.

The issue then arises of how to pay public providers (hospitals, stand-alone programmes—institutional or voluntary sector, and possibly independent individual providers such as psychiatrists) for the services they render. The simplest forms of payment are global budgets for facilities and programmes, which may be carried over from year to year with minor adjustments for inflation, and salaries for individual providers. These simple payment mechanisms have the advantage of administrative simplicity. At the same time, they have at least two important drawbacks. First, they provide no incentive for increasing either the quantity or the quality of service provision. Second, population shifts are likely to cause the demand for the services of different providers to evolve; without taking changes in local demand into account inequities in payment across providers are likely to emerge and grow over time. This in turn will compromise access to overburdened providers, while possibly resulting in overprovision (e.g. excessive lengths of stay) by other providers. Accordingly, countries with the technical and administrative capacity to introduce more complex payment systems should consider doing so.

For hospitals, a fairly simple alternative which is applicable where care is sectorized is to modulate budgets on the basis of the population of the facility's catchment area. Countries with the technical capacity to do so may wish to adjust the payment level per person on the basis of sociodemographic variables known to be related to the need for inpatient mental health care (e.g. poverty).

For hospitals that have overlapping catchment areas, a combination of prospective payment (payment on the basis of number of admissions) and retrospective payment (payment on the basis of bed-days actually provided) may be preferable to exclusive reliance on one or the other. Pure retrospective payment encourages overprovision of services; pure prospective payment, given the difficulty of assessing reliably the degree of need for care of a person admitted for a psychiatric condition, may encourage underprovision.

For stand-alone programmes or individual providers, the two main options beyond a fixed budget or a salary are fee-for-service and capitation. Fee-for-service payment encourages a higher volume of services without regard to outcomes. If certain services (e.g. prescription of medications) are paid at a higher rate per unit time than others (e.g. psychotherapy), then fee-for-service payment will also influence the mix of services provided. In addition, fee-for-service payment tends to maximize contacts with patients who are less ill, more compliant, and easier to treat. Difficult or more severely ill patients receive less care unless payments are adjusted by severity—so-called case-mix adjustments. Efficient uses of clinical time such as telephone or computer contacts are ignored because they are not reimbursed.

Capitation payment encourages increasing the number of people served. It may lead to greater accountability for the care of specific patients. In and of itself, however, unless there is competition for patients across providers, it provides no incentive for quality. Furthermore, programmes often fill up to capacity and have difficulty shifting patients to less intensive services.

Countries with the technical and administrative capacity (and political leeway) to do so should consider introducing incentives for increasing quality, for hospitals, programmes, or individual providers. Following Donabedian's seminal work, quality is commonly conceptualized as related to structure, process, and outcomes (Best & Neuhauser, 2004). Adjusting payments to hospitals, programmes, or individual providers on the basis of structure or process indicators (e.g. formal qualifications of staff, achievement of a certain score on a model fidelity scale) assumes that these indicators actually predict quality. To the extent that they do, providing incentives for achieving a high score on those indicators is likely to be beneficial, with a neutral effect on which types of patients the provider will seek to serve. Adjusting payments based on outcomes (e.g. physiological indicators of metabolic syndrome, rehospitalization rates, and employment rates) has the advantage of being directly related to a system's ostensible goals. It encourages, however, selection of less ill patients.

More research is needed on how to design effective systems for encouraging quality of community-orientated mental health care that are practicable in countries with more or less developed technical and administrative capabilities. In sum, payment systems influence patient selection, quality and amount of treatments, and outcomes, in more or less favourable ways, and different systems require varying degrees of technical and administrative capacity to be implemented successfully. Determining the optimal system or combination of systems for a particular health care system or locale probably depends heavily on history, infrastructure, financial resources, human resources, and other factors.

Human resources

Human resources are the most critical asset in mental health service provision. The gradual transformation to community-based care has resulted in changes in the ways human resources have been utilized (Institute of Medicine, 2013). The essential changes have been a reallocation of staff from hospital to community-based service settings, the need for a new set of competencies which include recovery and rehabilitation, and training of a wider range of workers, including informal community care workers, within the context of the practical needs of a country (Kakuma et al., 2011). Further, in many LMICs trained psychiatrists work under conditions of heavy and relentless clinical demands and may not have dedicated time during the week for any service development duties.

Another perspective to human resource development has been the increasing emphasis on integration of mental health into a primary care setting, thereby increasing access to the vast majority of the underserved. This has necessitated the training of general health staff in basic skills in mental health care such as detection of mental disorders, provision of basic care, and referral of complex problems to specialist care. Training and support for primary care providers often requires some form of collaborative care, defined as a system in which social work and psychiatric back-ups are regularly available to evaluate, review, and help with complex patients. In most developing countries, there has been a need for a well-rounded generalist who is capable of coping with most psychiatric problems with little access to any mental health practitioner. Further important issues include lack of insurance, out-of-pocket expenses, and the economic burden falling on families.

The broadening scope associated with the shift to community-based mental health services introduces greater levels of complexity, which affect the role of psychiatrists, broadening it to areas such as promotion and social inclusion. Psychiatrists need to work in more settings, with more staff groups. Planning and management will take a more prominent place. Psychiatrists are seen to possess a unique expertise, and occupy leading positions in most countries, functioning as advisers to governments and chairing drafting groups that are responsible for the production of policies and action plans. There are countries where such groups comprise only psychiatrists. They have, therefore, a unique opportunity to shape the process of reform in the best interest of patients, families, carers, the public, and staff.

While psychosocial rehabilitation is an important part of the overall process of successful management of chronic mental illnesses, its practice is still rare compared to the use of medicines intended to 'cure' mental illnesses. In many developing countries, training is scarce for occupational therapists, psychologists, or social workers. In countries with few psychiatrists, numerous medical, administrative, and leadership duties leave psychiatrists little time to work with rehabilitation units. Even so, in many LMICs other resources are available, such as strong family and community networks, faith groups, and informal employment opportunities, that might be mobilized to support the rehabilitation of people with longer-term mental illnesses.

Organizational development, quality assurance, and service evaluation

Starting the reform process is a challenge worldwide, in part due to difficulties in imagining how a new system will work. Thus, initiation of community mental health care services generally requires strong leadership among stakeholders based on community-orientated care concepts, including greater attention to social determinants of mental health. Focusing on the structures and processes, organizational development is necessary to increase the potential for an organization to accomplish its goals. It enhances the organization's awareness, knowledge, and techniques required for the changes. It is practical to learn from successful models by using basic tools including timetables, assessment methods, job descriptions, and operational policies.

As part of the process of establishing a new system, and of maintaining it subsequently, coaching and maintenance activities are needed to make services robust and sustainable: manualization of operational procedures, reference materials, ongoing supervision, fidelity reviews, and technical assistance are essential to help organizations achieve and maintain continuous quality improvement in their community services. As community-orientated care becomes established in several regions, service components are gradually standardized, and manualized standard care becomes available.

Quality assurance is feasible even in settings with limited resources. Quality monitoring can be incorporated into routine activities by selecting target services, collecting data, and using the results for system problem-solving and future direction. External evaluation takes place at different levels. Local government checks whether service providers meet the requirement of laws or acts; payers focus on examining the necessity of services provided. Professional peers and consumers also participate in independent evaluation.

Since the primary purpose of mental health services is to improve outcomes for individuals with mental illness, it is crucial to assess outcomes of treatments and services. Also, the results can be used to justify the use of resources. More research is therefore needed to provide the best possible services that produce better outcomes for those in need of care. It is also important to recognize the variety of ways in which countries of all resource levels have developed their systems of healthcare over decades or centuries. Some countries, such as the US, for example, are now at a post-institutionalization phase, but are also experiencing the consequences of not implementing universal health care, comprehensive community-based services, and socioeconomic supports for people who are poor and disadvantaged.

Information technology

Innovations in information technology are improving mental health services with a diverse set of valuable tools that address education, communication, innovative interventions, quality improvement, and sophisticated algorithms based on artificial intelligence. Digital resources can enhance the three fundamental pillars of evidence-based medicine: providers' access to and understanding of the research evidence, patients' knowledge of and preferences for care, and using clinical expertise to enhance shared decision-making. In the future, information technology will continue to expand access, capacity, quality, effectiveness, and efficiency in mental health care across countries worldwide. The following concepts have been reviewed in greater detail elsewhere in this textbook (see Chapter 25).

The internet and other electronic resources already provide primary sources of education to providers, people with mental illness, and family members. Providers increasingly access current evidence regarding diagnostic tools, interventions, and treatment algorithms through the internet. Point-of-contact information (e.g. regarding side effects and interactions between medications) is widely available in high-income countries. Professional organizations rely on digital tools to assure continuing education and practice standards. Computerized decision tools can summarize current treatment evidence and suggest treatments for practitioners, thereby enhancing clinical expertise and the use of research evidence. In addition, information systems are commonly used to check for medical errors, such as incorrect medication dosages and adverse medication interactions.

For people experiencing mental health symptoms, widely available information regarding psychiatric syndromes, illnesses, treatments, and services promotes understanding and even self-diagnosis, at least preliminarily. In many countries information technology also enhances personal agency and shared decision-making; people use the web to explore their symptoms and treatment options, consider personal preferences, and make decisions before they seek professional or non-professional help. Computerized information can also promote shared decision-making when providers and patients interact, potentially increasing engagement and treatment adherence (Finnerty et al., 2018). In many areas people can use technology systems to consider their options: for example, self-administration of care using apps, attending self-help groups, choosing among various psychosocial interventions, trying different medications, or some combination of these choices. Electronic service provision involves guided self-treatment, such as computerized cognitive behavioural treatment for anxiety, depression, or addiction. Early studies show outcomes that are equivalent to professionally delivered interventions. It is also important to note that as the amount of information about mental health increases on the internet, so it becomes ever more difficult to distinguish accurate from inaccurate information.

As computer literacy increases, people with mental illnesses in many settings have demonstrated willingness and ability to enter personal information on demographics, medical histories, family history, and current symptoms prior to visits with professionals. To address the problem of illiteracy, software can be easily adapted for aural and touchscreen use. Diagnoses can be confirmed or refined by professionals, but self-entry of data obviously increases the efficiency of assessment and reduces costs. For many reasons, including concerns regarding privacy, people want to own and control their own personal health records, including current diagnoses, treatments, and allergies. Electronic records facilitate this capacity. People can easily carry their medical information and treatment preferences on a small computer memory device.

Remote communications were increasing before the Covid-19 pandemic (Griffiths et al., 2006) and have expanded tremendously since 2020 (e.g. Suran, 2022), not only between providers, insurers, and systems of care but also between patients and providers. Benefits have accrued dramatically for patients living far from providers and those without transportation. Resistance to remote appointments, follow-ups, and decision-making has declined substantially among providers and patients, but the future of telehealth will depend on insurers, government regulations, and other factors, including research on efficacy and cost-effectiveness.

Despite the promise of information technology, its impact is limited for now in low-income settings. In Ethiopia, for example, illiteracy rates among rural women are 73%, health centres struggle even to have phone contact with district or regional services, and there are major problems arising from unreliable electricity supplies, low-quality hardware, and inadequate protection from computer viruses. Health care systems in the future will need to expand digital access to disadvantaged populations or they will become even more disadvantaged relative to high-income populations.

For quality assurance, electronic case registries can track amount and quality of treatment. Services received should be consistent with treatment plans and evidence-based practices; these quality assurance indicators can be monitored and summarized daily through electronic records. Even in remote areas, people can be served and monitored according to evidence-based guidelines through telemedicine and other electronic communications. Although few mental health programmes currently monitor outcomes in real time to assess the effectiveness of services in relation to established benchmarks, patient data entry via web-based systems can serve this purpose. When patients do not respond to treatment or when they reach other decision points, they should be considered for alternative interventions according to the best available evidence, personal preferences, and clinical judgement. Guidelines for making such decisions, called treatment algorithms, can be made available electronically at the point of decision-making.

Beyond the current interventions we have described, what might the future of information technology in mental health look like? We expect that mental health care will continue to be behind other areas of medical care (if only because the brain is so complex and our understanding is so primitive), but changes that are currently occurring in other areas of medicine will eventually influence mental health as well. Chief among these will be the expanded use of big data science, computerized algorithms, and artificial intelligence. Algorithms are already used to interpret imaging and other testing procedures, to identify appropriate treatments, to track practice patterns, and to monitor patients' progress. But major changes are coming. In cancer therapy, for example, the availability of genetic evidence and new immunotherapies are developing so rapidly that cancer doctors must rely on experts for assistance. Cancer programmes in major academic medical centres are collecting data on individual characteristics, medical histories, genetics, treatments, and efficacy from tens of thousands of patients so that machine algorithms can identify patterns of optimal response. Medical centres are also developing technical assistance algorithms, based on rapidly synthesized information, to provide local cancer doctors with current evidence. At the same time, specialists in other areas are developing bioengineering interventions, including brain implants, and interventions to modify genetic expression that will fundamentally alter the course of serious illnesses and injuries. Although the timing is uncertain, these changes will inevitably affect community mental health.

Covid-19 and mental health

To be set against some gains in the acceleration of remote consulting and the use of telemedicine during and after the Covid-19 pandemic, this global crisis has also had profoundly negative consequences for mental health. Many surveys have now identified that general population rates of depression or anxiety increased by about 25% over prior baseline rates during the pandemic, especially during the worst waves of infection (Chekole & Abate, 2021; Wu et al., 2021). Rates of mortality from Covid-19 among people with mental illness or intellectual disability have been several-fold higher than for the general population (Fond et al., 2021; Vai et al., 2021; Wang et al., 2021). The impact has been especially heavy upon health care workers (Saragih et al., 2021). Yet at a time when the prevalence of mental disorders and the rates of mental health needs were increasing, the supply of services diminished. An early rapid assessment by the WHO showed that in most of the countries surveyed, mental health service investment declined early in the pandemic to divert funds to physical health care related to Covid-19 (WHO, 2020). It therefore seems very likely that the overall impact of the Covid-19 pandemic has been to set back progress for improvements in mental health care (see Chapter 42).

Growing global appreciation of the challenge of mental illness

During the last decade there has been a steadily growing awareness by policymakers of the scale of the challenges posed to family, community, and society by mental health conditions. In part, the accumulating evidence of the impact of morbidity and mortality of these conditions accounts for these positive changes (Vigo et al., 2016; Whiteford et al., 2015). In addition, the emergence of precise estimates, for example, from the World Mental Health Surveys of how few people with mental health conditions receive any treatment or care, has helped (Alonso et al., 2018; Degenhardt et al., 2017; Thornicroft et al., 2017). At the same time, the WHO has made major contributions to assist national policymakers in knowing what to actually do by developing and disseminating practical treatment tools and guidelines such as the WHO mhGAP Intervention Guide (Dua et al., 2011). A significant emphasis in this work has been on building capacity among primary care staff, from whom most people with mental health-related distress seek help. There has been a growing influence of NGOs, such as the Global Mental Health Peer Network, in their direct contributions to policy formation and in their contributions to international consortia to press mental health ever higher on the policy agenda. Another major contribution to raising mental health on policy agendas has been the inclusion of mental health-related targets and indictors in the United Nations Sustainable Development Goals, especially Goal 3 related to health outcomes (Gureje & Thornicroft, 2015; United Nations, 2015). There is now ever-clearer evidence on how to reduce stigma and discrimination (Thornicroft et al., 2016b).

Conclusion

We have described here a series of commonly occurring challenges and obstacles to implementing a community-orientated system of mental health care. At the same time, we have identified related steps and solutions which may work in responding positively and effectively to these barriers (Thornicroft et al., 2011a), as set out in Table 45.1. We therefore recommend that people interested in planning and implementing systems of mental health care that balance community-based and hospital-based service components give careful consideration to anticipating the challenges identified here and to learning the lessons from those who have grappled with these issues so far (Thornicroft & Tansella, 2014).

The expert reviews across the whole field of mental health practice which are included in this textbook lead us to the following conclusions: the future of community mental health is as likely to be heavily contested as its recent past, and those advocating for more humane services must stand resolutely for greater social inclusion and respect for the human rights of people with mental health conditions; there needs to be relentless advocacy to achieve this by bringing together powerful consortia of stakeholders from many sectors, including those who have not until now been active in the field of mental health; evidence-based and ethically sound proposals need to be repeatedly brought forward to policymakers to fund the health

Table 45.1 Obstacles, challenges, lessons learned, and solutions in implementing community-orientated mental health care

Obstacles and challenges		Lessons learned and solutions
Society	1. Disregard for, or violation of, human rights of people with mental illness	• Oversight by civil society and service user groups, government inspectorates, international NGOs, professional associations • Increase population awareness of mental illness and of the rights of people with mental illness and available treatments
	2. Stigma and discrimination, reflected in negative attitudes of health staff	• Encourage consumer and family and carer involvement in policymaking, medical training, service provision (e.g. board member, consumer provider), service evaluation (consumer satisfaction survey)
	3. Need to address different models of abnormal behaviour	• Traditional and faith-based paradigms need to be amalgamated, blended, or aligned as much as possible with medical paradigms
Government	4. Low priority given by government to mental health	• Government task force on mental illness outlines mission as a public health agenda • Mission can encompass values, goals, structure, development, education, training, and quality assurance for community-oriented mental health system from a public health perspective • Establish cross-party political support for the national policy and implementation plan • Effective advocacy on mental health gap, global burden of disease, impact of mental health conditions, cost-effectiveness of interventions, reduce life expectancy, use of WHO and other international agencies for advocacy, linking with priority health conditions and funds, positive response of untoward events • Identifying champions within government who have administrative and financial authority • Importance of giving priority to identified public health priorities and evidence-based practices in the face of industry lobbying for corporate profits
	5. Absence or inappropriate mental health policy	• Advocate for and formulate policy based upon widespread consultation with the full range of stakeholder groups, incorporating a rationalized public health perspective based on population needs, integration of service components • Consumer involvement in policymaking
	6. Absent, old, or inappropriate mental health legislation	• Create powerful lobby and rationale for mental health law • Modernize mental health law formulated and implemented relevant to community orientated care • Watchdog or inspectorate to oversee proper implementation of mental health law
	7. Inadequate financial resources in relation to population-level needs	• Help policymakers to be aware of the gap between burden of mental illness and allocated resources, and that effective treatments are available, and affordable • Advocate for improved mental health expenditure using relevant information, arguments, and targets, e.g. Global Burden of Disease, mhGAP unmet needs • Recruit key political and governance champions to advocate for adequate funding of initiatives
	8. Lack of alignment between payment methods and expected services and outcomes	• Design a system that directly relates required service components and financially reimbursable categories of care, e.g. for evidence-based practices • Provide small financial incentives for valued outcomes • Create categories of reimbursement consistent with system strategy • Develop and use key performance indicators • Reserve transitional cost to reallocate hospital staff to move to community
	9. Need to address infrastructure	• Government to plan and finance efficient use of, e.g. buildings, essential supplies, and electronic information systems and other to direct, monitor, and improve the system and outcomes
	10. Need to address structure of community-oriented service system	• Design the mental health system from local primary care to regional care to central specialty care and fill in gaps with new resources as funding grows
	11. Inadequate human resources for delivery of mental health care in relation to the level of need in the population	• Assessment of population level needs for primary care and specialist mental health care services • Build capacity of health workers engaged in providing general health care and mental health care in community • Training current health and mental health professionals in community orientated mental health care
	12. Brain drain, failure to retain talent, staff retention, and weak career ladders	• UN agencies/international NGOs assure sustainability of their projects/programmes • Exchange programmes between countries • Set period of time medical students/registrars have to serve in their countries or rural area • Task shifting/function differentiating of the psychiatrist to use their ability in their area of speciality • Create financial incentives and reputation systems for psychiatrists who engage in community mental health • Train other (less 'brain drainable') health professionals to deliver mental health care • Payment for education may be attached to the allocation and preservation of resources to address equitable distribution and to prevent emigration without appropriate reimbursement
	13. Unsustainable, parallel programmes by international NGOs	• Close relations with ministries and other stakeholders and international NGOs • Mental health plan in place so NGOs can help achieve these goals sustainably • Government to be proactive in collaborating with NGOs and private–public partnership

(continued)

Table 45.1 Continued

Obstacles and challenges		Lessons learned and solutions
Organization of the local mental health system	14. Need to design, monitor, and adjust organization of mental health system	• This includes plan for local, regional, and central mental health services based on public health need, full integration with primary care, rational allocation of multidisciplinary workforce, development of information technology, funding, and use of existing facilities. All stakeholder groups can be involved in developing, monitoring, and adjusting plan • Set implementation plan with clear coordination between services • Development of policy/implementation plan with number of services needed per population (e.g. New Zealand service 'Blueprint') • Role differentiation of the hospital, community and primary care services, and private and public services, using catchment area/capitation system with flexible funding system • Prioritization of target groups, especially people with severe and persistent mental illness
	15. Lack of a feasible mental health programme or non-implementation of mental health programme	• Make programme highly practical by identifying resources available, tasks to be completed, allocation of responsibilities, timescales, reporting and accountability arrangements, progress monitoring/evaluation systems
	16. Need to specify developmental phases	• Planners and professional leaders to design 5- and 10-year plans
	17. Poor utilization of existing mental health facilities	• Improve awareness of benefits of facilities and services • Specify pathways to care • Inbuilt monitoring quality of care, especially process and outcome phases
	18. Need to include non-medical services	• Include families, faith-based social services, NGOs, housing services, vocational services, peer-support services, and self-help services: all stakeholders involved in designing system • Task shifting, i.e. moving key tasks such as initial assessment and prescribing using a limited and affordable formulary to specially trained staff who are available at the appropriate local level • Identify leaders to champion and drive the process • More involvement in planning, policymaking, and leadership and management • Include in psychiatrist training programmes
	19. Lack of multisectoral collaboration, e.g. including traditional healers, housing, criminal justice, or education sectors	• Development of clear policy/implementation plan by all stakeholders • Collaborate with other local service to identify and help people with mental illness • Provision of information/training to all practitioners • Establish multisectoral advisory and governance groups • Familiarization sessions between practitioners in the Western and in the local traditions
	20. Poor availability or erratic supplies of psychotropic medication	• Educate policymakers and funders about the cost/benefits of specific medications • Provide infrastructure for clozapine monitoring • Monitoring prescribing patterns of psychotropic medication • Drug revolving funds, public–private partnerships
Professionals and practitioners	21. Need for leadership	• Psychiatrists and other professionals need to be involved as experts in planning, education, research, and overcoming inertia and resistance in the current environment
	22. Difficulty sustaining in-service training/adequate supervision	• Training of the trainers by staff from other regions or countries • Task shifting of the psychiatric functions, e.g. prescribing to trained and available practitioners • Lobby hard to ensure this is a priority and integral to the mental health plan
	23. High staff turnover and burnout, or low staff morale	• Introduction of recovery-oriented services • Collect case examples of recovery • Build trust by involving staff leaders in oversight and decision-making committees • Sponsor social events to enable staff to team build in non-work situations • Emphasize career-long continuing training programmes • Training of supervisors • Provide opportunities for attending out-of-area professional meetings • Equip with sufficient skills and support
	24. Poor quality of care/concern about staff skills	• Ongoing training and supervision • Create and disseminate guidelines for professionals • Third-party evaluation • Encourage and reward quality by awards and similar processes
	25. Professional resistance, e.g. to community-orientated care and service user involvement	• Government and professional societies promote the importance of community-oriented care and service user involvement • Task shifting/function differentiating of psychiatrists to use their abilities more broadly in their area of speciality and work with a range of stakeholders including consumers and carers/families • Develop training in recovery-orientated psychosocial rehabilitation as part of training of new psychiatrists, including at medical schools in LMICs • Collect case examples of recovery and successfully implemented community mental health initiatives
	26. Dearth of relevant research to inform cost-effective services and lack of data on mental health service evaluation	• More funding on research, for both qualitative and quantitative evidence of successfully implemented examples of community-orientated care
	27. Failure to address disparities (e.g. by ethnic, economic groups)	• All key stakeholders involved; advocacy for underrepresented group to develop policies and implementation plans

Table 45.1 Continued

Obstacles and challenges		Lessons learned and solutions
Users, families, and other advocates	28. Need for advocacy	• Users and other advocates may be involved in all aspects of social change, planning, lobbying the government, monitoring the development and functioning of the service system, and improving the service system
	29. Need for self-help and peer support services	• Users to lead these movements
	30. Need for person-centred care	• Users and other advocates must demand at all levels that the system shifts to value the goals of users and families, that shared decision-making become the norm, and that person-centeredness becomes a central value in assessing services and outcomes • Continuing professional education on human rights and staff attitudes emphasizing paying attention to preferences of consumers and carers • Consumer involvement at all levels: national level, local level, and patient care level

services and systems described in this book; and at every stage the preferences, priorities, and voices of people with mental health conditions must be paramount.

REFERENCES

Alonso, J., Liu, Z., Evans-Lacko, S., Sadikova, E., Sampson, N., Chatterji, S., et al. (2018). Treatment gap for anxiety disorders is global: results of the world mental health surveys in 21 countries. *Depression and Anxiety*, **35**, 195–208.

Bartels, S. M., Haider, S., Williams, C. R., et al. (2022). Diversifying implementation science: a global perspective. *Global Health: Science and Practice*, **10**(4), e2100757. https://doi.org/10.9745/GHSP-D-21-00757

Best, M. & Neuhauser, D. (2004). Avedis Donabedian: father of quality assurance and poet. *Quality and Safety in Health Care*, **13**, 472–473.

Bond, G. R. & Drake, R. E. (2020). Assessing the fidelity of evidence-based practices: history and current status of a standardized measurement methodology. *Administration and Policy in Mental Health*, **47**, 874–884.

Chekole, Y. A. & Abate, S. M. (2021). Global prevalence and determinants of mental health disorders during the COVID-19 pandemic: a systematic review and meta-analysis. *Annals of Medicine and Surgery*, **68**, 102634.

Chisholm, D., Docrat, S., Abdulmalik, J., Alem, A., Gureje, O., Gurung, D., et al. (2019). Mental health financing challenges, opportunities and strategies in low- and middle-income countries: findings from the Emerald project. *BJPsych Open*, **5**, e68.

Collins, P. Y., Patel, V., Joestl, S. S., March, D., Insel, T. R., Daar, A. S., et al. (2011). Grand challenges in global mental health. *Nature*, **475**, 27–30.

Degenhardt, L., Glantz, M., Evans-Lacko, S., Sadikova, E., Sampson, N., Thornicroft, G., et al. (2017). Estimating treatment coverage for people with substance use disorders: an analysis of data from the World Mental Health Surveys. *World Psychiatry*, **16**, 299–307.

Drake, R. E., Rosenberg, S. D., Teague, G. B., Bartels, S. J., & Torrey, W. C. (2003). Fundamental principles of evidence-based medicine applied to mental health care. *Psychiatric Clinics of North America*, **26**, 811–820.

Dua, T., Barbui, C., Clark, N., Fleischmann, A., van Ommeren, M., Poznyak, V., et al. (2011). Evidence based guidelines for mental, neurological and substance use disorders in low- and middle-income countries: summary of WHO recommendations. *PLoS Medicine*, **8**, 1–11.

Esan, O., Appiah-Poku, J., Othieno, C., Kola, L., Harris, B., Nortje, G., et al. (2019). A survey of traditional and faith healers providing mental health care in three sub-Saharan African countries. *Social Psychiatry and Psychiatric Epidemiology*, **54**, 395–403.

Fekadu, A., Demissie, M., Birhane, R., Medhin, G., Bitew, T., Hailemariam, M., et al. (2022). Under detection of depression in primary care settings in low and middle-income countries: a systematic review and meta-analysis. *Systematic Reviews*, **11**, 21.

Fond, G., Nemani, K., Etchecopar-Etchart, D., Loundou, A., Goff, D. C., Lee, S. W., et al. (2021). Association between mental health disorders and mortality among patients with COVID-19 in 7 countries: a systematic review and meta-analysis. *JAMA Psychiatry*, **78**, 1208–1217.

Griffiths, L., Blignault, I., & Yellowlees, P. (2006). Telemedicine as a means of delivering cognitive-behavioural therapy to rural and remote mental health clients. *Journal of Telemedicine and Telecare*, **12**, 136–140.

Gronholm, P. C., Henderson, C., Deb, T., & Thornicroft, G. (2017). Interventions to reduce discrimination and stigma: the state of the art. *Social Psychiatry and Psychiatric Epidemiology*, **52**, 249–258.

Gureje, O., Nortje, G., Makanjuola, V., Oladeji, B., Seedat, S., & Jenkins, R. (2015). The role of global traditional and complementary systems of medicine in treating mental health problems. *Lancet Psychiatry*, **2**, 168–177.

Gureje, O. & Thornicroft, G. (2015). Health equity and mental health in post-2015 sustainable development goals. *Lancet Psychiatry*, **2**, 12–14.

Hailemariam, M., Fekadu, A., Medhin, G., Prince, M., & Hanlon, C. (2019). Equitable access to mental healthcare integrated in primary care for people with severe mental disorders in rural Ethiopia: a community-based cross-sectional study. *International Journal of Mental Health Systems*, **13**, 78.

Hanlon, C., Alem, A., Lund, C., Hailemariam, D., Assefa, E., Giorgis, T. W., & Chisholm, D. (2019). Moving towards universal health coverage for mental disorders in Ethiopia. *International Journal of Mental Health Systems*, **13**, 11.

Institute of Medicine (2013). *Strengthening Human Resources through Development of Candidate Core Competencies for Mental, Neurological, and Substance Use Disorders in Sub-Saharan Africa: Workshop Summary*. Washington, DC: The National Academies Press.

Kakuma, R., Minas, H., van, G. N., Dal Poz, M. R., Desiraju, K., Morris, J. E., et al. (2011). Human resources for mental health care: current situation and strategies for action. *Lancet*, **378**, 1654–1663.

Keynejad, R., Spagnolo, J., & Thornicroft, G. (2021). WHO mental health gap action programme (mhGAP) intervention guide: updated systematic review on evidence and impact. *Evidence-Based Mental Health*, **24**, 124–130.

Li, J., Fan, Y., Zhong, H. Q., Duan, X. L., Chen, W., Evans-Lacko, S., & Thornicroft, G. (2019). Effectiveness of an anti-stigma training on improving attitudes and decreasing discrimination towards people with mental disorders among care assistant workers in Guangzhou, China. *International Journal of Mental Health Systems*, **13**, 1.

Maulik, P. K., Devarapalli, S., Kallakuri, S., Tripathi, A. P., Koschorke, M., & Thornicroft, G. (2019). Longitudinal assessment of an anti-stigma campaign related to common mental disorders in rural India. *British Journal of Psychiatry*, **214**, 90–95.

Mehta, N., Clement, S., Marcus, E., Stona, A.-C., Bezborodovs, N., Evans-Lacko, S., et al. (2015). Evidence for effective interventions to reduce mental health-related stigma and discrimination in the medium and long term: systematic review. *British Journal of Psychiatry*, **207**, 377–384.

Patel, V., Saxena, S., Lund, C., Thornicroft, G., Baingana, F., Bolton, P., et al. (2018). The Lancet Commission on global mental health and sustainable development. *Lancet*, **392**, 1553–1598.

Potts, L. C. & Henderson, C. (2021). Evaluation of anti-stigma social marketing campaigns in Ghana and Kenya: Time to Change Global. *BMC Public Health*, **21**, 1–14.

Saragih, I. D., Tonapa, S. I., Saragih, I. S., Advani, S., Batubara, S. O., Suarilah, I., & Lin, C. J. (2021). Global prevalence of mental health problems among healthcare workers during the Covid-19 pandemic: a systematic review and meta-analysis. *International Journal of Nursing Studies*, **121**, 104002.

Slade, M. (2009). *Personal Recovery and Mental Illness. A Guide for Mental Health Professionals*. Cambridge: Cambridge University Press.

Suran, M. (2022). Increased use of medicare telehealth during the pandemic. *JAMA*. **327**(4), 313. doi:10.1001/jama.2021.23332

Thornicroft, G., Alem, A., Dos Santos, R. A., Barley, E., Drake, R. E., Gregorio, G., et al. (2010). WPA guidance on steps, obstacles and mistakes to avoid in the implementation of community mental health care. *World Psychiatry*, **9**, 67–77.

Thornicroft, G., Alem, A., Drake, R. E., Ito, H., Mari, J., McGeorge, P., et al. (2011a). *Community Mental Health: Putting Policy into Practice Globally*. London: Wiley-Blackwell.

Thornicroft, G., Chatterji, S., Evans-Lacko, S., Gruber, M., Sampson, N., Aguilar-Gaxiola, S., et al. (2017). Undertreatment of people with major depressive disorder in 21 countries. *British Journal of Psychiatry*, **210**, 119–124.

Thornicroft, G., Deb, T., & Henderson, C. (2016a). Community mental health care worldwide: current status and further developments. *World Psychiatry*, **15**, 276–286.

Thornicroft, G., Lempp, H., & Tansella, M. (2011b). The place of implementation science in the translational medicine continuum. *Psychological Medicine*, **41**, 2015–2021.

Thornicroft, G., Mehta, N., Clement, S., Evans-Lacko, S., Doherty, M., Rose, D., et al. (2016b). Evidence for effective interventions to reduce mental-health-related stigma and discrimination. *Lancet*, **387**, 1123–1132.

Thornicroft, G. & Sunkel, C. (2020). Announcing the Lancet Commission on stigma and discrimination in mental health. *Lancet*, **396**, 1543–1544.

Thornicroft, G. & Tansella, M. (2014). Community mental health care in the future: nine proposals. *Journal of Nervous and Mental Disease*, **202**, 507–512.

United Nations (2006). *Convention on the Rights of Persons with Disabilities*. New York: United Nations.

United Nations (2015). *The 2030 Agenda for Global Action and the Sustainable Development Goals*. New York: United Nations.

Vai, B., Mazza, M. G., Delli Colli, C., Foiselle, M., Allen, B., Benedetti, F., et al. (2021). Mental disorders and risk of COVID-19-related mortality, hospitalisation, and intensive care unit admission: a systematic review and meta-analysis. *Lancet Psychiatry*, **8**, 797–812.

Vigo, D., Thornicroft, G., & Atun, R. (2016). Estimating the true global burden of mental illness. *Lancet Psychiatry*, **3**, 171–178.

Walker, E. R., McGee, R. E., & Druss, B. G. (2015). Mortality in mental disorders and global disease burden implications: a systematic review and meta-analysis. *JAMA Psychiatry*, **72**, 334–341.

Wang, Q., Xu, R., & Volkow, N. D. (2021). Increased risk of COVID-19 infection and mortality in people with mental disorders: analysis from electronic health records in the United States. *World Psychiatry*, **20**, 124–130.

Whiteford, H. A., Ferrari, A. J., Degenhardt, L., Feigin, V., & Vos, T. (2015). The global burden of mental, neurological and substance use disorders: an analysis from the global burden of disease study 2010. *PLoS One*, **10**, e0116820.

Winkler, P., Krupchanka, D., Roberts, T., Kondratova, L., Machu, V., Hoschl, C., et al. (2017). A blind spot on the global mental health map: a scoping review of 25 years' development of mental health care for people with severe mental illnesses in central and eastern Europe. *Lancet Psychiatry*, **4**, 634–642.

World Health Organization (2010). *mhGAP Intervention Guide*. Geneva: World Health Organization.

World Health Organization (2016). *mhGAP Intervention Guide for Mental, Neurological and Substance Use Disorders in Non-Specialized Health Settings: Mental Health Gap Action Programme (mhGAP) (Version 2.0)*. Geneva: World Health Organization.

World Health Organization (2020). *The Impact of COVID-19 on Mental, Neurological and Substance Use Services: Results of a Rapid Assessment*. Geneva: World Health Organization.

World Health Organization (2022). *World Mental Health Report*. Geneva: World Health Organization.

Wu, T., Jia, X., Shi, H., Niu, J., Yin, X., Xie, J., & Wang, X. (2021). Prevalence of mental health problems during the COVID-19 pandemic: a systematic review and meta-analysis. *Journal of Affective Disorders*, **281**, 91–98.

Zisman-Ilani, Y., Barnett, E., Harik, J., Pavlo, A., & O'Connell, M. (2017). Expanding the concept of shared decision making for mental health: a systematic and scoping review of interventions. *Mental Health Review Journal*, **22**, 191–213.

Index

For the benefit of digital users, indexed terms that span two pages (e.g., 52–53) may, on occasion, appear on only one of those pages.
Note: Tables, figures and boxes are indicated by an italic *t*, *f* and *b* following the paragraph number.

abuse 115–16, 402
   child abuse 441–42
   in hospitals 210
   human rights 83–84, 298, 335, 421
   physical and mental 87
   at Whorlton Hall 200, 202
   at Winterbourne View hospital 200
acamprosate 175*t*
acceptability, in evidence-based practices 371
acceptance and commitment therapy 150, 371
accreditation
   Centre for Quality Improvement (CCQI) 202, 203
   in the United States 203
Accredited Accommodation Scheme (Wales) 135
ACT *see* assertive community treatment (ACT)
Action for Mental Health 24
active response models 161
acute day hospitals 118, 190–91
acute inpatient care 117
   alternatives to 118–19
   outside inpatient units 127
   pathway 136
   in the United Kingdom 198–99
acute medical health care, in the emergency department 127–29
acute services, home-based 131
acute wards 134–35, 198–99
ADAPTE collaboration 378
adherence, to drug treatment 353, 358
admission, threshold of 127, 132, 199
adolescents
   alcohol misuse 315
   first-episode psychosis (FEP) 143
   guidelines for improving depression care in 375
   parents as prevention agents for depression and anxiety disorders 315
   risk and protective factors for depression 315
Adult Psychiatric Morbidity Survey (2014) 74–75
adults
   acute psychiatric inpatient service 201
   general adult mental health care 116–17
   mental health services in the 1990s 197
advance directives 118, 306–7
advance statements 306
adverse selection 344
advocacy 176, 287, 335, 461, 462
ÆSOP study 75
aetiology 23–24, 419
affective disorder with psychosis 142
Afghanistan 462
Africa 46
   collective identity of a person 419
   cultural values towards mental illness 323–24

digital mental health in 262
healing practices based on Islam and Christianity 418
mental health-related stigma in 323
number of psychiatrists in 417–18
policies on traditional and CAM 422
self-help user-led movement 46
traditional healers 417–18, 419
African Americans 74, 76–77, 78
   group intervention 255
   supported employment 220–21
   underdiagnosis and undertreatment of 87
age
   of onset of
     anxiety disorders 99
     eating disorders 101
     mental ill health 97
     substance use disorders 102
aggression 202
agoraphobia 46–48
AGREE II instrument 377, 377*b*
Aladura Church Movement (Nigeria) 418
alcohol use disorders (AUD) 102, 175–76, 234
   burden of 471
   Counselling for Alcohol Problems (CAP) 431
   impact of PRIME MHCP on 430
   medical comorbidity 233*t*
   medication-assisted treatment (MAT) 175, 175*t*
   PRIME MHCP in Ethiopia and 428
algorithms 476
Allan Memorial Institute of Psychiatry 187
Alleged Lunatics' Friend Society 243
allostatic load 234–35
Alma Ata Declaration 464
almshouses 23
alternative healing systems 418
alternative practitioners 417–24
Alternatives Study 134
Alvi, Arif 452
American Academy of Child and Adolescent Psychiatry (AACAP) guidelines 376
American Diabetes Association 237
American Psychiatric Association (APA)
   App Advisor Initiative 264
   App Evaluation Model 264, 265
   guidelines 376
   Task Force on psychiatric emergency services 129
analytical techniques 365–66
anecdotal evidence 369
anger 225, 322
Annan, Kofi 293–94
anorexia nervosa 101, 184
anticholinergics, deprescribing 174

anticonvulsant mood stabilizers 172
antidepressants 149
anti-discrimination laws 325, 327
antipsychotics 27, 149, 353–54, 357
   bipolar disorder 149
   first-generation 149
   long-acting injectable 175
   second-generation 149, 235
   side effects 149, 150
   weight management in people on 237
anti-realists 364
antisocial behaviours, induced by use of illicit drugs 341
anxiety disorders 99–100, 148, 398
   age of onset 99
   coping strategies 247*t*
   course and prognosis 99
   delays to get professional help 313–14
   early detection 99
   early intervention 99–100
   epidemiology 99
   impact of Covid-19 pandemic on 454
   medical comorbidity 233*t*, 234
   minimally adequate treatment for 51, 52*t*, 53, 66*f*, 66
   prediction 99
   prevalence of 51
   screening 99
   self-help strategies 314–15
App Advisor Initiative, American Psychiatric Association 264
App Evaluation Model, American Psychiatric Association 264, 265
apps, engagement with local mood and anxiety-related 263
Argentina 46, 47*t*, 50*t*, 51–52, 54–55, 398
aripiprazole 149
Asia 46, 57, 81, 104
   EMERALD programme 456
   mental health stigma in 323
   national mental health plans 455
   social health insurance 343
Asian Americans 82
   communication styles of 85
   health disparities among 82
   provider–patient communication disparities 85
   reluctance to discuss mental health needs 85–86
assertive community treatment (ACT) 116–17, 161, 192, 301, 354, 358
   active engagement or coercion in 166
   adaptations of 371
   aims of 285
   co-occurring alcohol and drug use disorders (COD) 256

Index

assertive community treatment (ACT) (cont.)
 development of 162–63
 differences between standard community mental health services and 163–64, 163t
 effectiveness of 165–66, 165t
 efficacy trial 355–56
 in England 164–65
 evidence for 164, 167
 examples of 166
 flexible 167
 forensic 166
 inadequate fidelity of 165–66
 modelling studies 354
 privacy in 285
 specialist and adapted 166
assertive outreach 161
assertive outreach teams (AOTs) 131, 166
assessment, of outcomes of treatments and services 475
asylums 196
 experimentation in 13
 move to community care from 196–97
 renamed as 'mental hospitals,' 12–13
 see also public hospitals
asylum seekers
 mental disorders among 75
 mental health of 75
 specialist services for 78
attention deficit hyperactivity disorder 147, 148, 273–74
attitudes, about serious mental illness 243
atypical neuroleptic drugs 357
audits 356
Australia
 early intervention in psychosis (EIP) 141
 evidence for schizophrenia and other psychoses in 75
 inpatient beds in 198t
 Minimum Data Set of the Partners in Recovery (PIR) national programme in 69
 models of youth mental health 154
 public views on psychiatric medications 314
 Queensland Mental Health Alcohol and Other Drugs Strategic Plan 62
 revision of mental health legislation in 337
 young people accessing headspace in 98
Authentic Happiness theory 36
autism spectrum disorder 147, 148, 200, 393
AVON Mental Health Measure 67
axis II disorders 147

back-end work 362–63
balanced care model 114, 117, 119, 469–70
 barriers for developing 122t, 122
 enhanced 469–70, 470f
 evidence for a balance of hospital and community care 115–16
 implementing 115–19
 in low-, medium-, and high-resource settings 115–16, 115t
Banstead Hospital 197
bariatric surgery 237
barriers, to mental health care 122t, 122, 379, 457
Barton, Russell 15
baseline
 legal 302
 moral 302
BasicNeeds programme 404
bed reductions 197, 198
beginning-of-life situations 284
behavioural family treatment 227

behavioural health technologies and telehealth 261–69
behavioural tailoring 247, 250
behaviour therapy 356t
Belgium 46, 47t, 50t, 51–52
beliefs, about serious mental illness 243
Belmont Hospital, Industrial Neurosis Unit 14
beneficence 287
benevolent paternalism 288
benzodiazepines 149
bereavement 440
best interests 304
best practices 370
Bethlem, London 195–96
Better Services for the Mentally Ill 17
Beyond Blue (Australian organization) 316
bias
 in mental health systems 273
 in trials of community mental health services 355
Bimaristans 195
binge eating disorder 101
bioethics 283–84, 288
 beginning-of-life situations 284
 end-of-life situations 284
 overview of 284
 principlism 284
 risk/benefit-to-others situations 284
biogenetic factors 324
biogenetic models 324
bipolar disorder 141
 guidelines on acute care 127
 medical comorbidity 233–34, 233t
Black Americans 74
Black Caribbeans
 in the United Kingdom 75, 77, 82
 in the United States 74
BluePages 317
bootstrap method 357–58
borderline personality disorder 100, 353–54
 dialectical behaviour therapy (DBT) 249
Bradley Report 271–72
Brazil 46, 47t, 51–52
 12-month contact coverage for DSM-IV/CIDI disorders by severity of disorder 50t
 mental health reform 463–64
 World Psychiatric Association anti-stigma initiative 324–25
brief educational programmes 228, 230
brokerage model 161
budgets
 management of 121
 see also funding
Bulgaria 46
 12-month contact coverage for DSM-IV/CIDI disorders by severity of disorder 50t
 Bulgarian Epidemiological Study of common mental disorders EPIBUL 54–55
 National Survey of Health and Stress 47t
bulimia nervosa 101
buprenorphine 175–76, 175t
burden
 of alcohol use disorders (AUD) 426
 analysis of disease burden 389
 of disability 390
 of disease 417–18
 of mental, neurological, substance use disorders, and suicide (MNSS) 389–90
 of mental illness 389
 non-communicable disease 389
 objective 225
 subjective 225

burnout, among health care workers 442, 454
Bush, George W., 27

Camberwell Assessment of Need (CAN) 67–68, 69
 empirical findings from 68
Camberwell Assessment of Need for Developmental and Intellectual Disabilities (CANDID) 67
Camberwell Assessment of Need—Forensic (CANFOR) 67
Camberwell Assessment of Need for the Elderly (CANE) 67
Camberwell Assessment of Need Short Appraisal Schedule (CANSAS) 67, 69
CAMHS units 201
Canada 81–82, 130–31, 164, 165, 205, 212
 Access Open Minds 98
 digital technology 288
 early intervention in psychosis (EIP) 141, 153
 emergency psychiatry 129
 estimates of local housing needs 209t
 housing and quality of life 212, 213t
 'Housing First' model 213
 inpatient beds in 198t
 models of youth mental health 154
 population-level needs assessment 69
 psychiatric inpatient beds in 198t
 public housing 287
 public views
  on antidepressants 314
  on psychiatric medications 314
 supported housing residents in 213
Canadian App4Independence (A4i) 263
cancer, as major cause of death among Asian Americans 82
cancer therapy 476
CAN—Clinical (CAN-C) 67
CAN—Clinical (CAN-R) 67
Candomblé, in Afro-Caribbean countries 418
cannabidiol 149
cannabis 102, 234
cannabis use disorder 233t
CANSAS—Patient-rated (CANSAS-P) 67
capitation payments 473
Caracas Declaration of Mental Health and Human Rights 402–3
Cardinal Needs Schedule (CNS) 67
cardiovascular disease 235
care, continuity of 136
care ethics 284
caregivers, programmes to support family members and 225–32
Care in Action 17
care in the community, criticisms of 17
Care in the Community 17
care management, for patients with serious mental illness 176–77
Care Quality Commission (CQC), England 202, 207–8, 210
carers, informal 286
Carers and Users Experience of Services (CUES) 67
Carter, Jimmy 26
case analysis, negative (or deviant) 366
case management 116–17, 161, 285
 co-occurring alcohol and drug use disorders (COD) 256
 differences between community mental health services and 163–64, 163t
 evidence for 161–62
 impact of Covid-19 pandemic on 168
 intensive 161–62, 166

levels of intensity of 168
models of 161, 162t
types of 161
case managers 161
Cassel Hospital 12–13, 14
Castle, Barbara 17
categorical imperative 283–84
CATIE (Clinical Antipsychotic Trials of Intervention Effectiveness) trials 235
Central Hospital (Warwick) 14n.5
Centre for Quality Improvement (CCQI) 202
challenges
    integrating mental health care in primary health care (PHC) 465
    of mental illness 476
charitable donations 345t
Charlesworth, Edward 358–59
Chez Soi model 213, 214
child abuse 441–42
child adversity 148
Child Health Improvement through Computer Automation (CHICA) system for maternal depression 375
childhood, neuroses of 12
childhood trauma 453
child neglect 441–42
children 441–42
    first-episode psychosis (FEP) 143
    impacts of infectious diseases on general and mental health of 441
Children Act (1948) 16
Chile, female participation in labour force within 4 months of Covid-19 pandemic 441
CHIME framework 34
China, People's Republic of
    12-month contact coverage for DSM-IV/CIDI disorders by severity of disorder 50t
    Mental Health Survey 47t
Christianity, healing approaches based on 418
chronic care model 88, 88f
    in the United States 189
chronic diseases
    among Asian Americans 82
    relationship between trauma and 83, 84t
chronic metabolic diseases 176
civil and political rights 295
Claybury Hospital 14
Client Assessment of Strengths, Interests and Goals (CASIG) 67
Clinical High At Risk Mental State (CHARMS) 100
Clinical Interview for DSM-5 (SCID) 147
clinical practice in the community, dilemmas in 285–86
clinical recovery 33
    definitions of 33
    features of 33
clinical staging model 97
Clinton, Bill 29
Clinton administration health insurance reform 29
clonidine 175t
clozapine 149, 151, 256, 273
Clunis, Christopher 210
cluster randomization 355
Cochrane Collaboration (Cochrane) 356
Cochrane Effective Practice and Organisation of Care group 380
coding, multiple 365–66
coercion 77, 285, 301, 302
    in assertive community treatment 166
    coercive intervention 20, 202
    coercive proposal 302
    coercive threats 302

in mental healthcare 20
objective and subjective 303
reduction in level of perceived 307
used only when necessary 307
cognitive behavioural therapy (CBT) 149
    apps 263
    for first-episode psychosis (FEP) 150
    group based 99–100
cognitive difficulties, coping strategies for persistent symptoms 247t
cognitive therapy 356t
Collaborative Psychiatric Epidemiology Surveys 74
Colombia 46
    12-month contact coverage for DSM-IV/CIDI disorders by severity of disorder 50t
    National Study of Mental Health 47t, 54–55
Committee on the Rights of Persons with Disabilities (CRPD) 293
communicable diseases 462
communication barriers
    communication style of patients 85
    cultural differences 85
    for immigrants and refugees 84–85
    levels of health literacy 86
    limited English-language proficiency (LEP) 85–86
    provider–patient 85–86
    socioeconomic differences 85
community
    as the context for mental health care 472
    and control 17–18
    deficiencies in recognition of mental disorders 314
    difficulties dealing with persons with severe disorders in 25
    importance of support of 119
    involvement in mental health care 463
    psychiatric care in relation to the 286–87
    as therapy 13–15
community advisory board (CAB), in Ethiopia district mental health care plan 426, 427t
community-based crisis assessment and home treatment
    CORE fidelity scale for 133
    current evidence on 133
community gatekeepers 104, 430–31
community health extension workers 427t
community health workers (CHWs) 88
community knowledge, on mental health first aid 315
community mental health
    definition of 3–4
    in the future 469–80
    introduction to 3–7
    public health perspective 3
community mental health care
    definition of 3, 3b
    evolution of 3–4
    obstacles, challenges, lessons learned, and solutions in implementing 476, 477t
Community Mental Health Centers Act (1963) (US) 24
community mental health centres (CMHCs) 24–25, 27
Community Mental Health Common Assessment Project (CMHCAP), Ontario, Canada 69
community mental health services
    mistakes to avoid in implementing 472–73
    population needs, treatment coverage, and focusing 113–14
    staff attitudes towards

institutional and community perspectives 114, 114t
service users and models of care 114–15
therapeutic orientation between the institutional and community perspectives 114–15, 115t
time needed to progress from initiation to consolidation phase 121
community mental health teams (CMHTs) 116–18, 161, 276–77
    assertive community treatment (ACT) teams 117–18
    early intervention teams 118
community psychiatry 11
    beneficence 287
    digital technologies 288
    key dilemmas in 287–88
    obligation to advocate or to whistle-blow 287
    social justice and basic human rights 287
    understanding of ethics within legal frameworks 287–88
community rehabilitation units 199
community support systems 28, 29
community treatment orders 297
Compass Strategy 317
complementary and alternative medicine (CAM) 85, 418–19
    cosmologies, philosophies, and explanatory models 419–20
    evolution of 419
    examples of 418
    national policies on 422
    use of the term 418
    WHO definition of 418
complementary and alternative practitioners (CAPs) 417–24
    effectiveness of 421
    prevalence of use, reasons for, and pattern of patronage of 420
complex care 199
compliance 353
Comprehensive Assessment of At-Risk Mental States (CAARMS) 146
Comprehensive Mental Health Action Plan 402, 403t
comprehensive psychiatric emergency programme (CPEP) 129
compulsion 303
concealment, of mental illness 324
concordance 353
conduct disorder 398
confidentiality 271, 285
confinement 14
    damaging and anti-therapeutic effects of 15
confirmability 364
conflict of duty, to patient versus others 286
conflicts, mental health consequences of 335
Conolly, John 358–59
consensus for change 472
consent to treatment 297
consequentialism 283
Consolidated Framework for Implementation Research 379, 379f
consolidation phase of change 121
consumer and recovery movement 243–44
consumer-held records 326
consumer–survivor–ex-patient movement 57
contracts 132
    block contracts 346b
    cost-and-volume contracts 346b
    between purchasers and providers 346b
    spot and call-off contracts 346b
control group 358

Index

co-occurring alcohol and drug use disorders (COD) 257
  active treatment stage 255
  affects on communities 254
  case management 256
  complications related to 253–54
  comprehensive, longitudinal involvement 255
  contingency management 256
  course of 254
  engagement treatment stage 255
  family therapy 256
  functional analysis 254–55
  group intervention 255–56
  integrated treatment 254–55, 257
  interventions 255–57
  medications 256
  persuasion treatment stage 255
  psychotherapy 255
  recovery 254
  relapse prevention stage 255
  research 257
  residential interventions 256
  risk factors for 253
  shared decision-making 255
  social determinants 256
  treatment 254, 255
co-occurring physical disorders 233–42
co-occurring substance use disorders 253–60
  prevalence 253
  psychosocial risk factors 253
  underlying factors 253
coping strategies for persistent symptoms 245–46, 247t, 371
co-production 62
coronary heart disease 82
coronavirus disease *see* Covid-19 pandemic
cost, of providing care to psychotic patients 357f, 357–58
Cotton, Nathaniel 195
Council of Europe 292–93, 292n.3
Council of State Governments and Governors Conferences 24
Countdown Global Mental Health 2030 449, 455
coverage 66
  actual 45–46
  bottlenecks in 46
  cascade 46, 46f
  concept of 45–46
  contact 52
  for DSM-IV/CIDI disorders by severity of disorder in WMHS 49, 50t
  effective 46
  indicators of 45
  potential 45–46
  treatment profiles 49–51
  types of, for high- versus low- and middle-income countries 52, 53f
  users' perceptions of care 50–51, 51f
'COVID-19 and Life Stressors Impact on Mental Health and Well-being' (CLIMB) study 454
Covid-19 pandemic 327, 401–2, 439, 443, 449–50
  crisis assessment centres 130
  and digital health technology 261
  effectiveness of electronic mental health intervention during 444
  impact on
    case management 168
    mental health of children and young people 456
    migrants and refugees 84
  and mental health 84, 453, 476
  structural changes in the brain from infection 440
Cowper, William 195
criminal justice, unfairness and bias in 273
Criminal Justice and Court Services Act (2000) (England and Wales) 272
crisis and emergency services 127–40
  acute care outside the inpatient unit 127
  assessment following police contact 130–31
  community-based crisis assessment and home treatment 133
  community-based crisis residential services 133–34
  core interventions 132–33
  crisis family placements 135
  crisis houses 118, 134, 203
  emergency departments, acute mental health care in 127–29
  extended assessment and diversion 129
  home-based acute services 131
  outside the general hospital 129–30
crisis assessment
  following police contact 130–31
  outside the general hospital 129–30
crisis cafes 130
crisis cards 306
crisis intervention theory 129
crisis mental health service models 135
crisis plans 118, 326
crisis residential services, community-based 133–34
crisis resolution and home treatment teams (CRHTTs) 127
  CORE fidelity scale for 133
  core interventions delivered by 132–33, 133b
  evolution of 131
  implementation of 131–32
  organizational characteristics of 132, 132b
  principles and practice of 132
crisis resolution teams, 24-hour 162–63
crisis services, informal drop-in 130
cris resolution and home treatment teams (CRHTTs), working practices of 131
critical realists 364
CRPD *see* United Nations (UN) Convention on the Rights of Persons with Disabilities (CRPD)
cultural activation 60
cultural beliefs 77
cultural competence 77, 78
cultural issues 114
cultural tailoring 88
cultural values, towards mental illness 323–24
culture, definitions of 73
custodial institutions 15–16

Dartmouth assertive community treatment scale (DACTS) 162–63
data, individual- and population-level 69
databases, for mental health 377
day care centres 188, 192
  in the United States 189
day centres, in the United Kingdom 189
day hospitals
  history of 187
  and partial hospitalized programmes 187–94
  in the United Kingdom 189
  in the United States 189
day treatment programmes
  evaluations of 220
  in the United States 189
decentralization
  of mental health care from tertiary care to community care 465
  resistance to decentralization of health resources 463
deception 302
decision-making, political 336–37
decision-making capacity 304
decision tools 475
de-hospitalization 463
deinstitutionalization 25, 27, 131, 197, 347
  criticisms of 26
  in the early 1970s 25
  economics of 348
  influenced by qualitative research 363
  job security concerns and 463
  research on 212
  resistance to 463
dementia 380
demonic possession beliefs, as cause of mental illness 418
Denmark
  assertive community treatment (ACT) 167
  crisis family placements 135
  early intervention in psychosis (EIP) 141
  evidence for schizophrenia and other psychoses in 75
  FACT teams in 167
  headspace 98
  models of youth mental health 154
deontology 283
dependability 364
depot antipsychotic medication 151
depot progesterone 235
deprescribing, definition of 174
depression 99, 148, 262
  apps 263
  Beyond Blue (Australian organization) 316
  conceptual model of trauma, PTSD, physical health and 86, 87f
  coping strategies for persistent symptoms 247t
  European Alliance Against Depression 316
  genetic vulnerability to 234
  health impact of 83
  Healthy Activity Programme (HAP) for 431
  impact of PRIME MHCP on 430
  impact on family members 225
  Lancet–World Psychiatric Association Commission on depression 456–57
  in low- and middle-income countries 450
  medical comorbidity 233t
  minimally adequate treatment for 51, 52t
  outcomes of duration of untreated 314
  PRIME in Ethiopia 428
  risk and protective factors 315
  self-help strategies 314–15
  smartphone apps 263
  websites 316
design, of clinical trials of treatment interventions 355
Deutsch, Albert 15
developed countries, lessons from mental care in 456
diabetes 82, 83, 84, 148, 176
  depression and 233
  disease burden (DALYs) across the lifetime globally 394f
  genetic risks 234
  from medication side effects 235
  prevention and treatment of 237
  rates of non-treatment of 235
  in refugees 86, 86t

risk factors 235
and screening for eating disorders 102
Diagnostic and Statistical Manual of Mental Disorders, fifth edition (DSM-5) 144
diagnostic criteria 377
dialectical behaviour therapy (DBT) 249
dialogical bioethics 284, 286, 288
diet interventions 237
digital apps 263–64
digital literacy 264
digital technologies 261, 288
    access to 264
    attitudes towards use of 261
    challenges in 264–65
    current evidence on 262–63
    definition of 261–62
    implementation in routine mental health care settings 264–65
    innovations in delivery of 265
    in low- and middle-income countries 262–63
    and specific mental health conditions 263
    for supporting mental health 261
    technology-enabled clinical care 265
    technology specialists 265
    user engagement 264
disability
    -adjusted life years (DALYs) 389, 391*f*
    persons with 293
disadvantaged social groups 81
discharge planning 201
discrimination 60, 286–87, 323, 472
    as challenge to community involvement in advocacy 462
    global patterns of 323–24
    links to violations of human rights of people with mental health conditions 402
    racial 60
    in the workplace 325
Discrimination and Stigma Scale (DISC) 323
disease burden disability-adjusted life years (DALYs)
    across the lifetime globally 394*f*
    global distribution 391*f*
    of MNSS across the lifetime globally 395*f*
disease outbreaks 439
    examples of infectious 439
    long-lasting mental health consequences 440
    sources of economic hardship during 440
dissemination and implementation (phase 4) 356
district general hospitals 16–17, 196, 197
district-level mental health care plans (MHCPs) 425
    advantages of 435
    benefits of 428
    economic benefits 428
    impacts of 428
    treatment coverage 428
disulfiram 175*t*
divination 421
domestic violence 83, 87, 453
do no harm 271
donors, external 345*t*
double-blind trials 356
drop-in crisis services 130
drug dependency 409
drug therapy, treatment fidelity 358
dyslipidaemia 86*t*, 174, 235

early intervention
    across the lifespan 104–5
    for mental and substance use disorders 99–104
    mood and anxiety disorders 99–100

early intervention in psychosis (EIP) 97, 141–59
    aim of 141
    clinical high risk for psychosis (CHR-P) clinics 153
    community services/teams 153
    core clinical interventions in first-episode psychosis 153
    design of 152
    education campaigns to raise awareness and signpost for referrers 152–53
    funding and resources 154
    future challenges for 154
    hub and spoke model 152
    importance of 141–42
    improving front-end access to Early Intervention Service (EIS) 153
    key components of 152–54
    people targeted by 142–43
    reducing the duration of untreated psychosis 152–53
    reduction of duration of untreated psychosis (DUP) 152–53
    service evaluation, development, and research 154
    staffing, training, supervision, management and governance 154
early intervention services (EIS) 147, 154, 357
    CHR-P clinics 153
    core clinical interventions in first-episode psychosis 153
    focus of 152
    funding and resources 154
    goal of 97
    long-term outcomes 152
    models 152
    reduction of duration of untreated psychosis (DUP) 152–53
    service evaluation, development, and research 154, 154*t*
    staffing, training, supervision, management and governance 154
early mortality, reasons for 234*t*, 234–36
Early Psychosis Association 141
early psychosis inpatient services 153
early psychosis service model 98
East Africa 439
eating disorders 101–2
    course and prognosis 101–2
    day hospital versus outpatient care 184
    early detection 102
    early intervention 102
    early-stage 102
    epidemiology 101
    inpatient unit teams 201
    screening for 102
economic burden on society, mental health conditions 409
economic hardship 440
ECRI Guidelines Trust 376
education interventions 324
effectiveness trials 373
effect size 371–72
efficacious 354
efficacy 354
effort syndrome 14
Egypt, World Psychiatric Association anti-stigma initiative 324–25
elderly persons 23, 26–27, 198, 442
    Camberwell Assessment of Need for the Elderly (CANE) 67
    see also older adults
electroconvulsive therapy 201–2

electronic case registries 475–76
electronic records 475
emergency department
    acute inpatient beds and services in 135
    in the acute medical health care 127–29
    case management interventions 128–29
    extended assessment and diversion following attendance at 129
    psychosocial interventions 128–29
    specialist psychiatric personnel 128
    training for staff 128–29
emergency psychiatric assessment, treatment and healing (EmPATH) 129
emergency psychiatry 129
'Emerging mental health systems in LMICs' (EMERALD) research programme 413*b*, 456
emotional disorders, true prevalence of 113
emotional distress, in migrant and minority ethnic populations 76
emotional health 453
emotional reactions, towards mental illnesses 322–23
empirical knowledge 59
employment
    as avenue to social inclusion 219
    supported 219–24
empowerment 229
end-of-life situations 284
England
    assertive community treatment (ACT) in 164–65
    bed numbers in 197
    compulsory admissions 200
    development of residential care for people with mental health problems in 207
    forensic inpatient provision 272
    long-stay hospital beds 207
    Mental Capacity Act (2005) 298
    mental hospitals in the 1930s in 13
    models of youth mental health 154
    monitoring frameworks 207–8
    move towards a 'recovery- orientation,' 212
    Multi-Agency Public Protection Arrangements (MAPPA) 272
    National Health Service and Community Care Act 65
    National Service Framework for Mental Health 164
    National Service Framework for Mental Health 209
    number of prison places 209–10
    outpatient clinics 183
    patients in mental hospitals at the outbreak of the First World War 11–12
    public asylums during the first half of the 20th century 196
    public attitudes towards people with mental health problems living in the community 211–12
    regulation in 202
    residential alternatives 209
    residential care 209
    Youthspace and Forward Thinking 98
    see also United Kingdom (UK)
Enlight guidelines 264
ENMESH (European Network for Mental Health Service Evaluation) 357
entitlement programmes 28
entitlements 296–97
    statutory 302
environmental interventions 453

epidemics and pandemics
  mental health aspects of 439–48
  public health response to 443–44
  vulnerabilities to the mental health consequences of 440–43
  vulnerability of persons with pre-existing mental health conditions 443
epidemiological instruments 68
epilepsy 393
  benefits of mental health care plans (MHCP) for people with 428
escitalopram 99–100
ethical challenges, approaches to addressing 286
ethical decision-making 286
  capacity/best interests framework 286
  paternalism framework 286
ethical framework for community mental health 283–89
  ethical problems 288
  mental health care of individuals in the community 285
ethics
  community mental health care and 284–85
  definitions and central theories in 283–84
  within legal frameworks 287–88
Ethiopia 426–29, 475
  components of the district mental health care plan 426, 427t
  development of the district mental health care plan 426
  health care in 469
  impacts of the district mental health care plan 428
  implementation of the district mental health care plan 427–28
  involvement of service users in national planning in 405b
  mental health stigma in 323
  National Mental Health Strategic Plan (NMHSP) in 405b
  scalable district mental health care plan (MHCP) 426
  Sodo district 426
Ethiopian Mental Health Service Users Association (MHSUA) 405b
ethnic groups 60
  disadvantaged 406
  during disease outbreaks 441
  distribution of mental disorders by 74–75
  level of burden of communicable and non-communicable diseases 441
ethnicity
  characteristics of 73–74
  and cultural diversity 73–80
Europe
  assertive community treatment (ACT) 167
  ethnicity in 74
  forensic community mental health services 271
  H1N1 swine flu outbreak in 442
  immigrants and refugees in 81
  Islamic healers in 418
  Mental Health Declaration and Action Plan 327
  mental illness-related stigma 323
  outpatient care 183
  social health insurance 343
  walk-in crisis intervention services 129
European Alliance Against Depression 316
European Convention on Human Rights and Fundamental Freedoms (ECHR) 292–93
European Network for Mental Health Service Evaluation (ENMESH) 357

European Union (EU) 197, 292n.3, 316, 334
  anti-discrimination laws 327
  immigrants and refugees in 81
evaluation 353
  preclinical or theoretical phase (phase 0) 354
  modelling phase (phase 1) 354
  exploratory trial phase (phase 2) 355
  randomized controlled trials phase (phase 3) 355–56
  dissemination and implementation phase (phase 4) 356
  choice of, for different treatments 356–57
  stages of 354–56
evidence-based medicine 37, 354
  enhancement by digital resources 475
  factors of 37
evidence-based mental health care 471
evidence-based practices (EBPs) 114, 369–74, 471
  articulation of the problem 370–71
  criteria for 370
  development of 370–73
  identification of possible treatments 371
evil spirits (jinn) 418, 419–20
EVITA (Evidence to Policy Advocacy framework) 412
evolution of community mental health care 4–5
expertise, decentralization of 463
explanatory models 419
explanatory trials 355
exploitation 302, 303
expressed emotion 226–27

FACT see flexible ACT (FACT)
fairness, in financing mental health 344
faith healers/healing 417, 418
families
  caring for people with mental disability 195
  impact of mental illness on 225–26
  listening to experiences and perspectives of 121
  multifamily group therapy 227
  professional view of 5
  programmes to support caregivers and 225–32
family consultations 228–29, 230
family-focused treatment (FFT) programme 227
family involvement 230, 463, 464
  barriers to 230
  integrated community models for 230
family programmes 226–30
  clinic-based 226
  features of 226
  peer-delivered 226
  principles and goals of 226
family psychoeducation (FPE) 226–28, 230, 247, 248, 250
  benefits of 227
  effectiveness of 227
  features of 227
  impact on family outcomes 227
family sponsor homes 131, 134
family stress 247
family therapy, co-occurring alcohol and drug use disorders (COD) 256
feasibility, in evidence-based practices 371
Federal Employees Health Benefits (FEHB) programme 29
federal entitlement programmes 25, 27
federal Substance Abuse and Mental Health Services Administration 28
feedback 192, 375
fee for service 346, 473
Felix, Robert H., 24
fidelity 372

financing
  of mental health 462
  mental health care 344–45, 345t
Finland 134, 230
first-episode psychosis (FEP) 141, 230, 263
  antipsychotic medication regimen in 150f
  biological investigations 148, 148t
  clinical formulation and diagnosis 148
  comorbid axis I and II conditions 148
  core clinical interventions in 153
  core details in the clinical history 147b
  definition of 143–44
  diagnosed by Child and Adolescent Mental Health Services 143
  discharge and long-term follow-up 151–52
  distinguishing types of 144–45
  distribution 143f
  early intervention 373
  family interventions 150–51
  group programmes 151
  guidelines for assessment and treatment 146–48
  initial assessment, formulation, diagnosis, and treatment plan 146–47
  mental state examination 147
  monitoring for emerging psychotic symptoms 149
  pharmacotherapy 149–50
  physical examination and investigations 147–48
  psychological interventions 149, 150
  relapse following 151
  risk assessment and management plan 148
  specialist community services for 166
  specific medication interventions 149
  stage-specific interventions 148–51
  standardized assessment tools 147
  treatment guidelines in 150
  vocational/educational/psychosocial interventions 151
  work and school for people with 221
First World War 12
flexible ACT (FACT) 167
  plus videoconferencing 168
fluoxetine 99–100
focusing 66
FOCUS smartphone app 263
forensic community mental health services 271–79, 306
  community treatment under legal mandates 275–76
  forensic inpatient provision 272–73
  forensic inpatient services 199, 209–10
  information sharing 275
  integration and separate provision 276
  mentally disordered offenders and generic outpatient services 276
  provision of care 273–75
  psychotherapy treatment 274
  resource constraints 276
  risk assessment in community settings 274–75
  social context 271–73
  structure and goals of care 273
  tensions and controversies 275–76
  treatment with medication 273–74
Fountain House 243
France 46, 51–52
  12-month contact coverage for DSM-IV/CIDI disorders by severity of disorder 50t
  inpatient beds in 198t
  moral treatment 196
  outpatient clinics 183
FREED early intervention programme, for eating disorders 102

freedom 36–37, 296–97
'Friendship Bench' initiative, Zimbabwe 456
Friern Barnet Hospital, North London 197
front-end work 362–63
frontline workers, during infectious disease outbreaks 442
Fulbourn Hospital 14
full-time hospitalization 187
  cost-effectiveness of partial versus 190
  effectiveness of partial versus 189–90
funding 341–49, 473–74
  allocation to providers 345–46
  community-based mental health care 346–47
  fairness in 344
  incentive-based 346
  lack of 462
  prepayment mechanisms 344
  progressive 344
  regressive 344
  sources of 343–44
  transitional or dual 347

gatekeeping role 132, 132b
Geertz, Clifford 361
gender-based violence, among migrants 83
General Accounting Office 26
general hospital psychiatric units 196
generalizability 358
general medical sector 49, 50–51, 52–53
general standards 207–8
general taxation 343, 343t, 345, 345t
genetic factors 234
genetic risks, for medical morbidity and early mortality 234
Germany 46, 316
  12-month contact coverage for DSM-IV/CIDI disorders by severity of disorder 50t
  admissions to hospitals in 200
  crisis houses 134
  crisis resolution and home treatment team (CRHTT) model 132
  development of partial hospitalization in 187
  effectiveness of electronic mental health intervention during Covid-19, 444
  flexible ACT (FACT) 167
  inpatient beds in 198t
  Nuremberg Alliance Against Depression 316
  outpatient clinics 183
  public support for improving services 316
  public views on psychiatric medications 314
  World Mental Health Survey 47t
Ghana 418, 419
  Christian and Muslim herbalists 420
  collaboration between biomedical practitioners and traditional and faith healers 422
  prayer camps in 418
  traditional and faith healers (TFHs) 420
Global Assessment of Functioning (GAF) 48
global budgets for facilities and programmes 473
global burden of disease 389, 390, 462
  across the life course 390–93
  results tool 343
  studies 334
global mental health 6, 402, 403–4
Global Mental Health Peer Network 402–3, 476
GLP1 agonists 237
Gnawa cults (Morocco) 418
goals
  of interventions 371
  recovery 34–35, 36
  treatment 36
Goffman, Erving 15

good life, types of 36
governments, mental health policy 335
GPs
  beliefs about, as a source of help 314
  first-episode psychosis (FEP) patients seen by 146
Grading of Recommendations Assessment, Development and Evaluation (GRADE) 377
Greece, crisis resolution and home treatment team (CRHTT) model 132
group homes 116, 208, 208t
group intervention, co-occurring alcohol and drug use disorders (COD) 255–56
group therapy 201–2
Guatemala, American Indian shaman in 418
guidelines 375–85
  adaptation of existing 378
  adaptation of identified knowledge or research to the local context 377–79
  barriers to using knowledge 379
  catalogues of external 376
  clinical practice 375
  framework for implementation of 377, 378t
  identification of in bibliographic databases 376
  identification of problems that need addressing 375–76
  implementation of 377, 383
  monitoring knowledge use and evaluation of outcomes 380–81
  for psychiatric disorders 377
  review and selection of 376–77
  trustworthiness of 376

H1N1 swine flu outbreak in Europe (2009), psychological effect of 442
habits, strategies that can create new habits or disrupt old ones 380, 381f
half-way houses 15, 18
hallucinations, coping strategies for persistent symptoms 247t
haloperidol 149, 353–54
harm, preventing harm to others 286
HCR-20, risk measure for violence 148
headache disorders 393, 398
headspace model of care 98
health
  right to 296–97
  social determinants of 61, 114, 234–35
Health and Welfare: The Development of Community Care 16–17
health care, ethical problems in 283–84, 288
health care behaviours, of people with mental illness 235
health care ethics see bioethics
health care professionals 326
  attitudes towards mental illness 322–23
  on the frontline of disease outbreaks 442
health care workers, assessment of, during the Covid-19 pandemic 454
health disparities
  among Asian Americans 82
  definition of 81
health insurance
  characteristics of mechanisms of 343t
  coverage for treatment services for mental health conditions 29
health issues, relevant to national mental health plan 409
health literacy 86
hearing voices 323

helplines, for persons in need of mental health assistance 444
herbalists, Christian and Muslim 420
herbal medicines 422
high-income countries (HICs)
  burden caused by drug use disorders 393
  complementary and alternative medicine (CAM) 418
  contact coverage for major depressive disorder (MDD) in 53–54
  disease burden in 393
high-resource countries 120f, 469
Hill, Austin Bradford 355
Hill–Burton Act (1946) 24
Hippocratic oath 284
historical changes in mental health practice 11–22
  community and control 17–18
  community as therapy 13–15
  community psychiatry 15–16
  institutions, blurring the boundaries of 16–17
  psychiatry 11–13
HIV/AIDS programmes 462
Hogan, Michael F., 27
holocaust survivors, study of stress, coping and thriving among 363
'Home Chez Soi,' 213
home treatment/crisis resolution teams 118
homicides 17–18, 202
hospital abuse scandals 210
hospital hostels 211
hospitals
  payments to 473
  state sector responsibility for government-run 345
Hospital Services for the Mentally Ill 16–17
hostels 119
Host Families scheme, Hertfordshire 135
Hoult, John 131–32
housing, estimates of local housing needs 208, 209t
Housing First model 213, 214
Humanitarian Emergency Settings Perceived Needs (HESPER) scale 67
human resources 474
human rights 283, 287, 402, 404–5, 462
  abuse 83–84, 298, 335, 421
  and basic health care values 471
  international 291–300
  underpinning of community mental health 294–96
  violations 334
Hungary 134, 316
Hunt, Paul 296
hybrid services 134
hypercholesterolaemia 82, 148, 176, 235
hyperglycaemia 148
hyperlipidaemia 235, 379
hypertension 83, 148, 174, 235
  association between PTSD and 83t
  public knowledge and awareness 313
  in refugees 86t
hypertriglyceridaemia 235
hypothesis testing 362

identity 73–74, 419
ideology 27–28
'if … then' propositions 302
ignorance about mental illness 321–22
illness management and recovery (IMR) programme 248, 249–50
illness self-management programmes 243–52
  behavioural tailoring 250
  consumer and recovery movement 243–44

illness self-management programmes (cont.)
    coping strategies for persistent symptoms 245–46, 247t
    development of 243–44
    dialectical behaviour therapy (DBT) 249
    family psychoeducation (FPE) 247, 250
    goals of 244
    historical factors in the development of 243–44
    illness management and recovery (IMR) programme 248
    medication adherence strategies 244–45, 245t
    methods for improving 244–47
    methods of teaching 247
    peer support 246, 248
    psychoeducation 244, 245b, 247, 250
    relapse prevention training 245, 246b
    research 247–48, 250
    shared decision-making 244
    Social and Independent Living Skills (SILS) programme 248–49
    social skills training 246, 250
    standardized 248–49
    stress management 246
    Wellness Recovery Action Plan (WRAP) 249
immigrants
    communication barriers for 84–85
    health status in the United States 81–82
    magnitude of mental health and resettlement problems 81
    mental health challenges of 81–93
immigration, health impact of 82–83
Immigration Act (US) 81–82
implementation 114
implementation plans 471
implementation science 471–72
Improving Health Systems and Services for Mental Health 412
inappropriate care 77
India 324, 429–30, 449
    budget for mental health in 345–46
    mental health initiative 452
    National Mental Health Programme (NMHP) 455
    PRIME mental health care plan (MHCP) 429
    TELE-MANAS programme 452
Indigo Network 327
individual placement and support (IPS) 151, 219–24
    obtaining and retaining employment 36
individual placement and supported employment
    cognitive studies 221
    compared to traditional approaches 219, 220t
    cost studies 221
    dissemination 221–22
    employment outcomes 220
    implementation and fidelity 221
    IPS Fidelity Scale 221
    long-term trajectories 221
    model 371
    principles and practice of 219–20
    randomized controlled trials 220–21
    review of research 220–21
    success and barriers 222
individual therapies 14, 15, 150, 227
inducements
    problematic 303
    and threats 302–3
industrial therapy 196
inequalities 453
infectious disease outbreaks, overview of mental health in 439–40
informal carers 286

informal family involvement 229
information, how to find quality mental health 316
information collection and dissemination 337
information sharing, between health and justice agencies 275
information technology 475–76
    integration of psychiatric and medical care using 238
initiation stage of change 121
injuries 390, 393
inpatient care *see* inpatient treatment
inpatient services *see* inpatient treatment
inpatient treatment 195–205
    in the 21st century 198–99
    asylum movement 196
    from asylums to community care 196–97
    bed reductions across the world 197
    coercion and control 200
    concerns about 199–200
    definition of 195
    development of a positive ward culture 202
    in England 202–3
    failures of 200
    history of 195–96
    inpatient experience of service users 201
    inpatient wards 201–2
    international trends in 197–98
    issues facing 203
    moral treatment 196
    open door policy 200
    pathways 201
    quality assurance and quality improvement 202–3
    quality of 200
    regulation 202
    scientific literature on 203
    in the United States 199, 203
    use of in the UK local population 165
    use of 'out-of-area' beds in 200
    by World Bank income group 198t
inpatient units *see* inpatient treatment
insanity 12
Institute of Medicine 375
institutionalism 15
institutionalization, of community mental health services 121–22
institutional neurosis 15, 196
insurance agencies 346
insuring, mental illness 341–42
integrated and community-based care 406
intensive care model, in the United States 189
international collaborative programmes 456
International Covenant on Civil and Political Rights (ICCPR) 292, 295
International Covenant on Economic, Social and Cultural Rights 292, 296
international donors 344
international human rights
    and community mental health 291–300
    law 291–93
international networks, to train public mental health leaders 465
internet, as source for health information 316, 475
interpersonal leverage 301–2
interventions
    coercive 202
    'common-sense' approach for developing 379–80
    cost-effectiveness of mental health 462
    dropouts 371
    evaluation in randomized controlled trials 372–73

    financial 379–80
    implementation and process measures 373
    to improve physical health 236
    inpatient-specific 201–2
    issues to address 238
    mapping 380
    organizational 379–80
    overview of reviews 380, 382t
    patient-centred 236t
    pilot testing of 371–72
    professional 379–80
    provider-centred 236t
    REFOCUS 36
    regulatory 379–80
    standardization of manuals 372
    system-centred 236t
    targeting habits and routines 380
    target populations 371
    theory-based behavioural change 380
intervention science 5
interviews, in-depth 361, 365
intravenous drug use, medical comorbidity 233t
'in vivo'
    contacts 165–66, 167
    work 163–64, 163t, 165, 166
involuntary detention 378
Iran 398
Iraq 46, 49
    12-month contact coverage for DSM-IV/CIDI disorders by severity of disorder 50t
    Mental Health Survey 47t, 54–55
Ireland 316
    crisis resolution and home treatment team (CRHTT) model 132
    early intervention in psychosis (EIP) 141
    inpatient beds in 198t
    Jigsaw 98
    models of youth mental health 154
Islam, healing approaches based on 418
Israel 46
    12-month contact coverage for DSM-IV/CIDI disorders by severity of disorder 50t
    headspace 98
    National Health Survey 47t
issue entrepreneurs 335
Italy 46
    12-month contact coverage for DSM-IV/CIDI disorders by severity of disorder 50t
    acute inpatient care 117
    community resettlement in 212
    crisis care following Covid-19 pandemic 130
    European Study Of The Epidemiology Of Mental Disorders (ESEMeD) survey 47t
    health care professionals in 322–23
    inpatient beds in 197–98, 198t
    outpatient clinics 183
    patterns of care in Verona 121, 121f

Japan
    12-month contact coverage for DSM-IV/CIDI disorders by severity of disorder 50t
    Illness Management and Recovery Programme (IMR) 248
    inpatient beds in 197, 198t
    schizophrenia stigma in 323
    World Psychiatric Association anti-stigma initiative 324–25
Jenkin, Patrick 17
Joint Commission on Mental Illness and Health 24
joint crisis plans 118, 306
Journey to Wellness guide 62

Kamuli (Uganda) 433
Kant, Immanuel 283–84
Kennedy, John F., 24
Kenya 418, 419
    Christian and Muslim herbalists 420
    traditional and faith healers (TFHs) 420
knowledge to action process framework 376f
knowledge use, sustaining ongoing 381

labels, mental illness 314
Ladder of Co-Production 62
Lancet Commission on ending stigma and discrimination in mental health 327, 449, 450, 451
Lancet Commission on global mental health and sustainable development 402, 469–70
Lancet Initiative (2011) 455
Lancet–World Psychiatric Association Commission on depression 449, 456–57
Langsley, Donald G., 24–25
large outbreaks of infectious disease
    increase of mental health conditions during 440
    prevention strategies for mental health during 445
Latin America 81–82
    community-based mental health treatments and rehabilitation programmes 116
    social health insurance 343
Latino Americans 74, 76–77
leadership roles, for individuals with lived experience 62
learning disability 200
Lebanon 46, 323–24
    12-month contact coverage for DSM-IV/CIDI disorders by severity of disorder 50t
    Lebanese Evaluation of the Burden of Ailments and Needs of the Nation (LEBANON) 47t
legal capacity, right to 298
legal rights, of people who experience mental health conditions 4
legislation 407, 462
Lewis, Aubrey 19
LGBTQ communities, migrants from 83–84
life events 33
    traumatic 82–83, 86
limited English-language proficiency (LEP) 85–86
literacy of mental health *see* mental health literacy
lithium 149, 172, 235
lived experience
    of a mental health condition 59
    in practice 61–63
    role in education and research 62–63
Local Government Act (1929) 13n.3
local needs assessment 68
local opinion leaders 382t
local stakeholders 119
    engagement with 119, 403–4
lofexidine 175t
loneliness 453
long-stay community residential care, alternative types of 119
long-stay hospital beds, policy of closing 336–37
long-term community-based residential care 117
low- and middle-income countries (LMICs)
    contact coverage for MDD in 53–54
    experiences of 456
    explanatory models of mental illness 419
    financial resources 343b, 461–62
    funding for mental health services in 473
    gap between need for services and availability of resources to meet the needs 444
    historical developments in mental health services 455
    infectious disease outbreaks in 444
    mental health in 449–60
    mental health leaders in 464
    mental health treatment gaps in 417–18
    overcoming impediments to community mental health in 461–66
    pathways to mental health care 420
    progress in 457
    traditional and faith healers (TFHs) 420
lower supported accommodation 119
low-income countries (LICs)
    contact coverage for major depressive disorder (MDD) in 53–54
    disease burden during childhood 390–93
    fees for health services 343–44
low-resource settings 120f, 469
lunacy 12
lunatics 12–13

Macarthur Violence Risk Assessment Study 253–54
McMaster Mental Health Modules 375
mad doctors 195
madhouses 195
Madhya Pradesh (India) 429
    integration of health systems in 430
    scaling up of mental health services in 430
    sustainable financing of the mental health programme in 430
madness 16, 18
major depressive disorder (MDD)
    contact coverage for 52
    coverage for 51–52
    effective coverage 53, 389
    impact of Covid-19 pandemic on 454
    minimally adequate treatment for 51, 52t, 53–54, 171
Malaysia
    Covid-19 modifications for psychological intervention 444
    health services 344
Mandelbrote Hospital (Gloucester) 14n.5
Mapperly Hospital (Nottingham) 14n.5
mapping, of key drivers of population mental health 409
marital prospects, mental illness affecting 324
market failure 341–42
Marlborough Day Hospital (London) 187
Maslow, hierarchy of needs 65
maternal depression, screening for 375
Maudsley Family-Based Treatment, anorexia nervosa 102
Maudsley Hospital 12–13
measurement-based care 172
media, reporting of issues by 335–36
Medicaid 25, 26–27, 29
medical care, inadequate 235–36
medical comorbidity 233, 233t, 234
    interventions 236, 236t
    mental illness 233t
medical morbidity
    causes of 234t
    reasons for 234–36
Medical Research Council Needs for Care Assessment (NFCAS) 67
Medicare 26–27, 29
medication
    and recovery 39
    side effects 235
medication-assisted treatment (MAT)
    opioid and alcohol use disorders 175t
    substance use disorders 175–76
medication management
    assessment of adherence 174–75
    care coordination and management to support 176–77
    coordination with family and key support persons 177
    coordination with other providers 177
    deprescribing 174
    dose and duration of treatment 173–74
    guidelines for prescribers working in community mental health settings 171
    initiation and ongoing 173–75
    timely follow-up 174
medicine man 419
medium-resource settings 120f, 469
member checking 366
mental, neurological, substance use disorders, and suicide (MNSS) *see* MNSS (mental, neurological, substance use disorders, and suicide)
Mental Aftercare Association 196
Mental Capacity Act (2005) 304
Mental Health (Surgeon General) 27
Mental Health, Human Rights and Legislation: Guidance and Practice 403
Mental Health Act (1959) 16
Mental Health Atlas 2020 454–55
mental health first aid 315, 317
Mental Health Gap Action Programme 335, 403
mental health literacy 313, 322
    deficiencies in 318
    examples of 313
    links to behaviours that benefit mental health from 313, 313f
    of university students 317
    web-based interventions 317
mental health nurses 326
Mental Health Parity and Addictions Equity Act 29
mental health policies
    after the Second World War 23–24
    in Commonwealth countries 455
    concept of 'recovery' in 27
    in the early 19th century 23
    in the early 21st century 28–29
    in modern United States 23–31
    national 333–40
    strategies to overcome challenges 410–12
    in WHO member states 327
Mental Health Policy and Service Guidance 412
mental health professionals
    role of 18
    support of an individual's recovery 35–37
mental health programmes 471
mental health rehabilitation services 166
mental health service responses 78
mental health services
    acceptable and attractive to users 306
    access to, and use of 76–78
    availability and organization of 287
    components relevant to low-resource, medium-resource and high-resource settings 120f
    improving delivery of 336
    involvement of patients in planning their own care 306–7
    measurement of access to 66
    organization of 462–64
    outcome measures 336
    partnership between housing providers and 209
    patterns of, in Verona 121, 121f
    planning and implementing 425–37

mental health services (cont.)
   public support for improving 316
   recommended structures for 407–8
   remote access to 444
   scaling up for whole populations 471–72
   steps in planning and budgeting for 342, 342f
   transformation of 472
Mental Health Study Act (1955) 24
mental health systems, recommended structures for 407–8
Mental Health Systems Act 26
Mental Health Treatment Requirement (MHTR) 272
mental hospitals
   barriers in new admissions, in last third of the 20th century 25–26
   budgets and bed capacities 347
   community alternatives to, during the 1950s 24
   cost of maintaining 16
   decline in populations of, after 1955 25
   downsizing of 463
   by the early 20th century 27–28
   in England and Wales in the 1930s 13
mental hygiene 12, 13
'Mental Illness in General Health Care' project 455
mental illness self-management programmes *see* illness self-management programmes
mental incapacity 304
'Mentally Healthy Nation,' American Psychiatric Association 456
mental state examination 147
Mental Treatment Act (1930) 12–13, 196
metabolic conditions 176, 235
metabolic screening 236
meta-diagnostic concepts 100
metformin 237
methadone 175, 175t
Mexico 46, 52
   12-month contact coverage for DSM-IV/CIDI disorders by severity of disorder 50t
   anti-stigma intervention for psychiatrists 326
   migrants in US from 81–82
   National Comorbidity Survey (M-HCS) 47t
M-Health Index and Navigation Database (MIND) 264
microaggressions 323
Middle East 46, 418
middle-income countries *see* low- and middle-income countries (LMICs)
migrants
   gender-based violence among 83
   impact of the Covid-19 pandemic on refugees 84
   from LGBTQ communities 83–84
migration 73
Milbank Memorial Fund 24
mild mental illness 48
military neurosis centres 13–14
Millennium Development Goals (MDGs) 462
Mill Hill Neurosis Unit 14
mindfulness 150
mindLAMP 265
miniethnographies 78
minimally adequate treatment 46, 53
   for major depression, anxiety disorders, and substance use disorders 51, 52t, 53
minimally effective treatment, in high-, lower-middle and low-income countries 66f
ministry of health 412
minority ethnic groups, specialist services for 78
misdiagnosis
   inappropriate care and 77
   of psychoses 76

mixed drug and psychological therapies 356t
MNSS (mental, neurological, substance use disorders, and suicide)
   age-standardized burden of 393
   disability-adjusted life years (DALYs) 393
   disease burden of 390–93
   distribution of burden in men and women 393
   global disability 390
   ranking of sex-specific 393, 396t
   variation of disease burden across the life course 393
   during the working years 398
   years lived with disability (YLDs) 393
Mobile App Rating Scale (MARS) 264
mobile crisis services 131
moderate mental illness 48
monetary benefits, conditional access to 302
Mongolia 324
mood disorders 99–100
   course and prognosis 99
   early detection 99
   early intervention 99–100
   epidemiology 99
   prediction 99
   Programme for Mood Disorders 192
   screening 99
moodgym 317
mood stabilizers 151, 235, 378
   in acute manic psychosis 149, 150, 150f
   anticonvulsant 172
   lithium 235
   for reducing violent offending 273–74
   side effects 176, 235
   valproate 235
moral hazard 341–42, 343–44, 343t
moral injury 442
moral treatment 196
morbidity, surveys of population-based 68
Morocco
   Gnawa cults 418
   Mullah in 418
mortality
   among Asian Americans 82
   anorexia nervosa and bulimia nervosa 101
   borderline personality disorder 100
   Covid-19, 84
   medical morbidity and early 234–36, 234t
   MNSS 390
   people with psychosis 233–34
   psychotropic polypharmacy 174
   schizophrenia 148
   smoking-related 82–83
   substance use disorders 175, 234
mothers and pregnant women with mental health problems (CAN-M) 67
motivational interviewing 103, 371
Movement for Global Mental Health 402–3
Multi-Agency Public Protection Arrangements (MAPPA) 272
multidisciplinary teams 177, 219
multiple coding 365–66
multiple drug therapy 356t
musculoskeletal disorders 393

naloxone 175–76, 175t
naltrexone 175–76, 175t
narrative therapy 61
National Alliance on Mental Illness (NAMI)
   Family-to-Family programme 226, 229
   Homefront programme 226, 229
National Comorbidity Survey Replication study 113, 113t

National Confidential Inquiry into Suicide and Safety in Mental Health (NCISH) 202
National Health Service (NHS)
   funding of 343
   'Hospital Plan,' 207
National Health Service Act (1946) 16
National Health Service and Community Care Act (1990) 207
National Institute for Health and Care Excellence (NICE) 166
   guidelines 376
   psychosis treatment recommendations 273
National Institute of Mental Health (NIMH) 24
national insurance 343t, 348
National Mental Health Act (1946) 24
national mental health policy 333–40
   development of 336
   evaluation of 337–38
   factors influencing policy cycle 338–39, 338t
   implementation of 337
   mental health professionals and 339
   problem identifications 334–36
   support for adoption of 337
National Mental Health Strategic Plan (NMHSP), in Ethiopia 405b
national plans
   in LMICs 465
   National Plan on Chronic Mental Illness 29
National Service Framework for Mental Health 207
National Service Framework for Mental Health in England 164
natural disasters, mental health consequences of 335
needle exchange programmes 336
needs 74–76
   for action 66
   assessment 65, 68–69
   definition of 65
   epidemiological evidence 74–76
   ethnicity, culture, and diagnosis 75–76
   health and social care 65
   for improved health 65–66
   individual-level assessment measures 67
   measurement of 65–72
   needs-led care planning 66
   prevalence and incidence 74–75
   risk and protective factors 76
   for services 66
negative attitudes, towards mental illnesses 322–23
negative rights 295
negative spillover effects 341
negative symptoms, coping strategies for persistent symptoms 247t
Nepal 430–31
   Community Informant Detection Tool (CIDT) 431
   district mental health care plan (MHCP) 430
   female community health volunteers (FCHV) 431
   lessons learned 431
   mental health stigma in 323
   National Mental Health Policy (1996) 430
   non-governmental agencies driving the planning agenda in 412, 413b
   proactive case detection 431
   psychological interventions by community psychosocial counsellors 431
Netherlands 46, 47t
   @ease 98
   12-month contact coverage for DSM-IV/CIDI disorders by severity of disorder 50t
   assertive community treatment (ACT) 167

Cumulative Needs for Care Monitor (CNCM)
database 69
development of partial hospitalization in 187
evidence for schizophrenia and other
psychoses in 75
inpatient beds in 198t
Netherne Hospital 14n.5
neurocognitive disorders 393
neuroses 12
neurotics 13
New Economics Foundation 36
New Zealand
12-month contact coverage for DSM-IV/CIDI
disorders by severity of disorder 50t
early intervention in psychosis (EIP) 141
inpatient beds in 197, 198t
Mental Health Survey 47t
population-level needs assessment 69
well-being budget 347
nicotine 102
nicotine cessation treatment 176
nicotine use disorder 176, 237
Nigeria 46, 49, 324, 418, 419, 449
12-month contact coverage for DSM-IV/CIDI
disorders by severity of disorder 50t
Aladura Church Movement 418
Christian and Muslim herbalists 420
collaboration between biomedical practitioners
and traditional and faith healers 422
Mental Health Leadership and Advocacy
Programme 465
National Mental Health Act (2021) 452–53
Nigerian Survey of Mental Health and Wellbeing
(NSMHW) 47t
Pentecostal healers 418
traditional and faith healers (TFHs) 420
nocebo effect 356
non-communicable disorders, disease
burden of 390
non-governmental organizations (NGOs) 345, 463
non-governmental sector 344
non-psychotic disorders, in migrant and minority
ethnic populations 74
non-reflective processes 379
North America, psychiatric associations in 376
Northern Ireland 46, 47t, 50t
Northfield Military Hospital 14
Norway
adoption of the crisis resolution and home
treatment team (CRHTT) model 132
assertive community treatment (ACT) 167
'Mental Health is For Everyone' programme 317
Nuremberg Alliance Against Depression 316
Nuremberg Code 284
nursing homes 25

Obama, Barack 29
occupation 117
alternatives forms of 119
occupational and industrial therapies 15
occupational therapists 201–2
offenders
management of 272
with mental disorders 306
older adults
during disease outbreaks 442
fear of direct affects of highly transmissible
pathogens 442
first-episode psychosis (FEP) 143
inpatient services 201
omega-3 fish oils 149
Omnibus Budget Reconciliation Act 26

OneHealth Tool 343, 343b, 410
online clinical decision support tools 375
open dialogue (OD) approach 230
opioid use disorder 398
medications for 175, 175t, 176
oppression 286–87
optional protocols 292
organizational development 474
organization of community mental health
services 113–25, 443–44, 445
balanced care model, implementation of 115–19
barriers to change 122
lessons learned 119–22
lessons learned from 119–22
local stakeholders, engagement with 119
pre-conditions 113–15
other specific feeding and eating disorders 101
outcome measures 357–58
cost 357–58
generalizability 358
outcomes 377, 380–81
out-of-pocket spending 345t
outpatient/ambulatory clinics 116, 117
outpatient care *see* outpatient services
outpatient civil commitment 271
outpatient clinics *see* psychiatric outpatient clinics
outpatient commitment orders 303
outpatient services
compared to
community mental health teams 184
day hospital treatment 184
inpatient treatment 184
other settings 184
costs of 184–85
evaluation of 184
history of 183

pain disorder 389–90
Pakistan 449, 452, 463
*Palgrave Handbook of American Mental Health
Policy, The* (Goldman) 28
pandemics 439
mental health aspects of 439–48
panic disorder 46–48
partial hospitalization 187
advantages of 188
as alternative to acute inpatient care 189
comparison with inpatient and outpatient
services 188
as continuation of acute inpatient care 189
contraindications for 190
cost-effectiveness of partial versus full-time
hospitalization 190
day care or rehabilitation 189
definition of 188
development and further growth of 187–88
disadvantages of 188
effectiveness of
outpatient treatment versus 191
partial versus full-time hospitalization 189–90
evaluative research 189
as an extension to outpatient care 189, 192
functions of 189, 192
history of 187
and overnight hospitalization or backup
beds 191
respite programme 190
satisfaction with 190
target populations 188
therapeutic factors 191–92
treatment duration 190
typology of 188–89

participation, in the community 57–58
Partnership in Action 207
paternalism framework 304–5
patient-oriented research 381
patient preference trials 356
Patient Protection and Affordable Care Act 29
payment systems 473–74
'pay-as-you-go,' 348
prospective 473
retrospective 473
peer-led programmes 226, 229–30
peer-led services 61–62
peer providers 61–62
peer recovery support services 61–62
peer respite programmes 62
peer specialist training programmes 62
peer support 5, 36, 61–62, 201–2, 246
people-centred care 405–6
people with lived experience (PWLE) 402, 404, 413
Personal Assessment and Crisis Evaluation (PACE)
criteria 146
personal identity 35
personality-based interventions 103
personality disorders 100–1, 147
course and prognosis 100
day hospital versus outpatient care for people
with 184, 185
early detection 100
early intervention 100–1
effectiveness of outpatient, day hospital and
inpatient treatment in patients with 184
epidemiology 100
inpatient care for people with 199
partial hospitalization for patients with 192
prevalence of 100
personal medicine 39
balance between pill medicine and 39
personal recovery 33–35, 406
definitions of 34
and medication 39
treatment goals 36
personal recovery framework 35, 36f
personal weakness, mental illness perceived
as 324
person-centred care planning 37–39
based on person's strengths 38
centred on an individual person 37–38
change over time with person's evolving goals
and needs 38
encouragement and support of the person in
assuming control over their life 38–39
person's own role in their recovery 38
plans and services understandable to the
person 38
personhood 4
persuasion 301
pharmacotherapy 51
physical activity, in people with mental
illness 237
physical disability 402–3
physical disorders
people with psychosis and 233–34
relationships between mental illness and 233
physical distancing 440, 442
physical health
conceptual model of trauma, PTSD, depression
and 86, 87f
parity between mental health and 405
pill medicine 39
pilot testing, of interventions 371–72
placebo effect 356, 358
placebos 353–54

Index

planning national mental health care 401–15
  areas of action involved in 407
  collaboration with stakeholders 411
  contextualization of 410–11
  creation of a supportive network for a system change 411–12
  determination of
    costs and resources available and budget 410
    major activities 410
    strategies and time frames 410
  gaps in 404
  within the global policy context 402–4
  guidelines and materials 412
  indicators and targets 410
  key elements of 406–9
  monitoring and evaluation of 410
  multisectoral collaboration and action 408–9
  outline o 409–10
  preparatory steps 409
  recommendations for successful 413b
  relevance of mental health to national planners 401–2
  urgency of global action for 402
  vision for 407
pleasant life 36
point-of-contact information 475
Polak, Paul 131
Poland 46, 47t, 50t
police
  crisis intervention teams 272
  involvement in mental health crises 130
policy 462, 471
  change 356t
  cycle 333, 333f
  definition of 333
  level development 454–55
political interests, linking with reform of mental health care 473
polypharmacy 174
Portugal 46, 316
  12-month contact coverage for DSM-IV/CIDI disorders by severity of disorder 50t
  International Master in Mental Health Policy and Services 465
  National Mental Health Survey 47t
positionality 364
posteriori knowledge 59
post-modernists 364
post-traumatic stress disorder (PTSD) 82–83, 147
  conceptual model of trauma, depression, physical health and 86, 87f
  relationship between physical illness and 83, 83t
poverty 334, 402, 408
Powell, Enoch 16–17
power statements 39
pragmatic trials 353–54, 355
prayer camps, in Ghana 418
prejudices 322–23, 472
  gut level 322
  'hot,' 322
prescribed medications
  medication adherence strategies 244–45, 245t
  protocol for the initiation and follow-up of 379
Prescribing Observatory for Mental Health (POMH-UK) 203
pressure, used only when necessary 307
prevalence of mental health conditions
  estimates of 69
  relationship between true and treated 113, 113f
  treated 113
  true 113

prevention, of mental disorders 27–28, 236, 315, 408
primary care see primary health care
primary health care
  access to 86
  barriers for refugees accessing 87, 87b
  definition of 86
  mental health integration 406, 412, 464, 465, 474
  role of 86–88
  with specialist back-up 116
primary health care providers 87
PRIME 425–37, 456
  aim of 425
  in Ethiopia 426, 428
  intervention coordinator 427–28
  planning, implementation, and evaluation tools 435
PRIME India mental health care plan (MHCP)
  development of 429–30
  enabling packages 429
  functioning programme management package 429
  impacts of 430
  lessons learned 430
  service delivery packages 429
principlism 288
prisons
  community mental health input to 272
  people with mental illness in 209–10
privacy 285
private insurance companies 341–42
prodromal symptoms
  Scale of Prodromal Symptoms (SOPS) 146
  screening for individuals with 378–79
  Structured Interview for Prodromal Symptoms (SIPS) 146
professional attitudes, towards mental illness 196
professional help, knowledge of 314
Programme for Improving Mental health carE see PRIME
promotion, of mental health 408
protection of others 305–6
protocols 292
provision mixed economy, mental health care 344–45, 345t
psychiatric advance directives (PAD) 118–19, 306–7
  facilitated 307
psychiatric assessments, racial stereotyping in 76
psychiatric associations, in North America 376
psychiatric care, integration of medical and 237–38
psychiatric decision units 129
psychiatric emergency services (PESs), in general hospitals 129
psychiatric hospitals, societal attitudes towards conditions in 335
psychiatric institutions 463
psychiatric intensive care units 199
psychiatric interventions 11
psychiatric medications, public views on 314
psychiatric nursing 14–15
psychiatric outpatient clinics 183–86
  costs of 184–85
  definition of 183
  efficacy and effectiveness of 185
  evaluation of 184
  functions of 183–84
  history of 183
Psychiatric Services (journal) 28
psychiatric social work 16
psychiatric treatments
  evaluation in community psychiatry 356, 356t

forced 296–97
psychiatrists 326
  role of 465, 474
psychiatry
  scope in community mental health 19
  territory of 11–13
  World Psychiatric Association–Lancet Psychiatry Commission on the future of psychiatry 453
psychodynamic therapy 356t
psychoeducation 226, 250
  mental illness self-management programmes 244, 247
  outline of curriculum about psychiatric disorders 245b
psychological assessments 201–2
psychological services, to support people in or seeking work 326
psychological treatments
  application of 377
  treatment fidelity 358
psychopathology 11–12
psychopharmacology 15–16, 175–76
psychopharmacology assessment 171–72
  initial psychiatric evaluation 172
  testing, diagnosis, and target symptoms 172
psychosis
  affective 142, 144–45, 145f
  apps for 263
  benefits of mental health care plan (MHCP) for people with 428
  Camberwell Assessment of Need (CAN) 67–68
  clinical staging model of 145–46
  community-based rehabilitation ('RISE' trial) for people with 428
  delays to get professional help 313–14
  development timelines/trajectories and clinical staging of 145f
  duration of untreated psychosis and steps in the pathways to care 141–42, 142f
  early intervention 29, 97, 118, 141–59
  general population risk of and clinical staging 1–IV PACE 144f
  medical comorbidity 233t
  non-affective 144–45, 145f
  outcomes of duration of untreated 314
  outpatients under forensic care with 273
  partial hospitalization for patients with 192
  point prodrome ends and acute psychotic episode begins 144
  prevalence in migrant and minority ethnic populations 75, 76
  recovery rates in long-term follow-up studies of 34t
  screening for individuals with prodromal symptoms of 378–79
  stages
    asymptomatic at-risk group (stage 0) 145
    mild symptomatic clinical high-risk group (stage 1a) 145
    clinical high-risk group with subthreshold/prodromal symptoms (stage 1b) 146
    first-episode psychosis (stage 2) 146
    incomplete/partial remission and relapse (stage 3) 146
    severe, persistent, unremitting, treatment-refractory psychosis (stage 4) 146
  Treatment and Intervention in Psychosis (TIPS) 317
  treatment of 273
Psychosis Risk Syndrome 144
psychosocial disability 402–3

psychosocial interventions 356–57
psychosocial rehabilitation 474
psychosocial treatments 356
psychotherapy 24–25, 51
   based on relational frame theory 371
   co-occurring alcohol and drug use disorders (COD) 255
   in forensic community mental health services 274
psychotic disorders *see* psychosis
psychotics, pre-Second World War psychiatric population 13
psychotropic drugs 15, 24, 171, 172
psychotropic polypharmacy 174
PTSD *see* post-traumatic stress disorder (PTSD)
public advocacy 326
Public Health Service 24
public hospitals 27–28
public housing facilities 16
public knowledge and awareness about mental illness 313–19
   interventions based in educational institutions 317
   interventions to improve 316–17
   population interventions to improve 316–17
   prevention of mental disorders 315
   recognition of developing disorders which can guide early help-seeking 313–14
public mental health leaders, training courses for 465
public mental health leadership 464–65
public mental health systems, adaptions during large outbreaks of infectious diseases 443
public mental hospitals 196
public perceptions, regarding risks posed by people with mental illness 210
public policy 287
public policy cycle 333, 333f
public providers, funding of 473
Puras, Dainius 296

qualitative research 361–67
   aims of 361–62
   in community mental health 363
   confirmability 364
   credibility 364
   criteria of rigour in 364
   data analysis 362–63
   dependability 364
   in-depth interviews 361
   design and execution of 362–63
   differences between quantitative research and 362, 362t
   ensconced in existing literature 366
   ethnographic observation 361
   focus groups 361
   'front-end' work and 'back-end work,' 362–63
   published in journals 363
   relevance 364
   reliability 364
   residential care 213
   sample sizes in 365
   transferability 364
   trustworthiness 364
   validity 364
quality 471, 473–74
quality assurance 474–76
quality of care 211
   training and 210t, 211
quality of life 211
   factors in determining 211
   housing and 212

   for people with mental illness 334
quality outcome studies 212, 213t
quantitative research 362
   differences between qualitative research and 362, 362t
   'front-end' work and 'back-end work,' 362–63
quarantines during pandemics
   detrimental impacts of 440
   reducing the effects of 445
quasi-experimental design 370
Querido, Arie 131
quetiapine 149

race 60, 74
racism 60
   institutional 77–78
   structural 60
Randomised Evaluation of Assertive Community Treatment in North London (REACT) study 164–65, 166
randomized controlled trials (RCT) 355–56, 369, 370
   cluster 372–73
   comparison groups for 373
   conduction in real-world clinical settings 370
   effectiveness studies 373
   efficacy studies 373
   evaluation of interventions in 372–73
   individual 372–73
   outcome measures 373
   primary outcomes 373
   sample sizes 355
   secondary outcomes 373
rapid appraisal/rapid assessment techniques 69
Rawls, John 283–84
REACT study 164–65, 166
Reagan, Ronald 26
recognition, of mental disorders 314
recovery 27, 33–42
   being in recovery with a mental illness *see* personal recovery
   CHIME framework 34
   concept of 28
   definitions of 3–4, 33, 243–44
   as an integrative paradigm 34–35
   link with sociopolitical movements 35
   medication and 39
   and mental health professionals 35–37
   'from' mental illness *see* clinical recovery
   paradigm 35, 363
   person-centred care planning and 37–39
   principles of 208
   in residential care 212
Recovery-Oriented Decisions for Relatives' Support (REORDER) programme 229
Rees, John Rawlings 13–14
REFOCUS intervention 36
refugees
   common presenting health problems in 86, 86t
   communication barriers for 84–85
   health status in the United States 81–82
   magnitude of mental health and resettlement problems 81
   mental disorders among 75
   mental health challenges of 81–93
   mental health of 75
   specialist services for 78
regulation, in England 202
rehabilitation 117, 192, 199
   alternatives forms of 119
rehabilitation model, in the United States 189

rejection
   'cold' forms of 322
   emotional aspects of 322
relapse prevention training 245, 246b
relationships, fostering of 35–36
reliability 364
   internal 370–71
   inter-rater 364, 370–71
   test–retest 364, 370–71
religion 417
   connection between spirituality, mental health and 417
   healing practices informed by 422
   religious conversions 419
religiosity 454
religious, alternative, and complementary practitioners 417–18
   definitions of 418
religious groups 418
remote appointments 475
research
   community mental health 5
   engagement of service users in 19–20
   replication of 370
   on unmet needs 5
research assistants, posing as 'pseudopatients' at psychiatric hospitals 363
research designs, multiple baseline research design 370
research designs and evaluating treatment interventions 353–60
   choice of evaluations for different treatments 356–57
   outcome measures 357–58
   patient preference trials 356
   stages of evaluation 354–56
residential care 207–17
   24-hour 119, 212
   community-based crisis assessment and home treatment 213
   day-staffed 119
   estimation of needs 208–9
   forms of 208
   historical and policy background 207–8
   housing developments 214
   leaders in care teams 211
   lower supported accommodation 119
   outcomes 212–13, 214
   for people with disabilities 207
   planning and estimation of needs 214
   qualitative research 213, 214
   quality of the housing environment 211
   quantitative research 214
   recovery orientation 214
   rules and restrictions 211
   staff and staff training 210–11
   staffing and interventions 214
   transitional residential rehabilitation approach to 213
   types of 208, 208t
   user preferences 214
residential homes 119
residential interventions 256
resilience 39, 453
resource(s)
   decentralization of 463
   needs 342–43, 471–72
respondent validation 366
retention 371
revenue collection 343
'revolving door' patients 162–63, 209, 271, 433
rhetoric 27–28

Richmond Fellowship 15
right(s)
  to legal capacity 298
  to live in the community 297
  to treatment 335
rights-based approach 297, 404–5
rigour
  reflexivity as a criterion of 364
  techniques and strategies to enhance 365–66
risk 18
  assessment and management of 18, 271
  of harm to others 286
  high 18
  knowledge of risk factors that can be used to guide preventive action 315
  low 18
  management of, in the community 19
  medium 18
  poor mental health risk factors 402
risperidone 149
Robert Wood Johnson Foundation 28
Romania 46, 51–52
  12-month contact coverage for DSM-IV/CIDI disorders by severity of disorder 50t
  Mental Health Survey 47t
routines, strategies that can create new routines or disrupt old ones 380, 381f
Royal College of Psychiatrists 202
Royal Commission on Lunacy and Mental Disorder 12, 13n.3
Royal Commission on Mental Illness and Mental Deficiency 16
Rwanda 462

'Safer Services' toolkit 202
samidorphan 237
sampling 365
  by multidisciplinary teams 365
  nature and scope of samples 365
  sample sizes 362
SARS-CoV-2 pandemic see Covid-19 pandemic
satanic entities (shaytaan) 418
Saudi Arabia 46, 47t, 50t
Scale of Prodromal Symptoms (SOPS) 146
schizoaffective disorder, psychotropic polypharmacy in patients with 174
schizophrenia 141
  Accelerated Medicines Partnership (AMP) Schizophrenia (SCZ) programme 154
  apps targeting 263
  assumption of violent, unpredictable behaviour of people with 321–22
  attitudes towards discharge of patients with 196
  brief educational programmes 228
  and cardiovascular disease 234
  concept of recovery from 27
  day hospital versus outpatient care for people with 184
  families with high or low expressed emotion of people with 226–27
  family psychoeducation (FPE) 227–28
  guidelines on acute care 127
  lifespans for people with 148
  long-term outcome of 243–44
  medical comorbidity 233t
  in migrant and minority ethnic groups 75, 76
  needs assessment measures 67–68
  outpatient versus inpatient treatment for people with 184
  prescription of antipsychotic drugs in 356
  psychotropic polypharmacy in patients with 174
  rates of respiratory disorders in people with 233–34
  social skills training 247
  in utero exposure to 1918 flu and risk of developing 441
Schizophrenia Patient Outcomes Research Team (PORT) 127
Schizophrenia Proneness Instrument-Adult (SPIA) 146
schizophrenia spectrum disorders, Social and Independent Living Skills (SILS) programme 248–49
schools
  mental health literacy interventions in high schools 317
  as safe environment for children 441
scientific evidence 369
secondary prevention 236
Second World War 13
  mental health policy in the US following 29
secure services 210
Sehore, India 429
selective serotonin reuptake inhibitors 99–100
self-directed care 347
self-harm 104, 393
  course and prognosis 104
  early detection 104
  early intervention 104
  epidemiology 104
  postvention as prevention/early intervention 104
self-help groups 35–36
self-help movement 244
self-help strategies
  knowledge of 314–15
  public views on 315
self-help user-led movement 57
self-interest 472
Sen, Amartya 36–37
serendipity 371
serious mental disorder 25
serious mental illness 233
  inadequate medical care for people with 235
  prevalence of co-occurring alcohol and drug use disorders (COD) 253
  see also severe mental illness
services, population-level service planning 69
service users 57
  acting in the health interests of 286
  definition of 57
  involvement in national planning in Ethiopia 405b
  self-directed care financing 347
  stigmatization or marginalization of 58
  use of, in the design of mental health services 19
  wellness habits to manage trauma and mental challenges 61
severe mental disorders 393
severe mental illness
  definition of 48
  independent housing and support for people with 213
  rate of co-occurring alcohol and drug use disorders in people with 257
  see also serious mental illness
severity, of mental disorders 48
sex offenders 287–88
  psychotherapy for 274
  treatment of 274
shared care agreements 326
shared decision-making 172–73, 236, 244
  CommonGround program 173
  co-occurring alcohol and drug use disorders (COD) 255
  and family involvement 229
  goals and preferences related to psychiatric medications 172–73
  information regarding medication options 173
  information technology and 475
  joint decisions 173
Sheehan Disability Scales (SDS) 48
shell shock 12
Siberia 324
side effects, of psychiatric medications 176
Sierra Leone, barriers to mental health programmes during Ebola outbreak 444
single drug therapy 356t
Sitharaman, Nirmala 452
skin colour 74
sleep problems, coping strategies for persistent symptoms 247t
slums 453
smartphone apps 261, 262
smartphones 264
Social and Independent Living Skills (SILS) programme 248–49
social attainments 65
social behaviour 65–66
social contact, with people with mental illness 327
social determinants 406, 409, 473
  Covid-19 and 454
  of mental health 453–54
social disablement 65
social environment 35
social exclusion 324, 334
social functioning measures 65
social health insurance 343, 344
social identity 35
social inclusion 36–37, 58, 287, 325, 325t
social insurance 16, 343t, 345t
social isolation, during pandemics, effects of 440
social justice 57, 57t, 287
  through advocacy 57–58
social learning theory 371
social networks 453
Social Psychotherapy Centre (later Marlborough Day Hospital) (London) 187
social role performance measures 65
social services 463
social skills training 246, 247, 250, 371
social systems intervention 132–33
social welfare 23
socioeconomic status, low 440
soft paternalism 304
somatization 77
somatoform disorders 393
  with prominent pain 389–90
Soteria model 134
Soteria service (Loren Mosher) 134
South Africa 46, 47t, 431–33, 463
  12-month contact coverage for DSM-IV/CIDI disorders by severity of disorder 50t
  challenges for PRIME project 432
  Department of Health 432
  Department of Social Development 432
  development of the district mental health care plan 431–32
  impacts of the district mental health care plan 432–33
  implementation of the district mental health care plan 432
  lessons learned from PRIME programme 433
  multilevel planning for decentralized implementation 411, 411b

Primary Care 101 (Adult Primary Care) 431
PRIME programme in 431
Southern African Mental health INTegration (SMhINT) project 432
South Sudan 439
Spain 46, 47t
   12-month contact coverage for DSM-IV/CIDI disorders by severity of disorder 50t
   crisis resolution and home treatment team (CRHTT) model 132
   inpatient beds in 198t
'spatial' distancing 440
Spears, Britney 298
special education 295
specialist acute community teams, focus on preventing admissions 131
specialized mental health services 117–19
   community mental health teams (CMHTs) 117–18
   outpatient/ambulatory clinics 117
specific occupational groups, during disease outbreaks 442–43
spending, on mental health 347–48
spirituality 417
   healing practices informed by 422
staff, and staff training 210–11
stakeholders 336, 473
   local 119, 121b
standardization, of interventions 370
Stein, Leonard 131, 162–63
Stein and Test's (1980) 'Training in Community Living,' 162–63
stereotypes 322
Stevens–Johnson syndrome/toxic epidermal necrolysis 172
stigma 58–59, 211–12, 286–87, 314, 334, 341
   as challenge to community involvement in advocacy 462
   components of 321
   definition of 321
   and discrimination 6
      reducing 321–30
   education interventions to reduce 324
   elements of 321
   faced by patients with mental illness 176
   global patterns of 323–24
   health care professionals 326
   individual 58, 59
   interpersonal 58, 59
   Lancet Commission on stigma and discrimination in mental health 451
   links to violations of human rights of people with mental health conditions 402
   literature on 321
   local-level strategies to reduce 325
   national-level campaigns to reduce 324–25
   personal contact with persons with mental illness to reduce 324
   person-level interventions to reduce 325–26
   policy-level interventions to reduce 326–27
   protests, to reduce 324
   public-level interventions to reduce 324–25
   reduction of 472
   role in public policy 287
   self-stigma 59
   structural 58–59
   'thick description' of 361–62
   towards men with mental illness 323–24
'Strategies for Extending Mental Health Care' (1975–1981) 455
stress management 246

Structured Interview for Prodromal Symptoms (SIPS) 146
subclinical psychosis 143–44
sub-Saharan Africa 422, 469
   funds for mental health services in 462
   number of traditional and faith healers (TFHs) in 420
   pathways to mental health care 420
   traditional and faith healing in 419, 420, 421
substance abuse 25, 335
substance use
   early onset 103
   motives for 255
substance use disorders 102–3, 148, 393
   co-occurring 253–60
   course and prognosis 102–3
   early detection 103
   early intervention 103
   epidemiology 102
   medical comorbidity 234
   medication-assisted treatment for 175–76
   minimally adequate treatment for 51, 52t, 53
   outpatient treatment programme 372–73
   prevalence of 51
   treatment 237
substantial freedom 36–37
substitute decision-making 305
suicide/suicidality 75, 104, 335, 393
   associated with mental health problems 202
   course and prognosis 104
   early detection 104
   early intervention 104
   epidemiology 104
   postvention as prevention/early intervention 104
   in youth depression 99
supernatural aetiology, of mental illness 419
supervision, of researchers 365
supported employment 369–70
   Individual Placement and Support model 371
Surgeon General 29
   report 28
sustainable development goals 327
Sweden 75, 134
Switzerland 134
   crisis resolution and home treatment team (CRHTT) model 132
SWOT analysis, of policies 409
syndemics 406

talking to 'spirits,' 323
Tanahashi framework 45–46
Tanzania 439
TAPS study (London) 117, 211, 212
Tarasoff decisions 284
Tavistock Clinic 13–14
taxation, general 345, 345t
Team for the Assessment of Psychiatric Services (TAPS) study (London) 117, 211, 212
technology-enabled clinical care 265
telehealth 475
telemedicine 168
telepsychiatry 168, 261–62
tertiary prevention 236
Theoretical Domains Framework (TDF) 379, 380, 380t
therapeutic community 14, 196
'thick descriptions,' 361–62
   of life in asylums 363
   of life in the community for recently discharged people 363
threats 302
Time To Change campaign (England) 324–25

tobacco smoking 234
tobacco use disorder 233t
traditional and faith healers (TFHs) 418–19
   assessment, diagnosis, and treatment of mental disorders 421
   beliefs about the causation of mental illness 418
   collaboration between biomedical practitioners and 422
   harmful practices and human rights abuses 421
   implications for legislation, policy, research, training, and practice 421–22
   practice characteristics of 420
traditional healers 417–18, 419
traditional medicine 418
   national policies on 422
training 464
   of researchers 365
Training in Community Living service 131
'Transforming Care' programme 200
transient psychotic experiences 143
transinstitutionalization 198
trauma 148
   conceptual model of PTSD, depression, physical health and 86, 87f
   health impact for migrants 82–83
   relationship between chronic medical conditions and 83, 84t
treaties 292, 402–3
Treatment and Intervention in Psychosis (TIPS) 317
'treatment as usual' (TAU) group 358
treatment coverage see coverage
treatment exposure measures 373
treatment fidelity 358, 370
treatment guidelines 471–72
treatment manuals 372
treatment pressures 285, 301–3
   inducement and threats 302–3
   interpersonal leverage 301–2
   justification
      based on protection of others 305–6
      in the best interests of the patient 304–5
      for exercising 303–6
   persuasion 301
   reduction in the need for 306–7
treatments
   access to 5
   adherence to 303
   consent to 297
   cost-effectiveness of 354
   effectiveness of 353–54
   efficaciousness in practice 354
   fidelity 358
   knowledge of 314
   minimally adequate 51
   non-consensual 305
   patient preference trials 356
   pressures, coercion, and compulsion 301–9
triangulation
   investigator 365
   methodological 365
   participant 365
Tuke, Samuel 196

Uganda 433–35, 439
   community detection 434
   community sensitization and anti-stigma mobilization 433
   district mental health care plan 433
   impacts of the district mental health care plan 434
   lessons learned from district mental health care plan (MHCP) 434–35

Uganda (cont.)
  National Health Policy (2010–2015) 433
  National Health Policy Framework (2011–2030) 433
  packages of care at community level 433–34, 434t
  recovery package 434
  Village Health Teams 434
Ukraine 46, 47t, 50t
unemployment 58–59, 117
unfairness, in mental health systems 273
unipolar depressive disorders 234
United for Global Mental Health 455
United Global Mental Health initiative, 'Countdown,' 455
United Kingdom (UK)
  acute inpatient care 198–99
  Black Caribbeans in the 75, 77, 82
  day centres 189
  day hospitals 189
  inpatient beds in 198t
  see also England; Wales
United Nations (UN)
  Mental Illness Principles (1991) 294
  principle of universal health coverage 471
  Sustainable Development Goals (SDGs) 402–3, 403t, 404
United Nations (UN) Convention against Torture 295
United Nations (UN) Convention on the Rights of Persons with Disabilities (CRPD) 4, 20, 291, 293–94, 299, 305, 402–3, 471
  adoption of 293–94
  Article 12, 298
  Article 25, 296
  civil and political rights 295
  on consent to treatment 297
  definition of 'persons with disabilities,' 293
  disability mainstreaming provision 294
  economic, social and cultural rights 295
  general obligations on States to comply with provisions of 294
  guiding principles 294
  implementation of 293, 298
  raising awareness of 298–99
  reasonable accommodation concept 296
  reasons for existence of 293
  right to education 295
  right to health 296
  right to legal capacity 298
  right to live in the community 297
  right to relationships, to sexual activity, and to family life 295
  right to work and employment 295
United Nations High Commissioner for Refugees (UNHCR) 75, 81
United States (US)
  12-month contact coverage for DSM-IV/CIDI disorders by severity of disorder 50t
  accreditation of inpatient facilities in 203
  allcove youth mental health care 98
  Black Caribbeans in the 74
  chronic care model 189
  collaboration between criminal justice and mental health agencies 272
  crisis family placements 135
  crisis houses 134
  day care centre/chronic care model 189
  day care centres 189
  day hospital/intensive care model 189
  day hospitals 189
  day hospitals versus day treatment versus day care 189
  day treatment programme/rehabilitation model 189
  day treatment programmes 189
  day treatment programmes converting to individual placement and support (IPS) 221
  development of partial hospitalization in 187
  evidence for schizophrenia and other psychoses in 75
  foreign-born population in 81–82
  forensic assertive community treatment teams 271
  health status of immigrant/refugee populations in 81–82
  individual placement and supported employment 221–22
  inpatient beds in 197, 198t
  inpatient services in 199
  integrated care 237–38
  licensing of health care providers in 203
  mandatory psychiatric treatment 275–76
  mental health helpline '988,' 456
  mental health policies in 23–31
  mental health systems, in 2002 27
  mental illness coverage 344
  National Comorbidity Survey 171
  National Comorbidity Survey Replication (NCS-R) 47t
  National Healthcare Disparities Reports 85
  patient portals in 238
  population-level needs assessment 69
  President's New Freedom Commission on Mental Health 27, 28, 29
  Preventative Services Task Force 103
  services in the 203
  Surgeon General's review of research on culture and mental health 76–77
  White House Conference on Mental Health 29
universal health care policy 452
universal health coverage 344
unwelcome events 302
urbanization 453
user-led movements 57, 58
users
  listening to experiences and perspectives of 121
  mental health service 19
'Users' Guides to the Medical Literature' series 377
utilitarianism 283
  act utilitarianism 283
  rule utilitarianism 283

validity of research 364
valproate 235
values 4
van Veldhuizen, Remmers 167
Veterans Administration 29
Veterans Affairs Family Forum 230
vicarious traumatization 442
violence 202
  association between mental illness and 321–22
  Macarthur Violence Risk Assessment Study 253–54
  by people with mental illnesses 271
  prediction of serious 305
  risk assessment in community settings 274
  structural 61
violent premature death 236
virtue ethics 283
voluntary insurance 343, 343t, 345t
voluntary patients, alternative care for 117

Wales
  Accredited Accommodation Scheme, Powys, Wales 135
  forensic inpatient provision 272
  long-stay hospital beds 207
  Mental Capacity Act (2005) 298
  mental hospitals in the 1930s in 13
  monitoring frameworks 207–8
  Multi-Agency Public Protection Arrangements (MAPPA) 272
  number of prison places 209–10
  patients in mental hospitals at the outbreak of the First World War 11–12
  public asylums during the first half of the 20th century 196
  see also United Kingdom (UK)
Warlingham Park Hospital 14n.5, 197
websites, as source of mental health information 317
weight management 236–37
well-being 419
  promotion of 36
wellness 57, 57t, 60
  eight dimensions of 58f, 60, 60t, 61
Wellness Recovery Action Plan (WRAP) 249
Wellness Respite 62
Western medicine, evolution of 419
whistle-blowers 287
whistle-blowing 287
'whole-of-society' approach 406
Whorlton Hall 200, 202
Wing, John 15
Winterbourne View (hospital) 200
women, vulnerability to mental health impact of disasters 441
work 117
  alternatives forms of 119
workforce
  diversification of 465
  strengthening of 464
working professionals, reasonable adjustments 325
World Health Organization (WHO)
  Action Plan 404
  'Assessment Instrument for Mental Health Systems,' 412
  Atlas report 404
  Composite International Diagnostic Interview (CIDI) 46–48, 334–35
  Comprehensive Mental Health Action Plan 2013–2020 335
  Comprehensive Mental Health Action Plan 2013–2030 405, 412, 455
  Global Action Plan 407
  'Guidance on community mental health services,' 299, 412
  Mental Health Atlas 334, 403
  mental health Gap Action Programme Intervention Guide (mhGAP-IG) 337, 406, 407–8, 413b, 425, 426, 471–72, 476
  mental health policy and planning package 461
  pyramid of the optimal mix of services to deliver mental health 407–8, 408f
  QualityRights initiative 299, 334, 404–5
  recommendations by 404
  School Mental Health programme 452
  standards to guide countries in producing/revising mental health laws 326
  Tanahashi framework 45–46
  Thinking Healthy programme for mothers 452
  World Mental Health Report 456, 457
World Health Report 2001 455

World Mental Health (WMH) Surveys 46, 99, 334–35, 476
  mental disorders in 46–48
  sample characteristics 46, 47t
World Mental Health Day 2021 456
World Mental Health Report: Transforming Mental Health for All 449–50, 452
  key shifts to transform mental health for all 451f
  recommendations 452
  themes 450
  three transformative paths towards better mental health 450f
World Migration Report 73
World Psychiatric Association–Lancet Psychiatry Commission on the future of psychiatry 453
Worthing experiment 131

Yardley Psychiatric Emergency Team 131–32
years lived with disability (YLDs) 389, 393
  disease burden distribution globally 392f

years of life lost (YLLs) 389
York Retreat 196
young people
  affected by mental ill health 97
  early intervention in psychosis (EIP) 142
  integrated youth mental health care services 98, 98b
  screening for depression 99

Zimbabwe, 'Friendship Bench' initiative 456